EDITION

Linné & Ringsrud's

CLINICAL LABORATORY SCIENCE

CONCEPTS, PROCEDURES, *and* CLINICAL APPLICATIONS

MARY LOUISE TURGEON, EdD, MLS(ASCP)[CM]

Clinical Laboratory Education Consultant
Mary L. Turgeon & Associates
Boston, Massachusetts, and St. Petersburg, Florida

Adjunct Associate Professor
University of Texas Medical Branch
School of Health Professions
Department of Clinical Laboratory Sciences
Galveston, Texas

Associate Clinical Professor
Chair, Department of Medical Laboratory Sciences
Graduate and Undergraduate Programs Director (previous)
Northeastern University
Bouve College of Health Professions
Boston, Massachusetts

ELSEVIER

ELSEVIER

3251 Riverport Lane
St. Louis, Missouri 63043

LINNÉ & RINGSRUD'S CLINICAL LABORATORY SCIENCE: CONCEPTS, PROCEDURES, AND CLINICAL APPLICATIONS, EIGHTH EDITION

ISBN: 978-0-323-53082-8

International Standard Book Number 978-0-323-53082-8

Executive Content Strategist: Kellie White
Senior Content Development Manager: Ellen Wurm-Cutter
Publishing Services Manager: Julie Eddy
Senior Project Manager: Rich Barber
Designer: Patrick Ferguson

Printed in Canada

Last digit is the print number: 9 8 7 6 5 4 3 2

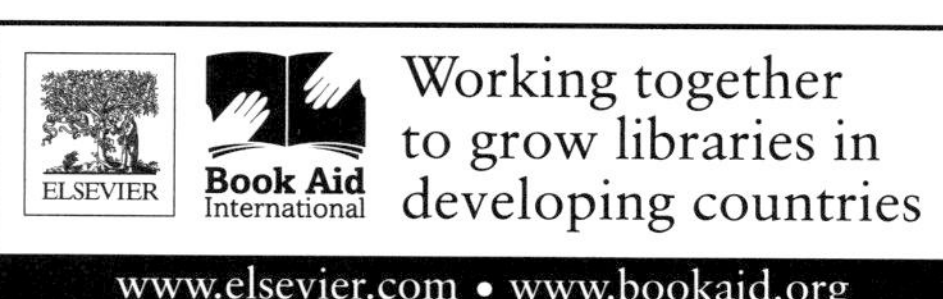

ABOUT THE AUTHOR

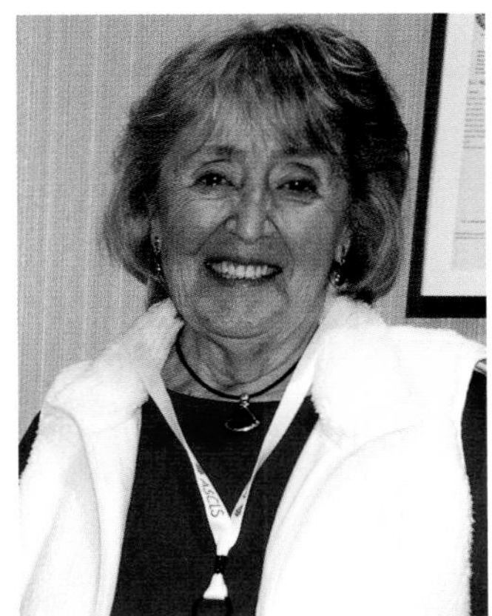

Mary Louise Turgeon, EdD, MT(ASCP)^{CM}, is an author, professor, and consultant in medical laboratory science. Her books are *Basic & Applied Clinical Laboratory Science,* ed 7 (2015); *Immunology and Serology in Laboratory Medicine,* ed 6 (2018); *Clinical Hematology,* ed 6 (2018); and *Fundamentals of Immunohematology,* ed 2. Foreign language editions have been published in Chinese, Spanish, and Italian.

Dr. Turgeon has 18 years of university and 15 years of community college teaching and program administration experience. Guest speaking, scientific presentations, and technical and educational workshops complement her teaching and writing activities. Her consulting practice focuses on new clinical laboratory science program development, curriculum revisions, course development, and increasing teaching effectiveness in the United States and internationally. She has volunteered as a laboratory educational consultant in Lesotho, South Africa, and Cambodia.

REVIEWERS

Maritza I. Cintron, MPA, BSMT(AMT)
MLT Program Director
Health Science Instructor
Marion Technical College
Ocala, Florida

Susan L. Conforti, EdD, MLS(ASCP)SBB
Associate Professor
Medical Laboratory Technology
Farmingdale State College
Farmingdale, New York

Amy Kapanka, MS, MT(ASCP)SC
MLT Program Director
Health Science
Hawkeye Community College
Waterloo, Iowa

Kyle P. Miller, B.S., MLS(ASCP)CM
Graduate Student
Clinical Laboratory Sciences
University of North Carolina
Chapel Hill, North Carolina
Medical Laboratory Scientist
Covenant Health
Crossville, Tennessee

Angela Njoku, MS, MT(ASCP)
Assistant Professor
Clinical Laboratory Technology
St. Louis Community College
St. Louis, Missouri

Patricia Raphiel-Brown, MA, CLS(AMT)
Assistant Professor
Program Director, Phlebotomy/Medical Laboratory Technology
Southern University at Shreveport
Shreveport, Louisiana

Julie Zemplinski, MSH, MS, MLS(ASCP)CM
Clinical Laboratory Science Program Director
Health Sciences
Florida Gulf Coast University
Fort Myers, Florida

Every New Day Should be a Learning Adventure

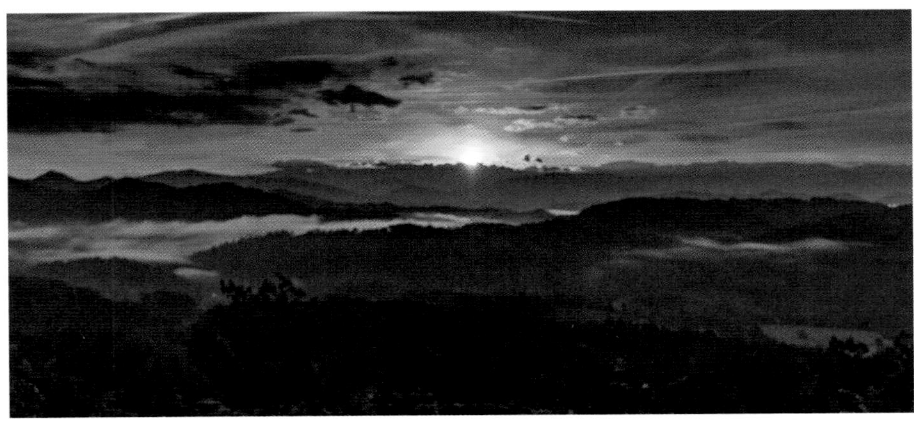

This edition is dedicated to the home team of Dick and Murphy.

PREFACE

The intention of this eighth edition of *Clinical Laboratory Science: Concepts, Procedures, and Clinical Applications* is to continue to fulfill the need for a basic, comprehensive textbook that can be used by students and instructors for career preparation in many different courses throughout the entire medical laboratory science curriculum.

Multiple sources are used to revise content in each new edition of *Clinical Laboratory Science*. These sources include tracking emerging information in journals, participating in professional meetings and expositions, and consulting peer reviewers. The newest Entry Level Curriculum Updates for workforce entry published by the American Society for Clinical Laboratory Science (ASCLS) and the American Society for Clinical Pathology (ASCP) Board of Certification Exam Content Outlines serve as additional content reference sources.

A solid, robust foundation exists for each new edition of *Clinical Laboratory Science* because of feedback on previous editions following field testing by instructors and undergraduate medical laboratory technician (MLT) and medical laboratory science (MLS) students in the classroom and laboratory. Dynamic interaction continues to strengthen the clarity and organization of content presented in *Clinical Laboratory Science*.

The purpose of this edition continues to be to integrate and apply basic and emerging concepts in laboratory medicine, to outline the underlying theory of routine laboratory procedures done in clinical laboratories of varying sizes and geographic locations, and to present applicable case studies to help students critically assess theory and practice.

The organization of *Clinical Laboratory Science* begins with key terms and a topical outline. Learning outcomes are differentiated into MLT and MLS levels. Different levels of outcomes are reflected in the verbs used for each learning objective. Learning outcomes and an extensive number of end-of-chapter review questions are organized and coordinated under major topical headings.

Fully developed laboratory exercises focus on representative student laboratory procedures and consistently use the Clinical and Laboratory Standards Institute (CLSI) format. Laboratory exercises have associated learning outcomes and review questions. Case studies with critical thinking group-discussion questions are included in relevant chapters.

A comprehensive bank of end-of-chapter review questions appears in each chapter. Illustrations, full-color photographs, tables, and boxes are used throughout *Clinical Laboratory Science* to visually clarify concepts and arrange detailed information to complement the learning preferences of today's digital learners.

WHAT'S NEW IN THE EIGHTH EDITION OF *CLINICAL LABORATORY SCIENCE*?

Clinical Laboratory Science is divided into two main sections: Part I, Basic Laboratory Techniques, and Part II, Clinical Laboratory Specializations. The entire book has been thoroughly reviewed and revised, as needed, to introduce new concepts and practices and to eliminate any outdated content.

Part I: Basic Laboratory Theory and Techniques

Chapter 1–Chapter 9

Content in this section addresses traditional core content related to fundamental principles and practices in the laboratory. In addition, foundation knowledge continues to be refined and expanded in each new edition.

The "new face" of laboratory practice is reflected in an increased emphasis on safety, patient considerations, quality, and delivery of testing. Innovative laboratory testing techniques are included in Chapter 8, Basic and Contemporary Techniques in the Clinical Laboratory, and Chapter 9, Laboratory Testing: From Point of Care to Total Automation.

Examples of What's New in Part I

- Presentation of the newest concept of a designated laboratory safety officer supported by laboratory safety coaches as the critical "safety eyes" and "safety ears" to implement surveillance of correct safety practices.
- Assessment of the real net clinical value of a laboratory result in balancing the benefits that a test delivers against any harm that it may cause to a patient.
- Comparison of proficiency testing and alternate assessment of quality. Alternative methods include external split samples, internal split samples, audit samples, and the use of government and university inter-laboratory comparisons.
- Introduction of a system for managing analytical quality based on the concept of *total analytic error* (TAE).
- Explanation of The Joint Commission's National Patient Safety Goals and the newest American Hospital Association Patient Care Partnership document.
- Investigation of the concepts of patient-centric laboratory testing, personal direct-to-consumer genetic testing. and emerging patient-centric technologies.
- Inclusion of new evacuated blood-collection tubes and bar codes.
- Clarification of various levels of water purity.
- Evaluation of lateral and vertical flow immunoassays and alternative labeling technologies.
- Comparison of the technology of the latest handheld point-of-care instruments.

Part II: Clinical Laboratory Specializations

Chapter 10–Chapter 17

This section of the book addresses the principles of testing, physiology, analysis by laboratory methods, and applicable diseases or disorders and provides related case studies with critical thinking group-discussion questions in each chapter. The emphasis in each clinical chapter is on new or emerging point-of-care testing methods and automated laboratory testing.

Examples of What's New in Part II

- Introduction of additional information related to Ca^{2+}, calculation of the estimated glomerular filtration rate, and the newest cardiovascular disease risk factors and assessment strategies.
- Discussion of new methods for determination of the erythrocyte sedimentation rate.
- Presentation of new automated hematology instruments.
- Assessment of new point-of-care testing instruments for international normalized ratio (INR) testing.
- Presentation of new automated urine and body fluid analyzers.
- Explanation of magnetic resonance spectroscopy testing.
- Description of fetal lung maturity assessment and prediction of risk of respiratory distress syndrome.
- Comparison of the relationship of expected microbiota, host microbiota, and the immune system in maintaining tissue homeostasis in healthy individuals.
- Discussion of probiotics.
- Introduction of matrix-assisted laser desorption ionization time-of-flight mass spectrometer (MALDI-TOF) technology in microbiology.
- Comparison of laboratory safety measures for Zika and Ebola viruses.
- Assessment of fetomaternal hemorrhage and Rh prophylaxis with calculation of the required number of vials of RhIg.

WAYS TO USE THIS BOOK

The eighth edition of *Clinical Laboratory Science* can be used as a primary or supplementary textbook from the beginning to the end of the entire clinical laboratory science curriculum for Medical Laboratory Science, MLS, and Medical Laboratory Technology, MLT) students.

The majority of chapters in Clinical Laboratory Science feature case studies to enhance critical thinking skills. Narrative answers are provided for instructors to guide a discussion of case study related critical thinking group discussion questions. Applicable chapters have related Student Procedure Worksheets to reinforce classroom content. Appropriate courses to consider for *Clinical Laboratory Science* adoption are as follows:

- Introduction to Medical Laboratory Science
- Laboratory Techniques, including Microscopy
- Phlebotomy
- Urinalysis
- Lab Math
- Core Clinical Laboratory Theory and Practice
- Laboratory Instrumentation
- Immunology and Serology
- Hematology*
- Clinical Chemistry*
- Microbiology*
- Blood Banking/Transfusion Medicine*
- Comprehensive Course and Certification Examinations Review

Comments from clinical laboratory students and instructors are always welcome.

Mary L. Turgeon
Boston, Massachusetts
St. Petersburg, Florida
Turgeonbooks@gmail.com

*All semesters—MLT; first semester—MLS.

ACKNOWLEDGMENTS

My objective in writing *Clinical Laboratory Science: Concepts, Procedures, and Clinical Applications,* Eighth Edition, is to continue to integrate and apply concepts, theory, and applications of clinical laboratory science. This book provides me with a challenging opportunity to share classic and emerging laboratory science information with students and educators.

Thanks to Ellen Wurm-Cutter, Senior Content Development Manager. We have worked together on three previous editions of *Clinical Laboratory Science* and multiple previous editions of *Immunology and Serology in Laboratory Medicine.* Working with her is always a pleasure.

Additional thanks to Kellie White, Executive Content Strategist, who is my editor for this edition of *Clinical Laboratory Science* and was my editor for *Immunology and Serology in Laboratory Medicine*, ed 6. Thank you to Alexandra York, Associate Content Development Specialist, for her efforts associated with this edition.

Finally, a big thank you to Rich Barber for his patience and extreme concern for the highest level of quality in this book.

Ellen, Kellie, and Rich, I sincerely appreciate all of your efforts on my behalf and your friendships.

Mary L. Turgeon

CONTENTS

1 Fundamentals of the Clinical Laboratory

http://evolve.elsevier.com/Turgeon/clinicallab

CHAPTER CONTENTS

LEARNING OUTCOMES

Clinical laboratory science

- Name and differentiate the functions of various professional organizations.
- Compare the characteristics of individual professional certifications, including the newest professional degree, and licensure.

Clinical laboratory overview

- Distinguish between various clinical laboratory staffing levels and functions.

Clinical laboratory improvement amendments (CLIA) of 1988

- Differentiate the classification of laboratory testing by complexity of the test: waived, moderately complex, highly complex, and provider-performed microscopy based on CLIA '88 regulations.
- Name the three most frequent inspection deficiencies over time for all CLIA-approved laboratories.
- Define the acronyms and explain the purpose of OSHA, CLIA '88, CMS, TJC, and CAP.

Laboratory departments

- Name the typical departments of a clinical laboratory and briefly describe the functions of each department.
- Name the types of testing that is typically performed in a core laboratory.
- Explain the advantages of molecular testing, the newest direction in laboratory testing.

Health care organizations

- Diagram and describe the organizational structure of a health care organization.

Primary accrediting organizations

- Name and compare at least three different primary laboratory accrediting organizations.

External government laboratory accreditation and regulation

- Describe the importance of federal, state, and institutional regulations concerning the quality and reliability of laboratory work.

Alternate sites of testing

- Compare and contrast the uses of various sites for laboratory testing: central laboratory, point of care, physician office laboratory, and reference laboratory.
- Categorize the features of alternate sites of laboratory testing.

Medical-legal issues

- Define the abbreviation HIPAA, and assess the major points of the legislation.

Medical ethics

- Define the term *ethics*, and discuss medical applications.

Case Studies

❖ Critically analyze and formulate an opinion related to each of the medical ethics case studies at the end of this chapter.

Review Questions

- Demonstrate comprehension of this chapter content by completing the end-of-chapter review questions with a grade of 80% or higher.

Note:

- indicates MLT and MLS core content

❖ indicates MLT (optional) and MLS advanced content

KEY TERMS

algorithm
analytes
body fluids
chain of custody
ethics
informed consent
pathogens
point-of-care testing (POCT)
waived testing

CLINICAL LABORATORY SCIENCE

Rudimentary examinations of human body fluids date back to the Greek physician Hippocrates, about 300 BC. Not until 1896, however, was the first clinical laboratory opened in a small room equipped at a cost of $50 at Johns Hopkins Hospital, Baltimore, Maryland. The diagnostic and therapeutic value of laboratory testing was not yet understood. Many physicians viewed clinical laboratories simply as an expensive luxury that consumed both valuable space and time.

Discovery of the causative agents of devastating epidemics such as tuberculosis, diphtheria, and cholera in the 1880s and the subsequent development of tests for their detection in the late 1890s highlighted the importance on laboratory testing.

Clinical laboratory testing plays a crucial role in the detection, diagnosis, and treatment of disease. The medical laboratory scientist (MLS) and medical laboratory technician (MLT) collect and process specimens and perform chemical, biological, hematologic, immunologic, microscopic, molecular diagnostic, and microbial testing. They may also collect and prepare blood for transfusion.

After collecting and examining a specimen, laboratory professionals analyze and communicate results to physicians or other primary care providers. In additional to routine testing, duties in the clinical laboratory include developing and modifying procedures and monitoring programs to ensure the accuracy of test results.

CLINICAL LABORATORY SCIENCE AS A PROFESSION

The U.S. Bureau of Labor Statistics *Occupational Outlook Handbook* for clinical laboratory technologists and technicians states, "About half of all medical laboratory technologists and technicians were employed in hospitals in 2016. Employment of medical laboratory technologists and technicians is projected to grow 13 percent from 2016–2026, much faster than the average for all occupations. An increase in the aging population will lead to a greater need to diagnose medical conditions, such as cancer or type 2 diabetes, through laboratory procedures."[1]

Original Credentialing and Professional Organizations

The American Society for Clinical Pathology (ASCP) created the Board of Registry (BOR) in 1928 to certify laboratory professionals. Individuals who passed the BOR's registry examination were referred to as *medical technologists*, identified by the acronym MT (ASCP).

In 1933 the American Society of Clinical Laboratory Technicians was formed, currently known as the *American Society for Clinical Laboratory Science (ASCLS)*. The catalyst for establishment of ASCLS was the desire for greater autonomy and control over the direction of the profession by nonphysician laboratory professionals. ASCLS is proud to champion the profession and ensure that other members of the health care field—as well as the public—fully recognize the contributions of clinical laboratory professionals.[2]

In 1973, as a result of pressure from the U.S. Office of Education and the National Commission on Accrediting, the National Accrediting Agency for Clinical Laboratory Sciences (NAACLS) was formed.

Individual Professional Recognition

During the 1960s, new categories of laboratory professionals joined generalist medical technologists in performing the daily work of the clinical laboratory. These categories were created to help cope with an increased workload. The category of the now-discontinued certified laboratory assistant was developed as a 1-year certificate program; the category of MLT was developed as a 2-year associate degree program. Simultaneously, specialist categories in chemistry, microbiology, hematology, and blood banking were created. Specialists certified in cytotechnology, histotechnology, laboratory safety, and molecular pathology/molecular biology have evolved as well. Technicians certified as donor phlebotomists or phlebotomy technicians are part of the laboratory team. Pathologists' assistants are another category of specialty certification. Certification as a Diplomat in Laboratory Management is available.[3]

Additional Individual Professional Certification and Licensure

Many employers prefer, or are required by, the Clinical Laboratory Improvement Amendments of 1988 (CLIA '88) regulations to hire laboratory staff who are certified by a recognized professional association. In addition to those previously listed, the American Medical Technologists also offer certification.

Numerous states and U.S. territories currently require licensure (Box 1.1), with other states considering licensure. The requirements for licensure vary by state and specialty. Information is available from state departments of health or boards of occupational licensing for laboratory professionals.

Newest Professional Recognition

In September 2009, a historic step was taken in professional recognition. ASCP and the now-defunct National Credentialing Agency joined together in credentialing laboratory professionals under the auspices of the BOR. Generalists are now referred to as *medical laboratory scientists (MLSs)*. The similar technician-level designation continued to be designated as *medical laboratory technicians (MLTs)*. The appropriate professional credentialing is MLS(ASCP) and MLT(ASCP).

Continuing education is now a requirement for certified professionals to maintain certification. Continuing education is always part of a laboratory's program for ensuring high-quality service and maintaining the morale of the laboratory staff. Programs are offered at professional meetings as well as online. The acknowledgment of continuing certification is expressed as MLS (ASCP)^{CM} and MLT(ASCP)^{CM}.

In 2012 a new postbaccalaureate degree, the doctorate in clinical laboratory science (DCLS), was approved in the United States. This credential is beyond that of the entry-level generalist and represents the terminal advanced-practice degree in the profession. The DCLS professionals will assume roles as consultants, educators, and administrators to contribute to the common goals of decreasing medical errors, reducing health care costs, and improving patient outcomes. NAACLS categorizes the responsibilities of the DCLS into five areas in which these roles are utilized: patient care management, education, research applications, health care policy development, and health care services delivery and access.[4]

BOX 1.1 States and U.S. Commonwealth Territories with Licensure of Laboratory Professionals

States

California	Nevada
Florida	New York
Georgia	North Dakota
Hawaii	Rhode Island
Louisiana	Tennessee
Montana	West Virginia

U.S. Commonwealth Territories

Guam
Northern Mariana Islands
Puerto Rico

(From American Society for Clinical Laboratory Science (ASCLS). www.ascls.org/educator and www.ascls.org. Accessed May 25, 2013.)

CLINICAL LABORATORY OVERVIEW

Functions

Appropriate utilization of the clinical laboratory is critical to the practice of laboratory medicine (see Chapter 3). It is important that the laboratory serve to educate the physician and other health care providers so that the information available through the reported test results can be used appropriately. When tests are being ordered, the clinical laboratory should assume a role of leadership and education in assisting the physician to understand the most useful pattern of ordering, for example, to serve the best interest of the patient, improve the clinical decision-making process for the physician, and consider the costs involved.

Hundreds of different laboratory tests are readily available in the larger laboratories (http://labtestsonline.org/), but typically only a small percentage of these tests are routinely ordered. When the results of these tests are used appropriately in the context of the patient's clinical case, physical examination findings, and medical history, clinical decision making will be improved. It is unusual for the results from a single laboratory assay to provide a diagnosis. Certain additional laboratory tests may be needed to take decision making to the next step. Generally, a small number of appropriately chosen laboratory tests (a panel of tests) or a reflective testing algorithm is sufficient to confirm or rule out one or more of the possibilities in a differential diagnosis.

Staffing

Clinical laboratory professionals are an essential component of the medical team. In some laboratories, personnel are cross-trained to work in core laboratories (laboratories with high volume hematology and chemistry instrumentation) but other laboratories may have specialists in certain areas of the laboratory.

Laboratory Directors

Most clinical laboratories are operated under the direction of a pathologist or PhD. Pathologists have training in both anatomic and clinical pathology, although research can be substituted for the clinical pathology portion of the pathology residency program. The anatomic pathologist is a licensed physician, usually trained for an additional 4 to 5 years after graduating from medical school, to examine (grossly and microscopically) all the surgically removed specimens from patients, which include frozen sections, tissue samples, and autopsy specimens. Examination of Pap smears and other cytologic and histologic examinations are also generally done by an anatomic pathologist. A clinical pathologist is also a licensed physician with additional training in clinical pathology or laboratory medicine. Under the direction of the clinical pathologist, many common laboratory tests are performed on blood and urine. Consultation with physicians is also important; any information gained concerning the patient's case is actually the result of collaborative activity between the laboratory and the attending physician.

A person with a PhD in a scientific discipline, such as clinical microbiology or biochemistry, may be recognized as a laboratory director. Such individuals may oversee an entire laboratory or a specialty section of a large laboratory.

The leaders and managers of the clinical laboratory must be certain all legal operating regulations have been met and all persons working in the laboratory setting are fully aware of the importance of compliance with these regulations. Those in leadership positions in a clinical laboratory must have expertise in medical, scientific, and technical areas as well as a full understanding of regulatory matters. All laboratory personnel must be aware of these regulatory considerations, but the management is responsible for ensuring that this information is communicated to everyone who needs to know.

Laboratory Supervisor or Manager

Typically, a laboratory has a supervisor or manager who is responsible for the technical aspects of managing the laboratory. This person is most often an MLS with additional education and experience in administration. In very large laboratories, a technical manager may supervise the technical aspects of the facility (issues involving assay of analytes), including quality control programs, off-site testing, and maintenance of the laboratory instruments. In addition, a business manager may be hired to handle administrative details.

The supervisor or administrative manager may also be the technical manager in the case of smaller laboratories. Section-supervising technologists are in place as needed, depending on the size and workload of the laboratory. A major concern of administrative technologists, regardless of the job titles used, is ensuring that all federal, state, and local regulatory mandates are being followed by the laboratory. Persons in leadership and management positions in the clinical laboratory must be certain all legal operating conditions have been met and that these conditions are balanced with the performance of work in a cost-effective manner.

It is important that the people serving in a supervisory position be able to communicate in a clear, concise manner, both to the persons working in their laboratory settings and to the physicians and other health care workers who utilize laboratory services.

Technologists, Technicians, and Specialists

Depending on the size of the laboratory and the numbers and types of laboratory tests performed, various levels of trained personnel are needed. CLIA '88 regulations set the standards for personnel, including their levels of education and training. Generally, the level of training or education of the laboratory professional will be taken into consideration in the roles assigned in the laboratory and the types of laboratory analyses performed.

The responsibilities of MLSs and MLTs vary but may include performing some of the same laboratory assays, supervising other staff, or teaching. Some are engaged in research. An important aspect of clinical laboratory science education is to understand the science behind the tests being performed so that problems can be recognized and solved. Troubleshooting is a constant consideration in the clinical laboratory. Because of in-depth knowledge of technical aspects, principles of methodology, and instrumentation used for the various laboratory assays, the laboratory professional is able to correlate and interpret the data.

Other laboratory professionals may be assigned to specific sections of the laboratory. Although MLSs and MLTs may collect blood specimens at smaller facilities, phlebotomists collect blood specimens in larger hospitals. Laboratory professionals may also work in a specimen-processing section of the laboratory.

CLINICAL LABORATORY IMPROVEMENT AMENDMENTS (CLIA) OF 1988

Much of how clinical laboratories perform their work is delineated by federal regulations or other external policies. CLIA '88 regulations govern most of the activities of a particular laboratory, although federal laboratories (such as Veterans Affairs hospitals/medical centers) are not regulated by CLIA requirements.[3,4] The goals of these amendments are to ensure that the laboratory results reported are of high quality regardless of where the testing is done: small laboratory, physician's office, large reference laboratory, or patient's home. CLIA '88 regulations include aspects of proficiency testing programs, management of patient testing, quality assessment programs, use of quality control systems, personnel requirements, inspections and site visits, and consultations. Several federal agencies govern practices in the clinical laboratory. These regulatory agencies or organizations are primarily concerned with setting standards, conducting inspections, and imposing sanctions when necessary.

CLIA Requirements for Personnel

The personnel section of the CLIA regulations defines the responsibilities of persons working in each of the testing sites where tests of moderate or high complexity are done, along with the educational requirements and training and experience needed. Minimum education and experience needed by testing personnel to perform the specific laboratory tests on human specimens are also regulated by CLIA '88. These job requirements are listed in the CLIA '88 final regulations, along with their amendments published from 1992 to 1995.[5]

There are no CLIA regulations for testing personnel who work at sites performing only waived tests. For laboratories where only tests of moderate complexity are performed, the minimum requirement for testing personnel is a high school diploma or equivalent, provided there is documented evidence of an amount of training sufficient to ensure that the laboratory staff has the skills necessary to collect, identify, and process the specimen and perform the laboratory analysis.

For tests of the highly complex category, the personnel requirements are more stringent. Anyone who is eligible to perform highly complex tests can also perform moderate-complexity testing. The U.S. Occupational Safety and Health Administration (OSHA) requires that training in handling chemical hazards, as well as training in handling infectious materials (Standard Precautions), be included for all new testing personnel. The laboratory director is ultimately responsible for all personnel working in the laboratory.

Levels of General Laboratory Testing

External standards have been set to ensure that all laboratories provide the best, most reliable information to the physician and the patient. This is the goal of CLIA'88.

CLIA regulations divide laboratories into categories based on the "complexity" of the tests being performed by the laboratory, as follows:

- Waived tests
- Moderately complex tests
- Highly complex tests
- Provider-Performed Microscopy

This tiered grouping has been devised with varying degrees of regulation for each level. The criteria for classification include the following:

1. Risk of harm to the patient
2. Risk of an erroneous result
3. Type of testing method used
4. Degree of independent judgment and interpretation needed
5. Availability of the particular test in question for home use

Waived Tests

The law contains a provision to exempt certain laboratories from standards for personnel and from quality control programs, proficiency testing, or quality assessment programs. These laboratories are defined as those that perform only simple, routine tests considered to have an insignificant risk of an erroneous result. Laboratories that receive a "certificate of waiver" can perform waived testing.

As currently defined, waived laboratory tests or procedures are those cleared by the U.S. Food and Drug Administration (FDA) for home use, which employ simple methodologies unlikely to cause erroneous results and pose no reasonable risk of harm to the patient if the test is performed incorrectly. The list of waived tests continues to expand. Waived tests include dipstick urinalysis and blood glucose by FDA-approved monitoring devices specifically made for home use.[5]

Moderate and High Complexity Testing

The two additional categories are moderate-complexity and high-complexity levels of testing. These levels are more regulated, with some minimal personnel standards required, as well as proficiency testing and quality assessment programs.

Provider-Performed Microscopy

Another category of specialized laboratory testing is Provider-Performed Microscopy (PPM) testing, generally performed by the physician in the office setting; this category is also exempt from some of the CLIA requirements but there are requirements for personnel who perform provider performed microscopy (PPM) (CFR 493.1351 to 493.1365). Personnel requirements include director qualifications and responsibilities and testing personnel responsibilities.

To meet the criteria for inclusion in the PPM category, procedures must follow the following specifications:

1. The examination must be personally performed by the practitioner (defined as a physician, a midlevel practitioner under the supervision of a physician, or a dentist).
2. The procedure must be categorized as moderately complex.
3. The primary instrument for performing the test is the microscope (limited to brightfield or phase-contrast microscopy).
4. The specimen is labile.
5. Control materials are not available.
6. Specimen handling is limited.

As currently defined, the PPM category includes all direct wet mount preparations for the presence or absence of bacteria, fungi, parasites, and human cellular elements in vaginal, cervical, or skin preparations; all potassium hydroxide preparations; pinworm examinations; fern tests; postcoital direct qualitative examinations of vaginal or cervical mucus; urine sediment examinations; nasal smears for granulocytes (eosinophils); fecal leukocyte examinations; and qualitative semen analysis (limited to the presence or absence of sperm and detection of motility).

LABORATORY DEPARTMENTS

The organization of a particular clinical laboratory depends on its size, the number of tests done, and the facilities available. Larger laboratories tend to be departmentalized; a separate area is designated for each of the various divisions. Fig. 1.1 shows a typical system for the organization of a traditional clinical laboratory. The current trend is to have a more "open" design or a *core laboratory* where hematology, urinalysis, hemostasis/coagulation, and clinical chemistry share workspace. Cross-training is important in a core laboratory model. In addition to the traditional areas already mentioned, the disciplines of cytogenetics, toxicology, flow cytometry, and other specialized divisions (such as molecular diagnostics) are present in larger laboratories.

Traditional Departments of a Clinical Laboratory

Laboratory medicine, or clinical pathology, is the medical discipline in which clinical laboratory science and technology are applied to the care of patients. With either the more traditional

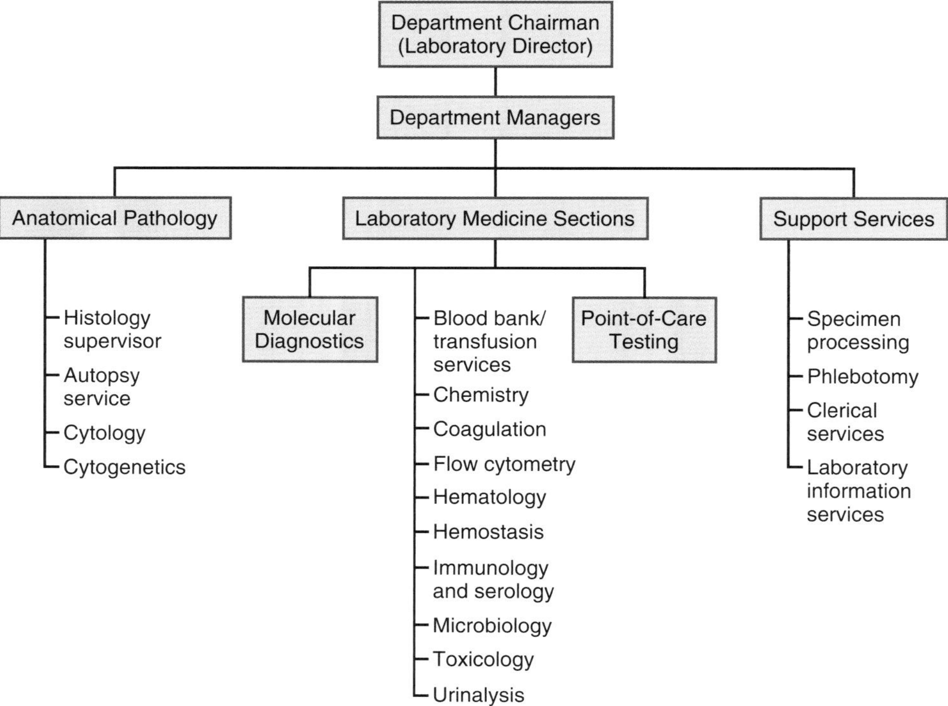

Fig. 1.1 Organization of a Clinical Laboratory. (Modified from Kaplan LA, Pesce AJ: *Clinical chemistry: theory, analysis and correlations,* ed 5, St Louis, 2010, Mosby.)

divisions by separate areas or the open model, there are still several distinct departments or divisions in the organization of the clinical laboratory. Anatomic pathology, including cytology and histology, is part of the overall clinical laboratory but usually functions independently.

A working clinical laboratory is traditionally organized into several major scientific disciplines: blood banking/transfusion medicine, clinical chemistry, hematology and hemostasis, immunology and serology, microbiology, and urinalysis. Each of these disciplines of laboratory medicine is described in more detail in Part II of this book.

Many changes are taking place in the clinical laboratory and are already affecting the types of tests and the locations where tests are being conducted. The core laboratory configuration combines routine hematology, hemostasis and blood coagulation, and clinical chemistry. Each specialty department focuses on a different area of laboratory medicine.

Blood Banking/Transfusion Medicine

Blood products for transfusion are studied and prepared in this laboratory section.

Clinical Chemistry

The clinical chemistry laboratory section performs quantitative analysis of constituents (such as glucose) on blood serum, urine, and body fluids. This department may include toxicology to analyze drugs.

Flow Cytometry

Specimens are studied for cell identification markers.

Hematology and Hemostasis

The hematology laboratory studies the formed elements of blood (such as red and white blood cells, platelets) and performs blood coagulation tests.

Immunology and Serology

The immunology and serology laboratory section focuses on testing of antigens and antibodies in blood serum. Procedures based on these principles may be conducted in clinical chemistry and other departments.

Microbiology

Microorganisms that cause disease, pathogens, are detected in the microbiology laboratory section. The microorganisms can be bacteria, parasites, fungi, or viruses.

Urinalysis

The body fluid urine is examined by chemical analysis and microscopically in the urinalysis section of the laboratory.

Core Laboratory

Many medium to large size laboratories have developed a central testing area with a cluster of instruments devoted to high volumes of test samples. These laboratories usually function 24/7.

Examples of the types of testing performed in a core laboratory are complete blood counts, urinalysis, and blood chemistries.

Expanded Directions of Laboratory Testing: Molecular Diagnostics

Molecular diagnostics, an application of biotechnology, applies the principles of basic molecular biology to the study of human diseases. Molecular diagnostics provides information related to molecular genetics research as real-time information for applications such as gene therapy, genetic screening, stem cell research, cloning, and cell culture.

New approaches to human disease assessment are being developed by clinical laboratories because of the new information about the molecular basis of disease processes in general. Traditional laboratory analyses give results based on a description of events currently occurring in the patient (such as blood cell counts, infectious processes, and blood glucose concentration). However, molecular biology introduces a predictive component: findings from these tests can be used to anticipate events that may occur in the future, when patients may be at risk for a particular disease or condition. More than ever, this predictive component reinforces the importance of how laboratory test results are used and emphasizes ethical considerations and the need for genetic counseling.

Genetics was in its infancy in the 1850s with the publication of Darwin's *On the Origin of Species* and Mendel's experiments of inheritance factors in pea plants. A milestone in genetics came in 1994 when the FDA approved the FlavrSavr tomato, the first genetically engineered food to go on the market.

In the 21st century, molecular diagnosis is the hottest topic in the clinical laboratory. The release of a complete mapping of the human genome in 2003 created an explosion of new testing. The Human Genome Project transformed biological science, changed the future of genetic research, and opened new doorways into the diagnosis and treatment of disease. The finished sequence covers 99% of the genome and is accurate to 99.99%.

For health care and information-solution providers, development in the expansive field of molecular diagnostics is currently driving change in each specialty in laboratory medicine.

The fundamentals of clinical laboratory practice have expanded in recent years to incorporate massive amounts of data related to recent revolutionary discoveries in molecular biology.

HEALTH CARE ORGANIZATIONS

Modern health care organizations have many different configurations, depending on the geographic region and market, mix of patients (such as age), overall size, and affiliations. The size of health care organizations ranges from the very large tertiary care–level teaching hospitals, to community hospitals, to freestanding specialty clinics or phlebotomy drawing stations.

A common organizational structure for a hospital includes the chief executive officer and the board of trustees, who set policy and guide the organization (Fig. 1.2). The chief operating officer is responsible for implementing policies and daily activities. Other high-level positions can include the chief financial officer, chief information officer, and chief technology officer, depending on the size of a health care organization. A variable number of vice presidents (VPs) have several departments reporting to them. Organizations usually have VPs of Nursing, Clinical Services, General Services, and Human Resources. The VP of Clinical Services oversees the managers of the clinical laboratory as well as radiology and pharmacy.

PRIMARY ACCREDITING ORGANIZATIONS

In current laboratory settings, many governmental regulations, along with regulations and recommendations from professional,

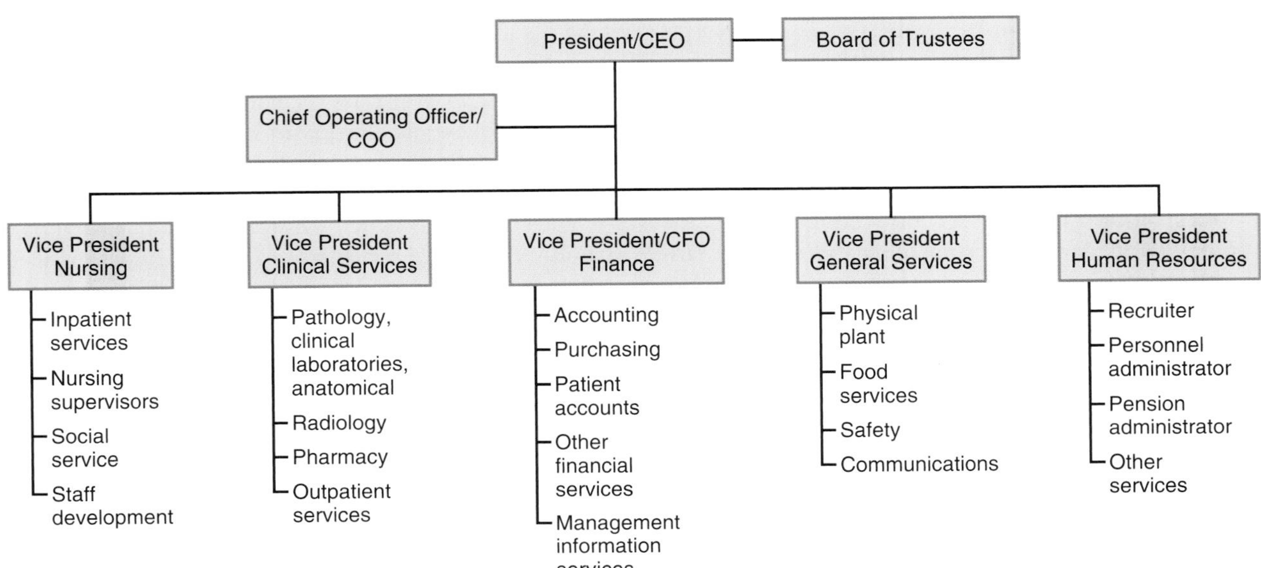

Fig. 1.2 Hospital Organizational Chart. (Modified from Kaplan LA, Pesce AJ: *Clinical chemistry: theory, analysis and correlations,* ed 5, St Louis, 2010, Mosby.)

state, and federal accreditation agencies and commissions of various types, govern the activities of the laboratory.

In the United States, there are approximately 15,697 accredited laboratories,[6] 97% of which are inspected by three primary accrediting organizations: Commission on Office Laboratory Accreditation (COLA), College of American Pathologists (CAP), and The Joint Commission (TJC).[2]

Commission on Office Laboratory Accreditation

The COLA accredits 6566 facilities.[6] COLA was founded in 1988 as a private alternative to help laboratories stay in compliance with the new CLIA regulations. In 1993 the U.S. Health Care Financing Administration (HCFA), now the Centers for Medicare and Medicaid Services (CMS), granted COLA deeming authority under CLIA. In 1997 The Joint Commission on Accreditation of Health Care Organizations, now TJC, also recognized COLA's laboratory accreditation program.

Since the increased government scrutiny of survey organizations, COLA was the first to be renewed and was given permission to accredit laboratories for the next 6 years to help these meet CLIA requirements. The increase in oversight by CMS was driven by a government investigation in 2006 into how some highly publicized laboratory errors had occurred and could have been prevented. COLA will incorporate new standard program requirements that coincide with updated CLIA requirements and are closely aligned with quality systems methodology. The new standard program requirements are a compilation of 75 new or revised criteria to the existing 299 questions. Some of the new program features for laboratories in 2007 include the following:

- Revised quality control requirements
- Increased attention to laboratory information systems
- New focus on quality assessments activities that span all phases of laboratory testing
- Incorporation of quality systems processes to all categories of the laboratory's path of workflow

College of American Pathologists

The CAP accredits 5670 facilities.[6] The CAP Laboratory Accreditation Program is an internationally recognized program and the only one of its kind that utilizes teams of practicing laboratory professionals as inspectors. Designed to go well beyond regulatory compliance, the program helps laboratories achieve the highest standards of excellence to positively impact patient care. The CAP Laboratory Accreditation Program meets the needs of a variety of laboratory settings. Now granted deeming authority by CMS, the CAP Laboratory Accreditation Program is also recognized by TJC and can be used to meet many state certification requirements.

The Joint Commission

TJC accredits 2409 facilities[6] and has been evaluating and accrediting hospital laboratory services since 1979 and freestanding laboratories since 1995. Laboratories eligible for accreditation include the following:

- Laboratories in hospitals, clinics, long-term care facilities, home care organizations, behavioral health care organizations, ambulatory sites, and physician offices
- Reference laboratories
- Freestanding laboratories, such as assisted reproductive technology laboratories
- Blood transfusion and donor centers
- Public health laboratories, including Indian Health Service laboratories
- Laboratories in federal facilities (such as Department of Veterans Affairs, and Department of Defense)
- Point-of-care testing (POCT) sites, including blood gas laboratories providing services to patients in emergency departments, surgical suites, cardiac catheterization laboratories, and other patient care areas

Other Agencies

Other specialty organizations, including the American Association of Blood Banks, American Society of Histocompatibility and Immunogenetics, and American Osteopathic Association, accredit more than 455 facilities.[6]

EXTERNAL GOVERNMENT LABORATORY ACCREDITATION AND REGULATION

Regulations and standards are designed specifically to protect staff working in the laboratory, other health care personnel, patients treated in the health care facility, and society as a whole. Federal regulations exist to meet these objectives. Certain regulatory mandates have been issued externally, such as CLIA '88. Others are internal, and some are both external and internal.[5,7,8] In addition to CLIA '88 regulations, other state and federal regulations are in place to regulate chemical waste disposal, use of hazardous chemicals, and issues of laboratory safety for personnel, including handling of biohazardous materials and application of Standard Precautions, previously called *Universal Precautions*.

A laboratory that wants to receive payment for its services from Medicare or Medicaid must be certified under the Public Health Service Act (42CFR493.1-Basis and Scope). To be certified, the laboratory must meet the conditions for participation in those programs. CMS has the administrative responsibility for both the Medicare and CLIA '88 programs. Facilities accredited by approved private accreditation agencies such as CAP must also follow the regulations for licensure under CLIA '88. States with equivalent CLIA '88 regulations are reviewed individually as to possible waiver for CLIA '88 licensure.

The U.S. Department of Health and Human Services (HHS) has also established regulations to implement CLIA '88. Different accreditation processes are used by TJC, CAP, and other organizations, but all of these requirements are based on CLIA requirements. CLIA Document Control Requirements state: 1. All laboratory procedures must be made available to laboratory personnel, and initial and subsequent versions of each procedure must be authorized by the laboratory director. 2. A copy of each procedure, date of first use, and date of discontinuance must be retained for at least 2 years after a procedure has been removed from service. Any facility performing quantitative, qualitative, or screening test procedures or examinations on materials derived from the human body is regulated by CLIA '88. This includes hospital laboratories of all sizes; physician office laboratories; nursing home facilities; clinics; industrial laboratories; city, state, and county laboratories; pharmacies, fitness centers, and health fairs; and independent laboratories.

As of December 29, 1993, HCFA approved the accreditation program developed by the COLA for the physician office laboratory (POL). This means that COLA accreditation requirements are recognized by HCFA as being equivalent to those established by CLIA. The COLA accreditation established a peer review option in place of the CLIA regulatory requirements. COLA-accredited laboratories are surveyed every 2 years to ensure that they meet requirements developed by their peers in family practice, internal medicine, or pathology.

The Clinical Laboratory Standards Institute (CLSI) is a nonprofit, educational organization created for the development, promotion, and use of national and international laboratory standards. CLSI recommendations, guidelines, and standards follow the CLIA '88 mandates.

Through labor laws such as the 1990 Americans with Disabilities Act (ADA) and the ADA Amendments Act of 2008 (ADAAA) as well as environmental regulations, laboratory workers can know that they are in a safe atmosphere and that every precaution has been taken to maintain that safe atmosphere. The new ADAAA has its greatest impact in the employment context, requiring employers with 15 or more employees covered by the ADA to adjust their policies and procedures to comply with the ADAAA. OSHA has been involved in setting these practices into motion.

Other external controls include standards mandated by public health laws and reporting requirements through the U.S. Centers for Disease Control and Prevention and through certification and licensure requirements issued by the FDA. State regulations are imposed by Medicaid agencies, state environmental laws, and state public health laws and licensure laws. Local regulations include those determined by building codes and fire prevention codes.

Two certifying agencies, CAP and TJC, have been given deemed status to act on the federal government's behalf (see previous discussion). From an external source, guidelines and standards have also been set by these organizations to govern safe work practices in the clinical laboratory. Independent agencies also have influence over practices in the clinical laboratory through accreditation policies or other responsibilities, including CAP, TJC, and other specific proficiency testing programs.

ALTERNATE SITES OF TESTING

Another change in laboratory testing has been the move from tests being done in a centralized laboratory setting to POCT. Alternative testing sites—the patient's bedside, in operating rooms or recovery areas, or even home testing—are extensions of the traditional clinical laboratory site.

The traditional setting for performance of diagnostic laboratory testing has been a centralized location in a health care facility (hospital) where specimens from patients are sent to be tested. The centralized laboratory setting remains in many institutions, but the advent of near-testing, bedside testing, or POCT has changed the organization of many laboratories. In POCT the laboratory testing actually comes to the bedside of the patient. Any changes to implement the use of POCT should show a significant improvement in patient outcome and a total financial benefit to the patient and the institution, not only a reduction in the costs of equipment and supplies.

Point-of-Care Testing

Decentralization of testing away from the traditional laboratory setting can greatly increase the interaction of laboratory personnel with patients and with other members of the health care team. POCT is an example of an interdisciplinary activity that crosses many boundaries in the health care facility. POCT is not always performed by laboratory staff. Other health care personnel, including nurses, respiratory therapists, anesthesiologists, operating room technologists, and physician assistants, often perform near-patient testing. Even in these cases, however, the CLIA '88 regulations associated with clinical laboratory testing must be followed for POCT, even if nonlaboratory staff members are actually performing the tests.

CLIA regulations are considered "site neutral." This means that all laboratory testing must meet the same standards for quality of work done, personnel, proficiency testing, and quality control, whether in a central laboratory or at the bedside of the patient. Regulation of the clinical laboratory (waived tests, tests of moderate or high complexity, PPMs) also applies to POCT. If performed in a facility that is accredited by TJC or CAP, these tests are regulated in essentially the same way as tests performed in a centralized laboratory.

Qualifications for POCT personnel are also set by federal, state, and local regulations.[5] The level of training varies with the analytical system being employed and the background of the individual involved, which can range from a requirement for a high school diploma with no experience to a bachelor of science degree with 2 years of experience. The director of the laboratory is responsible for setting additional requirements, provided the federal CLIA '88 regulations are also being followed.

Because results can be reported immediately and the patient's case management depends on these results, it is essential that POCT devices have built-in quality control and quality assessment systems to prevent erroneous data from being reported to the physician. POCT has been found to provide cost-effective improvements in medical care. In a hospital setting, POCT provides immediate assessment and management of the critically ill patient; this is its most significant use for this setting. Tests usually included in POCT are based on criteria of immediate medical need, including blood gases, prothrombin time coagulation test, partial thromboplastin time coagulation or activated blood-clotting time test, red blood cell measurements (such as hematocrit, hemoglobin), and glucose. POCT attempts to meet the demands of intensive care units (ICUs), operating rooms, and emergency departments for faster reporting of test results. Other benefits of POCT may include improved therapeutic turnaround times, less trauma and more convenience for the patient (when blood is collected and analyzed at the bedside), decreased preanalytical errors (formerly errors caused by specimen collection, transportation, and handling by the laboratory), decreased use of laboratory personnel (use of cross-training, whereby nurses can perform the laboratory analysis, eliminating a laboratorian for this step), more collaboration of clinicians with the laboratory, and shorter ICU stays. Certain tests, such as the fecal screen for blood and the routine chemical screening of urine by reagent strips, can often be done more easily on the nursing unit, if the assays are properly performed and controlled using quality assessment protocol.

In outpatient settings, POCT provides the ability to obtain test results during the patient's visit to the clinic or the physician's office, enabling diagnosis and subsequent case management in a timelier manner.

When central laboratory testing is compared with POCT, consideration must be given to which site of testing will provide the most appropriate testing mechanism. Centralized laboratories can provide "stat" testing capabilities, which can report results in a timely manner. Some laboratories develop a laboratory satellite that is set up to function at the point of need, such as a laboratory located near or in the operating room or a laboratory that is portable and can be transported on a cart to the point of need.

Reference Laboratories

When a laboratory performs only routine tests, specimens for the more complex tests ordered by the physician must be sent to a reference laboratory for analysis. It is often more cost-effective for a laboratory to perform only certain common, repetitive tests and to send the others to an outside laboratory. These reference laboratories can then perform the more complex tests for many patients, giving good turnaround times; this is their service to their customers. It is important to select a reference laboratory where the mechanisms for specimen transport and results reporting are managed well. The turnaround time is important and is often a function of how well the specimens are handled by the reference laboratory. There must be a good means of communication between the reference laboratory and its customers. The reference laboratory should be managed by professionals who both recognize the importance of providing quality results and, when needed, can provide the patient's clinician information about utilizing the results. Messengers or couriers are engaged to transport or drive specimens within a fixed, reasonable geographic area. The various commercial delivery systems are used for transport out of the area.

Physician Office Laboratories

A POL is a laboratory where the tests performed are limited to those done for the physician's own patients coming to the practice, group, or clinic. Because of the concern that quality work was lacking in some laboratories, the CLIA '88 regulations included POLs. Before CLIA, the POLs were largely unregulated. Most POLs perform only the waived tests or PPM, as set by CLIA. Tests most often performed in POLs are visually read reagent strip urinalysis, blood glucose, occult fecal blood, rapid streptococcus A in throats, hemoglobin/hematocrit, urine pregnancy, and cholesterol.

The convenience to the patient of having laboratory testing done in the physician's office is a driving force for physicians to include a laboratory in their office or clinic. Manufacturers of laboratory instruments have accommodated the clinic or office setting with a modern generation of instruments that require less technical skill by the user. However, the improved turnaround times for test results and patient convenience must be balanced with cost-effectiveness and the potential for physicians to be exposed to problems outside their expertise or training. Laboratory staff, including pathologists, must be available to act as consultants when the need arises.

A POL must submit an application to HHS or its designee. This application form includes details about the number of tests done, methodologies used for each measurement, and the qualifications of each of the testing personnel employed to perform the tests. Certificates are issued for up to 2 years, and any changes in tests done or methodologies used, personnel hired, and so forth must be submitted to HHS within 30 days of the change. This application may also be made through an accreditation agency whose requirements are deemed by HHS to be equal to or more stringent than the HHS requirements. Accreditation requirements from COLA have been recognized by CMS as being equivalent to the CLIA requirements.

When a POL performs only waived tests or PPM tests, there are no CLIA personnel requirements. The physician is responsible for the work done in the POL. When moderately or highly complex testing is done in a POL, the more stringent CLIA personnel requirements must be followed for the testing personnel; these POLs must also adhere to a program of quality assessment, including proficiency testing.

MEDICAL-LEGAL ISSUES

Informed Consent

For laboratories, an important responsibility is obtaining **informed consent** from the patient. Informed consent means that the patient is aware of, understands, and agrees to the nature of the testing to be done and what will be done with the results reported. Generally, when a patient enters a hospital, there is an implied consent to the many routine procedures that will be performed while the patient is in the hospital. Venipuncture is one of the routine tests that carry this implied consent. The patient must sign specific consent forms for more complex procedures, such as bone marrow aspiration, lumbar puncture for collection of cerebrospinal fluid, and fine-needle biopsy, as well as for nonurgent transfusion of blood or its components.

The patient should be given sufficient information about the reasons why the informed consent is needed and must be given the opportunity to ask questions. In the event the patient is incapable of signing the consent form, a guardian's consent should be obtained, as when the patient is a minor, legally not competent, physically unable to write, hearing impaired, or does not speak English as the first language. Health care institutions have policies in place for handling these situations.

Health Insurance Portability and Accountability Act

Any results obtained for specimens from patients must be kept strictly confidential. The Health Insurance Portability and Accountability Act (HIPAA) of 1996 requires the privacy of patient information.[9] Any information about the patient, including the types of measurements being done, must also be kept in confidence. Only authorized persons should have access to the information about a patient, and any release of this information to non–health care persons (such as insurance personnel, lawyers, and friends of patient) can be done only when authorized by the patient. It is important to discuss a particular patient's situation only in the confines of the laboratory setting and not in public places (such as elevators or hospital coffee shops).

With the passage of the HIPAA, laboratory information systems (LIS) security received new emphasis. Communications from the LIS should meet HIPAA compliance for encryption and methodology. Users should be prompted to log on and off the software to ensure that unauthorized access is prevented. The LIS should have full transaction capture, to track any manipulation of patient results data.

Public Law 104-191 (HIPAA) establishes a minimum standard for security of electronic health information to protect the confidentiality, integrity, and availability of protected patient information. HHS published the Privacy Rule on December 28, 2000, and adopted modifications on August 14, 2002. This rule set national standards for the protection of health information by health plans, health care clearinghouses, and health care providers who conduct certain transactions electronically. The HIPAA Privacy Rule established for the first time a foundation of federal protections for the privacy of protected health information. The rule does not replace federal, state, or other laws that grant individuals even greater privacy protections, and covered entities are free to retain or adopt more protective policies or practices.

Most portions of HIPAA are relevant to electronic information and the electronic interchange of information. HIPAA rules apply to any health information that can be linked to a person by name, social security number, employee number, hospital identification number, or other identifier. These provisions cover protected health information, regardless of whether it is or has been in electronic form or relates to any past, present, or future health care or payments. HIPAA legislation has a direct effect on the LIS. It includes requirements for the laboratory to collect diagnosis codes from the ordering provider on outpatient testing reimbursed by Medicare, a requirement under the Balanced Budget Act of 1997.

New Patient Access Regulations

A new final rule by CMS grants patients direct access to their laboratory results. The new rule revises CLIA '88 and HIPAA privacy rules to require laboratories to give a patient, or a person designated by the patient or his or her "personal representative," access to the patient's completed test reports on the patient's or the representative's request. Generally, the rule requires that laboratories provide individuals with access to their laboratory test reports within 30 days of the request. The rule does provide clinical laboratories with the flexibility to determine the process that allows them to fulfill the patient's request, including the process of verifying the identity of the patient.

The new final rule does not require that laboratories interpret test results for patients. Patients merely have the right to inspect and receive a copy of their completed test reports and other individually identifiable health information maintained in a designated record set by a HIPAA-covered laboratory. Laboratories may continue to refer patients with questions about test results back to their ordering or treating health care providers.

Chain of Custody

When specimens are involved in possible medicolegal situations, certain specimen-handling policies are required. Medicolegal or forensic implications require that any data pertaining to the specimen in question be determined in such a way that the information will be recognized by a court of law.

Laboratory test results that could be used in a court of law, such as at a trial or judicial hearing, must be handled in a specific manner. For evidence to be admissible, each step of the analysis, beginning with the moment the specimen is collected and transported to the laboratory, to the analysis itself and the reporting of the results, must be documented; this process is known as "maintaining the chain of custody." The links between specimen collection and presentation in court must establish certainty that the material or specimen tested had not been altered in any way that would change its usefulness as admissible evidence. Any specimen that has potential evidentiary value should be labeled, sealed, and placed in a locked refrigerator or other suitable secure storage area.

For drug testing, it is the course of action of documenting the management and storage of a specimen from the moment a donor gives the specimen to the collector to the final destination of the specimen and the review and reporting of the final result.[10] Blood specimens for alcohol level determination, specimens collected from rape victims, specimens for paternity testing, and specimens submitted from the medical examiner's cases are the usual types requiring chain-of-custody documentation.

Chain-of-custody documentation must be signed by every person who has handled the specimens involved in the case in question. The actual process may vary in different health care facilities, but the general purpose of this process is to make certain that any data obtained by the clinical laboratory will be admissible in a court of law, and that all the proper steps have been taken to ensure the integrity of the information produced.

Other Legal Considerations

Health care organizations and their employees are obliged to provide an acceptable standard of care, defined as the degree of care a reasonable person would take to prevent an injury to another. When a hospital or other health care provider, or a physician or other medical professional, does not treat a patient with the proper quality of care, resulting in serious patient injury or death, the provider has committed medical negligence. As a result, perceived negligence may lead to legal action or a lawsuit or tort. A tort is an act that injures someone in some way and for which the injured person may sue the "wrongdoer" for damages. Legally, torts are called *civil wrongs.* Medical personnel working directly with patients (such as phlebotomists) are more likely than laboratory bench staff to encounter legal issues.

MEDICAL ETHICS

What is **ethics**? According to *Merriam-Webster's Collegiate Dictionary*, the definition of ethics includes "the discipline dealing with what is good and bad" as well as "a set of moral principles." Personal ethics are based on values or ideals and customs that are held in high regard by an individual or group of people. For example, many people value friendship, hard work, and loyalty.

Ethics also encompasses the principles of conduct of a group or individual, such as professional ethics. ASCLS endorses a professional code of ethics (Box 1.2), which states that all laboratory professionals have a responsibility for proper conduct toward the patient, their colleagues and the profession, and society. In addition, ASCLS has a pledge to the profession (Box 1.3).

BOX 1.2 American Society for Clinical Laboratory Science Code of Ethics

Preamble

The Code of Ethics of the American Society for Clinical Laboratory Science sets forth the principles and standards by which clinical laboratory professionals practice their profession.

I. Duty to the Patient

Clinical laboratory professionals are accountable for the quality and integrity of the laboratory services they provide. This obligation includes maintaining individual competence in judgment and performance and striving to safeguard the patient from incompetent or illegal practice by others.

Clinical laboratory professionals maintain high standards of practice. They exercise sound judgment in establishing, performing, and evaluating laboratory testing.

Clinical laboratory professionals maintain strict confidentiality of patient information and test results. They safeguard the dignity and privacy of patients and provide accurate information to other health care professionals about the services they provide.

II. Duty to Colleagues and the Profession

Clinical laboratory professionals uphold and maintain the dignity and respect of our profession and strive to maintain a reputation of honesty, integrity, and reliability. They contribute to the advancement of the profession by improving the body of knowledge, adopting scientific advances that benefit the patient, maintaining high standards of practice and education, and seeking fair socioeconomic working conditions for members of the profession.

Clinical laboratory professionals actively strive to establish cooperative and respectful working relationships with other health care professionals, with the primary objective of ensuring a high standard of care for the patients they serve.

III. Duty to Society

As practitioners of an autonomous profession, clinical laboratory professionals have the responsibility to contribute from their sphere of professional competence to the general well-being of the community.

Clinical laboratory professionals comply with relevant laws and regulations pertaining to the practice of clinical laboratory science and actively seek, within the dictates of their consciences, to change those which do not meet the high standards of care and practice to which the profession is committed.

(Reprinted with permission of the American Society for Clinical Laboratory Science, 2013. www.ascls.org/)

BOX 1.3 Pledge to the Profession

As a clinical laboratory professional, I strive to:

- Maintain and promote standards of excellence in performing and advancing the art and science of my profession
- Preserve the dignity and privacy of others
- Uphold and maintain the dignity and respect of our profession
- Seek to establish cooperative and respectful working relationships with other health professionals
- Contribute to the general well-being of the community

I will actively demonstrate my commitment to these responsibilities throughout my professional life.

(Reprinted with permission of the American Society for Clinical Laboratory Science, 2013. www.ascls.org/)

Situational ethics is a system of ethics by which acts are judged within their context instead of by categorical principles. Hospitals have ethics committees to evaluate situational ethics cases and to offer consultation services. Individual laboratory professionals may need to make decisions based on personal or professional values.

In the realm of health care, it is difficult to hold rules or principles that are "absolute." Many variables exist in the context of medicine, with several principles that seem to be applicable in many situations. Even though these are not considered absolute, the rules and principles serve as powerful action guides in medicine. Over the years, moral principles have won a general acceptance as applicable in the analysis of ethical issues in medicine.

The first prominent medical ethics committee in the United States was at the University of Washington.[11] The first task of this committee was to help clinicians determine which people should receive hemodialysis. In the late 1960s, hemodialysis was considered to be experimental, and the University of Washington hospital could care for only limited numbers of patients. The decisions of the committee meant life or death for patients in need of renal dialysis. The problem of allocating hemodialysis to patients in need was not solved until the U.S. government began to finance the treatment for anyone who required hemodialysis in the 1970s.

Ethics committee members usually represent major clinical services and other stakeholders in health care delivery. All members of the ethics committee take responsibility for learning techniques of ethical analysis and the arguments addressing volatile issues in medicine.

Hospital ethics committees usually have the major functions: responsibility of providing clinical ethics consultation, developing and/or revising policies pertaining to clinical ethics and hospital policy (such as advance directives, withholding and withdrawing life-sustaining treatments, informed consent, and organ procurement), and promoting education in medical ethics.

CASE STUDIES

CASE STUDY 1.1

G.G. is an unmarried 19-year-old college student. She has not been feeling well lately and went to see a primary care provider at the college health service. G.G. has an active sexual relationship with her boyfriend but practices safe sex. Blood was drawn for a complete blood count and monospot test. Urine was collected for routine examination and a pregnancy test.

M.M. is a work-study student at the college health service. His job is to schedule appointments and transmit follow-up testing results to the primary care provider. When G.G.'s blood and urine results were sent to the health service, M.M. noticed that her total white blood count was extremely elevated and her red blood count was very low. A notation was made on the report that follow-up testing was required to rule out leukemia or rule out other red or white blood cell disorders.

The next day, M.M. saw G.G. in their history class. G.G. asked him if her lab test results were back yet. He said that the results were received late the previous afternoon. G.G. then asked, "How were my results?"

Note: Narrative answers on instructor EVOLVE website.

Multiple Choice Question (Answer in Appendix A)

1. In this situation, M.M. is ethically responsible to:
   a. Only share the actual blood cell measurement results.
   b. Tell G.G. that he doesn't know the results.
   c. Share his interpretation of the results with G.G., the patient.
   d. Advise G.G., the patient, to contact her healthcare provider for her results.

Critical Thinking Group Discussion Questions

1. How should M.M. answer G.G.'s question? Should he say that he does not know, when he does know? Or, should he tell G.G. that he is not authorized to give test results to patients unless specifically told to do so by the primary care provider?
2. How would you handle a similar situation with a classmate?

CASE STUDY 1.2

Patricia was completing her clinical internship at the local hospital. At the end of the day, several patients were brought to the emergency department as the result of a car crash. Patricia recognized a patient's name on a tube of blood as one of her hometown neighbors. When she completed her assigned work, she was finished with her shift.

Note: Narrative answers on instructor EVOLVE website.

Multiple Choice Question (Answer in Appendix A)

1. In this situation, Patricia should:
   a. Take personal responsibility for her neighbor's laboratory testing.
   b. Recheck all of the patient's laboratory results for accuracy.
   c. Remain calm and do not interfere with the neighbor's care at the hospital.
   d. Wait for her neighbor to be transferred to ICU and then visit her.

Critical Thinking Group Discussion Questions

1. Should Patricia call her parents to tell them that a neighbor had been in a serious car crash and was in the hospital?
2. Should Patricia return to the hospital to visit the patient?
3. Should Patricia ask the nurse about the patient's status when she goes to work the next day?

REFERENCES

1. Bureau of Labor Statistics, U.S. Department of Labor, Occupational Outlook Handbook, Medical and Clinical Laboratory Technologists and Technicians, on the Internet at https://www.bls.gov/ooh/healthcare/medical-and-clinical-laboratory-technologists-and-technicians.htm (visited June 28, 2018).
2. Delwiche FA: Mapping the literature of clinical laboratory science, *J Med Libr Assoc* 91(3):303–310, 2003.
3. American Society of Clinical Pathologists. www.ascp.org (Accessed 18.08.09).
4. Nadder TS: The development of the doctorate in clinical laboratory science in the U.S., *J Int Federation Clin Chem Lab Med* 24(1), 2013.
5. U.S. Health Care Financing Administration, Department of Health and Human Services: Clinical laboratory improvement amendments of 1988, Fed Regist, April 24, 1995 (Final rules with comment).
6. Yost J: CLIA—2012 update, Centers for Medicare and Medicaid Services, Baltimore, Md. www.pointofcare.net (Accessed 01.06.13).
7. U.S. Health Care Financing Administration, Department of Health and Human Services: Clinical laboratory improvement amendments of 1988, Fed Regist, Feb 28, 1992 (CLIA '88; Final Rule. 42 CFR. Subpart K, 493.1201).
8. U.S. Health Care Financing Administration, Department of Health and Human Services: Clinical laboratory improvement amendments of 1988, Fed Regist, Sept 15, 1995 (Proposed rules).
9. Health Insurance Portability and Accountability Act of 1996 (HIPAA): Privacy and security rules. www.hhs.gov (Accessed 04.09.14).
10. Drug testing: what is chain of custody? http://www.drugtestingusa.com/documents/what_is_chain_of_custody.pdf (Accessed 04.09.14).
11. University of Washington School of Medicine: Ethics in medicine: ethics committees, programs and consultation. https://depts.washington.edu (Accessed 01.06.13).

BIBLIOGRAPHY

Americans with Disabilities Act and Amendments, 2010. www.ada.gov. Retrieved May 31, 2013.

Berger D: Medicare, government regulation, and competency certification: a brief history of medical diagnosis and the birth of the clinical laboratory. Part 3, MLO Med Lab Obs 31(10), www.ncbi.nlm.nih.gov (Accessed 12.02.09).

Clinical and Laboratory Standards Institute (CLSI), National Committee for Clinical Laboratory Standards: *Clinical laboratory technical procedure manuals: approved guideline,* ed 4, Pa, 2006, Wayne GP2–A5.

Hakim G: What is on the molecular diagnostics horizon? Part 5b. A brief history of medical diagnosis and the birth of the clinical laboratory, *MLO Med Lab Obs* 40(3), 2008.

Malone B: ISO accreditation comes to America, *Clin Lab News* 35(1):3–4, 2009.

Scott K: Using an electronic control document program, *Clin Lab News* 43(7), 2017.

Turgeon ML: *Immunology and serology in laboratory medicine,* ed 6, St Louis, 2017, Elsevier/Mosby.

REVIEW QUESTIONS (ANSWERS IN APPENDIX A)

Clinical Laboratory Science

1. The correct designation for a generalist laboratory professional with a bachelor's degree certified by the American Society for Clinical Pathology is:
   a. Medical laboratory technician
   b. Medical laboratory scientist
   c. Medical technician
   d. Medical technologist

Overview of the Clinical Laboratory

2. The role of the laboratory supervisor or manager is to:
   a. Supervise technical aspects of testing.
   b. Supervise business functions of testing.
   c. Examine surgically removed organs.
   d. Screen cytology for Pap smears.

Clinical Laboratory Improvement Amendments (CLIA) of 1988

3. Which of the following acts, agencies, or organizations was created to make certain the quality of work done in the laboratory is reliable?
   a. Centers for Medicare and Medicaid Services (CMS)
   b. Occupational Safety and Health Administration (OSHA)
   c. Clinical Laboratory Improvement Amendments of 1988 (CLIA '88)
   d. Centers for Disease Control and Prevention
4. Laboratories performing which of the following types of tests need to be enrolled in a CLIA-approved proficiency testing program?
   a. Waived
   b. Moderately complex
   c. Highly complex
   d. Both b and c
5. The role of provider-performed microscopy (PPM) is the:
   a. Continuation of the process of evaluating and monitoring all aspects of the laboratory to ensure accuracy of test results
   b. Specific microscopic tests (wet mounts) performed by a physician for his or her own patients
   c. Means by which quality control between laboratories is maintained
   d. Process of performing laboratory testing at the bedside of the patient and a means of decentralizing some of the laboratory testing

Laboratory Departments

6. The newest direction for laboratory testing procedures is:
   a. Larger automated instruments
   b. Networked systems for point-of-care testing
   c. Molecular diagnostic techniques in various laboratory departments
   d. Robotic specimen handling

Health Care Organizations

7. A hospital chief operating officer is responsible for:
   a. Implementing policies and oversight of daily activities
   b. Finances
   c. Setting policy and guiding the organization
   d. Overseeing the hospital information system

Primary Accrediting Organizations

8. What is the best description of the purpose of the College of American Pathologists (CAP) pertaining to the clinical laboratory?
   a. Sets accreditation requirements for physician office laboratories (POLs)
   b. Administers both CLIA '88 and Medicare programs
   c. CMS has given CAP deemed status to act on the government's behalf to certify clinical laboratories
   d. Nonprofit educational group that establishes consensus standards for maintaining a high-quality laboratory organization

External Government Laboratory Accreditation and Regulation

9. What is the best description of the purpose of the Commission on Office Laboratory Accreditation (COLA) pertaining to the clinical laboratory?
   a. Sets accreditation requirements for physician office laboratories (POLs)
   b. Administers both CLIA '88 and Medicare programs
   c. CMS has given COLA deemed status to act on the government's behalf to certify clinical laboratories
   d. Nonprofit educational group that establishes consensus standards for maintaining a high-quality laboratory organization
10. What is the best description of the purpose of the Centers for Medicare and Medicaid Services (CMS) pertaining to the clinical laboratory?

a. Sets accreditation requirements for physician office laboratories (POLs)
b. Administers both CLIA '88 and Medicare programs
c. CMS has given itself deemed status to act on the government's behalf to certify clinical laboratories
d. Nonprofit educational group that establishes consensus standards for maintaining a high-quality laboratory organization

Alternate Sites of Testing

11. The role of point-of-care testing (POCT) compared with in-laboratory testing is the:
   a. Continuation of the process of evaluating and monitoring all aspects of the laboratory to ensure accuracy of test results
   b. Specific microscopic tests (wet mounts) performed by a physician for his or her own patients
   c. Means by which quality control between laboratories is maintained
   d. Process of performing laboratory testing at the bedside of the patient and a means of decentralizing some of the laboratory testing

Medical-Legal Issues

12. Sally is seeing her new primary care provider for the first time. When she signs in, she is asked to sign papers for the release of medical records, including her laboratory results. According to the Health Insurance Portability and Accountability Act (HIPAA), she must authorize release of records before ________ would be permitted to receive and review her records.
   a. Her insurance company
   b. Her attorney
   c. Her husband
   d. Any of the above
13. In which of the following laboratory situations is a verbal report permissible?
   a. When the patient is going directly to the physician's office and wants to have the report available
   b. When the report cannot be found at the nurse's station
   c. When preoperative test results are needed by the anesthesiologist
   d. None of the above
14. All the following characteristics are accurate for the influence of Health Insurance Portability and Accountability Act (HIPAA) *except*:
   a. Replaces federal, state, or other laws that grant individuals even greater privacy protections than HIPAA
   b. Covers entities that are free to retain or adopt more protective policies or practices
   c. Establishes a minimum standard for security of electronic health information and the electronic interchange of information
   d. Directly effects the laboratory information system (LIS)
15. In order to perform a venipuncture on a newly admitted hospital patient, a phlebotomist needs to:
   a. Ask for the patient's written permission to perform the procedure.
   b. Verify that the patient has specifically named the drawing of blood in the admissions papers.
   c. Realize that an admitted hospital patient has given implied consent to routine procedures such as phlebotomy.
   d. Verify with the patient's primary care provider that phlebotomy is covered as a routine procedure.
16. Chain-of-custody procedures must be followed for:
   a. Blood specimens for alcohol level determination
   b. Routine urinalysis for glucose and ketones
   c. Therapeutic drug threshold determinations
   d. Throat swabs of group A beta streptococcus screening

Medical Ethics

17. Medical ethics:
   a. Has strict guidelines
   b. Applies to laboratory professionals
   c. Includes situational ethics
   d. Both b and c
18. *Bonus Challenge Question:* Answer this question based on the following laboratory situation:
   Lisa works in the laboratory at a small community hospital in a small Midwestern town. She received orders to draw blood from a newly admitted patient for a complete blood count (CBC) and a metabolic chemistry panel. When Lisa arrived in the patient's room, she discovered that the patient was Carla, her best friend's mother. She chatted with Carla for a bit and then headed back to the lab to complete testing on the samples. Thirty minutes later, Betsy, who is one of Carla's friends, called the lab to talk with Lisa. Apparently, Carla posted on a social media site that Lisa had drawn her blood and Betsy was calling to get all of the details. "I called Carla to find out what's going on, but she's being evasive. I'm watching her dog so I need to know the real scoop...."

What should Lisa do?
   a. It is acceptable to share information with Betsy because Carla stated on social media that she was in the hospital.
   b. Politely tell Betsy she cannot comment on patients in the hospital.
   c. Thank Betsy for her concern and tell her that Carla seemed "okay."
   d. Politely tell Betsy she cannot talk about work with people who are not employed at the hospital.

2

Safety: Patient and Clinical Laboratory Practices

http://evolve.elsevier.com/Turgeon/clinicallab/

CHAPTER CONTENTS

LEARNING OUTCOMES

Patient safety

- Analyze the six goals for health care delivery, and provide examples of the important issues in each goal category.
- Explain why medical euphemisms are a bad habit and what negative outcomes can be generated by their use.
- Evaluate a strategy to mitigate patient risk during an information technology outage, and assess potential high priorities in a strategy.

Safety Standards and Governing Agencies

- Name the two agencies responsible for laboratory safety in the United States.
- Describe the general functions of various governmental and professional agencies.
- Describe the laboratory-related goals of the National Healthcare Safety Network.
- Examine and compare the general safety regulations governing the clinical laboratory, including components of the OSHA-mandated plans for chemical hygiene and for occupational exposure to bloodborne pathogens, the importance of the safety manual, and general emergency procedures.

Avoiding transmission of infectious diseases

- Define a laboratory-acquired infection (LAI) and name the top 10 microorganisms causing LAIs.
- Name the three most common viral causes of LAIs.

Bloodborne Pathogens

- Name three mandated OSHA bloodborne safety standard practices.
- Describe four specific factors that carry a higher risk of HIV transmission due to percutaneous injury.

Safe work practices for infection control

- Contrast the basic aspects of infection control policies, including how and when to use personal protective equipment or devices (such as gowns, gloves, and goggles), and evaluate the reasons for using Standard Precautions.
- Explain proper decontamination of a work area at the beginning and end of a routine workday, as well as when a hazardous spill has occurred.
- Describe nine safety practices to reduce the risk of inadvertent contamination with blood or certain body fluids.
- Explain the three required contents of a laboratory Safety Manual.

Specimen Handling and Shipping Requirements

- Name government agency that specifies the requirements for shipping clinical specimens.

Prevention of disease transmission

- Assess preexposure and postexposure prophylactic measures for handling potential occupational transmission of certain pathogens, especially hepatitis B virus (HBV) and human immunodeficiency virus (HIV).

Additional laboratory hazards

- Evaluate how to take the necessary precautions to avoid exposure to the many potentially hazardous situations in the clinical laboratory: biohazards; chemical, fire, and electrical hazards; and certain supplies and equipment (such as broken labware).
- Explain successful implementation of chemical hazards "right-to-know" rules.

Final decontamination of waste materials

- Explain the process of properly segregating and disposing of various types of waste products generated in the clinical laboratory, including use of sharps containers for used needles and lancets.

Safety audit

- Summarize the top six safety audit issues and choose resolutions to each of the issues.

Basic first-aid procedures

- List and describe the basic steps of first aid
- Perform each laboratory exercise and summarize the purpose and sources of error of each exercise.

Case Study

❖ Analyze the patient history, clinical signs and symptoms, and laboratory data for the stated case studies, answer the related critical thinking questions, and conclude the most likely diagnosis.

Review Questions

- Demonstrate comprehension of the chapter content by completing the end-of-chapter review questions with a grade of 80% or higher.

Note:

• indicates MLT and MLS core content

❖ indicates MLT (optional) and MLS advanced content

KEY TERMS

biohazard
disinfection
Hazard Communication Standard (HCS)
iatrogenic
infectious waste
necrosis
nosocomial
Occupational Exposure to Bloodborne Pathogens
pathogens
personal protective equipment (PPE)
safety data sheet (SDS)
sepsis
Standard Precautions

PATIENT SAFETY

The Agency for Healthcare Research and Quality defines patient safety as "freedom from accidental or preventable injuries produced by medical care."[1] Each year the ECRI Institute publishes the Top 10 safety issues. Two of the identified errors are patient identification errors and test reporting with follow up. Errors related to laboratory testing are discussed in chapter 3, Quality Assessment and Quality Control in the Clinical Laboratory.[2]

According to 2018 The Joint Commission (TJC): Laboratory National Patient Safety Goals[3], three goal areas have specific applications for laboratory services. These goals relate to correctly identifying a patient by using two ways to identify a patient, improving staff communication to get important test results to the correct staff person in a timely manner, and preventing infection by using CDC or WHO hand cleaning guidelines.

In "Crossing the Quality Chasm: a New Health System for the 21st Century," the U.S. Institute of Medicine[4] presents the multiple ways in which patient care in the United States falls short of expectations. The Institute outlines six goals for health care delivery to improve the quality of care, as follows:

1. *Safety.* This goal focuses on avoiding injuries from care delivered to the patient. The applicability of this goal in the laboratory is centered on avoiding preevaluation, evaluation, and postevaluation errors.
2. *Timeliness.* This goal addresses reduction in the length of time or delays in providing or receiving care. Laboratory examples of improving timeliness can be found by incorporating point-of-care testing and focusing on improving the turnaround time of testing that supports improved patient outcomes.
3. *Effectiveness.* This goal category stresses the avoidance of underuse, overuse, and misuse of laboratory testing. The laboratory can impact this goal by performing an analysis of underused, overused, and misused assays. Additionally, outdated procedures can be retired using evidence-based practice knowledge. In this way, patients who could benefit from laboratory tests receive appropriate care, and those who are not likely to benefit avoid nonbeneficial testing.
4. *Efficiency.* This goal aims to reduce or avoid waste. Waste may be in the form of materials and supplies or wasted time. Examples of waste can be identified in the three phases of laboratory analysis: preevaluation (preanalytic), evaluation (analytic), and postevaluation (postanalytic).
5. *Equitable treatment.* This goal addresses the need to provide consistent quality of care regardless of gender, ethnicity, socioeconomic class, or geographic location. The laboratory can influence success in this goal category by expanding outpatient hours and sites of specimen collection, providing multilanguage information about laboratory testing, and documenting consistency of quality between in-house and POCT procedures.
6. *Patient-centered focus.* This final category of quality improvement spotlights the need to provide respectful care that is responsive to diversified patients. Laboratory professionals can be instrumental in facilitating this goal by answering patient questions and communicating pertinent information to them.

The American Society for Clinical Laboratory Science provides patient safety indicators (Table 2.1) and a seven-step procedure to evaluate patient safety in the clinical laboratory (Table 2.2).

TABLE 2.1 Examples of ASCLS Patient Safety Indicators

Testing Phase	Category	Representative Examples
Preanalytical	Patient identification	Failure to use two patient identifiers
	Phlebotomy-associated negative events	Lapse in infection prevention/hand hygiene
		Skin reaction to tape/bandage/latex
		Sharps (needles or lancets) left in patient bed
	Specimen identification	Unlabeled specimen
		Mislabeled specimen
	Order entry	Test(s) ordered on the wrong patient
		Incorrect test or procedure ordered
	Specimen integrity	Insufficient volume of specimen
		Lost or destroyed sample
		Improper temperature maintained while transporting or storing
	Effective use of the clinical laboratory	Failure to order the appropriate test
		Test requested at inappropriate time
Analytical	Verification of the accuracy of abnormal results	Failure to recognize specimen-processing errors that affect test results
		Failure to verify abnormal or critical point-of-care results with the clinical laboratory
Postanalytical	Communication of test results	Critical values not reported within defined time frame to clinician
		Failure of timeliness in communication of results to clinician
	Effective use of test results	Incorrect interpretation of test results
		Failure to order follow-up test(s)
	Outcomes of laboratory testing	Failure of provider to notify patient of abnormal test results and required next steps

Modified from American Society for Clinical Laboratory Science (ASCLS) with permission: ASCLS Patient Safety Indicators. www.ascls.org. Retrieved May 16, 2013.

TABLE 2.2 ASCLS Seven-Step Procedure to Evaluate Patient Safety in Laboratory Testing

Step	Description	Comments
1	Determine areas of risk	Identify the Patient Safety Indicators that pose the greatest risk of harm to patients (see Table 2-1).
2	Collect data	Based on selection of the indicators with the greatest risk, select a few indicators, either all in one phase or spread across all three phases of the Total Testing Process. It is important to incorporate the entire scope of testing services (such as chemistry) and the spectrum of practice sites (such as hospital, clinic, outpatient drawing centers).
3	Determine the denominator to calculate the error rate	It is important to convert the absolute number of errors that occur into an error rate in order to achieve consistency in comparing different laboratories. Error rate for nonhospital labs should calculate error rate on an event per patient encounter basis. The denominator will be the number of patient encounters for the evaluation time frame. Error rate for hospital labs should calculate error rate per adjusted patient day, which includes inpatient and outpatient services. The denominator is adjusted patient days.
4	Capture data	The length of time for collecting data is dependent on how often the process error occurs. The time frame can range from weekly to annual.
5	Data analysis	Factors to consider include acceptability of rate of errors, impact of the error, trending of data, and patient outcomes.
6	Design intervention	After root cause(s) and other results of data analysis, an intervention should be developed with a pilot study. Measurements methods must be the same pre- and post-intervention.
7	Follow-up	Once acceptable error rates have been achieved, an indicator should be monitored periodically or as a spot check.

Modified from American Society for Clinical Laboratory Science (ASCLS) with permission, ASCLS procedure to evaluate aspects of Clinical Laboratory Services Total Testing Process that impact patient safety. www.ascls.org. Retrieved May 16, 2013.

TABLE 2.3 Medical Euphemisms

Euphemism	Meaning
Adverse event	A patient was harmed due to a problem in medical care.
Incident	An event has come into being and is not good.
Near miss	A patient was nearly harmed. A more accurate euphemism would be "near hit."
Occurrence	An event that has come into being.
Potential adverse event	A patient was nearly harmed due to a problem in medical care.
Sentinel event	A patient died or was severely harmed due to a problem in medical care, most likely a preventable error.
Variance	A movement away from our desired norm.

From Astion M: Clear communication and patient harm events, *Clin Lab News* 38(1):13, 2012.

Communications

The need for clear communication is imperative. Avoiding direct communication of an error that harmed a patient is unacceptable.[5] Avoidance lowers or removes the urgency for quality improvement. *Medical euphemisms* are commonly used in clinical laboratories to describe medical errors that harm patients (Table 2.3). The use of euphemisms is a bad habit thought to be rooted in the desire to avoid painful, complex quality improvement issues as well as the extra work that improvement strategies create. Taking time to communicate will help ensure patient safety.

Mitigating Patient Risk

A critical area of concern related to patient safety is the mitigation of patient risk during information technology (IT) outages.[6] This is a universal challenge for clinical laboratories and health care systems. Laboratories need to be prepared for two types of total or partial IT downtime: (1) planned outages for updates or upgrades and (2) unexpected failures or impairments with an unknown length of downtime. In the current highly automated laboratory environment, affected services can impact test ordering, specimen collection and labeling, specimen processing and testing, and the reporting of results.

The initial step toward managing IT downtime is to have a clear activation and communications plan with established guidelines for initiating downtime protocols. Downtime protocols may differ depending on the IT systems affected. For effective downtime implementation, plans should be shared with patient care areas to ensure that laboratory personnel lead a team effort to provide testing. A single laboratory contact creates an organized approach to information management. Some form of mass communication should briefly state that laboratory results will be delayed because of IT issues. An estimated length of downtime may be included.

Laboratory staff members need to know the time frames for initiating alternate testing protocols. "Stat" testing from the emergency department, intensive care unit (ICU), or critical care unit must receive the highest priorities. Clearly labeled specimens from patients in these designated high-preference areas should be used. Reporting of critical results should be a special focus of risk mitigation during IT outages. During these times, laboratory personnel must identify critical results and report these to care providers. Command centers or designated service pagers for receiving data on critical results are of utmost importance to high-quality patient care during these emergencies. When the crisis has been resolved, communication with end users is essential; this step closes the communications loop. Lastly, a critique of the processes and events during the IT outage needs to be conducted. This critique will contribute to a better workflow in the event of future IT outages.

SAFETY STANDARDS AND GOVERNING AGENCIES

The importance of safety and correct first-aid procedures cannot be overemphasized. Many accidents do not just happen; they are caused by carelessness, lack of attention to detail, or lack of proper communication. For this reason, the practice of safety should be uppermost in the mind of all persons working in a clinical laboratory. Most laboratory accidents are preventable by exercising good technique, staying alert, and using common sense.

Laboratory safety includes Occupational Safety and Health Administration (OSHA) standards and Centers for Disease Control and Prevention (CDC) guidelines designed to protect laboratory personnel from potential hazards in the clinical laboratory. Safety in the clinical laboratory encompasses bloodborne pathogen protection and chemical, fire, and electrical safety.

Ergonomics is a safety issue. Ergonomics studies human capabilities in relationship to the work demands placed on an individual while at work. Clinical laboratories have multiple ergonomic stressors, such as back strain from an uncomfortable chair or aching feet from walking or standing on hard floors. Repetitive actions such as pipetting or typing are potential sources of motion injuries (such as carpal tunnel syndrome). The term musculoskeletal disorders (MSDs) is used to describe the most common physical ergonomic stressors where muscles, nerves, tendons, joints, or discs are affected. MSDs include carpal tunnel syndrome, rotator cuff syndrome, tendinitis, and sciatica. Any type of stressor likely to lead to an MSD is called a "work-related musculoskeletal disorder hazard." To improve working conditions in the clinical laboratory, a periodic ergonomic assessment should be conducted. Stressors with injury potential include repetition, posture, force or pressure associated with hard surfaces, vibration, and ambient temperature. Engineering changes can improve ergonomic conditions. Working conditions (such as shift length) and educational interventions on prevention of unfavorable conditions can reduce the threat of ergonomic injury.

Safety standards for patients and clinical laboratories are initiated, governed, and reviewed by the following federal agencies and professional organizations[7–11]:

1. OSHA, U.S. Department of Labor
2. Clinical and Laboratory Standards Institute (CLSI)
3. CDC, U.S. Department of Health and Human Services, Public Health Service (PHS)
4. College of American Pathologists (CAP)
5. The Joint Commission. TJC has established National Patient Safety Goals, three apply specifically to laboratory services.

National Healthcare Safety Network

The National Healthcare Safety Network (NHSN). This voluntary system integrates a number of surveillance systems and provides data on devices, patients, and staff. The NHSN expands legacy patient and health care personnel safety surveillance systems managed by the Division of Healthcare Quality Promotion at CDC. NHSN also includes a new component for hospitals to monitor adverse reactions and incidents associated with receipt of blood and blood products. Enrollment is open to all types of health care facilities in the United States.

The National Nosocomial Infections Surveillance System of the CDC performed a survey from October 1986 to April 1998. The highest rates of infection occurred in the burn ICU, the neonatal ICU, and the pediatric ICU. Within hours of admission, colonies of hospital strains of bacteria develop in the patient's skin, respiratory tract, and genitourinary tract. Risk factors for the invasion of colonizing pathogens can be categorized into the following three areas:

- Iatrogenic risk factors include pathogens on the hands of medical personnel, invasive procedures (such as intubation and extended ventilation, indwelling vascular lines, and urine catheterization), and antibiotic use and prophylaxis.
- Organizational risk factors include contaminated air-conditioning systems, contaminated water systems, and staffing and physical layout of the facility (such as nurse-to-patient ratio and open beds close together).
- Patient risk factors include the severity of illness, underlying immunocompromised state, and length of stay.

Nosocomial infections are estimated to occur in 5% of all acute care hospitalizations. In the United States the incidence of hospital-acquired infection is more than 2 million cases per year. Nosocomial infections are caused by viral, bacterial, and fungal pathogens. In pediatric patient units surveyed between 1992 and 1997, the incidence of nosocomial invasive bacterial and fungal infections was highest in bloodstream infections, with coagulase-negative staphylococci found in the majority of cases. Infections caused by methicillin-resistant *Staphylococcus aureus* (MRSA) are not worse than those caused by susceptible *S. aureus*. MRSA requires treatment with different families of antibiotics. Although the pathogenicity does not generally differ from that of susceptible strains of *S. aureus*, MRSA strains that carry the loci for Panton-Valentine leukocidin can be hypervirulent and can cause lymphopenia, rapid tissue necrosis, and severe sepsis.

Many hospitals have reorganized the physical layout of handwashing stations and have adopted patient cohorting to prevent the spread of pathogens. They have also restricted or rotated the administration of many antibiotics that are used to combat nosocomial infections. A special concern in regard to bacterial agents is that multiresistant organisms, such as vancomycin-resistant enterococci, glycopeptide-resistant *S. aureus*, and inducible or extended-spectrum beta-lactamase gram-negative organisms, are a constant threat.

Occupational Safety and Health Administration Acts and Standards

To ensure that workers have safe and healthful working conditions, the U.S. Federal Government created a system of safeguards and regulations under the Occupational Safety and Health Act of 1970 and in 1988 expanded the Hazard Communication Standard[8] (HCS; revised in 2012) to apply to hospital staff. Occupational Safety and Health Act regulations apply to all businesses with one or more employees and are administered by the U.S. Department of Labor through OSHA. The programs deal with many aspects of safety and health protection, including compliance arrangements, inspection procedures, penalties for noncompliance, complaint procedures, duties and responsibilities for administration and operation of the system, and how the many standards are set. Responsibility for compliance is placed on both the administration of the institution and the employee.

Both OSHA and CDC have published numerous safety standards and regulations that are applicable to clinical laboratories. Ensuring safety in the clinical laboratory includes the following measures:

- A formal safety program
- Specifically mandated plans (such as chemical hygiene and bloodborne pathogens)
- Identification of various hazards (such as fire, electrical, chemical, and biological)
- Safety officer and safety coaches

A designated laboratory safety officer and laboratory safety coaches are a critical part of a laboratory safety program, including "safety eyes" and "safety ears" to implement surveillance of correct safety practices including compliance with existing regulations affecting the laboratory and staff, correct labeling of chemicals and the proper handling and disposal of waste.

The safety officer is responsible for initial orientation of staff and the periodic updating of staff (Table 2.4). Safety coaches are volunteers who assume additional job responsibilities. These volunteers represent all laboratory departments and shifts, and job roles. Safety coaches have six important functions:

1. Communicator of safety habits
2. Educator of safety habits
3. Role model of safety habits
4. Observer of safety habits

TABLE 2.4 Recommended Safety Training Schedule

Topic	Who Needs to be Trained	Frequency
All laboratory safety policies and procedures	All laboratory staff	Upon employment
Fire extinguisher practice	All laboratory staff	Upon employment
Spill cleanup	All technical staff	Upon employment
Fire prevention and preparedness	All laboratory staff	Annually
Fire drill evacuation	All laboratory staff	Annually
Chemical safety	All staff who handle or transport chemicals	Annually
Biological hazard	All laboratory staff	Annually
Infection control	All laboratory staff	Annually
Radiation safety	Only employees who use or transport radioactive materials	Annually
Specimen packaging and shipping procedures	Staff who package specimens for shipping by ground or air	Every 24 months

From Gile TJ: *Complete guide to laboratory safety,* Marblehead, Mass, 2004, HCPro.

5. Storyteller to implement positive change
6. Change agent for maximum compliance with correct safety habits

Safety coaches can facilitate safety habits for prevention of errors by paying attention to details, communicating clearly, and having a questioning attitude. These volunteers must recognized that barriers such as peer resistance and time constraints need to be overcome.

OSHA-Mandated Plans

In 1991, OSHA mandated that all clinical laboratories must implement a chemical hygiene plan (CHP) and an exposure control plan. As part of the CHP, a copy of the **safety data sheet (SDS)** must be on file and readily accessible and available to all employees at all times.

Chemical Hygiene Plan

A CHP is the core of the OSHA safety standard. Existing safety and health plans may meet the CHP requirements. A written CHP is to be developed by each employer and must specify the following:

- The training and information requirements of the OSHA standard
- Designation of a chemical hygiene officer and committee
- Appropriate work practices
- A list of chemicals in inventory
- Availability of SDSs
- Labeling requirements
- Record-keeping requirements
- Standard operating procedures and housekeeping requirements
- Methods of required engineering controls, such as eyewashes and safety showers
- Measures for appropriate maintenance and list of protective equipment
- Requirements for employee medical examinations
- Special precautions for working with particularly hazardous substances
- Information on waste removal and disposal
- Other information deemed necessary for safety assurance

Hazard Communication Standard

The OSHA HCS (29 CFR 1910.1200[g]), revised in 2012, requires that the chemical manufacturer, distributor, or importer provide SDSs, formerly material safety data sheets (MSDSs), for each hazardous chemical to downstream users to communicate information on these hazards. The information contained in the SDS is largely the same as the MSDS, except now the SDSs are required to be presented in a consistent, user-friendly, 16-section format (Box 2.1).

As with the current standard, the new HCS requires chemical manufacturers and importers to evaluate the chemicals they produce or import and provide hazard information to employers and workers by putting labels on containers and preparing SDSs. The modified standard provides a single set of harmonized criteria for classifying chemicals according to their health and physical hazards and specifies hazard communication elements

BOX 2.1 Safety Data Sheet (SDS) Format in OSHA Hazard Communication Standard (HCS)

Section 1: Identification

This section identifies the chemical on the SDS as well as the recommended uses. It also provides the essential contact information of the supplier. The required information consists of:

- Product identifier used on the label and any other common names or synonyms by which the substance is known.
- Name, address, phone number of the manufacturer, importer, or other responsible party, and emergency phone number.
- Recommended use of the chemical (such as a brief description of what it actually does, for example with flame retardant) and any restrictions on use (including recommendations given by the supplier).

Section 2: Hazard(s) Identification

This section identifies the hazards of the chemical presented on the SDS and the appropriate warning information associated with those hazards. The required information consists of:

- The hazard classification of the chemical (such as flammable liquid, category[1]).
- Signal word.
- Hazard statement(s).
- Pictograms (the pictograms or hazard symbols may be presented as graphical reproductions of the symbols in black and white or be a description of the name of the symbol (such as skull and crossbones or flame)).
- Precautionary statement(s).
- Description of any hazards not otherwise classified.
- For a mixture that contains an ingredient(s) with unknown toxicity, a statement describing how much (percentage) of the mixture consists of ingredient(s) with unknown acute toxicity. Please note that this is a total percentage of the mixture and not tied to the individual ingredient(s).

Section 3: Composition/Information on Ingredients

This section identifies the ingredient(s) contained in the product indicated on the SDS, including impurities and stabilizing additives. This section includes information on substances, mixtures, and all chemicals where a trade secret is claimed. The required information consists of:

Substances

- Chemical name.
- Common name and synonyms.
- Chemical Abstracts Service (CAS) number and other unique identifiers.
- Impurities and stabilizing additives, which are themselves classified and which contribute to the classification of the chemical.

Mixtures

- Same information required for substances.
- The chemical name and concentration (i.e., exact percentage) of all ingredients which are classified as health hazards and are:
  Present above their cutoff/concentration limits *or*
  Present a health risk below the cutoff/concentration limits.
- The concentration (exact percentages) of each ingredient must be specified, except concentration ranges may be used in the following situations:
  A trade secret claim is made,
  There is batch-to-batch variation, *or*
  The SDS is used for a group of substantially similar mixtures.

Chemicals where a trade secret is claimed

- A statement that the specific chemical identity and/or exact percentage (concentration) of composition has been withheld as a trade secret is required.

Section 4: First-Aid Measures

This section describes the initial care that should be given by untrained responders to an individual who has been exposed to the chemical. The required information consists of:

- Necessary first-aid instructions by relevant routes of exposure (inhalation, skin and eye contact, and ingestion).
- Description of the most important symptoms or effects, and any symptoms that are acute or delayed.
- Recommendations for immediate medical care and special treatment needed, when necessary.

Section 5: Fire-Fighting Measures

This section provides recommendations for fighting a fire caused by the chemical. The required information consists of:

- Recommendations of suitable extinguishing equipment, and information about extinguishing equipment that is not appropriate for a particular situation.
- Advice on specific hazards that develop from the chemical during the fire, such as any hazardous combustion products created when the chemical burns.
- Recommendations on special protective equipment or precautions for firefighters.

Section 6: Accidental Release Measures

This section provides recommendations on the appropriate response to spills, leaks, or releases, including containment and cleanup practices to prevent or minimize exposure to people, properties, or the environment. It may also include recommendations distinguishing between responses for large and small spills where the spill volume has a significant impact on the hazard. The required information may consist of recommendations for:

- Use of personal precautions (such as removal of ignition sources or providing sufficient ventilation) and protective equipment to prevent the contamination of skin, eyes, and clothing.
- Emergency procedures, including instructions for evacuations, consulting experts when needed, and appropriate protective clothing.
- Methods and materials used for containment (such as covering the drains and capping procedures).
- Cleanup procedures (such as appropriate techniques for neutralization, decontamination, cleaning or vacuuming; adsorbent materials; and/or equipment required for containment/cleanup).

Section 7: Handling and Storage

This section provides guidance on the safe handling practices and conditions for safe storage of chemicals. The required information consists of:

- Precautions for safe handling, including recommendations for handling incompatible chemicals, minimizing the release of the chemical into the environment, and providing advice on general hygiene practices (such as eating, drinking, and smoking in work areas is prohibited).
- Recommendations on the conditions for safe storage, including any incompatibilities. Provide advice on specific storage requirements (such as ventilation requirements).

Section 8: Exposure Controls/Personal Protection

This section indicates the exposure limits, engineering controls, and personal protective measures that can be used to minimize worker exposure. The required information consists of:

- OSHA Permissible Exposure Limits (PELs), American Conference of Governmental Industrial Hygienists (ACGIH) Threshold Limit Values (TLVs), and any other exposure limit used or recommended by the chemical manufacturer, importer, or employer preparing the safety data sheet, where available.
- Appropriate engineering controls (for example, use local exhaust ventilation, or use only in an enclosed system).
- Recommendations for personal protective measures to prevent illness or injury from exposure to chemicals, such as personal protective equipment (PPE) (for example, appropriate types of eye, face, skin, or respiratory protection needed based on hazards and potential exposure).

Continued

BOX 2.1 Safety Data Sheet (SDS) Format in OSHA Hazard Communication Standard (HCS)—cont'd

- Any special requirements for PPE, protective clothing, or respirators (such as type of glove material, as in PVC or nitrile rubber gloves; and breakthrough time of the glove material).

Section 9: Physical and Chemical Properties

This section identifies physical and chemical properties associated with the substance or mixture. The minimum required information consists of:

- Appearance (physical state, color, etc.)
- Odor
- Odor threshold
- pH
- Melting point/freezing point
- Initial boiling point and boiling range
- Flash point
- Evaporation rate
- Flammability (solid, gas)
- Upper/lower flammability or explosive limits
- Vapor pressure
- Vapor density
- Relative density
- Solubility(ies)
- Partition coefficient: n-octanol/water
- Auto-ignition temperature
- Decomposition temperature
- Viscosity

The SDS may not contain every item on the above list because information may not be relevant or is not available. When this occurs, a notation to that effect must be made for that chemical property. Manufacturers may also add other relevant properties, such as the dust deflagration index (Kst) for combustible dust, used to evaluate a dust's explosive potential.

Section 10: Stability and Reactivity

This section describes the reactivity hazards of the chemical and the chemical stability information. This section is broken into three parts: reactivity, chemical stability, and other. The required information consists of:

Reactivity

- Description of the specific test data for the chemical(s). These data can be for a class or family of the chemical if such data adequately represent the anticipated hazard of the chemical(s), where available.

Chemical Stability

- Indication of whether the chemical is stable or unstable under normal ambient temperature and conditions while in storage and being handled.
- Description of any stabilizers that may be needed to maintain chemical stability.
- Indication of any safety issues that may arise should the product change in physical appearance.

Other

- Indication of the possibility of hazardous reactions, including a statement whether the chemical will react or polymerize, which could release excess pressure or heat, or create other hazardous conditions. Also, a description of the conditions under which hazardous reactions may occur.
- List of all conditions that should be avoided (such as static discharge, shock, vibrations, or environmental conditions that may lead to hazardous conditions).
- List of all classes of incompatible materials (such as classes of chemicals or specific substances) with which the chemical could react to produce a hazardous situation.
- List of any known or anticipated hazardous decomposition products that could be produced because of use, storage, or heating. (Hazardous combustion products should also be included in Section 5: Fire-Fighting Measures of the SDS.)

Section 11: Toxicological Information

This section identifies toxicological and health effects information or indicates that such data are not available. The required information consists of:

- Information on the likely routes of exposure (inhalation, ingestion, skin and eye contact).
- The SDS should indicate if the information is unknown.
- Description of the delayed, immediate, or chronic effects from short- and long-term exposure.
- The numerical measures of toxicity (for example, acute toxicity estimates such as the LD50 (median lethal dose)—the estimated amount [of a substance] expected to kill 50% of test animals in a single dose.
- Description of the symptoms. This description includes the symptoms associated with exposure to the chemical including symptoms from the lowest to the most severe exposure.
- Indication of whether the chemical is listed in the National Toxicology Program (NTP) Report on Carcinogens (latest edition) or has been found to be a potential carcinogen in the International Agency for Research on Cancer (IARC) Monographs (latest editions) or found to be a potential carcinogen by OSHA.

Section 12: Ecological Information (non-mandatory)*[2]

This section provides information to evaluate the environmental impact of the chemical(s) if it were released to the environment. The information may include:

- Data from toxicity tests performed on aquatic and/or terrestrial organisms, where available (such as acute or chronic aquatic toxicity data for fish, algae, crustaceans, and other plants; toxicity data on birds, bees, and plants).
- Whether there is a potential for the chemical to persist and degrade in the environment either through biodegradation or other processes, such as oxidation or hydrolysis.
- Results of tests of bioaccumulation potential, making reference to the octanol-water partition coefficient (Kow) and the bioconcentration factor (BCF), where available.
- The potential for a substance to move from the soil to the groundwater (indicate results from adsorption studies or leaching studies).
- Other adverse effects (such as environmental fate, ozone layer depletion potential, photochemical ozone creation potential, endocrine disrupting potential, and/or global warming potential).

Section 13: Disposal Considerations (non-mandatory)*

This section provides guidance on proper disposal practices, recycling or reclamation of the chemical(s) or its container, and safe handling practices. To minimize exposure, this section should also refer the reader to Section 8 (Exposure Controls/Personal Protection) of the SDS. The information may include:

- Description of appropriate disposal containers to use.
- Recommendations of appropriate disposal methods to employ.
- Description of the physical and chemical properties that may affect disposal activities.
- Language discouraging sewage disposal.
- Any special precautions for landfills or incineration activities.

Continued

BOX 2.1 Safety Data Sheet (SDS) Format in OSHA Hazard Communication Standard (HCS)—cont'd

Section 14: Transport Information (non-mandatory)*

This section provides guidance on classification information for shipping and transporting of hazardous chemical(s) by road, air, rail, or sea. The information may include:

- UN number (i.e., four-figure identification number of the substance)[3]
- UN proper shipping name
- Transport hazard class(es)
- Packing group number, if applicable, based on the degree of hazard
- Environmental hazards (such as identifing if it is a marine pollutant according to the International Maritime Dangerous Goods Code [IMDG Code])
- Guidance on transport in bulk according to Annex II of MARPOL 73/78,[4] and the International Code for the Construction and Equipment of Ships Carrying Dangerous Chemicals in Bulk (International Bulk Chemical Code [IBC Code]).
- Any special precautions which an employee should be aware of or needs to comply with, in connection with transport or conveyance either within or outside their premises (indicate when information is not available).

Section 15: Regulatory Information (non-mandatory)*

This section identifies the safety, health, and environmental regulations specific for the product that is not indicated anywhere else on the SDS. The information may include:

- Any national and/or regional regulatory information of the chemical or mixtures (including any OSHA, Department of Transportation, Environmental Protection Agency, or Consumer Product Safety Commission regulations).

Section 16: Other Information

This section indicates when the SDS was prepared or when the last known revision was made. The SDS may also state where the changes have been made to the previous version. You may wish to contact the supplier for an explanation of the changes. Other useful information also may be included here.

Employer Responsibilities

Employers must ensure that the SDSs are readily accessible to employees for all hazardous chemicals in their workplace. This may be done in many ways. For example, employers may keep the SDSs in a binder or on computers as long as the employees have immediate access to the information without leaving their work area when needed and a backup is available for rapid access to the SDS in the case of a power outage or other emergency. Furthermore, employers may want to designate a person(s) responsible for obtaining and maintaining the SDSs. If the employer does not have an SDS, the employer or designated person(s) should contact the manufacturer to obtain one.

Modified from Occupational Safety and Health Administration, 29 CFR 1910.1200(g) and Appendix D. Globally Harmonized System of Classification and Labeling of Chemicals (GHS), third revised edition, United Nations, 2009. http://www.osha.gov/dsg/hazcom/index.html

[1]Chemical, as defined in the HCS, is any substance, or mixture of substances.

[2]Because other agencies regulate this information, OSHA will not be enforcing Sections 12 through 15.

[3]Found in the most recent edition of the United Nations Recommendations on the Transport of Dangerous Goods.

[4]MARPOL 73/78 means the International Convention for the Prevention of Pollution from Ships, 1973, as modified by the Protocol of 1978 relating thereto, as amended.

for labeling and SDSs. Employers must ensure that SDSs are readily accessible to employees.

The major changes to the HCS include the following:

1. **Hazard classification:** Chemical manufacturers and importers are required to determine the hazards of the chemicals they produce or import. Hazard classification under the new, updated standard provides specific criteria to address health and physical hazards as well as classification of chemical mixtures.
2. **Labels:** Chemical manufacturers and importers must provide a label (Fig. 2.1) that includes a signal word, pictogram (Fig. 2.2), hazard statement, and precautionary statement for each hazard class and category.
3. **Safety data sheets:** The new SDS format requires 16 specific sections, ensuring consistency in presentation of important protection information (see Box 2.1).
4. **Information and training:** To facilitate understanding of the new system, the new standard requires that workers be trained by December 1, 2013, and beyond for specified requirements (Table 2.5).

New changes to OSHA's HCS are bringing the United States into alignment with the Globally Harmonized System of Classification and Labeling of Chemicals (GHS), further improving safety and health protections for America's workers. The new system is being implemented throughout the world by countries that include Canada, the European Union, China, Australia, and Japan. Building on the success of OSHA's current HCS, the GHS is expected to prevent injuries and illnesses, save lives, and improve trade conditions for chemical manufacturers. The HCS in 1983 gave the workers the "right to know," but the new GHS gives workers the "right to understand."

Exposure Control Plan

The OSHA-mandated program, Occupational Exposure to Bloodborne Pathogens, became law in March 1992. This regulation requires that laboratories:

- Develop, implement, and comply with a plan that ensures the protective safety of laboratory staff to potential infectious bloodborne pathogens.
- Manage and handle medical waste in a safe and effective manner.

Government regulations require that all employees who handle hazardous material and waste must be trained to use and handle these materials. Chemical hazard education sessions must be presented to new employees and conducted annually for all employees. Each laboratory is required to evaluate the effectiveness of its plan at least annually and to update it as necessary. The written plan must be available to employees. A laboratory's written plan must include the purpose and scope of the plan, references, definitions of terms and responsibilities, and detailed procedural steps to follow.

The CDC also recommends safety precautions concerning the handling of all patient specimens, known as Standard Precautions, previously called *Universal Precautions.* OSHA has also issued guidelines for the laboratory worker in regard to protection from bloodborne diseases spread through contact

SAMPLE LABEL

PRODUCT IDENTIFIER

CODE ____________________

Product Name ____________________

SUPPLIER IDENTIFICATION

Company Name ____________________
Street address ____________________
City ____________ State ________
Postal Code ________ Country ________
Emergency Phone Number ________

PRECAUTIONARY STATEMENTS

Keep container tightly closed. Store in cool, well ventilated place that is locked.
Keep away from heat/sparks/open flame. No smoking.
Only use non-sparking tools.
Use explosion-proof electrical equipment.
Take precautionary measure against static discharge.
Ground and bond container and receiving equipment.
Do not breathe vapors.
Wear Protective gloves.
Do not eat, drink or smoke when using this product.
Wash hands thoroughly after handling.
Dispose of in accordance with local, regional, national, international regulations as specified.

In Case of Fire: use dry chemical (BC) or Carbon dioxide (CO_2) fire extinguisher to extinguish.

First Aid
If exposed call Poison Center.
If on skin (on hair): Take off immediately any contaminated clothing. Rinse skin with water.

HAZARD PICTOGRAMS

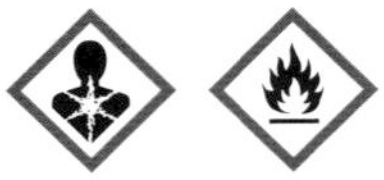

SIGNAL WORD
Danger

HAZARD STATEMENT

Highly flammable liquid and vapor.
May cause liver and kidney damage.

SUPPLEMENTAL INFORMATION

Directions for use
____
____
____

Fill weight: ____________ Lot Number ______
Gross weight: __________ Fill Date: ________
Expiration Date: ____________________

Fig. 2.1 Hazard Communication Standard Labels. (From www.osha.gov. Accessed June 10, 2014.)

Health Hazard • Carcinogen • Mutagenicity • Reproductive Toxicity • Respiratory Sensitizer • Target Organ Toxicity • Aspiration Toxicity	**Flame** • Flammables • Pyrophorics • Self-Heating • Emits Flammable Gas • Self-Reactives • Organic Peroxides	**Exclamation Mark** • Irritant (skin and eye) • Skin Sensitizer • Acute Toxicity (harmful) • Narcotic Effects • Respiratory Tract Irritant • Hazardous to Ozone Layer (Non-Mandatory)
Gas Cylinder • Gases Under Pressure	**Corrosion** • Skin Corrosion/Burns • Eye Damage • Corrosive to Metals	**Exploding Bomb** • Explosives • Self-Reactives • Organic Peroxides
Flame Over Circle • Oxidizers	**Environment (Non-Mandatory)** • Aquatic Toxicity	**Skull and Crossbones** • Acute Toxicity (fatal or toxic)

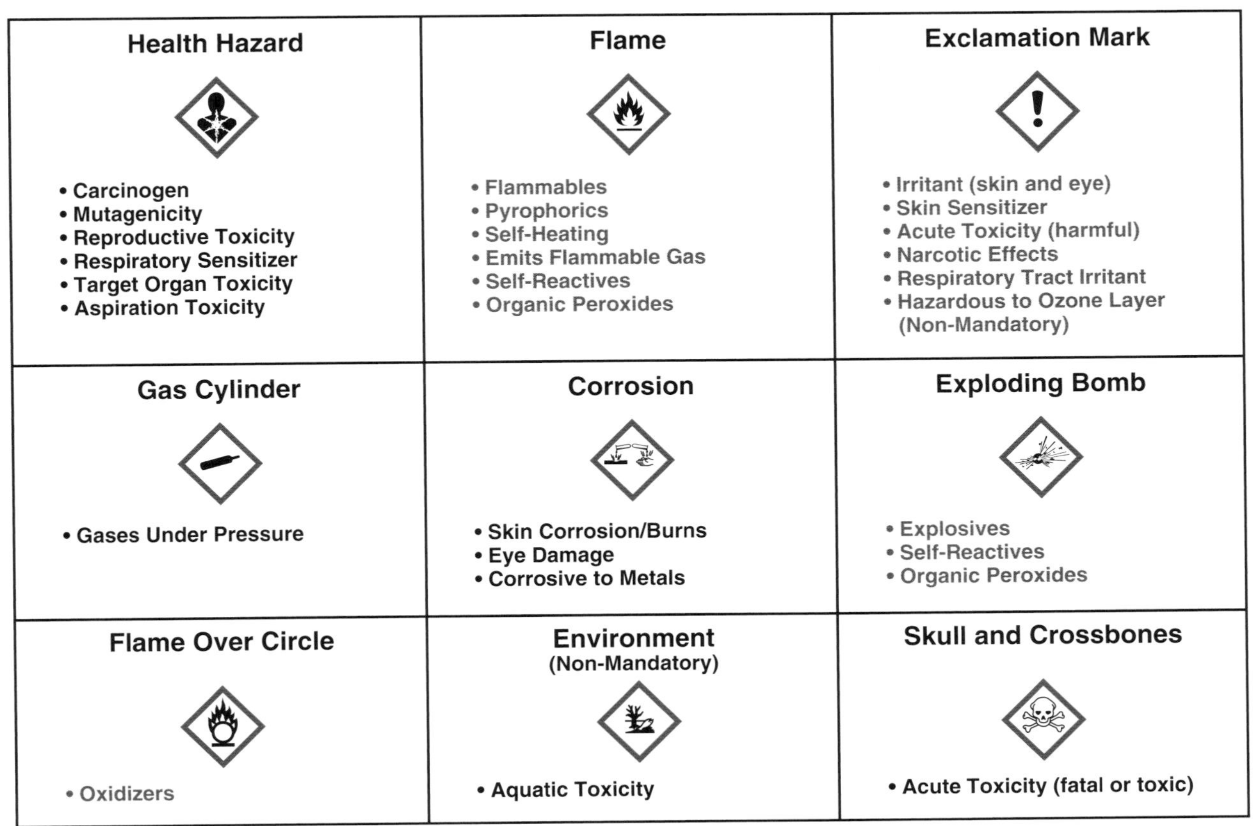

Fig. 2.2 Hazard Communication Standard Pictogram. (From www.osha.gov. Accessed June 10, 2014.)

TABLE 2.5 Effective Completion Dates for Hazard Communications Standard

Date	Requirement(s)	Who
December 1, 2013	Train employees on the new label elements and safety data sheet (SDS) format.	Employers
June 1, 2015 December 1, 2015	Comply with all modified provisions of this final rule, except: Distributors may ship products labeled by manufacturers under the old system until December 1, 2015.	Chemical manufacturers, importers, distributors, and employers
June 1, 2016	Update alternative workplace labeling and hazard communication program as necessary, and provide additional employee training for newly identified physical or health hazards.	Employers
Transition period	Comply with either 29 CFR 1910.1200 (this final standard) or the current standard, or both.	All chemical manufacturers, importers, distributors, and employers

TABLE 2.6 Safety Standards for Bloodborne Pathogens

Category	Comments
Training	Annual bloodborne pathogen training is required regardless of an employee's prior training or education. Annual training should concur within a reasonable time from an employee's annual hire date. The language used for bloodborne training should be understandable to non-English-speaking or limited-English-speaking employees.
Infectious disease prevention	The need to comply with personal protective equipment (PPE) should be determined by an employer. Eye protection (such as safety glasses, face mask, or protective shield) must be used while working to prevent spraying or splashing of potentially contaminated specimens. Every employer must have a written, dated record of each dose of hepatitis B vaccination.
Laboratory practices	Blood specimen tubes should be covered with gauze to prevent accidental exposure. Urine containers that do not contain visible blood do not need to be disposed of in a biohazard container (red bag waste).
First aid	First-aid services must be available within 3 to 4 minutes whether using in-house or outside emergency services.

Data from www.osha.gov. Retrieved May 17, 2013.

with patient specimens (Table 2.6). In addition, CDC provides recommendations for treatment after occupational exposure to potentially infectious material. These agencies are working to reduce the risk of exposure of health care workers to bloodborne pathogens.

AVOIDING TRANSMISSION OF INFECTIOUS DISEASES

Because many hazards in the clinical laboratory are unique, a special term, **biohazard**, was devised. This word is posted throughout the laboratory to denote infectious materials or agents that present a risk or even a potential risk to the health of human beings or animals in the laboratory. The potential risk can be either through direct infection or through the environment. Infection can occur during the process of specimen collection or from handling, transporting, or testing the specimen. Safe collection and transportation of specimens to the laboratory must take priority in any discussion of safety in the laboratory.

Risk is defined as the probability that a health effect will occur after an individual has been exposed to a specified amount of a hazard. Risk assessment is a process of gathering all available information on a hazardous substance and evaluating it to determine the possible risks associated with exposure. This is followed by determining the mitigation strategies necessary to provide protection.

Bioterrorism agents are a concern to laboratories. These agents are divided into categories A, B, and C (Box 2.2 and Table 2.7). The OSHA categories of risk classifications are now obsolete.

Biosafety and Biosafety Levels

Biosafety means reducing the risk of unintentional exposure to pathogens and toxins or their accidental release. A biosafety

BOX 2.2 Categories and Characteristics of Bioterrorism Agents

Category A

Pathogens that are rarely seen in the United States. These agents have the highest priority; organisms in this category pose a risk to national security because they:

- Can be easily disseminated or transmitted from person to person
- Result in high mortality rates and have the potential for major public health impact
- Might cause public panic and social disruption
- Require special action for public health preparedness

Category B

These agents have the second-highest priority and include pathogens that:

- Are moderately easy to disseminate
- Result in moderate morbidity rates and low mortality rates
- Require specific enhancements of the CDC's diagnostic capacity and enhanced disease surveillance

Category C

These agents have the third-highest priority and include emerging pathogens that could be engineered for mass dissemination in the future because of:

- Availability
- Ease of production and dissemination
- Potential for high morbidity and mortality rates and major health impact

Modified from Centers for Disease Control and Prevention: Bioterrorism agents/diseases (website). http://www.bt.cdc.gov/agent/agentlist-category.asp. Accessed February 2005.

TABLE 2.7 Examples of Bioterrorism Agents and Diseases

Agent	Disease
Category A	
Anthrax	*Bacillus anthracis*
Botulism	*Clostridium botulinum* toxin
Plague	*Yersinia pestis*
Smallpox	Variola major
Tularemia	*Francisella tularensis*
Viral Hemorrhagic Fevers	
Filoviruses	Ebola, Marburg
Arenaviruses	Lassa, Machupo
Category B	
Brucellosis	*Brucella* species
Epsilon toxin	*Clostridium perfringens*
Food contaminants	*Salmonella* species, *Escherichia coli* 0157:H7, *Shigella*
Glanders	*Pseudomonas (Burkholderia) mallei*
Melioidosis	*Pseudomonas (Burkholderia) pseudomallei*
Psittacosis	*Chlamydia psittaci*
Q fever	*Coxiella burnetii*
Ricin toxin	*Ricinus communis* (castor beans)
Staphylococcal Enterotoxin B	
Typhus fever	*Rickettsia prowazekii*
Viral encephalitis	Alphaviruses (such as Venezuelan equine encephalitis, Eastern equine encephalitis, and Western equine encephalitis)
Water safety threats	*Vibrio cholerae, Cryptosporidium parvum*

Modified from Centers for Disease Control and Prevention: Bioterrorism agents/diseases (website). www.bt.cdc.gov/agent/agentlist-category.asp. Retrieved February 2005.

management plan addresses the laboratory practices and procedures designed or intended to reduce risks associated with potential biological safety hazards.

Biosafety practices apply safety precautions that reduce a laboratory staff member's risk of exposure to a potentially infectious microorganism and limit contamination of the work environment and, ultimately, the community. Fig. 2.3 shows the symbol used to denote the presence of biohazards.

Biosafety is not an add-on task in the laboratory; it is a critical activity. A strong safety culture produces a reduction in exposure incidents and management of medical waste. A strong safety culture results from positive employee attitudes, effective policies and procedures, action to correct unsafe behaviors, and employee training and involvement in safety practices.

There are four biosafety levels (see Box 2.3). Each level has specific controls for containment of microorganisms and biological agents. Risk assessment is an important part of biosafety. The primary risks that determine levels of containment are infectivity, severity of disease, transmissibility, and the nature of the work conducted. In addition, the origin of the microorganism or agent in question, and the route of exposure is important.

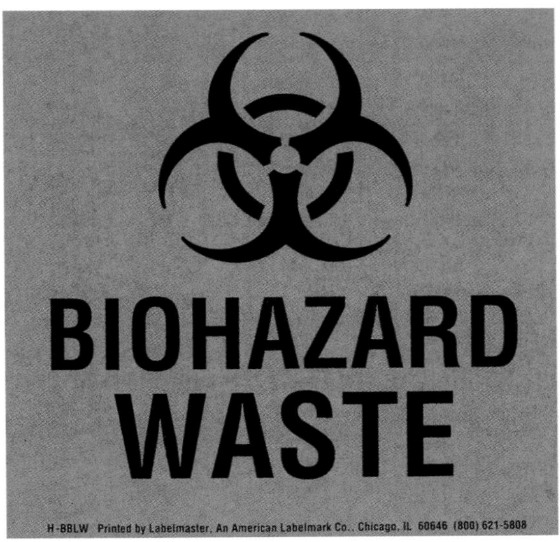

Fig. 2.3 Biohazard symbol. (From Rodak BF, Fritsma GA, Keohane EM: *Hematology: clinical principles and applications,* ed 4, St Louis, 2012, Elsevier/Saunders.)

Biosafety Level 1(BSL 1) is the least hazardous level. The risk of disease in healthy adults presents minimal potential hazard to staff and the environment. An example of a microorganism that is typically studied in a BSL-1 laboratory is a nonpathogenic strain of *E. coli.*

Biosafety Level 2 (BSL-2) builds upon BSL-1 requirements. A BSL-2 laboratory poses moderate hazards to laboratory staff and the environment. Encountered microorganism are typically indigenous and associated with diseases of varying severity. An example of a microorganism is typically worked with at a BSL-2 laboratory is *Staphylococcus aureus.*

When working with Zika virus in the laboratory, Zika virus preparations may be handled under BSL-2 precautions. Laboratories should perform a risk assessment to determine if there are certain procedures or specimens that may require higher levels of biocontainment, e.g., use of a biosafety cabinet for potential aerosol generating activities or suspicion that the specimen may contain a pathogen that requires BSL-3 precautions.

Biosafety Level 3 (BSL-3) builds upon the requirements of BSL-2. Microorganisms that can be encountered in a designated BSL-3 laboratory can be either indigenous or exotic. They can cause serious or potentially lethal disease through respiratory transmission. One example of a microbe that is typically worked with in a BSL-3 laboratory is *Mycobacterium tuberculosis.*

Biosafety Level 4 (BSL-4) builds upon the containment requirements of BSL-3 and is the highest level of biological safety. There are only a small number of BSL-4 labs in the United States and globally. Microrganisms encountered in a BSL-4 lab are dangerous and exotic, posing a high risk of aerosol-transmitted infections. Infections caused by these microbes are frequently fatal and are without treatment or vaccines. Two examples of microbes encountered in a BSL-4 laboratory include Ebola and Marburg viruses.

BOX 2.3 Biosafety Levels

Biosafety Level 1 (BSL-1)

Laboratory Practices

- Standard microbiological practices are followed.
- Work can be performed on an open lab bench or table.

Safety Equipment

- Personal protective equipment (PPE), (lab coats, gloves, eye protection) are worn as needed.

Laboratory Construction

- A sink must be available for hand washing.
- The laboratory should have doors to separate the working space with the rest of the facility.

Biosafety Level 2 (BSL-2)

In addition to BSL-1 considerations, BSL-2 laboratories have the following requirements:

Laboratory Practices

- Access to the laboratory is restricted when work is being conducted.

Safety Equipment

- Appropriate personal protective equipment (PPE) is worn, including lab coats and gloves. Eye protection and face shields can also be worn, as needed.
- All procedures that can cause infection from aerosols or splashes are performed within a biological safety cabinet (BSC).
- An autoclave or an alternative method of decontamination is available for proper disposals.

Facility Construction

- The laboratory has self-closing doors.
- A sink and eyewash are readily available.

Biosafety Level 3 (BSL-3)

In addition to BSL-2 considerations, BSL-3 laboratories have the following containment requirements:

Laboratory Practices

- Laboratorians are under medical surveillance and might receive immunizations for microbes they work with.
- Access to the laboratory is restricted and controlled at all times.

Safety Equipment

- Appropriate PPE must be worn, and respirators might be required.
- All work with microbes must be performed within an appropriate BSC.

Facility Construction

- A hands-free sink and eyewash are available near the exit.
- Exhaust air cannot be recirculated, and the laboratory must have sustained directional airflow by drawing air into the laboratory from clean areas towards potentially contaminated areas.
- Entrance to the laboratory is through two sets of self-closing and locking doors.

Biosafety Level 4 (BSL-4)

In addition to BSL-3 considerations, BSL-4 laboratories have the following containment requirements:

Laboratory Practices

- Change clothing before entering.
- Shower upon exiting.
- Decontaminate all materials before exiting.

Safety Equipment

- All work with the microbe must be performed within an appropriate Class III Biological Safety Cabinet or by wearing a full body, air-supplied, positive pressure suit.

Facility Construction

- The laboratory is in a separate building or in an isolated and restricted zone of the building.
- The laboratory has dedicated supply and exhaust air, as well as vacuum lines and decontamination systems.

Reference: https://www.cdc.gov/training/quicklearns/biosafety/ retrieved August 14, 2017.

Risk assessment is an important part of biosafety. Laboratories should perform a risk assessment to determine if there are certain procedures or specimens that may require higher levels of biocontainment. Risk is defined as the probability that a health effect will occur after an individual has been exposed to a specified amount of a hazard. Risk assessment is a process of gathering all available information on a hazardous substance and evaluating it to determine the possible risks associated with exposure. This is followed by determining the strategies necessary to provide protection.

Laboratory-Acquired Infections

Before 2014, laboratories never had a patients in the United States with Ebola virus. Fear of infection from Ebola resulted in some laboratories refusing to test any samples from suspected Ebola patients and some instrument manufacturers refusing to service instrument used to test patients suspected of having Ebola. This occurrence renewed the focus on laboratory-acquired infections (LAIs).

A laboratory-acquired infection (LAI) is defined as an infection acquired through laboratory or laboratory-related activities regardless of whether they are symptomatic or asymptomatic in nature. Common LAIs encountered in the laboratory are presented in Box 2.4. The most frequent routes of exposure and accidental inoculation are as follows:

- Inhalation (accidental aspiration of infectious material such as aerosols sprays from syringes, aerosols from the uncapping of specimen tubes, and centrifuge accidents)
- Percutaneous inoculation (such as needle and syringe, cuts or abrasions from contaminated items, and animal bites, accidental inoculation with contaminated needles or syringes)
- Contact between mucous membranes and contaminated material (such as hands and surfaces)
- Ingestion (such as aspiration through a pipette, smoking, and eating)

The majority of reported LAIs are caused by disregarding biosafety practices, followed by bio-incidents caused by human errors (such as spills and needlesticks).

Although the data is not very good, the incidence of LAI ranges from 1.4-3.5 infections per 1,000 employees. The most commonly implicated bacteria causing LAI include *Brucella* spp., *Coxiella burnetii*, *Salmonella typhi*, *Francisella tularensis*,

BOX 2.4 Risk Groups for Infectious Diseases

Risk Group 1 (no or low individual and community risk). A microorganism that is unlikely to cause human beings disease or animal disease.
Risk Group 2 (moderate individual risk, low community risk). A pathogen that can cause human or animal disease but is unlikely to be a serious hazard to laboratory workers, the community, livestock, or the environment. Laboratory exposures may cause serious infection, but effective treatment and preventive measures are available and the risk of spread of infection is limited.
Risk Group 3 (high individual risk, low community risk). A pathogen that usually causes serious human or animal disease and may present a serious hazard to laboratory personnel. Could present a risk if spread in the community or the environment. Effective treatment and preventive measures are usually available.
Risk Group 4 (high individual and community risk). A pathogen that usually causes serious human or animal disease and present a serious hazard to laboratory personnel. Can be readily transmitted from an one animal or to another human being, directly or indirectly. Effective treatment and preventive measures are not usually available.

Source: Centers for Disease Control and Prevention/National Institute of Health *Biosafety in Microbiological and Biomedical Laboratories Manual*, 5th edition, 2009.

and Mycobacterium tuberculosis complex. Bloodborne pathogens hepatitis B virus (HBV), hepatitis C virus (HCV), and human immunodeficiency virus (HIV) account for the majority of the reported viral infections.

BLOODBORNE PATHOGENS

Transmission of various bloodborne pathogens has always been a concern for laboratory staff, but with the identification of HIV, a new awareness was created. Specific regulations in regard to the handling of blood and body fluids from patients suspected or known to be infected with a bloodborne pathogen were originally issued in 1983.

Current safety guidelines for the control of infectious disease are based on the original CDC 1987 recommendations and 1988 clarifications. Safety practices were further clarified by OSHA in 1991. The purpose of the standards for bloodborne pathogens and occupational exposure is to provide a safe work environment. OSHA mandates that an employer do the following:

1. Educate and train all health care workers in Standard Precautions and preventing bloodborne infections.
2. Provide proper equipment and supplies, such as gloves.
3. Monitor compliance with the protective biosafety policies.

HIV has been isolated from blood, semen, vaginal secretions, saliva, tears, breast milk, cerebrospinal fluid, amniotic fluid, and urine, but only blood, semen, vaginal secretions, and breast milk have been implicated in transmission of HIV to date. Evidence for the role of saliva in transmission of the virus is unclear; however, Standard Precautions do not apply to saliva uncontaminated with blood.

The latest statistics on acquired immunodeficiency syndrome (AIDS) and HIV in the United States were published for 2016 by the CDC.[12] Since the beginning of the HIV/AIDS epidemic, health care workers across the world have become infected with HIV. The main cause of infection in occupational settings is exposure to HIV-infected blood via a percutaneous injury. Such exposures may come from needles, instruments, or bites that break the skin. Occupational transmission of HIV to health care workers is extremely rare. The average risk for HIV transmission after such exposure to infected blood is low, about 3 per 1000 injuries, but it remains an area of considerable concern for many health care workers.

Specific factors may mean a percutaneous injury carries a higher risk of HIV transmission and include the following:

- A deep injury
- Late-stage HIV disease in the source patient
- Visible blood on the device that caused the injury
- Injury with a needle that had been placed in a source patient's artery or vein

In a small number of cases, HIV has been acquired through contact with nonintact skin or mucous membranes (such as splashes of infected blood in the eye). Research suggests that the risk of HIV infection after mucous membrane exposure is less than 1 in 1000 infections. Scientists estimate that the risk of infection from a needlestick is less than 1%, based on the findings of several studies of health care workers who received punctures from HIV-contaminated needles or were otherwise exposed to HIV-contaminated blood.

Blood is the single most important source of HIV, HBV, and other bloodborne pathogens in the occupational setting. HBV may be stable in dried blood and blood products at 25° C for up to 7 days. HIV retains infectivity for more than 3 days in dried specimens at room temperature and for more than 1 week in an aqueous environment at room temperature.

Both HBV and HIV may be indirectly transmitted. Viral transmission can result from contact with inanimate objects such as work surfaces or equipment contaminated with infected blood or certain body fluids. If the virus is transferred to the skin or mucous membranes by hand contact between a contaminated surface and nonintact skin or mucous membranes, it can produce viral exposure.

Medical personnel should be aware that HBV and HIV are totally different diseases caused by completely unrelated viruses. The most feared hazard of all, the transmission of HIV through occupational exposure, is among the least likely to occur. The modes of transmission for HBV and HIV are similar, but the potential for transmission in the occupational setting is greater for HBV than HIV.

The risk of transmission of HBV and **HCV** from an occupational exposure is significantly greater than the risk of HIV transmission. The average risk of HBV infection ranges from 1% to 30% depending on the presence of hepatitis e antigen (HBe antigen + average risk is 22.0%-30%; HBe antigen − average risk is 1.0%-6%). The risk of HCV infection following a needlestick is 1.8%.[13]

Since the late 1980s, the incidence of acute hepatitis B has declined steadily. During 1990 to 2002, the incidence of acute hepatitis B declined 67%. Although the number of cases has sharply declined since hepatitis B vaccine became available, unvaccinated health care workers can become infected with HBV following occupational exposure.

The likelihood of infection after exposure to blood infected with HBV or HIV depends on a variety of factors, including:

- The concentration of HBV or HIV virus; viral concentration is higher for HBV than for HIV.
- The duration of the contact.
- The presence of skin lesions or abrasions on the hands or exposed skin of the health care worker.
- The immune status of the health care worker for HBV.

Both HBV and HIV may be directly transmitted by various portals of entry. In the occupational setting, however, the following situations may lead to infection:

1. Percutaneous (parenteral) inoculation of blood, plasma, serum, or certain other body fluids from accidental needlesticks.
2. Contamination of the skin with blood or certain body fluids without overt puncture, caused by scratches, abrasions, burns, weeping, or exudative skin lesions.
3. Exposure of mucous membranes (oral, nasal, conjunctival) to blood or certain body fluids as the direct result of pipetting by mouth, splashes, or spattering.
4. Centrifuge accidents or improper removal of rubber stoppers from test tubes, producing droplets. If these aerosol products are infectious and come in direct contact with mucous membranes or nonintact skin, direct transmission of virus can result.

OSHA estimates that 5.6 million workers in the health care industry and related occupations are at risk of occupational exposure to bloodborne pathogens. An *occupational exposure* is defined as a percutaneous injury (such as needlestick or cut with a sharp object) or contact by mucous membranes or nonintact skin (especially when the skin is chapped, abraded, or affected with dermatitis or the contact is prolonged or involves an extensive area) with blood, tissues, blood-stained body fluids, body fluids to which Standard Precautions apply, or concentrated virus. Blood is the most frequently implicated infected body fluid in HIV and HBV exposure in the workplace.

Most exposures do not result in infection. The risk not only varies with the type of exposure, but also may be influenced by other factors, such as the amount of infected blood in the exposure, the length of contact with infectious material, and the amount of virus in the patient's blood, body fluid, or tissue at the time of exposure.

SAFE WORK PRACTICES FOR INFECTION CONTROL

Standard Precautions represent an approach to infection control used to prevent occupational exposures to bloodborne pathogens. This approach eliminates the need for separate isolation procedures for patients known or suspected to be infectious. The application of Standard Precautions also eliminates the need for warning labels on specimens. According to the CDC concept of Standard Precautions, all human blood and other body fluids are treated as potentially infectious for HIV, HBV, and other bloodborne microorganisms that can cause disease in human beings. The risk of nosocomial transmission of HBV, HIV, and other bloodborne pathogens can be minimized if laboratory personnel are aware of and adhere to essential safety guidelines.

Personal Protective Equipment

OSHA requires laboratories to have a personal protective equipment (PPE) program and defines PPE as specialized clothing or equipment worn by an employee for protection against a hazard. Putting on and taking off PPE properly (Figs. 2.4, 2.5 and 2.6) is essential to the control of infections.

Implementing appropriate safety measures and adhering to a well-structured personal protective equipment program can reduce exposures to infectious material and improve overall safety condition in clinical laboratories. In clinical laboratories, laboratory-acquired infections are a particularly significant concern.

General work clothes (such as uniforms, pants, shirts, or blouses) not intended to function as protection against a hazard are not considered PPE. The components of this regulation include the following:

- A workplace hazard assessment with a written hazard certification
- Proper equipment selection
- Employee information and training, with written competency certification
- Regular reassessment of work hazards

Laboratory personnel should not rely solely on devices for PPE to protect themselves against hazards. They also should apply PPE standards when using various forms of safety protection. A clear policy on institutionally required Standard Precautions is needed. For usual laboratory activities, PPE consists of gloves and a laboratory coat or gown. Other equipment, such as masks, would normally not be needed.

Standard Precautions are intended to supplement rather than replace handwashing recommendations for routine infection control. The risk of nosocomial transmission of HBV, HIV, and other bloodborne pathogens can be minimized if laboratory personnel are aware of and adhere to essential safety guidelines.

Selection and Use of Gloves

Gloves for phlebotomy and laboratory work are made of vinyl or latex. There are no reported differences in barrier effectiveness between intact latex and intact vinyl gloves. Either type is usually satisfactory for phlebotomy and as a protective barrier when performing technical procedures. Latex-free gloves should be available for personnel with sensitivity to the typical glove material.

Care must be taken to avoid indirect contamination of work surfaces or objects in the work area. Gloves should be properly donned and removed (Fig. 2.7) or covered with an uncontaminated glove or paper towel before answering the telephone, handling laboratory equipment, or touching doorknobs. Guidelines for the use of gloves during phlebotomy procedures are as follows:

1. Gloves must be worn when performing fingersticks or heelsticks on infants and children.
2. Gloves must be worn when receiving phlebotomy training.
3. Gloves should be changed between each patient contact.

HOW TO PUT ON AND TAKE OFF

Personal Protective Equipment (PPE)

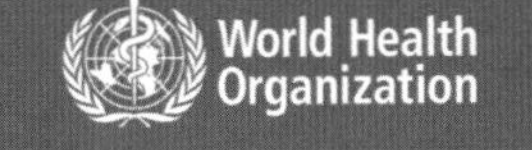

How to put on PPE (when all PPE items are needed)

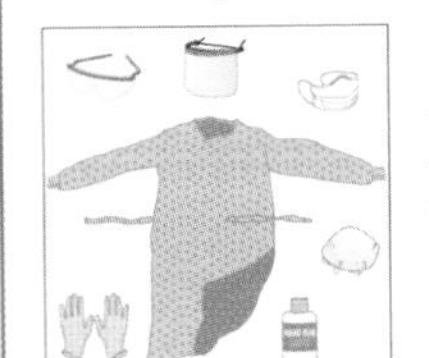

Step 1
- Identify hazards & manage risk. Gather the necessary PPE.
- Plan where to put on & take off PPE.
- Do you have a buddy? Mirror?
- Do you know how you will deal with waste?

Step 2
- Put on a gown.

Step 3a
- Put on face shield.

OR

Step 3b
- Put on medical mask and eye protection (e.g. eye visor/goggles)

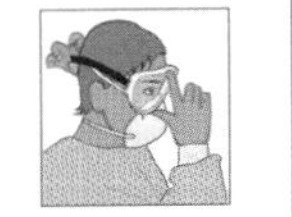

Note: If performing an aerosol-generating procedure (e.g. aspiration of respiratory tract, intubation, resuscitation, bronchoscopy, autopsy), a particulate respirator (e.g. US NIOSH-certified N95, EU FFP2, or equivalent respirator) should be used in combination with a face shield or an eye protection. Do user seal check if using a particulate respirator.

Step 4
- Put on gloves (over cuff).

How to take off PPE

Step 1
- Avoid contamination of self, others & the environment
- Remove the most heavily contaminated items first

Remove gloves & gown
- Peel off gown & gloves and roll inside, out
- Dispose gloves and gown safely

Step 2
- Perform hand hygiene

Step 3a
If wearing face shield:
- Remove face shield from behind
- Dispose of face shield safely

Step 3b
If wearing eye protection and mask:
- Remove goggles from behind
- Put goggles in a separate container for reprocessing
- Remove mask from behind and dispose of safely

Step 4
- Perform hand hygiene

Fig. 2.4 How To Put On and Take Off Personal Protective Equipment (PPE) (From World Health Organization, Geneva, August 2017.)

Steps to **put on** personal protective equipment (PPE)

1 Always put on essential required PPE when handling either a suspected, probable or confirmed case of viral haemorragic fever.

2 The dressing and undressing of PPE should be supervised by another trained member of the team.

3 Gather all the necessary items of PPE beforehand. Put on the scrub suit in the changing room.

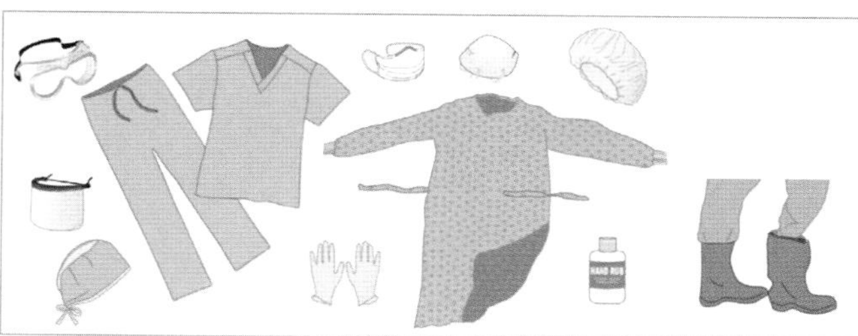

4 Put on rubber boots. If not available, make sure you have closed, puncture and fluid resistant shoes and put on overshoes.

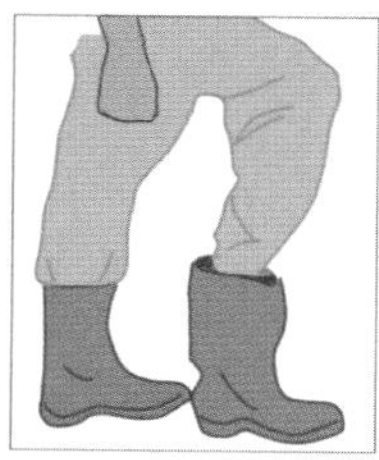

OR, IF BOOTS UNAVAILABLE

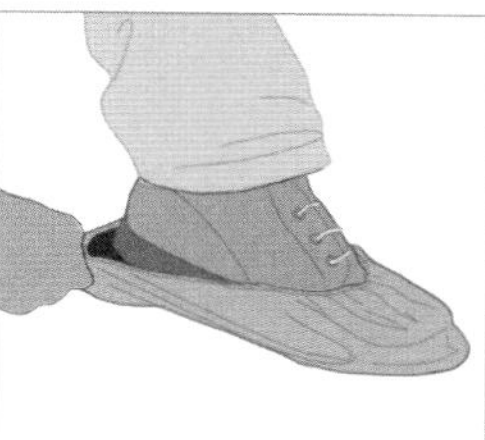

5 Place the impermeable gown over the scrubs.

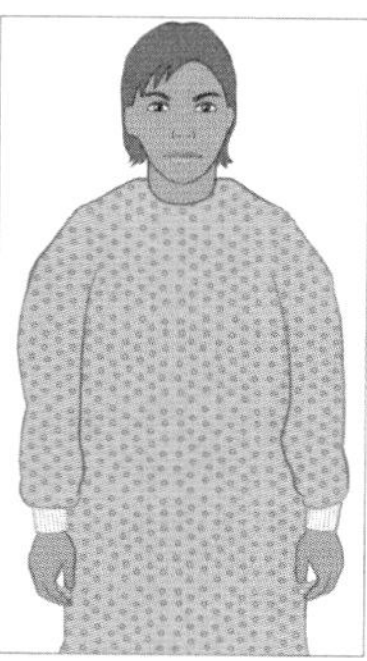

6 Put on face protection:

6a Put on a medical mask.

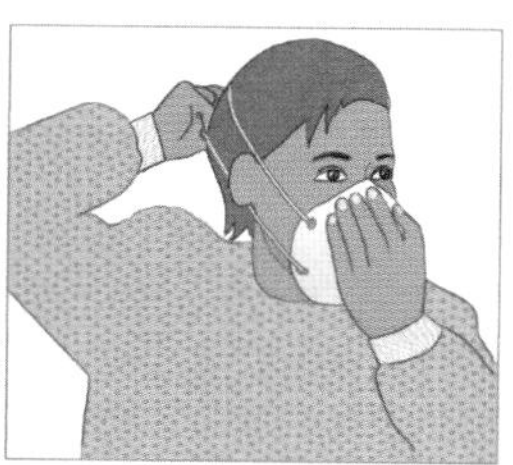

6b Put on goggles or a face shield.

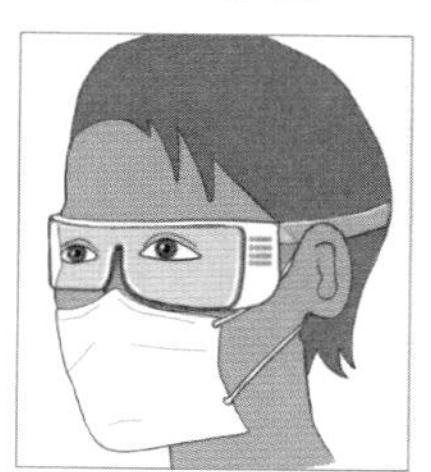

7 If available, put a head cover on at this time.

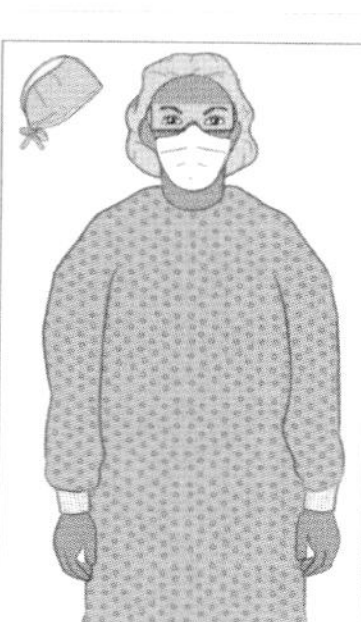

8 Perform hand hygiene.

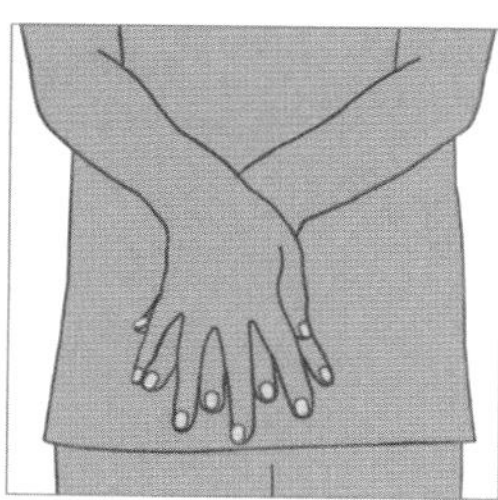

9 Put on gloves* (over cuff).

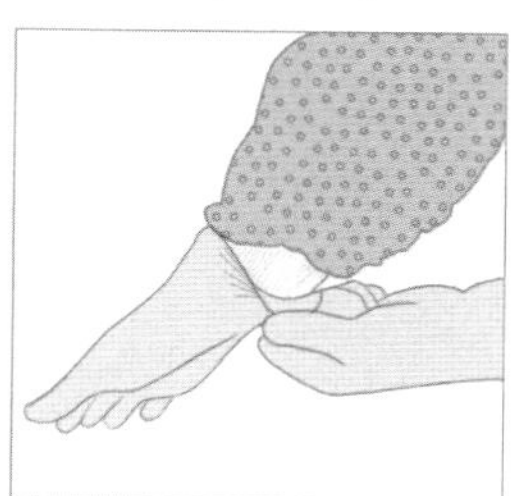

10 If an impermeable gown is not available, place waterproof apron over gown.

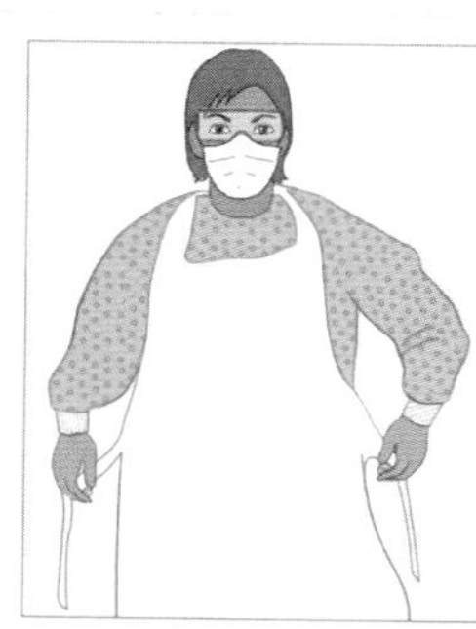

While wearing PPE:

- Avoid touching or adjusting PPE
- Change gloves between patients
- Remove gloves if they become torn or damaged
- Perform hand hygiene before putting on new gloves

* Use ***double gloves*** if any strenuous activity (e.g. carrying a patient or handling a dead body) or tasks in which contact with blood and body fluids are anticipated. Use ***heavy duty/rubber gloves*** for environmental cleaning and waste management.

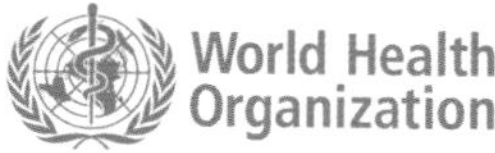

Fig. 2.5 How To Put On Personal Protective Equipment (PPE) (From World Health Organization, Geneva, August 2017.)

Steps to **remove** personal protective equipment (PPE)

1 Remove waterproof apron and dispose of safely. If the apron is to be reused, place it in a container with disinfectant.

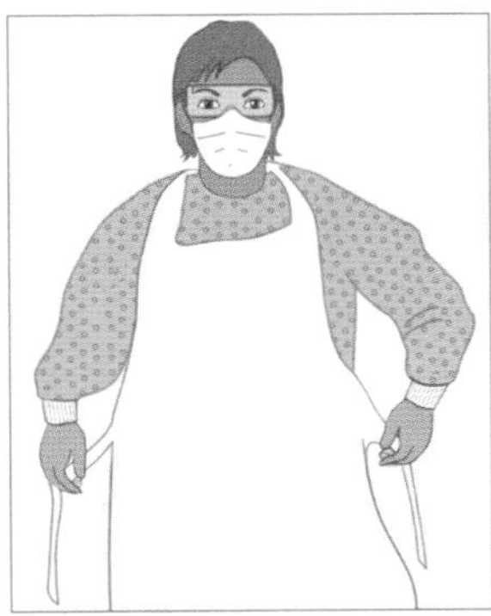

2 If wearing overshoes, remove them with your gloves still on (If wearing rubber boots, see step 4).

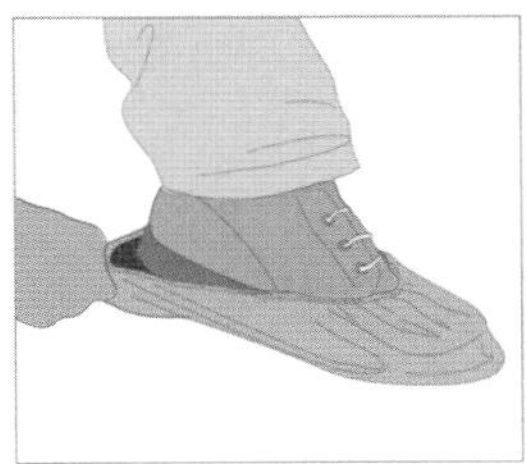

3 Remove gown and gloves and roll inside-out and dispose of safely.

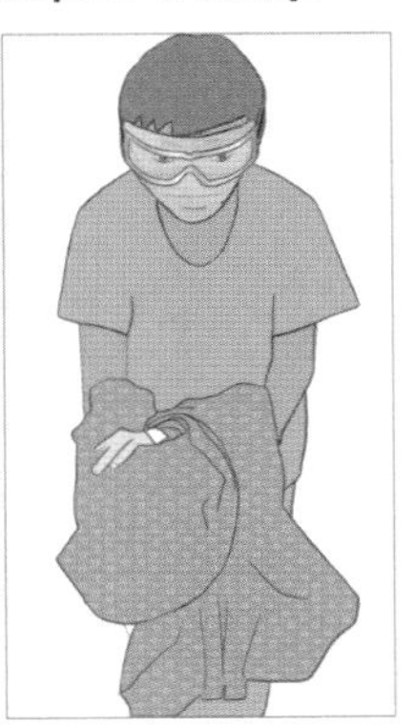

4 If wearing rubber boots, remove them (ideally using the boot remover) without touching them with your hands. Place them in a container with disinfectant.

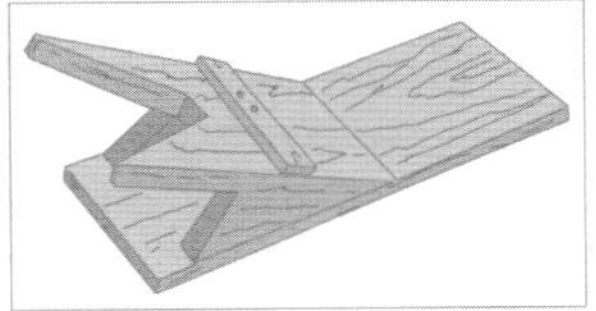

5 Perform hand hygiene.

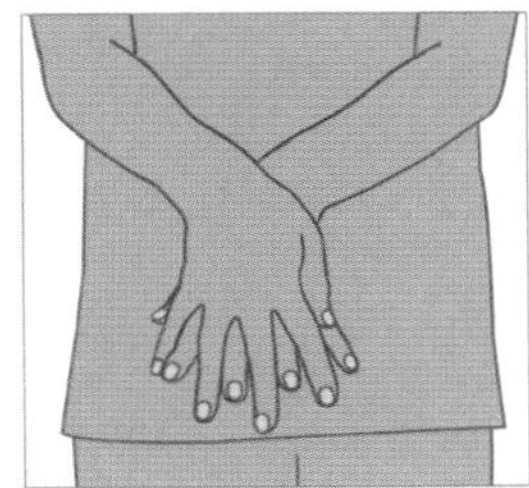

6 If wearing a head cover, remove it now (from behind the head).

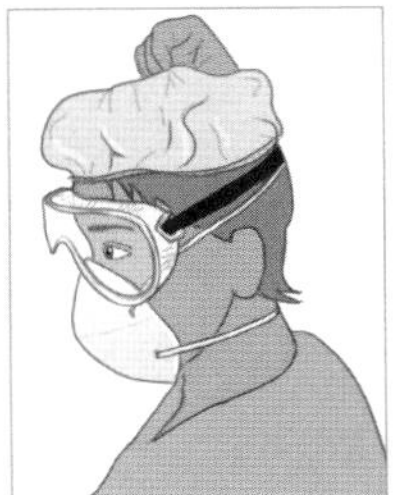

7 Remove face protection:

7a Remove face shield or goggles (from behind the head). Place eye protection in a separate container for reprocessing.

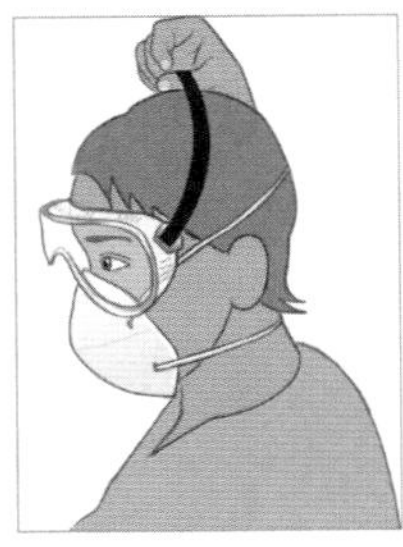

7b Remove mask from behind the head. When removing mask, untie the bottom string first and the top string next.

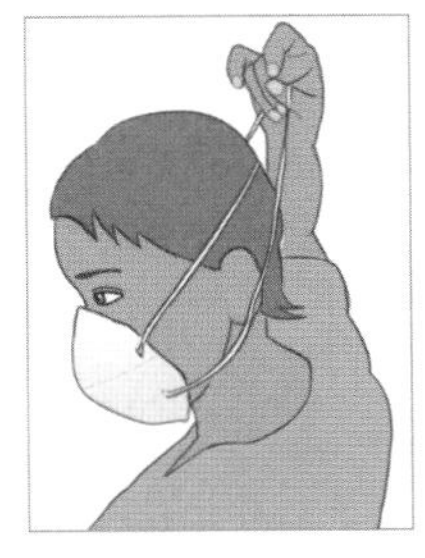

8 Perform hand hygiene.

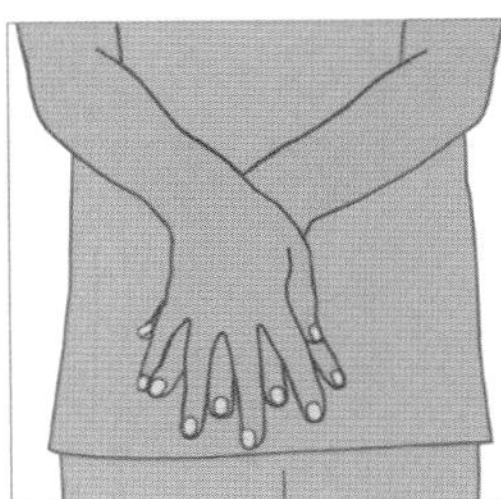

Source: Modified from Clinical Management of Patients with Viral Haemorrhagic Fever: A pocket Guide for the Front-line Health Worker. World Health Organization, 2014

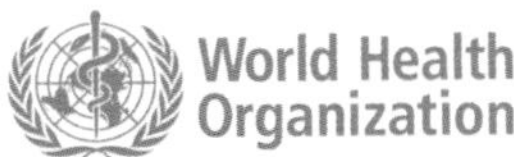

Fig. 2.6 How To Take Off Personal Protective Equipment (PPE) (From World Health Organization, Geneva, August 2017.)

When the hand hygiene indication occurs before a contact requiring glove use, perform hand hygiene by rubbing with an alcohol-based handrub or by washing with soap and water.

I. How to don gloves:

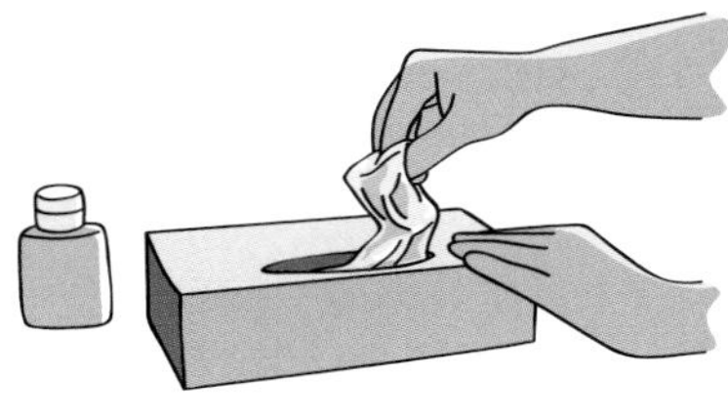

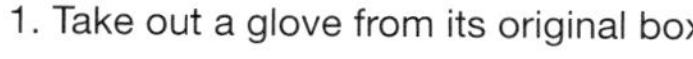

1. Take out a glove from its original box

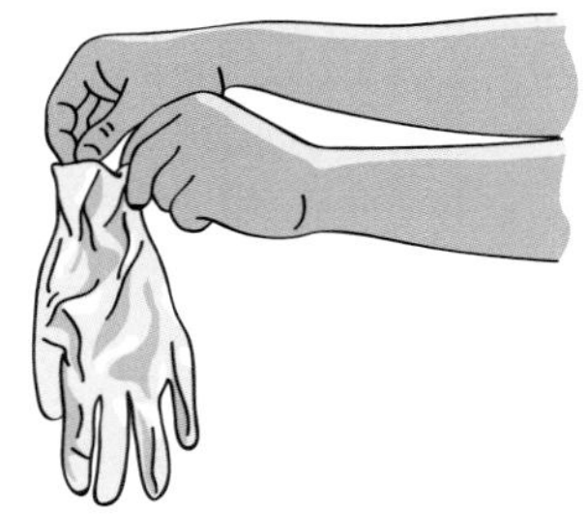

2. Touch only a restricted surface of the glove corresponding to the wrist (at the top edge of the cuff)

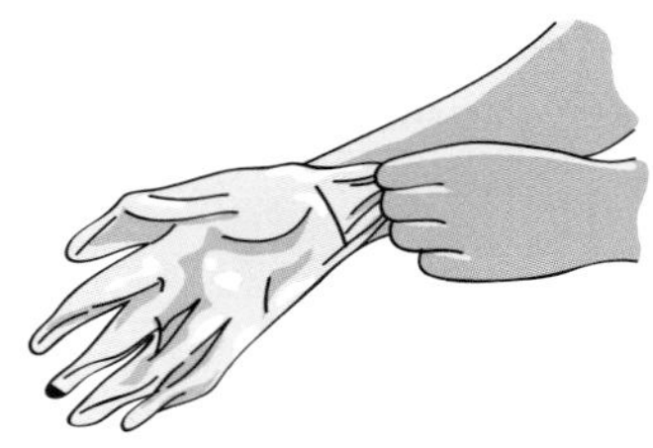

3. Don the first glove

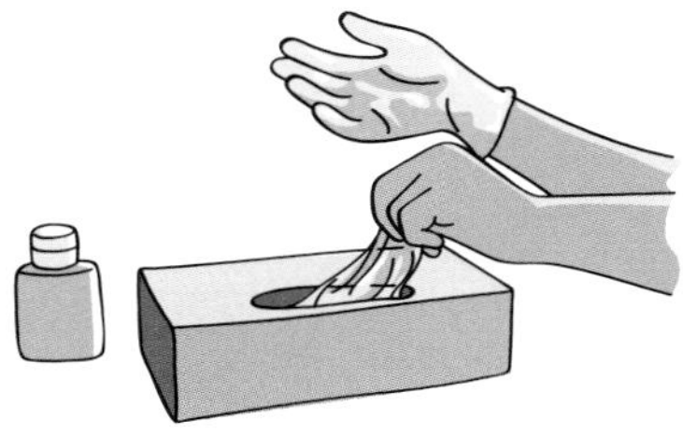

4. Take the second glove with the bare hand and touch only a restricted surface of glove corresponding to the wrist

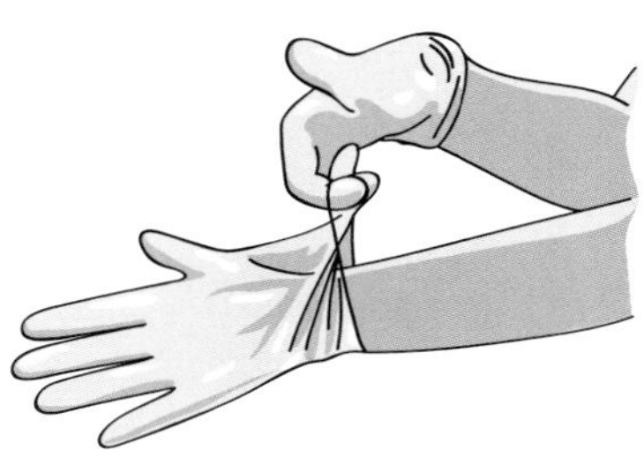

5. To avoid touching the skin of the forearm with the gloved hand, turn the external surface of the glove to be donned on the folded fingers of the gloved hand, thus permitting to glove the second hand

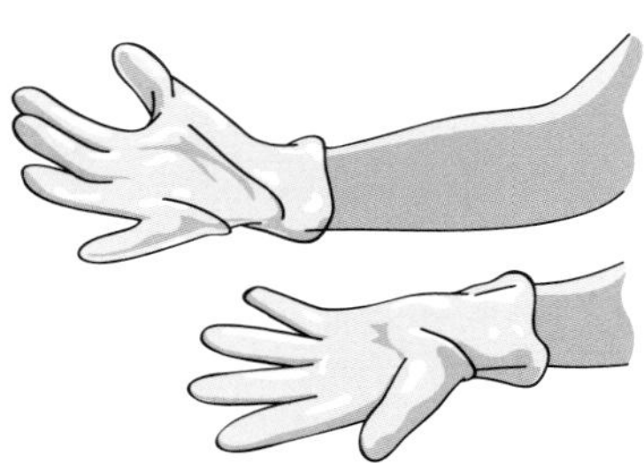

6. Once gloved, hands should not touch anything else that is not defined by indications and conditions for glove use

II. How to remove gloves:

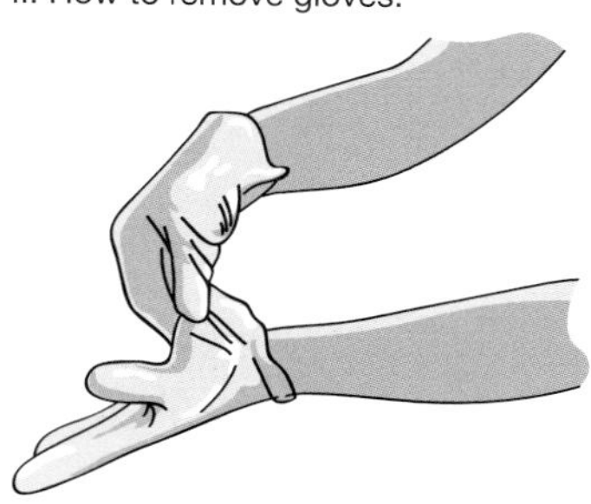

1. Pinch one glove at the wrist level to remove it, without touching the skin of the forearm, and peel away from the hand, thus allowing the glove to turn inside out

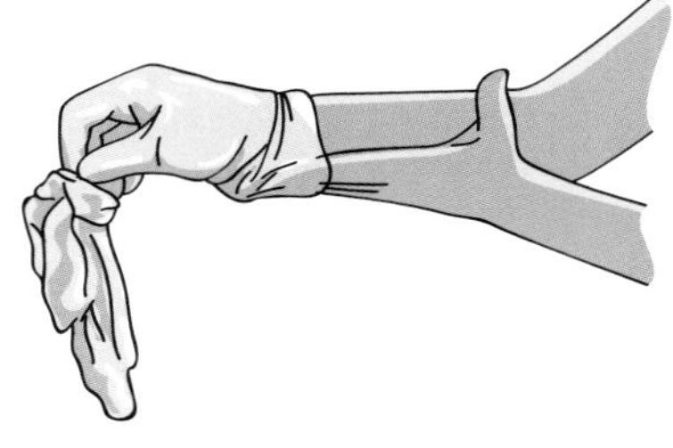

2. Hold the removed glove in the gloved hand and slide the fingers of the ungloved hand inside between the glove and the wrist. Remove the second glove by rolling it down the hand and fold into the first glove

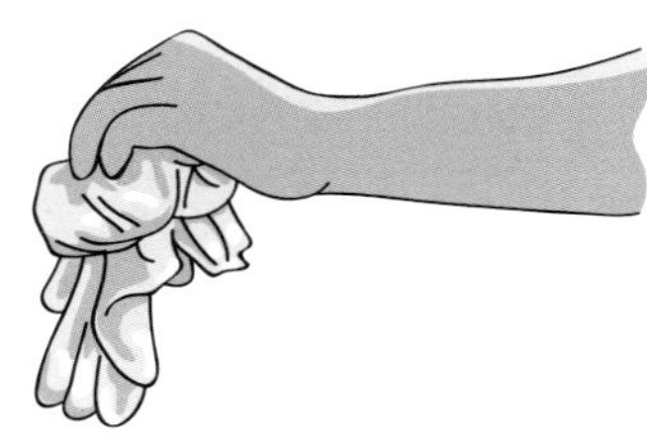

3. Discard the removed gloves

4. Then, perform hand hygiene by rubbing with an alcohol-based handrub or by washing with soap and water.

Fig. 2.7 Technique for donning and removing nonsterile examination gloves. (From World Health Organization: Glove use information leaflet, Geneva, August 2009, WHO.)

Facial Barrier Protection and Occlusive Bandages

Facial barrier protection should be used if there is a potential for splashing or spraying of blood or certain body fluids. Masks and facial protection should be worn if mucous membrane contact with blood or certain body fluid is anticipated. All disruptions of exposed skin should be covered with a water-impermeable occlusive bandage. This includes defects on the arms, face, and neck.

Laboratory Coats or Gowns as Barrier Protection

A color-coded, two–laboratory coat or equivalent system should be used whenever laboratory personnel are working with potentially infectious specimens. The coat worn in the laboratory must be changed or covered with an uncontaminated coat when leaving the immediate work area. If a lab coat becomes grossly contaminated with blood or body fluids, it should be changed immediately to prevent seepage through street clothes to the skin. Contaminated coats or gowns should be placed in an appropriately designated biohazard bag for laundering.

Disposable laboratory coats are available. A problem with coats during dry weather is the buildup of static electricity. Static electricity can create problems with laboratory equipment and computers. Coats constructed of antistatic material are preferable. A new type of lab coat overcomes the problem of being hot (DenLine Uniforms, Quincy, Illinois). These coats have a lightweight back with air permeability.

Disposable plastic aprons are recommended if blood or certain body fluids might be splashed. Aprons should be discarded into a biohazard container.

Nail Care

According to the CDC, to promote infection control, nails should be no longer than ¼ inch beyond the tip of the finger. Longer nails do not fit into gloves properly and can cause problems with blood collection and analysis.

Shoes

According to CLSI document GP17-A2, shoes worn in the clinical laboratory and phlebotomy services should be rubber-soled and cover the entire foot. Unless covered with shoe covers, canvas shoes are not recommended. Fluid-impermeable material (such as leather or synthetic) is recommended.

Electronic Devices

Electronic devices (such as smart phones and tablet computers) should not be exposed to potential sources of infectious contamination.

Handwashing

Frequent handwashing is an important safety precaution.[14] It should be performed after contact with patients and laboratory specimens. Gloves should be used as an adjunct to, not a substitute for, handwashing. The Association for Professionals in Infection Control and Epidemiology reports extreme variability in the quality of gloves, with leakage in 4% to 63% of vinyl gloves and 3% to 52% of latex gloves.

BOX 2.5 Guidelines for Handwashing and Hand Antisepsis in Health Care Settings

Use an alcohol-based waterless antiseptic agent for routine decontamination of hands, if not visibly soiled. Waterless antiseptic agents are highly preferable, but hand antisepsis using antimicrobial soap may be considered in certain circumstances. Wash hands with a nonantimicrobial soap and water or an antimicrobial soap and water when hands are visibly dirty or contaminated with proteinaceous material.

Decontaminate hands:

1. After removing gloves.
2. After completing laboratory work and before leaving the laboratory.
3. After accidental skin contact with blood, body fluids, or tissues.
4. After contact with patient's skin.
5. After contact with inanimate objects in the immediate vicinity of a patient.
6. If moving from a contaminated area to clean body site during patient care.
7. Before eating, drinking, applying makeup, and changing contact lenses, and before and after using the bathroom.
8. Before all activities that involve hand contact with mucous membranes or breaks in the skin.

Modified from Centers for Disease Control and Prevention: Guideline for hand hygiene in health care settings, *MMWR* 51(RR-16):1, 2002.

The efficacy of handwashing in reducing transmission of microorganisms has been demonstrated (see Student Procedure Worksheet 2.1). At the very minimum, hands should be washed with soap and water or by hand antisepsis with an alcohol-based handrub even if hands are not visibly soiled. Handwashing in other situations is described in Box 2.5. An important point when decontaminating hands with a waterless antiseptic agent (such as alcohol-based foam) is to apply 1.5 to 3 mL (or manufacturer's recommended amount) of the alcohol gel or foam to the palm of one hand and then rub hands together, covering all surfaces of hands and fingers, including fingernails. Rubbing should continue until the alcohol dries, about 15 to 25 seconds, until hands are dry.

Decontamination of Work Surfaces, Equipment, and Spills

Disinfection[15] describes a process that eliminates many or all pathogenic microorganisms, except bacterial spores, on inanimate objects. In health care settings, objects usually are disinfected by liquid chemicals or wet pasteurization. Factors that affect the efficacy of both disinfection and sterilization include the following:

- Prior cleaning of the object
- Organic and inorganic load present
- Type and level of microbial contamination
- Concentration of and exposure time to the germicide
- Physical nature of the object (such as crevices, hinges, and lumens)
- Presence of biofilms
- Temperature and pH of the disinfection process
- In some cases, relative humidity of the sterilization process (such as ethylene oxide)

The effective use of disinfectants is part of a multibarrier strategy to prevent health care–associated infections. Surfaces are considered noncritical items because they contact intact skin. Use of noncritical items or contact with noncritical surfaces carries minimal risk of causing an infection in patients or staff.

Disinfecting Solutions

Hypochlorites, the most widely used of the chlorine disinfectants, are available in liquid (such as sodium hypochlorite) or solid (such as calcium hypochlorite) forms. The most prevalent chlorine products in the United States are aqueous solutions of 5.25% to 6.15% sodium hypochlorite, usually called *household bleach.* They have a broad spectrum of antimicrobial activity, do not leave toxic residues, are unaffected by water hardness, are inexpensive and fast acting, remove dried or fixed organisms and biofilms from surfaces, and have a low incidence of serious toxicity. Sodium hypochlorite at the concentration used in household bleach can produce ocular irritation or oropharyngeal, esophageal, and gastric burns. The U.S. Environmental Protection Agency (EPA) has determined the currently registered uses of hypochlorites will not result in unreasonable adverse effects to the environment.

Hypochlorites are widely used in health care facilities in a variety of settings. Inorganic chlorine solution is used for spot disinfection of countertops and floors. A 1:10 to 1:100 dilution of 5.25% to 6.15% sodium hypochlorite (i.e., household bleach) or an EPA-registered tuberculocidal disinfectant has been recommended for decontaminating blood spills. For small spills of blood (i.e., drops) on noncritical surfaces, the area can be disinfected with a 1:100 dilution of 5.25% to 6.15% sodium hypochlorite or an EPA-registered tuberculocidal disinfectant. Because hypochlorites and other germicides are substantially inactivated in the presence of blood, large spills of blood require that the surface be cleaned before an EPA-registered disinfectant or a 1:10 (final concentration) solution of household bleach is applied. If a sharps injury is possible, the surface initially should be decontaminated, then cleaned and disinfected (1:10 final concentration).

An important issue concerning use of disinfectants for noncritical surfaces in health care settings is that the contact time specified on the label of the product is often too long to be practically followed. The labels of most products registered by EPA for use against HBV, HIV, or *Mycobacterium tuberculosis* specify a contact time of 10 minutes. Such a long contact time is impractical for disinfection of environmental surfaces in a health care setting, because most health care facilities apply a disinfectant and allow it to dry (~1 minute). Multiple scientific papers have demonstrated significant microbial reduction with contact times of 30 to 60 seconds.

Hypochlorite solutions in tap water at a pH above 8 stored at room temperature (23° C) in closed, opaque plastic containers can lose up to 40% to 50% of their free available chlorine level over 1 month. Sodium hypochlorite solution does not decompose after 30 days when stored in a closed brown bottle.

Disinfecting Procedure

While wearing gloves, employees should clean and sanitize all work surfaces at the beginning and end of their shift with a 1:10 dilution of household bleach. Instruments such as scissors or centrifuge carriages should be sanitized daily with a diluted solution of bleach. It is equally important to clean and disinfect work areas frequently during the workday as well as before and after the workday. Studies have demonstrated that HIV is inactivated rapidly after being exposed to common chemical germicides at concentrations that are much lower than those used in practice. Disposable materials contaminated with blood must be placed in containers marked "Biohazard" and properly discarded.

Neither HBV (or HCV) nor HIV has ever been documented as being transmitted from a housekeeping surface (such as countertops). However, an area contaminated by either blood or body fluids must be treated as potentially hazardous, with prompt removal and surface disinfection. Strategies differ for decontaminating spills of blood and other body fluids; the cleanup procedure depends on the setting (such as the porosity of the surface) and volume of the spill. The following protocol is recommended for managing spills in a clinical laboratory:

1. Wear gloves and a laboratory coat.
2. Absorb the blood with disposable towels. Remove as much liquid blood or serum as possible before decontamination.
3. Using a diluted bleach (1:10) solution, clean the spill site of all visible blood.
4. Wipe down the spill site with paper towels soaked with diluted bleach.
5. Place all disposable materials used for decontamination into a biohazard container.

Decontaminate nondisposable equipment by soaking overnight in a dilute (1:10) bleach solution and rinsing with methyl alcohol and water before reuse. Disposable labware or supplies that have come in contact with blood should be autoclaved or incinerated.

General Infection Control Safety Practices

All laboratories need programs to minimize risks to the health and safety of employees, volunteers, and patients. Suitable physical arrangements, an acceptable work environment, and appropriate equipment should be available to maintain safe operations (see Student Procedure Worksheet 2-2).

Laboratories should adhere to the following safety practices to reduce the risk of inadvertent contamination with blood or certain body fluids:

1. All devices in contact with blood and capable of transmitting infection to the donor or recipient must be sterile and nonreusable.
2. Food and drinks should not be consumed in work areas or stored in the same area as specimens. Containers, refrigerators, or freezers used for specimens should be marked as containing a biohazard.
3. Specimens needing centrifugation should be capped and placed into a centrifuge with a sealed dome.
4. Rubber-stoppered test tubes must be opened slowly and carefully with a gauze square over the stopper to minimize aerosol production (introduction of substances into the air).
5. Autodilutors or safety bulbs should be used for pipetting. Pipetting of any clinical material by mouth is strictly forbidden (see following discussion).
6. No tobacco products can be used in the laboratory.

7. No manipulation of contact lenses or teeth-whitening strips should be done with gloved or potentially infectious hands.
8. No lipstick or makeup should be applied in the laboratory.
9. All personnel should be familiar with the location and use of eyewash stations and safety showers.

Pipetting Safeguards: Automatic Devices

Pipetting must be done by mechanical means, either mechanical suction or aspirator bulbs. Another device, a bottle top dispenser, can be used to deliver repetitive aliquots of reagents. It is designed as a bottle-mounted system that can dispense selected volumes in an easy, precise manner. It is usually trouble free and requires minimal maintenance.

Safety Manual

Each laboratory must have an up-to-date safety manual. This manual should contain a comprehensive listing of approved policies, acceptable practices, and precautions, including Standard Precautions. Specific regulations that conform to current state and federal requirements (such as OSHA regulations) must be included in the manual. Other sources of mandatory and voluntary standards include TJC, CAP, and CDC.

Sharps Safety and Needlestick Prevention

The control measures required by OSHA[16,17] include the use of puncture-resistant sharps containers (Fig. 2.8). These containers must have the following characteristics:

- Closable, puncture resistant, and leakproof on sides and bottom
- Accessible, maintained upright, and not allowed to overfill
- Labeled or color-coded according to 29 CFR 1910.1030(g)(1)(i)
- Colored red or labeled with the biohazard symbol
- Labeled in fluorescent orange or orange-red, with lettering and symbols in a contrasting color (29 CFR 1910.1030[g][1][i][C]) (Red bags or containers may be substituted per 29 CFR 1910.1030[g][1][i][E].)

The primary purpose of using these containers is to eliminate the need for anyone to transport needles and other sharps while looking for a place to discard them. Sharps containers are to be located in patient areas as well as conveniently placed in the laboratory. Phlebotomists should carry these red, puncture-resistant containers in their collection trays. Needles should not be overfilled and should not project from the top of the container. Overfilling can result in a needle bouncing back at the employee and potential needlestick injury. To discard, sharps containers are closed and placed in the biohazard waste.

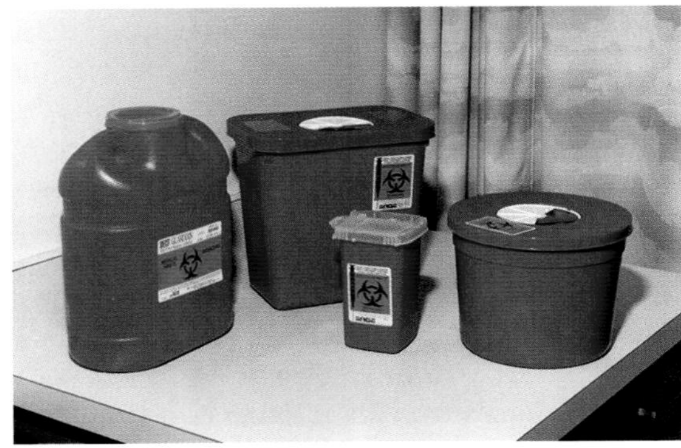

Fig. 2.8 Sharps containers. (From Kinn ME, Woods M: *The medical assistant: administrative and clinical,* ed 8, Philadelphia, 1999, Saunders.)

Use of the special sharps container permits quick disposal of a needle without recapping and safe disposal of other sharp devices that may be contaminated with blood. This supports the recommendation against recapping, bending, breaking, or otherwise manipulating any sharp needle or lancet device by hand. Most needlestick accidents have occurred during recapping of a needle after a phlebotomy. Injuries also can occur to housekeeping personnel when contaminated sharps are left on a bed, concealed in linen, or disposed of improperly in a waste receptacle. Most accidental disposal-related exposures can be eliminated by the use of sharps containers. An accidental needlestick must be reported to the supervisor or other designated individual.

To help laboratories make informed decisions about sharps safety, needlestick prevention, and device selection, ECRI (www.ecri.org), formerly the Emergency Care Research Institute, a nonprofit health services research agency, conducts comparative ratings of available protective devices. This service assists laboratories in determining whether and to what degree a product can protect staff from injury without compromising the patient's safety or comfort.

Transport and Handling of Diagnostic Specimens

Specimens should be transported to the laboratory in plastic leakproof bags. Protective gloves should always be worn for handling any type of biological specimen.

Substances can become airborne when the stopper (cap) is popped off a blood-collecting container, a serum sample is poured from one tube to another, or a serum tube is centrifuged. When the cap is being removed from a specimen tube or a blood collection tube, the top should be covered with a disposable gauze pad or a special protective pad. Gauze pads with an impermeable plastic coating on one side can reduce contamination of gloves. The tube should be held away from the body and the cap gently twisted to remove it. Snapping off the cap or top can cause some of the contents to aerosolize. When not in place on the tube, the cap should be kept in the gauze, not placed directly on the work surface or countertop.

Specially constructed plastic splash shields are used in many laboratories for the processing of blood specimens. Tube caps are removed behind or under the shield, which acts as a barrier between the person and the specimen tube. This is designed to prevent aerosols from entering the nose, eyes, or mouth. Laboratory safety boxes are commercially available and can be used to remove stoppers from tubes or perform other procedures that might cause spattering. Splash shields and safety boxes should be periodically decontaminated.

When specimens are being centrifuged, the tube caps should always be kept on the tubes. Centrifuge covers must be used and left on until the centrifuge stops. The centrifuge should be allowed to stop by itself and should not be manually stopped by the worker.

Another step that should be taken to control the hazard from aerosols is to exercise caution in handling pipettes and other equipment used to transfer human specimens, especially pathogenic materials. These materials should be discarded properly and carefully.

Zika Precautions

Specimens from individuals suspected of having Zika virus infection should be handled in accordance with the Healthcare Infection Control Practices Advisory Committee Standard Precautions Standard. These include the use of gloves, a laboratory gown or coat, and eye protection when handling these specimens. In general, Biosafety Level 2 precautions are appropriate for the handling of these specimens.

SPECIMEN HANDLING AND SHIPPING REQUIREMENTS

Proper handling of blood and body fluids is critical to the accuracy of laboratory test results, and the safety of all individuals who come in contact with specimens must be guaranteed.

If a blood specimen is to be transported, the shipping container must meet OSHA requirements for shipping clinical specimens (*Federal Register* 29, CAR 1910.1030). Shipping containers must meet the packaging requirements of major couriers and U.S. Department of Transportation hazardous materials regulations. Approved reclosable plastic bags for handling biohazardous specimens (Fig. 2.9) and amber bags for specimens for analysis of light-sensitive drugs are available. Approved bags have bright-orange and black graphics that clearly identify bags as holding hazardous materials. Some products have an additional marking area that allows phlebotomists to identify contents that must be kept frozen, refrigerated, or at room temperature.

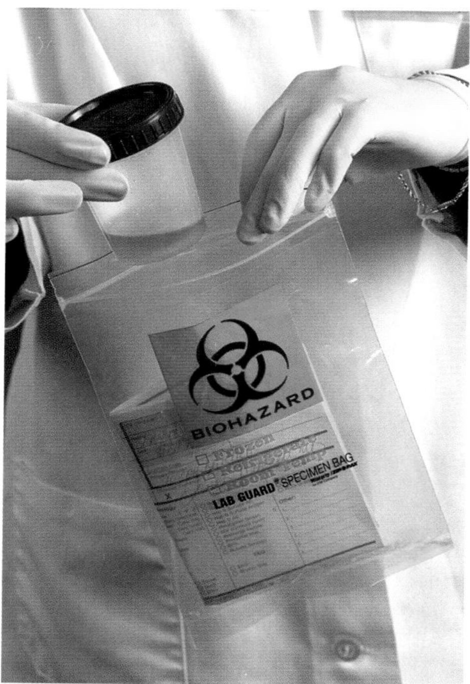

Fig. 2.9 Approved plastic bag for handling biohazardous materials. (From Warekois RS, Robinson R: *Phlebotomy: worktext and procedures manual*, ed 3, St Louis, 2012, Elsevier/Saunders.)

Maintaining specimens at the correct preanalytical temperature is extremely important. Products such as the Insul-Tote (Palco Labs, Scotts Valley, California) are convenient for specimen transport from the field to the clinical laboratory. This particular product has a reusable cold gel pack that keeps temperatures below 70° F for 8 hours even if the exterior temperature is above 100° F. Many laboratory courier services use common household coolers. Blood specimen collection and processing should conform to the current checklist requirements adopted by CAP. Errors in specimen collection and handling are a significant cause of incorrect patient results.

Once the specimen has been collected and properly labeled, it must be transported to the laboratory for processing and analysis. In many institutions, a specimen container is placed in a leakproof plastic bag as a further protective measure to prevent pathogen transmission—the implementation of the Standard Precautions policy and the use of barriers. The request form must be placed on the outside of this bag; many transport bags have a special pouch for this purpose.

Zika Precautions

Cultures of Zika virus and specimens collected from individuals for Zika virus studies may be transferred within the U.S. as Category B Biological substances in accordance with Department of Transportation Hazardous Materials Regulations (49 CFR Part 171-180). Guidance for packaging samples in accordance with Category B Biological substance requirements can be found in the CDC/NIH Publication *Biosafety in Microbiological and Biomedical Laboratories*, 5th edition.

PREVENTION OF DISEASE TRANSMISSION

Immunization/Vaccination

A well-planned and properly implemented immunization program is an important component of a health care organization's infection prevention and control program. When planning these programs, valuable information is available from the Advisory Committee on Immunization Practices, the Hospital Infection Control Practices Advisory Committee, and the CDC. Major considerations include the characteristics of the health care workers employed, the individuals served, and the requirements of regulatory agencies and local, state, and federal regulations.

Preemployment health profiles with baseline screening of students and laboratory staff should include an immune status evaluation for hepatitis B, rubella, and measles at a minimum. It is important to identify those employees whose maintenance of immune status is important; this includes laboratory staff. Individuals are recognized for being at risk for exposure to, and possible transmission of, diseases that can be prevented by immunizations.

Recommendations are divided into the following three categories:

- Immunizing agents strongly recommended for health care workers
- Other immunologics that are or may be indicated for health care workers
- Other vaccine-preventable diseases

All health care organizations should include those immunizations that are strongly recommended. To determine whether or not to include those immunologics that may or may not be included, the incidence of the vaccine-preventable diseases within the community served needs to be reviewed. Also, comparing the demographics of the workforce pool with the disease pattern within the community will determine which of these immunologics are indicated for the specific organization's program. Some vaccines may not be routinely administered but may be considered after an injury or exposure incident or for immunocompromised or older health care workers. Box 2.6 lists vaccines recommended for teens and college students.

Hepatitis B

Any worker who reasonably anticipates having contact with blood or other potentially infectious materials during performance of his or her job is considered to have "occupational exposure" and to be at risk of being infected. Hepatitis vaccine[18,19] must be offered after the worker is trained and within 10 days of initial assignment to a job where there is occupational exposure, unless the worker has previously received the vaccine series, antibody testing has revealed that the worker is immune, or the vaccine is contraindicated for medical reasons. A written opinion from a licensed health care professional within 15 days of the evaluation for vaccination must express the opinion as to whether hepatitis B vaccination is indicated for the worker and if the worker has received the vaccination. Employees who decline vaccination must sign a declination form.

Before the advent of the hepatitis B vaccine, the leading occupationally acquired infection in health care workers was hepatitis B. OSHA issued a federal standard in 1991 mandating employers to provide the hepatitis B vaccine to all employees who have or may have occupational exposure to blood or other potentially infective materials. The vaccine is to be offered at no expense to the employee, and if the employee refuses the vaccine, a declination form must be signed.

Influenza

Influenza has been shown to be transmitted in health care facilities during community outbreaks of this disease. Annual influenza vaccination programs are carried out in the fall. Programs that immunize both the health care worker and the individuals served have been extremely effective in reducing morbidity and mortality and staff absenteeism. It has been demonstrated that when the vaccine is available free to the health care worker and at a convenient location and time, the number of recipients increases significantly.

In addition to the annual flu vaccine, a newly developed H1N1 flu vaccine became available in Fall 2009. The general populations, including health care workers and students, are advised to receive this vaccination.

BOX 2.6 Vaccines Recommended for Teens and College Students

- Tetanus-diphtheria-pertussis vaccine
- Meningococcal vaccine
- Human papillomavirus (HPV) vaccine series
- Hepatitis B vaccine series
- Polio vaccine series
- Measles-mumps-rubella (MMR) vaccine series
- Varicella (chickenpox) vaccine series
- Influenza vaccine
- Pneumococcal polysaccharide (PPV) vaccine
- Hepatitis A vaccine series
- Annual flu + H1N1 flu shot

Note: Changes in the 2017 adult immunization schedule from the previous year's schedule include new or revised ACIP recommendations for influenza, human papillomavirus, hepatitis B, and meningococcal vaccines.

Influenza vaccination Live Attenuated Virus vaccine (LAIV) (FluMist, MedImmune) should not be used because of low effectiveness. Adults with a history of egg allergy who have only hives after exposure to egg should receive age-appropriate inactivated influenza vaccine (IIV) or recombinant influenza vaccine (RIV). Adults with a history of egg allergy with symptoms other than hives may receive age-appropriate vaccine but the selected vaccine should be administered in an inpatient or outpatient medical setting and supervised by a health care provider who is able to recognize and manage severe allergic conditions.

Human papillomavirus vaccination. Healthy adolescents who start their human papillomavirus (HPV) vaccination series before age 15 years are recommended to receive 2 doses of HPV vaccine. Adults and adolescents who did not start their HPV vaccination series before age 15 years should receive 3 doses of HPV vaccine. Changes in recommendations in the adult immunization schedule include updates regarding HPV vaccination for adults who did not complete the HPV vaccination series as adolescents.

Hepatitis B vaccination. Adults with chronic liver disease, including, but not limited to, hepatitis C virus infection, cirrhosis, fatty liver disease, alcoholic liver disease, autoimmune hepatitis, and an alanine aminotransferase (ALT) or aspartate aminotransferase (AST) level greater than twice the upper limit of normal should receive a HepB series.

Meningococcal vaccination. There are two changes in meningococcal vaccination recommendations for 2017. First, the ACIP recommended that adults with human immunodeficiency virus (HIV) infection receive a 2-dose primary series of serogroups A, C, W, and Y meningococcal conjugate vaccine (MenACWY). Second, the ACIP provided updated dosing guidance for one of the serogroup B meningococcal vaccines (MenB) (MenB-FHbp [Trumenba, Pfizer]). Young adults aged 16 through 23 years (preferred age range is 16 through 18 years) who are healthy and not at increased risk for serogroup B meningococcal disease may receive either MenB-4C (2 doses administered at least 1 month apart) or MenB-FHbp (3 doses administered at 0, 1–2, and 6 months) for short-term protection against most strains of serogroup B meningococcal disease.

Source: Advisory Committee on Immunization Practices Recommended Immunization Schedule for Adults Aged 19 Years or Older — United States, 2017, MMWR, 66(5);136–138, Feb, 2017 www,cdc.gov.
Full ACIP recommendations for each vaccine https://www.cdc.gov/vaccines/hcp/acip-recs/index.html.

Measles

Although ongoing measles transmission was declared eliminated in the United States in 2000 and in the World Health Organization Region of the Americas in 2002, approximately 20 million cases of measles occur each year worldwide. However, measles is one of the leading causes of death among young children even though a safe and cost-effective vaccine is available. In 2016, there were 89,780 measles deaths globally – making this the first time in history that deaths fell below 100,000/year.

Measles vaccination resulted in a 84% drop in measles deaths between 2000 and 2016 worldwide. In 2016, about 85% of the world's children received one dose of measles vaccine by their first birthday through routine health services – up from 72% in 2000. During 2000–2016, measles vaccination prevented an estimated 20.4 million deaths making measles vaccine one of the best buys in public health.[20]

As a result of a successful U.S. vaccination program, measles elimination, defined as an interruption of endemic measles transmission, was declared in the United States in 2000.

Sporadic outbreaks underscore the ongoing risk for measles among unvaccinated persons and the importance of maintaining high levels of vaccination. Outbreaks of measles cases serve as a reminder that measles is still imported into the United States and can result in outbreaks unless population immunity remains high through vaccination.

Mumps

Mumps transmission has been reported in medical settings. Programs that ensure that the worker is immune to mumps are easily linked to measles and rubella control.

Rubella

Vaccination programs have significantly decreased the overall risk for rubella transmission in all age groups. All workers who are likely to have contact with pregnant women should be immune to rubella. Because it is not harmful for people who are already immune to measles, mumps, or rubella to receive the vaccine, the trivalent MMR (measles, mumps, rubella) vaccine should be given rather than the monovalent vaccine.

Varicella

Postexposure procedures to address varicella-zoster virus are usually costly and disruptive to a health care organization. A program that (1) identifies susceptible workers, patients, and visitors; (2) applies restrictions when necessary; and (3) provides the immunization can help prevent the need to manage such exposure incidents.

Optional Immunizations

Hepatitis A

Standard Precautions are recommended and often a part of the isolation practices of U.S. health care facilities. When these are followed, nosocomial transmission of the hepatitis A virus (HAV) is rare.[3] Also, most patients hospitalized with hepatitis A are admitted when they are beyond the point of peak infectivity, which is after the onset of jaundice. Health care workers have not demonstrated an elevated prevalence of HAV compared with other occupational groups who were serologically tested. In communities that have high rates of hepatitis A or that are experiencing an outbreak, immunizing the health care worker population may need to be considered in certain settings. This vaccine has also been recommended for preexposure prophylaxis for the following groups who may be included in a health care worker population[3]:

- Those who travel to an endemic country
- Household and sexual contacts of HAV-infected people
- Those who have contact with active cases
- Laboratory workers who handle live HAV; workers and attendees at day care centers where attendees wear diapers; food handlers, staff, and residents of institutions for mentally handicapped patients; chronic carriers of hepatitis B; and people with chronic liver diseases

Meningococcal Disease

Routine vaccination of health care workers against meningococcal disease is not recommended. If an outbreak of serogroup C meningococcal disease is identified, use of the meningococcal vaccine may be warranted.

Pertussis

No vaccine against pertussis is licensed for use in an adult population. If one becomes available in the future, booster doses of adult formulations may be recommended because pertussis is highly contagious.

Typhoid

Typhoid vaccine should be administered to workers in microbiology laboratories who frequently work with *Salmonella typhi*.

Vaccinia

Vaccinia vaccine should be administered to the few people who work with orthopoxviruses, such as the laboratory workers who directly handle cultures or animals contaminated or infected with vaccinia.

Other Immunizations

Other vaccine-preventable diseases include diphtheria, pneumococcal disease, and tetanus. Because health care workers are not at increased risk for acquiring these diseases over the general population, they should seek these immunizations from their primary care provider.

Screening Tests

Tuberculosis: Purified Protein Derivative (Mantoux) Skin Test

If health care workers have recently spent time with and been exposed to someone with active tuberculosis (TB), their TB skin test reaction may not yet be positive. They may need a second skin test 10 to 12 weeks after the last time they had contact with the infected person. It can take several weeks after infection for the immune system to react to the TB skin test. If the reaction to the second test is negative, the worker probably does not have latent TB infection. Workers who have strongly positive reactions, a skin test diameter greater than 15 mm, and symptoms suggestive of TB should be evaluated clinically and microbiologically. Two sputum specimens collected on successive days should be investigated for TB by microscopy and culture.

QuantiFERON TB Gold (QFT) is a blood test used to determine if a person is infected with TB bacteria. The QFT measures the response to TB proteins when they are mixed with a small amount of blood. Currently, few health departments offer the QFT. If the worker's health department does offer the QFT, only one visit is required, at which time the person's blood is drawn for the test.

Rubella

All phlebotomists and laboratory staff need to demonstrate immunity to rubella. If antibody is not demonstrable, vaccination is necessary.

Hepatitis B Surface Antigen

All phlebotomists and laboratory staff need to demonstrate immunity to hepatitis B. If antibodies are not demonstrable, vaccination is necessary.

Prophylaxis, Medical Follow-up, and Records of Accidental Exposure

If accidental occupational exposure occurs, laboratory staff members should be informed of options for treatment. Because a needlestick can trigger an emotional response, it is wise to think about a course of action before an actual incident occurs. If a "source patient" can be identified, part of the workup could involve testing the patient for various infectious diseases. Laws addressing the patient's rights in regard to testing of a source patient can vary from state to state.

Although the most important strategy for reducing the risk of occupational HIV transmission is to prevent exposure, plans for postexposure management of health care personnel should be in place. Occupational exposures should be considered urgent medical concerns by the employee and health department.

The CDC has issued guidelines for the management of health care personnel exposure to HIV and recommendations for postexposure prophylaxis (PEP).[21] Considerations include whether personnel should receive PEP and which type of PEP regimen to use.

Hepatitis B Virus Exposure

After skin or mucosal exposure to blood, immunoprophylaxis depends on several factors. If an individual has not been vaccinated, hepatitis B immune globulin (HBIG) is usually given, within 24 hours if practical, and concurrently with hepatitis B vaccine postexposure injuries. HBIG contains antibodies to HBV and offers prompt but short-lived protection.

Recommendations for HBV postexposure management include initiation of the hepatitis B vaccine series for any susceptible, unvaccinated person who sustains an occupational blood or body fluid exposure. PEP with HBIG and hepatitis B vaccine series should be considered for occupational exposures after evaluation of the hepatitis B surface antigen (HBsAg) status of the source and the vaccination and vaccine response status of the exposed person. The specific protocol for these measures is determined by the institution's infection control division. Postvaccination testing for the development of antibody to HBsAg, for persons at occupational risk who may have had needlestick exposures necessitating PEP, should be done to ensure that the vaccination has been successful.

Hepatitis C Virus Exposure

Immune globulin and antiviral agents (such as interferon with or without ribavirin) are not recommended for PEP of hepatitis C. For **HCV** postexposure management, the HCV status of the source and the exposed person should be determined. For health care personnel exposed to an HCV-positive source, follow-up HCV testing should be performed to determine if infection develops. After exposure to blood of a patient with (or with suspected) HCV infection, immune globulin should be given as soon as possible. No vaccine is currently available.

In special circumstances (such as delayed exposure report, unknown source person, pregnancy in exposed person, resistance of source virus to antiretroviral agents, and toxicity of PEP regimen), consultation with local experts and the National Clinicians' Post-Exposure Prophylaxis Hotline (PEPline, 1-888-448-4911) is recommended.

Human Immunodeficiency Virus

Transmission of HIV is believed to result from intimate contact with blood and body fluids from an infected person. Casual contact with infected persons has not been documented as a mode of transmission. If there has been occupational exposure to a potentially HIV-infected specimen or patient, the antibody status of the patient or specimen source should be determined if allowed by law and not already known. If the source is a patient, voluntary consent should be obtained, if possible, for testing for HIV antibodies as soon as possible. High-risk exposure prophylaxis includes the use of a combination of antiretroviral agents to prevent seroconversion. For most HIV exposures that warrant PEP, a basic 4-week, two-drug regimen is recommended. For HIV exposures that pose an increased risk of transmission, a three-drug regimen may be recommended. Special circumstances (such as delayed exposure report, unknown source person, pregnancy in exposed person, resistance of source virus to antiviral agents, and toxicity of PEP regimens) are discussed in the CDC guidelines.

The PEP guidelines from the CDC are based on the determined risks of transmission (stratified as "highest," "increased," and "no risk"). Highest risk has been determined to exist when there has been occupational exposure both to a large volume of blood (as with a deep percutaneous injury or cut with a large-diameter hollow needle previously used in the source patient's vein or artery) and to blood containing a high titer of HIV (known as a *high viral load*), to fluids containing visible blood, or to specific other potentially infectious fluids or tissue, including semen, vaginal secretions, and cerebrospinal, peritoneal, pleural, pericardial, and amniotic fluids.

If a known or suspected parenteral exposure takes place, a technician or technologist may request follow-up monitoring for HIV (or HBV) antibodies. This monitoring and follow-up counseling must be provided free of charge. If voluntary informed consent is obtained, the source of the potentially infectious material and the technician/technologist should be tested immediately. The laboratory technologist should also be tested at intervals after exposure. An injury report must be filed after parenteral exposure.

An enzyme immunoassay screening test is used to detect antibodies to HIV. Before any HIV result is considered positive, the result is confirmed by Western blot (WB) analysis. A negative antibody test for HIV does not confirm the absence of virus. There is a period after infection with HIV during which detectable antibody is not present. In these cases, detection of antigen is important; a polymerase chain reaction (PCR) assay for HIV deoxyribonucleic acid (DNA) can be used for this purpose, and a p24 antigen test is used for screening blood donors for HIV antigen.

If the source patient is seronegative, the exposed worker should be screened for antibody again at 3 and 6 months. If the source patient is at high risk for HIV infection, more extensive follow-up of both the worker and the source patient may be needed.

If the source patient or specimen is HIV positive (HIV antibodies, WB assay, HIV antigen, or HIV DNA by PCR), the blood of the exposed worker should be tested for HIV antibodies within 48 hours if possible. Exposed workers who are initially seronegative for the HIV antibody should be tested again 6 weeks after exposure. If this test is negative, the worker should be tested again at 12 weeks and 6 months after exposure. Most reported seroconversions have occurred between 6 and 12 weeks after exposure. PEP should be started immediately and according to policies set by the institution's infection control program. A policy of "hit hard, hit early" should generally be in place.

During the early follow-up period after exposure, especially the first 6 to 12 weeks, the worker should follow CDC recommendations regarding the transmission of AIDS, including the following:

1. Refrain from donating blood or plasma.
2. Inform potential sex partners of the exposure.
3. Avoid pregnancy.
4. Inform health care providers of their potential exposure so they can take necessary precautions.
5. Do not share razors, toothbrushes, or other items that could become contaminated with blood.
6. Clean and disinfect surfaces on which blood or body fluids have spilled.

The exposed worker should be advised of the risks of infection and evaluated medically for any history, signs, or symptoms consistent with HIV infection. Serologic testing for HIV antibodies should be made available to all health care workers who are concerned they may have been infected with HIV.

Occupational exposures should be considered urgent medical concerns to ensure timely postexposure management and administration of HBIG, hepatitis B vaccine, and HIV PEP.

Respirators or Masks for Tuberculosis Control

A person must be exposed to *Mycobacterium tuberculosis* to be infected with TB. This occurs through close contact over time, when contaminated droplet nuclei from an infected person's respiratory tract enter another person's respiratory tract.

A commonsense way to control transmission of these contaminated droplets is to cover the mouth during coughing and to use tissues. In addition, specialized types of masks or respirators are now OSHA-mandated measures[22] for use by persons who are occupationally exposed to patients with suspected or confirmed cases of pulmonary TB. A "Special Respiratory Precautions" sign should identify rooms where there are patients fitting this criterion. Health care personnel caring for these patients must be fitted with and trained to use the proper respirator.

Protection from Aerosols

Biohazards are generally treated with great respect in the clinical laboratory. The adverse effects of pathogenic substances on the body are well documented. The presence of pathogenic organisms is not limited to the culture plates in the microbiology laboratory. Airborne infectious particles, or aerosols, can be found in all areas of the laboratory where human specimens are used.

Biosafety Cabinets

Biosafety cabinets are protective workplace devices used to control the presence of infectious agents in the air. Microbiology laboratories selectively use biological safety cabinets for performing procedures that generate infectious aerosols. Several common procedures in the processing of specimens for culture—grinding, mincing, vortexing, centrifuging, and preparation of direct smears—are known to produce aerosol droplets. Air containing the infectious agent is sterilized by heat or ultraviolet light or, most often, by passage through a high-efficiency particulate air filter. Biosafety cabinets not only remove air contaminants through a local exhaust system but also provide an added measure of safety by confining the aerosol contaminant within an enclosed area, thereby isolating it from the worker.

Negative-Pressure Isolation Rooms

Another infectious disease control measure is the use of negative-pressure isolation rooms. This type of room is used to control the direction of airflow between the room and adjacent areas, preventing contaminated air from escaping from the room into other areas of the facility. The minimum pressure difference necessary to achieve and maintain negative pressure that will result in airflow into the room is very small (0.001 inch of water), but higher pressures ($>$ 0.001 inch of water) are satisfactory. Negative pressure in a room can be altered by changing the ventilation system operation or by opening and closing the room's doors, corridor doors, or windows. When an operating configuration has been established, it is essential that all doors and windows remain properly closed in the isolation room and other areas (such as doors in corridors that affect air pressure), except when persons need to enter or leave the room or area.

ADDITIONAL LABORATORY HAZARDS

It cannot be overemphasized that clinical laboratories present many potential hazards simply because of the nature of the work done there. In addition to biological hazards, other hazards present in the clinical laboratory include open flames, electrical equipment, labware, chemicals of varying reactivity, flammable solvents, and toxic fumes.

In addition to the safety practices common to all laboratory situations, such as the proper storage of flammable materials, certain procedures are mandatory in a medical laboratory. Proper procedures for the handling and disposal of toxic, radioactive, and potentially carcinogenic materials must be included in the safety manual. Information regarding the hazards of particular substances must be addressed both as a safety practice and to comply with the legal right of workers to know about the hazards associated with these substances. Some chemicals (such as benzidine) previously used in the laboratory are now known to be carcinogenic and have been replaced with safer chemicals.

Chemical Hazards

Proper storage and use of chemicals are essential to avoid a potential fire hazard and other health hazards resulting from inhalation of toxic vapors or skin contact. Fire and explosion are a concern when flammable solvents (such as ether or acetone) are used. These materials should always be stored in special OSHA-approved metal storage cabinets that are properly ventilated. Storage of organic solvents is regulated by OSHA rules.

Organic solvents should be used in a fume hood. Proper precautions must be taken to avoid vaporization. Disposal of flammable solvents in sewers is prohibited. Chemical waste must be deposited in appropriately labeled receptacles for eventual disposal.

Specific Hazardous Chemicals

Specific chemicals must be handled with care because of potential hazards associated with their use and include the following:

- ***Sulfuric acid:*** At a concentration above 65%, may cause blindness; may produce burns on the skin; if taken orally, may cause severe burns, depending on the concentration.
- ***Nitric acid:*** Gives off yellow fumes that are extremely toxic and damaging to tissues; overexposure to vapor can cause death, loss of eyesight, extreme irritation, itching, and yellow discoloration of the skin; if taken orally, can cause extreme burns, may perforate the stomach wall, or cause death.
- ***Acetic acid:*** Severely caustic; continuous exposure to vapor can lead to chronic bronchitis.
- ***Hydrochloric acid:*** Inhalation of vapors should be avoided; any acid on the skin should be washed away immediately to prevent a burn.
- ***Sodium hydroxide:*** Extremely hazardous in contact with the skin, eyes, or mucous membranes (mouth), causing caustic burns; dangerous even at very low concentrations; any contact necessitates immediate care.
- ***Phenol*** (a disinfectant): Can cause caustic burns or contact dermatitis even in dilute solutions; wash off skin with water or alcohol.
- ***Carbon tetrachloride:*** Damaging to the liver even at an exposure level with no discernible odor.
- ***Trichloroacetic acid:*** Severely caustic; respiratory tract irritant.
- ***Ethers:*** Cause depression of central nervous system.

Select Carcinogens

OSHA regulates select substances as carcinogens. Carcinogens are any substances that cause the development of cancerous growths in living tissue. Carcinogens are considered hazardous to personnel working with these substances in laboratories. When possible, substances that are potentially carcinogenic have been replaced by less hazardous substances. If necessary, with the proper safeguards in place, potentially carcinogenic substances can be used in the laboratory. Lists of potential carcinogens used in a particular laboratory must be available to all personnel who work there; these lists can be long.

Protective Measures

When any potentially hazardous solution or chemical is being used, protective equipment for the eyes, face, head, and extremities, as well as protective clothing or barriers, should be used. Volatile or fuming solutions should be used under a fume hood. In case of accidental contact with a hazardous solution or a contaminated substance, quick action is essential. The laboratory should have a safety shower where quick, "all-over" decontamination can take place immediately. Another essential safety device in all laboratories is a face or eye washer that streams aerated water directly onto the face and eyes to prevent burns and loss of eyesight. Any such action must be undertaken immediately, so these safety devices must be present in the laboratory area.

Measures to limit exposure to hazardous chemicals must be implemented. All personnel must use appropriate work practices, emergency procedures, and PPE. Many of the measures taken are also those needed for protection from biological hazards, as discussed previously (see Personal Protective Equipment). These measures include the use of gloves, keeping the work area clean and uncluttered, proper and complete labeling of all chemicals, and use of proper eye protection, fume hood, respiratory equipment, and any other emergency or protective equipment as necessary.

General equipment (such as safety showers and eyewashes) must be present in each laboratory. Routine verification of equipment operation and maintenance must be established.

Electrical Hazards

Shock or fire hazards from electrical apparatus in the clinical laboratory can be a source of injury. OSHA regulations stipulate that the requirements for grounding electrical equipment published in the National Fire Protection Association's (NFPA's) National Electrical Code must be met. Some local codes are more stringent.

All electrical equipment must be Underwriters Laboratories (UL) approved. Regular inspection of electrical equipment decreases the likelihood of electrical accidents. Grounding of all electrical equipment is essential. Personnel should not handle electrical equipment and connections with wet hands, and electrical equipment should not be used after liquid has been spilled on it. Any equipment used in an area where organic solvents are present must be equipped with explosion-free fittings (such as outlets and plugs).

Fire Hazards

The NFPA and OSHA publish standards related to fire safety. In addition, NFPA also publishes the National Fire Codes, which may be adopted instead of OSHA regulations.

Personnel need to be trained in the use of safety equipment and procedures. Annual retraining is mandatory. Each laboratory must have equipment to extinguish or confine a fire in laboratory as well as on an individual's clothing. Safety showers are essential. Fire blankets must be easily accessible in wall-mounted cabinets.

Fires are classified into five different basic types, as follows:

Class A: Ordinary combustibles
Class B: Flammable liquids and gases
Class C: Electrical equipment
Class D: Powdered metal (combustible) material
Class E: Cannot be extinguished

Fires can be classified as a combination of A, B, and C classes (Fig. 2.10). The type of recommended extinguisher is determined by the class of fire. There are four different types or classes of fire extinguishers, each of which extinguishes specific types of fire. Newer fire extinguishers use a picture/labeling system to designate the types of fire for which an extinguisher should be used. Older fire extinguishers are labeled with colored geometric shapes and letter designations. Additionally, class A and class B fire extinguishers have a numeric rating based on UL-conducted tests and are designed to determine the extinguishing potential for each size and type of extinguisher.

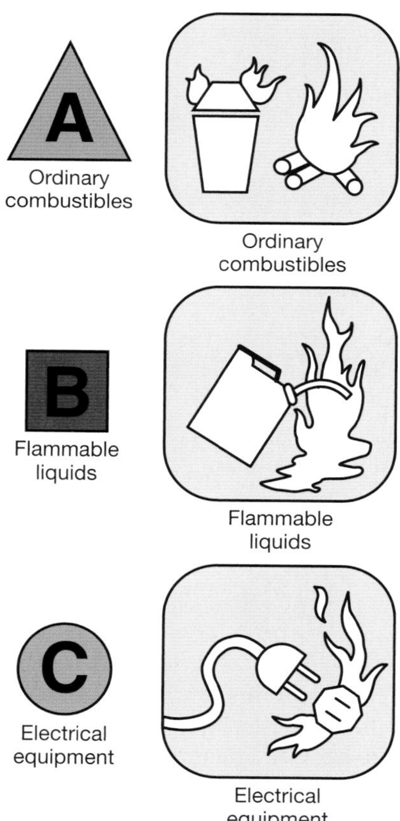

Fig. 2.10 Classes of fire extinguisher with corresponding types of fire.

Many extinguishers currently available can be used on different types of fires and will be labeled with more than one designator, such as A-B, B-C, or A-B-C. Class D and E fires should be handled only by trained personnel. Many clinical laboratories are installing computerized systems to minimize fire damage in temperature- and humidity-controlled rooms.

The various types of fire extinguishers are water, carbon dioxide, Halon 1211 or 1301 foam, loaded steam, dry chemical, and triplex dry chemical. Dry chemical extinguishers are the most common all-purpose extinguishers.

The local fire marshal determines where the equipment will be stored, the locations of fire alarms, and maps of evacuation routes. A fire extinguisher should be located near each laboratory door and also at the end of the room opposite the door in large laboratories. Fire extinguishers must be tested by qualified personnel at intervals specified by the manufacturer. Even though extinguishers come in various shapes and sizes, they all operate in a similar manner. An easy acronym for use of fire extinguishers is PASS: pull, aim, squeeze, and sweep.

Labware Hazards

Many forms of labware are basic implements in the clinical laboratory. Caution must be used to prevent unnecessary or accidental breakage. Most labware currently used is discarded when broken. Any broken or cracked labware should be discarded in a special container for broken glass, not thrown in the regular waste container. Common sense should be used in storing labware, with heavy pieces placed on lower shelves and tall pieces placed behind smaller pieces. Shelves should be installed at reasonable heights; labware should not be stored out of reach.

Infectious Waste

The purpose of waste disposal control is to confine or isolate any possible hazardous material from all workers, laboratory personnel as well as custodial and housekeeping personnel. CLSI has also published guidelines on management of clinical laboratory waste.

OSHA Standards

OSHA standards provide for the implementation of a waste disposal program. On the federal level, the storage and management of medical waste is primarily regulated by OSHA. Laws and statutes are defined by the Occupational Health and Safety Act and Clean Air Act. For more information, refer to www.fedcenter.gov.

States often expand the definition of medical waste or blood to include animals. State-by-state guidance concerning regulated medical waste and mercury issues can be found at www.encap.org. The OSHA regulations only apply to human blood, human infectious waste, and human pathologic waste, and include the following:

- Contaminated reusable sharps must be placed in containers that are closeable, puncture resistant, labeled or color-coded, and leakproof on the sides and bottom (see Fig. 2.8). Reusable sharps that are contaminated with blood or other potentially infectious materials must not be stored or processed in a manner that requires employees to reach by hand into the containers.
- Specimens of blood or other potentially infectious material are required to be placed in a container that is labeled and color-coded and closed before being stored, transported, or shipped. Contaminated sharps must be placed in containers that are closeable, puncture resistant, leakproof on sides and bottoms, and labeled or color-coded (see Fig. 2.8).
- Regulated wastes (liquid or semiliquid blood or other potentially infectious materials).
- Contaminated items that would release blood or other potentially infectious materials in a liquid or semiliquid state if compressed.
- Items that are caked with dried blood or other potentially infectious materials and are capable of releasing these materials during handling.
- Contaminated sharps.
- Pathologic and microbiological wastes containing blood or other potentially infectious materials must be placed in containers that are closeable, constructed to contain all contents and prevent leakage of fluids, labeled or color-coded, and closed before removal (see following discussion of biohazard containers and biohazard bag).
- All bins, pails, cans, and similar receptacles intended for reuse that are likely to become contaminated with blood or other potentially infectious materials are required to be inspected and decontaminated on a regularly scheduled basis. Waste containers must be easily accessible to personnel and must be located in laboratory areas where they are typically used. Containers for waste should be constructed so that their contents will not be spilled if the container is tipped over accidentally.
- Labels affixed to containers of regulated wastes, refrigerators and freezers containing blood or other potentially infectious materials, and other containers used to store, transport, or ship blood or other potentially infectious materials must include the biohazard symbol; must be fluorescent orange or orange-red or predominantly so, with lettering and symbols in contrasting color; and must be affixed as closely as possible to the container by adhesive or wire to prevent loss or removal.

Biohazard Containers

Body fluid specimens, including blood, must be placed in well-constructed biohazard containers with secure lids to prevent leakage during transport and for future disposal. Contaminated specimens and other materials used in laboratory tests should be decontaminated before reprocessing for disposal, or they should be placed in special impervious bags for disposal in accordance with established waste removal policies. If outside contamination of the bag is likely, a second bag should be used.

Hazardous specimens and potentially hazardous substances should be tagged and identified as such. The tag should read "Biohazard," or the biological hazard symbol should be used. All persons working in the laboratory area must be informed about the meaning of the tags and the precautions that should be taken for each tag.

Contaminated equipment must be placed in a designated area for storage, washing, decontamination, or disposal. With the increased use of disposable protective clothing, gloves, and other PPE, the volume of waste for discard will also increase.

Biohazard Bags

Plastic bags are appropriate for disposal of most infectious waste materials, but rigid, impermeable containers should be used for disposal of sharps and broken labware (see Fig. 2.9). Plastic bags with the biohazard symbols and lettering prominently visible can be used in secondary metal or plastic containers. These containers can be decontaminated or disposed of on a regular basis or immediately when visibly contaminated. These biohazard containers should be used for all blood, body fluids, tissues, and other disposable materials contaminated with infectious agents and should be handled with gloves.

FINAL DECONTAMINATION OF WASTE MATERIALS

The Medical Waste Tracing Act is a law that requires hospitals to establish a "cradle-to-grave" waste-tracking system for both chemical and biohazard waste streams.[23] Currently an amended bill seeking to improve the Medical Waste Management Act is under discussion by the U.S. Congress. Most laboratories usually generate at least three major types of waste streams:

1. Nonregulated waste
2. Regulated medical waste (RMW)
3. Chemical waste

The RMW is divided into two groups:

- Biohazard waste
- Biohazard sharps

The control of infectious, chemical, and radioactive waste is regulated by a variety of government agencies, including OSHA and the U.S. Food and Drug Administration. Legislation and regulations that affect laboratories include the Resource Recovery and Conservation Act, Toxic Substances Control Act, clean air and water laws, and chemical hazard communication laws. Laboratories should implement applicable federal, state, and local laws that pertain to hazardous material and waste management by establishing safety policies. Safety policies should be reviewed and signed annually or whenever a change is instituted. Employers are responsible for ensuring that personnel follow the safety policies.

Infectious Waste

It is important to know how to separate and handle each type of waste because disposing of sharps RMW can cost up to eight times more than nonsharps RMW. Items such as gloves, disposable lab coats, and plastic transfer pipettes that are not grossly or visibly contaminated with blood can be disposed of in the regular trash. Generally, urine specimens are not considered to be RMW unless visibly bloody or known to contain blood. As such, urine specimens or specimen containers can be disposed of in the regular trash.

Infectious waste, such as contaminated gauze squares and test tubes, must be discarded in proper biohazard containers. These containers should have the following characteristics:

1. Conspicuously marked "Biohazard" and bear the universal biohazard symbol.
2. Display the universal color: orange, orange and black, or red.
3. Rigid, leakproof, and puncture resistant; cardboard boxes lined with leakproof plastic bags are available.
4. Used for blood and certain body fluids, as well as for disposable materials contaminated with blood and fluids.

If the primary infectious waste containers are red plastic bags, these should be kept in secondary metal or plastic cans. Extreme care should be taken not to contaminate the exterior of these bags. If it does become contaminated on the outside, the entire bag must be placed into another red plastic bag. Secondary plastic or metal cans should be decontaminated regularly and immediately after any grossly visible contamination, with an agent such as a 1:10 freshly prepared solution of household bleach.

Since enactment of the U.S. Clean Air Act Amendments in 1990, many incinerators previously used to dispose of RMW have been shut down, and other methods of disposal have been developed. The current approaches to processing RMW are chemical disinfection, enzymatic processing, irradiation, and steam sterilization. Once treated, RMW can be placed into municipal solid-waste landfills with nonregulated wastes. This type of disposal reduces the need for segregated hazardous landfills. Recycling of sharps containers also reduce biohazard waste.

Radioactive Waste

The Nuclear Regulatory Commission regulates the methods of disposal of radioactive waste. Radioactive waste associated with the radioimmunoassay (RIA) laboratory must be disposed of with special caution. In general, low-level RIA radioactive waste can be discharged in small amounts into the sewer with copious amounts of water. This practice will probably be illegal in the future; therefore the best method of disposal is to store the used material in a locked, marked room until the background count is down to 10 half-lives for radioiodine (^{125}I). It can then be disposed with other refuse. Meticulous records are required to document the amounts and methods of disposal.

SAFETY AUDIT

A comprehensive safety audit should be conducted in every laboratory each year. This audit should include the six leading laboratory safety issues, as follows.

1. ***Laboratory coats.*** Clean coats must be separated from coats that are being used.
2. ***Fire extinguishers.*** Extinguishers should be in date and not expired.
3. ***Biosafety cabinets and hoods.*** This equipment needs to be certified annually.
4. ***Eyewash stations and safety showers.*** This equipment needs to be within 100 feet or no more than a 10-second walk from hazardous chemicals.
5. ***Chemicals.*** Chemicals must be inventoried annually.
6. ***Safety data sheets.*** SDSs need to be available as hard copy or electronically within 5 minutes of a request.

BASIC FIRST-AID PROCEDURES

Because of the many potential hazards in a clinical laboratory, knowledge of basic first aid should be an integral part of any educational program in the clinical laboratory. The first priority should be removal of the accident victim from further injury, followed by definitive action or first aid to the victim. By definition, *first aid* is the immediate care of a person who has been injured or acutely ill. Any person who attempts to perform first aid before professional treatment can be arranged should remember that such assistance is only temporary. Stop bleeding, prevent shock, and then treat the wound—in that order.

A rule to remember in dealing with emergencies in the laboratory is to keep calm. This is not always easy but is important to the victim's well-being. Keep crowds of people away, and give the victim plenty of fresh air. Because many injuries may be extreme, and because immediate care is critical with such injuries, all laboratory personnel must thoroughly understand the application of the proper first-aid procedures. Every student or person working in the medical laboratory should learn the following more common emergencies and appropriate first-aid procedures:

Alkali or acid burns on the skin or in the mouth. Rinse thoroughly with large amounts of running tap water. If the burns are serious, consult a physician.

Alkali or acid burns in the eye. Wash out eye thoroughly with running water for a minimum of 15 minutes. Help the victim by holding the eyelid open so water can make contact with the eye. An eye fountain is recommended for this purpose, but any running water will suffice. Use of an eyecup is discouraged. A physician should be notified immediately, while the eye is being washed.

Heat burns. Apply cold running water (or ice in water) to relieve the pain and stop further tissue damage. Use a wet dressing of 2 tablespoons of sodium bicarbonate in 1 quart of warm water. Apply the bandage securely but not tightly. In the case of a third-degree burn (skin is burned off), do not use ointments or grease, and consult a physician immediately.

Minor cuts. Wash the wound carefully and thoroughly with soap and water. Remove all foreign material (such as glass) that projects from the wound, but do not gouge for embedded material. Removal is best accomplished by careful washing. Apply a clean bandage if necessary.

Serious cuts. Apply direct pressure to the wound area to control the bleeding, using the hand over a clean compress covering the wound. Call for a physician immediately.

For victims of serious laboratory accidents such as burns, medical assistance should be summoned while first aid is being administered. With general accidents, competent medical help should be sought as soon as possible after the first-aid treatment has been completed. In cases of chemical burns, especially when the eyes are involved, speed in treatment is most essential.

Remember that first aid is useful not only in your working environment, but also at home and in your community. It deserves your earnest attention and study.

CASE STUDY

CASE STUDY 2.1

Charlie is a laboratory technologist on the midnight shift at a 125-bed rural community hospital. He has worked at this institution for 25 years, always on the midnight shift. He is known for taking shortcuts to get his work done faster, but he is reliable, and management is reluctant to counsel him. It is difficult to find qualified employees in the rural areas. The work is done quickly, and Charlie has ample time to work in a stress-free environment.

Tonight Charlie is updating the chemical inventory. His supervisor has asked him to collect any chemicals that are out of date or no longer used and to box them up for disposal. As he scans the shelves, Charlie notices that there is a liter of glacial acetic acid on the top shelf that has been in the lab for years. He is not sure when it was opened because the date is missing, but he knows the chemical is no longer used, and he puts it in the box for disposal. He also finds a small bottle of sodium azide and puts it in the disposal box as well. He continues to check the inventory, and all chemicals on the list are accounted for in the upper cabinets in the lab. There are two new chemicals that come with the chemistry kits, but he does not add these to the list, leaving that for the day shift.

Evaluation time is next month, and Charlie wants to make a good impression on his supervisor. Charlie decides to save the laboratory some money and dispose of the acetic acid and sodium azide himself by pouring them down the drain. Charlie knows that lab packs are expensive, and the "stuff just goes into the septic tanks used by the hospital."

Charlie's supervisor left him a note to change a compressed gas tank. Charlie removes the valves and replaces the tank. He leaves the empty tank sitting beside the newly installed tank. Because he is in a hurry, Charlie leaves a note requesting that someone on the next shift complete the installation of the new

Continued

CASE STUDY 2.1—cont'd

tank. His supervisor also asked him to check the eyewash; Charlie was supposed to do this 2 weeks ago but forgot. He removes the eyewash caps, turns the water on and off quickly, and replaces the caps.

At 6:45 AM, Charlie puts on his lab coat again as the day shift arrives. At 7:30 AM, he hangs the coat up with the lab coats that have just been delivered from the laundry and hurries out the door, happy to be heading home.

CASE STUDY 2.1 MULTIPLE CHOICE QUESTIONS (ANSWERS IN APPENDIX A)

1. Charlie is unsure of how to correctly dispose of any of the old or unused chemicals. He should:
   a. ask his supervisor
   b. dump all of the liquids down the sink while running water
   c. consult the SDS sheets
   d. pack all of the chemicals for incineration
2. What should Charlie have done for the replacement of the new compressed gas tank?
   a. secured the new tank upright on the wall.
   b. store the new tank with other flammables materials until he could get to replacing the old tank.
   c. drag the new tank to an out-of-the-way location until he could get to doing the replacement of the old tank.
   d. remove safety covers from the regulators of the new gas tank.

CRITICAL THINKING GROUP DISCUSSION QUESTIONS

1. What safety violations has Charlie committed?
2. As a laboratory administrator, identify the issues and how you would handle the situation.

Note: Narrative answers are published on the EVOLVE instructor site.

REFERENCES

1. Agency for Healthcare Research and Quality. Patient safety network glossary. https://psnet.ahrq.gov/glossary/p (Accessed November 20, 2017).
2. Tierman BF: The role of lab automation in reducing diagnostic errors, MLO Med Lab Obs 49(10):28,30, 2017.
3. The Joint Commission: Laboratory National Patient Safety Goals, www.jointcommission.org, 2018, (Accessed June 23, 2018).
4. US Institute of Medicine: *Crossing the quality chasm: a new health system for the 21st century*, March 2001. www.iom.edu.
5. Astion M: Clear communication and patient harm events, *CL Lab News* 38(1):13, 2012.
6. Baumann N: Mitigating patient risk during IT outages, *CL Lab News* 39(4):15, 2012.
7. Occupational Safety and Health Administration, US Department of Labor: Occupational exposure to bloodborne pathogens: final rule, *Fed Regist* 56(235), 1991 (29 CFR 1910.1030, 64003-64182; Part 1910 to title 29 of Code of Federal Regulations).
8. Occupational Safety and Health Administration, US Department of Labor: Hazard communication final rule, *Fed Regist* 77(58): P17574, 2012.
9. Clinical and Laboratory Standards Institute (CLSI): *Protection of laboratory workers from infectious disease transmitted by blood, body fluids, and tissue: approved guideline*, ed 4, 2014 Wayne, PA, CLSI, M29-A4.
10. Centers for Disease Control and Prevention, US Department of Health and Human Services: Update: universal precautions for prevention of transmission of human immunodeficiency virus, hepatitis B virus, and other bloodborne pathogens in health-care settings, *MMWR* 37(24):377, 1988.
11. Centers for Disease Control and Prevention: *Guidelines for environmental infection control in health-care facilities*, Washington, DC, 2003, US Department of Health and Human Services.
12. Centers for Disease Control and Prevention, US Department of Health and Human Services: HIV Surveillance Report, vol. 28, 2016. www.cdc.gov (Accessed July 10, 2018).

13. Centers for Disease Control and Prevention, US Department of Health and Human Services: Recommendations for prevention of HIV transmission in healthcare settings, *MMWR Morb Mortal Wkly Rep* 36(Supp):3s, 1987.
14. Centers for Disease Control and Prevention, US Department of Health and Human Services: Guideline for hand hygiene in health care settings, *MMWR* 51(RR-16):1–44, 2002.
15. Rutala WA, Weber DJ, Hospital Infection Control Practices Advisory Committee (HICPAC): Guideline for disinfection and sterilization in health care facilities, www.cdc.gov, 2008 (Accessed 16.08.09).
16. Occupational Safety and Health Administration, US Department of Labor: Healthcare wide hazards: needlestick/sharps injuries. www.osha.gov/SLTC/etools/hospital/hazards/sharps/sharps.html (Accessed 14.03.14).
17. Occupational Safety and Health Administration, US Department of Labor: Sharps containers (29 CFR 1910.1030(d)(4)(iii)(A)(1)). www.cdc.gov (Accessed 14.03.14).
18. Zingman BS: Occupational exposures to hepatitis B and C in HIV prophylaxis following occupational exposure: guideline and commentary, *Medscape,* 2013. January 30, www.medscape.com/viewarticle/778035. Accessed 14.03.14.
19. Centers for Disease Control and Prevention, US Department of Health and Human Services: CDC guidance for evaluating health-care personnel for hepatitis B virus protection and for administering postexposure management, *MMWR* 62(10), 2013.
20. World Health Organization (WHO): Measles, http://www.who.int/news-room/fact-sheets/detail/measles, retrieved June 23, 2018.
21. Kuhar DT, et. al.: Updated US Public Health Service Guidelines for the Management of Occupational Exposures to Human Immunodeficiency Virus and Recommendations for Postexposure Prophylaxis, Inf Control and Hosp Epi 34(9), 2013.
22. Roark J: HICPAC revises isolation and TB guidelines. www.infectioncontroltoday.com (Accessed May 2005).
23. Occupational Safety and Health Administration, US Department of Labor: Standards for the tracking and management of medical waste, *Fed Regist* 54(107):24310–24311, 1989.

BIBLIOGRAPHY

All you ever wanted to know about fire extinguishers. (Accessed 10.09.14).

American Society for Clinical Laboratory Science (ASCLS): Procedure to evaluate aspects of Clinical Laboratory Services Total Testing Process that impact patient safety. www.ascls.org (Accessed May 16, 2013).

Astion M: Convincing Providers and Patients to Keep Testing Within Your Hospital and Laboratory's Utilization Management System, *Clin Lab News* 43(4), 2017.

Burtis CA, Ashwood ER, Bruns DE: *Tietz fundamentals of clinical chemistry,* ed 6, St Louis, 2008, Saunders.

Cannons A, Snyder JW: *Promoting Biosafety: "How far have we come," Making Your Core Lab Safe from Ebola and Zika, University Workshop,* San Diego, CA, 2017, AACC Annual Meeting.

Centers for Disease Control and Prevention, US Department of Health and Human Services: Protection against viral hepatitis: recommendations of the Immunization Practices Advisory Committee, *MMWR* 39:1, 1990.

Centers for Disease Control and Prevention, US Department of Health and Human Services: Provisional public health service recommendations for chemoprophylaxis after occupational exposure to HIV, *MMWR* 45:468, 1996.

Centers for Disease Control and Prevention, US Department of Health and Human Services: MMWR Updated US Public Health Service guidelines for the management of occupational exposure to HIV and recommendations for postexposure prophylaxis. www.cdc.gov (Accessed April 2006).

Centers for Disease Control and Prevention, US Department of Health and Human Services: Updated CDC recommendations for the management of hepatitis B virus–infected health-care providers and students, *MMWR* 61:3, 2012.

Golemboski K: Laboratory safety and patient safety—do you know the difference? *ASCLS Today* 27(3):1–12, 2013.

McDaniel G: Ergonomic issues in the clinical lab, *ADVANCE Med Lab Professionals* 25(2):6–7, 2013.

Rose J: Building an effective PPE program, *MLO Med Lab Obs* 49(5):24, 26, 2017.

Rothenberg IZ: Achieving a culture of safety with competency and commitment, *MLO Med Lab Obs* 49(10):26, 28, 2017.

Scungio DJ: Eco-friendly waste management, *MLO Med Lab Obs* 45(6):32–33, 2013.

Snyder J: *Biosafety and Biosecurity: "Where Do the Non-public Health Clinical Laboratories Fit in This Puzzle?" Making Your Core Lab Safe from Ebola and Zika, University Workshop,* San Diego, CA, 2017, AACC Annual Meeting.

Van BL: Assembling a Biosafety Toolkit To Keep Your Lab Safe. In *Making Your Core Lab Safe from Ebola and Zika, University Workshop,* San Diego, CA, 2017, AACC Annual Meeting.

Wyer LA: *Driving Quality through a Culture of Safety, 22nd Annual Management Sciences and Patient Safety Leadership Seminar,* San Diego, CA, 2017, AACC Annual Meeting.

REVIEW QUESTIONS (ANSWERS IN APPENDIX A)

Patient Safety

1. When reviewing the goals of national patient safety goals, the laboratory application of related goals is to:
   a. Improve accuracy of patient identification
   b. Identify analytical errors before releasing results
   c. Decrease the laboratory turn-around time
   d. All the above
2. A medical euphemism is associated with which of the following?
   a. A desire to avoid painful, complex quality improvement issues
   b. A desire to avoid extra paperwork that improvement strategies create
   c. Not being used to describe medical errors
   d. Both a and b
3. In developing a plan to manage information technology (IT) downtime, the initial planning step is to:
   a. Have a clear activation and communications plan.

b. Establish the estimated downtime.
c. Set up a command center.
d. Critique the processes and events during an IT outage.

Safety Standards and Governing Agencies

4. CDC is an abbreviation for the:
 a. College of DC Clinicians
 b. Centers for Disease Control and Treatment
 c. Centers for Disease Control and Prevention
 d. Communicable Disease Center
5. Which of the following is primarily responsible for safeguards and regulations to ensure a safe and healthful workplace?
 a. Health Care Finance Administration
 b. Occupational Safety and Health Administration
 c. Clinical Laboratory Improvement Act of 1988
 d. Centers for Disease Control and Prevention
6. Safety in the clinical laboratory includes:
 a. Educating and training all health workers in Standard Precautions
 b. Providing disposable gloves
 c. Monitoring compliance with protective biosafety policies
 d. All the above
7. Where appropriate, the OSHA standards provide:
 a. Provisions for warning labels
 b. Exposure control procedures
 c. Implementation of training and education programs
 d. All the above
8. To comply with various federal safety regulations, each laboratory must have which of the following?
 a. A chemical hygiene plan
 b. A safety manual
 c. Biohazard labels in place
 d. All the above

Avoiding Transmission of Infectious Diseases

9. Microorganisms included in the top 10 laboratory-acquired infections are:
 a. Hepatitis B virus
 b. Hepatitis C virus
 c. Human immunodeficiency virus
 d. Both a and b

Bloodborne Pathogens

10. The most common source of human immunodeficiency virus (HIV) in the occupational setting is:
 a. Saliva
 b. Urine
 c. Blood
 d. Cerebrospinal fluid
11. The CDC Bloodborne Pathogen Standard and the OSHA Occupational Exposure Standard mandate:
 a. Education and training of all health care workers in Standard Precautions
 b. Proper handling of chemicals
 c. Calibration of equipment
 d. Fire extinguisher maintenance
12. The term *Standard Precautions* refers to:
 a. Treating all specimens as if they are infectious
 b. Assuming that every direct contact with a body fluid is infectious
 c. Treating only blood or blood-tinged specimens as infectious
 d. Both a and b

Questions 13 and 14: Choose the correct terms to fill in the blanks from the choices below.

Transmission to medical personnel of (13) ________________ is more probable than (14) ________________ in unvaccinated individuals.

13. **a.** Human immunodeficiency virus (HIV)
 b. Hepatitis B virus (HBV)
 c. Hepatitis C virus (HCV)
 d. Malaria
14. **a.** Human immunodeficiency virus (HIV)
 b. Hepatitis B virus (HBV)
 c. Hepatitis C virus (HCV)
 d. Malaria

Safe Work Practices for Infection Control

15. Gloves for use in the clinical laboratory are:
 a. Sterile
 b. Nitrile or latex
 c. Used more than once, if no visible signs of blood contamination
 d. All the above
16. Decontaminate hands after:
 a. Contact with patient's skin
 b. Contact with blood or body fluids
 c. Removing gloves
 d. All the above
17. All work surfaces should be sanitized at the end of the shift with a solution of:
 a. 5% bleach
 b. 5% phenol
 c. 10% bleach
 d. Concentrated bleach
18. Each laboratory should have a manual containing approved mandatory and voluntary regulations or standards from:
 a. OSHA
 b. the city
 c. the hospital
 d. the county

Specimen Handling and Shipping Requirements

19. Containers for shipping blood specimens must meet ________ requirements.
 a. UPS
 b. Fed Ex
 c. OSHA
 d. the state

Prevention of Disease Transmission

20. Clinical laboratory personnel need to have demonstrable immunity to:
 a. Rubella
 b. Polio
 c. Hepatitis B
 d. Both a and c

21. Sue and her manager Jane are finishing their shift doing outpatient phlebotomy and specimen processing. Sue has just finished putting a paper clip on a requisition with a couple of blood drops on it. As she pushes the requisition into a pneumatic tube holder with the specimen of patient's blood, the paper clip sticks her finger through her gloved hand. What action does Jane need to initiate *first*?
    a. Take Sue to emergency department for initiation of the hepatitis B vaccine series.
    b. Immediately have Sue's vaccination status and vaccine response status determined.
    c. Determine the hepatitis B surface antigen status of the source patient.
    d. File an incident report with the Occupational Health Office and assure Sue that everything will be okay.

Additional Laboratory Hazards

22. Joe is a new employee assigned to inventory chemicals stored in clinical chemistry. While conducting his inventory, Joe notices that many of the labels have a red square with the letter B in the middle of the square. Conscious of safety practices, Joe checks the expiration date of the fire extinguisher in the immediate area of the chemicals and sees it is in date and labeled as a Class B extinguisher. Is this the appropriate class of fire extinguisher for dealing with Joe's chemical inventory?
    a. Yes; he needs an extinguisher for ordinary combustibles.
    b. Yes; he needs an extinguisher for flammable liquids and gases.
    c. No; he needs an extinguisher for powdered-metal (combustible) material.
    d. No; he needs an extinguisher for a fire that cannot be extinguished.
23. The origin of a Class A fire is:
    a. Paper
    b. Electrical
    c. Gasoline
    d. Hazardous chemicals
24. The OSHA Hazard Communication Standard, the "right-to-know" rule, is designed for what purpose?
    a. To avoid lawsuits
    b. To protect laboratory staff
    c. To protect patients
    d. To establish safety standards
25. A triangle with an outline of a person inside the triangle in the hazards identification system indicates which type of hazard?
    a. Flammability
    b. Reactivity-stability hazard
    c. Special hazard information
    d. Health hazard
26. The simplest, most important step in proper handling of any hazardous substance is:
    a. Wearing disposable gloves
    b. Wearing safety glasses
    c. Properly labeling containers
    d. Using a biosafety hood
27. The term *biohazard* denotes:
    a. Infectious materials that present a risk to the health of human beingss in the laboratory
    b. Infectious materials that present a *potential* risk to the health of human beings in the laboratory
    c. Agents that present a chemical risk or potential risk to the health of human beings in the laboratory
    d. Both a and b
28. Infectious sharps waste must be discarded into containers with all the following features *except*:
    a. Made of sturdy cardboard for landfill disposal
    b. Has a standard symbol
    c. Orange, orange and black, or red
    d. Marked "Biohazard"

Final Decontamination of Waste Materials

29. Terminal waste of infectious material can be processed by autoclaving or by:
    a. Incineration
    b. Soaking in bleach
    c. Ethylene dioxide gas
    d. Normal garbage disposal

Safety audit

30. A safety audit should consist of all the following considerations *except*:
    a. Laboratory coats
    b. Fire extinguishers
    c. Incubators
    d. Eyewash stations and safety shower

Basic first-aid procedures

31. Immediate first aid for acid burns on the skin is:
    a. Ice
    b. Running water
    c. Petroleum jelly
    d. Butter

Bonus Challenge Questions

Answer questions 32 to 34 based on the following laboratory situation:

Bess, a 21-year-old medical laboratory science student in her last year of training, is completing her morning phlebotomy rounds. Her final patient is a 16-year-old girl diagnosed with type 1 diabetes mellitus. The order is for a fasting blood sugar and a CBC, so Bess collects samples via venipuncture. After performing the venipuncture, Bess cleans up the equipment and trash from the patient's bed. In doing so, she pokes a gloved finger with the used needle because she failed to engage the safety cover correctly. Even though she is distraught, Bess keeps herself composed and exits the patient's room. Bess immediately goes and washes her hands with soap and warm water and then heads back to the laboratory.

32. What is the first thing Bess should do?
    a. Go to break; coffee is in order after this ordeal.
    b. Inform her supervisor.
    c. Go home sick; she cannot effectively work the rest of the day.
    d. She was wearing gloves, so it is not a major concern.

33. Bess meant to, but has not yet been vaccinated against hepatitis B virus (HBV). The source patient has consented to postexposure testing. What should be done to help protect Bess?
a. HBV testing is performed every other day, so wait and see if patient is positive or negative first.
b. Bess should receive HBIG immediately.
c. Bess should be vaccinated for HBV.
d. Nothing should be done until the patient results are available.

34. What are the next steps for Bess in her postexposure care plan?
a. Nothing; the patient was negative for HIV and HBV.
b. Bess should be given an antiretroviral agent.
c. A confirmatory HIV test should be performed on the source patient and on Bess.
d. Bess should be screened for HIV at 3 months and 6 months after exposure.

Turgeon: Linné & Ringsrud's Clinical Laboratory Science, 8th Edition

STUDENT PROCEDURE WORKSHEET 2-1

Handwashing

Read Chapter 2 in *Linné & Ringsrud's Clinical Laboratory Science: Concepts, Procedures, and Clinical Applications,* 8th edition, for a complete discussion of this topic.

Student Learning Outcomes
After reading Chapter 2, and at the completion of this laboratory exercise and the review questions, the student will be able to:

- Correctly wash hands before wearing and after removing disposable gloves.
- Complete the end-of-procedure review questions with a grade of 80% or higher.

Equipment and Supplies

1. Antiseptic soap
2. Sink with running warm water
3. Paper towels in a dispenser

Instructions for the Procedure
Read the list of required equipment and supplies and the procedural steps. Follow the procedural steps in exact order.

SEQUENCE	PROCEDURAL STEP	INSTRUCTOR-OBSERVED ACCEPTABLE PERFORMANCE (CHECK IF ACCEPTABLE)
1	Remove all jewelry from hands and wrists and deposit in a safe place.	
2	Turn on faucet, and adjust water to desired warm water temperature.	
3	Holding hands down under the running water, wet hands with water. Avoid having the water travel up the arms.	
4	Apply approximately 3-5 mL of antiseptic liquid soap to the hands and mid-forearms. The soap should be applied to the skin with 10 circular motions of the hands.	
5	Circular motions are used with suds soap as it is applied to palms of the hands, backs of the hands, and forearms.	
6	Fingers should be washed by interfacing fingers and rubbing them back and forth with friction about 10 times or for 15 seconds. Clean fingernails with a brush, if necessary.	
7	Lower hands and forearms under running water and rinse until no more soap is observable on the skin.	
8	Repeat steps 1-7 once.	
9	Gently dry hands and forearms with a paper towel.	
10	Use a clean paper towel to turn off the water faucet. The water faucet is considered to be contaminated.	
11	Inspect hands for any skin abrasions or cuts. If any skin is disrupted or if hangnails are present, cover with an adhesive strip.	
12	Put on new disposable gloves.	
13	After removing gloves and properly disposing of contaminated gloves, repeat steps 1-10.	

(Continued)

Turgeon: Linné & Ringsrud's Clinical Laboratory Science, 8th Edition

STUDENT PROCEDURE WORKSHEET 2-1

Review Questions

1. What is the purpose of properly washing your hands after specific conditions or before certain activities? What does handwashing do?

2. Why is it important to cover the skin thoroughly with antiseptic soap and rub it into the skin for at least 15 seconds?

3. Why wouldn't you turn off the faucet with your clean hand, after completing a proper handwashing?

Procedural Evaluation

Student's Name ______________________ Grade ________

Instructor's Signature ______________________ Date ________

Comments:

Turgeon: Linné & Ringsrud's Clinical Laboratory Science, 8th Edition

STUDENT PROCEDURE WORKSHEET 2-2

Practicing Clinical Laboratory Safety

Read Chapter 2 in *Linné & Ringsrud's Clinical Laboratory Science: Concepts, Procedures, and Clinical Applications,* 8th edition, for a complete discussion of this topic.

Student Learning Outcomes

After reading Chapter 2 and at the completion of this laboratory exercise and the review questions, the student will be able to:

- Use general laboratory safety equipment correctly.
- Dispose of biohazardous material in the clinical laboratory.
- Complete the end-of-procedure review questions with a grade of 80% or higher.

Equipment and Supplies

1. Antiseptic soap
2. Biohazard "red bag" waste bags
3. Biohazard sharps container
4. Disposable gloves
5. Disposable laboratory coats
6. Face shield or safety glasses
7. Fire extinguisher
8. Hand disinfectant (alcohol based)
9. Lancets (wrapped) or evacuated tube holder with unused needle
10. MSDS binder
11. Paper towels
12. Safety hood (chemical or laminar flow)
13. Safety shower
14. Sink with warm running water
15. Surface disinfectant

Instructions for the Procedure

Read the list of required equipment and supplies and the procedural steps. Follow the procedural steps in exact order.

SEQUENCE	PROCEDURAL STEP	INSTRUCTOR-OBSERVED ACCEPTABLE PERFORMANCE (CHECK IF ACCEPTABLE)
1	Locate or collect all of the listed equipment.	
2	Wash and dry hands (see Student Procedure Worksheet 2-1) or use hand sanitizer properly.	
3	Put on disposable gloves.	
4	Assemble and properly put on all additional personal protective equipment.	
5	Remove all safety equipment except the gloves.	
6	Pour a small amount of water on the floor to simulate a biohazardous spill (such as blood).	
7	Properly clean up the spill with disinfectant and paper towels.	
8	Dispose of the contaminated paper towels in biohazardous red bag waste.	
9	Remove contaminated gloves properly, disinfect hands with foam hand disinfectant, and put on clean gloves.	
10	Dispose of a lancet or evacuated tube needle holder with needle in the biohazard sharps container.	
11	Disinfect laboratory bench surfaces and specimen storage cart surfaces with surface disinfectant.	
12	Check to be sure all of the work area is clean without any biohazardous safety violations.	
13	Remove gloves, and disinfect hands with foam hand disinfectant.	
14	Place a bucket under the safety shower and test.	
15	Check the expiration date of the fire extinguisher.	
16	Check the chemical or laminar flow hood for acceptable fan operation and door access.	

(Continued)

Turgeon: Linné & Ringsrud's Clinical Laboratory Science, 8th Edition

STUDENT PROCEDURE WORKSHEET 2-2

Review Questions

1. Describe how to clean up a laboratory spill properly when a tube of blood is accidentally dropped.

2. Describe how you would properly disinfect a laboratory bench (when, what type of solution, disposable of potentially contaminated cleanup supplies).

3. Why is it important to put sharps in a plastic container rather than in "red bag" garbage bags?

Procedural Evaluation

Student's Name ______________________ Grade ________

Instructor's Signature ______________________ Date ________

Comments:

3

Quality Assessment and Quality Control in the Clinical Laboratory

http://evolve.elsevier.com/Turgeon/clinicallab/

CHAPTER OUTLINE

LEARNING OUTCOMES

The Value of Quality
- Name five effects of clinical laboratory testing.

Patient Specimens
- Name six types of specimens that can be analyzed in the laboratory in addition to body tissues.

Clinical Laboratory Improvement Amendments
- Describe the purpose of the CLIA '88 quality control requirements and the categories of testing that are regulated.

Voluntary Accrediting Organizations
- Name two voluntary accrediting agencies.

ISO 15189 Standards in Clinical Laboratories
- Assess the applicability and benefit of complying with ISO 15189.

Lean and Six Sigma
- Compare the focus of Lean to Six Sigma in the clinical laboratory.

Quality Assessment
- Explain who can certify a clinical laboratory.

Quality Assessment—Error Analysis
- Contrast active errors versus latent errors.

Quality Assessment—Phases of Testing
- Give at least two examples in each of the phases of testing: preanalytical, analytical, and postanalytical.
- Explain influencing factors in each of the nine nonanalytical factors in quality assessment.

Proficiency Testing
- Explain the requirements for proficiency testing for nonwaived and waived laboratory assays.
- Describe the process of proficiency testing.

Alternate Assessment
- Name and describe four alternate assessment methods for proficiency testing.

Accuracy in Reporting Results and Documentation
- Define the term *Delta check.*
- Explain the role of documentation of laboratory testing.

Quality Control
- Describe the role of quality control in quality laboratory testing.
- ❖ Compare the purpose of internal versus external quality control.
- Define the terms *systematic error* and *random error.*

Control Specimens
- Name the major functions of control specimens in laboratory testing.
- Define the terms *dispersion, drift,* and *trends.*

Quality Assessment Descriptors
- Define terms used in quality assessment: *accuracy, calibration, control, precision,* and *standards.*
- Define and compare sensitivity and specificity of a test and predictive values.

Quality Control Statistics
- Define the statistical terms of *mean, median, mode, standard deviation, standard deviation index, confidence intervals, total analytic error, coefficient of variation.*
- Describe the use of reference values, including using the mean and standard deviation in determining reference range.
- Identify sources of variance or error in a procedure.

Total Analytical Error
- Define the total analytical concept.

Monitoring Quality Control
- Evaluate Levey-Jennings charts and Westgard Rules for monitoring quality control.
- Identify factors contributing to questionable validity of the reference ranges of laboratory assays.

Other QC Rules
- Name and describe the eight nonanalytical factors in quality assessment.

Testing Outcomes
- Define the terms *reference values* and *normal values.*

Case Study
- ❖ Analyze the patient history, clinical signs and symptoms, and laboratory data for the stated case studies, answer the related critical thinking questions, and conclude the most likely diagnosis.

Review Questions
- Demonstrate comprehension of the chapter content by completing the end-of-chapter review questions with a grade of 80% or higher.

Note:
- indicates MLT and MLS core content
- ❖ indicates MLT (optional) and MLS advanced content

KEY TERMS

accuracy
calibration
coefficient of variation (CV)
confidence intervals
control specimens
continuous quality improvement (CQI)
Delta check system
dispersion
drift
Levey-Jennings (Shewhart) QC charts
precision
predictive value
proficiency testing (PT)
quality assessment (QA)
quality control (QC)
reliability
sensitivity
specificity
standard deviation (SD)
trends
variance
Westgard Rules

THE VALUE OF QUALITY

Quality outcomes are of the utmost importance in a clinical laboratory. Every year more than 10 billion clinical laboratory assays are performed in the United States. These diagnostic laboratory test results play a decisive role in decision-making related to individual patient care, public health policy, and research decisions.

Testing a patient's tissues or body fluids provides the necessary data for health care providers to make informed medical decisions. Laboratory testing affects multiple aspects of patient care including screening, diagnosis, staging, treatment, and monitoring of disease. But the real net clinical value[1] of a laboratory testing result involves balancing the benefits that a test delivers against any harm that it may cause a patient. Harm can be caused by:

- Ordering an inappropriate test,
- Not ordering an appropriate test,
- Not using an appropriate test result properly,
- Delaying or missing a test result from an appropriate test,
- Reporting an incorrect or inaccurate test result.

Quality management works at the organizational level to implement an overall quality policy. Formalized systems document processes, procedures, and responsibilities for achieving quality policies and objectives. The quality management system Six Sigma[2] defines the components critical to quality as the key measurable characteristics of a product or process whose performance requirements or specification limits must be met to satisfy the customer.

Quality management encompasses *quality assurance* and *quality control.* To achieve a 99% level of quality means accepting a 1% error rate. Key components of providing high- quality laboratory results include an educated laboratory and extended specimen collection staff; appropriate, validated testing methods; properly functioning instruments; quality assurance and quality control processes; and peer-referenced proficiency testing.

PATIENT SPECIMENS

Clinical laboratory professionals work with many types of specimens. Blood and urine specimens are the most often tested, but examinations can be conducted also on body tissues and other

TABLE 3.1 Top 10 CLIA Deficiencies in Clinical Laboratories

Rank	Regulatory Cite	Deficiency	% of All Labs With Deficiency
1	493.1252(b)	The laboratory must define criteria for those conditions that are essential for proper storage of reagents and specimens, accurate and reliable test system operation, and test result reporting. These conditions must be monitored and documented.	5.1
2	493.1289(a)	The laboratory must establish and follow written policies and procedures for an ongoing mechanism to monitor, assess, and when indicated, correct problems identified in the analytic systems specified in 493.1251 through 493.1283.	4.9
3	493.1251(b)	The procedure manual must include the requirements for specimen acceptability, microscopic examination, step-by-step performance of the procedure, preparation of materials for testing, etc.	4.6
4	493.1236(c)(1)	At least twice annually, the laboratory must verify the accuracy of any test or procedure it performs that is not included in subpart I or this part (General Lab Systems)	4.4
5	493.1291(c)	The test report must indicate the following: for positive patient identification, either the patient's name and identification number, or a unique patient identifier and identification number, the name and address of the laboratory location where the test was performed, and other requirements specified in 493.1291(c).	4.3
6	493.1235	As specified in the personnel requirements in subpart M, the laboratory must establish and follow written policies and procedures to assess employee and, if applicable, consultant competency.	3.9
7	493.1252(a)	Test systems must be selected by the laboratory. The testing must be performed following the manufacturer's instructions and in a manner that provides test results within the laboratory's stated performance specifications for each test system as determined under 493.1253	3.6
8	493.1252(d)	Reagents, solutions, culture media, control materials, calibration materials, and other supplies must not be used when they have exceeded their expiration date, have deteriorated, or are of substandard quality.	3.4
9	493.1254(a)(1)	Maintenance as defined by the manufacturer and with at least the frequency specified by the manufacturer.	3.3
10	493.1255(b)	The laboratory must perform and document calibration verification instructions using the criteria verified or established by the laboratory at least once every 6 months and whenever certain instances occur.	3.2

Total number of laboratories surveyed = 17,120; total number of physician office laboratories (POLs) surveyed = 10,857. Data based on the most recent survey.
Source: CLIA UPDATE Division of Laboratory Services, Centers for Medicare and Medicaid Services: Top 10 Deficiencies in the Nation—CMS CLIA Data Base, January 2017.

body fluids, including synovial, cerebrospinal, seminal, peritoneal, and pericardial fluids. The purpose of the clinical laboratory is to provide information regarding the assay results for the specimens analyzed; it is most important that the specimens be properly identified and collected. In the testing process, analytes or constituents are measured by using only very small amounts of the specimens collected. In interpreting the results, it is assumed that the results obtained represent the actual concentrations of the analytes in the patient. Only by using the various quality assessment (QA) systems can the reliability of results be ensured. No matter how carefully a laboratory assay has been carried out, valid laboratory results can be reported only when preanalytical quality control (QC) has also been ascertained. Special patient preparation for some specimen collections, along with proper transportation to and handling in the laboratory before the actual analytical assay, is very important. Examples of patient-related physiologic factors include fasting and the influence of food and alcohol intake.

Appropriate QA programs must be in place in the laboratory to make certain that each patient specimen is given the best analysis possible and that the results reported will benefit the patient in the best possible way.

CLINICAL LABORATORY IMPROVEMENT AMENDMENTS

In 1988 the U.S. Congress enacted the Clinical Laboratory Improvement Amendments of 1988 (CLIA '88) in response to concerns about laboratory testing errors.[3] The final CLIA rule,[4] Laboratory Requirements Relating to Quality Systems and Certain Personnel Qualifications, was published in 2003. Enactment of CLIA established a minimum threshold for all aspects of clinical laboratory testing.

The introduction of routine QC in the clinical laboratory was a major advance in improving the accuracy and reliability of clinical laboratory testing. Various agencies monitor laboratory quality and have commonality in many of the noted top 10 deficiencies (Table 3.1). Effective in 2003, all laboratories must meet and follow the final QC requirements. These regulations established minimum requirements with general QC systems for all nonwaived testing. In addition, a controversial 2004 regulation allows the Centers for Medicare and Medicaid Services (CMS) to consider acceptable alternative approaches to QC practices, called *equivalent quality control,* for laboratory testing.

VOLUNTARY ACCREDITING ORGANIZATIONS

The public's focus on health care delivery is relevant to most areas of work done in clinical laboratories. Standards have been set by The Joint Commission (TJC), formerly the Joint Commission on Accreditation of Healthcare Organizations, reflecting the Commission's focus on QA programs. TJC requires hospital laboratories to be accredited by TJC itself, the Commission on Office Laboratory Accreditation (COLA), or the College of American Pathologists (CAP).

As announced by TJC, a periodic performance review (PPR) will be required for the laboratory accreditation program.[5] The PPR is a formal standards evaluation tool intended to support continuous compliance and is being added to the accreditation process at the request of accredited laboratories. Effective January 1, 2006, a laboratory must participate in either the full PPR or in one of the three approved PPR options. Laboratories in complex organizations (such as a hospital and laboratory) are required to participate in the PPR using the same methodology or selection of submission choice as the primary program. For example, if the primary program completes the full PPR, the laboratory will also complete the full PPR. Laboratories in TJC-accredited organizations that are accredited by a cooperative partner (such as CAP or COLA) are not required to complete the laboratory PPR. These laboratories need to participate in an equivalent intracycle assessment process. For TJC-accredited organizations that provide only waived-testing laboratory services, the standard requirements are addressed in the organizational PPR.

BOX 3.1 Overview of ISO 15189

Management requirements	Technical requirements
Organization and management	Personnel
Quality management system	Accommodation and environmental conditions
Document control	Laboratory equipment
Review of contracts	Preexamination procedures
Examination by referral laboratories	Examination procedures
External services and supplies	Assuring quality of examination procedures
Advisory services	Postexamination procedures
Resolution of complaints	Reporting of results
Identification and control of nonconformities	
Corrective action	
Preventive action	
Continual improvement	
Quality and technical records	
Internal audits	
Management review	

From Malone B: ISO accreditation comes to America, *Clin Laboratory News* 35:1–4, 2009.

ISO 15189 STANDARDS IN CLINICAL LABORATORIES

The International Organization for Standardization (International Standards Organization; ISO) is the world's largest developer and publisher of international standards. ISO is a network of 159 national standards institutes, with one member per country and a Central Secretariat in Geneva, Switzerland, that coordinates the system. ISO is a nongovernmental organization that forms a bridge between the public and private sectors. It enables problem solving by consensus building on solutions that meet both the requirements of business and the needs of society.

As the second largest laboratory accrediting organization, CAP recently adopted an optional accreditation program based on the ISO 15189 standards for medical laboratories.[6] The 15189 standards, designed specifically for medical laboratories, covers 15 management requirements and eight technical requirements that focus on areas such as technical competency. The basic benefit to using ISO 15189 is the use of a comprehensive and highly structured approach for quality management that allows laboratories to use tools such as Six Sigma. The process uses actual assessment by certified assessors, who educate people about the expectation and the intent of the standard.

In the ISO 15189 accreditation program, one of the most important steps is the *gap analysis* that occurs after a laboratory has purchased the 15189 document from ISO and conducted a preliminary internal audit of its processes. In the gap analysis, assessors look carefully at where the laboratory does not meet the ISO standard. This analysis reveals what facets of day-to-day operations warrant improvement. A preassessment from CAP may take place. Once a laboratory passes the final accreditation assessment, a 3-year cycle begins. During this period, two surveillance assessments are scheduled, and an on-site reaccreditation is required.

One caution about using 15189 is that it is considered to be too general and, in some cases, not as stringent or specific as CLIA regulations. Therefore ISO standards are not acceptable to the U.S. government.

Requirements for quality and competence in ISO 15189 are unique because considerations include the specific requirements of the medical environment and the importance of the medical laboratory to patient care (Box 3.1). ISO 15189:2007 is for use by medical laboratories in developing their quality management systems and in assessing their own competence, and, by accreditation bodies in confirming or recognizing the competence of medical laboratories. ISO 15189 contains the general requirements for testing and calibration laboratories. This working group included advice to users of the laboratory service and requirements for the collection of patient samples, the interpretation of test results, acceptable turnaround times, testing in a medical emergency, and the laboratory's role in the education and training of health care staff.[7]

CAP 15189 is a voluntary, nonregulated accreditation to the ISO 15189:2007 Standard. CAP 15189 requires a steadfast commitment to the laboratory management system and all interacting departments. CAP 15189 does not replace CAP's CLIA-based Laboratory Accreditation Program, but rather complements CAP accreditation and other quality systems by optimizing processes to improve patient care, strengthen the deployment of quality standards, reduce errors and risk, and control costs. CAP 15189 promotes sustainable quality by looking beyond individual procedures and discovering ways to improve continuously the structure and function of laboratory operations. As a management philosophy, CAP 15189 raises the bar on quality as it drives decisions throughout an entire institution.

LEAN AND SIX SIGMA

Pioneering clinical laboratories in the United States that use management systems such as *Lean* (Box 3.2), which focuses on reducing waste, and *Six Sigma*, a metric and methodology that focuses on reducing variability, can achieve immediate

BOX 3.2 Key LEAN Lessons

- It is not possible to overcommunicate.
- Continuously focus on improvement.
- Engage all facets of an organization, not just a core team.
- Actions speak louder than words.
- Ideas flow from the bottom up.
- Be respectful to every individual. Listen to and seriously consider everyone's ideas.
- A feedback loop is critical to overcoming challenges.
- To achieve success, staff must be accountable.

From Coons J, Courtois H: LEAN laboratory puts patient safety first, *MLO Med Laboratory Obs* 41:35, 2009.

and recognizable results when these systems are properly applied. When either of these systems was used to redesign workflow in high-volume core hematology and chemistry laboratories, a 50% reduction in average test turnaround time, a 40% to 50% improvement in labor productivity, and a comparable improvement in the quality of results were observed.[8]

Lean principles of reduction of unnecessary and non–value-added activities to decrease total production time and effort can be appropriately applied in all sections of the laboratory (such as urinalysis). Lean tools focus on identifying steps in a procedure that are error prone. If these steps cannot be eliminated, they must be controlled. Lean principles support the concept of performing tasks correctly the first time, with minimal wasted time and effort. One highly effective tool in applying Lean principles is a process map of external and internal activities related to a specific laboratory assay. This mapping allows for a step-by-step analysis. Knowledge of a detailed process allows for improvement in outcomes.[8]

QUALITY ASSESSMENT

External standards have been set to ensure the quality of laboratory results reported through QA, as imposed by CLIA '88 and administered by CMS. A clinical laboratory must be certified by CMS, by a private certifying agency, or by a CMS-approved state regulatory agency. Once certified, the laboratory is scheduled for regular inspections to determine compliance with the federal regulations, including CLIA '88.

QA programs are now also a requirement in the federal government's implementation of CLIA '88. The standards mandated are for all laboratories, with the intent that the medical community's ability to provide good-quality patient care will be greatly enhanced. Included in the CLIA '88 provisions are requirements for QC and QA, for the use of **proficiency testing (PT)**, and for certain levels of personnel to perform and supervise the work in the laboratory.

According to CLIA '88 regulations, QA activities in the laboratory must be documented and must be an active part of the ongoing organization of the laboratory. Dedication of sufficient planning time to QA and to implementation of the program in the total laboratory operation is critical. All clinical laboratory personnel must be willing to work together to make the quality of service to the patient their top priority. It is important to develop a comprehensive program to include all levels of laboratory staff.

Local programs must be in place to carry out the external mandates. Internal regulation comes also from the need to ensure quality performance and reporting of results for the many laboratory tests being done—a process of QA. It is the responsibility of the clinical laboratory, to both patient and physician, to ensure that the results reported from that laboratory are reliable and that the physician is provided with an estimate of what constitutes the reference or "normal" range for an analyte being measured. Internal QA monitoring programs may be a component of total quality management or **continuous quality improvement (CQI)**, each of which is designed to monitor and improve the quality of services provided by the laboratory.

QUALITY ASSESSMENT—ERROR ANALYSIS

Two types of errors occur in error analysis[9]: active error and latent error. An active error is obvious. It occurs at the interface between a health care worker and the patient (Box 3.3). In comparison, a latent error is less obvious. Latent failures are related to the organization or design of a laboratory (Box 3.4).

Ways to improve overall errors include at least three strategies:

1. Formal patient safety training, including discussion of disconnect between laboratory personnel and the patient
2. Enhanced communication between patients and laboratory staff and providers directly caring for patients

BOX 3.3 Examples of Active Errors

- Failing to identify a patient before phlebotomy
- Missing a blood vessel during phlebotomy
- Errors with anticoagulants in collection tubes
- Errors with the transportation system (such as a pneumatic tube)
- Errors with data entry
- Errors with an instrument or computer (such as ignoring an instrument flag)

Modified from Astion M: Latent errors in laboratory services, *Clin Laboratory News* 35:15, 2009.

BOX 3.4 Examples of Latent Errors

- Staffing problems (such as chronic shortages)
- Information technology (such as no interface with technology)
- Equipment malfunctions (such as old error-prone analyzers)
- Work environment (such as multitasking, poor laboratory layout, and disconnect between laboratory and patients)
- Policy and procedures (such as the relabeling of mislabeled or unlabeled tubes and laboratory requisition variation)
- Teamwork factors (such as poor communication between shifts and departmental "silos")
- Management/organization (such as when profit is a goal, patient safety is ignored, incident reports are deemphasized, and interventions based on analysis are minimized)

Modified from Astion M: Latent errors in laboratory services, Clin Laboratory News 35:15, 2009.

3. Quality improvement projects that involve patient outcomes data and feedback of the data to laboratory staff, with an analysis of the consequences of high-quality and low-quality work

QUALITY ASSESSMENT—PHASES OF TESTING

The total testing process (TTP) serves as the primary point of reference for focusing on quality in the clinical laboratory.[10] TTP is defined by activities in three distinct phases related to workflow outside and inside the laboratory:

1. Preanalytical (preexamination)
2. Analytical (examination)
3. Postanalytical (postexamination)

Currently, the majority of laboratory errors are related to the preexamination or postexamination phases of testing rather than to the examination phase. Specimen-related errors continue to be a major problem[2] (Fig. 3.1).

The preanalytical phase of testing is particularly error prone. A major reason that the preanalytical phase is so error prone is that it is especially susceptible to human error. Frequently, specimen collection is performed outside of the laboratory and involves nonlaboratory personnel, who may not be properly trained. One[11] study reported that the majority of laboratory errors now occur in the preanalytical phase. To reduce and potentially eliminate laboratory errors, a QA program is mandated. A QA program can be divided into two major components: nonanalytical factors and the analysis of quantitative data (QC). CAP[6] includes a variety of considerations in QA management (Box 3.5). The Institute for Quality in Laboratory Medicine (IQLM)[11] has developed 12 measures to evaluate quality in the laboratory, based on the phase of testing (Boxes 3.6–3.7).

BOX 3.5 CAP Quality Assessment Considerations

- Supervision
- Procedure manual
- Specimen collection and handling
- Results reporting
- Reagents, calibration, and standards
- Controls
- Instruments and equipment
- Personnel
- Physical facilities
- Laboratory safety

From College of American Pathologists (CAP): Chemistry-coagulation, chemistry and toxicology, and point-of-care checklists, revised October 2005. www.cap.org

BOX 3.6 Examples of Errors in Laboratory Testing

Preanalytical (Preexamination) Phase

- Test order inaccuracy
- Error in order entry
- Wrong patient identification
- Blood culture contamination
- Type of evacuated tube used for blood collection
- Specimen labeling errors
- Improper specimen handling
- Adequacy of specimen information

Analytical Phase (Examination)

- Poor quality control
- Accuracy of point-of-care testing
- Instrument malfunction
- Analysis inference, e.g., hemolysis, lipemia
- Incorrect results resulting from drug interference

Postanalytical (Postexamination) Phase

- Failure in critical value reporting
- Increased turnaround time
- Missing laboratory test results resulting from discontinuity of care
- Incorrect interpretation of results
- Lack of clinician follow-up

From IQLM Proposed Quality Assessment Measures Institute for Quality Laboratory, Medicine (IQLM). www.phppo.cdc.gov

PROFICIENCY TESTING (PT)

Requirements

PT is required by CLIA (42 CFR 493 for Subpart H Participation in Proficiency Testing for Laboratories Performing Nonwaived Testing) for nonwaived tests, or as part of verification for tests and/or as part of process improvement, and it identifies the specialties, subspecialties, and specific analytes or tests that require testing participation.[3] CLIA regulations apply to moderate-complexity or high-complexity assays cleared and approved by the U.S. Food and Drug Administration (FDA) and to moderate-complexity or high-complexity assays *not* cleared or approved by the FDA. If a laboratory performs moderate-complexity or high-complexity tests for which no PT is available, it must have a system for verifying the accuracy and reliability of its test results at least twice a year (Box 3.8).

If a laboratory performs only waived tests, it is not required to participate in a PT program. However, it must apply for and be given a certificate of waiver from the U.S. Department of Health and Human Services. Many point-of-care testing (POCT) assays are waived and do not fall under the CLIA regulations, but some nonwaived assays may be performed in

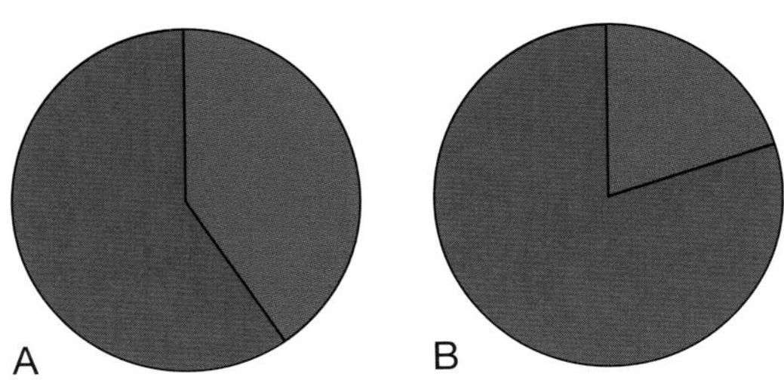

Fig. 3.1 Clinical laboratory testing errors. (A) Preanalytical errors are 46% to 68.2% of total errors. (B) Postanalytical errors are 18.5% to 47% of total errors. (From Plebani M: Errors in clinical laboratories or errors in laboratory medicine? *Clin Chem Laboratory Med* 44:750–759, 2006.)

BOX 3.7 Examples of Potential Preanalytical, Analytical, and Postanalytical Errors

Preanalytical (Preexamination)

Incorrectly ordered assay
Specimen obtained from wrong patient
Specimen procured at the wrong time
Specimen collected in the wrong tube or container
Blood specimens collected in the wrong order
Incorrect labeling of specimen
Improper processing of specimen

Analytical (Examination)

Oversight of instrument flags
Out-of-control quality control results
Wrong assay performed

Postanalytical (Postexamination)

Reporting the wrong result
Verbal reporting of results
Instrument: laboratory information system incompatibility error
Confusion about reference ranges

BOX 3.8 Requirements for Twice-Annual Laboratory Accuracy Verification[1]

Any test or procedure it performs that is not included in subpart I of this part.

Any test or procedure listed in subpart I of this part for which compatible proficiency testing samples are not offered by a CMS-approved proficiency testing program.

[1]U.S. Health Care Financing Administration, Department of Health and Human Services: Clinical laboratory improvement amendments of 1988, Fed Regist, Feb 28, 1992 (CLIA '88; Final Rule. 42 CFR. Subpart K, 493.1236 2(c)

satellite laboratories or patient care areas and are considered POCT testing. Such testing sites have accreditation and regulatory implications, and the location of the testing is not relevant. It is important to ensure that these locations are included in a PT program.

According to CLIA '88, a laboratory must establish and follow written QC procedures for monitoring and evaluating the quality of the analytical testing process of each method to ensure the accuracy and reliability of patient test results and reports. Participation in a PT program involves receiving identical specimen samples periodically. PT programs are available through CAP, the Centers for Disease Control and Prevention (CDC), and through the health departments in some states.

PT requires sending a patient specimen for assay of a specific analyte to another laboratory for testing, where the sample is analyzed using the same procedure as that used for the patient sample. Subsequently, the PT results are sent to a provider for evaluation of the results by method or procedure. Results of the assays are graded for each participating laboratory according to designated evaluation limits, and the results are compared with those of other laboratories participating in the same PT program. The PT provider informs the laboratory of the results, and the laboratory reviews the PT results and makes any necessary corrections, if a problem is identified. This process is intended to achieve standardized laboratory results.

Challenges

PT programs evolve over time. Programs can be affected by new technologies and methods, and increased automation. This rapid development of new factors offers a challenge to PT. Laboratory automation has both a potential positive and negative effect on PT. As a result of automation, factors such as inclusion of all instruments from same or different manufacturers, testing of the same analyte on different types of instruments, testing of all analytes that may require multiple survey panels, and testing of all staff must be ensured. A positive effect of automation is that it may mitigate some of the effect of PT failure associated with inexperienced staff or testing that is not done routinely. Factors that may have a negative effect include the number of the same manufacturer's instruments in a laboratory and the number of instruments from different manufacturers that perform the same tests.

ALTERNATE ASSESSMENT

If a PT program is not available for a specific analyte, an alternate assessment of quality is needed. Several methods exist:

- External Split Sample: participate with another laboratory using the same method or another method
- Internal Split Sample: reexamine a specific patient sample using a different method or a different technologist
- Audit Sample: analyze the same sample over time to assess reproducibility and stability of a method
- Use government and university interlaboratory comparisons

ACCURACY IN REPORTING RESULTS AND DOCUMENTATION

Appropriate communication is critical to high-quality patient care. In most situations, laboratory reports are recorded and sent to the appropriate patient area rather than conveyed by telephone; the risk for error is too great when depending on verbal reports alone. In emergency ("stat") situations, verbal reports may be necessary but must be followed by written reports as soon as possible. It is equally important in reporting results to be on the alert for clerical errors, particularly transcription errors. The introduction of computer-interfaced, online reporting is useful in communicating information correctly and efficiently.

The **Delta check system** monitors individual patient results. The difference between a patient's current laboratory result and consecutive previous results that exceed a specified cutoff value is referred to as a *Delta check*. That specified cutoff value represents the maximal allowable change that is acceptable for a laboratory procedure. The cutoff value may be presented as an absolute change, percent change, rate of change, or rate of percent change. An abrupt change, high or low, can trigger a computer-based warning system and should be investigated before reporting a patient result. Delta checks are investigated by the laboratory internally to rule out mislabeling, clerical error, or possible analytical error.

The most common true positive Delta check flags results from incorrect specimen collection in a tube as a result of an insufficient quantity of blood, specimen contamination with intravenous (IV) fluid, or an evacuated blood collection tube with the wrong anticoagulant for the assay.

The ongoing process of making certain the correct laboratory result is reported for the right patient in a timely manner and at the correct cost is known as *continuous quality improvement (CQI)*. This process assures the clinician ordering the test that the testing process has been done in the best possible way to provide the most useful information in diagnosing or managing the particular patient. QA indicators are evaluated as part of the CQI process to monitor the laboratory's performance. Each laboratory will set its own indicators, depending on the specific goals of the laboratory. Any QA indicators should be appreciated as a tool to ensure that reported results are of the highest quality.

An important aspect of QA is documentation. CLIA regulations mandate that any problem or situation that might affect the outcome of a test result be recorded and reported. All such incidents must be documented in writing, including the changes proposed and their implementation, and follow-up must be monitored. Reportable incidents can involve specimens that are improperly collected, labeled, or transported to the laboratory or problems concerning prolonged turnaround times for test results. There must be a reasonable attempt to correct the problems or situation, and all steps in this process must be documented.

Another valuable QA technique is to examine relationships in the data generated for each patient, including the mathematical association between anions and cations in the electrolyte report, the correlation between protein and casts in urine, and the relationship between hemoglobin and hematocrit and the appearance of the blood smear in hematologic studies.

Laboratory computer systems and electronic information processing expedite record keeping. QA programs require documentation, and computer record-keeping capability assists in this effort. When control results are within the acceptable limits established by the laboratory, these data provide the necessary link between the control and the patient data, thus giving reassurance that the patient results are reliable, valid, and reportable. This information is necessary to document that uniform protocols have been established and are being followed. The data can also support the proper functioning capabilities of the test systems being used at the time patient results are produced.

QUALITY CONTROL

The components of QC include avoiding the report of wrong testing results and complying with regulatory guidelines. Whereas quality assurance verifies the three phases of laboratory testing, QC evaluates only the analytical part of the process. Specific goals of QC include detecting and correcting errors and generating high-quality results that are accurate, precise, and reliable. The ultimate goal of QC is to monitor the analytical performance of a measurement procedure and to alert analysts to problems that might limit the usefulness of a test result.

There are two types of QC:

- Internal QC, or statistical QC, which evaluates the daily precision of assay measurements
- External QC, which evaluates the accuracy of assay measurements. This type of QC uses data generated from voluntary submission of internal QC control assay results (peer-groups) and data generated from required submission of specific control specimens (PT)

In QC, two types of errors can occur: systematic and random. Systematic error is caused by the same factor regularly producing reproducible error in one direction from the true value, which can be detected and corrected. Systematic error is the most commonly encountered laboratory testing error. In contrast, random error can be reduced but not completely eliminated. A random error is a result of an accidental cause that can be difficult to identify. This type of error causes imprecision of assay results.

CONTROL SPECIMENS

A QC program for the laboratory makes use of **control specimens**, which are or resemble a serum sample with a known concentration of the analyte being measured in the testing procedure. Most clinical laboratories use multiconstituent controls because these require less storage space, offer ease of inventory, and increase manufacturer services through peer laboratory comparisons. Lyophilized (freeze-dried) and liquid control materials offer good stability and reasonable expiration dating. Liquid controls may offer greater reproducibility between bottles because, unlike lyophilized controls, no pipetting error is added on reconstitution. Suppliers often offer to sequester a specific quantity (estimated usage) of control material to be sent to the laboratory at the customer's request. This ensures that the customer can continue to receive the same lot over time.

QC oversees each procedure for an established protocol to ensure the quality of the results. Usually, normal and abnormal control samples are analyzed at the same time patient specimens are analyzed. In-house and commercial QC approaches can be used by clinical laboratories. The use of in-house QC specimens is more economical and offers a matrix, which consists of the components of a specimen other than the analyte of interest and which more closely resembles the patient specimen. The "matrix effect" can have a considerable effect on the quality of results. In comparison, commercially prepared QC specimens are more stable and have assigned concentration values available at normal and abnormal values.

A control specimen must be carried through the entire test procedure and treated in exactly the same way as any unknown specimen; it must be affected by all the variables that affect the unknown specimen. Control specimens are used because repeated determinations on the same or different portions (or aliquots) of the same sample will not, as a rule, give identical values for any particular constituent. Many factors can produce variations in laboratory analyses. With a properly designed control system, it is possible to monitor testing variables.

According to CLIA regulations, a minimum of two control specimens (negative or normal and positive or increased) must be run in every 24-hour period when patient specimens are being run. Alternately, when automated analyzers are in use, the bi-level controls are run once every 8 hours of operation (or once per shift).[3]

The use of QC specimens is an indication of the overall reliability of the results reported by the laboratory, a part of the QA process. If the value of the QC specimen for a particular method is not within the predetermined acceptable range, it must be assumed that the values obtained for the unknown specimens are also incorrect, and the results are not reported. After the procedure has been reviewed for any indication of error, and after the error has been found and corrected, testing must be repeated until the control value falls within the acceptable range. In controlling the reliability of laboratory determinations, the objective is to reject results when there is evidence that more than the permitted amount of error has occurred. The clinical laboratory has several ways of controlling the reliability of its reported results.

Assaying control specimens and standards along with patient specimens serves the major functions of:

1. Detecting errors in equipment, reagents, or individual technique.
2. Confirming the stability and accuracy of testing compared with reference values.
3. Detecting an increase in the frequency of both high and low minimally acceptable values (**dispersion**).
4. Detecting any progressive **drift** of values to one side of the average value for at least 3 days (**trends**). Slow deterioration of reagents, controls, or light source can produce this type of systematic error.
5. Demonstrating an abrupt shift or change from the established average value for 3 days in a row (shift).

As mentioned earlier, QC consists of procedures used to detect errors that result from test system failure, adverse environmental conditions, variation in operator performance, and procedures to monitor the accuracy and **precision** of test performance over time.[10] Accrediting agencies require the monitoring and documenting of QA records. CLIA states, "The laboratory must establish and follow written QC procedures for monitoring and evaluating the quality of the analytical testing process of each method to assure the accuracy and reliability of patient test results and reports."[3] For tests of moderate complexity, CLIA states that laboratories must comply with the more stringent of the following requirements:

- Perform and document control procedures using at least two levels of control material each day of testing.
- Follow the manufacturer's instructions for QC.

QC activities include monitoring the performance of laboratory instruments, reagents, other testing products, and equipment. A written record of QC activities for each procedure or function should include details of deviation from the usual results, problems, or failures in functioning or in the analytical procedure and any corrective action taken in response to these problems.

Documentation of QC includes preventive maintenance records, temperature charts, and QC charts for specific assays. All products and reagents used in the analytical procedures must be carefully checked before actual use in testing patient samples. Use of QC specimens, PT, and standards depends on the specific requirements of the accrediting agency.

In addition to performing in-house QC, laboratories may be asked to assist other departments in the health care facility in their QC measures. This can include checking the effectiveness of autoclaves in surgery or in the laundry, or providing aseptic checks for the pharmacy, blood bank, or dialysis service.

QUALITY ASSESSMENT DESCRIPTORS

The ability of the reported laboratory results to substantiate a diagnosis, lead to a change in diagnosis, or provide follow-up on patient management is what makes laboratory assays useful to the clinician. The diagnostic usefulness of a test and its procedure is assessed by using statistical evaluations, such as descriptions of the accuracy and reliability of the test and its methodology. To describe the reliability of a particular procedure, two terms are often used: *accuracy* and *precision*. The reliability of a procedure depends on a combination of these two factors, although they are different and are not dependent on each other. **Variance** is another general term that describes the factors or fluctuations that affect the measurement of the substance in question. Statistical methods available can assess also the usefulness of a test result in terms of its **sensitivity**, **specificity**, and **predictive value (PV)**.

Other Quality Descriptors Are:

1. **Accuracy** describes how close a test result is to the true value. Reference samples and standards with known values are needed to check accuracy.
2. **Calibration** is the comparison of an instrument measure or reading to a known physical constant.
3. **Control** (noun) represents a specimen with a known value that is similar in composition, for example, to the patient's blood. The value of a control specimen is known. Control specimens are tested in exactly the same way as the patient specimen is tested, and control specimens are tested daily or in conjunction with the unknown (patient) specimen. Controls are the best measurements of precision and may represent normal or abnormal test values.
4. Precision describes how close the test results are to one another when repeated analyses of the same material are performed. Precision refers to the reproducibility of test results. It is important to make a distinction between precision and accuracy. The term accuracy implies freedom from error; the term precision implies freedom from variation.
5. **Standards** are highly purified substances of a known composition. A standard may differ from a control in its overall composition and in the way it is handled in the test. Standards are the best way to measure accuracy. Standards are used to establish reference points to construct graphs (such as the manual hemoglobin curve) or to calculate a test result.

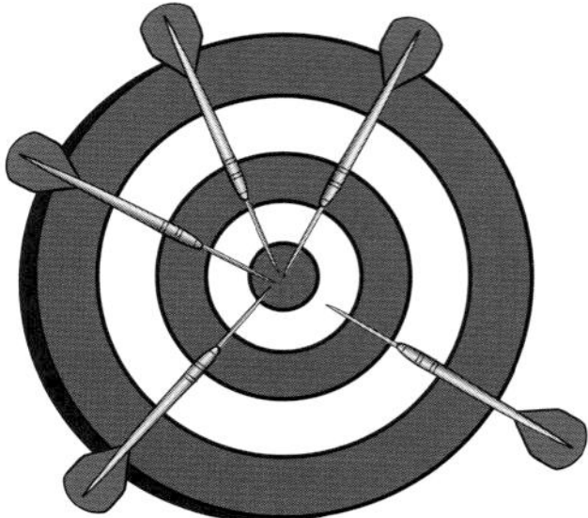

Fig. 3.2 Accuracy. (From Doucette LJ: *Basic mathematics for the health-related professions,* Philadelphia, 2000, Saunders.)

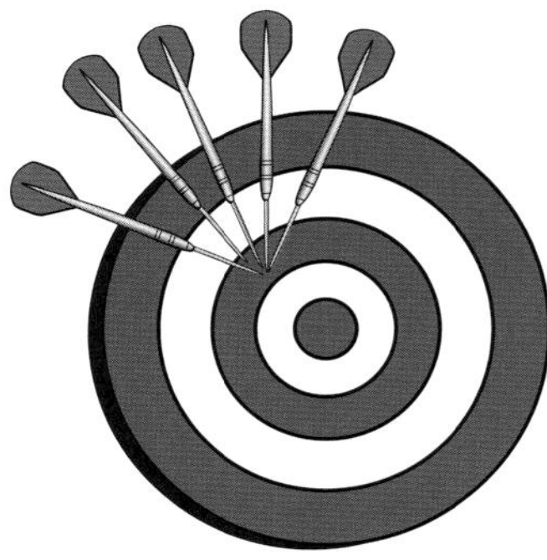

Fig. 3.3 Precision. (From Doucette LJ: *Basic mathematics for the health-related professions,* Philadelphia, 2000, Saunders.)

Accuracy Versus Precision

The accuracy of a procedure refers to the closeness of the result obtained to the true or actual value (Fig. 3.2), whereas precision refers to repeatability, or reproducibility, in obtaining the same value in subsequent tests on the same sample (Fig. 3.3). It is possible to have great precision, with all laboratory personnel who perform the same procedure arriving at the same answer, but without accuracy if the answer does not represent the actual value being tested. The precision of a test, or its reproducibility, may be expressed as standard deviation (SD) or as the derived coefficient of variation (CV). A procedure may be extremely accurate but so difficult to perform that laboratory personnel are unable to arrive at values close enough to be clinically meaningful.

In general terms, accuracy can be aided by the use of properly standardized procedures, statistically valid comparisons of new methods with established reference methods, the use of samples of known values (controls), and participation in PT programs.

Precision can be ensured by the proper inclusion of standards, reference samples, or control solutions; statistically valid replicate determinations of a single sample; and duplicate determinations of sufficient numbers of unknown samples. Day-to-day and between-run precision are measured by inclusion of control specimens.

Sensitivity and Specificity of a Test

Laboratory results that give medically useful information, including the specificity and sensitivity of the tests being ordered and reported, are important. Both specificity and sensitivity are desirable characteristics for a test, but in different clinical situations, one is generally preferred over the other.

BOX 3.9 Common Avoidable Causes of False-Positive and False-Negative Results

- Use of a test at an inappropriate time
- Use of an obsolete test
- Use of a test with inherently poor sensitivity or specificity
- Use of a test on a patient population with low or high prevalence of the disease under consideration
- Use of a test that lacks extensive clinical validation
- Use of a test on a patient population that differs from the intended or studied population

From Jackson B: The dangers of false-positive and false-negative test results: false-positive results as a function of pretest probability, *Clin Laboratory Med* 28:306, 2008.

BOX 3.10 Potential Consequences of False-Positive and False-Negative Results

- No effect in some cases
- Cascade of increasingly expensive or invasive follow-up testing
- Lengthened hospital stay
- Additional office visits
- Inappropriate therapy
- Psychological trauma caused by false belief of having a disease

From Jackson B: The dangers of false-positive and false-negative test results: false-positive results as a function of pretest probability, *Clin Laboratory Med* 28:306, 2008.

For assessing the sensitivity and specificity of a test, four categories are needed: tests positive, tests negative, disease present (positive), and disease absent (negative). True positives are those patients who have a positive test result and who also have the disease in question. True negatives represent those who have a negative test result and who do not have the disease. False positives are those patients who have a positive test result but do not have the disease. False negatives are those who have a negative test result but do have the disease.

Every assay in the clinical laboratory is subject to false-positive and false-negative results. Boxes 3.9 and 3.10 present common avoidable causes and potential consequences of false positives and false negatives.

Sensitivity

The sensitivity of a test is defined as the proportion of cases with a specific disease or condition that give a positive test result (i.e., the assay correctly predicts with a positive result), as follows:

$$\text{Sensitivity\%} = \frac{\text{True positives}}{\text{True positives} + \text{False negatives}} \times 100$$

Practically, sensitivity represents how much of a given substance is measured; the more sensitive the test, the smaller the amount of assayed substance that is measured.

Specificity

The specificity of a test is defined as the proportion of cases with absence of the specific disease or condition that gives a negative test result (i.e., the assay correctly excludes with a negative result), as follows:

$$\text{Specificity\%} = \frac{\text{True negatives}}{\text{False positives} + \text{True negatives}} \times 100$$

Practically, specificity represents what is being measured. A highly specific test measures only the assay substance in question; it does not measure interfering or similar substances.

Predictive Values

To assess the PV for a test, the sensitivity, specificity, and prevalence of the disease in the population being studied must be known. The prevalence of a disease is the proportion of a population that has the disease. This is in contrast to the incidence of a disease, which is the number of people found to have the disease within a defined period, such as a year, in a population of 100,000.

A positive PV for a test indicates the number of patients with an abnormal test result who have the disease, compared with all patients with an abnormal result, as follows:

$$\text{Positive predictive value} = \frac{\text{Number of patients with disease and with abnormal test results}}{\text{Total number of patients with abnormal test results}}$$

$$\text{Positive predictive value} = \frac{\text{True positives}}{\text{True positives} + \text{False positives}}$$

A negative PV for a test indicates the number of patients with a normal test result who do not have the disease, compared with all patients with a normal (negative) result, as follows:

$$\text{Negative predictive value} = \frac{\text{True negatives}}{\text{True negatives} + \text{False negatives}}$$

QUALITY CONTROL STATISTICS

Statistically, the reference range for a particular measurement in most cases is related to a normal bell-shaped curve[12–14] (Fig. 3.4). This Gaussian curve or Gaussian distribution has been shown to be correct for virtually all types of biological, chemical, and physical measurements. A statistically valid series of individuals who are thought to represent a normal healthy group are measured, and the average value is calculated. This mathematical average is defined as the mean (*x*, called the *x-bar*). The distribution of all values around the average for the particular group measured is described statistically by the SD.

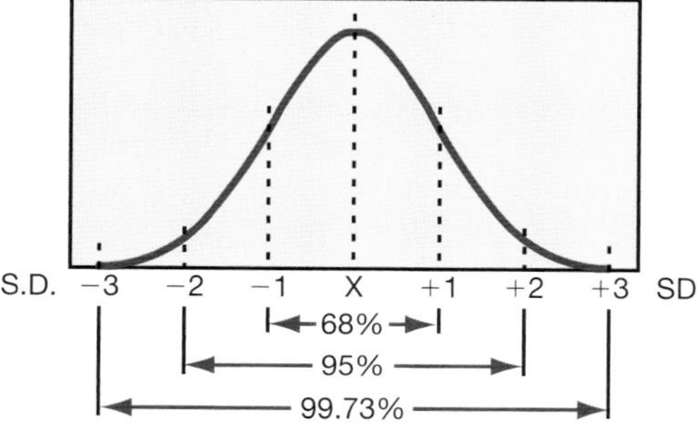

Fig. 3.4 Normal bell-shaped Gaussian curve. *SD,* Standard deviation.

Mean, Median, and Mode

Often used in laboratory measurements, the mean is the mathematical average calculated by taking the sum of the values and dividing by the number of values in the list. The Clinical and Laboratory Standards Institute (CLSI) describes several methods for estimating the mean and precision for a control level.[13] CLSI recommends that at a minimum, 20 data points from 20 or more separate testing runs be obtained to determine an estimate of mean and precision. If 20 runs cannot be completed, a minimum of seven runs (three replicates per run) may be used to set provisional ranges. A mean and SD can be calculated and used to set provisional ranges. The mean and limits derived from the abbreviated data collection should be replaced by a new mean and limits calculated when data from 20 separate runs become available.

The *median* is the middle value of a body of data. If all the variables are arranged in order of increasing magnitude in a body of data, the median is the variable that falls halfway between the highest and the lowest variables. The median equals the middle value. To find the median, the list of numbers must first be ranked according to magnitude, such as 2, 2, 3, 4, 5, 6, 7. The median number is the middle value in the list; in this example, of the seven numbers in the list, the median is 4.

The mode is the value most frequently occurring in a list of numbers. In the example of 2, 2, 3, 4, 5, 6, 7, the mode is 2.

Standard Deviation

Standard deviation (SD) is a measure of the spread, or variability, in a data set. Most scientific calculators contain a feature for calculating SD.

The SD is the square root of the variance of the values in any one observation or in a series of test results. In any normal population, 68% of the values will be clustered above and below the average and defined statistically as falling within the first SD (±1 SD). The second SD represents 95% of the values falling equally above and below the average (±2 SD), and 99.7% will be included within the third SD (±3 SD). (Again, variations occur equally above and below the average value [or mean] for any measurement.) Thus in determining reference values for a particular measurement, a statistically valid series of people are chosen and assumed to represent a healthy population. These people are then tested, and the results are averaged. The term *reference range* therefore means the range of values that includes 95% of the test results for a healthy reference population. This term replaces "normal values" or "normal range." The limits (or range) of normal are defined in terms of the SD from the average value.

In evaluating an individual's state of health, values outside the third SD value are considered clearly abnormal. When the distribution is Gaussian, the reference range closely approximates the mean ±2 SD. Values within the first (68%) and second (95%) SD limits are considered normal, whereas those between the second (95%) and third (99.7%) SD limits are questionable. The reference values are stated as a range of values. This stated range is in terms of SD units.

The SD index (SDI) is a measurement of bias or the proximity of your measured assay value to the target value. The SDI expresses bias as increments of the SD. The Bio-Rad Unity™ Interlaboratory Program uses the consensus group value as the target value.

$$\text{SDI} = \frac{\text{Laboratory Mean} - \text{Consensus Group Mean}}{\text{Consensus Group Standard Deviation}}$$

The SDI is a clinically important statistical tool to control the bias that is likely with a predefined probability (commonly $p < 0.05$) and to influence the clinical decision between health and disease if studied in the context of all the other uncertainty components involved, including biological variation. The target SDI is 0.0, which indicates that there is not any difference between the laboratory mean and the consensus group mean. Bias increases or decreases the percentage of patients outside the defined reference limit. A value of ≤ 1.25 is an acceptable value, but a maximum SDI value of ≥ 2.0 is an unacceptable value.

Confidence Intervals

When the reference range is expressed using 2 SD on either side of the mean, with 95% of the values falling above and below the mean, the term **confidence intervals (CI)** or *confidence limits* is used. This interval should be kept in mind when there are day-to-day shifts in values for a particular analytical procedure.

The 95% CI is used in part to account for certain unavoidable errors caused by sampling variability and imprecision of the methods themselves. For example, in a population study, the 95% CI can be interpreted in the following way. If the procedure or experiment is repeated many times and 95% CI is constructed each time for the parameter being studied, 95% of these intervals will actually include the true population parameter, and 5% will not.

The manufacturer's stated reference ranges give an indication of where a laboratory's mean and ranges may be established. Individual laboratories must establish an appropriate mean and QC limits based on the patient population. New lots of control material should be analyzed for each analyte in parallel with the control material in current use.

TOTAL ANALYTIC ERROR

The goal of laboratory testing is to provide accurate and useful information for health care providers to use in making patient diagnostic and treatment decisions. One system for managing analytical quality is based on the concept of *total analytic error (TAE),* a useful metric both to assess laboratory assay quality and to set quality goals for assays.

Previously, a quantitative approach for judging the acceptability of method performance was to evaluate precision (imprecision) and accuracy (inaccuracy, bias) as separate sources of errors and to evaluate their acceptability individually. Today it is recognized that the analytical quality of a test result depends on the overall or total effect of a method's precision and accuracy, the TAE concept. Using TAE, the acceptability of a method's performance is judged on the magnitude of the observed errors relative to a defined *allowable total error (ATE).* A direct estimation of TAE can be obtained by using a comparison with a reference method or the CLSI 2016 publication, *Evaluation of Total Analytical Error for Quantitative Medical Laboratory Measurement Procedures,* ed 2. A document that uses this approach.

The FDA currently recommends that manufacturers evaluate TAE as the combination of errors from all sources, both systematic and random, often expressed in terms of an interval that contains a specified proportion (e.g., 95%) of the observed differences between the working method and the comparative method. In comparison, clinical laboratories must make individual estimates of precision and bias to verify manufacturers' claims, with the exception of tests categorized by the FDA as waived. For nonwaived tests, which comprise the majority of testing in clinical laboratories, CLIA regulations also require that laboratories verify manufacturers' performance claims for precision and bias, implement a minimum SQC procedure with two levels of controls per day, and successfully perform in periodic PT surveys. For waived tests, the FDA requires manufacturers to define ATE and to estimate TAE, but the CLIA regulations do not require laboratories to verify or validate method performance or to perform QC, unless specified in the manufacturer's directions.

For clinical laboratories to meet CLIA regulations, the CMS recommends a minimum of 20 control samples to estimate precision and the same number of patient samples to verify a manufacturer's claim for bias. Consequently, it is more practical to make an initial estimate of TAE by combining results by replication and comparison of methods. Laboratories may also choose to make ongoing estimates by using long-term QC data and periodic estimates of bias from PT or external QA surveys.

Although the original recommendation for a total error criterion was ATE $\geq$ bias + 2 SD, today the recommendation is that ATE $\geq$ bias + 4 SD and, with the adoption of Six Sigma concepts, suggested ATE $\geq$ bias + 5 SD and ATE $\geq$ bias + 6 SD. The higher the sigma metric, the better the quality of the testing process.

Coefficient of Variation

The CV in percent (%CV) is equal to the SD divided by the mean. The CV normalizes the variability of a data set by calculating the SD as a percent of the mean (Box 3.11). The CV can be used to compare SDs of two samples. SDs cannot be compared directly without considering the mean. The %CV is helpful in comparing precision differences that exist among assays and assay methods.

BOX 3.11

Example of Coefficient of Variation Percent (%CV)

$$\%CV = \frac{SD \times 100}{x} = \frac{0.36 \times 100}{3.14} = 11.5\%$$

SD, Standard deviation = 0.36; Mean = 3.14.

After estimating the mean and total precision (SD) of the analytical measuring system, the next step is to set control limits as some multiple of the total precision around the mean. In many laboratories, the standard procedure is to set these control limits at ±2 SD; however, setting limits at ±2 SD can lead to certain problems. It is evident that ±2 SD ranges result in unnecessarily high false rejection rates. CLIA '88 does not explicitly recommend a method for determining when a system is "out of control," but this federal law does explain that laboratories must establish written procedures for monitoring and evaluating analytical testing processes (see Monitoring Quality Control).

With strict ±2 or ±3 SD limits, an out-of-control condition is marked by one QC value falling outside the limit of 2 or 3 SD. A ±2 SD limit offers a method that is sensitive to detecting a change but that also presents a problem for a laboratory: a high rate of false rejection.

Determination of Control Range

Once a control solution has been purchased unassayed, it is necessary for the laboratory to determine the acceptable control range for a particular analysis, and there are various ways of establishing it. One method to establish a control range is to assay an aliquot of the control serum with the regular batch of assays for 15 to 25 days. In testing the control sample, it is important to treat it exactly like an unknown specimen; it must not be treated any more or less carefully than the unknown specimen.

Repeated determinations on different aliquots of the same sample often will not give identical values for any particular constituent. It has been shown that if a sufficient number of repeated determinations are made, the values obtained will fall into a normal bell-shaped curve. When a statistically sufficient number of determinations have been run (the number is different for averaged duplicate determinations and single tests), the mathematical mean (x) or average value can be calculated. The acceptable limits or variation from the mean for the control solution are then calculated on the basis of the SD from the mean, using statistical formulas. Most laboratories use 2 SD above and below the mean as the allowable range of the control specimen, whereas others use this range as a warning limit. According to the normal bell-shaped curve, setting 2 SD as the allowable range for the control sample means that 95% of all determinations on that sample will fall within the allowable range and that 5% will be out of control. It may not be desirable to disallow this many batches, however, and the third SD may be chosen as the limit of control. Once the range of acceptable results has been established, one of the control specimens is included in each batch of determinations. If the control value is not within the limits established, the procedure must be repeated, and no patient results may be reported until the control value is acceptable.

It is important to remember that CLIA requires laboratories to establish written procedures for monitoring and evaluating analytical testing processes, including procedures for resolving an out-of-control situation. Control procedures may include the following:

1. Review the procedures used.
2. Search for recent events that could cause change, such as a new reagent kit or lot, component replacement, or environmental condition (such as temperature and humidity).
3. Prepare new control materials.
4. Follow the manufacturer's troubleshooting guide.
5. Contact manufacturers of instruments, reagent materials, and controls.

Sources of Variance or Error

In general, it is impossible to obtain exactly the same result each time a determination is performed on a particular specimen. This may be described as the variance, or error, of a procedure. These factors include limitations of the procedure itself and limitations related to the sampling mechanism used.

Sampling Factors

One of the major difficulties in guaranteeing reliable results involves the sampling procedure. Sources of variance that involve the sample include the time of day when the sample is obtained, the patient's position (lying down or seated), the patient's state of physical activity (in bed, ambulatory, or physically active), the interval since last eating (fasting or not), and the time interval and storage conditions between the collection of the specimen and its processing by the laboratory. The aging of the sample is another source of error.

Procedural Factors

Other sources of variance involve aging of chemicals or reagents, personal bias or limited experience of the person performing the determination, and laboratory bias because of variations in standards, reagents, environment, methods, or apparatus. There may also be experimental error resulting from changes in the method used for a particular determination, changes in instruments, or changes in personnel.

MONITORING QUALITY CONTROL

Levey-Jennings Charts

Most laboratories plot the daily control specimen values on a QC chart. Currently, many instruments automatically generate QC charts on each day of testing. Out-of-control specimen results are automatically flagged. If an instrument does not generate QC charts, the laboratory professional must perform this task (Student Procedure Worksheet 3.1).

Levey-Jennings (Shewhart) QC charts[15] have traditionally been used to identify unacceptable runs and then to evaluate the source and magnitude of the deviation to decide whether results are to be released to patient charts (Fig. 3.5). Software designed for laboratory information systems and personal computers is available to automate the plotting of control values. The software's complexity and capabilities (for multiple QC options) will vary among suppliers, but all types typically provide a graphical presentation of data using the traditional Levey-Jennings chart. The main purpose for control charting in the clinical laboratory is to aid in maintaining stability of the analytical measuring system (Fig. 3.6).

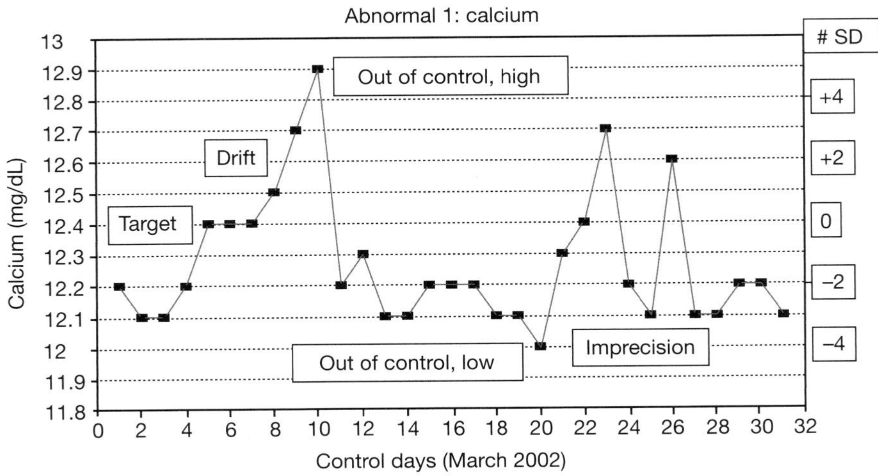

Fig. 3.5 **Levey-Jennings quality control chart.** (From Kaplan LA, Pesce AJ: *Clinical chemistry: theory, analysis, correlation,* ed 5, St Louis, 2010, Elsevier/Mosby.)

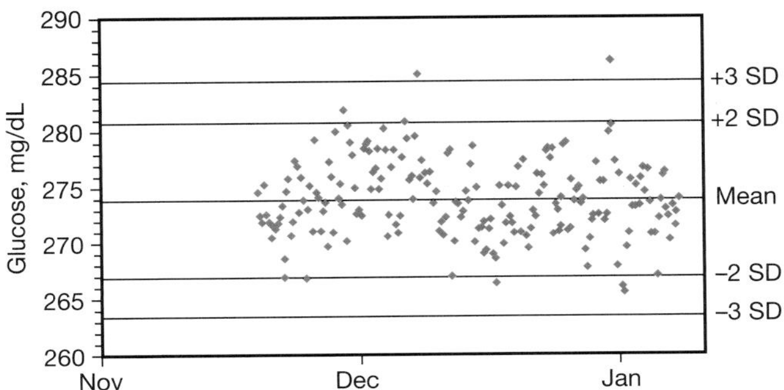

Fig. 3.6 **Levey-Jennings graph for glucose level.** (From McPherson RA, Pincus MR: *Henry's clinical diagnosis and management by laboratory methods,* ed 21, Philadelphia, 2006, Saunders.)

QC uses at least two different control samples for a specific analyte (such as total protein). Normal and abnormal control specimens are used. Each manufacturer's lot with an expiration date has an insert sheet with a mean value and ±2 SD of the assayed value.

The mean value for the determination in question is then indicated on the chart, in addition to the limits of acceptable error. Control limits are generally set at ±2 SD or ±3 SD on either side of the mean. The 2- and 3-SD values can be set as indicators with the 2-SD value as a warning limit and the 3-SD value as an action limit. Each day the control value is plotted on the chart, and any value falling "out of control" can easily be seen. The control chart serves as visual documentation of the information derived from using control specimens. A different control chart is plotted for each substance being determined. It is possible to observe trends and drift (see later discussion) leading toward trouble by plotting the control values daily. When procedural changes are made (such as the addition of new reagents, standards, or instruments), these are also noted on the control chart.

Appropriate Testing Methods

Another part of the QC program concerns the way new procedures are validated before they are included among the methods routinely used by the laboratory. Each laboratory must determine the reproducibility (or confidence limits) for each procedure used and establish acceptable limits of variation for control specimens. The QC program includes calculation of the mean (or average value) and SD and the generation of control charts for each procedure. To detect problems, each laboratory must have an assessment routine for all procedures performed on a daily, weekly, or monthly basis. When such problems are indicated, these must be corrected as soon as possible and before patient results are reported.

Shifts, Trends, and Dispersion

Regular visual inspection of the control chart is useful for observing a shift, trend, or increased dispersion of results in the assay results of the control specimen. A shift is defined as a sudden and sustained change in one direction in control sample values (Fig. 3.7). A trend or drift is a gradual change in the control sample results (Fig. 3.8). A systematic drift or trend is displayed when the control value direction moves progressively in one direction from the mean for at least 3 days. By comparison, dispersion is observed when random error or lack of precision increases. Each type of change is indicative of particular problems. A shift or abrupt change may be observed with the sudden malfunction of an instrument. A trend error suggests a progressive problem with the testing system or control sample, such as deterioration of reagents or control specimen. Dispersion may indicate instability problems. Fig. 3.9 presents the frequency of various error conditions.

Westgard Rules

Westgard rules are often formulated to analyze data in control charts based on statistical methods[16] (Figs. 3.10–3.12). These rules define specific performance limits for a particular assay and can be used to detect both random and systematic errors. If QC is out of control, testing must stop until the problem is identified and remediated. Patient results cannot be reported until control specimens meet performance requirements.

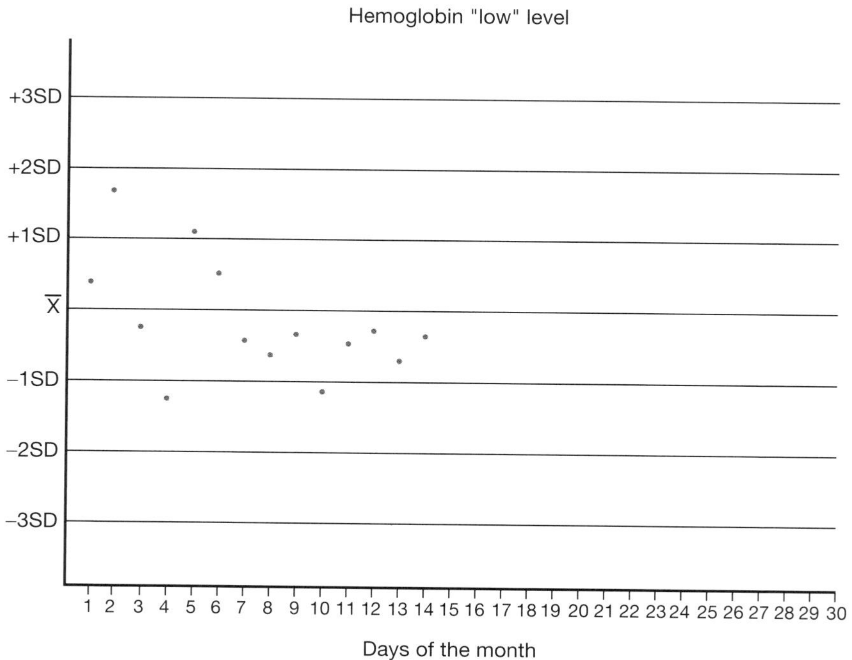

Fig. 3.7 Shift. (From Doucette LJ: *Basic mathematics for the health-related professions,* Philadelphia, 2000, Saunders.)

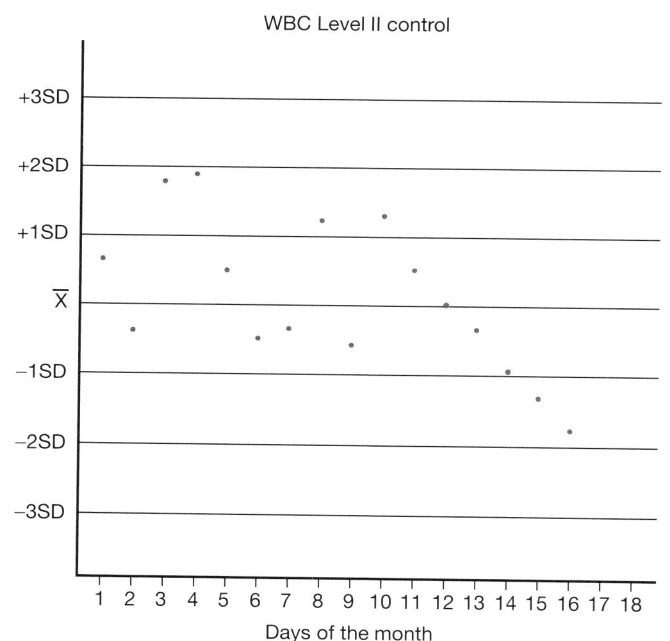

Fig. 3.8 Trend. (From Doucette LJ: *Basic mathematics for the health-related professions,* Philadelphia, 2000, Saunders.)

A Levey-Jennings chart can be interpreted using the Westgard rules, Two single rules are usually applied: 1_{2s}or 1_{3s}

The 1_{2s} in Box 3.12 refers to the control rule that is commonly used with a Levey-Jennings chart when the control limits are set as the mean ±2 SD. This rule is used as a warning to trigger careful inspection of the control data by the following the rejection rules. There is a false-alarm problem with a 1_{2s} rule, as is shown in the Levey-Jennings chart with 2s control limits; when $N = 2$, it is expected that 9% of good test runs will be falsely rejected.

The 1_{3s} refers to a control rule that is commonly used with a Levey-Jennings chart when the control limits are set as the mean + 3 SD and the mean − 3 SD. A Levey-Jennings chart with 3s control limits has a very low false rejection rate, only 1%. The false-alarm problem with $N = 3$ is even higher than with $N = 2$, at about 14%. False rejections waste a lot of time and materials in the laboratory, but the problem with the 1_{3s} control rule is that medically important errors may not be detected.

Westgard Multi-Rules

Multirule QC procedures are obviously more complicated than single-rule procedures, so that's a disadvantage, but they often provide better performance than the commonly used 1_{2s} and 1_{3s} single-rule QC procedures. The rationale for applying Westgard multirules includes reducing the false rejections made when only the 1_{2S} rule is applied and increasing error detection as compared with when only the 1_{3S} rule is applied for run rejection; the rules also detect and distinguish random and systematic errors; e.g., 1_{3S} and R_{4S} to detect random error and 2_{2S}, 4_{1S}, and 10_x to detect systematic error. The advantages of multirule QC procedures are that false rejections can be kept low while a high level of error detection is maintained simultaneously. This is done by selecting individual rules that have very low levels of false rejection, then building up the error detection by using these rules together. A multirule QC procedure uses two or more statistical tests (control rules) to evaluate the QC data, then rejects a run if any one of these statistical tests is positive.

The Westgard Multi-Rule Procedure is designed to improve the power of QC methods using ±3 SD limits to detect trends

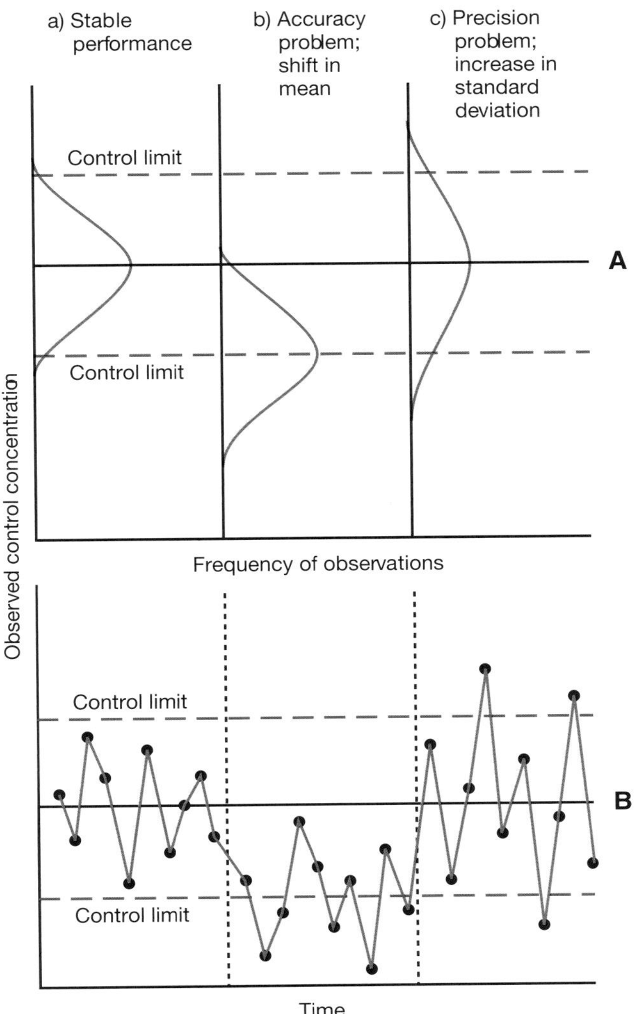

Fig. 3.9 Conceptual basic of control charts. (A) Frequency distributions of control observations for different error conditions. (B) Display of control values representing those distributions for which concentration is plotted versus time on a control chart. (From Burtis CA, Bruns DE: *Tietz fundamentals of clinical chemistry*, ed.7, St. Louis, 2015, Elsevier/Saunders.)

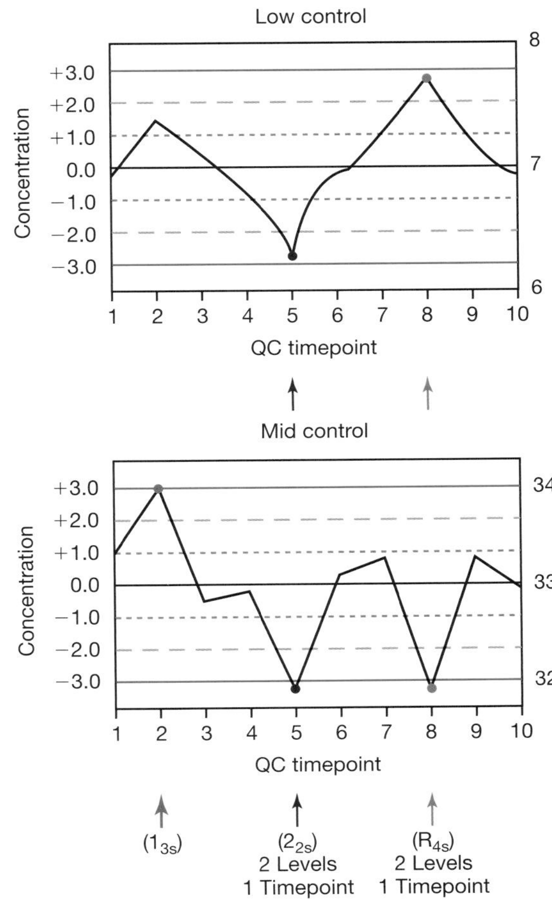

Fig. 3.10 Westgard Multi-Rule Procedure. Example for 1_{3S}, 2_{2S}, and R_{4S}. *QC,* Quality control.

or shifts. While maintaining a low false rejection rate, the Westgard procedure examines individual values and determines the status of the measuring system. Proper use of the Westgard Multi-Rule Procedure can substantially reduce the incidence of false rejection by as much as 88% compared with strict ±2 SD limits.

The N_x Multi Rule is violated if 7, 8, 9, 10, or 12 values from the assay of the same control are on the same side of the mean. If the rule is violated within a control level, it indicates systemic bias in a single area of the method curve. If the rule is violated across control levels, it indicates systematic error over a wide range of concentrations of the analyte being assayed.

Different Westgard rule configurations are possible for the same set of rules. When selecting a set of rules, the key is to understand how they perform statistically. Many software packages allow a laboratory to tailor a multirule set to each type of analyte assayed. This automated monitoring of QC makes the Westgard Multi-Rule Procedure much easier to apply correctly. Automated instruments can be interfaced with Bio-Rad Unity Real Time Software. Reports generated by the software have a detailed statistical analysis.

OTHER QC RULES

The four QC rules in addition to the Westgard rules are as follows:

1. Moving average rule uses patient test results to judge the performance of a laboratory testing process and to identify changes in the stability of an assay.
2. Risk-based QC relies on patient risk–based assessment or on a risk-based approach to monitoring laboratory testing. Risk can be defined as a measure of the severity of the effect of a potential error, multiplied by the probability that the error will occur, and by the ability to detect the error if it should occur. Risk management consists of a sequential process of:
   a. Risk identification: identifying potential errors
   b. Risk assessment: evaluating errors to determine the effect on patient test results
   c. Risk mitigation: controlling errors to make residual risk manageable

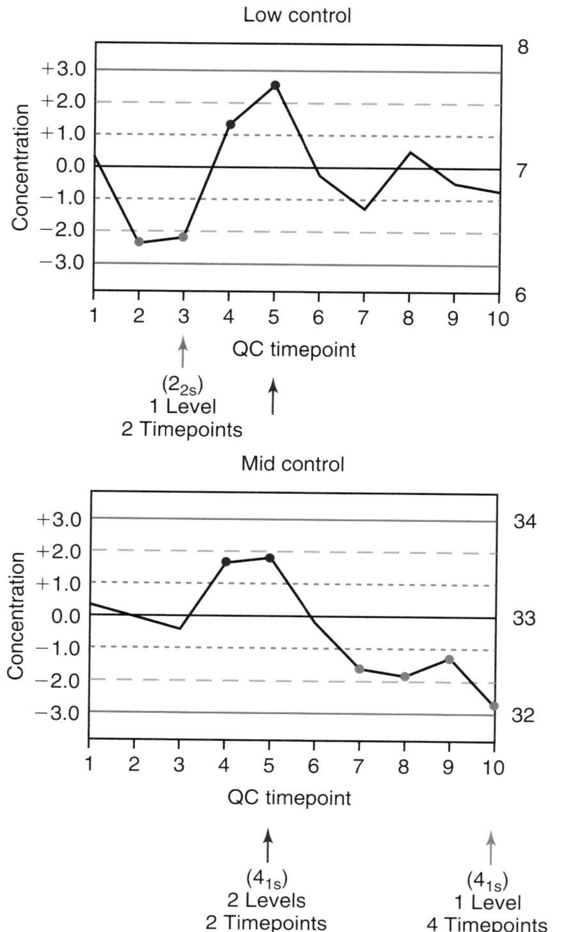

Fig. 3.11 **Westgard Multi-Rule Procedure.** Example for 2_{2S}, 4_{1S} (across two levels), and 4_{1S} (across one level). *QC*, Quality control.

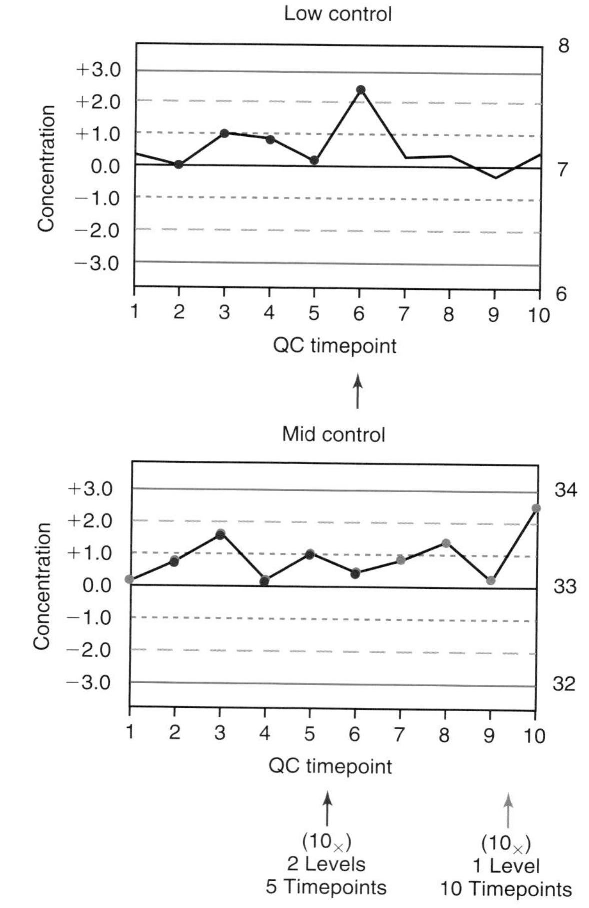

Fig. 3.12 **Westgard Multi-Rule Procedure.** Examples for $10\times$ across two levels and $10\times$ for one level. *QC*, Quality control.

3. Six Sigma is a process that uses medical cutoffs as tolerance limits. This method expects 99.99966% of all opportunities to be free of defects.
4. Individualized QC Plan (IQCP) is CLIA's QC procedure for an alternate QC option allowed by 42CFR493.1250. IQCP permits the laboratory to customize its QC plan according to test method and use, environment, and personnel competency while providing for equivalent quality testing. This approach includes risk assessment, a QC plan, and QA.

Nonanalytical Factors in Quality Assessment

To guarantee the highest-quality laboratory results and to comply with CLIA regulations, a variety of preanalytical and postanalytical factors must be considered. Nonanalytical factors that support quality testing include the following:

1. Qualified personnel
2. Established laboratory policies
3. Laboratory procedure manual
4. Test requisitioning
5. Patient identification, specimen procurement, and labeling
6. Proper procedures for specimen collection and storage
7. Specimen transportation and processing
8. Preventive maintenance of equipment
9. Appropriate methodology

1. Qualified Personnel

The competence of personnel is an important determinant of the quality of the laboratory result.[17] Only properly certified personnel can perform nonwaived assays. CLIA '88 requirements for laboratory personnel in regard to levels of education and experience or training must be followed for laboratories doing moderately complex or highly complex testing.

In addition to the actual performance of analytical procedures, competent laboratory personnel must be able to perform QC activities, maintain instruments, and keep accurate and systematic records of reagents and control specimens, equipment maintenance, and patient and analytical data. For new laboratory personnel, a thorough orientation to the laboratory procedures and policies is vital.

Periodic opportunities for personal upgrading of technical skills and for obtaining new, relevant information should be made available to all persons working in the laboratory. This can be accomplished by offering in-service training classes and opportunities to attend continuing education courses, and by encouraging independent study habits by means of scientific journals and audiovisual materials.

BOX 3.12 Westgard Rules for Analysis of Quality Control Charts

Warning Rule

Westgard 1_{2S}

This rule is violated when one of two control results falls outside of ±2 SD

- Alerts technologist to possible problem with control data
- Not a cause for rejecting a run of specimens. False rejections lead to unnecessary repeat testing of patient specimens, waste of time and materials, and unnecessary delay of patient results.
- Must then evaluate the 1_{3S} rule

Westgard 1_{3S}

This rule is violated when any QC result falls outside of ±3 SD

- Identifies random error or possibly the beginning of a large systematic error
- May be statistically significant but may not be biologically or medically relevant

Westgard 2_{2S}

This rule is violated when two consecutive control values for the same level fall outside of ±2 SD in the same direction, or when both control levels in the same test batch exceed ±2 SD.

- Detects systematic error only
- Patient results cannot be reported
- Requires immediate corrective action

Note: 1_{3s} refers to a control rule that is commonly used with a Levey-Jennings chart when the control limits are set as the mean plus 3s and the mean minus 3s.

Westgard 3_{1S} and 4_{1S} Rules

These rules are violated when 3 or 4 consecutive control results are greater than 1 SD and on the same side of the mean.

- Within a control level, indicates systematic bias in a single area of the method curve.
- Across control levels, indicates systematic error over a broader range of concentrations.

Westgard 4_{1S} Rule

This rule is broken when four consecutive QC results for one level of control are outside ±1 SD, or when both levels of control have consecutive results that are outside of ±1 SD

- Requires control data from previous assay runs

Westgard R_{4S} Rule

This rule is broken when one control measurement exceeds the +2 SD and the other exceeds the −2 SD control limit. This represents at least a 4 SD difference between control values within a single run. The 4-SD deviation consists of a +2 SD deviation, and the other consists of a −2 SD deviation.

- Identifies random error
- Applied only within a current assay batch run, not within the same run
- Results of assay run are rejected

Westgard 10x Rule

This rule is broken when 10 consecutive QC results for one level of assay control are on one side of the mean, or both levels of control have five consecutive results that are on the same side of the mean.

- Results of assay run are rejected
- Requires control data from previous assay runs

Westgard N_x Rules

These rules are violated when 7, 8, 9, 10, or 12 control results are on the same side of the mean.

- Within a control level, indication of systematic bias in a single area of the method curve
- Across control levels, indication of systematic error over a broader range of concentrations

QC, quality control; *SD*, Standard deviation.
Goldsmith B: How to Implement Quality Control, Adding Value to Patient Care Using Quality Control, AACC Global Laboratory Quality Initiative, San Diego, CA, July 30, 2017.

Personnel performance should be monitored with periodic evaluations and reports. QA demands that a supervisor monitor the results of daily work and that all analytical reports produced during a particular shift be evaluated for errors and omissions.

2. Established Laboratory Policies

Laboratory policies should be included in a laboratory reference manual available to all hospital personnel. Each laboratory must have an up-to-date safety manual. This manual contains a comprehensive listing of approved policies, acceptable practices, and precautions, including standard blood and body fluid precautions. Specific regulations that conform to current state and general requirements, such as Occupational Safety and Health Administration regulations, must be included in the manual. Other sources of mandatory and voluntary standards include TJC, CAP, and the CDC.

3. Laboratory Procedure Manual

A complete laboratory procedure manual for all analytical procedures performed within the laboratory must be provided. The manual must be reviewed regularly, in some cases annually, by the supervisory staff and updated as needed.

The CLSI[18] recommends that the organization of the procedures in these manuals follow a specific pattern. Each assay done in the laboratory must be included in the manual. The minimal components are as follows:

- Title of the assay
- Principle of the procedure and statement of clinical applications
- Protocol for specimen collection and storage
- QC information
- Reagents, supplies, and equipment
- Procedural protocol
- Reference ranges
- Technical sources of error
- Limitations of the procedure
- Proper procedures for specimen collection and storage

4. Test Requisitioning

A laboratory test can be requested by a primary care provider or, in some states, by the patient. The request, either hard copy or electronic, must include the patient identification data, time and date of specimen collection, source of the specimen, and analyses to be performed. The information on the accompanying specimen container must match exactly the patient identification on the test request. The information needed by the physician to assist in ordering tests must be included in a database or handbook.

5. Patient Identification, Specimen Procurement, and Labeling

Patients must be carefully identified. For outpatients, identification may be validated with two forms of identification. Once obtained from the patient, the clinical specimens must be properly labeled or identified using established information requirements. Computer-generated labels help ensure that proper patient identification is noted on each specimen container sent to the laboratory. An important rule to remember is that the analytical result can only be as good as the specimen received (see Specimen Collection, Chapter 4).

6. Proper Procedures for Specimen Collection and Storage

Maintaining an electronic database or handbook of specimen requirement information is one of the first steps in establishing a QA program for the clinical laboratory. Current information about obtaining appropriate specimens, special collection requirements for various types of tests, ordering tests correctly, and transporting and processing specimens appropriately should be included in the database.

7. Specimen Transportation and Processing

Correct storage of specimens is critical to obtaining accurate results.

Specimens must be efficiently transported to the laboratory. Some assays require special handling conditions, such as placing the specimen on ice immediately after collection. Some analyses require that specimens be refrigerated or frozen immediately or kept out of direct light.

Specimens should be tested promptly, preferably within 2 hours of collection, to produce accurate results.

Documenting specimen arrival times in the laboratory, along with other specific test request data, is an important aspect of the QA process. It is important that the specimen status can be determined at any time—that is, where in the laboratory processing system a given specimen can be found.

8. Preventive Maintenance of Equipment

Monitoring the temperatures of heat blocks and refrigerators is important to the quality of test performance. Microscopes, centrifuges, and other pieces of equipment must be cleaned regularly and checked for accuracy. A preventive maintenance schedule should be followed for all automated equipment. Failure to monitor equipment regularly can produce inaccurate test results and lead to expensive repairs.

Manufacturers will recommend a calibration frequency determined by measurement system stability and will communicate in product inserts the specific criteria for mandatory recalibration of instrument systems. These may include the following:

- Reagent lot change
- Major component replacement
- Instrument maintenance
- New software installation

Clinical laboratories must follow the requirements set by CLIA or the manufacturer for instrument calibration frequency, whichever is more stringent. CLIA requires that laboratories recalibrate an analytical method at least every 6 months.

9. Appropriate Methodology

When a new method is introduced, it is important to check the procedure for accuracy and variability. Replicate analyses using control specimens are recommended to check for accuracy and to eliminate factors such as day-to-day variability, reagent variability, and differences between technologists.

TESTING OUTCOMES

It is important to realize that reference values will vary with innumerable factors, but especially between laboratories and between geographic locations. Each laboratory must provide the physician with information on the range of reference values for that particular laboratory. The values will be related to an overall reference range, but the values may be more refined or narrow and may be skewed in the particular situation in question.

Before physicians can determine whether a patient has a disease, they must know what is acceptable for a representative population of similar patients (such as being the same age, same gender, or same ethnicity) and the analytical method used for an assay. To complicate matters, an individual may show daily, circadian, or physiologic variations.

Biometrics, the science of statistics applied to biological observations, is a rapidly expanding field that attempts to describe these variations. The selection of a group on which to base "reference groups" is another problem confronting the individual laboratory.

Traditionally, reference ranges have been defined by testing such groups as blood donors, persons who are working and "feeling healthy," medical students, student nurses, and medical technologists.[13] Many established reference ranges reported in the medical literature have questionable validity because of factors such as poor sampling techniques, questionable selection of the normal group, and questionable use of clinical methods. In developing reference values previously referred to as *normal values,* the proper statistical tools of sampling, selecting the comparison group, and analyzing data must be used.

CASE STUDY

CASE STUDY 3.1

Macy works within the Chemistry department in her first job out of a Medical Laboratory Science program. Today has been a typically busy day for her as she loads samples into instruments and checks results. Macy loaded two levels of quality control (QC) materials prior to a large run of patients and on checking the results for the QC, she noticed that one of the levels was outside the range that had been established.

1. What is Macy's next step?
   a. Testing should be suspended until the issue is resolved.
   b. It depends on how far "out" the QC level is.
   c. There are a number of stat tests in the run, and she should report them "out."
   d. She should repeat running the QC level that is out until it falls within range.

As part of Macy's investigation into the QC issue, she notices that a scheduled preventive maintenance (PM) activity was not performed yesterday. Macy completes the PM and then recalibrates the test that is having QC issues. After recalibration, the QC level is now in range. Macy documents the missed PM and her resolution within the binder kept with that machine.

2. Are Macy's actions considered part of a quantitative QC program?
   a. No; a quantitative QC program involves the use of only two levels of control material for each day of testing.
   b. Yes; a quantitative QC program encompasses both equipment and reagents.
   c. No; the most important aspect of a quantitative QC program is the assurance of reliability.
   d. Yes; calibration is the most important part of a quantitative QC program.

Critical Thinking Group Discussion Questions

1. What is the difference between a 1_{2s} and a 1_{3s}?
2. What is the significance of a 1_{2s} versus a 1_{3s} value?

Note: Answers to narrative questions are posted on the EVOLVE instructor website.

REFERENCES

1. Hallworth M: *The (True) Value of Laboratory Medicine,* The Pathologist, Issue 1015, 2015. www.thepathologist.com.
2. Six Sigma: http://www.isixsigma.com/sixsigma/six_sigma.asp. Accessed October 2005.
3. U.S. Department of Health and Human Services: Medicare, Medicaid, and CLIA programs: regulations implementing the Clinical Laboratory Improvement Amendments of 1988 (CLIA), *Final rule, Fed Regist* 57(7002), 1992.
4. U.S. Department of Health and Human Services, Centers for Medicare and Medicaid Services: Laboratory requirements relating to quality systems and certain personnel qualifications. Final Rule, 42CFR Part 405 et al. (16:3640), Fed Regist, 2003.
5. Joint Commission on Accreditation of Healthcare Organizations: Periodic performance review (PPR) for laboratories. www.jcaho.org (Accessed October 2005).
6. College of American Pathologists: Checklists, revised 10/06/2005. www.cap.org (Accessed October 2005).
7. Ford A: *Labs on the brink of ISO 15189 approval,* November 2008, CAP News.
8. Smith TJ: Tracking the trends, *Advance for the Laboratory* 33–40:344–346, 2006.
9. Astion M: Latent errors in lab services, *Clin Lab News* 35:15–17, 2009.
10. Becton Dickinson: Accuracy from bedside to lab, Franklin Lakes, NJ, 2003, BD Inc.
11. Nutting PA, Main DS, Fischer PM, et al: Problems in laboratory testing in primary care, *JAMA* 275(8):635–639, 1996.
12. Clinical and Laboratory Standards Institute: *Statistical Quality Control for Quantitative Measurement Procedures: Principles and Definitions; Approved Guideline,* ed. 4, 2016. C24-A3.
13. Clinical and Laboratory Standards Institute: *How to define and determine reference intervals in the clinical laboratory: approved guideline,* ed 2, 2000. Wayne, Pa, C28-A2.
14. Clinical and Laboratory Standards Institute: *Evaluation of precision performance for clinical chemistry devices: approved guideline,* ed 2, 2004. Wayne, Pa, EP5-A2.
15. Levey S, Jennings ER: The use of control charts in the clinical laboratory, *Am J Clin Pathol* 20:1059, 1950.
16. Westgard JO, Barry PL, Hunt MR, et al: A multi-rule Shewhart chart for quality control in clinical chemistry, *Clin Chem* 27:493, 1981.
17. Clinical and Laboratory Standards Institute: *Training and competence assessment: approved guideline,* ed 4, 2016. Wayne, Pa, QMS 03.
18. Clinical and Laboratory Standards Institute: *Quality Management System: Development and Management of Laboratory Documents,* ed 6, 2013. Wayne, Pa, QMS02.

BIBLIOGRAPHY

American Society of Clinical Pathology (ASCP): Continuing education module: proficiency testing as a quality improvement tool. www.ascp.org (Accessed December 2012).

American Society of Clinical Pathology (ASCP): Continuing education module: unannounced surveys—new requirements. www.ascp.org (Accessed December 2012).

ASQ hospitals see benefits of Lean and Six Sigma: ASQ releases benchmark study results, March 17, 2009. www.asq.org (Accessed 19.08.09).

Astion M: Reducing errors in manual processes, *CL Lab News* 12, January 2014.

Astion ML, Shojania KG, Hamill TR, et al: Classifying laboratory incident reports to identify problems that jeopardize safety, *Am J Clin Pathol* 120:18, 2003.

Bostic G, Thompson R, Atanasoski S, et al: Quality Improvement in the Coagulation Laboratory: Reducing the Number of Insufficient Blood Draw Specimens for Coagulation Testing, *Lab Medicine* 46(4):347–355, 2015.

Boone DJ: A history of the QC gap in the clinical laboratory, *Lab Med* 36(10):611, 2005.

Campbell JB, Campbell JM: *Laboratory mathematics: medical and biological applications,* ed 5, St Louis, 1997, Mosby.

Chawla R, Goswami B, Tayal D, Mallika V: Identification of the types of preanalytical errors in the clinical chemistry laboratory: 1-year study at G.B. Pant Hospital, *Lab Med* 41(2):89–92, 2010.

Chittiprol S, Bornhorst J, Kiechle F: Top Laboratory deficiencies, *Cl Lab News* 44(6):32–42, 2018.

Clinical and Laboratory Standards Institute: Using Proficiency Testing and Alternative Assessment to Improve Medical Laboratory Quality, *Approved Guideline,* ed. 3, 2016. QMS24-ED3.

Clinical and Laboratory Standards Institute: *Use of Delta Checks in the Medical Laboratory,* ed.1, 2016. EP33.

Clinical and Laboratory Standards Institute: *Evaluation of Total Analytical Error for Quantitative Medical Laboratory Measurement Procedures,* ed.2, 2016. EP21.

COLA: Troubleshooting recurring problems with hemolyzed blood specimens, *MLO Med Lab Obs* 49(2):3, 2017.

Daugherty K: Pre-analytical errors: working with manufacturers to help improve quality, *MLO Med Lab Obs* 46(2):18–24, 2014.

Dawson J: What's Your Cost of Poor Quality, AACC 2017 Annual Meeting Bio-Rad Laboratories Industry Workshop, www.QCNet.com.

Elbireer A, Gable AR, Jackson JB: Cost of quality at a clinical laboratory in a resource-limited country, *Lab Med* 41(7):429–433, 2010.

Elston DM: Opportunities to improve quality in laboratory medicine, *Clin Lab Med* 28(2):173–177, 2008.

Goldsmith B: How to Implement Quality Control. In *Adding Value to Patient Care Using Quality Control*, San Diego, CA, July 30, 2017, AACC Global Lab Quality Initiative.

Hamilton LH: Lean, Lean Six Sigman, and the clinical laboratory, *MLO Med Lab Obs* 52(2):42–43, 2018.

Hilborne LH: Choosing tests wisely turns U.S. medicine inside out, *Crit Values* 6(2):19–21, 2013.

Hill E: Using Sigma metrics and measurement Uncertainty in QC, *MLO Med Lab Obs* 49(8):70–72, 2017.

Hill E: The role of Six Sigma in a modern quality management strategy, *Med Lab Obs* 50(8):46–47, 2018.

Kampfrath T: Delta Checks Checkup: Optimizing cutoffs with lab-specific inputs, *Cl Lab News* 43(8):4–5, 2017.

Kantartjis M, et al: Increased Patient Satisfaction and a Reduction in Pre-Anlytical Errors Following Implementation of an Electronic Specimen Collection Module in Outpatient Phlebotomy, *Lab Med* 48(3):277–281, 2017.

Kurec A: Proper patient preparation, specimen collection, and sample handling are critical to quality care, *MLO Med Lab Obs* 49(1):22–24, 2017.

Lasky FD: Technology variations: strategies for assuring quality results, *Lab Med* 36(10):617, 2005.

Lesher S: Incorporating Big Data into daily laboratory QC, *MLO Med Lab Obs* 49(8):76–78, 2017.

Lippi G, Mattiuzzi C, Plebani M: Event reporting in laboratory medicine, *MLO Med Lab Obs* 41(3):23, 2009.

Malone B: The race to reduce readmissions, *CL Lab News* 39(4):2–4, 2013.

Mathias PC, Turner EH, Scroggins SM: Applying Ancestry and Sex Computation as a Quality Control Tool in Targeted Next-Generation Sequencing, *Am J Clin Pathol* 145(3):308–315, 2016.

Meng Q: Quality Control Rules/Westgard Rules. In *Adding Value to Patient Care Using Quality Control*, San Diego, CA, July 30, 2017, AACC Global Lab Quality Initiative.

Orton S: Proficiency testing today, *MLO Med Lab Obs* 49(3):24–26, 2017.

Parvin CA, Jones JB: QC design: it's easier than you think, *MLO Med Lab Obs* 45(12):18–22, 2013.

Romero A, et al: Integrating Research Techniques to Improve Quality and Safety in the Preanalytical Phase, *Lab Med* 49(2):179–189, 2018.

Rothenberg IZ: Achieving a culture of safety with competency and commitment, *MLO Med Lab Obs* 49(10): 26,28, 2017.

Algeciras-Schimnich A: What is Quality Control? Why is it important?. In *Adding Value to Patient Care Using Quality Control*, San Diego, CA, July 30, 2017, AACC Global Lab Quality Initiative.

Scott K: Taking Quality to a Higher Level, *Cl Lab News* 44(4):20–24, 2018.

Shires GW: Allowable measurement error associated with quality management plans, *MLO Med Lab Obs* 45(2):20–22, 2013.

Strathmann F: Defining, Implementing, and Monitoring an Effective QC Strategy, AACC 2017 Annual Meeting Bio-Rad Laboratories Industry Workshop, www.QCNet.com.

Westgard JO, Westgard SA: Equivalent quality testing versus equivalent QC procedures, *Lab Med* 36(10):626, 2005.

Wians FH: Clinical laboratory tests: which, why, and what do the results mean? *Lab Med* 40(2):105, 2009.

Yost J, Mattingly P: CLIA and equivalent quality control: options for the future, *Lab Med* 36(10):614, 2005.

Yundt-Pacheco J, Parvin CA: The impact of QC frequency on patient results, *MLO Med Lab Obs* 40(9):24–26, 2008.

Zhang V: Best Practices in Quality Control. In *Adding Value to Patient Care Using Quality Control*, San Diego, CA, July 30, 2017, AACC Global Lab Quality Initiative.

REVIEW QUESTIONS (ANSWERS IN APPENDIX A)

The Value of Quality

1. Quality management consists of:
   - **a.** Quality assurance
   - **b.** Quality control
   - **c.** Peer-Reviewed Proficiency Testing
   - **d.** Both a and b

Patient Specimens

2. In addition to blood and urine, the major types of body fluid specimens that can be tested by the clinical laboratory include:
   - **a.** Synovial fluid, cerebrospinal fluid
   - **b.** Peritoneal fluid, pericardial fluid
   - **c.** Sweat, seminal fluid
   - **d.** a, b or c

Clinical Laboratory Improvement Amendments

3. The CLIA'88 Amendment regulations established minimum requirements with general QC systems for:
   - **a.** All nonwaived testing
   - **b.** Some nonwaived testing
   - **c.** All waived testing
   - **d.** Only waived testing

Voluntary Accrediting Organizations

4. The abbreviation TJC stands for an organization that:
   - **a.** Accredits hospitals and inspects clinical laboratories
   - **b.** Accredits physician laboratories
   - **c.** Determines waived and nonwaived categories of assays
   - **d.** Accredits only hospital laboratories

5. The abbreviation CAP stands for an organization that:
   a. Accredits hospitals and inspects clinical laboratories
   b. Accredits physician laboratories
   c. Determines waived and nonwaived categories of assays
   d. Accredits only hospital laboratories
6. The abbreviation COLA stands for an organization that:
   a. Accredits hospitals and inspects clinical laboratories
   b. Accredits physician laboratories
   c. Determines waived and nonwaived categories of assays
   d. Accredits only hospital laboratories
7. The abbreviation CLIA stands for an organization that:
   a. Accredits hospitals and inspects clinical laboratories
   b. Accredits physician laboratories
   c. Determines minimum QC requirements for nonwaived assays
   d. Accredits only hospital laboratories

ISO 15189 Standards in Clinical Laboratories

8. ISO 15189 is intended for use in:
   a. Biological research laboratories
   b. Medical laboratories
   c. Pharmaceutical research laboratories
   d. In vitro fertilization laboratories

Lean and Six Sigma

9. Six Sigma management focuses on:
   a. Reduction of waste
   b. Reduction of variability in laboratory results
   c. Reduction of nonvalue added activities
   d. Identifying steps in a procedure that are error prone

Quality Assessment

10. CLIA'88 requires
    a. Posting of quality control data in the laboratory
    b. Participation in proficiency testing
    c. Recertification of laboratory personnel
    d. Continuing education for laboratory supervisors

Quality—Error Analysis

11. If the incorrect anticoagulant is in a blood collection tube, it is:
    a. An active error
    b. A latent error
    c. A safety violation
    d. Not an obvious problem

Quality Assessment—Phases of Testing

12. An example of a preanalytical (preexamination) error is:
    a. Malfunction of a microprocessor that affects accuracy in testing
    b. Incorrect identification of a patient
    c. Transposition of a numeric critical value in transmitting a report
    d. Verbally reporting a laboratory result over the telephone
13. An example of an analytical (examination) error is:
    a. Malfunction of a microprocessor that affects accuracy in testing
    b. Incorrect patient identification
    c. Transposition of a numeric critical value in transmitting a report
    d. Use of the wrong anticoagulant in the patient sample tube
14. An example of a postanalytical (postexamination) error is:
    a. Malfunction of a microprocessor that affects accuracy in testing
    b. Incorrect patient identification
    c. Transposition of a numeric critical value in transmitting a report
    d. Use of the wrong anticoagulant in the patient sample tube
15. Blood from the wrong patient is an example of a/an:
    a. Preanalytical (preexamination) error
    b. Analytical (examination) error
    c. Postanalytical (postexamination) error
    d. Either a or b
16. Specimen collected in the wrong tube is an example of a/an:
    a. Preanalytical (preexamination) error
    b. Analytical (examination) error
    c. Postanalytical (postexamination) error
    d. Either a or b
17. Quality control outside of acceptable limits is an example of a/an:
    a. Preanalytical (preexamination) error
    b. Analytical (examination) error
    c. Postanalytical (postexamination) error
    d. Either a or c

Proficiency Testing

18. Proficiency testing is required by CLIA for:
    a. Nonwaived tests
    b. Many waived tests
    c. FDA cleared and approved moderate-complexity or high-complexity assays
    d. Both a and c

Alternate Assessment

19. If proficiency testing (PT) is not available fro a specific analyte, one alternate assessment method is:
    a. Send to a reference laboratory
    b. Internal split-sample analysis
    c. Calculate 2 S.D.s of a repeat test
    d. No alternate assessment needs to be conducted.

Accuracy in Reporting Results and Documentation

20. The Delta check cutoff value may be presented as:
    a. Absolute change
    b. Percent change
    c. Rate of change
    d. Any of the above

Quality Control

21. Quality control evaluates the ____________ phase of testing.
   a. Preanalytical
   b. Analytical
   c. Postanalytical
   d. Overall management
22. Systematic error:
   a. Is the most commonly encountered laboratory testing error.
   b. Can be reduced but cannot be completely eliminated.
   c. Is caused by an accidental cause that can be difficult to identify.
   d. Causes imprecision of assay results.

Control Specimens

23. The “matrix “ of a specimen
   a. Has the components of a specimen other than the analyte of interest
   b. More closely resembles the patient specimen
   c. Is the analyte to be assayed
   d. Both a and b

Quality Assessment Descriptors

24. Accuracy is defined as:
   a. How close results are to one another
   b. How close a test result is to the true value
   c. Specimen that is similar to patient’s blood; known concentration of constituent
   d. Comparison of an instrument measure or reading to a known physical constant
25. Calibration is defined as:
   a. How close results are to one another
   b. How close a test result is to the true value
   c. Specimen that is similar to patient’s blood; known concentration of constituent
   d. Comparison of an instrument measure or reading to a known physical constant
26. A control is defined as:
   a. How close a repeated assay test result is to the true value
   b. Specimen that is similar to patient’s blood; known concentration of constituent
   c. Comparison of an instrument measure or reading to a known physical constant
   d. Measurement of a highly purified substance of known composition
27. Precision is defined as:
   a. How close results are to one another
   b. How close a test result is to the true value
   c. Comparison of an instrument measure or reading to a known physical constant
   d. Measurement of a highly purified substance of known composition
28. Standards are defined as:
   a. How close a test result is to the true value
   b. Specimens that are similar to patient’s blood; known concentration of constituent
   c. Comparison of an instrument measure or reading to a known physical constant
   d. Highly purified substances of known composition
29. Sensitivity is:
   a. Cases with a specific disease or condition that produce a positive result
   b. Cases without a specific disease or condition that produce a negative result
   c. Cases with a specific disease or condition that produce a negative result
   d. Cases without a specific disease or condition that produce a positive result
30. Specificity is:
   a. Cases with a specific disease or condition that produce a positive result
   b. Cases without a specific disease or condition that produce a negative result
   c. Cases with a specific disease or condition that produce a negative result
   d. Cases without a specific disease or condition that produce a positive result

Quality Control Statistics

31. The mean is:
   a. Another term for the average
   b. Most frequently occurring number in a group of values
   c. Number that is midway between the highest and lowest values
   d. A representation of a true analyte value
32. The median is:
   a. Another term for the average
   b. Most frequently occurring number in a group of values
   c. Number that is midway between the highest and lowest values
   d. A representation of a true analyte value
33. The mode is:
   a. Another term for the average
   b. Most frequently occurring number in a group of values
   c. Number that is midway between the highest and lowest values
   d. A representation of a true analytic value
34. The standard deviation is:
   a. Equal to SD divided by the mean
   b. Measure of variability
   c. The same as the mean value
   d. An exact measurement of an analytic value
35. The coefficient of variation is:
   a. Equal to SD divided by the mean
   b. Measure of variability
   c. The same as the mean value
   d. An exact measurement of an analytic value

Total Analytical Error

36. Total Analytical Error depends on:
   a. A method’s precisions
   b. A method’s accuracy
   c. Both a and b
   d. Being within 2 SDs of the mean

Monitoring Quality Control

37. Levey-Jennings plots:
- **a.** Show values on a chart
- **b.** Have three warning rules
- **c.** Have three mandatory rules
- **d.** All the above

38. The 1_{2S} refers to the control rule that is commonly used with a Levey-Jennings chart,
- **a.** When the control limits are set as the mean ±1 SD
- **b.** When the control limits are set as the mean ±2 SD
- **c.** When the control limits are set as the mean ±3 SD
- **d.** When the control limits are set as the mean ±4 SD

Other QC Rules

39. When a specimen is transported to the laboratory, the optimum time for testing is:
- **a.** Immediately
- **b.** Within 1 hour of collection
- **c.** Within 2 hours of collection
- **d.** Within 8 hours of collection

Testing Outcomes

40. Biometrics is:
- **a.** The science of statistics applied to biological observations
- **b.** Measurement of ethnic differences
- **c.** Tracking of disease outbreaks
- **d.** Application of molecular diagnostics to disease transmission

Turgeon: Linné & Ringsrud's Clinical Laboratory Science, 8th Edition

STUDENT PROCEDURE WORKSHEET 3-1

Preparing a Levey-Jennings Control Chart

See Chapter 3 in *Linné & Ringsrud's Clinical Laboratory Science: Concepts, Procedures, and Clinical Applications,* 8th edition, for a complete discussion of this topic.

Student Learning Outcomes
After reading Chapter 3, and at the completion of this laboratory exercise and the review questions, the student will be able to:

- Gather control sera data and compute standard deviations.
- Draw the standard deviations on graph paper and enter daily results.
- Correctly complete the end-of-procedure review questions with a grade of 80% or greater.

Equipment and Supplies (for Manual Method)
NOTE: A Levey-Jennings chart can be constructed using Excel.

1. Calculator
2. Pen and paper
3. Standard graph paper
4. Data: assay results for normal and abnormal control sera for a specific procedure, such as cholesterol.

Instructions for the Procedure
Read the list of required equipment and supplies and the procedural steps. Follow the procedural steps in exact order.

SEQUENCE	PROCEDURAL STEP	INSTRUCTOR-OBSERVED ACCEPTABLE PERFORMANCE (CHECK IF ACCEPTABLE)
1	Record daily values from the same lot of normal and abnormal control samples, respectively.*	
2	Visually inspect the data for continuity in data.	
3	Calculate the mean value for both the normal and the abnormal samples.	
4	Calculate the standard deviation (SD).	
5	Determine the values for 2 SD and optionally 3 SD.	
6	Chart the results on graph paper. Use two sheets of graph paper, one for each chart of the normal and abnormal control values. a. **Label charts.** Include the name of the test and the name of the control material. The measurement unit may be included in the label for the *y*-axis. Other data typically included on the chart are the name of the analytical system, the lot number of the control material, the current mean and standard deviation, and the time period covered by the chart. b. **Scale and label *x*-axis.** The horizontal axis or *x*-axis represents time and is typically set for 30 days per month or 30 runs per month. c. **Scale and label *y*-axis.** The vertical axis or *y*-axis represents the measured control value. It is set to the scale to accommodate the lowest and highest results expected. d. **Draw lines for mean and control limits.** On the *y*-axis, locate the values that correspond to the mean, and draw a green horizontal line (such as at 200 mg/dL for control 1). Locate the values that correspond to the mean + 2 s and the mean – 2 s and draw yellow horizontal lines (for example at 192 and 208 for control 1).	

*The rule of thumb is to collect at least 20 measurements over at least 2 weeks or 10 working days, and preferably over at least 4 weeks or 20 working days.

(Continued)

Turgeon: Linné & Ringsrud's Clinical Laboratory Science, 8th Edition

STUDENT PROCEDURE WORKSHEET 3-1

Preparing a Levey-Jennings Control Chart

Review Questions

Student's Name ______________________ Date __________

1. What is the general purpose of preparing a Levey-Jennings Chart?

2. What phase of testing does the control chart aim to investigate?

3. What are the control limits of Levey-Jennings chart? What is the value of the control limits?

Procedural Evaluation

Student's Name ______________________ Grade__________

Instructor's Signature ______________________ Date__________

Comments:

4

Phlebotomy: Collecting and Processing Patient Blood Specimens

http://evolve.elsevier.com/Turgeon/clinicallab/

CHAPTER OUTLINE

LEARNING OUTCOMES

Quality Assessment

- Identify eight factors that should be monitored by quality assessment methods.
- Demonstrate the knowledge and skills needed to interact with patients when collecting specimens.
- Explain the Patient Care Partnership and its importance.
- Compare the characteristics of patients in various age groups.

Infection control

- Interpret the principles and applications of Standard Precautions.

Specimen Collection
- Describe the role of a phlebotomist.
- Describe the equipment used for venous blood collection.
- Arrange the proper steps in the collection technique for venous blood and analyze the outcomes if the sequence of steps is incorrect.
- Identify the color codes of evacuated tubes with the additives contained in the tubes.
- Compare common anticoagulants and additives used to preserve blood specimens and describe the general use of each type of anticoagulant.
- Describe the mode of action of ethylenediaminetetraacetate (EDTA) and heparin.
- Identify the major potential type of error in specimen collection.

Venous Blood Collection (Phlebotomy)
- Assess the cause and formulate a solution to correct five specific situations that could complicate venipuncture site selection.
- Name some typical phlebotomy problems, and describe the solution for each problem.
- Explain some techniques for obtaining blood from small or difficult veins.

Specimens: General Preparation
- State examples of types of unacceptable blood specimens and their effects on test results.
- Describe the preserving and storing of specimens.

Capillary or Peripheral Blood Collection by Skin Puncture
- Describe special blood collection considerations for pediatric and geriatric patients.
- Categorize the symptoms of potential phlebotomy complications and propose treatment for each type of complication.

Capillary Blood Collection
- Demonstrate and describe the proper technique for collecting a capillary blood specimen.

Case Studies
❖ Analyze the patient history, clinical signs and symptoms, and laboratory data for the stated case studies, answer the related critical thinking questions, and conclude the most likely diagnosis.

Review Questions
- Demonstrate comprehension of the chapter content by completing the end-of-chapter review questions with a grade of 80% or higher.

Note:
- indicates MLT and MLS core content
❖ indicates MLT (optional) and MLS advanced content

KEY TERMS

anticoagulant	hematoma	phlebotomy
capillary	hemolysis	plasma
dialysis	iatrogenic anemia	postprandial
edema	icteric	serum
fibrinogen	lipemic	venipuncture

QUALITY ASSESSMENT

The term *quality assessment,* or the alternate term *quality assurance,* encompasses policies that maintain and control processes involving the patient and laboratory analysis of specimens. Quality assessment includes monitoring the following specimen collection measures:
- Preparation of a patient for any specimens to be collected
- Collection of valid samples
- Proper specimen transport
- Performance of the requested laboratory analyses
- Validation of test results
- Recording and reporting the assay results
- Transmitting test results to the patient's medical record
- Documentation, maintenance, and availability of records describing quality assessment practices and quality control measures

The accuracy of laboratory testing begins with the quality of the specimen received by the laboratory. This quality depends on how a specimen was collected, transported, and processed. A laboratory assay will be no better than the specimen on which it is performed. If a preanalytical error occurs, the most perfect analysis is invalid and cannot be used by the physician in diagnosis or treatment.

Venous or arterial blood collection, **phlebotomy**, and **capillary** blood collection remain an error-prone phase of the testing cycle. In the United States it is estimated that more than 1 billion **venipunctures** are performed annually, and errors occurring within this process may cause serious harm to patients, either directly or indirectly (Table 4.1). Leading causes of preanalytical errors include the following[1]:
1. Specimen collection tube not filled properly
2. Patient identification error
3. Inappropriate specimen collection tube or container
4. Test request error

Other types of potential preanalytical errors include hemolyzed specimens, blood clots caused by inadequate mixing of evacuated collection tubes containing **anticoagulant**, and other factors that affect the volume of blood collected in an evacuated tube. Underfilling an evacuated tube containing an anticoagulant changes the ratio of blood to anticoagulant and can interfere with accurate test results. For example, if a blue-top evacuated tube is >90% full, it will typically prolong the prothrombin time (PT), activated partial thromboplastin time

TABLE 4.1 Examples of Phlebotomy Preanalytical Errors

Before Phlebotomy	Phlebotomy Procedure	After Phlebotomy
Misidentified patient	Excess tourniquet time	Improper transport or storage conditions
Wrong evacuated specimen tubes	Incorrect order of draw of specimen	Hemolysis caused by improper mixing of blood with the additive (shaking)
Inadequate fasting conditions	Failure to gently invert specimen collection tubes several times, if the tube contains an anticoagulant or additive	Incorrect specimen-handling directions (such as improper centrifugation or clot contact time)
Not coordinated with medication	Underfilling evacuated tubes	

Modified from Ernst DJ: *Applied phlebotomy,* Philadelphia, 2005, Lippincott Williams & Wilkins, p. 62.

(APTT), and thrombin (TT). It may underestimate fibrinogen and D-dimer assay results as well.

Because the tubing is attached to a butterfly needle, the first tube collected will underfill as a result of in the tubing. If a winged blood collection device (butterfly) is used to collect a light-blue top tube for coagulation studies, a waste tube should be drawn first. This waste tube is drawn first to remove the air in the tubing of the winged collection device. Once blood flows through the tubing, the waste tube can be removed and discarded. The waste tube does not need to be completely filled. Once complete, other evacuated tubes needed for diagnostic purposes can then be drawn following the standard order of draw.

Patient Care Partnership

The delivery of health care involves a partnership between patients and physicians and other health care professionals. When collecting blood specimens, it is important that the phlebotomist consider the rights of the patient at all times. The American Hospital Association[2] has developed the *Patient Care Partnership* document, which replaces the former Patient's Bill of Rights. This document stresses the following:

- High-quality hospital care
- A clean and safe environment
- Involvement by patients in their care
- Protection of patients' privacy
- Help for patients when leaving the hospital
- Help for patients with billing claims

Patients themselves or another person chosen by the patient can exercise these patient rights. A proxy decision maker can act on the patient's behalf if the patient lacks decision-making ability, is legally incompetent, or is a minor.

The partnership nature of health care requires that patients—or their families or surrogates—take part in their care. As such, patients are responsible for providing an accurate medical history and any written advance directives, following hospital rules and regulations, and complying with activities that contribute to a healthy lifestyle.

Pediatric Patients

When working with children, it is important to be gentle and compassionate. Attempt to interact with the pediatric patient, realizing that both the patient and the parent (if present) may have anxiety about the procedure and may be unfamiliar with the clinical setting. Acknowledge both the parent and the child.

Do not hurry; allow enough time for the procedure. It is important to take extra time to gain a child's confidence before proceeding with specimen collection. When working with pediatric patients, it is important to bolster their morale as much as possible. Ask for help in restraining a very small or uncooperative child. Older children may be more responsive when permitted to "help" (for example by holding the gauze).

In the nursery, each hospital will have its own rules, but a few general precautions apply. After working with an infant in a crib, the crib sides must be returned to the precollection position. If an infant is in an incubator, the portholes should be closed as much as possible. When oxygen is in use, do not forget to close the openings when the collection process is completed. Dispose of all waste materials properly.

Adolescent Patients

When obtaining a blood specimen from an adolescent, it is important to be relaxed and alert to possible anxiety. Adolescents may mask their anxiety. General interaction techniques include allowing enough time for the procedure, establishing eye contact, and allowing the patient to maintain a sense of control.

Adult Patients

Adult patients must be told briefly what is expected of them and what the test involves. Complete honesty is important. The patient should be greeted in a friendly and tactful manner. Without becoming overly familiar, a pleasant conversation can be started. The patient should be told about the purpose of the blood collection. Any personal information revealed by the patient is told in confidence and must be kept confidential. The patient's religious beliefs should be respected, and laboratory reports must be kept confidential. Information about other patients or physicians is always kept confidential. If the same patient is seen frequently, the phlebotomist may become familiar with the patient's interests, hobbies, or family and use these as topics of conversation. Many patients in the hospital are lonely; kindness is greatly appreciated. Occasionally, especially if extremely ill, the patient will not want to talk at all, and this should be respected. It is important to be honest but also to attempt to boost the patient's morale as much as possible.

Even if the patient is disagreeable, the phlebotomist should remain pleasant. A smile can often work miracles. It is important to be firm when the patient is unpleasant, to remain cheerful, and to express confidence in the work to be done.

In a hospital setting, before leaving the patient's room, the area should be checked to see that everything is in place in the laboratory tray and that the room has been left as it was found. The tray holding the blood collection supplies and equipment should always be kept out of reach of the patient. All sharps and supplies should be disposed of properly.

Geriatric Patients

It is extremely important to treat geriatric patients with dignity and respect and not demean them. It is best to address the patient with a more formal title, such as Mrs., Ms., or Mr., rather than by his or her first name. As with patients in general, older patients may enjoy a short conversation. Keep a flexible agenda so enough time is allowed. If a patient appears to be having difficulty hearing, speak slightly slower and louder.

Phlebotomy Challenges

Obstacles can be encountered when trying to collect a patient's blood specimen. A phlebotomist must never proceed with a procedure until any obstacles have been remediated.

Difficulties can include simply finding a patient or identifying a patient under difficult circumstances, e.g., in the emergency department. The presence of physicians, clergy, or visitors can impede blood collection.

Patients themselves can present challenges. A sleeping or unconscious patient may be difficult to wake up for the phlebotomy procedure. Patients who are apprehensive require extra time and assurance before attempting a venipuncture. Some patients may not understand the phlebotomist's explanation of the phlebotomy procedure because of language barriers.

Occasionally, a patient will be combative. This may be the result of alcohol ingestion, drug use, or a psychiatric condition. In some of these cases, such as with mentally challenged patients, the phlebotomist needs the written permission of a parent, guardian, or conservator. This is the same requirement as for drawing blood from a minor—a patient younger than 18 years of age. Because both the patient and the phlebotomist could be injured during a phlebotomy, a supervisor should be consulted. The supervisor could consult with the patient's physician regarding how to proceed with this patient.

INFECTION CONTROL

The chain of infection requires a continuous link of three primary factors:

1. Reservoir: an infected symptomatic or nonsymptomatic host
2. Means of transmission: a contaminated object, food, or water.
3. Susceptible host: a patient, a health care worker, or a visitor.

In addition to these factors, other links in the chain of infection include a portal of exit for an infectious agent and a portal of entry into the host.

Isolation as a Safety System

Isolation was once understood as the separation of a seriously ill patient to stop the spread of infection to others or to protect the patient from irritating factors. The term *isolation* has changed from meaning a special set of precautions performed by a few health care providers for a select few patients to a safety system that is practiced by everyone in the course of routine patient care. Isolation precautions are now a routine part of the everyday work process.

Modern isolation techniques incorporate a broad-based theory that addresses the needs of both patients and employees to ensure that the safest possible environment is maintained throughout the health care facility. Current guidelines use the two-tiered strategy to create this safety system.

Standard and Additional Precautions

A two-tiered system has been developed, the goal of which is to minimize the risk for infection and to maximize the safety level within the health care facility's environment.

The first tier of infection control is the practice of Standard Precautions. The Standard Precautions theory recognizes the need to reduce the risk for microbial transmission, including human immunodeficiency virus (HIV), from both identified and unidentified sources of infection. These precautions require that protective protocols be followed whenever contact is made with blood and body fluids.

A second tier of an infection control system was developed to provide additional precautions to control the transmission of infectious agents under special circumstances when Standard Precautions alone may not be enough. Transmission-based precautions are divided into three basic categories: contact, airborne, and droplet.

Contact Precautions

Contact precautions are designed to stop the spread of microorganisms through direct contact, such as skin-to-skin contact, and indirect contact, which is usually the result of a person making contact with a contaminated inanimate object. Contact precautions include wearing gloves when making contact with the patient's skin or with inanimate objects that have been in direct contact with the patient. The use of gowns may be mandated when the health care worker's clothing is likely to come in contact with the patient or items in the patient's room.

Droplet Precautions

Droplet precautions protect health care workers, visitors, and other patients from droplets that may be expelled during coughing, sneezing, or talking. Guidelines include using a mask when working close to the patient. Guidelines for patient placement, whether in a private room or a room with special air-handling capabilities, should be implemented as well. Specific guidelines for transport and placement of patients and the environmental management of equipment should be implemented according to each category's requirements. Droplet precautions are particularly important when influenza or whooping cough is present.

Airborne Precautions

Airborne precautions are designed to provide protection from airborne bacteria or dust particles, which may be suspended in the air for an extended period. Guidelines include the use of respiratory protection (such as N95 respirator) and the use of special air-handling systems to control airborne bacteria. Airborne precautions must be observed when patients have measles or tuberculosis.

SPECIMEN COLLECTION

Blood is the type of specimen most frequently analyzed in the clinical laboratory. Urine specimens, body fluids, and stool specimens are also frequently analyzed. Other specimens such as throat cultures and swabs from wound abscesses are sent to the microbiology laboratory for study.

Knowledge of proper collection, preservation, and processing of specimens is essential. A properly collected blood specimen is crucial to quality performance in the laboratory. In addition to specimen procurement, related areas of specimen transportation, handling, and processing must also be fully understood by anyone who collects or handles blood specimens.

Strict adherence to the rules of specimen collection is critical to the accuracy of any test. The major potential sources of error include identification errors, both of the patient and the specimen.

The Phlebotomist

Blood specimens may be collected by health care personnel with several different educational backgrounds, depending on the facility. In some institutions, blood specimen collection is done by the clinical laboratory scientist/medical technologist or the clinical laboratory technician/medical laboratory technician. In other institutions, specially trained individuals, phlebotomists, perform blood collections.

The phlebotomist is a critically important member of the laboratory team. In fact, the phlebotomist represents the laboratory to patients. It is important that the phlebotomist project a professional image by wearing a clean white laboratory coat with a visible name badge. Hair should be short or tied back with no dangling jewelry, nails should be short and clean, and proper shoes must be worn for safety reasons (see Chapter 2). The collection tray or work cubicle must be immaculate (see Specimen Collection).

The role of the phlebotomist has never been more important to the patient and the laboratory. Phlebotomists in the hospital, clinic, or drawing station have a major effect on the impression that patients develop of the entire laboratory. Phlebotomists are laboratory ambassadors. These members of the health care team must demonstrate professionalism by their conduct, appearance, composure, and communication skills. Critical thinking skills are essential for phlebotomists. They must make effective decisions and solve problems, frequently under conditions of stress.[3]

One specific area of improvement in laboratory test results is in the blood sample collection and analysis process. The majority of laboratory errors are caused by mistakes before testing, or preanalytical errors. Errors in the preanalytical phase involving phlebotomists can be reduced through appropriate professional training and constant vigilance in testing.

The phlebotomist is expected to deliver unexcelled customer satisfaction. It is important to understand and know the patient's expectations, manage unrealistic expectations through patient education, and be diplomatic with patient complaints. If a patient is dissatisfied, the phlebotomist should listen with interest, express genuine concern, and make an attempt to resolve the issue of concern. If the phlebotomist is directly at fault, an apology would be appropriate.

Blood Collection Variables

Most clinical laboratory determinations are done on whole blood, plasma, or serum. Blood specimens may be drawn from fasting or nonfasting patients. The fasting state is defined as having no food or liquid other than water for 8 to 12 hours before blood collection. Fasting specimens are not necessary for most laboratory determinations. Blood from fasting patients is usually drawn in the morning before breakfast.

Blood collected directly after a meal is described as a **postprandial** specimen. In the case of blood glucose, a sample may be collected 2 hours postprandially. After 2 hours, blood glucose levels should return to almost fasting levels in patients who are not diabetic. Blood should not be collected while intravenous (IV) solutions are being administered, if possible.

Food intake, medication, activity, and time of day can all influence the laboratory results for blood specimens. It is critically important to control preanalytical variables such as timed drawing of a specimen, peak and trough drug levels, and postmedication conditions. Other controllable biological variations in blood include the following:

- Posture (whether the patient is lying in bed or standing up)
- Immobilization (such as resulting from prolonged bed rest)
- Exercise
- Circadian/diurnal variations (cyclical variations throughout the day)
- Recent food ingestion (such as caffeine effect)
- Smoking (nicotine effect)
- Alcohol ingestion

Blood Collection Procedures

There are two general sources of blood for clinical laboratory tests: venous blood and peripheral (or capillary) blood. The Clinical and Laboratory Standards Institute (CLSI) has set standards for the collection of venous blood (venipuncture or phlebotomy) and capillary blood (finger prick or skin puncture).[4,5] Arterial blood may be needed to perform specific procedures such as blood gas analysis.

Layers of Normal Anticoagulated Blood

In vivo (in the body) the blood is in a liquid form, but in vitro (outside the body) it will clot in a few minutes. Blood that is freshly drawn into a glass tube appears as a translucent, dark-red fluid. In minutes it will start to clot, or coagulate, forming a semisolid, jellylike mass. If left undisturbed in the tube, this mass will begin to shrink, or retract, in about 1 hour. Complete retraction normally takes place within 24 hours.

Whole blood that is allowed to clot normally produces a pale-yellow fluid called **serum** that separates from the clot and appears in the upper portion of the tube. During the process of coagulation, certain factors present in the original blood

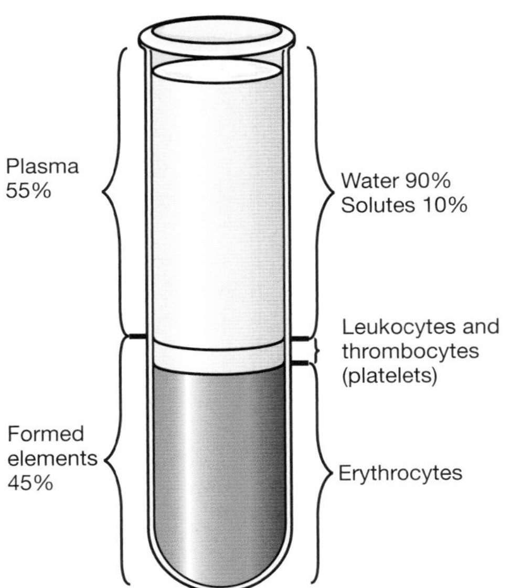

Fig. 4.1 Composition of blood. (Redrawn from Applegate E: *The anatomy and physiology learning system*, ed 4, St Louis, 2011, Elsevier/Saunders.)

sample are depleted, or used up. Fibrinogen is one important substance found in circulating blood (in the plasma portion) that is necessary for coagulation to occur. Fibrinogen is converted to fibrin when clotting occurs, and the fibrin lends structure to the clot in the form of fine threads in which the red blood cells (RBCs, erythrocytes) and the white blood cells (WBCs, leukocytes) are embedded. To assist in obtaining serum, collection tubes with a separator gel additive are used. Serum is used extensively for chemical, serologic, and other laboratory testing and can be obtained from the tube of clotted blood by centrifuging.

When fresh whole blood is mixed with a substance that prevents blood clotting, called an anticoagulant, the blood can be separated into plasma, a straw-colored fluid, and the cellular components: erythrocytes, leukocytes, and platelets (thrombocytes). When an anticoagulated blood specimen is allowed to stand for a time, the components will settle into three distinct layers (Fig. 4.1), as follows:

1. Plasma, the top layer, a liquid that normally represents about 55% of the total blood volume
2. Buffy coat, a grayish-white cellular middle layer composed of WBCs and platelets, normally about 1% of the total blood volume
3. Erythrocytes, the bottom layer, consisting of packed RBCs and normally about 45% of the total blood volume

Environmental Factors Associated With Evacuated Blood Collection Tubes

A variety of environmental factors can affect the quality of evacuated tubes used to collect blood. These factors can then influence the published expiration dates of the evacuated tubes.[6] Environmental factors affecting evacuated tubes include the following:

- Ambient temperature
- Altitude
- Humidity
- Sunlight

Ambient Temperature

If an evacuated tube is stored at low temperature, the pressure of the gas inside the tube decreases, leading to an increase in draw volume. Conversely, higher temperatures can cause reductions in draw volume.

Increased temperatures in evacuated tubes also can have a negative effect on the stability of certain tube additives, such as biochemicals or gel. Gel is a compound that potentially can degrade when exposed to high temperatures.

Altitude

In situations where blood is drawn at high altitudes (>5000 feet), the draw volume may be affected. Because the ambient pressure at high altitude is lower than at sea level, the pressure of the residual gas inside the tube will reach this reduced ambient pressure during filling earlier than if the tube were drawn at sea level. The resulting draw volume will be lower.

Humidity

The effect of storage at various levels of humidity can affect only plastic evacuated tubes because of the greater permeability of these materials to water vapor relative to glass. Conditions of extremely high humidity could lead to the migration of water vapor inside a tube that contains a moisture-sensitive material, such as a lyophilized additive. Conditions of extremely low humidity could hasten the escape of water vapor from a tube containing a wet additive. Such storage conditions may compromise the accuracy of clinical results.

Light

A special additive mixture for coagulation testing that is sensitive to light and found only in glass evacuated tubes is called *CTAD* (citric acid, theophylline, adenosine, and dipyridamole). The CTAD mixture minimizes platelet activation after blood collection. Normally, this additive has a slightly yellow appearance that becomes clear when no longer viable. These tubes are generally packaged in small quantities to minimize exposure to light.

Expiration Dates of Evacuated Tubes

Expiration dates (see Table 4.2) are determined by testing shelf life under known environmental conditions. *Shelf life* of an evacuated tube is defined by the stability of the additive and vacuum retention. Most evacuated tubes on the market have at least a 12-month shelf life. It is important that tubes be stored under recommended conditions.

The expiration dates of glass tubes are generally limited by the shelf life of the additives, because vacuum and water vapor losses are minimal over time. Exposure to irradiation during sterilization of tubes and to moisture or light during the shelf life of the product can limit the stability of biochemical additives. The expiration dates of evacuated plastic tubes are also limited by the same factors that affect glass tubes. Evacuated plastic tubes do sustain a measurable loss of vacuum over time, and some evacuated plastic blood collection tubes may have

TABLE 4.2 Evacuated Tube Volumes and Shelf Life

Evacuated Tube Description	Old Draw Volume (mL)	New Draw Volume (mL)	Old Shelf Life (months)	New Shelf Life (months)
VACUETTE® tube LH lithium heparin separator; 13×75 green cap, yellow ring; nonridged	4.0	3.5	18	15
VACUETTE® tube K2E K_2EDTA separator; 13×75 lavender cap, yellow ring; nonridged	4.0	3.5	18	15
VACUETTE® tube Z serum separator clot activator; 13×75 red cap, yellow ring; nonridged	4.0	3.5	18	15
VACUETTE® tube Z serum separator clot activator; 13×75 gold cap, gold ring, black label; nonridged	4.0	3.5	18	15

Greiner Bio-One North America, Inc. Product Modification: Draw Volume and Shelf Life Changes of VACUETTE® Tubes, Monroe, NC, June 13, 2017.

their expiration dates determined by their ability to ensure a known draw volume.

It is important to understand that evacuated blood collection tubes are not completely evacuated. There is a small amount of gas (air) still residing in the tube, at low pressure. The higher the pressure of the gas inside the tube on the date of manufacture, the lower the intended draw volume will be for a tube of a given size. The draw volume specified for a given tube is achieved by manufacturing the tube at a designated evacuation pressure.

The dynamics of blood collection inside the tube are based on the ideal gas law:

$$PV = nRT$$

where P is the pressure inside the tube, V is the volume that the gas occupies, n is the number of moles of gas inside the tube, R is the universal gas constant, and T is the temperature inside the tube.

According to the equation, if the moles of gas and the temperature do not change, the product of pressure and volume is a constant. When blood starts filling the tube, the residual gas inside is confined into a decreasing volume, causing the pressure of the gas to increase. When the pressure of this gas reaches ambient pressure, the collection process is completed for that tube.

The inability of an evacuated tube to fill correctly, referred to as a "short draw" or quantity-not-sufficient specimen, is a cause of rejection of a blood specimen. In fact, underfilling has been cited as the second most frequent cause of specimen rejection, with a rate of underfilling of 16% to 21%. To reduce the number of rejected specimens as a result of underfilling because of an expired shelf life, a laboratory can initiate a *kaizen* ("good change" in Japanese) to improve the inventory. A strategy that can be implemented is to survey the inventory in all phlebotomy supply centers.

Changes in Shelf Life

Temperatures during transport and storage often cannot be monitored. To improve sample quality in these conditions, adjustment can be made to the draw volume of a 13 × 75 mm, 4-mL VACUETTE® gel separator tube, for example, which will draw 0.5 mL less blood and have a shelf life of 15 months. Change will increase the amount of headspace in tubes to reduce the potential effect of vacuum pressure on the sample.

Evacuated Blood Tubes

Evacuated blood collection tubes without an *anticoagulant* are used to yield *serum* (or are used as a discard tube), whereas many types of evacuated tubes contain some type of anticoagulant or additive (Tables 4.3 and 4.4 and back cover). The additives range from those that promote faster clotting of the blood

TABLE 4.3 Examples of BD Stopper Colors for Venous Blood Collection[a]

Color	Additive
Lavender	K_2EDTA (spray-coated plastic tube) K_3EDTA (liquid in glass tube)
Pink	K_2EDTA (spray-coated plastic tube)
Light green/marbled green	Sodium heparin, lithium heparin, ammonium heparin
Light blue or clear (Hemogard closure)	Buffered sodium citrate, CTAD
White[b]	K_2EDTA with gel
Red/light gray[c] or clear (Hemogard closure)	None (plastic)
Red	Silicone coated (glass) Clot activator, silicone coated (plastic)
Red/gray	
Gold/marbled red	Clot activators and gel
Gray	Sodium fluoride
Yellow	SPS: blood culture (Hemogard closure) Acid citrate dextrose: HLA studies (color stopper)
Royal blue	No additives for toxicology, trace metals (Hemogard)
Orange/marbled yellow	Thrombin
Black	Sodium citrate
Tan	Sodium heparin

CTAD, Citric acid, theophylline, adenosine, and dipyridamole; *HLA,* human leukocyte antigen; *K_2EDTA,* dipotassium ethylenediaminetetraacetate; *K_3EDTA,* tripotassium ethylenediaminetetraacetate; *SPS,* sodium polyanethol sulfonate.

[a]See inside book cover for the comprehensive venous blood collection tube guide, including additives, inversions of blood collection, and laboratory use.

[b]New tube for use in molecular diagnostic test methods.

[c]New red/light gray for use as a discard tube or secondary specimen tube.

Modified from BD Vacutainer venous blood collection tube guide, Becton Dickinson.

TABLE 4.4 Examples of VACUETTE® Cap Color Codes for Venous Blood Collection

Description of Plastic Tubes	Additive	SAFETY Cap Color	Cap Inner Ring Color
No-additive tubes	None	White	Black
Coagulation tubes	3.2% sodium citrate	Light blue	Black
	3.8% sodium citrate	Light blue	Black
Serum tubes	Clot activator	Red	Black
	Clot activator with gel	Red or gold	Yellow or gold
Heparin tubes	Lithium heparin	Green	Black
	Lithium heparin with gel	Green	Yellow
	Sodium heparin	Green	Green
EDTA tubes	K_2EDTA	Lavender	Black
	K_2EDTA with gel	Lavender or white	Yellow
	K_3EDTA	Lavender	Black
Glycolytic inhibitor tubes	NaF/KO	Gray	Black
Trace-element tubes	Sodium heparin	Royal blue	Black
ESR tubes (not available in United States)	3.2% sodium citrate	Black standard stopper	—

EDTA, Ethylenediaminetetraacetate; *ESR,* erythrocyte sedimentation rate; *K_2EDTA,* dipotassium ethylenediaminetetraacetate; *K_3EDTA,* tripotassium ethylenediaminetetraacetate; *KO,* potassium oxalate; *NaF,* sodium fluoride. Note: Tubes with a *white* inner cap ring refer to smaller draw volumes of 2 mL. *Black* rings identify standard draw and *yellow* rings identify gel tube. VACUETTE® Greiner Bio-One North America, Inc., Monroe, NC.

to those that preserve or stabilize certain analytes (such as glucose) or cells. The inclusion of additives at the proper concentration in evacuated tubes greatly enhances the accuracy and consistency of test results and facilitates faster turnaround times in the laboratory.

Anticoagulants

The several types of additives used as anticoagulants in blood collection tubes include inorganic additives (see inside back cover), biochemical additives and gel. Some frequently used anticoagulants are tripotassium ethylenediaminetetraacetate (K_3EDTA), dipotassium ethylenediaminetetraacetate (K_2EDTA), sodium citrate, and heparin. Each type of anticoagulant prevents the coagulation of whole blood. The proper proportion of anticoagulant to whole blood is important to avoid the introduction of errors into test results. The specific type of anticoagulant needed for a procedure should be stated in the laboratory procedure manual.

EDTA. The International Council for Standardization in Haematology (ICSH) and CLSI recommend the salts of the chelating (calcium-binding) agent EDTA as the anticoagulant of choice for blood cell counting and sizing, because EDTA produces less shrinkage of RBCs and less of an increase in cell volume on standing. EDTA is spray-dried on the interior surface of evacuated plastic tubes. The proper ratio of EDTA to whole blood is important because some test results will be altered if the ratio is incorrect. Excessive EDTA produces shrinkage of erythrocytes, thus affecting tests such as the manually performed packed cell volume (microhematocrit).

K_2EDTA and K_3EDTA are found in evacuated tubes. The mode of action of this anticoagulant is that it removes ionized calcium (Ca^{2+}) through the process of chelation. This process forms an insoluble calcium salt that prevents blood coagulation.

EDTA is the most frequently used anticoagulant in hematology for the complete blood cell count (CBC) or any of its component tests: hemoglobin, packed cell volume, total leukocyte count and leukocyte differential count, and platelet count. The modified Westergren erythrocyte sedimentation rate (ESR) method uses EDTA as the anticoagulant of choice. In addition, EDTA is used routinely for testing in blood banking such as blood grouping, Rh typing, and antibody screening.

K_2EDTA with gel is used for testing plasma in molecular diagnosis. K_3EDTA may be used for viral marker testing.

Sodium citrate. Sodium citrate solutions are available in concentrations of 3.2% and 3.8%. Sodium citrate removes calcium from the coagulation system by precipitating it into an unusable form. Sodium citrate is effective as an anticoagulant because of its mild calcium-chelating properties. It is used as an anticoagulant for APTT and PT testing and for the classic Westergren ESR. The correct ratio of one part anticoagulant to nine parts whole blood in blood collection tubes is critical. An excess of anticoagulant can alter the expected dilution of blood and produce errors in the results. Because of the dilution of anticoagulant to blood, sodium citrate is generally unacceptable for most other hematology tests.

Heparin. Heparin is used as an in vitro and in vivo anticoagulant. Heparin acts as an antithrombin, or substance that inactivates the blood-clotting factor thrombin and factor Xa. This inactivation of thrombin is caused by the complexing of heparin with the antithrombin III molecule, catalyzing the inhibition of thrombin.

Lithium heparin is the recommended form of heparin for use in laboratory testing because it is least likely to interfere when performing tests for other ions. The in vitro formation of fibrin in heparinized plasma opposes the anticoagulation action of heparin and can result in the subsequent formation of fibrin in the plasma. Several specimen-processing steps are recommended to help ensure a good-quality heparinized plasma sample to aid in minimizing the formation of latent fibrin.

Heparin is the only anticoagulant that should be used for the determination of pH, blood gases, electrolytes, and ionized calcium. Heparin is used to coat "micro" (capillary blood) collection tubes for use in certain hematology or clinical chemistry procedures.

Heparin is an inappropriate anticoagulant for many hematologic tests, including Wright-stained blood smears, because the smear will stain too blue.

Additives

Clot activators. The presence of a clot activator promotes blood coagulation. One type of additive is thrombin, an enzyme that converts fibrinogen to fibrin. Thrombin tubes are often used for "stat" serum testing because of the short clotting time. Glass or silica also promotes clotting by providing more surface area for platelet activation.

Clot activators may coat the inside of a tube and require gentle inversion of the tube five times to allow the whole blood to come in contact with the activator.

Serum separators. The function of additive polymer gel is to provide a physical and chemical barrier between the serum or plasma and the cells. Its use offers significant benefits in collecting, processing, and storing the specimen in the primary tube.

Separator gels are capable of providing barrier properties because of the way they respond to applied forces. After blood is drawn into the evacuated gel tube, and once centrifugation begins, the *g*-force applied to the gel causes its viscosity to decrease, enabling it to move or flow. Materials with these flow characteristics are often called *thixotropic.* Once centrifugation ceases, the gel becomes an immobile barrier between the supernatant and the cells. The composite nature of gels gives these gel tubes a perpetual shelf life.[6]

Preservative. Sodium fluoride (NaF), which is both a dry additive and a weak anticoagulant, is used primarily to preserve blood glucose specimens by preventing glycolysis, or destruction of glucose (see Chapter 10).

Adverse effects of additives. The additives chosen for specific determinations must not alter the blood components or affect the laboratory tests to be done. The following are some adverse effects of using an improper additive or of using the wrong amount of additive:

- *Interference with the assay.* The additive may contain a substance that is the same, or reacts in the same way, as the substance being measured; for example, use of sodium oxalate as the anticoagulant for a sodium determination.
- *Removal of constituents.* The additive may remove the constituent to be measured, for example, use of an oxalate anticoagulant for a calcium determination; oxalate removes calcium from the blood by forming an insoluble salt, calcium oxalate.
- *Effect on enzyme action.* The additive may affect enzyme reactions; for example, use of NaF as an anticoagulant in an enzyme determination; NaF destroys many enzymes.
- *Alteration of cellular constituents.* An additive may alter cellular constituents; for example, use of an older anticoagulant additive, oxalate, in hematology. Oxalate distorts the cell morphology; RBCs become crenated (shrunken), vacuoles appear in the granulocytes, and bizarre forms of lymphocytes and monocytes appear rapidly when oxalate is used as the anticoagulant. Another example is the use of heparin as an anticoagulant for blood to be used in the preparation of blood films that will be stained with Wright stain. Unless the films are stained within 2 hours, heparin gives a blue background with Wright stain.
- *Incorrect amount of anticoagulant.* If too little additive is used, partial clotting of whole blood will occur. This interferes with cell counts. By comparison, if too much liquid anticoagulant is used, it dilutes the blood sample and thus interferes with certain quantitative measurements.

Color-Coded Evacuated Tubes

The presence or absence of additives in evacuated tubes is indicated by the color of the tube top. Evacuated tubes and Microtainer tubes have various color-coded stoppers determined by the manufacturer. The stopper color denotes the type of anticoagulant or additive, or the presence of a gel separator. Increasingly, glass collection tubes are being replaced with safer plastic tubes.

Storage temperature for blood collection tubes should be between 40°F and 77°F (4°C–25°C). If plastic tubes reach higher temperatures, they may lose their vacuum or implode. Evacuated tubes are intended for one-time use.

Usually, the name of a laboratory test is indicated on the patient requisition, and the phlebotomist must choose the appropriate tube (see Box 4.1). When collecting multiple tubes of blood, a specified "order of draw" protocol should be followed to diminish the possibility of cross-contamination between tubes caused by the presence of various additives (Table 4.5). Errors in the order of draw can affect laboratory test results.

Venipuncture Procedure

Safe Blood Collection: Equipment and Supplies

Safe blood collection requires sterile needles, which come in a range of sizes. Besides length, needles are classified by gauge size: The higher the gauge number, the smaller the inner diameter, or bore. An increased emphasis on safety has led to new product development by various companies.

For blood collection with a syringe or evacuated blood collection tube, a 21-gauge needle is the standard size. Butterfly

BOX 4.1 Examples of Color-Coded Evacuated Tube Uses

Gray
Used for fasting blood sugar, lactic acid, and alcohol level assays.

Lavender
Used for complete blood count, sedimentation rate, and routine immunohematology testing, e.g., ABO blood grouping.

Light Blue
Used for coagulation assays.

Pink
Used for blood bank testing with a label and closure that meet the American Association of Blood Banks standards.

Red
Used for testing in blood bank, chemistry, and serology.

Tan
Used for blood lead level assay.

Yellow
Used for blood culture collection.

TABLE 4.5 Order of Draw of Multiple Evacuated Tubes Collections[a]

Order	Closure Color	Type of Tube	Mix by Inverting BD Tubes[b]	Mix by Inverting Greiner Tubes[c]
1	Yellow	Blood cultures: SPS—aerobic and anaerobic	8–10×	
2	Light blue	Citrate tube[d]	3–4×	4×
3	Gold or red/gray	BD Vacutainer SST gel separator tube	5×	
	Red	Serum tube (plastic)	5×	5–10×
	Red	Serum tube (glass)	None	
	Orange	BD Vacutainer RST	5–6×	
4	Light green or green/gray	PST gel separator tube with heparin	8–10×	5–10×
	Green	Heparin	8–10×	5–10
5	Lavender	EDTA	8–10×	5–10
6	White	PPT separator tube K_2EDTA with gel	8–10×	8–10×
7	Gray	Fluoride (glucose) tube	8–10×	

EDTA, Ethylenediaminetetraacetate; *K_2EDTA,* dipotassium ethylenediaminetetraacetate; *PPT,* plasma preparation tube; *PST,* plasma serum tube; *RST,* rapid serum tube; *SPS,* sodium polyanethol sulfonate; *SST,* serum separator tube.

[a]The order of draw has been revised to reflect the increased use of plastic evacuated collection tubes. Plastic serum tubes containing a clot activator may cause interference in coagulation testing. Some facilities may continue using glass serum tubes without a clot activator as a waste tube before collecting special coagulation assays. Reflects change in CLSI recommended order of draw (H3-A5, 23[32], 8.10.2).

[b]Modified from Becton Dickinson, 2010.

[c]Modified from Greiner Bio-One

[d]If a winged blood collection set for venipuncture is used, a discard tube should be drawn first. The blood flowing through the tubing into the discard tube displaces air in the tubing. This ensures a proper fill of blood into the evacuated tube with a proper blood anticoagulant ratio. The discard tube does not need to be completely filled.

needles are being used more frequently as the acuity of patients increases. The collecting needle is double pointed; the longer end is for insertion into the patient's vein, and the shorter end pierces the rubber stopper of the discard and collection tubes. It is important to use an evacuated tube as a discard tube to remove the air from the tubing attached to the butterfly needle.

The specially designed holder used to secure the needle is for one-time use only. It is no longer acceptable to wash and reuse the plastic needle holder device.[7] For example, the BD Vacutainer one-use holder is a clear plastic needle holder prominently marked with the words "Do Not Reuse" and "Single Use Only." Once a venipuncture is completed, the entire needle and holder assembly is disposed of in a sharps container. The needle should not be removed from the holder. No change in venipuncture technique is required with a single-use holder.

The Needlestick Safety and Prevention Act of 2000:

- Requires health care employers to provide safety-engineered sharps devices and needleless systems to employees to reduce the risk for occupational exposure to HIV, hepatitis C, and other bloodborne disease.
- Expands the definition of engineering controls to include devices with engineered sharps injury protection.
- Requires that exposure control plans document consideration and implementation of safer medical devices designed to eliminate or minimize occupational exposure. Plans must be reviewed and updated at least annually.
- Requires each health care facility to maintain a sharps injury log, with detailed information regarding percutaneous injuries.
- Requires employers to solicit input from health care workers when identifying and selecting sharps and document process.

The U.S. Occupational Safety and Health Administration (OSHA) posted a Safety and Health Information Bulletin (SHIB) in 2003 to clarify the OSHA position on reusing tube holders during blood collection procedures, a clarification of the OSHA Bloodborne Pathogens Standard [29 CFR 1910.1030 (d)(2)(vii)(A)]. The standard prohibits the removal of a contaminated needle from a medical device. Prohibition of needle removal from any device is addressed in the 1991 and 2001 standards, the OSHA compliance directive (CPL 2–2.69), and in a 2002 letter of interpretation. Blood collected into the syringe would then need to be transferred into a tube before disposal of the contaminated syringe. In these situations, a syringe with an engineered sharps injury prevention feature should be used whenever possible, along with safe work practices. Transfer of the blood from the syringe to the test tube must be done using a needleless blood transfer device.

As with any OSHA rule or regulation, noncompliance may result in the issuance of citations by an OSHA compliance officer after the completion of on-site inspection. It is the responsibility of each facility to evaluate its work practices, implement appropriate engineering controls, and institute all other applicable elements of exposure control to achieve compliance with current OSHA rules and regulations. The OSHA SHIB provides a step-by-step Evaluation Toolbox for a facility to follow (Box 4.2).

Preattached blood collection needle and holder. A preattached needle holder provides additional protection from tube holder–end needlestick injuries that virtually eliminates a phlebotomist's exposure to a contaminated needle. The risks associated with reusing a needle holder are well recognized. The National Phlebotomy Association (NPA) found that 99% of sampled reusable holders were contaminated with blood, creating an unnecessary risk for exposure to HIV, hepatitis C virus, hepatitis B virus, and other bloodborne pathogens for health care workers and patients. (The complete statement, along with more information about the NPA, is available at www.nationalphlebotomy.org.)

A study of various types of safety-engineered devices to prevent needlestick injuries concluded that automatic (passive) safety-engineered devices are more effective than semiautomatic or manually activated devices in reducing needlestick injuries.[7] Passive devices with automatic safety caused a needlestick injury at a rate of 0.06 per 100,000 uses.

BOX 4.2 OSHA Safety and Health Information Bulletin: Evaluation Toolbox

1. Employers must first evaluate, select, and use appropriate engineering controls (such as sharps with engineered sharps injury protection), which include single-use blood tube holders with sharps with engineered sharps injury protection (SESIP) attached.
2. The use of engineering and work practice controls provides the highest degree of control to eliminate potential injuries after performing blood draws. Disposing of blood tube holders with contaminated needles attached after the activation of the safety feature affords the greatest hazard control.
3. In very rare situations, needle removal is acceptable.
   - If the employer can demonstrate that no feasible alternative to needle removal is available (such as the inability to purchase single-use blood tube holders because of a supply shortage of these devices).
   - If the removal is necessary for a specific medical or dental procedure.
   - In these rare cases, the employer must ensure that the contaminated needle is protected by a SESIP before disposal. In addition, the employer must ensure that a proper sharps disposal container is located in the immediate area of sharps use and is easily accessible to employees. This information must be clearly detailed and documented in the employer's Exposure Control Plan.
4. If it is necessary to draw blood with a syringe, a syringe with engineered sharps injury protection must be used, in which the protected needle is removed using safe work practices, and transfer of blood from the syringe to the tube must be done using a needleless blood transfer device.

From Occupational Safety and Health Administration: Disposal of contaminated needles and blood tube holders used for phlebotomy. Safety and Health Information Bulletin, October 2003. http://www.osha.gov/dts/shib/shib101503.html

A blood collection system consists of a collection needle, a nonreusable needle holder, and a tube containing enough vacuum to draw a specific amount of blood (Fig. 4.2).

Syringe Technique

Disposable plastic syringes are used for special cases of venous blood collection. If a patient has particularly difficult veins, or if other special circumstances exist, the syringe technique may be used. Some facilities recommend an order of draw with a syringe that varies from the evacuated-tube protocol. Currently, it is more common to use wing-tip (butterfly) blood collection sets for difficult patients or some pediatric patients.

General Protocol

1. Phlebotomists should pleasantly introduce themselves to the patient and clearly explain the procedure to be performed. It is always a courtesy to speak a few words in a patient's native language if English is not his or her first language. Ethnic populations vary geographically, but many patients are now Spanish speaking. If a patient doesn't understand English and the phlebotomist is not fluent in the patient's native language, an interpreter should be requested.
2. Patient identification is the critical first step in blood collection. Patient misidentification errors are potentially associated with the worst clinical outcomes because of the possibility of misdiagnosis and mishandled therapy.[1]

   It is necessary to have the patient state and speak his or her name. If a patient cannot provide this information, he or she

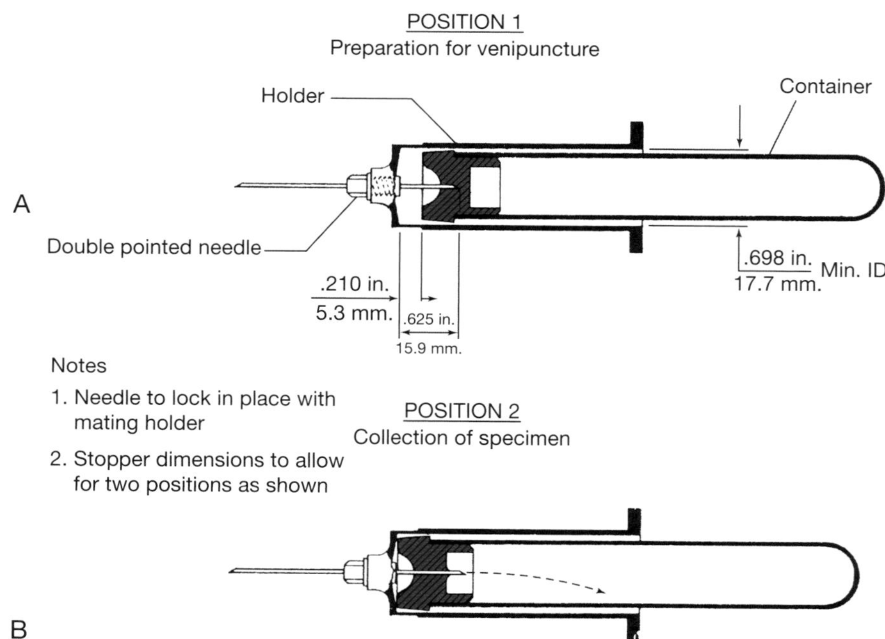

Fig. 4.2 Standard double-ended blood-collecting needle with holder using vacuum tube system. (A) Preparation for venipuncture. (B) Collection of specimen. (NCCLS H1-A4: Evacuated tubes and additives for blood specimen collection—fourth edition; approved standard, 1996.)

must provide some form of identification or must be identified by a family member or caregiver. Check the identification band that is physically attached to the patient. Wristbands with unique bar-coded patient identifiers have great potential for reducing patient misidentification. Unfortunately, wristband errors do occur. A study conducted by the College of American Pathologists (CAP) identified six major types of wristband errors, as follows:

- Absent wristband
- Wrong wristband
- More than one wristband with different information
- Partially missing information on the wristband
- Erroneous information on the wristband
- Illegible information on the wristband

When the patient is unable to give his or her name, or when identification is attached to the bed or is missing, nursing personnel should be asked to identify the patient physically. Any variations in protocol should be noted on the test requisition. A CAP recommendation is that phlebotomists should refuse to collect blood from a patient when a wristband error is detected.

The current requirement for two patient identifiers usually includes the patient stating his or her full name and the date of birth. The name of the patient's physician should be verified to avoid any possible confusion when test results are sent to the ordering physician.

3. The patient should be asked if he or she is taking any medications, including over-the-counter medications such as aspirin. It is particularly important that patients inform personnel if they are taking an anticoagulant such as warfarin (Coumadin). When therapeutic drug levels are being determined, it is important to ask when the last dose of a medication was consumed.
4. Test requisitions should be checked and the appropriate evacuated tubes assembled. All specimens should be properly labeled immediately after the specimen is drawn. Prelabeling is unacceptable.
5. The patient's name, unique identification number, room number or clinic, and date and time of collection are usually found on the label. In some cases, labels must include the time of collection of the specimen and the type of specimen. A properly completed request form should accompany all specimens sent to the laboratory.

NOTE: Capillary blood collection is performed with a sterile, disposable lancet. These lancets should be properly discarded in a puncture-proof container after a single use.

Labels

Quality assessment policies are implemented in the clinical laboratory to protect the patient from any mistakes resulting from errors caused by an improperly handled specimen, beginning with the collection of that specimen. Laboratory quality assessment and accreditation require that specimens be properly labeled at the time of collection. All specimen containers must be labeled by the person doing the collection to ensure that the specimen was actually collected from the patient whose identification is on the label. Additional labeling requirements, such as a separate blood banking wristband and identification of the phlebotomist, are enforced for routine blood bank testing such as red cell grouping, Rh typing, and antibody screening.

An unlabeled container or one labeled improperly should not be accepted by the laboratory. Specimens are considered improperly labeled when there is incomplete or no patient identification on the tube or container holding the specimen. Many specimen containers are transported in leakproof plastic bags. It is unacceptable practice for only the plastic bags to be labeled; the container actually holding the specimen must be labeled as well. If the identification is illegible, the specimen is unacceptable. A specimen is also unacceptable if the specimen container identification does not match exactly the identification on the request form for that specimen.

Bar Codes

The AUTO12 system addresses location and orientation of bar code identifiers and bar code symbols. The U.S. Centers for Disease Control and Prevention identified use of bar codes as a best practice for reducing specimen identification errors. In many laboratories, labels are computer generated, which helps ensure that the proper identification information is included for each patient. Bar-coded labels facilitate this process. One automated computer system, the BD.id Patient Identification System, eliminates mislabeling because the system reads the patient's bar-coded wristband. The software indicates the tests, appropriate tubes, and quantity of tubes required for the patient, then generates bar-coded laboratory labels for tube identification at the patient's bedside. Each laboratory has a specific protocol for the handling of mislabeled or "unacceptable" specimens.

Clinical laboratory professionals developed the CLSI document "AUTO12-A, Specimen Labels: Content and Location, Fonts, and Label Orientation." The adoption of standardized bar-coded labels requires a small investment but subsequently becomes "the gift that goes on giving."[8] This investment provides a return in cost savings from a reduction in errors, a factor that is particularly important when laboratory budgets are shrinking. Mislabeling error rates in the United States have been reported to range from 0.1% to 5%.[9]

In the Laboratory Services category of the 2018 National Patient Safety Goals set by TJC,[10] the first goal is improving the accuracy in patient identification. This goal requires two identifiers on each patient specimen, with the directive that all specimens must be labeled in the presence of the patient. AUTO12 covers specimen labeling from the time of collection through all phases of laboratory processing and testing. Labeling errors most often can be divided into three categories: unlabeled, mislabeled, and mismatched specimen to requisition. All efforts should result in a decrease in labeling errors. The effect of these errors is significant in causing negative patient outcomes.

VENOUS BLOOD COLLECTION (PHLEBOTOMY)

Supplies and Equipment

The following is a list of supplies and equipment that will be needed in venipuncture (Student Procedure Worksheet 4.1):

- Test requisition

- Tourniquet and disposable gloves
- Sterile disposable needles and needle holder
- Various evacuated blood tubes
- Alcohol (70%) and gauze square or alcohol wipes
- Any special equipment
- Adhesive plastic strips

Special Blood Collection: Blood Cultures

A serious avoidable error is blood culture contamination. Contamination can cause false-positive results, diagnostic errors, and increased cost and length of hospitalization. The American Society for Microbiology (ASM) benchmark for contaminated cultures is no greater than 3%. The ASM recommends that two to four sets of blood cultures be collected. If only one specimen is positive, the physician can conclude that it is a contaminated culture. Reduction in contamination rate can be achieved if personnel are properly trained and managed. Some institutions have blood culture collection teams.

The ASM target rate or lower can be achieved by following a strict protocol for blood collection, banning repalpation of the venipuncture site, and avoiding drawing blood from an indwelling IV line. To prevent contamination, blood-drawing site preparation is the first step in the protocol.

The CLSI in its guidelines has discontinued the traditional technique of preparing the venipuncture site with a circular motion because it is not an evidence-based practice in infection control. An antiseptic such as alcohol, tincture of iodine, chlorhexidine, or povidone-iodine (Betadine) is left on the skin for 30 seconds of contact time to destroy bacteria. After preparation, the site must not be repalpated. If the phlebotomist must repalpate, the skin must be prepared as it was originally. A practice allowed by ASM guidelines is to apply antiseptic to the gloved finger before repalpating. Moreover, the venipuncture should enter the vein directly, not through an inserted IV line (see Chapter 15 for further discussion of blood culture collection and related topics).

Other special blood collection situations include timed blood collections, e.g., glucose tolerance testing or therapeutic drug testing. Patient symptoms can dictate the collection of blood smears in suspected malaria cases.

Special Site-Selection Situations

Five specific situations may result in a difficult venipuncture or may be sources of preanalytical error: IV lines, edema, scarring or burn patients, dialysis patients, and mastectomy patients.

Intravenous Lines

A limb with an IV line running should not be used for venipuncture because of contamination to the specimen. The patient's other arm or an alternate site should be selected.

Edema

Edema is the abnormal accumulation of fluid in the intracellular spaces of the tissue.

Scarring or Burn Patients

Veins are very difficult to palpate in areas with extensive scarring or burns. Alternate sites or capillary blood collection should be used.

Dialysis Patients

Blood should never be drawn from a vein in an arm with a cannula (temporary dialysis access device) or fistula (permanent surgical fusion of vein and artery). A trained staff member can draw blood from a cannula. The preferred venipuncture site is a hand vein or a vein away from the fistula on the underside of the arm.

Mastectomy Patients

If a mastectomy patient has had lymph nodes removed adjacent to the breast, venipuncture should not be performed on the same side as the mastectomy.

Phlebotomy Problems

Occasionally, a venipuncture is unsuccessful. Do not attempt to perform the venipuncture more than twice. If two attempts are unsuccessful, notify the phlebotomy supervisor. Problems encountered in phlebotomy can include the following:

1. Refusal by the patient to have blood drawn
2. Difficulty obtaining a specimen because the bore of the needle is against the wall of the vein or is going through the vein
3. Movement of the vein
4. Sudden movement by the patient or phlebotomist that causes the needle to come out of the arm prematurely
5. Needle angles that result in missing the vein
6. Problems with collapse of a vein
7. Hematoma that results from the needle bevel being halfway into the vein with the other half still in the tissue
8. Inadequate amount of blood in an evacuated tube
9. Fainting or illness subsequent to venipuncture

Phlebotomy Complications

Patients can experience complications resulting from a phlebotomy procedure. These complications can be divided into the following seven major categories:

1. **Vascular complications.** Bleeding from the site of the venipuncture and hematoma formation are the most common vascular complications.
2. **Infections.** The second most common complication of venipuncture is infection.
3. **Loss of consciousness or nausea and vomiting.** If patients lose consciousness, it is important to guard against a fall. An emergency protocol should be developed for these severe complications.
4. **Anemia.** Iatrogenic anemia is also known as *nosocomial anemia, physician-induced anemia,* or *anemia resulting from blood loss for testing.* This can be a particular problem with pediatric patients.
5. **Neurologic complications.** Postphlebotomy patients can exhibit some neurologic complications, including convulsions or pain.
6. **Cardiovascular complications.** Cardiovascular complications include orthostatic hypotension, syncope, shock, and cardiac arrest.
7. **Dermatologic complications.** The most common dermatologic consequence of phlebotomy is an allergic reaction to iodine in the case of blood donors.

SPECIMENS: GENERAL PREPARATION

Accurate chemical analysis of biological fluids depends on proper collection, preservation, and preparation of the sample, in addition to the technique and method of analysis used. The most quantitatively perfect determination is of no use if the specimen is not properly handled in the initial steps of the procedure.

Processing Blood Specimens

Blood specimens must be properly handled after collection. Blood samples should be analyzed as promptly as possible. Institutional protocol should be followed for conditions of storage (such as room temperature, refrigerated, or frozen), depending on the analyte to be measured. In general, specimens should be analyzed within 24 hours of collection. It is important that the proper evacuated tube be used, especially if a specimen is being analyzed for glucose, which requires a preservative.

If no anticoagulant is used, the blood will clot, and serum is obtained. The serum is then removed from the clot by centrifugation. To prevent excessive handling of biological fluids, many laboratory instrumentation systems can now use the serum directly from the centrifuged tube, without another separation step and without removing the stopper.

It is important to remove the plasma or serum from the remaining blood cells, or clot, as soon as possible. Because biological specimens are being handled, the need for certain safety precautions is stressed. The Standard Precautions policy should be used because all blood specimens should be considered infectious and must be handled with gloves. The outside of the tubes may be bloody, and initial laboratory handling of all specimens necessitates direct contact with the tubes.

To separate the serum and plasma from blood cells or a blood clot, tubes must have stoppers for centrifugation. When a stopper must be removed from the tube to obtain plasma or serum, it must be removed carefully and not popped off, because this could cause infection by inhalation or by contact of the infectious aerosol with mucous membranes. Stoppers should be twisted gently while being covered with protective gauze to minimize the risk from aerosolization. This processing step can be done using a protective plastic shield to prevent direct splashes.

It is generally best to test specimens as quickly as possible. Specimens should be processed to the point where they can be properly stored so that the constituents to be measured will not be altered. It must be guaranteed that specimens collected at stations away from the testing laboratory are delivered in less than 2 hours from collection, and that they have been stored properly, with refrigeration or freezing, if necessary. Testing laboratories provide specific instructions on the collection, processing, and delivery requirements for all assays that they perform.

Centrifuging the Specimens

After clotting has taken place, the tube is centrifuged with its cap on (Fig. 4.3). It is important to use Standard Precautions, which require all persons handling specimens to wear gloves. When necessary, stoppers must be carefully removed from blood collection tubes to prevent aerosolization of the specimen. Centrifuges must be covered and placed in a shielded area. When serum or plasma samples must be removed from the blood cells or clot, mechanical suction is used for pipetting, and all

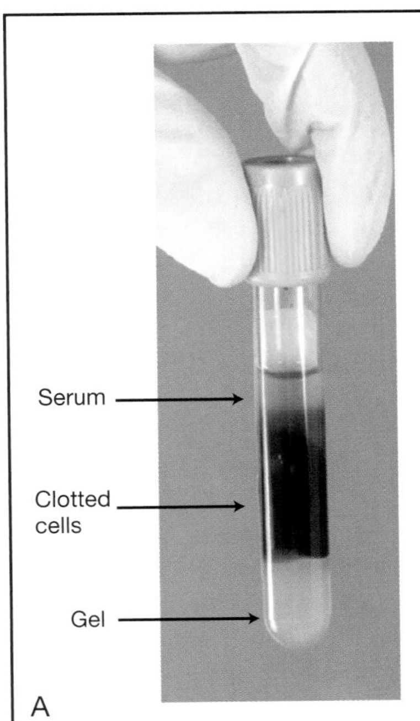

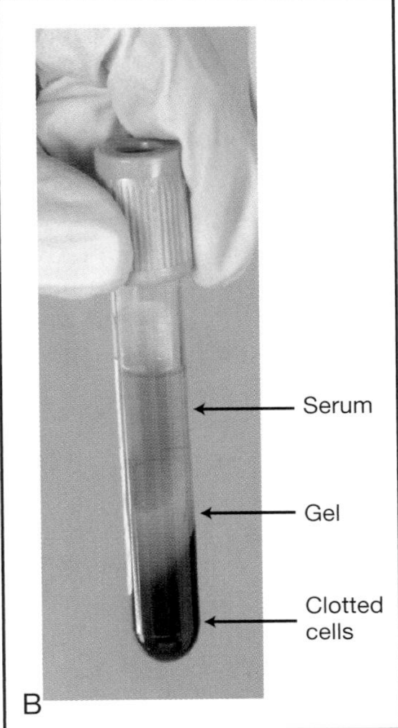

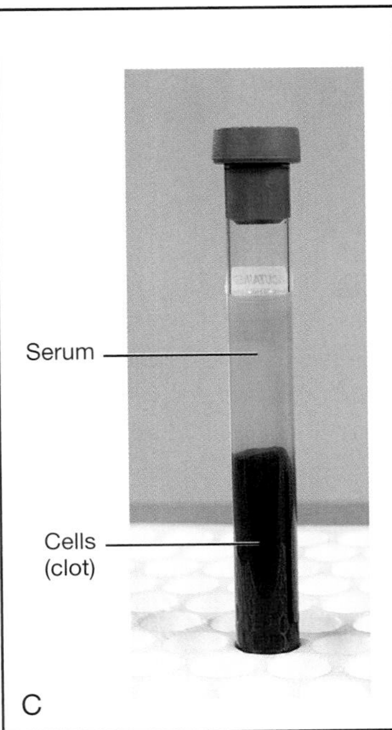

Fig. 4.3 (A) Gold serum separator tube centrifugation. Note the position of the gel on the bottom. (B) Gold serum separator tube after centrifugation. Note that the gel now separates the serum from the clotted cells. (C) Centrifuged red-topped "clot" tube with no gel or clotting additive. (Modified from Bonewit-West K: *Clinical procedures for medical assistants,* ed 6, Philadelphia, 2004, Saunders.)

specimen tubes and supplies must be discarded properly in biohazard containers.

With automated analyzers, the primary collection tube can often be used for the analysis itself. In these cases, the primary blood tube is centrifuged with its cap on, and the serum is aspirated directly into the analyzer.

Unacceptable Specimens

Various conditions render a blood specimen unsuitable for testing. Clotted specimens are not suitable for cell counts because the cells are trapped in the clot and cannot be counted. A cell count on a clotted sample will be falsely low.

Hemolyzed Specimens

Hemolysis in specimens is the most common cause of an abnormal appearance. Hemolyzed serum or plasma is unfit as a specimen for various assays, including coagulation testing and chemistry assays (such as potassium and hemoglobin measurements), blood banking, and immunology testing.

A specimen that is hemolyzed appears red (usually clear red) because the RBCs have been lysed and the hemoglobin has been released into the liquid portion of the blood. Often the cause of hemolysis in specimens is the technique used for venipuncture. A poor venipuncture with excessive trauma to the blood vessel can result in a hemolyzed specimen. Other causes include inappropriate needle bore size and contact with alcohol on the skin. Hemolysis of blood can also result from freezing, prolonged exposure to warmth, or the serum or plasma remaining on the cells too long before testing or removal to another tube. A determination of whether the hemolysis is in vitro or in vivo is also useful. Although relatively rare, in vivo hemolysis is a clinically significant finding.

Hemolyzed serum or plasma is unsuitable for several chemistry determinations because substances that are usually present within cells (such as potassium) can be released into the serum or plasma if the serum is left on the cells for a prolonged period. In addition, several other constituents, including the enzymes acid phosphatase, lactate dehydrogenase, and aspartate transaminase (or aminotransferase [AST]; formerly glutamic oxaloacetic transaminase), are present in large amounts in RBCs, so hemolysis of red cells will significantly elevate the value obtained for these substances in serum. Hemoglobin is released during hemolysis and may directly interfere with a reaction, or its color may interfere with photometric analysis of the specimen. The procedure to be performed should always be identified to determine whether abnormal-looking specimens can be used.

Icteric Specimens

Icteric (yellow) serum or plasma is another specimen with an abnormal appearance. When serum or plasma takes on an abnormal brownish-yellow color, there has most likely been an increase in bile pigments (i.e., bilirubin). Excessive intravascular destruction of RBCs, obstruction of the bile duct, or impairment of the liver leads to an accumulation of bile pigments in the blood, and the skin becomes yellow. Those performing clinical laboratory determinations should note any abnormal appearance of serum or plasma and record it on the report form. The abnormal color of the serum can interfere with photometric measurements.

Lipemic Specimens

Lipemic plasma or serum takes on a milky white color. The presence of lipid, or fats, in serum or plasma can cause this abnormal appearance. Often the lipemia results from collecting the blood from the patient too soon after a meal. Use of a lipemic serum specimen does not interfere with some laboratory determinations, but others may be affected (such as triglyceride assay and nephelometric assays).

Drug Effect on Specimens

Blood drawn from patients taking certain types of medication can result in invalid chemistry results for some constituents. Drugs can alter several chemical reactions and can affect laboratory results in two general ways:

1. Some action of the drug or its metabolite can cause an alteration (in vivo) in the concentration of the substance being measured.
2. Some physical or chemical property of the drug can alter the analysis directly (in vitro).

The number of drugs that affect laboratory measurements is increasing.

Logging and Reporting Processes

As part of the processing and handling of laboratory specimens, a careful, accurate logging and recording process must be in place in the laboratory, regardless of the size of the facility. A log sheet and a printed report form are vital to the operation of any laboratory. The log sheet documents on a daily basis the various patient specimens received in the laboratory. Log sheets and result reports are generated by laboratory information systems when used.

Items to be listed on the log sheet are the patient's name, identification number, type of specimen collected (description of the specimen and its source), date and time of specimen collection, and laboratory tests to be done. The log sheet should also indicate the time when the specimen arrived in the laboratory and may include a column for test results and the date when the tests are completed. Results can be documented by hand, by use of laboratory instrument–printed reports, or by computer printouts. The log sheet data are part of the permanent record of the laboratory and must be stored and available for future reference.

A printed report is often sent to the physician, with the vital data pertaining to the test results. Result reports are also available electronically in many facilities. The following information should be included in the report: patient's name, identification number, date and time of specimen collection, description and source of specimen, the initials of the person who collected the specimen, tests requested, the name of the physician requesting the tests, the test results, and the initials or signature of the person who performed the test. The fasting or nonfasting status of the patient, the name and time of the last dose of medication taken, and the appearance of a sample (such as icteric or hemolyzed) should be noted.

Much of this documentation of data is being done with the use of computerized laboratory information systems. Copies of this laboratory report may be sent to the medical records department and to the accounting office for patient billing purposes.

Preserving and Storing Specimens

Some chemical constituents change rapidly after the blood is removed from the vein. The best policy is to perform tests on fresh specimens. When the specimen must be preserved until the test can be done, there are ways to impede alteration. For example, NaF can be used to preserve blood glucose specimens because it prevents glycolysis.

With few exceptions, the lower the temperature, the greater the stability of the chemical constituents. Furthermore, the growth of bacteria is considerably inhibited by refrigeration and completely inhibited by freezing. Room temperature is generally considered to be 18°C to 30°C, refrigerator temperature about 4°C, and freezing about 5°C or less. Refrigeration is a simple and reliable means of impeding alterations, including bacteriologic action and glycolysis, although some changes still take place. Refrigerated specimens must be brought to room temperature before chemical analysis. Removing cells from plasma and serum is another means of preventing some changes. Some specimens needed for certain assays, such as bilirubin, must be shielded from the light or tested immediately. Bilirubin is a light-sensitive substance.

Serum or plasma may be preserved by freezing. Whole blood cannot be frozen satisfactorily because freezing ruptures the RBCs (hemolysis). Freezing preserves enzyme activities in serum and plasma. Serum and plasma freeze in layers with different concentrations, and therefore these specimens must be well mixed before use in a chemical determination.

If the results are to be meaningful, every precaution must be taken to preserve the chemical constituents in the specimen from the time of collection to testing in the laboratory. In general, tubes for collecting blood for chemical determinations do not need to be sterile, but tubes should be chemically clean. Serum is usually preferred to whole blood or plasma when the constituents to be measured are relatively evenly distributed between the intracellular and extracellular portions of the blood.

Storage of Processed Specimens

Sample stability may also depend on the type of tube used for blood collection (including any separation gels, anticoagulants, and other additives present), on the pretesting storage temperature, and on the laboratory method used for determination. Stability is particularly relevant in relation to hemostasis.

The mode of transporting samples to the laboratory may be relevant as well. Rapid sample delivery by pneumatic tube transportation is attractive for reducing transport times and is an acceptable method of sample transport for some types of laboratory tests. In cases such as blood gas measurement, however, at least some pneumatic transfer systems may be unsuitable.

The processing of individual serum or plasma tubes will depend on the analysis to be done and the time that will elapse before analysis. Serum or plasma may be kept at room temperature, refrigerated, frozen, or protected from light, depending on the circumstances and the determination to be done. Some specimens must be analyzed immediately after they reach the laboratory (such as blood gases, pH).

Blood specimens for hematology studies can be stored in the refrigerator for 2 hours before being used in testing. After storage, anticoagulated blood, serum, or plasma must be thoroughly mixed after it has reached room temperature.

There is no consensus on the stability of PT or APTT after collection in an appropriately filled 3.2% citrate tube. It is good practice to centrifuge the specimen as soon as it arrives in the laboratory, leaving the plasma on top of the cells, and to analyze the specimen promptly. CLSI[11] recommends that a PT test be completed within 24 hours from the time of collection if stored at room temperature, between 18°C and 24°C. Other investigators have reported that PT is stable for 24 hours if the plasma is stored at room temperature or on ice (4°C), although room-temperature storage for a maximum of 6 and 8 hours has been recommended by others.

As already noted, plasma and serum often can be frozen and preserved satisfactorily until a determination can be done, but whole blood cannot because RBCs rupture on freezing. Freezing preserves most chemical constituents in serum and plasma and provides a method of sample preservation for the laboratory. In general, refrigerating specimens impedes alterations of many constituents. With all biological specimens, however, preservation should be the exception rather than the rule. A laboratory determination is best done on a fresh specimen.

CAPILLARY OR PERIPHERAL BLOOD COLLECTION BY SKIN PUNCTURE

Capillary blood (see Fig. 4.4) can be used in a variety of testing locations and for a range of laboratory assays, including point-of-care testing (POCTs). Fingerprick POCT is ideal for limited-resource countries because of factors that include its simplicity and the low cost of supplies. Even in the United States, certain low-resource settings, including inner cities, drug clinics, and Native American reservations, benefit from an alternative to centralized laboratory testing. POCT also offers diabetic patients the benefit of in-home testing for glucose.

Because of the small sample size with capillary blood compared with venous blood, testing it presents some trade-offs, including the following:

- Accepting the inaccuracy of finger prick blood as a trade-off for easy blood collection,
- Collecting, reading, and averaging multiple drops to improve accuracy even if this requires more cost and time,
- If high accuracy is required, collecting and analyzing venous blood instead of capillary blood.

Blood Spot Collection for Neonatal Screening Programs

Most states have passed laws requiring that newborns be screened (see Fig. 4.5) for certain diseases that can result in serious abnormalities, including mental retardation, if they are

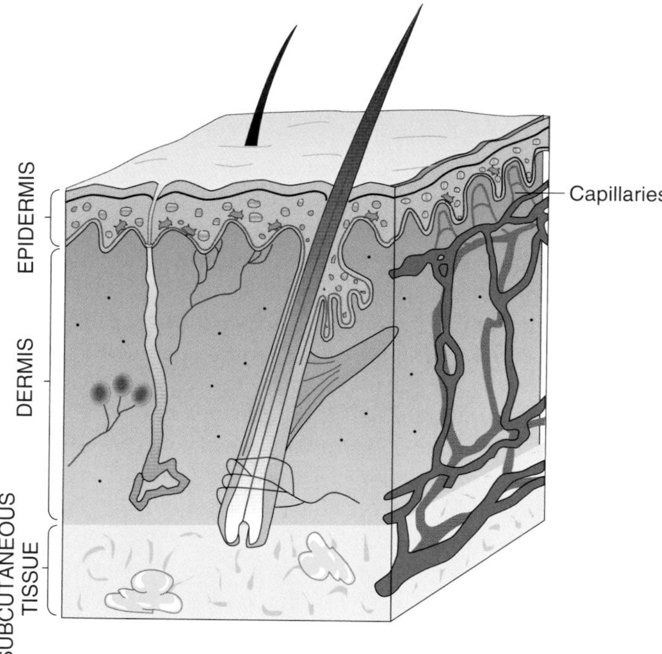

Fig. 4.4 The proper sites for capillary collection are those that provide an adequate capillary bed and sufficient clearance from underlying bone. (From VanMeter KC, Hubert RJ: *Gould's pathophysiology for the health professions,* ed 5, St Louis, Saunders, 2015. In Warekois RS, Robinson R: *Phlebotomy: worktext and procedures manual,* ed 4, St Louis, 2016, Saunders.)

not diagnosed and treated early. These diseases include phenylketonuria (PKU), galactosemia, hypothyroidism, and hemoglobinopathies. CLSI[12] has set standards for filter paper collection, or blood spot collection, of blood for these screening programs. Blood should be collected 1 to 3 days after birth, before the infant is discharged from the hospital, and at least 24 hours after birth and after ingestion of food for a valid PKU test. There is an increased chance of missing a positive test result when an infant is tested for PKU before 24 hours of age. When infants are discharged early, however, many physicians prefer to take a sample early rather than risk having no sample at all.

In most neonatal screening programs, the specimen is collected on filter paper and sent to the approved testing laboratory for analysis. Special collection cards with a filter paper portion are supplied by the testing laboratory; these are kept in the hospital nursery or central laboratory. These cards have a section where, as for any other request form, all information requested must be provided. The filter paper section of the card contains circles designed to identify the portion of the paper onto which the specimen should be placed, where the filter paper will properly absorb the amount of blood necessary for the test.

Collection is usually done by heel puncture following the accepted procedure for the institution. When a drop of blood is present, the circle on the filter paper is touched against the drop until the circle is completely filled. A sufficiently large drop should be formed so that the process of filling the circle can be done in only one step. The filter paper is allowed to air-dry and then is transported to the testing laboratory in a plastic transport bag or other acceptable container. The procedure established by the testing laboratory should be followed for the collection step.

Capillary Blood for Testing at the Bedside (Point-of-Care Testing)

Capillary blood samples for glucose testing and other assays are used frequently in many health care facilities for bedside testing, or POCT. Quantitative determinations for glucose are made available within 1 or 2 minutes, depending on the system employed.

Many diabetic outpatients also perform POCT for glucose at home by using their own blood and one of several glucose-measuring devices. It is important for diabetic patients, especially those with insulin-dependent diabetes mellitus, to monitor their own blood glucose levels several times a day and to be able to adjust their dosage of insulin accordingly to maintain good glucose control.

For the diabetic inpatient, POCT is also a valuable tool for diabetes management. The blood glucose level is often unstable in these patients, a situation that may necessitate frequent adjustments of insulin dosage. POCT provides results that are immediate, so dosages can be adjusted more quickly. Ordering and collecting venous blood specimens for glucose tests done by a central laboratory, with the necessary frequency and rapidity of reporting required, are often impractical, making POCT much more useful. Good quality control programs must be used to ascertain the reliability of the POCT results. Whole-blood samples should be collected by puncture from the heel (for infants only), finger, or flushed heparinized line, using policies for Standard Precautions. Arterial or venous blood should not be used unless the directions from the manufacturer of the POCT device specify the appropriateness of these alternative blood specimens. The POCT instrument should be calibrated and the test performed according to the manufacturer's directions. Results should be recorded permanently in the patient's medical record in a manner that distinguishes between bedside test results and central laboratory test results.

It is critical to understand and consider the specific limitations of each POCT detection system, as described by the manufacturer, so reliable results are obtained. A quality assessment program is mandatory to ensure reliable performance of these procedures. The use of POCT for measuring glucose in diabetic patients, whether bedside testing or self-testing, is intended for management only, not initial diagnosis. POCT is used only as a supplement, not to replace the standard laboratory tests for glucose.

Several commercial instruments are available, and with each product, a meter provides quantitative determination of glucose present when used with an accompanying reagent strip. A drop of capillary blood is touched to the reagent strip pad and, according to the specific procedure, read in the meter. The instrument provides an accurate and standardized reading when used according to the manufacturer's directions. The reagent strips must be handled with care and used within their proper shelf life. The strips are specific only for glucose. The meters are packaged in convenient carrying cases and are small enough to be placed in a pocket or briefcase.

DO NOT WRITE IN BLUE SHADED AREAS–DO NOT WRITE ON BARCODE

CC040H1088462C

ALL INFORMATION MUST BE PRINTED

Birthdate: [ ] [ ] [ ] MM/DD/YY Time [ ] [ ] (Use 24 hr time only)
Baby/s name: (last, first)
Hospital provider number: (mandatory)
Hospital name:
Mother's name: (last, first, Initial)
Mother's ID: Baby's ID:
Mother's address:
Mother's phone: ( ) -
Specimen date [ ] [ ] [ ] MM/DD/YY Time [ ] [ ] (Use 24 hr time only)
Physician's name:
Physician's address:
City: Ohio zip
Physician's phone: ( ) - ODH COPY
Physician's provider number: (mandatory)
ODH COPY: [ ] SPECIAL:

TEST RESULTS
[ ] Screening test normal for PKU, HOM, GAL, Hypothyroidism
[ ] Screening test normal for PKU and HOM only
[ ] Screening test normal
[ ] PKU [ ] HOM [ ] GAL
[ ] Hypothyroidism
[ ] Screening test abnormal
See footnote __________ on back
[ ] Specimen rejected for reason:

Baby sex: [ ] Male [ ] Female
Birth weight: grams
Premature: [ ] Yes [ ] No
Antibiotics: [ ] Yes [ ] No
Transfusion: [ ] Yes [ ] No
Specimen: [ ] First [ ] Second
Submittor: [ ] Hospital
[ ] Physician
[ ] Health department
[ ] Other (name below)

HEA 2518 __________

FILL ALL CIRCLES WITH BLOOD
BLOOD MUST SOAK COMPLETELY THROUGH
DO NOT APPLY BLOOD TO THIS SIDE

A

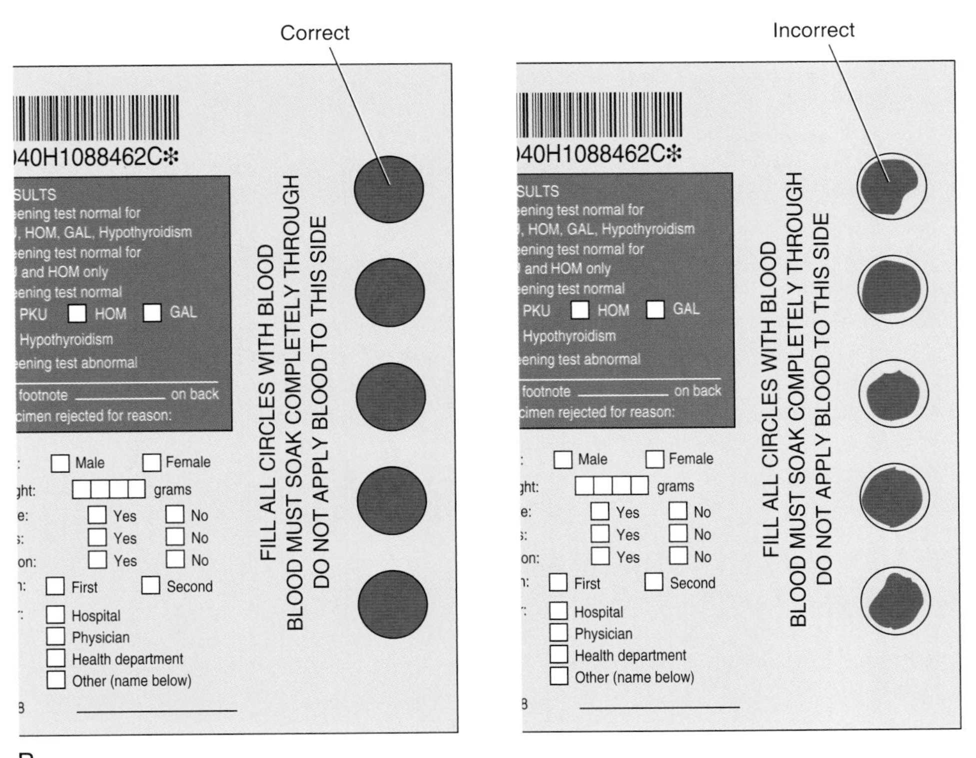

Fig. 4.5 Neonatal screening tests. (A) An example of filter paper used in neonatal screening. (B) Correct and incorrect ways to fill in the circles. (Modified from Bonewit-West K: *Clinical procedures for medical assistants,* ed 7, Philadelphia, 2008, Saunders.)

CAPILLARY BLOOD COLLECTION

Supplies and Equipment

The following is a list of supplies and equipment that will be needed in capillary blood collection (Student Procedure Worksheet 4.2):

- Alcohol (70%) and gauze squares or alcohol wipes
- Disposable gloves and sterile small gauze squares
- Sterile disposable blood lancets
- Equipment specific to the test ordered (such as glass slides for blood smears, micropipette and diluent for CBCs, and microhematocrit tubes)

Special Capillary Blood Collection

The BD Unopette collection system is no longer available, but equivalent products are manufactured by Bioanalytic GmbH. Now approved by the U.S. Food and Drug Administration (FDA), these products have been on the European market since 1978 (www.bioanalytic.de).

A product insert describes the collection and processing procedure used in special capillary blood collection.

Capillary Blood for Slides

To collect capillary blood for slides, a finger or heel puncture is made, and after the first drop is wiped away, the glass slide is touched to the second drop formed. The slide is placed on a flat surface, and a spreader slide is used to prepare the smear (see Chapter 11). After being allowed to air-dry, the slide is properly labeled and transported to the laboratory for examination.

Collecting Microspecimens

At times, only a small amount of capillary blood can be collected (Box 4.3), and many laboratory determinations have been devised for testing small amounts of sample. In general, the same procedure is followed as for any other drawing of capillary blood. For chemistry procedures, blood can be collected in a capillary tube or in microcontainers (Figs. 4.6–4.8) by touching the tip of the tube to a large drop of blood while the tube is held in a slightly downward position. The blood enters the collection unit by capillary action. Several tubes can be filled from a single skin puncture, if needed. Tubes are capped and brought to the laboratory for testing. Careful centrifugation technique must be used if serum is needed. Microcontainers are available with various additives, including serum separator gels (Table 4.6).

BOX 4.3 Order of Draw for Capillary Specimens

1. Blood gases
2. Ethylenediaminetetraacetate tubes
3. Other additive minicontainers
4. Serum

Order of draw for capillary blood collection is different from blood specimens drawn by venipuncture.

From Clinical and Laboratory Standards Institute: *Procedures and devices for the collection of diagnostic blood specimen by skin puncture: approved standard,* ed 6, Wayne, Pa, 2008, H4-A6.

BD Diagnostics: Lab Notes 20(1):2, 2009, Becton Dickinson.

NOTE: If multiple specimens are collected by heelstick or fingerstick puncture (capillary blood collection), anticoagulant tubes must be collected first to avoid the formation of tiny clots resulting from prolonged collection time. Blood gases should be collected first if the phlebotomy team is responsible for collection of these specimens.

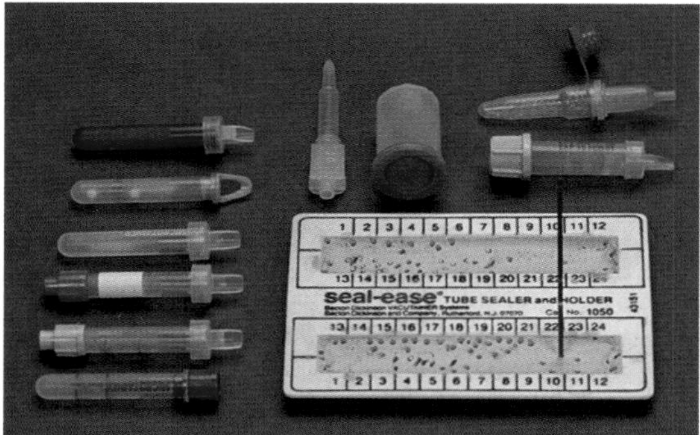

Fig. 4.6 Microtainer tube system. (From Warekois RS, Robinson R: *Phlebotomy: worktext and procedures manual,* ed 3, St Louis, 2012, Elsevier/Saunders.)

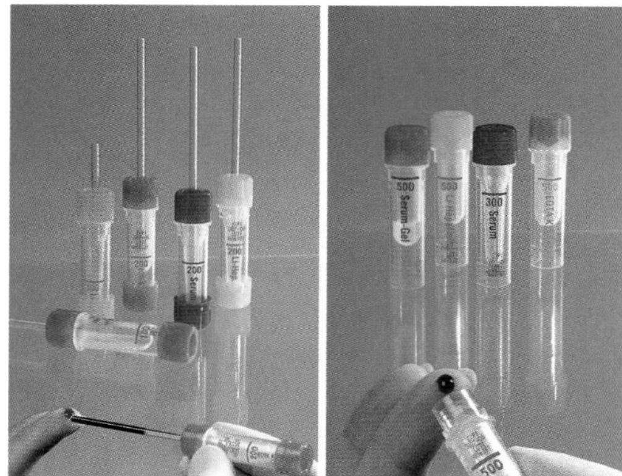

Fig. 4.7 Microvette® capillary blood collection system. (Courtesy Sarstedt Inc., Newton, NC.)

TABLE 4.6 Order of Draw for BD Microtainer Tubes With BD Microgard Closure

Order	Closure Color	Additive	Mix by Inverting
1	Lavender	K_3EDTA	10×
2	Green	Lithium heparin	10×
3	Mint green	Lithium heparin and gel for plasma separation	10×
4	Gray	NaF	
	Na_2EDTA	10×	
5	Gold	Clot activator and gel for serum separation	5×
6	Red	No additive	0×

K_3EDTA, Tripotassium ethylenediaminetetraacetate; *Na_2EDTA,* disodium ethylenediaminetetraacetate; *NaF,* sodium fluoride.

NOTE: Hold tube upright, gently invert 180 degrees and back, and repeat movement as recommended. If not mixed properly, tubes with anticoagulants will clot and specimen often will need to be recollected.

Modified From BD Diagnostics: *LabNotes* 20(1):7, 2009, Becton Dickinson.

Laser Equipment

Laser technology is the first radical change in phlebotomy in more than 100 years. Revolutionary devices received approval from the FDA in 1997. The Lasette (Cell Robotics, Albuquerque, New Mexico) and the Laser Lancet (Transmedica International, Little Rock, Arkansas) can draw blood without the use of sharp objects (Fig. 4.8).

A laser device emits a pulse of light energy that lasts a fraction of a second. The laser concentrates on a very small portion of skin, literally vaporizing the tissue about 1 to 2 mm to the capillary bed. The device can draw a 100-μL blood sample, a sufficient amount for certain tests. The laser process is less painful and heals faster than when blood is drawn with traditional lancets. The patient feels a sensation more like heat than the prick of a sharp object.

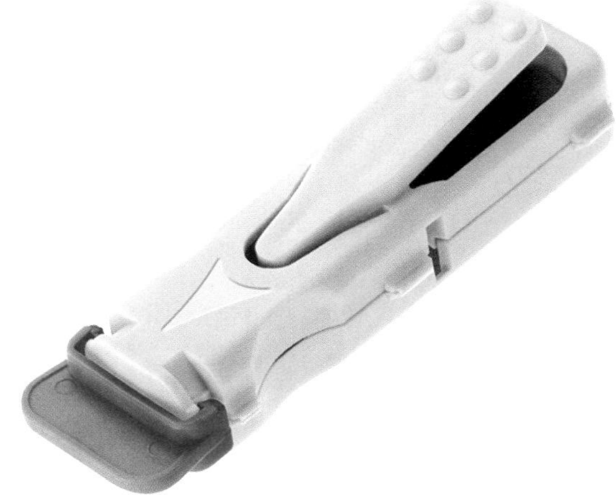

Fig. 4.8 OneTouch lancing device. (Courtesy LifeScan, Milpitas, CA.)

CASE STUDIES

CASE STUDY 4.1

Sarah works as a phlebotomist in a local hospital. Her neighbor John Englant shows up to have his blood drawn. Because Sarah knows him, she glances at the specimen labels she's been given, but does not notice the labels say *England, John.* Sarah proceeds with the venipuncture procedure. First, she dons her gloves and visually inspects both arms. She applies the tourniquet, finds a site, and cleanses it with 70% alcohol. Next, Sarah inserts the needle into the skin and draws blood into a lavender-top tube. As soon as blood flows into the tube, Sarah releases the tourniquet and removes the needle once the tube is full. She applies pressure to the site with a gauze pad, mixes the tube, and labels the tube as required by the laboratory.

1. What adverse outcome is the most probable as a result of this venipuncture procedure?
   a. Infection
   b. incorrect results
   c. Hematoma
   d. Blood loss
2. A second error occurred during this procedure. What was it?
   a. Patient was subjected to unnecessary pain.
   b. Phlebotomist did not wear gloves.
   c. The wrong anticoagulant tube was drawn.
   d. The tourniquet was removed prematurely.

Critical Thinking Group Discussion Questions

1. How could the patient have had a better experience?
2. How can the errors that occured in this case be avoided in the future?

Note: Narrative answers are posted on the instructor EVOLVE website.

CASE STUDY 4.2

Andy is working second shift, and it is almost time for him to go home. He goes into a patient's room to perform a routine venipuncture for a chemistry profile, which requires a green top. Andy properly identifies the patient and assembles all the necessary equipment. Next, he inspects both arms and thinks he has a good vein within the antecubital area of the right arm. He applies the tourniquet and inserts the needle into the skin and draws blood into a green-top tube. As soon as blood flows into the tube, Andy releases the tourniquet and removes the needle once the tube is full. He applies pressure to the site with a gauze pad, mixes the tube, and labels the tube as required by the laboratory.

1. What adverse outcome is the most probable as a result of this venipuncture procedure?
   a. Infection
   b. incorrect results
   c. Hematoma
   d. Blood loss
2. A second error occurred during this procedure. What was it?
   a. Patient was subjected to unnecessary pain.
   b. Phlebotomist did not wear gloves.
   c. The wrong anticoagulant tube was drawn.
   d. The tourniquet was removed prematurely.

Critical Thinking Group Discussion Questions

1. How could the patient have had a better experience?
2. How can the errors that occured in this case be avoided in the future?

Note: Narrative answers are posted on the instructor EVOLVE website.

CASE STUDY 4.3

Meg has been performing venipunctures all day, and her tray is depleted of supplies. She decides to draw one more patient before she takes a break, so she calls back the next patient and asks him to take a seat. Meg notices she is out of regular venipuncture needles, but she does have a butterfly needle available. The order is for a CBC. Meg dons her gloves and visually inspects both arms. She applies the tourniquet just above the patient's wrist, finds a site in his hand, and cleanses it with 70% alcohol. Next, Meg inserts the needle into the skin and draws blood into a purple-top tube. Meg removes the needle once the tube is full and applies pressure to the site with a gauze pad, but forgets to remove the tourniquet. As she mixes the tube and prepares to label it as required by the laboratory, the patient points out that the tourniquet is still on his arm.

1. What potential adverse outcome may occur as a result of this venipuncture procedure?
   a. Infection
   b. Incorrect results
   c. Hematoma
   d. Bruising of the skin
2. A second error occurred during this procedure. What was it?
   a. Patient was subjected to unnecessary pain.
   b. Phlebotomist did not wear gloves.
   c. The wrong tube was drawn.
   d. The wrong venipuncture site was chosen.

Critical Thinking Group Discussion Questions

1. How could the patient have had a better experience?
2. How can the errors that occured in this case be avoided in the future?

Note: Narrative answers are posted on the instructor EVOLVE website.

REFERENCES

1. Carraro P, Plebani M: Errors in a state laboratory: types and frequencies 10 years later, *Clin Chem* 53:1338–1342, 2007.
2. American Hospital Association: Patient care partnership. www.aha.org (Accessed January 2014).
3. Ogden-Grable H: *Phlebotomy A to Z: using critical thinking and making ethical decisions, Chicago,* 2008, American Society for Clinical Pathology.
4. Clinical and Laboratory Standards Institute: *Procedures and devices for the collection of diagnostic capillary blood specimens,* ed 6, Pa, 2008, Wayne. GP42.
5. Clinical and Laboratory Standards Institute: *Tubes and additives for venous and capillary blood specimen collection,* ed 6, Pa, 2010, Wayne. GP39.
6. Bush V, Cohen R: The evolution of blood collection tubes, *Lab Med* 34:304–310, 2003.
7. Tosini W, Ciotti C, et al: Needlestick injury rates according to different types of safety-engineered devices: rsult of a French multicienter study, *Infect Control Hosp Epidemiol* 31(4):402–407, 2010.
8. Michel R: Standard bar code labels can reduce lab errors, The Dark Report, *May* 6, 2013.
9. Hawker CD: Bar codes may have poorer error rates than commonly believed, *Clin Chem* 56(10):1513–1514, 2010.
10. The Joint Commission 2018 Laboratory National Patient Safety Goals, www.jointcommission.org. (Accessed June 30, 2018).
11. Clinical and Laboratory Standards Institute: *Collection of diagnostic venous blood specimens,* ed 7, Pa, 2017, Wayne. GP-41.
12. Clinical and Laboratory Standards Institute: *Blood collection on filter paper for newborn screening programs,* ed 6, Pa, 2013, Wayne. NBS01.

BIBLIOGRAPHY

Armstrong M: Blood sample processing: clinical perspectives on recent developments in technology and laboratory operations, *Lab Med* 43:8–10, 2012.

Bond MM, Richards-Kortum RR: Drop-to-drop variation in the cellular components of fingerprick blood: implications for point-of-care diagnostic development, *Am J Pathol* 144(6):885–894, 2015.

Bostic G, Thompson R, Atanasoski S, et al: Quality Improvement in the Coagulation Laboratory: Reducing the Number of Insufficient Blood Draw Specimens for Coagulation Testing, *Lab Medicine* 46(4):347–355, 2015.

Burtis CA, Ashwood ER, editors: *Tietz fundamentals of clinical chemistry,* ed 6, St Louis, 2008, Elsevier/Saunders.

Bush V: Why doesn't my heparinized plasma specimen remain anticoagulated? *Lab Notes* 13(2):9–10, 2003.

Bush V, Mangan L: The hemolyzed specimen: causes, effects and reduction, *Lab Notes* 13(1):1–5, 2003.

CLSI: *Essential Elements of a Phlebotomy Training Program 1st edition. CLSI Guideline GP48,* Wayne, PA, 2017, Clinical Laboratory Standards Institute.

Clinical Laboratory Standards Institute (CLSI): Laboratory Quality Control Based on Risk Management, EP23, 1st Edition, 2011.

COLA: Troubleshooting recurring problems with hemolyzed blood specimens, *MLO Med Lab Obs* 49(2):3, 2017.

Dale JC: Phlebotomy complications. In *Paper presented at Mayo Laboratory's Phlebotomy Conference, Boston,* 1996. August.

Daugherty K: Best practices in phlebotomy, *MLO Med Lab Obs* 44(4):20–22, 2012.

Duesman K, Duncan RJ: Safer sharps in a dangerous world, *MLO Med Lab Obs* 44(12):30–33, 2012.

DeLong C: The future of fingerprick testing, *CLN Clin Lab News* 43(11):8–10, 2016.

Faber V: Phlebotomy and the aging patient, *Adv Med Lab Prof* 29:24, 1998.

Forbes BA, Sahm DF, Weissfeld A: *Bailey & Scott's diagnostic microbiology,* ed 12, St Louis, 2007, Elsevier/Mosby.

Foubister V: Quick on the draw: coagulation tube response, *CAP Today* 16:38, 2002.

Gerberding JL: Occupational exposure to HIV in health care settings, *N Engl J Med* 348:826, 2003.

Haraden L: Pediatric phlebotomy: great expectations, *Adv Med Lab Prof* 28:12, 1997.

Hawker CD: Lab guidelines & standards: what constitutes a correctly labeled specimen? *Lab Med* 42(10):630, 2011.

Hurley TR: Considerations for the pediatric and geriatric patient. In *Paper presented at Mayo Laboratory's Phlebotomy Conference, Boston.* 1996. August.

Latshaw J: Laser takes sting out of phlebotomy, *Adv Med Lab Prof* 28:40, 1997.

Lee F, Lind N: *Isolation guidelines.* www.infectioncontroltoday.com/articles/051col5.html (Accessed May 2005).

Magee LS: Preanalytical variables in the chemistry laboratory, *Lab Notes* 15(1):1–4, 2005.

Norberg A, et al: Contamination rates of blood cultures obtained by dedicated phlebotomy vs intravenous catheter, *JAMA* 289:726, 2003.

Occupational Safety and Health Administration, US Department of Labor: *Disposal of contaminated needles and blood tube holders used in phlebotomy, Safety and Health Information Bulletin.* www.osha.gov/dts/shib/shib101503.html. (Accessed May 2005).

Occupational Safety and Health Administration, US Department of Labor: *Best practice: OSHA's position on the reuse of blood collection tube holders, Safety and Health Information Bulletin.* www.osha.gov/dts/shib/shib101503.html. (Accessed May 2005).

Ogden-Grable H, Gill GW: Preventing phlebotomy errors: potential for harming your patients, *Lab Med* 36:430, 2005.

Seaver C, Gray AJ: Drawing extra blood tubes in the ED: re-examining a common practice, *MLO Med Lab Obs* 44(12):38–40, 2012.

Sidhu D, Naugler C: Fasting time and lipid levels in a community-based population: a cross-sectional study, https://doi.org/10.1001/archinternmed.2012.3708, 2012.

Turgeon M: *Clinical hematology: theory and procedures,* ed 6, Philadelphia, 2018, Lippincott Williams & Wilkins, p 18.

Understanding additives: heparin, *Lab Notes* 14(1):7, 2004. (Accessed May 2005). www.bd.com/vacutainer/labnotes/2004winterspring/additives_heparin.asp.

REVIEW QUESTIONS (ANSWERS IN APPENDIX A)

Quality Assessment

1. One of the top five causes of a Pre-Phlebotomy preanalytical errors is:
   a. Improperly filled blood collection tube
   b. Patient incorrectly identified
   c. Hemolysis
   d. All the above

Infection Control

2. Which transmission-based infection control precaution stops direct spread of bacteria by touching?
   a. Contact precautions
   b. Airborne precautions
   c. Droplet precautions
   d. Standard Precautions
3. Which transmission-based infection control precaution stops agents dispersed by talking, coughing, or sneezing?
   a. Contact precautions
   b. Airborne precautions
   c. Droplet precautions
   d. Standard Precautions
4. Which transmission-based infection control precaution provides protection from dust particles?
   a. Contact precautions
   b. Airborne precautions
   c. Droplet precautions
   d. Standard Precautions

Specimen Collection

5. When the coagulation of fresh whole blood is prevented through the use of an anticoagulant, the straw-colored fluid that can be separated from the cellular elements is:
   a. Serum
   b. Plasma
   c. Whole blood
   d. Platelets
6. Which characteristic is inaccurate with respect to the anticoagulant dipotassium ethylenediaminetetraacetic acid (K_2EDTA)?
   a. Removes ionized calcium (Ca^{2+}) from fresh whole blood by the process of chelation
   b. Is used for most routine coagulation studies
   c. Is the most often used anticoagulant in hematology
   d. Is conventionally placed in lavender-stoppered evacuated tubes
7. Heparin inhibits the clotting of fresh whole blood by neutralizing the effect of:
   a. Platelets
   b. Ionized calcium (Ca^{2+})
   c. Fibrinogen
   d. Thrombin

Questions 8 through 11: Fill in the blanks with the correct letters to the colors below.

8. An evacuated tube with EDTA has a ________________ colored stopper.
9. An evacuated tube with heparin has a ________________ colored stopper.
10. An evacuated tube with sodium citrate has a ________________ colored stopper.
11. An evacuated tube with no anticoagulant has a ________________ colored stopper.
   a. Red
   b. Lavender
   c. Blue
   d. Green

Venous Blood Collection (Phlebotomy)

12. The first category of steps in performing a venipuncture includes:
    a. Selecting an appropriate site and preparing the site.
    b. Identifying the patient, checking test requisitions, assembling equipment, washing hands, and putting on clean gloves.
    c. Removing the tourniquet, removing the needle, applying pressure to the site, and labeling all tubes.
    d. Introducing yourself and briefly explaining the procedure to the patient.
13. The second category of steps in performing a venipuncture includes:
    a. Selecting an appropriate site and preparing the site.
    b. Identifying the patient, checking test requisitions, assembling equipment, washing hands, and putting on gloves.
    c. Removing the tourniquet, removing the needle, applying pressure to the site, and labeling all tubes.
    d. Introducing yourself and briefly explaining the procedure to the patient.

14. The third category of steps in performing a venipuncture includes:
    a. Selecting an appropriate site and preparing the site.
    b. Identifying the patient, checking test requisitions, assembling equipment, washing hands, and putting on gloves.
    c. Removing the tourniquet, removing the needle, applying pressure to the site, and labeling all tubes.
    d. Introduce yourself and briefly explain the procedure to the patient.
15. The fourth of five steps in performing a venipuncture includes:
    a. Selecting an appropriate site and preparing the site.
    b. Identifying the patient, checking test requisitions, assembling equipment, washing hands, and putting on gloves.
    c. Removing the tourniquet, removing the needle, applying pressure to the site, and labeling all tubes.
    d. Reapplying the tourniquet and performing the venipuncture.
16. The final category of steps in performing a venipuncture includes:
    a. Selecting an appropriate site and preparing the site.
    b. Identifying the patient, checking test requisitions, assembling equipment, washing hands, and putting on gloves.
    c. Removing the tourniquet, removing the needle, applying pressure to the site, and labeling all tubes.
    d. Reapplying the tourniquet and performing the venipuncture.
17. The appropriate veins for performing a routine venipuncture are the:
    a. Cephalic, basilic, and median cubital
    b. Subclavian, iliac, and femoral
    c. Brachiocephalic, jugular, and popliteal
    d. Saphenous, suprarenal, and tibial
18. A blood sample is needed from a patient with intravenous (IV) fluid lines running in one arm. Which of the following is an acceptable procedure?
    a. Any obtainable vein is satisfactory.
    b. Disconnect the IV line.
    c. Obtain sample from the other arm.
    d. Do not draw a blood specimen from this patient.
19. How should the bevel of the needle be held during a venipuncture?
    a. Sideways
    b. Upward
    c. Downward
    d. In any direction
20. A hematoma can form if:
    a. Improper pressure is applied to a site after the venipuncture.
    b. The patient suddenly moves, and the needle comes out of the vein.
    c. The needle punctures both walls of the vein.
    d. All the above.
21. Phlebotomy problems can include:
    a. The use of improper anticoagulants
    b. Misidentification of patients
    c. Inadequate filling of an evacuated tube containing anticoagulant
    d. All the above

Specimens: General Preparation

22. Blood specimens are unacceptable for laboratory testing when:
    a. There is no patient name or identification number on the label.
    b. The label on the request form and the label on the collection container do not match.
    c. The wrong collection tube has been used (for example, anticoagulant additive instead of tube for serum).
    d. All the above.
23. If serum is allowed to remain on the clot for a prolonged period, which of the following effects will be noted?
    a. Elevated level of serum potassium
    b. Decreased level of serum potassium
    c. Elevated level of glucose
    d. None of the above
24. A red-pink appearance of serum/plasma can be caused by:
    a. Elevated bilirubin (jaundice; icteric serum)
    b. Lysis of red blood cells (hemolyzed serum)
    c. Presence of lipids or fat (lipemic serum)
    d. Dehydration
25. A dark-yellow appearance of serum/plasma can be caused by:
    a. Elevated bilirubin (jaundice; icteric serum)
    b. Lysis of red blood cells (hemolyzed serum)
    c. Presence of lipids or fat (lipemic serum)
    d. Dehydration
26. A milky white appearance of serum/plasma can be a result of:
    a. Elevated bilirubin (jaundice; icteric serum)
    b. Lysis of red blood cells (hemolyzed serum)
    c. Presence of lipids or fat (lipemic serum)
    d. Dehydration

Capillary or Peripheral Blood Collection

27. Which of the following area(s) is (are) acceptable for the collection of capillary blood from an infant?
    a. Previous puncture site
    b. Posterior curve of the heel
    c. The arch
    d. Medial or lateral plantar surface
28. The proper collection of capillary blood includes:
    a. Wiping away the first drop of blood
    b. Occasionally wiping the site with a plain gauze pad to avoid the buildup of platelets
    c. Avoiding the introduction of air bubbles into the column of blood in a capillary collection tube
    d. All the above

Turgeon: Linné & Ringsrud's Clinical Laboratory Science, 8th Edition

STUDENT PROCEDURE WORKSHEET 4-1

Venipuncture: Evacuated Tube Technique

See Chapter 4 of *Linné & Ringsrud's Clinical Laboratory Science: Concepts, Procedures, and Clinical Applications,* 8th edition, for a complete discussion of this procedure.

Student Learning Outcomes

After reading Chapter 4, and at the completion of this laboratory exercise and the review questions, the student will be able to:

- Correctly perform a venipuncture.
- Complete the end-of-procedure review questions with a grade of 80% or higher.

Reagents, Supplies, and Equipment

1. Test requisition
2. Tourniquet
3. Disposable gloves
4. Sterile disposable safety needle in needle holder
5. Various evacuated blood collection tubes
6. Alcohol (70%) disposable prep pads or alcohol and sterile gauze squares
7. Adhesive plastic strips
8. *Optional:* Model practice arm

Instructions for the Procedure

Read the list of required equipment and supplies and the procedural steps. Follow the procedural steps in exact order.

SEQUENCE	PROCEDURAL STEP	INSTRUCTOR-OBSERVED ACCEPTABLE PERFORMANCE (CHECK IF ACCEPTABLE)
Initiation of the Venipuncture Procedure		
1	Properly identify the patient. Ask patient to spell his or her name. See General Protocol, #2.	
2	Assemble all necessary equipment and evacuated tubes at the patient's bedside.	
3	Put on disposable gloves using proper technique (see Fig. 2-4).	
4	The plastic shield on a needle is to remain on the needle until immediately before the venipuncture.	
5	The evacuated tube is placed into the holder and gently pushed until the top of the stopper reaches the guideline on the holder. Do not push the tube all the way into the holder, or a loss of vacuum will result.	
Selection of an Appropriate Site Obtaining a blood specimen from an intravenous (IV) line should be avoided because it increases the risk of mixing the fluid with the blood sample and producing incorrect test results.		
6	Visually inspect both arms. Choose a site that has not been repeatedly used for phlebotomy. In the arm, three veins are typically used for venipuncture: the cephalic, basilic, and median cubital (Fig. 4.9).	

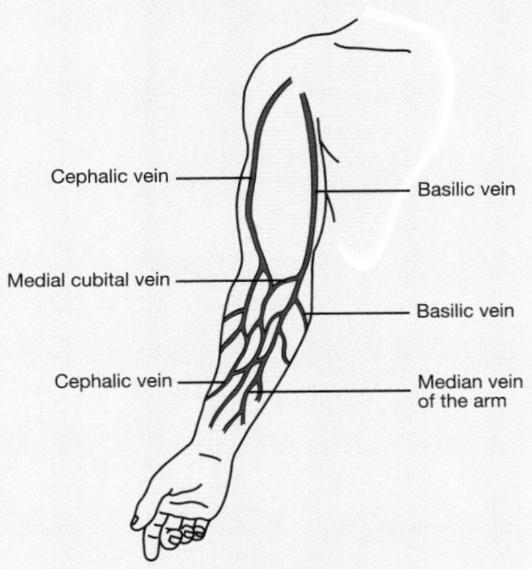

Fig. 4.9 Anatomy of major veins of the arm.

(Continued)

Turgeon: Linné & Ringsrud's Clinical Laboratory Science, 8th Edition

STUDENT PROCEDURE WORKSHEET 4-1

SEQUENCE	PROCEDURAL STEP	INSTRUCTOR-OBSERVED ACCEPTABLE PERFORMANCE (CHECK IF ACCEPTABLE)
7	Apply the tourniquet (Fig. 4.10). Do not leave the tourniquet on for more than 1 minute. Prolonged tourniquet application can elevate certain blood chemistry analytes, including albumin, aspartate transaminase (AST), calcium, cholesterol, iron, lipids, total bilirubin, and total protein.	

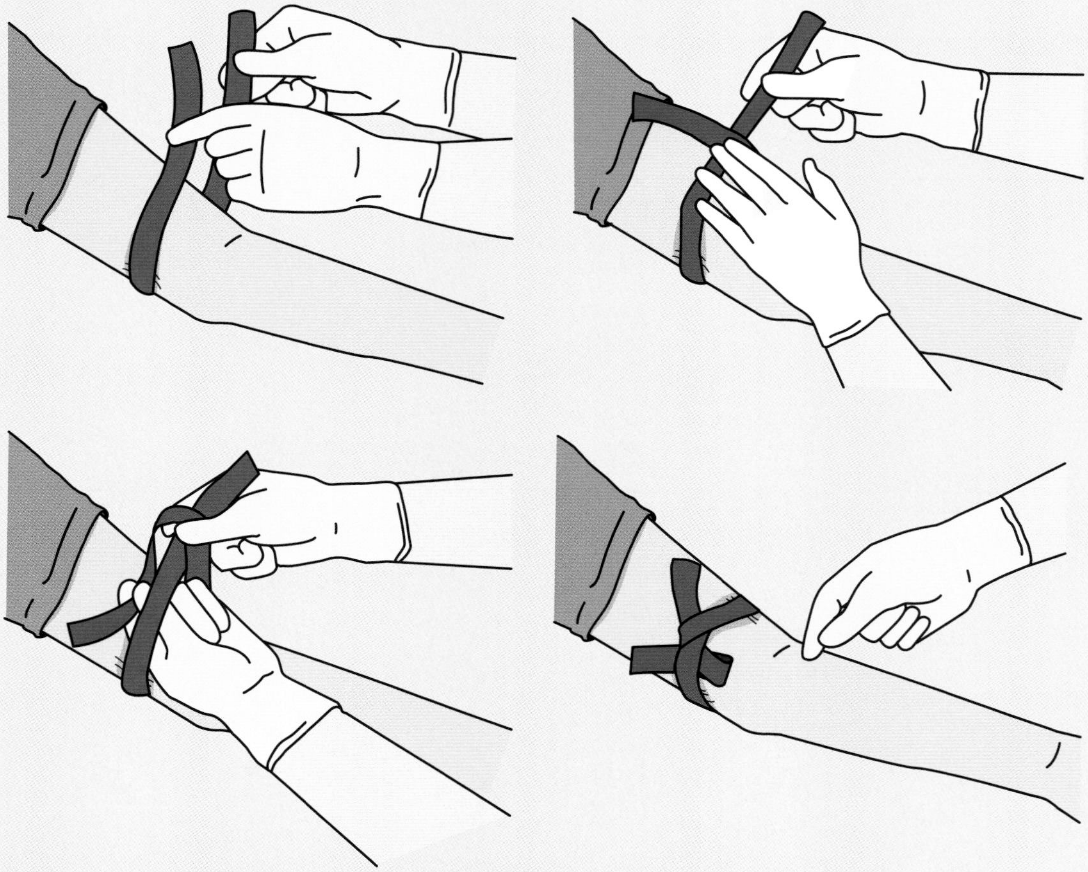

Fig. 4.10 Selection of appropriate venipuncture site.

SEQUENCE	PROCEDURAL STEP	INSTRUCTOR-OBSERVED ACCEPTABLE PERFORMANCE (CHECK IF ACCEPTABLE)
8	To make the veins more prominent, ask the patient to make a fist. With the index finger, palpate (feel) for an appropriate vein. The ideal site is generally near or slightly below the bend in the arm.	
Preparation of the Venipuncture Site		
9	After an appropriate site has been chosen, release the tourniquet.	

(Continued)

Turgeon: Linné & Ringsrud's Clinical Laboratory Science, 8th Edition

STUDENT PROCEDURE WORKSHEET 4-1

SEQUENCE	PROCEDURAL STEP	INSTRUCTOR-OBSERVED ACCEPTABLE PERFORMANCE (CHECK IF ACCEPTABLE)
10	Using an alcohol pad saturated with 70% alcohol, cleanse the skin in the area of the venipuncture site. Using a circular motion, clean the area from the center and move outward. Do not go back over any area of the skin once it has been cleansed.	
11	Allow the site to air-dry.	
Performing the Venipuncture Avoid touching the cleansed venipuncture site.		
12	Use one hand to hold the evacuated tube assembly. Position the patient's arm in a slightly downward position. Use one finger or thumb of the opposite hand to secure the skin area of the forearm below the intended venipuncture site. This will tighten the skin and secure the vein.	
13	Hold the safety needle with attached holder about 1 to 2 inches below and in a straight line with the intended venipuncture site. Position the blood-drawing unit at an angle of about 20 degrees. The bevel of the needle should be upward (Fig. 4.11).	

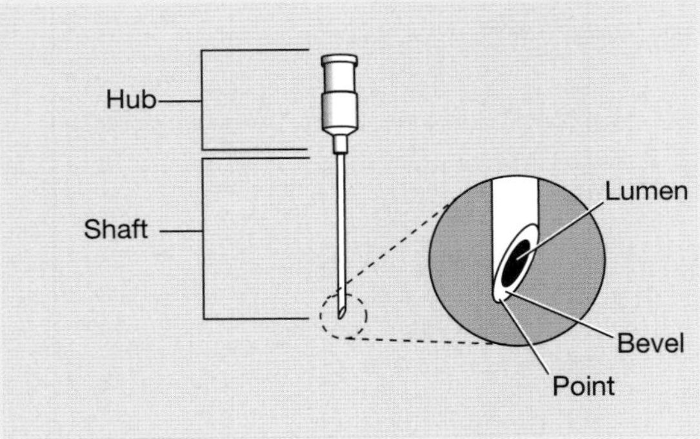

Fig. 4.11 Parts of a needle.

SEQUENCE	PROCEDURAL STEP	INSTRUCTOR-OBSERVED ACCEPTABLE PERFORMANCE (CHECK IF ACCEPTABLE)
14	Insert the needle through the skin and into the vein. This insertion motion should be smooth. One hand should steady the needle holder unit while the other hand pushes the tube to the end of the plastic holder. It is important to hold the needle steady during the phlebotomy to avoid interrupting the flow of blood.	
15	Multiple samples can be drawn by inserting each additional tube as soon as the tube attached to the needle holder has filled.	
16	If required, gently invert tubes with anticoagulant or additive to mix.	
Termination of the Procedure		
17	The tourniquet can be released as soon as the blood begins to flow into the evacuated tube or syringe or immediately before the final amount of blood is drawn.	
18	Ask the patient to open the hand.	

(Continued)

Turgeon: Linné & Ringsrud's Clinical Laboratory Science, 8th Edition

STUDENT PROCEDURE WORKSHEET 4-1

SEQUENCE	PROCEDURAL STEP	INSTRUCTOR-OBSERVED ACCEPTABLE PERFORMANCE (CHECK IF ACCEPTABLE)
19	Withdraw the blood-collecting unit with one hand, and immediately press down on the gauze pad with the other hand after the desired amount of blood has been drawn.	
20	If possible, have the patient elevate the entire arm and press on the gauze pad with the opposite hand. If the patient is unable to do this, apply pressure until bleeding ceases.	
21	Place a nonallergenic adhesive spot or strip over the venipuncture site. Failure to apply sufficient pressure to the venipuncture site could result in a hematoma (a collection of blood under the skin that produces a bruise).	
22	Mix tubes with anticoagulant by inverting the tubes several times (see manufacturer's requirements in Table 4-5). Do not shake the tubes. Discard the used equipment into an appropriate sharps puncture-proof container.	
23	Label all test tubes as required by the laboratory.	
24	Clean up supplies from the work area and phlebotomy tray, remove gloves (see Fig. 2-4 for correct method of glove removal), dispose of them in a biohazard container, and wash hands (see Chapter 2).	
25	If the patient is an outpatient, wait a few minutes after the venipuncture is complete, and check to be sure the patient does not feel dizzy or nauseated before discharge. Disinfect the work area.	

(From Warekois RS, Robinson R: *Phlebotomy: worktext and procedures manual*, ed 3, St Louis, 2012, Saunders.)

(Continued)

Turgeon: Linné & Ringsrud's Clinical Laboratory Science, 8th Edition

STUDENT PROCEDURE WORKSHEET 4-1

Venipuncture: Evacuated Tube Technique

Review Questions

1. How would you select an appropriate vein for a venipuncture procedure?

2. What is the proper order of draw for evacuated blood collection tubes?

3. Why is it important to gently mix evacuated blood tubes with anticoagulants or additives?

Procedural Evaluation

Student's Name ______________________________ Grade__________

Instructor's Signature ___________________________ Date__________

Comments:

Turgeon: Linné & Ringsrud's Clinical Laboratory Science, 8th Edition

STUDENT PROCEDURE WORKSHEET 4-2

Blood Collection: Capillary Puncture

See Chapter 4 of *Linné & Ringsrud's Clinical Laboratory Science: Concepts, Procedures, and Clinical Applications,* 8th edition, for a complete discussion of this procedure.

Student Learning Outcomes

After reading Chapter 4, and at the completion of this laboratory exercise and the review questions, the student will be able to:

- Correctly perform a capillary puncture.
- Complete the end-of-procedure review questions with a grade of 80% or higher.

Reagents, Supplies, and Equipment

1. Test requisition
2. Disposable gloves
3. Sterile disposable blood lancets
4. Alcohol (70%) disposable prep pads
5. Sterile gauze squares
6. Adhesive plastic strips
7. Equipment specific for the test ordered: glass slides for blood smears, microhematocrit tubes, microcollection vials
8. *Optional:* Practice model of foot

Instructions for the Procedure

Read the list of required equipment and supplies and the procedural steps. Follow the procedural steps in exact order.

SEQUENCE	PROCEDURAL STEP	INSTRUCTOR-OBSERVED ACCEPTABLE PERFORMANCE (CHECK IF ACCEPTABLE)
1	Assemble equipment and supplies.	
2	Wash your hands and put on gloves and eye protection as directed.	
Selection of an Appropriate Site		
3	Usually the fingertip of the third or fourth finger, and the heel are appropriate sites for the collection of small quantities of capillary blood. The earlobe may be used as a site of last resort in adults. NOTE: Do not puncture the skin through previous sites, which may be infected. The plantar surface (sole) of the heel is an appropriate site in infants or in special cases such as burn victims. The ideal site in infants is the medial or lateral plantar surface of the heel, with a puncture no deeper than 2 mm beneath the plantar heel skin surface and no more than half this distance at the posterior curve of the heel (Fig. 4.12). CLSI recommendations are *not* to use fingers of infants. The back of the heel should never be used because of the danger of injuring the heel bone, cartilage, and nerves in this area. **Fig. 4.12 Sites for heel puncture in infants.** (From Warekois RS, Robinson R: *Phlebotomy: worktext and procedures manual,* ed 4, St Louis, 2016, Saunders.)	

(Continued)

Turgeon: Linné & Ringsrud's Clinical Laboratory Science, 8th Edition

STUDENT PROCEDURE WORKSHEET 4-2

SEQUENCE	PROCEDURAL STEP	INSTRUCTOR-OBSERVED ACCEPTABLE PERFORMANCE (CHECK IF ACCEPTABLE)
4	The site of blood collection must be warm to ensure the free flow of blood.	
Preparation of the Site		
5	Hold the area to be punctured with the thumb and index finger of a gloved hand.	
6	Wipe the area with a 70% alcohol pad and allow to air-dry.	
7	Wipe the area with a dry gauze square. If the area is not dry, the blood will not form a rounded drop and will be difficult to collect.	
Puncturing the Skin		
8	Use a disposable sterile lancet once, and discard it properly in a puncture-proof container.	
9	Securely hold the area, and puncture once (perpendicular) with a firm motion (Fig. 4.13). NOTE: The incision must be perpendicular to the fingerprint or heelprint.	
10	Wipe away the first drop of blood, because the first drop of blood is mixed with lymphatic fluid and possibly alcohol.	
11	Apply gentle pressure to the area to obtain a suitable specimen.	
12	Discard used lancets in a sharps container and discard gauze and other contaminated supplies into a red bag biohazard container.	
13	Remove gloves and discard into biohazard container.	
14	Wash hands using proper procedure. *Optional:* Clean any unused equipment and return to proper storage. If procedure is not performed bedside, clean work area with disinfectant solution.	

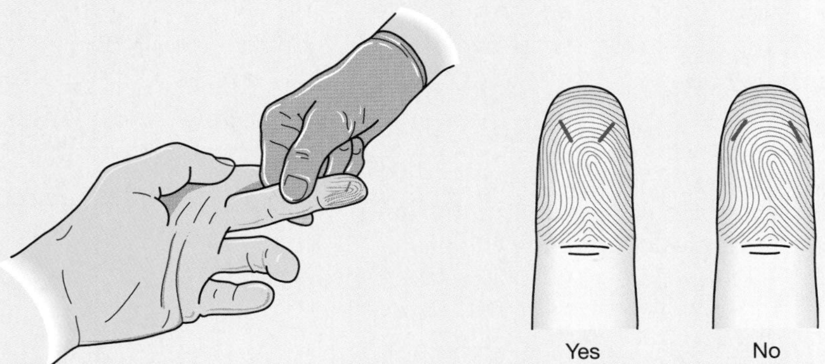

Fig. 4.13 Sites for finger puncture. (From Warekois RS, Robinson R: *Phlebotomy: worktext and procedures manual,* ed 4, St Louis, 2016, Saunders.)

(Continued)

Turgeon: Linné & Ringsrud's Clinical Laboratory Science, 8th Edition

STUDENT PROCEDURE WORKSHEET 4-2

Review Questions

1. Describe appropriate sites for collection of capillary blood.

2. Why is the first drop of blood wiped away from the puncture site?

3. If a baby's heel feels cold, what can you do to promote blood circulation in the foot?

Procedural Evaluation

Student's Name ______________________________ Grade__________

Instructor's Signature __________________________ Date__________

Comments:

5

The Microscope

http://evolve.elsevier.com/Turgeon/clinicallab/

CHAPTER OUTLINE

LEARNING OUTCOMES

Description
- Define the terms *numerical aperture* and *resolution.*

Parts of the Microscope
- Compare the magnification strengths and applications of low-power, high-power, and oil-immersion lenses.
- Identify the parts of the microscope.
- Name and explain the components of the illumination and magnification systems of a microscope.
- Define *parfocal,* and describe how it is used in microscopy.
- Correlate various positions of the microscope condenser with different types of objectives.

Care and Cleaning of the Microscope
- Describe the proper cleaning of a microscope.

Use of the Microscope
- Define alignment, and describe the process of aligning a microscope.
- Explain the procedure for correct light adjustment to obtain maximum resolution with sufficient contrast.
- Arrange the required steps in focusing the microscope to examine a slide specimen.
- Prioritize the steps required to troubleshoot problems with using the microscope.

Other Types of Microscopes (Illumination Systems)
- Name the components of a phase-contrast microscope, and explain how they differ from the components of a brightfield microscope.
- Identify the components of the compensated polarized microscope, and describe their locations and functions.
- Compare and differentiate darkfield, fluorescence, and electron microscopy.

Digital Microscopy
- Describe the function and applications of artificial neural networks.

Review Questions
- Demonstrate comprehension of the chapter content by completing the end-of-chapter review questions with a grade of 80% or higher.

Note:
- indicates MLT and MLS core content

❖ indicates MLT (optional) and MLS advanced content

KEY TERMS

artificial neural network (ANN)	diopter adjustment	ocular
body tube	electron microscopy	parcentric
brightfield illumination	fluorescence microscopy	parfocal
condenser	focal length	phase-contrast microscopy
confocal	interpupillary distance	polarized light microscopy
darkfield microscopy	magnification	resolution
diaphragm	microscope objectives	working distance
digital microscopy	numerical aperture (NA)	

The microscope is probably the piece of equipment that receives the most use (and misuse) in the clinical laboratory. Microscopy is a basic part of the work in many areas of the laboratory, including hematology, urinalysis, and microbiology. Because the microscope is a precision instrument and such an important piece of equipment, it must be kept in excellent condition, optically and mechanically. It must be kept clean, and it must be kept aligned.

DESCRIPTION

In simple terms, a microscope is a magnifying glass. The compound light microscope, or the brightfield microscope—the type used in most clinical laboratories—consists of two magnifying lenses, the objective, and the eyepiece (ocular). It is used to magnify an object to a point where it can be seen with the human eye.

The total magnification observed is the product of the magnifications of these two lenses. In other words, the magnification of the objective times the magnification of the ocular equals the total magnification. For example, the total magnification of an object seen with a 10 × ocular and a 10 × objective is 100 times (100 ×). Magnification units are in terms of diameters, so 10 × means the diameter of an object is magnified to 10 times its original size. The object itself or its area is not magnified 10 times; only the diameter of the object is magnified.

Because of the manner in which light travels through the compound microscope, the image seen is upside down and reversed. The right side appears as the left, the top as the bottom, and vice versa. Keep this in mind when moving the slide (or object) that is being observed.

As with magnification, resolution is a basic term in microscopy. Resolution indicates how small and how close individual objects (dots) can be and still be recognizable. Practically, the resolving power is the limit of usable magnification. Further magnification of two dots that are no longer resolvable would be "empty magnification" and would result in a dumbbell appearance, as shown in Fig. 5.1.

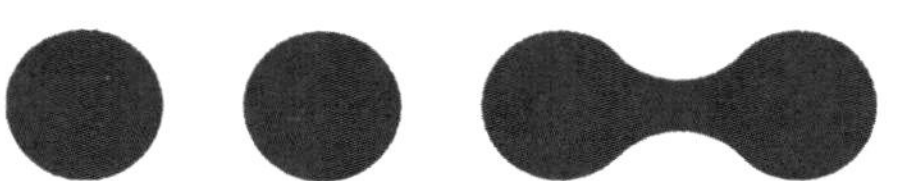

Fig. 5.1 Resolution versus empty magnification.

The relative resolving powers of the human eye, the light microscope, and the electron microscope are as follows (nm = nanometer; mm = millimeter; m = meter):

Human eye

0.25 mm 0.25×10^3 m 0.00025 m

Light microscope

0.25 mm 0.25×10^6 m 0.00000025 m

Electron microscope

0.5 nm 0.5×10^9 m 0.0000000005 m

Another term encountered in microscopy is numerical aperture (NA). The light-gathering ability of a microscope objective is quantitatively expressed in terms of the NA, which is a measure of the number of highly diffracted image-forming light rays captured by the objective. Higher NA values allow increasingly oblique rays to enter the objective front lens, producing a more highly resolved image.

As the NA increases, objects can be positioned closer and still be distinguished from each other; that is, the greater the NA, the greater the resolving power of a lens. Any particular lens has a constant-rated NA, and this value depends on the radius of the lens and its focal length—the distance from the object being viewed to the lens or the objective—but decreasing the amount of light passing through a lens will decrease the actual NA. The importance of this becomes apparent in the later discussion of proper light adjustments with the microscope. The magnification and NA are inscribed on each lens as a number (Table 5.1).

PARTS OF THE MICROSCOPE

The structures basic to all types of compound microscopes fall into four main categories[1–3] (Fig. 5.2):

1. Framework
2. Illumination system
3. Magnification system
4. Focusing system

TABLE 5.1 Typical Numerical Aperture Values

Magnification	Term	Numerical Aperture value
4 ×	Scanning	0.1
10 ×	Low power	0.25
40 ×	High power	0.65
100 ×	Oil immersion	1.25

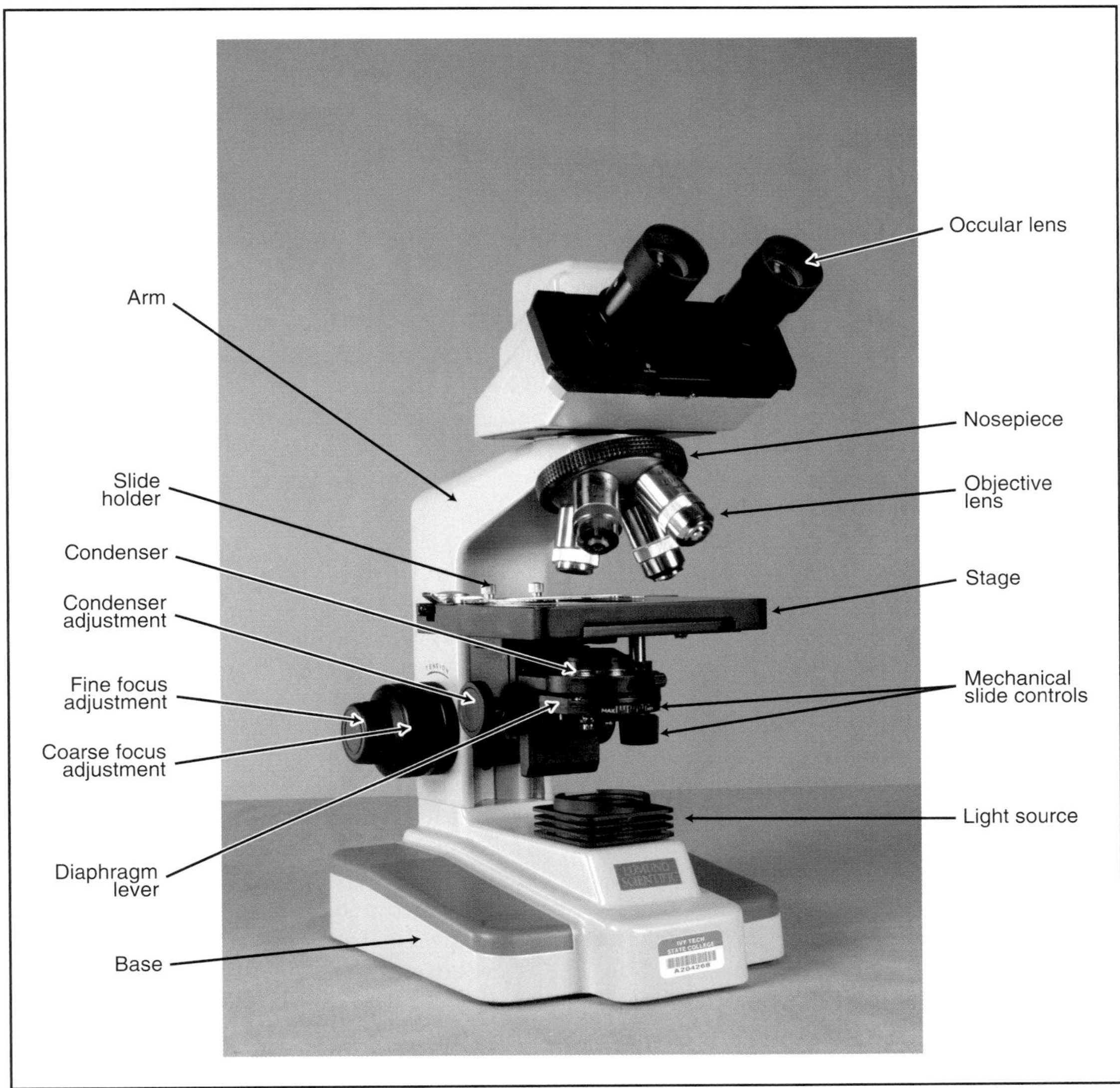

Fig. 5.2 Parts of the binocular microscope. (Courtesy Zack Bent; from Garrels M, Oatis CS: *Laboratory testing for ambulatory settings: a guide for health care professionals,* Philadelphia, 2006, Saunders.)

Framework

The framework of the microscope consists of several units. The *base* is a firm, horseshoe-shaped foot on which the microscope rests. The *arm* is the structure that supports the magnifying and adjusting systems. The arm is also the handle by which the microscope can be carried without damaging the delicate parts. The *stage* is the horizontal platform, or shelf, on which the object being observed is placed. Most microscopes have a mechanical stage, making it much easier to manipulate the object being observed.

Illumination System

Good microscope work cannot be accomplished without proper illumination. The illumination system is an important part of the compound light microscope. **Brightfield illumination** is the common type of illumination for general laboratory work. Different illumination techniques or systems are useful in special applications in the clinical laboratory and include the following:

1. Phase contrast
2. Interference contrast
3. Polarized and compensated polarized
4. Fluorescence
5. Darkfield
6. Electron

The illumination system begins with a source of light. The clinical microscope most often has a built-in light source (or bulb). The bulb is turned on with an on/off switch (or in some cases by a rheostat, which turns on the bulb and adjusts the intensity of the light). The light intensity is controlled by a rheostat, dimmer switch, or slide, ensuring both adequate illumination and comfort for the microscopist. When there is a separate on/off switch, to lengthen the life of the bulb, the light intensity should be lowered before the bulb is turned off. The light source is located at the base of the microscope, and the light is directed upward. It is important that the bulb be positioned correctly for proper alignment of the microscope. Proper alignment means that the parts of the microscope are adjusted so that the light path from the source of light through the microscope and the ocular is physically correct. Microscopes are designed such that the light bulb filament is centered when the bulb is installed properly. Many styles or types of bulbs are available, generally tungsten or tungsten-halogen, and it is important that the bulb designed for a particular microscope is used.

Condenser

Another part of the illumination system is the condenser. Microscopes generally use a substage *Abbé-type condenser.* The condenser directs and focuses the beam of light from the bulb onto the material under examination. Suitable for *Köhler illumination,* the Abbé condenser is a lens system that is conical with the point planed off (it actually consists of two lenses) (Fig. 5.3). The condenser position is adjustable; it can be raised and lowered beneath the stage by means of an adjustment knob on the side of the microscope. It must be appropriately positioned while focusing on the image of the field diaphragm to focus the light correctly on the material being viewed. When it is correctly positioned, the image field is evenly lighted.

When the microscope is properly used, the apparent NA of the condenser should be equal to or slightly less than the rated NA of the objective being used. The apparent or actual NA of the condenser can be varied by changing its position; as it is lowered, the apparent NA is reduced. To maximize the light focus and the resolving power of the microscope, the condenser position must be adjusted with each objective used. When the apparent NA of the condenser is decreased to below that of the rated NA of the objective, contrast and depth of field are gained and resolution is lost. This manipulation is often necessary in the clinical laboratory when wet, unstained preparations are being observed, such as urine sediment. In this case to gain contrast when a specimen is being scanned, the condenser is lowered (or the aperture iris diaphragm partially closed), thus reducing the apparent NA of the condenser. Preferably, the condenser should be left in a generally uppermost position, at most only 1 or 2 mm below the specimen, and the light adjusted primarily by opening or closing the aperture iris diaphragm located in the condenser. The practice of "racking down" the condenser when one is looking at wet preparations is not acceptable.

Some microscopes are equipped with a condenser element that is used in place for low-power work and that swings out for high power. Other models employ an element that swings out for low-power work and is used in place for higher magnification. This changes the apparent NA of the condenser, matching it with that of the objective. Other illumination systems employ different types of condensers, such as phase-contrast, differential interference-contrast (DIC), and darkfield condensers.

Aperture Iris Diaphragm

The aperture iris diaphragm also controls the amount of light passing through the material under observation. It is located at the bottom of the condenser, under the lenses but within the condenser body, as seen in Fig. 5.4. This aperture diaphragm consists of a series of horizontally arranged interlocking plates with a central aperture. It can be opened or closed as necessary to adjust the intensity of the light by means of a lever or dial. The size of the aperture, and consequently the amount of light permitted to pass, is regulated by the microscopist. Such regulation of the light affects the apparent NA of the condenser, decreasing the size of the field under observation, with the iris diaphragm decreasing the apparent NA of the condenser. Thus proper illumination techniques involve a combination of proper light intensity regulation, condenser position, and field-size regulation.

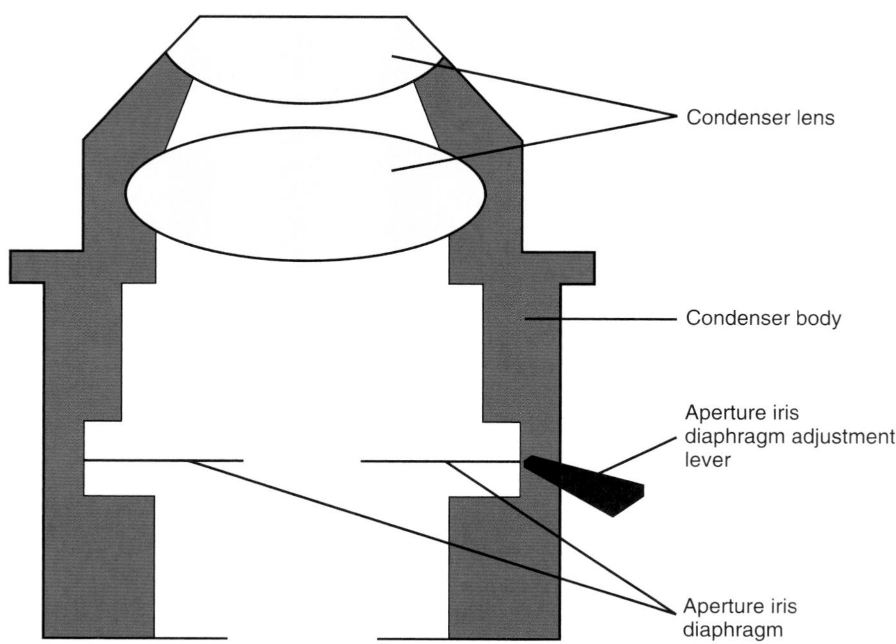

Fig. 5.3 Abbé-type substage condenser with aperture iris diaphragm.

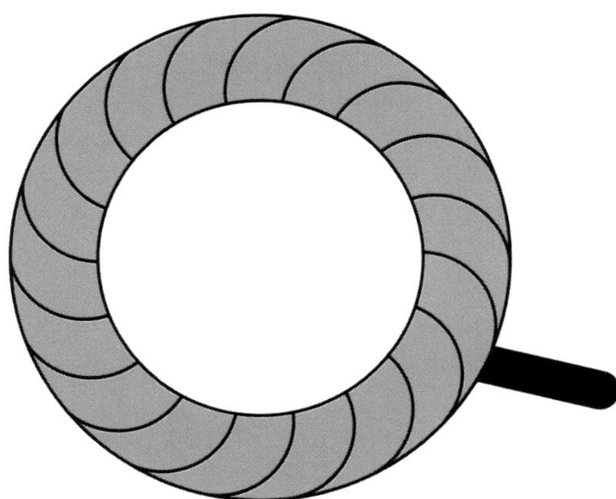

Fig. 5.4 Aperture iris diaphragm. By opening or closing the aperture iris diaphragm, more or less light is let into the field of view.

Field Diaphragm

Better microscopes have a field iris diaphragm, located in the light port in the base of the microscope, through which light passes up to the condenser. The field diaphragm controls the area of the circle of light in the field of view when the specimen and condenser have been properly focused. It is also used in the alignment of the microscope.

Magnification System

The magnification system contains several important parts. It plays an extremely important role in the use of the microscope.

Ocular (Eyepiece)

The ocular, or eyepiece, is a lens that magnifies the image formed by the objective. The usual magnification of the ocular is 10 (10 ×); however, 5 × and 20 × oculars are generally also available. Most microscopes have two oculars and are called *binocular microscopes.* Some microscopes have only one ocular and are called *monocular microscopes.* The magnification produced by the ocular, when multiplied by the magnification produced by the objective, gives the total magnification of the object being viewed. The distance between the two oculars (interpupillary distance) is adjustable, as is the focus on one of the oculars (diopter adjustment).

Objectives

Microscope objectives are probably the most important components of an optical microscope. Objectives are responsible for primary image formation and play a central role in determining the quality of images the microscope is capable of producing. Objectives are also instrumental in determining the magnification of a particular specimen and the resolution under which fine specimen detail can be observed in the microscope.

Three critical design characteristics of the objective set the ultimate resolution limit of the microscope. These include the wavelength of light used to illuminate the specimen, the angular aperture of the light cone captured by the objective, and the refractive index in the object space between the objective front lens and the specimen.

TABLE 5.2 Passage of Light Through the Microscope

Sequence	Equipment	Description
1	Lamp condenser	Lens projects an image of the light source onto the plane of the condenser diaphragm.
2	Substage lens system	Once the light has passed through the lamp condenser and the field diaphragm, it passes through the condenser aperture and lens system below the specimen stage. The substage condenser functions to concentrate the light onto the specimen.
3	Objective lens	Most important lens of the microscope lens system. Function of objective lens is to gather light passing through a specimen and to project an image into the body tube. This is the beginning of the magnification process.
4	Ocular lens (eyepiece)	The eyepiece magnifies the virtual image created by the objective lens a second time and creates a virtual image that can be seen as if viewed close to the eye.

Light passing through the condenser is organized into a cone of illumination that emanates onto the specimen and then is transmitted into the objective front lens element as a reversed cone (Table 5.2). The size and shape of the illumination cone is a function of the combined NAs of the objective and condenser.

When a manufacturer's set of matched objectives, such as all achromatic objectives of various magnifications, are mounted on the nosepiece, they are usually designed to project an image to approximately the same plane in the body tube. Thus changing objectives by rotating the nosepiece usually requires only minimal use of the fine-adjustment knob to reestablish sharp focus. Such a set of objectives is described as being parfocal, a useful convenience and safety feature. Matched sets of objectives are also designed to be parcentric, so that a specimen centered in the field of view for one objective remains centered when the nosepiece is rotated to bring another objective into use.

Objective lenses are inscribed with certain information, including type of lens, magnification, rated NA, body tube length, and coverglass thickness or requirement for immersion oil. Most microscopes have three, or sometimes four, objectives. With three objectives, the magnifying powers are 10 ×, 40 ×, and 100 ×. The objectives are mounted on the nosepiece, which pivots to enable a quick change of objectives.

Objectives are described or rated according to focal length, which is inscribed on the outside of the objective. Microscopes used in the clinical laboratory most often have 16-mm, 4-mm, and 1.8-mm objectives. The focal length is a physical property of the objective lens and is slightly less than the distance from the object being examined to the center of the objective lens. Practically speaking, the focal length of a lens is very close in value to the working distance, the distance from the bottom of the objective to the material being studied. The greater the magnifying power of a lens, the smaller is the focal length and thus the working distance. This becomes very important when the microscope is being used, because the working distance is very short for the 40 × (4-mm) and 100 × (1.8-mm) objectives. For this reason, correct focusing habits are necessary to prevent damaging the objectives against the slide on the stage.

Achromatic and Planachromatic Objectives. Generally, two types of objectives are available in clinical microscopes: achromats and planachromats. The least expensive and most common objectives used on most laboratory microscopes are the achromatic objectives, which correct for color (chromatic) aberrations. Although achromats are adequate for most laboratory work, the center of the field of view will be in sharp focus, but the edges appear out of focus, and the field does not appear to be flat. Achromatic objectives yield their best results with light passed through a green filter (often an interference filter). The lack of correction for flatness of field further hampers achromat objectives.

Most manufacturers provide flat-field corrections for achromat objectives and call these corrected objectives planachromats. Planachromatic objectives, although more expensive, are more appropriate for high-magnification work using a 40 × or 100 × objective, because the field of view is in focus and flat throughout.

Apochromatic objectives also are available. This type of objective corrects for chromatic and spherical aberrations. These are the finest lenses available and may be necessary for photomicroscopy. Because these are significantly more expensive, however, apochromats are unnecessary for routine laboratory microscopy (Table 5.3).

Low-Power Objective. The low-power objective is usually a 10 × lens with a 16-mm working distance. This objective is used for the initial scanning and observation in most microscope work. For example, blood films and urine sediment are routinely examined using the low-power objective first. This is also the lens employed for the initial focusing and light adjustment of the microscope. Some routine microscopes also have a very-low-power 4 × magnification lens. This is used in the initial scanning in the morphologic examination of histologic sections.

A term often used in discussing microscopes is *parfocal,* which means that if one objective is in focus and a change is made to another objective, the focus will not be lost. Thus if the microscope is focused under low power and then changed to the high-power or oil-immersion objective (by rotating the nosepiece), it will still be in focus, except for fine adjustment.

The rated NA of the low-power objective is significantly less than that of the condenser on most microscopes; for the 10 × objective, the NA is approximately 0.25; for the condenser, it is approximately 0.85. To achieve focus, the NAs must be more closely matched by reducing the light to the specimen. This is done by focusing or lowering the condenser slightly (1 or 2 mm below the specimen) and then reducing the size of the field of light to about 70% to 80% with the aperture iris diaphragm.

High-Power Objective. The high-power objective, or high-dry objective, is usually a 40 × lens with a 4-mm working distance. This objective is used for more detailed study; the total magnification with a 10 × eyepiece is 400 × as compared with the 100 × of the low-power system. The high-power objective is used to study histologic sections and wet preparations (such as urine sediment) in more detail. The working distance of the 4-mm lens is quite short, so care must be taken in focusing. The NA of the high-power lens is fairly close to (although slightly less than) that of most frequently used condensers (for most high-power objectives, NA = 0.65; for the condenser, NA = 0.85). Therefore the condenser should generally be all the way up (or very slightly lowered) and the light field slightly closed, with the aperture iris diaphragm adjusted for maximum focus.

Oil-Immersion Objective. The oil-immersion objective is generally a 100 × lens with a 1.8-mm working distance. This is a very short focal length and working distance. In fact, the objective lens almost rests on the microscope slide when the microscope is in use. An oil-immersion lens requires that a special grade of oil called *immersion oil* be placed between the objective and the slide or coverglass. Oil is used sparingly to increase the NA and thus the resolving power of the objective. Because the focal length of this lens is so small, there is a problem in providing enough light from the microscope field to the objective. Light travels through air at a greater speed than through glass, and light travels through immersion oil at the same speed as through glass. Thus to increase the effective NA of the objective, oil is used to slow down the speed at which light travels, increasing the gathering power of the lens.*

Because the NA of the oil-immersion objective is greater than that of the condenser in most systems (for the 100 × objective, NA = 1.2; for the condenser, NA = 0.85), the condenser should be used in the uppermost position, and the aperture iris diaphragm generally should be open. Practically speaking, however, partially closing the iris diaphragm may be necessary. The oil-immersion lens, with a total magnification of 1000 × when used with a 10 × eyepiece, is generally the limit of magnification with the light microscope.

TABLE 5.3 Examples of Objective Correction for Optical Aberration

Objective Type	Spherical Aberration	Chromatic Aberration	Field Curvature
Achromat	1 color	2 colors	No
Planachromat	1 color	2 colors	Yes
Apochromat	3 or 4 colors	4 or 5 colors	Yes

Modified from Nikon Microscopy U. www.microscopyu.com. Accessed July 8, 2009.

*The speed at which light travels through a substance is measured in terms of the refractive index. The refractive index is calculated as the speed at which light travels through air divided by the speed at which it travels through the substance. The refractive index of air is therefore 1.00. The refractive index of glass is 1.515; immersion oil, 1.515; and water, 1.33.

The oil-immersion lens is routinely used for morphologic examination of blood films and microbes. The short working distance requires dry films. Wet preparations (such as urine sediment) cannot be examined under an oil-immersion lens.

The high-power lens is also referred to as a *high-dry lens* because it does not require the use of immersion oil. Other objectives that might be present on a microscope in the clinical laboratory are a lower-power 4 × scanning lens and a 50 × or 63 × oil-immersion lens.

Focusing System

Oculars are a component of the focusing system. There is an interocular adjustment and an adjustment for the left ocular to focus for the left eye.

The body tube is the part of the microscope through which the light passes to the ocular. The tube length from the eyepiece to the objective lens is generally 160 mm. This is the tube that actually conducts the image. The required body tube length is also inscribed on each objective.

The adjustment system enables the body tube to move up or down for focusing the objectives. This usually consists of two adjustments: coarse and fine. The coarse adjustment gives rapid movement over a wide range and is used to obtain an approximate focus. The fine adjustment provides very slow movement over a limited range and is used to obtain exact focus after coarse adjustment.

CARE AND CLEANING OF THE MICROSCOPE

The microscope is a precision instrument and must be handled with great care.[4] When it is necessary to transport the microscope, it should always be carried with both hands; one hand should carry the microscope by its arm, and the other hand should provide support under the base. When not in use, the microscope should be covered and put away in a microscope case or in a desk or cupboard. It should be left with the low-power (10 ×) objective in place and the body tube barrel adjusted to the lowest possible position.

Cleaning the Microscope Exterior

The surface of most microscopes is resistant to most laboratory chemicals, so it may be washed with a neutral soap and water. To clean the metal and enamel, a gauze or soft cloth should be moistened with the cleaning agent and rubbed over the surface with a circular motion. The surface should be dried immediately with a clean, dry piece of gauze (or Kimwipe), which should never be used to clean the optical parts of the microscope.

Cleaning Optical Lenses

The glass surfaces of the ocular, the objectives, and the condenser are hand-ground optical lenses. These lenses must be kept meticulously clean (see Student Procedure Worksheet 5.1). Optical glass is softer than ordinary glass and should never be cleaned with paper tissue or gauze; these materials will scratch the lens. To clean the lenses of the microscope, use lens paper. Before polishing with lens paper, take care that nothing is present that will scratch the optical glass in the polishing process. Such potentially abrasive dirt, dust, or lint can easily be blown away before polishing. Cans of compressed air are commercially available, or an air syringe can be made simply by fitting a plastic eyedropper or a 1-mL plastic tuberculin syringe with the tip cut off into a rubber bulb of the type used for pipetting. This air syringe is used to blow away dust or lint that otherwise might scratch the optical glass in the polishing process.

Cleaning the Objectives

Oil must be removed from the oil-immersion (100 ×) objective immediately after use by wiping with clean lens paper. If not removed, oil may seep inside the lens or dry on the outside surface of the objective. The high-dry (40 ×) objective should never be used with oil, but if this or any other objective or microscope part comes into contact with oil, it should be cleaned immediately. If especially dirty, a lens may be cleaned with a small amount of commercial lens cleaner, methanol, or manufacturer-recommended solution applied to lens paper and then wiped across the surface. Xylene should not be used; it can damage the lens mounting if allowed beyond the front seal, and its fumes are toxic.

To clean the oil-immersion lens properly, first lower the stage and then rotate the objective to the front and wipe gently with clean lens paper. Clean off the immersion oil with lens paper dampened with special lens cleaner. Alternatively, the cleaning agent may be applied to a wooden applicator stick wrapped with cotton or lens paper and moistened with the cleaning agent. Do not use a plastic applicator stick; it will be dissolved by the solvent, ruining the objective. Apply the cleaning agent by blotting and using a circular motion, beginning at the center and moving outward. Repeat with new, dampened lens paper as necessary. Finally, blot dry with clean lens paper. Do not rub; this may scratch the surface of the lens.

Lenses should never be touched with the fingers. Objectives must not be taken apart because even a slight alteration of the lens setting may ruin the objective. Merely clean the outer surface of the lens as described. An especially dirty objective may be removed (unscrewed) from the nosepiece, then held upside down and checked for cleanliness by using the ocular (removed from the body tube) as a magnifying glass. Dust or lint also can be removed from the rear lens of the objective by blowing it away with an air syringe. Such removal of the objective from the nosepiece is not a routine cleaning procedure. The final step after using the microscope should always be to wipe off all objectives with clean lens paper.

Cleaning the Ocular

The ocular, or eyepiece, is especially vulnerable to dirt because of its location on the microscope and contact with the observer's eye. Mascara presents a constant cleaning problem. Dust can be removed from the lens of the ocular with an air syringe or camel's hair brush; air is probably easier to use and more efficient. The lens should then be polished with lens paper. The ocular can be checked for additional dirt by holding it up to a light and looking through it. When looking into the microscope, one can see that dirt on any part of the ocular will rotate with the ocular when it is turned. The ocular should not be removed for more than a few minutes; dust can collect in the body tube and settle on the rear lens of an objective.

Cleaning the Condenser

The light source and condenser should also be free of dust, lint, and dirt. First, blow away the dust with an air syringe or camel's hair brush; then polish the light source and condenser with lens paper. It may be necessary to clean these parts further with lens paper moistened with a commercial lens cleaner or methanol before polishing them with lens paper.

Cleaning the Stage and Adjustment Knobs

The stage of the microscope should be cleaned after each use by wiping with gauze or a tissue. After it has been cleaned thoroughly, the stage should be wiped dry.

The coarse and fine adjustments occasionally need attention, as does the mechanical stage adjustment mechanism. When there is unusual resistance to any manipulation of these knobs, force must not be used to overcome it. Such force might damage the screw or rack-and-pinion mechanism. Instead, the cause of the problem must be found. A small drop of oil may be needed.

It is best to call in a specialist to repair the microscope when a serious problem occurs. In addition, the microscope should be cleaned at least once a year by a professional microscope service company.

USE OF THE MICROSCOPE

When a microscope is being used, two conditions must be met: The microscope must be clean, and it must be aligned. The cleaning procedure is described in the previous section; alignment is discussed next (see Student Procedure Worksheet 5.2).

This process should require about 30 seconds. Touch up the two irises while moving from one section of the sample to another or from one magnification to another. Because many confocal sections are highly scattering, settings may only be able to be approximated, but putting in a lot of effort will greatly help the quality of images and results.

Alignment

When properly aligned, the microscope is adjusted in such a way that the light path through the microscope, from the light source to the eye of the observer, is correct. This is referred to as *Köhler illumination.* If a microscope is misaligned, the field of view will seem to swing—a very uncomfortable situation, often described as making the observer feel seasick. This can be corrected by properly aligning or adjusting the light path through the microscope. Many microscopes produced for student use are aligned by the manufacturer, and realignment requires special knowledge and experience because the field diaphragm, condenser-centering adjustment screws, and removable eyepieces are not present. In such microscopes, realignment should be done by a professional microscope service company.

If the microscope has a field diaphragm, it is used in the alignment procedure. A field diaphragm is an iris diaphragm that is part of the built-in illuminator. With the low-power objective in place, close down the field diaphragm to a minimum; then focus the condenser by adjusting the condenser height with the condenser focus knob until the image of the field diaphragm is sharply visible in the field of view (Fig. 5.5A). Next, bring the image of the field diaphragm into the center of the field by means of the centering screws located on the condenser (Fig. 5.5B). Open the field diaphragm until it is contained just within the field of view (Fig. 5.5C). At this point, it may be necessary to repeat the centering procedure. Finally, open the diaphragm until the leaves are just out of view.

Light Adjustment

With the low-power objective in position, the object to be examined, usually on a glass microscope slide, is placed on the stage and secured. Care must be taken to avoid damaging the objective when the specimen is placed on the stage. The slide is positioned so the portion of the slide containing the specimen to be examined is in the light path, directly over the condenser lens.

The greatest concern in learning how to use a microscope is the lighting and fine-adjustment maneuvers. The user must be certain that the light source, condenser, and aperture iris diaphragm are in correct adjustment. Light adjustment is made before any focusing is done. The power supply is turned on, and the light intensity is adjusted to a bright but comfortable level. Light adjustment is further accomplished by raising and lowering the condenser and opening and closing the aperture iris diaphragm. At the start of this initial light adjustment, the low-power (10 ×) objective should be in place. The condenser

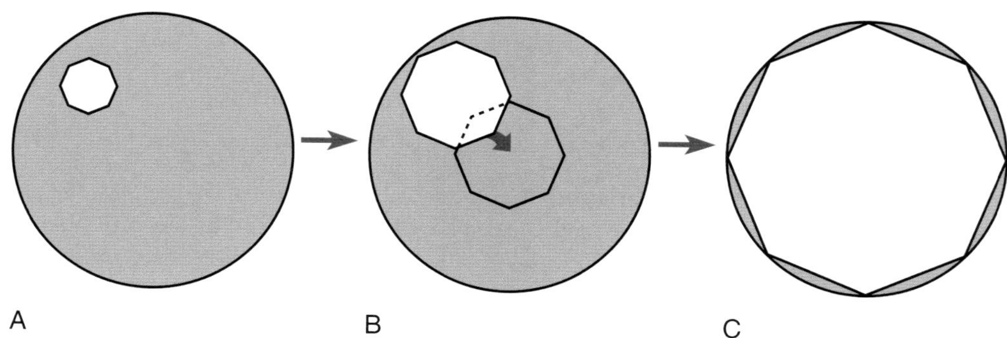

Fig. 5.5 **Microscope alignment; condenser centration.** (A) Stopped-down field diaphragm image, off center or misaligned. (B) Field diaphragm image widened and moved toward center by means of condenser adjustment knobs. (C) Field diaphragm image diameter widened and centered.

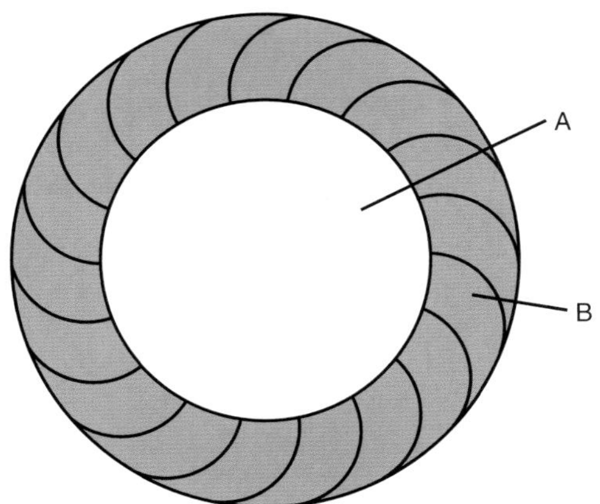

Fig. 5.6 Adjusting the aperture iris diaphragm. (A) From 70% to 80% of light is presented to objective. (B) From 20% to 30% of light is restricted by stopping down the aperture iris diaphragm.

should be near its highest position, no more than 1 to 2 mm below the slide, with the aperture and field diaphragms open all the way and the body tube down so that the lens is approximately 16 mm from the slide, the working distance for the low-power lens. If the microscope is equipped with a field diaphragm, the condenser height should be adjusted so as to bring the field diaphragm into sharp focus, as described in the alignment procedure.

To adjust the aperture iris diaphragm (Fig. 5.6), look through the ocular while closing the diaphragm until the light is just barely reduced. Alternately, if possible, remove the eyepiece and darken out approximately 20% to 30% of the light by closing the iris diaphragm while looking down the body tube. Further closing of the iris diaphragm (or lowering of the condenser), although it may increase contrast and depth of focus, will reduce resolution.

Focusing

Focusing is the next technique to be mastered (Student Procedure Worksheet 5.3). If using a binocular microscope, adjust the interpupillary distance between the oculars so that the left and right fields merge into one. With the object to be examined on the stage, and while watching from the side, bring the low-power (10 ×) objective down as far as it will go so it almost meets the top of the specimen. Use the coarse adjustment for this procedure. The objective must not be in direct contact with the specimen. Watch from the side to avoid damaging the objective. Once the objective is just at the top of the specimen, slowly focus upward, using the coarse-adjustment knob and looking through the ocular. When the object is almost in focus, bring it into clear focus with the fine-adjustment knob. Perform this procedure with the right eye, and then set the ocular diopter to the left eye by rotating until the left eye is in clear focus; the object should now be in focus for both eyes.

Further light adjustment can now be made to ensure maximum focus and resolution. Adjust the light intensity with the brightness control so the background light is sufficiently bright (white) but comfortable. Next, adjust the iris diaphragm by opening it completely and then slowly closing it until the light intensity just begins to be reduced. Alternatively, remove the eyepiece and close the aperture iris diaphragm until about 80% of the body tube is filled with light.

When changing to another objective, changing the barrel distance is unnecessary. As noted, most microscopes are parfocal. The only adjustment necessary should be made with the fine-adjustment knob. It is essential to remember that fine adjustment is used continuously during microscopic examination, especially when wet preparations such as urine sediment are being examined.

When greater magnification is needed, more light is necessary. It is obtained by repositioning the condenser and aperture iris diaphragm in the manner previously described. In general, the condenser will be raised and the aperture iris diaphragm opened as the objective magnification increases. When the oil-immersion lens is used, the condenser should be raised to its maximum position.

Additional light is provided by the use of immersion oil, which is placed on the viewing slide when the oil-immersion (100 ×) objective is used. The oil directs the light rays to a finer point, reducing spherical aberration. When the oil-immersion lens is to be used, first find the desired area on the slide by using the low-power (10 ×) objective. Once this area is located, pivot the objective out of position, place a drop of immersion oil on the slide, and pivot the oil-immersion lens into the oil while observing it from the side. Next, move the objective from side to side to ensure contact with the oil and to avoid the presence of air bubbles. To prevent damage to the objective, the nosepiece rather than the objective itself should be grasped when lenses are being changed. The ocular should not be looked through during this adjustment procedure. After the initial adjustment has been made, adjust the fine focus while looking through the ocular. After the study has been completed, clean off the oil remaining on the objective with lens paper, as described earlier.

OTHER TYPES OF MICROSCOPES (ILLUMINATION SYSTEMS)

With few exceptions, brightfield microscopy illumination has been the primary type of microscope illumination system used in the routine clinical laboratory. Alternate types of microscopy with various characteristics have been developed (Table 5.4). The basic principles of microscopy and rules for usage apply to all these variations. The primary difference from brightfield microscopy is the character of light delivered to the specimen and illuminating the microscope.

Darkfield Microscope

With darkfield microscopy, a special substage condenser is used that causes light waves to cross on the specimen (oblique angles) rather than pass in parallel waves through the specimen. Only light that is scattered by the specimen can reach the objective lens. When only deflected scattered light is seen, the resulting image has a black background, and only the objects appear light.

Any brightfield microscope may be converted to a darkfield microscope with the use of a special darkfield condenser in place of the usual condenser.

TABLE 5.4 Comparison of Alternate Types of Microscopy

Type	Use
Darkfield	Uses scattered light to view objects that appear light on a dark background.
Differential interference contrast	Gives objects a three-dimensional appearance.
Digital	Automatically locates and preclassifies blood cells into categories. Digitizes images for electronic retrieval and sharing.
Electron	Provides greater magnification and resolution than conventional light microscopy.
Fluorescence	Used to observe molecules that fluoresce when molecules are coupled to antibodies for specific fluorescent labeling.
Phase contrast	Used to increase the contrast in unstained specimens.
Polarized light	Used to identify crystals in body fluids (such as synovial or joint)

The darkfield microscope has long been used in the routine clinical laboratory to observe spirochetes in exudates from leptospiral or syphilitic infections. A more recent use, facilitated by newer microscope design technology, is as a low-power scanner for urine sediment. A darkfield effect may be achieved by using a mismatched phase annulus and phase objective, such as a low-power phase objective with a high-power phase annulus.

Differential Interference-Contrast Microscope

In DIC microscopy, the viewer sees a three-dimensional (3D) image of the object under study. The resulting image has higher contrast than the image obtained with a normal light microscope. DIC microscopy is also referred to as *Nomarski microscopy.*

For conversion to a DIC microscope, the brightfield microscope is modified with the addition of a special beam-splitting (Wollaston) prism to the condenser. The two split beams are then polarized; one passes through the specimen, which alters the amplitude (or height) of the light wave, and the other (which serves as a reference) does not pass through the specimen. The two dissimilar light beams then pass separately through the objective and are recombined by a second Wollaston prism. This recombination of light waves gives the 3D image to the additive or subtractive effects of the light waves as they are combined.

As with phase-contrast microscopy, DIC microscopy is especially useful for wet preparations (such as urine sediment), showing finer details without the need for special staining techniques.

Electron Microscope

In general, the principle of the electron microscope is the same as for the light microscope. Electrons traveling in a stream will have wave properties just as light does. The limit of magnification with any of the variations of the light microscope is about 1500 × to 2000 ×. Above this, there is decreased resolving power. For magnification of up to about 50,000 ×, the electron microscope may be used with good resolution. There are two types of **electron microscopy**: transmission and scanning.

The electrons are accelerated by a high-voltage potential and pass through a condenser lens system, usually composed of two magnetic lenses. The electron beam is concentrated onto the specimen, and the objective lens provides the primary magnification. The final image is not visible and cannot be viewed directly; rather, it is projected onto a fluorescent screen or a photographic plate. This is the principle of transmission electron microscopy (TEM).

Scanning electron microscopy (SEM) focuses on the surface of the specimen and produces a 3D image by striking the sample with a focused beam of electrons. Electrons emitted from the surface of the sample, in addition to electrons deflected from the focused beam of electrons, are focused onto a cathode ray tube or photographic plate and visualized as a 3D image.

In both TEM and SEM, specimens need special preparation not done in routine clinical laboratories. Specimens must be extremely thin. With TEM, the electron beam must pass through the specimen, and electrons have very poor penetrating power. With SEM, the specimen can be slightly thicker because the beam of electrons does not pass through the specimen. In either case, it is impossible to study living cells with electron microscopy because of the high vacuum to which the specimen is subjected, and because the electron beam itself is highly damaging to living tissue. Despite this limitation, electron microscopy has provided much information about cell structure and function.

Fluorescence Microscope

Electrons from some compounds can be excited by high-energy wavelengths of light, usually blue, violet, and ultraviolet wavelengths. As these electrons lose the energy they absorbed from the high-energy wavelengths, they emit light of lower energy, such as green, red, or yellow light. Compounds that fluoresce are often coupled to specific antibodies for use in the clinical laboratory.

The transmitted-light fluorescence microscope is a further refinement, basically a darkfield microscope with wavelength selection. In **fluorescence microscopy** with transmitted light and a compound microscope, the darkfield condenser is preceded by a special exciter filter that allows only shorter-wavelength blue light to pass and cross on the specimen plane. If the specimen contains an object that fluoresces, either naturally or because of staining or labeling with certain fluorescent dyes, it will absorb the blue light and emit light of a longer yellow or green wavelength. A special barrier filter is placed in the microscope tube or eyepiece. This barrier filter will pass only the desired wavelength of emitted light for the particular fluorescence system, so the fluorescence technique shows only the presence or absence of the fluorescing object. The barrier filter used must be carefully chosen so that only light of the desired wavelength will be passed through the microscope to the observer. Objects in the specimen that do not fluoresce will not emit light of that wavelength and will not be seen.

Fluorescence techniques are especially useful in the clinical laboratory. Historically, this technique has been used in the clinical microbiology laboratory. Various fluorescent antibody techniques may be used in primary identification of microorganisms or in the final identification of bacteria such as group A streptococci, replacing older serologic methods. Such techniques have the advantage of saving time and allowing earlier diagnosis for the patient, and they are often more sensitive than other methods. Fluorescence techniques may also be useful in identifying organisms that cannot be cultured (such as *Treponema pallidum*).

Today, fluorescence microscopy is being used in the rapidly expanding fields of cellular and molecular biology. New techniques have spurred the development of more sophisticated microscopes, with widefield and confocal fluorescence illumination becoming one of the techniques of choice.

Phase-Contrast Microscope

Another extremely useful illumination system is the phase-contrast microscope. A disadvantage of brightfield illumination is that it is necessary to stain (or dye) many objects to give sufficient contrast and detail. Phase-contrast microscopy uses a hollow cone of light instead of the solid cone of light normally used in light microscopy. The cone of light must be aligned with special rings in the objective lenses to produce the best contrast. The principle of phase-contrast microscopy is that light slows down as it passes through the specimen. The phase rings in the objective lenses change the phase of the light, converting the slower light speed to an intensity that increases the contrast of the specimen.

A phase-contrast microscope is basically a brightfield microscope with changes in the objective and the condenser. An annular diaphragm, or ring, is put into (or below) the condenser. This condenser annulus is designed to let a hollow cone or "doughnut" of light pass through the condenser to the specimen. A corresponding absorption ring is fitted into the objective. Each phase objective must have a corresponding condenser annulus (Fig. 5.7). In microscopes with multiple phase objectives, the annular diaphragms are usually placed in a rotating condenser arrangement (Fig. 5.8). Use of each phase objective requires an adjustment of the condenser to "match" the annular diaphragm and the phase absorption ring.

The phase-contrast microscope may also be used as a brightfield microscope by setting the condenser to a standard brightfield (or open) position, which contains no annulus. Because the phase objective blocks out a ring of light, the resolution or detail that can be achieved when using phase objectives is compromised for brightfield examination. For more exact work, an additional brightfield objective should be employed in the microscope.

The annulus and absorption ring must be perfectly aligned or adjusted so they are concentric and superimposed; a problem with the phase-contrast microscope is the need for perfect alignment. The microscope must first be aligned for brightfield work. To align the phase annulus, match the phase objective to the corresponding phase annulus in the condenser by rotating the phase turret. Incorporate the aperture viewing unit either by inserting it into the body tube or by inserting a phase telescope into an ocular tube. Focus the viewing apparatus until the phase annulus (seen as a white ring of light) is in focus. There will be a bright (white) ring and a dark ring, which should be superimposed (Fig. 5.9). If not perfectly superimposed, the phase annulus can be repositioned by means of the annulus-centering knobs located on the condenser. Each microscope will have a slightly different means of adjustment, and the operation directions for that microscope should be followed.

However, all phase-contrast microscopes require the same alignment as for brightfield, plus alignment of the phase annulus to the matching phase objective.

The net effect of phase contrast is to slow down the speed of light by one-fourth of a wavelength. This diminution of the speed of light makes the system very sensitive to differences in refractive index. Objects with differences in refractive index, shape, and absorption characteristics show added differences in the intensity and shade of light passing through them. The end result is that the viewer can observe unstained wet preparations with good resolution and detail, as shown in Fig. 5.10. In the clinical laboratory, phase contrast is especially useful for

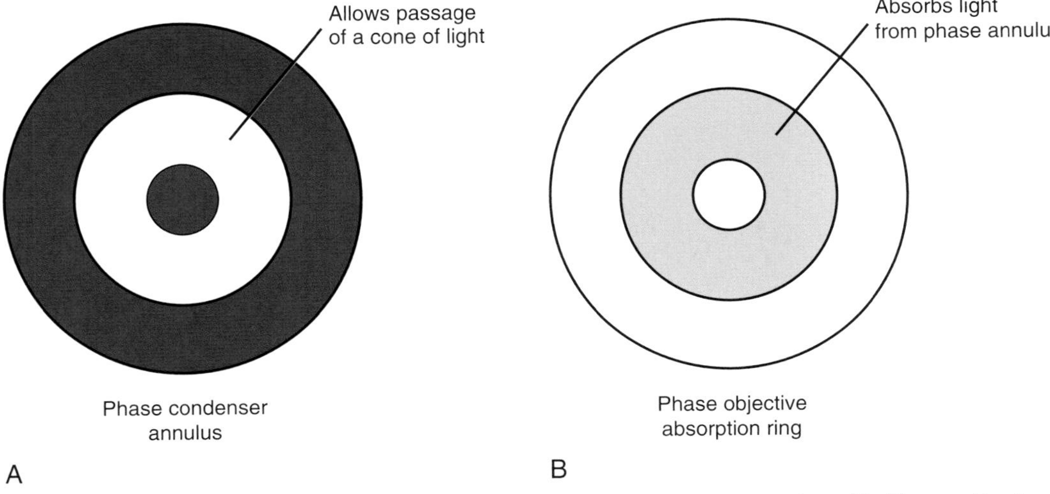

Fig. 5.7 Phase annulus and absorption ring. (A) Phase condenser annulus. (B) Phase objective absorption ring.

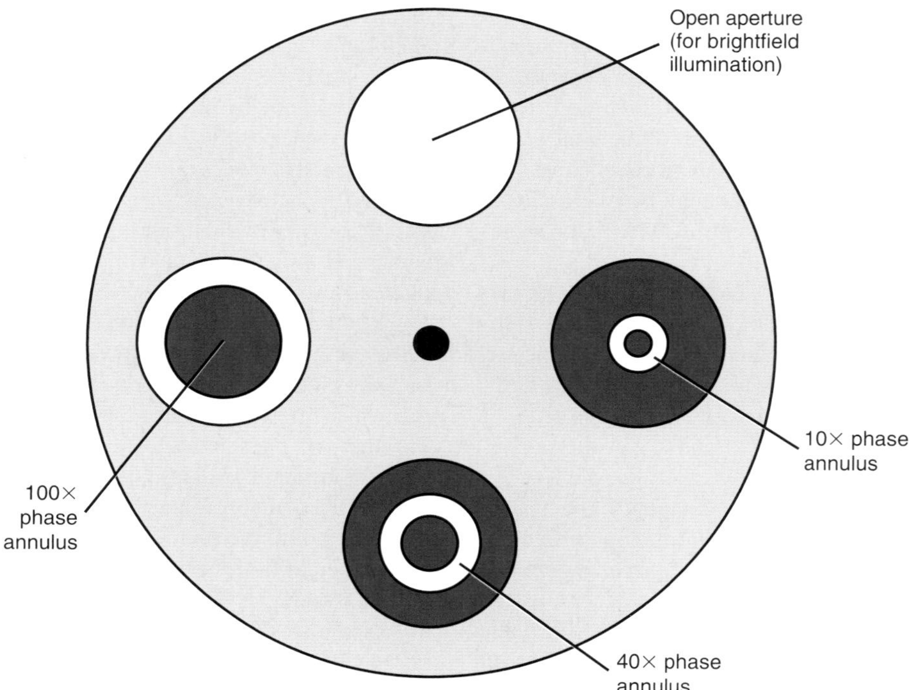

Fig. 5.8 Rotating phase condenser. Settings are for brightfield, low power (10 ×), high power (40 ×), and oil immersion (100 ×).

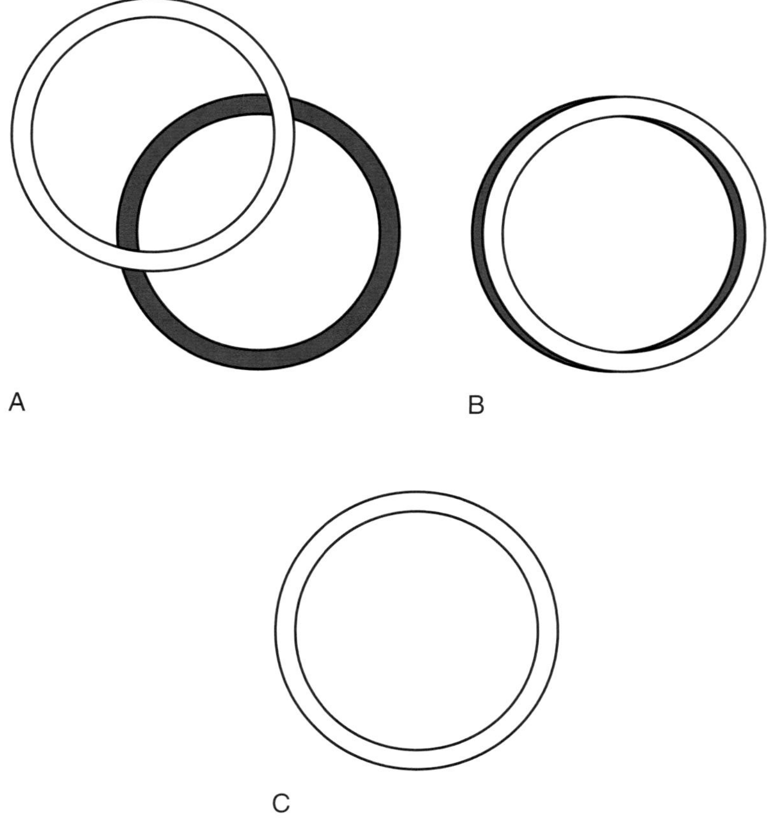

Fig. 5.9 Alignment of phase annulus to phase absorption ring. (A) Before alignment, phase annulus is out of phase adjustment. (B) Phase annulus moved so that it is nearly aligned. (C) Alignment: Phase annulus is superimposed on phase absorption ring.

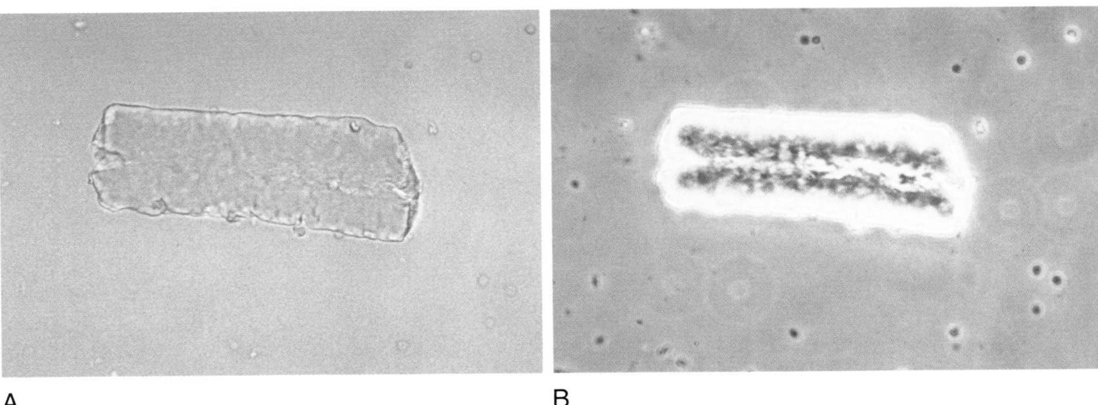

Fig. 5.10 Brightfield versus phase-contrast illumination. (A) Waxy cast with brightfield illumination, 100×. (B) Same field with phase-contrast illumination, 100×. Note the central fissure and increased detail. (From Brunzel NA: *Fundamentals of urine and body fluid analysis,* ed 2, Philadelphia, 2004, Saunders.)

counting platelets and for observing cellular structures and casts in wet preparations of urine sediment and vaginal smears. Because of its superior visualization and ease of operation, the phase-contrast microscope has become a common tool in routine urinalysis. However, the microscopist must be proficient in changing from brightfield to phase contrast, because in a given specimen some structures are better visualized with phase contrast and others with brightfield.

Phase contrast facilitates the study of unstained structures, which can be alive, because wet preparations of cells or organisms are observed without prior dehydration and staining. As the name implies, the structures observed with this system show added contrast in comparison with those seen with the brightfield microscope.

Polarized and Compensated Polarized Microscopes

Another useful adaptation of brightfield microscopy is polarized light microscopy. As light passes through the specimen, some objects (such as crystals) can rotate the light. When another filter is placed above the specimen at a different orientation, light that has not been rotated by the specimen cannot pass through the filter because the orientation of the filter above the specimen is different from that of the filter below the specimen.

A *polarizer* (or polarizing filter) may be defined as a sieve that takes ordinary light waves, which vibrate in all orientations (or directions), and allows only light waves of one orientation (north-south or east-west) to pass through the filter (Fig. 5.11A). In a polarizing microscope, a polarizing filter is placed between the light source (bulb) and the specimen. A second polarizing filter (called an *analyzer*) is placed above the specimen, between the objective and the eyepiece (either at some point in the microscope tube or in the eyepiece). One of the polarizers is then rotated until the two are at right angles to each other (Fig. 5.11B). When the viewer is looking through the eyepieces, this will be seen as the extinction of light (viewer sees a dark or black field), because all light is blocked out of the light path when the polarizing filters are at right angles to each other. However, certain objects have a property termed *birefringence,* which means that they rotate (or polarize) light. An object that polarizes bends light so that it can be visualized when viewed through crossed polarizers. Objects that do not bend light will not be observed in the microscope. An object that polarizes light (or is birefringent) will appear light against a dark background.

A further modification of the polarizing microscope involves the use of compensated polarized light. A compensator, also referred to as a *first-order red plate* (filter) or *full-wave retardation plate,* is placed between the two crossed polarizing filters and positioned 45 degrees to the crossed polarizer and analyzer (Fig. 5.11C and D). With this addition, the field background appears red or magenta, whereas objects that are birefringent (polarize light) appear yellow or blue in relation to their orientation to the compensator and their optical properties.

The compensated polarized microscope is especially useful clinically for differentiating between monosodium urate and calcium pyrophosphate dihydrate crystals in synovial fluid. It is also becoming useful in the routine study of urine sediment and in some histologic work. Polarizing microscopy is often used in geology for particle analysis and in forensic medicine clinically. With the polarizing microscope, the optical properties of an object can be determined.

DIGITAL MICROSCOPY

Performing blood and body fluid differentials using manual microscopy is a laborious and time-consuming laboratory procedure that is highly dependent on the availability of experienced technologists and technicians. Advances in artificial neural networks (ANN), image analysis, and slide handling have been combined to produce instruments that automate manual differentials in unique ways. Integration of digital imaging with automated blood cell counting produces faster results with higher specificity and sensitivity than manual microscopic examination[5].

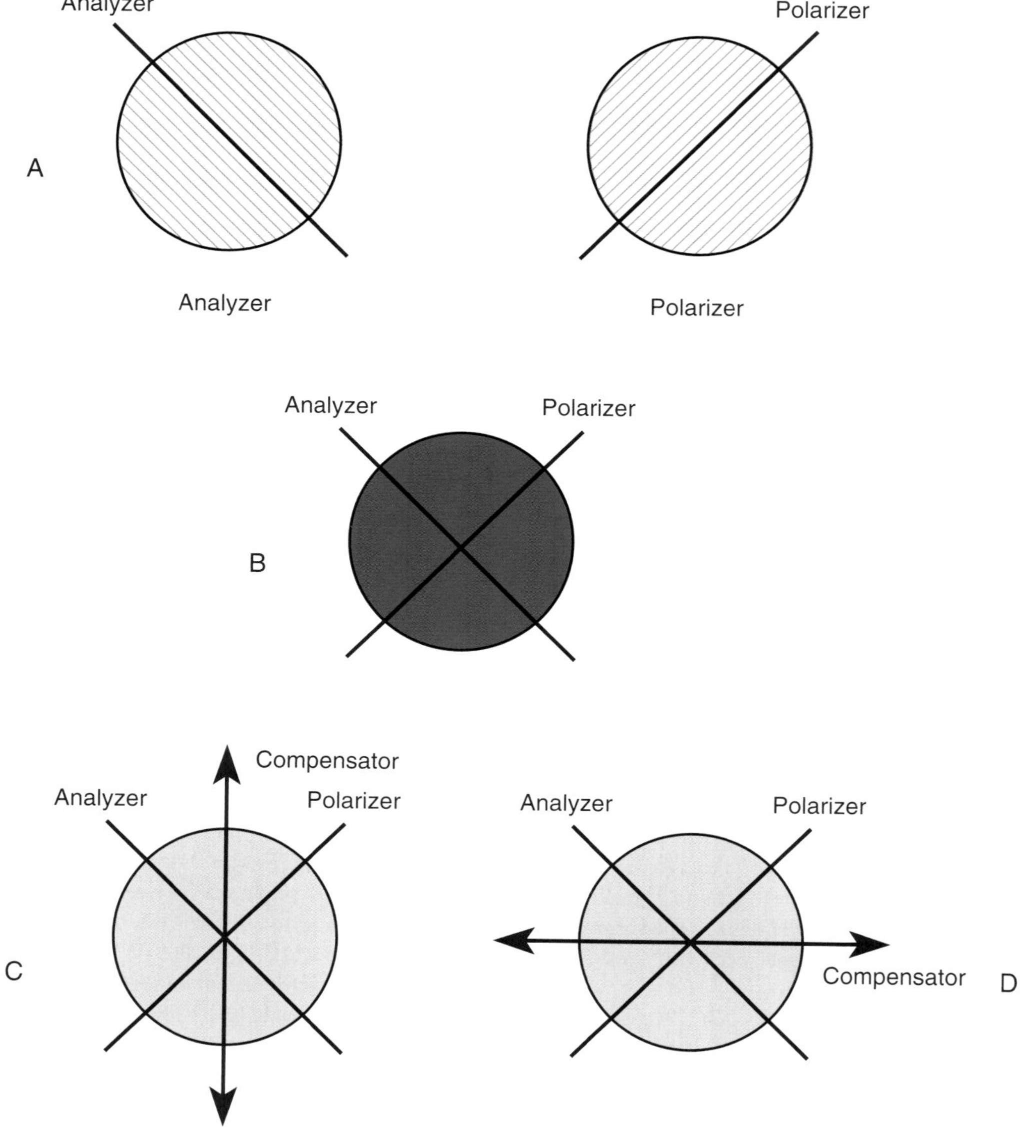

Fig. 5.11 Principle of polarized light and compensated polarized light. (A) Polarizing lenses or filters. Polarizer is placed between light source and specimen; analyzer is placed between specimen and eye of the observer. (B) Polarized light, obtained by placing analyzer and polarizer at right angles to each other. Position of analyzer is fixed, and polarizer is rotated until light is extinguished (seen as a black or dark background). (C) Compensated polarized light. Compensator is placed at 45 degrees to the crossed polarizers, resulting in a red or magenta background color. Here, direction of slow wave of compensation is in north-south (N-S) orientation. (D) Compensated polarized light. Here, direction of slow wave of compensation is in east-west (E-W) orientation.

In its simplest form, automated digital cell morphology is a process that automatically locates and pre-classifies peripheral blood cells and five types of leukocytes in body fluids. Digital mages of these cells are stored in a database and can be shared electronically.

This new technology, referred to as **digital microscopy** or automated digital cell morphology,[6] provides distinct advantages that include (5):

- Improved efficiency as an automated process that saves times and workforce energy,
- Enhanced quality of results because of consistency and standardization of morphological examination of cells,
- Increased opportunities for connectivity that facilitates virtual microscopy collaboration and remote analysis within and between laboratories throughout the world,
- Advanced learning opportunities to promote enhanced technical proficiency and competency assessment.

Artificial Neural Networks

An ANN is an information-processing model that simulates the way the human brain processes information. ANN emulates the neural structure of the brain, which is composed of a large number of highly interconnected processing elements (neurons) working together to solve specific problems. ANNs are the result of research in artificial intelligence (AI) and its attempt to mimic the capacity to learn, as seen in biological neural systems. AI systems resulted in the development of so-called expert systems. Although very useful in some applications, AI failed to capture key aspects of the human brain's ability to critically compare and contrast complex objects. ANNs have been known since the 1940s, but it was not until the mid-1980s that algorithms became sophisticated enough and computers powerful enough for general applications to develop. Applications of ANNs in which their pattern-recognition capabilities are used include speech recognition and analysis, handwriting, fingerprints, faces, and cellular morphology.

Digital Cell Morphology and Workflow

Digital morphology uses digital images and software algorithms to classify peripheral blood cells or body fluid leukocytes. Classification without manual intervention is defined as pre-classification. After review and subsequent possible re-classification by an expert technologist is defined as post-classification. The results can be released to a laboratory information system (LIS) and hospital information system (HIS) after validation by an experienced technologist.

In 2000, the CellaVision company initially launched a digital microscope that uses a digital camera capable of generating high-resolution images of peripheral blood cells. The system consisting of a digital microscope with a 100 × objective; a stepper motor and light control unit. A digital microscope can generate high-resolution images with enhanced features, extract information, or modify images. A progressive three-chip CCD color camera is connected to a computer with ANA software that assesses cellular size, shape and nuclear characteristics for classification of blood cells. In addition to detecting peripheral blood or body fluid cells, the software can subsequently classify the cells and present the data results in both absolute numbers and percentages.

Unlike earlier attempts by other manufacturers, a CellaVision instrument processes wedged smears that are stained according to the Wright, Wright-Giemsa, or May Grünwald–Giemsa staining protocols and uses ANNs trained on a large database of cells. It was the first image analysis system to locate and preclassify cells into 15 different categories and automatically precharacterize six red blood cell morphologic characteristics. Platelet estimates and erythrocyte precharacterization are performed in an overview image corresponding to eight high-power fields (100 ×).

Advanced Applications

The latest 2017 Cellavision software innovation enables a more comprehensive review of erythrocytes in conjunction with morphological examination of peripheral blood smears. Pre-characterization is based on 21 morphological characteristics. This software allows for single cell filtering and grouping. Erythrocytes can be viewed as groups arranged by shape, size, color, and inclusions. In addition, characteristics can be highlighted in a selected cell category. Additionally, change grading manually if re-characterization is needed.

Body fluids are another specimen type that can be analyzed by automated analysis. Cerebrospinal fluid analysis exhibits good and clinically acceptable accuracy between automated and manual examination. However, the lack of recognition of some defined categories of cells such as possible tumor cells and mesothelial cells is a significant drawback. Additional refinement is required before body fluids can be analyzed routinely by digital methods.

REFERENCES

1. Basic concepts and formulas in microscopy, Nikon. www.microscopyU.com (Accessed May 31, 2013).
2. Microscopy resource center, Olympus. www.olympusmicro.com (Accessed May 31, 2012).
3. Basics in microscopy, Leica. www.leica-microsystems.com (Accessed May 31, 2013).
4. Gill GW: Microscope cleaning tips, techniques and timing, *Lab Med* 36(8):460, 2005.
5. Hagner R, Wilson P: Automated digital cell morphology: taking the "manual" out of the manual differential. In Ward-Cook KM, Lehmann CA, Schoeff LE, Williams RH, editors: *Clinical diagnostic technology—the total testing process: Vol 3, the post-analytical phase*, Washington, DC, 2006, AACC Press.
6. CellaVision, Why Automate A Manual Differential, www.cellavision.com, 2018.

BIBLIOGRAPHY

Brueggeman MS, Swinehart C, Yue MJ, et al.: Implementing virtual microscopy improves outcomes in a hematology morphology course, Clin Lab Sci 25(3):149–155, 2012, Summer.

CellaVision. http://www.cellavision.com, 2018.

Riedl J: Digital imaging/morphology is the next chapter in hematology, Med Lab Obs 50(3):28,30,32, 2018.

Schwartz S: Trends in digital bioscience imaging, *Bio-It World* 4(7):48, 2005.

Virtual microscope. http://www.udel.edu/biology/ketcham/microscope/scope.html.

REVIEW QUESTIONS (ANSWERS IN APPENDIX A)

Description

1. The magnification of 40 × matches the:
   a. Oil-immersion objective
   b. High-power objective
   c. Low-power objective
   d. Scanning objective
2. The magnification of 10 × matches the:
   a. Oil-immersion objective
   b. High-power objective
   c. Low-power objective
   d. Scanning objective

3. The magnification of 100 × matches the:
   a. Oil-immersion objective
   b. High-power objective
   c. Low-power objective
   d. Scanning objective
4. The common numerical aperture for the oil-immersion objective is:
   a. 0.25 NA
   b. 0.65 NA
   c. 1.25 NA
   d. 1.80 NA
5. The common numerical aperture for the high-power objective is:
   a. 0.25 NA
   b. 0.65 NA
   c. 1.2 NA
   d. 1.80 NA
6. The common numerical aperture for the low-power objective is:
   a. 0.25 NA
   b. 0.65 NA
   c. 1.2 NA
   d. 1.8 NA

Parts of the Microscope

7. The ocular of the microscope can also be called the:
   a. Iris field diaphragm
   b. Eyepiece
   c. Objectives
   d. Condenser
8. How should the condenser be positioned, assuming that the NA of the condenser is 0.85 with the oil-immersion objective?
   a. Highest position possible or very slightly decreased (lowered)
   b. Highest (uppermost) position possible
   c. Decrease to 1 or 2 mm below the slide (lowering condenser slightly)
   d. Lowest possible position
9. How should the condenser be positioned, assuming that the NA of the condenser is 0.85 with the low-power objective?
   a. Highest position possible or very slightly decreased (lowered)
   b. Highest (uppermost) position possible
   c. Decrease to 1 or 2 mm below the slide (lowering condenser slightly)
   d. Lowest possible position

Care and Cleaning of the Microscope

10. Cleaning the objective lens should be done with:
    a. Camel's hair brush
    b. Tissue paper
    c. Facial tissue
    d. Lens paper
11. If you are unable to focus the microscope to achieve a sharp view of a specimen, the correct sequence of steps to be taken is:
    a. Replace the objective with one from another microscope, clean the oculars, clean the stage, and clean the objectives.
    b. Clean the oculars, clean the stage, clean the objectives, and replace the objective with one from another microscope.
    c. Clean the objectives, clean the oculars, and replace the objectives with a new set of objectives.
    d. Clean the objectives, replace the objective with one from another microscope, clean the ocular, and clean the stage.

Use of the Microscope

12. What objective must you always use when you first start looking at a slide?
    a. High power
    b. 100 ×
    c. 40 ×
    d. 10 ×
13. Which focusing adjustment do you use first when you begin looking at a slide?
    a. Small focusing knob
    b. Coarse focus
    c. Fine focus
    d. 4 × objective
14. Which objective allows you to see the largest area of the object you are viewing?
    a. 4 ×
    b. 10 ×
    c. 100 ×
    d. 40 ×
15. Describe how to decrease light intensity.
    a. Lower the condenser.
    b. Close the aperture iris diaphragm.
    c. Adjust the dimmer switch.
    d. All of the above are possible ways to decrease light intensity.
16. What do you adjust if you can see through one ocular and not the other?
    a. The fine focus
    b. The coarse focus
    c. Change to a different objective
    d. The other ocular
17. What do you adjust if you can see two overlapping circles, with part of the object in each circle?
    a. The focus
    b. The iris diaphragm
    c. The width of the oculars
    d. Change to a different objective
18. How do you increase depth of field?
    a. Close the aperture of the iris diaphragm.
    b. Open the aperture of the iris diaphragm.
    c. Use fine focusing.
    d. Both a and c.
19. Which focusing knob do you use with the 10 × and 40 × objectives?
    a. Fine focusing knob
    b. Coarse and fine focusing knobs, respectively
    c. Both fine focusing knob and the iris diaphragm

d. Coarse focusing knob

20. How much are you magnifying something when you are using 10 × oculars and the 40 × objectives?
    a. 40 ×
    b. 400 ×
    c. 4000 ×
    d. Cannot calculate without additional information

Other Types of Microscopes (Illumination Systems)

21. An adaptation of the brightfield microscope is the:
    a. Polarizing microscope
    b. Electron microscope
    c. Fluorescence microscope
    d. Darkfield microscope
22. A scanning electron microscope focuses on the surface of the specimen and produces a:
    a. One-dimensional image
    b. Two-dimensional image
    c. Three-dimensional image
    d. Four-dimensional image

Digital Microscopy and Workflow

23. Which of the following describes a characteristic representative of digital microscopy?
    a. Digital microscopy is driven by an artificial neural network that simulates the way the human brain processes information.
    b. Digital microscopy allows for preclassifying leukocytes and erythrocytes.
    c. Digital microscopy produces platelet estimates.
    d. All the above are representative characteristics of digital microscopy.

Bonus Challenge Questions

24. You are reviewing a hematology slide under the low-power (10 ×) objective. Which step should be completed first to scan the slide?
    a. Use the coarse-focus adjustment, followed by the fine-focus adjustment.
    b. Use the fine-focus adjustment, followed by the coarse-focus adjustment.
    c. Add oil to the slide.
    d. Adjust the light intensity until the background light is bright but comfortable to view.
25. You are reviewing a hematology slide under the 100 × oil-immersion objective, but the specimen is not in focus. What should you do to resolve the issue?
    a. Use the coarse-focus adjustment, followed by the fine-focus adjustment.
    b. Use the fine-focus adjustment, followed by the coarse-focus adjustment.
    c. Add oil to the slide.
    d. Adjust the light intensity until the background light is bright but comfortable to view.
26. You have completed a review of a hematology slide using the 100 × oil-immersion objective. What should you do before leaving the workstation?
    a. Turn off the light and put the slide away.
    b. Wipe the oil from the objective using a tissue, turn off the light, and put the slide away.
    c. Remove the oil from the objective with lens paper, turn off the light, and put the slide away.
    d. Wipe the oil from the objective with a clean, dry piece of gauze (or Kimwipe).

Turgeon: Linné & Ringsrud's Clinical Laboratory Science, 8th Edition

STUDENT PROCEDURE WORKSHEET 5-1

Cleaning the Microscope

Read Chapter 5 in *Linné & Ringsrud's Clinical Laboratory Science: Concepts, Procedures, and Clinical Applications,* 8th edition, for a complete discussion of this topic.

Student Learning Outcomes

After reading Chapter 5, and at the completion of the laboratory exercise and review questions, the student will be able to:

- Correctly clean a microscope.
- Complete the end-of-procedure review questions with a grade of 80% or higher.

Purpose

Regular cleaning is important not only in maintaining the life of the microscope and lenses but also in obtaining good-quality images. Lens cleaning in particular requires great care. All glass surfaces should be cleaned in the sequence described in the procedure.

Supplies and Equipment

1. Microscope
2. Lens paper
3. Lens cleaner
4. Compressed air
5. Gauze pieces (or Kimwipes)

Instructions for the Procedure

Read the list of required equipment and supplies and the procedural steps. Follow the procedural steps in exact order.

SEQUENCE	PROCEDURAL STEP	INSTRUCTOR-OBSERVED ACCEPTABLE PERFORMANCE (CHECK IF ACCEPTABLE)
1	Remove microscope from storage area and remove dust cover.	
2	Clean the oculars with lens paper.	
3	**Blowing:** Use air source to blow dust off lenses. This removes all larger particles of dust that could scratch the lens in the later cleaning stages. **Brushing:** Use clean, soft camel's hair or sable brush to remove particles of dust that blowing does not displace.	
4	**Wiping:** Gently clean each objective with lens paper. Use only clean lens paper to wipe lenses. Lens paper is specially made with soft fibers that will not scratch the glass. Moisten the lens paper with water or lens cleaner and wipe carefully; moistening further softens the paper fibers. Never use alcohol as a cleaning agent, because some lens adhesives are soluble in alcohol. CAUTION: Care should be taken to use a separate lens paper for dry and oil objectives so there is no transfer of oil, which may ruin the objectives.	
5	Clean the condenser with lens paper.	
6	Clean the stage and knobs with moistened pieces of gauze (or Kimwipes). Either water or a small amount of alcohol can be used.	
7	To conclude this procedure, position the lowest power (i.e., 10×) over the microscope stage. Center the stage mechanism. Turn the light source off. Be sure that a specimen slide has been removed. Cover the microscope with a dust cover. Return to storage, if it is not stored on the laboratory benchtop.	

Procedural Evaluation

Student's Name ______________________ Grade ________

Instructor's Signature ______________________ Date ________

Comments:

Turgeon: Linné & Ringsrud's Clinical Laboratory Science, 8th Edition

STUDENT PROCEDURE WORKSHEET 5-1

Cleaning the Microscope

Review Questions

Student's Name ______________________________ Date __________

1. Why is it important to use lens paper to clean the objective lens rather than Kimwipe or other types of tissue?

2. Why is alcohol not acceptable in cleaning the objective lens?

3. What parts of the microscope can be cleaned with a soft cleaning cloth (or Kimwipes)?

Turgeon: Linné & Ringsrud's Clinical Laboratory Science, 8th Edition

STUDENT PROCEDURE WORKSHEET 5-2

Aligning the Microscope

See Chapter 5 in *Linné & Ringsrud's Clinical Laboratory Science: Concepts, Procedures, and Clinical Applications*, 8th edition, for a complete discussion of this procedure.

Student Learning Outcomes
After reading Chapter 5, and at the completion of the laboratory exercise and review questions, the student will be able to:
- Correctly align the microscope.
- Complete the end-of-procedure review questions with a grade of 80% or higher.

Purpose
For the best performance, a microscope should be correctly aligned.

Equipment
Microscope

Instructions for the Procedure
Read the list of required equipment and supplies and the procedural steps. Follow the procedural steps in exact order.

Turgeon: Linné & Ringsrud's Clinical Laboratory Science, 8th Edition

STUDENT PROCEDURE WORKSHEET 5-2

SEQUENCE	PROCEDURAL STEP	INSTRUCTOR-OBSERVED ACCEPTABLE PERFORMANCE (CHECK IF ACCEPTABLE)
1	**NOTE**: For optimal results, set the alignment each time you sit down at the microscope and "touch up" the focus from one area of the sample to another. Assemble equipment and supplies. Remove dust cover and clean microscope (see Student Procedure Worksheet 5-1). Turn on the light source.	
2	Wash your hands and put on gloves as directed.	
3	Eyepieces/oculars (preliminary step): The eyepieces have focus rings on them (turn the very top). Set the "0" to the white dot.	
4	Objective: Bring the objective into focus for the sample by "focusing away." Start by looking outside the microscope at the distance between the front of the objective and the sample. Rotate the coarse focus knob away from you to raise the stage as close as possible to the objective. Then, while looking in the microscope, rotate the knob gently toward you until the image comes into sharp focus. Touch up with the fine focus.	
5	Condenser: Look under the stage for the small focusing knob for the condenser carrier. Raise the condenser until it is almost touching the back of the slide. Note which direction you turned the knob to raise the condenser. a. Close the field iris diaphragm. While watching in the microscope, gently rotate the condenser focus in the other direction until the dark edges of the field iris image come into focus. b. Open the field iris just outside the field of view. **NOTE**: If you have a highly scattering sample, try moving the feature of interest to the center of the field and leaving the field iris mostly closed. c. Adjust the condenser aperture iris until you have clean, crisp edges and as clear a background as possible.	
6	Final setting for eyepieces: Leave the microscope controls set for the dominant eye, and adjust the eyepiece focus to bring the image into focus for the other eye.	
Summary Set the eyepieces to "0." Focus away with the coarse focus to obtain a sharp image of the specimen. Bring the condenser up to the top using its own focus. Close the field iris, and while looking in the microscope, focus away to obtain a sharp image of the field iris superimposed on the image of the specimen. Set the field iris (usually just outside the field of view). Set the aperture iris (sharp, crisp, clean image). For final setting of eyepiece, focus for nondominant eye.		
7	Clean equipment and return to proper storage.	
8	Clean work area.	

Procedural Evaluation

Student's Name ______________________________ Grade__________

Instructor's Signature ___________________________ Date__________

Comments:

(Continued)

Turgeon: Linné & Ringsrud's Clinical Laboratory Science, 8th Edition

STUDENT PROCEDURE WORKSHEET 5-2

Aligning the Microscope

Review Questions

Student's Name ______________________ Date:__________

1. Briefly explain the alignment of the oculars, objectives, and condenser.

2. Once the oculars have a final setting, how do you achieve a sharp image of a specimen?

Turgeon: Linné & Ringsrud's Clinical Laboratory Science, 8th Edition

STUDENT PROCEDURE WORKSHEET 5-3

Using the Microscope

Read Chapter 5 in *Linné & Ringsrud's Clinical Laboratory Science: Concepts, Procedures, and Clinical Applications,* 8th edition, for a complete discussion of this procedure.

Student Learning Outcomes

After reading Chapter 5, and at the completion of the laboratory exercise and review questions, the student will be able to:

- Operate a microscope correctly.
- Complete the end-of-procedure review questions with a grade of 80% or higher.

Purpose

To achieve a sharp image for high-quality microscopic examination of specimens, it is important to know how to operate a microscope properly.

Supplies and Equipment

1. Microscope
2. Lens paper
3. Gauze pieces (or Kimwipes)
4. Immersion oil

Instructions for the Procedure

Read the list of required equipment and supplies and the procedural steps. Follow the procedural steps in exact order.

SEQUENCE	PROCEDURAL STEP	INSTRUCTOR-OBSERVED ACCEPTABLE PERFORMANCE (CHECK IF ACCEPTABLE)
1	Remove the microscope dust cover and clean (see Student Procedure Worksheet 5-1).	
2	Turn on light source. Rotate the low-power (10×) objective lens slowly until an audible click is heard. NOTE: Always begin initially focusing with the low-power objective.	
3	Look at the microscope from the side to increase the working distance as far as possible with the coarse adjustment.	
4	Put on gloves as directed. Select a specimen slide and place on the microscope stage. Secure with clamp on the stage.	
5	Center the slide on the stage by rotating the stage knobs located under the stage.	
6	On the ocular, turn the diopter ring to the middle of the adjustment range. While looking through the right eyepiece, slowly turn the coarse adjustment to bring the specimen into focus. Once in focus, use the fine adjustment knob to make a sharper image adjustment.	
7	While looking through the left eyepiece, turn the diopter adjustment ring to focus the specimen.	
8	Adjust the interpupillary distance of the eyepieces until both left and right fields of vision coincide completely. The image should appear as one single field with a sharply focused image. The image should remain in sharp focus if either eye is closed. NOTE: Lift out one eyepiece and adjust aperture diaphragm to about three-fourths full. Specific adjustments are 0.25 for 10×, 0.65 for 40×, and 1.3 for 100×. Replace eyepiece.	
9	After the specimen slide is in focus, open the iris diaphragm in the substage condenser to its widest adjustment. Set the light source intensity control to about two-thirds maximum output. A blue filter may be needed to reduce yellow emissions from the light source.	
10	If the condenser has a swing-out lens, position this lens in the light path.	
11	Lower the condenser and close the field iris diaphragm. Raise the condenser until the image of the circle of light is in sharp focus.	
12	Center the field iris diaphragm by manipulating the two centering screws on the compensating lens. note: To check, open the field iris diaphragm until its image touches the perimeter of the field of view. If the image is not precisely in the field of view, center again.	
13	Open the field iris diaphragm until the edge of the leaves disappear from your field of vision.	

(Continued)

Turgeon: Linné & Ringsrud's Clinical Laboratory Science, 8th Edition

STUDENT PROCEDURE WORKSHEET 5-3

SEQUENCE	PROCEDURAL STEP	INSTRUCTOR-OBSERVED ACCEPTABLE PERFORMANCE (CHECK IF ACCEPTABLE)
14	Select and position the objective lens of choice. Adjust the iris diaphragm until the appropriate amount of light is available. The amount of light is also controlled by the light source. **NOTE**: Less light is needed for 10x and the most amount of light is needed when using the oil-immersion objective (100x) lens. The amount of light needs to be adjusted each time a new objective lens is selected.	
15	Use the fine adjustment knob to refocus to the sharpest image. With parfocal objectives, once an image is in focus with 10×, it will remain in focus when higher power objectives (40×, 100×) are selected. If 100× lens is selected, move the slide slightly sideways and place a drop of immersion oil direct on the slide over the area to be observed. Return the slide to the appropriate viewing area. **CAUTION**: Always begin focusing with the low-power objective (10×).	
16	Following examination of a specimen slide, remove the slide and clean the microscope by wiping off the objective lens with lens paper. Be careful to clean the oil immersion lens last.	
17	Return the low-power objective (10×) to the viewing position, and completely decrease the working distance by lowering the objective to the lowest possible position.	
18	Cover the microscope and return to storage, if it is not stored on the laboratory benchtop.	

Procedural Evaluation

Student's Name ______________________ Grade __________

Instructor's Signature ______________________ Date __________

Comments:

Turgeon: Linné & Ringsrud's Clinical Laboratory Science, 8th Edition

STUDENT PROCEDURE WORKSHEET 5-3

Using the Microscope

Review Questions

Student's Name ______________________________ Date ________________

1. Describe how to begin to properly focus a specimen slide under the microscope.

2. If you examine a slide using low power, what is the total magnification?

3. If you examine a slide using high power, what is the total magnification?

4. If you examine a slide using oil immersion, what is the total magnification?

5. The use of which objective requires the most amount of light?

6

Systems of Measurement, Laboratory Equipment, and Reagents

http://evolve.elsevier.com/Turgeon/clinicallab/

CHAPTER OUTLINE

LEARNING OUTCOMES

Systems of Measurement
- Convert metric units of measurement for weight, length, and volume to English units and English units to metric units.

International System (SI System)
- Calculate temperatures from degrees Celsius to degrees Fahrenheit.
- Convert temperatures from degrees Fahrenheit to degrees Celsius.

Labware
- Describe the various types of and uses for laboratory volumetric glassware, the techniques for their use, and the various types of glass used to manufacture them.
- Explain how laboratory volumetric glassware is calibrated, how the calibration markings are indicated on the glassware, and proper cleaning protocol.
- Evaluate the advantages and use of micropipettes, volumetric pipettes, and serologic pipettes.

Laboratory Balances
- Discuss the characteristics of common laboratory balances.

Laboratory Centrifuges
- Compare various types and uses of laboratory centrifuges.

Laboratory Reagent Water
- Contrast various forms and grades of water used in the laboratory and their preparation methods.

Reagents Used in Laboratory Assays
- List and describe the various grades of chemicals used in the laboratory, including their levels of quality and their purpose.
- Define the terms solute and solvent, and calculate problems related to these constituents.
- Identify the components of a properly labeled container used to store a laboratory reagent or solution.

Review Questions
- Demonstrate comprehension of the chapter content by completing the end-of-chapter review questions with a grade of 80% or higher.

Note
- • indicates MLT and MLS core content
- ❖ indicates MLT (optional) and MLS advanced content

KEY TERMS

analytical balance
buffer
international units (SI)
meniscus
precipitate
reagent
safety data sheet (SDS)
solute
solvent
supernatant

If the results of laboratory analyses are to be useful to the physician in diagnosing and treating patients, the tests must be performed accurately. Many factors contribute to the final laboratory result for a single determination.

To unify physical measurements worldwide, the International System of Units (SI units) has been adopted. Many of these units also relate to the metric system. A coherent system of measurement units is vital to precise clinical laboratory analyses. This chapter discusses SI units of measure and the use of metric measurements in the laboratory; Chapter 7 discusses other laboratory calculations.

The use of high-quality analytical methods and instrumentation is essential to laboratory work. The importance of knowing the correct use of the various pieces of glassware must be thoroughly appreciated. The three basic pieces of volumetric glassware—*volumetric flasks, graduated measuring cylinders,* and *pipettes*—are specialized designs, with each having its own particular use in the laboratory. Many different pieces of laboratory equipment are used in performing clinical determinations, and knowledge of the proper use and handling of this equipment is an important part of any laboratory work. Use of balances and measurement of volume using pipettes are important basic analytical procedures in the clinical laboratory. Centrifuges also have a variety of uses in the laboratory.

The accuracy of laboratory analyses depends to a great extent on the accuracy of the **reagent**, a solution used for performing a chemical test. Traditional preparation of reagents makes use of balances and volumetric measuring devices such as pipettes and volumetric flasks—examples of fundamental laboratory apparatus. When reagents and standard solutions are being prepared, it is imperative that only the purest water supply be used in the procedure. Chapter 7 discusses the calculation of required constituents of solutions.

SYSTEMS OF MEASUREMENT

The ability to measure accurately is the keystone of the scientific method, and anyone engaged in performing clinical laboratory

TABLE 6.1 Common Conversions Between English and Metric Systems

ENGLISH (U.S.) TO METRIC CONVERSIONS	
English	**Metric**
1 inch	2.56 centimeters
1 foot	0.3 meter
1 yard	0.9 meter
1 quart	0.9 liter
1 gallon	3.79 liter
1 pound	0.5 kilogram
METRIC TO ENGLISH CONVERSIONS	
Metric	**English**
1 centimeter	0.39 = inches
1 meter	3.3 feet
1 meter	1.1 yards
1 liter	0.264 gallons
1 liter	1.05 quarts
1 kilogram	2.2 pounds

analyses must have a working knowledge of measurement systems and units of measurement. It is also necessary to understand how to convert units of one system to units of another system. Systems of measurement included here are the English, metric, and SI systems.

English and Metric Systems

The metric system has not been widely used in the United States, except in the scientific community. Because the English system is common in everyday use, English/metric system equivalents are presented in Table 6.1.

Traditionally, measurements in the clinical laboratory have been made in metric units. The metric system is based on a decimal system, a system of divisions and multiples of tens. The meter (m) is the standard metric unit for measurement of length, the gram (g) is the unit of mass, and the liter (L) is the unit of volume. Multiples or divisions of these reference units constitute the various other metric units.

INTERNATIONAL SYSTEM (SI SYSTEM)

Another system of measurement, **international units** (from Système International d'Unités) or **SI**), has been adopted by the worldwide scientific community as a coherent, standardized system based on seven base units. In addition, derived units and supplemental units are used as well. The SI base units describe seven fundamental but independent physical quantities. The derived units are calculated mathematically from two or more base units.

The SI system was established in 1960 by international agreement and is now the standard international language of measurement. The National Institute of Standards and Technology (NIST), formerly the National Bureau of Standards (NBS), an agency of the U.S. Department of Commerce, in conjunction with the International Bureau of Weights and Measures, is responsible for maintaining the standards on which the SI system of measurement is based.

The term *metric system* generally refers to the SI system, and for informational purposes, metric terms that remain in common usage are described here as needed.

Base Units of SI System

In the SI system, the base units of measurement are the metre (meter), kilogram, second, mole, ampere, kelvin, and candela (Table 6.2). All SI units can be qualified by standard prefixes that serve to convert values to more convenient forms, depending on the size of the object being measured (Table 6.3).

Various rules should be kept in mind when combining these prefixes with their basic units and using the SI system. An *s* should not be added to form the plural of the abbreviation for a unit or for a prefix with a unit. For example, 25 millimeters should be abbreviated as 25 mm, not "25 mms." Do not use periods after abbreviations (use mm, not "mm."). Do not use compound prefixes; instead, use the closest accepted prefix. For example, 24×10^{-9} gram (g) should be expressed as 24 nanograms (24 ng) rather than "24 millimicrograms." In the SI system, commas are not used as spacers in recording large numbers, because they are used in place of decimal points in some countries. Instead, groups of three digits are separated by spaces. When recording in the Kelvin scale, omit the degree sign. Therefore 295 kelvins should be recorded as 295 K, not "295° K." However, the symbol for degrees Celsius is ° C, and 22 degrees Celsius should be recorded as 22° C. Multiples and submultiples should be used in steps of 10^3 or 10^{-3}. Only one

TABLE 6.2 Basic Units of the SI System

Measurement	Unit Name	Abbreviation
Length	metre[a]	m
Mass	kilogram	kg
Time	second	s
Amount of substance	mole	mol
Electric current	ampere	A
Temperature	kelvin[b]	K
Luminous intensity	candela	cd

[a]The spelling *meter* is used in the United States and in this book.
[b]Although the basic unit of temperature is the kelvin, the degree Celsius is regarded as an acceptable unit, because the use of kelvins may be impractical in many cases. Celsius is used more often in the clinical laboratory.
SI, International System of Units.

TABLE 6.3 Prefixes of the SI System

Prefix	Symbol	Factor	Decimal
Tera	T	10^{12}	1 000 000 000 000
Giga	G	10^{9}	1 000 000 000
Mega	M	10^{6}	1 000 000
Kilo	K	10^{3}	1 000
Hecto	D	10^{2}	100
Deka	Da	10^{1}	10
Deci	D	10^{-1}	0.1
Centi	C	10^{-2}	0.01
Milli	m	10^{-3}	0.001
Micro	μ	10^{-6}	0.000 001
Nano	n	10^{-9}	0.000 000 001
Pico	p	10^{-12}	0.000 000 000 001
Femto	f	10^{-15}	0.000 000 000 000 001
Atto	a	10^{-18}	0.000 000 000 000 000 001

SI, International System of Units.

slash (/) is used when indicating per or a denominator: thus meters per second squared (m/s^2), not meters per second per second (m/s/s), and millimoles per liter-hour (mmol/L hour), not millimoles per liter per hour (mmol/L/hour). Finally, although the preferred SI spellings are "metre" and "litre," the spellings meter and liter remain in common usage in the United States and are used in this book.

The base units of measurement that are used most often in the clinical laboratory are those for length, mass, and volume.

Length

The standard unit for the measurement of length or distance is the meter (m). The meter is standardized as 1,650,763.73 wavelengths of a certain orange light in the spectrum of krypton-86. One meter equals 39.37 inches (in), slightly more than a yard in the English system. There are 2.54 centimeters in 1 inch.

Using the system of prefixes previously discussed, further common divisions and multiples of the meter follow. One-tenth of a meter is a decimeter (dm), one-hundredth of a meter is a centimeter (cm), and one-thousandth of a meter is a millimeter (mm). One thousand meters equals 1 kilometer (km). The following examples show equivalent measurements of length:

25 mm = 0.025 m
10 cm = 100 mm
1 m = 100 cm
1 m = 1000 mm

Other units of length that were in common usage in the metric system but that no longer are recommended in the SI system are the angstrom and the micron. The micron (μ), which is equal to 10^{-6} m, has been replaced by the micrometer (μm).

Mass (and Weight)

Mass denotes the quantity of matter, whereas weight takes into account the force of gravity and should not be used in the same sense as mass. These terms are often used interchangeably.

The standard unit for the measurement of mass in the SI system is the kilogram (kg). This is the basis for all other mass measurements in the system. One kilogram weighs approximately 2.2 pounds (lb) in the English system. The kilogram is divided into thousandths, called grams (g). One thousand grams equals 1 kg. The gram is used much more often than the kilogram in the clinical laboratory. The gram is divided into thousandths, called milligrams (mg). Grams and milligrams are units commonly used in weighing substances in the clinical laboratory. The following are examples of weight measurement equivalents:

10 mg = 0.01 g
0.055 g = 55 mg
25 g = 25,000 mg
1.5 kg = 1500 g

Volume

In the clinical laboratory the standard unit of volume is the liter (L). It was not included in the list of base units of the SI system, because the liter is a derived unit. The standard unit of volume in the SI system is the cubic meter (m^3). However, this unit is quite large, and the cubic decimeter (dm^3) is a more convenient size for use in the clinical laboratory. In 1964 the Conférence Générale des Poids et Mesures (CGPM) accepted the litre (liter) as a special name for the cubic decimeter. Previously, the standard liter was the volume occupied by 1 kg of pure water at 4° C (the temperature at which a volume of water weighs the most) and at normal atmospheric pressure. On this basis, 1 L equals 1000.027 cubic centimeters (cm^3), and the units, milliliters and cubic centimeters, were used interchangeably, although there is a slight difference between them. One liter is slightly more than 1 quart (qt) in the English system (1 L = 1.06 qt).

The liter is divided into thousandths, called *milliliters* (mL); millionths, called *microliters* (μL); and billionths, called *nanoliters* (nL). The following examples show volume equivalents:

500 mL = 0.5 L
0.25 L = 250 mL
2 L = 2000 mL

Because the liter is derived from the meter (1 L = 1 dm^3), it follows that 1 cm^3 is equal to 1 mL and that 1 millimeter cubed (mm^3) is equal to 1 mL. The former abbreviation for cubic centimeter (cc) has been replaced by cm^3. Although this is a common means of expressing volume in the clinical laboratory, milliliter (mL) is preferred.

Amount of Substance

The standard unit of measurement for the amount of a (chemical) substance in the SI system is the mole (mol). The *mole* is defined as the quantity of a chemical equal to that present in 0.0120 kg of pure carbon-12. A mole of a chemical substance is the relative atomic or molecular mass unit of that substance. Formerly, the terms *atomic weight* and *molecular weight* were used to describe the mole (see later discussion).

Temperature

Three scales are used to measure temperature: the Kelvin, Celsius, and Fahrenheit scales. The Celsius scale is sometimes referred to as the *centigrade scale,* which is an outdated term.

The basic unit of temperature in the SI system is the kelvin (K). The use of the kelvin may be impractical in many cases. The Celsius scale is used most often in the clinical laboratory. The Kelvin and Celsius scales are closely related, and conversion between them is simple because the units (degrees) are equal in magnitude. The difference between the two scales is that each has a different zero point. The zero point on the Kelvin scale is the theoretical temperature of no further heat loss, which is absolute zero. The zero point on the Celsius scale is the freezing point of pure water. Remember, however, that the magnitude of the degree in the two scales is equal. Therefore because water freezes at 273 kelvins (273 K), it follows that 0 degrees Celsius (0° C) equals 273 kelvins (273 K) and that 0 kelvin (0 K) equals minus 273 degrees Celsius (−273° C). Thus to convert from kelvins to degrees Celsius, add 273; to convert from degrees Celsius to kelvins, subtract 273, as follows:

K = ° C + 273
°C = K − 273

Because the Celsius scale was devised so that 100° C is the boiling point of pure water, the boiling point on the Kelvin scale is 373 K.

Converting from Celsius to Fahrenheit is not as simple, because the degrees are not equal in magnitude on these two scales. The Fahrenheit scale was originally devised with the

TABLE 6.4 Common Reference Points on the Three Temperature Scales

Reference Point	Degrees Fahrenheit	Kelvin	Degrees Celsius
Boiling point of water	212	373	100
Body temperature	98.6	310	37
Room temperature	68	293	20
Freezing point of water	32	273	0
Absolute zero[a]	−459.67	0	−273.15

[a]Coldest possible temperature.

BOX 6.2 Sample Temperature Conversion Problems

What is 50° F in degrees Celsius?

$°C = {}^5/_9\,(°\,F - 32)$

$x = {}^5/_9\,(50°\,F - 32)$

$x = {}^5/_9\,18°\,F$

$x = 10°\,C$

What is 18° C in degrees Fahrenheit?

$°F = {}^9/_5\,(°\,C) + 32$

$x = {}^9/_5\,(18°\,C) + 32$

$x = 32.4 + 32$

$x = 64.4°\,F$

zero point at the lowest temperature attainable from a mixture of table salt and ice, and the body temperature of a small animal was used to set 100° F. Thus on the Fahrenheit scale, the freezing point of pure water is 32° F, and the temperature at which pure water boils is 212° F. It is rare that readings on one of these scales must be converted to the other, because almost always, readings taken and used in the clinical laboratory are on the Celsius scale.

Table 6.4 provides examples of comparative readings of the three temperature scales, with common reference points.

It is possible to convert from one scale to the other. The most common conversions are between Celsius and Fahrenheit, and vice versa (Box 6.1). The basic conversion formulas are as follows:

To convert Fahrenheit to Celsius:

$$°C = {}^5/_9(°F - 32)$$

To convert Celsius to Fahrenheit:

$$°F = {}^9/_5(°C) + 32$$

Box 6.2 provides sample calculations between Celsius and Fahrenheit.

Non-SI Units

Several non-SI units are relevant to clinical laboratory analyses, such as minutes (min), hours (hr), and days (d). These units of time have such historic use in everyday life that it is unlikely new SI units derived from the second (the base unit for time in the SI system) will be implemented. Another non-SI unit is the liter (L), as already discussed with the base SI units of volume. Pressure is expressed in *millimeters of mercury (mm Hg)* and enzyme activity in *international units (IU)*. One unit (U) is defined as the amount of enzyme that will catalyze the transformation of 1 μmol of substrate per minute, or 1 unit (U) is the amount of enzyme that catalyzes the reaction of 1 nmol of substrate per minute.

Reporting Results in SI Units

To give a meaningful laboratory result, it is important to report both the numbers and the units by which the result is measured. The unit expresses or defines the dimension of the measured substance—concentration, mass, or volume—and is an important part of any laboratory result. Table 6.5 shows conversions between metric and SI units.

TABLE 6.5 Examples of Conversions Between Metric and SI Units

	Metric Unit ×	Factor =	SI units
Gram	g/mL	10^{15} MW	pmol/L
	g/100 mL	10	g/L
	g/100 mL	10^4 MW	mmol/L
Microgram	mcg/100 mL	10 MW	μmol/L
Milligram	mg/100 mL	10^{-2}	g/L
Milliliter	mL/100 g	10	mL/kg

mmol, Millimoles; *MW*, molecular weight; *mmol*, micromoles; *pmol*, picomoles; *SI*, International System of Units.

BOX 6.1 Temperature Conversions

From Fahrenheit to Celsius

To convert from degrees Fahrenheit to degrees Celsius, subtract 32° from the temperature and multiply by ${}^5/_9$:

Fahrenheit	0	10	20	30	40	50	60	70	80	90	100
Celsius	−18	−12	−7	−1	6	10	16	21	27	32	38

From Celsius to Fahrenheit

To convert from degrees Celsius to degrees Fahrenheit, multiply the temperature by 1.8 (${}^9/_5$) and add 32°:

Celsius	−10	−5	0	5	10	15	20	25	30	35	40
Fahrenheit	14	23	32	41	50	59	68	77	86	95	104

LABWARE

The general laboratory supplies described in this chapter are used for storage, measurement, and containment. Regardless of composition, most laboratory supplies must meet certain tolerances of accuracy. Those that satisfy NIST specifications are categorized as Class A. Vessels holding or transferring liquid are designed either "*to contain*" *(TC)* or "*to deliver*" *(TD)* a specified volume. Most labware can be divided into two main categories according to use:

- Containers and receivers (such as beakers, test tubes, Erlenmeyer flasks, and reagent bottles)
- Volumetric ware (such as automatic and manual pipettes, volumetric flasks, graduated cylinders, and burets)

Plasticware

The clinical laboratory has benefited greatly from the introduction of plasticware. It is less expensive and more durable, but glassware may be preferred because of its chemical stability and clarity. Plastic is unbreakable, which is its greatest advantage. It is preferred for certain analyses in which glass can be damaged by chemicals used in the testing. Alkaline solutions must be stored in plastic.

The disadvantages of plastic are that there is some leaching of surface-bound constituents into solutions, some permeability to water vapor, some evaporation through breathing of the plastic, and some absorption of dyes, stains, or proteins. Because evaporation is a significant factor in using plasticware, small volumes of reagent should never be stored in oversized plastic bottles for long periods.

Glassware

Although disposable plasticware has largely replaced glassware because of high resistance to corrosion and breakage, clinical and research laboratories still use glassware for analytical work. Certain types of glass can be attacked by reagents to such an extent that the determinations made in them are not valid. It is therefore important to use the correct type of glass for the testing being done.

Types of Glass

Clinical laboratory glassware can be divided into several types: glass with high thermal resistance, high-silica glass, glass with a high resistance to alkali, low-actinic glass, and standard flint glass.

Thermal-Resistant (Borosilicate) Glass. Glass with high thermal resistance is usually a borosilicate glass with a low alkali content. This type of glassware is resistant to heat, corrosion, and thermal shock and should be used whenever heating or sterilization by heat is employed. Borosilicate glass, known by the commercial name *Pyrex* (Corning Glass Works, Corning, NY), or *Kimax* (Kimble Glass Co., Vineland, NJ) is used widely in the laboratory because of its high qualities of resistance. Laboratory apparatus such as beakers, flasks, and pipettes are usually made from borosilicate glass. Other brands of glassware are made from lower-grade borosilicate glass and may be used when a high-quality borosilicate glass is not necessary. One or more of these brand names will be found on many different types of glassware in the laboratory. It is essential to choose glassware that has a reliable composition and will be resistant to laboratory chemicals and conditions. In borosilicate glassware, mechanical strength and thermal and chemical resistance are well balanced.

Alumina-Silicate Glass. Alumina-silicate glass has a high silica content, which makes it comparable to fused quartz in its heat resistance, chemical stability, and electrical characteristics. It is strengthened chemically rather than thermally. Corex (Corning) is made from alumina-silica. This type of glassware is used for high-precision analytical work; it is radiation resistant and can also be used for optical reflectors and mirrors. It is not used for the general type of glassware found in the laboratory.

Acid-Resistant and Alkali-Resistant Glass. Glass with high resistance to acids or alkali was developed particularly for use with strong acid or alkaline solutions. It is boron free. It is often referred to as *soft glass* because its thermal resistance is much less than that of borosilicate glass, and it must be heated and cooled very carefully. Its use should be limited to times when solutions of, or digestions with, strong acids or alkalis are made.

Low-Actinic (Amber Colored) Glass. Low-actinic glassware contains materials that usually impart an amber or red color to the glass and reduce the amount of light transmitted through to the substance in the glassware. It is used for substances that are particularly sensitive to light, such as bilirubin and vitamin A.

Flint Glass. Standard flint glass, or soda-lime glass, is composed of a mixture of the oxides of silicon, calcium, and sodium. It is the least expensive glass and is readily made into a variety of types of glassware. This type of glass is much less resistant to high temperatures and sudden changes in temperature, and its resistance to chemical attack is only fair. Glassware made from soda-lime glass can release alkali into solutions and can therefore cause considerable errors in certain laboratory determinations. For example, manual pipettes made from soda-lime glass may release alkali into the pipetted liquid.

Disposable Glassware. The widespread use of relatively inexpensive disposable glassware has greatly reduced the need to clean glassware. Disposable glassware is made to be used and discarded, and no cleaning is necessary either before or after use in most cases. Disposable glass and plastic are used to manufacture many laboratory supplies, including test tubes of all sizes, pipettes, slides, Petri dishes for microbiology, and specimen containers.

Containers and Receivers

This category of labware includes many of the most frequently used and most common pieces of glassware in the laboratory. Containers and receivers must be made of good-quality glass. These are not calibrated to hold a particular or exact volume, but rather are available for various volumes, depending on the use desired. Beakers, Erlenmeyer flasks, test tubes, and reagent bottles are made in many different sizes (Fig. 6.1). This glassware, as with the volumetric glassware, has certain information indicated directly on the vessel. The volume and the brand (trade) name (or trademark) are two pieces of information found on items such as beakers and test tubes. Containers

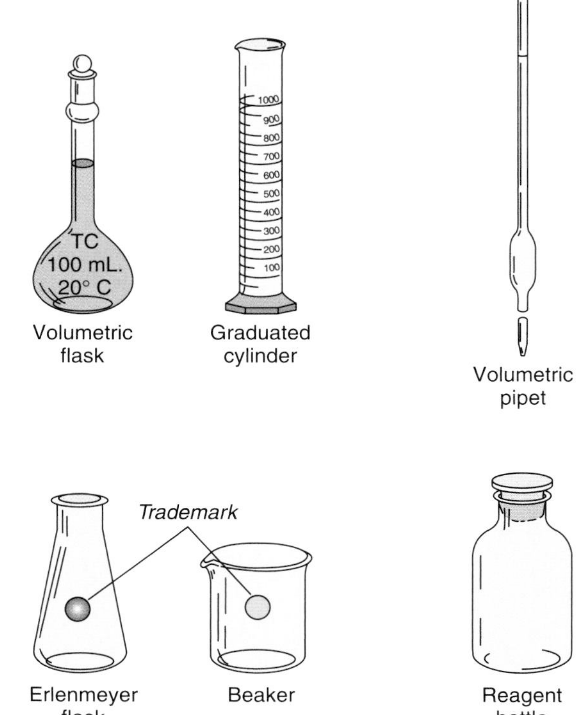

Fig. 6.1 Laboratory glassware. *TC,* To contain.

and receivers are not as expensive as volumetric glassware because the process of exact volume calibration is not necessary.

Beakers. Beakers are wide, straight-sided cylindrical vessels and are available in many sizes and in several forms. The most common form used in the clinical laboratory is known as the *Griffin low form.* Beakers should be made of glass that is resistant to the many chemicals used in beakers and also resistant to heat. Beakers are used along with flasks for general mixing and reagent preparation.

Erlenmeyer Flasks. Erlenmeyer flasks are often used in the laboratory for preparing reagents and for titration procedures. As with beakers, these flasks come in various sizes and must be made from a resistant form of glass.

Test Tubes. Test tubes come in many sizes, depending on the use for which they are intended. Test tubes without lips are the most satisfactory because there is less chance of chipping and eventual breakage. Disposable test tubes are used for most laboratory purposes. Because chemical reactions occur in test tubes used in the chemistry laboratory, test tubes intended for such use should be made of borosilicate glass, which is resistant to thermal shock.

Reagent Bottles. All reagents should be stored in reagent bottles of some type. These can be made of glass or some other material; some of the more common bottles are now made of plastic. Reagent bottles come in various sizes. The size used should meet the needs of the particular situation.

Volumetric Glassware

Volumetric glassware must go through a rigorous process of volume calibration to ensure the accuracy of the measurements required for laboratory determinations. In very precise work, it is never safe to assume that the volume contained or delivered by any piece of equipment is exactly that indicated on the equipment. The calibration process is lengthy and time-consuming, so the cost of volumetric glassware is relatively high compared with the cost of uncalibrated glassware.

Calibration of Volumetric Glassware. Calibration is the means by which glassware or other apparatus used in quantitative measurements is checked to determine its exact volume. To *calibrate* is to divide the glassware or mark it with graduations (or other indices of quantity) for the purpose of measurement. Calibration marks will be seen on every piece of volumetric glassware used in the laboratory. Specifications for the calibration of glassware are regulated by NIST.[1–3] High-quality volumetric glassware is calibrated by the manufacturer; this calibration can be checked by the laboratory that is using the glassware.

Each piece of volumetric glassware must be checked and must comply with these specifications before it can be accurately used in the clinical laboratory. Pipettes, volumetric flasks, and other types of volumetric glassware are supposed to hold, deliver, or contain a specific amount of liquid. This specified amount, or volume, is known as the *units of capacity* and is indicated by the manufacturer directly on each piece of glassware.

Volumetric glassware is usually calibrated by weight using distilled water. Water is typically used as the liquid for calibration because it is readily available and similar in viscosity and speed of drainage to the solutions and reagents used in the clinical laboratory. The units of capacity determined will therefore be the volume of water contained in, or delivered by, the glassware at a particular temperature. The manufacturer knows what the weights of various amounts of distilled water are at specific temperatures. This information is used in the manual calibration of volumetric glassware. If a manufacturer wants a volumetric flask to contain 100 mL, a sensitive balance such as an analytical balance is used. Weights corresponding to what 100 mL of distilled water weighs at a specific temperature are placed on one side of the balance. The flask to be calibrated is placed on the other side of the balance, and distilled water is gradually added to it until equilibrium is achieved. The manufacturer then makes a permanent calibration mark on the neck of the flask at the bottom of the water meniscus level. This flask is then calibrated to contain 100 mL. Other sizes and types of volumetric glassware are similarly calibrated.

The volume of a particular piece of glassware varies with the temperature. For this reason, it is necessary to specify the temperature at which the glassware was calibrated. Glass will swell or shrink with changes in temperature, and the volume of the glassware will therefore vary. Most volumetric glassware for routine clinical use is calibrated at 20° C. This means that the calibration process and checking took place at a controlled temperature of 20° C. On all volumetric glassware, the inscription "20° C" will be seen. Although 20° C has been almost universally adopted as the standard temperature for calibration of volumetric glassware, each piece of glassware will have the temperature of calibration inscribed on it. The volume of a volumetric flask is smaller at a low temperature than at a high temperature.

A 50-mL volumetric flask that was calibrated at 20° C would contain less than 50 mL at 10° C.

Because the laboratory depends so greatly on the quality of its glassware to produce reliable results, it is necessary to be certain that the glassware is of the best quality. The glass used for volumetric glassware must meet certain standards of quality. It must be transparent and free from striations and other surface irregularities. It should have no defects that would distort the appearance of the liquid surface or the portion of the calibration line seen through the glass.

The design and workmanship for volumetric glassware are also specified by NIST. The shape of the glassware must permit complete emptying and thorough cleaning, and it must stand solidly on a level surface.

Volumetric Flasks

Volumetric flasks are flasks with a round bulb at the bottom. This tapers to a long neck on which the calibration mark is found. The NIST specifications apply to all volumetric glassware and therefore to volumetric flasks[1] (see Fig. 6.1). Volumetric flasks are calibrated *to contain* a specific amount or volume of liquid, and therefore the letters *TC* are inscribed somewhere on the neck of the flask. Many different sizes of volumetric flasks are available for the different volumes of liquid used. Sizes in which volumetric flasks can be purchased include 10, 25, 50, 100, and 500 mL, and 1 and 2 L.

Volumetric flasks have been calibrated individually "to contain" the specified volume at a specified temperature; they are not calibrated "to deliver" this volume. For each size of volumetric flask, there are certain allowable limits within which its volume must lie. These limits are called the *tolerance* of the flask. All volumetric glassware has a specific tolerance, the *capacity tolerance,* which depends on the size of the glassware. For example, if a 100-mL volumetric flask has a tolerance of 0.08 mL, conditions are controlled during the calibration of a 100-mL volumetric flask to guarantee these limits. A tolerance of 0.08 mL indicates that the allowable limits for the volume of a 100-mL volumetric flask are from 99.92 to 100.08 mL. A tolerance of 0.05 mL for a 50-mL volumetric flask indicates allowable limits of 49.95 to 50.05 mL for the volume of the flask. Volumetric flasks are used in the preparation of specific volumes of reagents or laboratory solutions. They should be used with reagents or solutions at room temperature. Solutions diluted in volumetric flasks should be repeatedly mixed during the dilution so that the contents are homogeneous before they are made up to volume. In this way, errors caused by the expansion or contraction of liquids during mixing become negligible. An important factor in the use of any volumetric apparatus is an accurate reading of the meniscus level (see later discussion on pipetting technique).

Graduated Measuring Cylinders

A graduated measuring cylinder is a long, straight-sided cylindrical piece of glassware with calibrated markings. Graduated cylinders are used to measure volumes of liquids when a high degree of accuracy is not essential. They can be made from plastic or polyethylene or from glass. Graduated cylinders come in various sizes according to the volumes they measure: 10, 25, 50, 100, 500, and 1000 mL. A 100-mL graduated cylinder can measure 100 mL or a fraction of this amount, depending on the calibration, or graduation, marks on it. Most graduated cylinders are calibrated *to deliver,* as indicated directly on the glassware by the inscription "TD." The letters *TD* can be found on many types of volumetric glassware, especially on the numerous pipettes used in the laboratory.

Graduated cylinders can be used to measure a specified volume of a liquid, such as water, in the preparation of laboratory reagents. The calibration marks on the cylinder indicate its capacity at different points. If 450 mL of water is to be measured, the most satisfactory cylinder to use would be one with a capacity of 500 mL. Graduated cylinders are not calibrated as accurately as volumetric flasks. Therefore the capacity tolerance for graduated cylinders allows a greater variation in volume. The capacity tolerance is greater for the larger graduated cylinders. A 100-mL graduated cylinder (TD) has a tolerance of 0.40 mL, meaning that the allowable limits are 99.60 to 100.40 mL.

Pipettes

Pipettes are another type of volumetric glassware used to measure fluids (Fig. 6.2). Although many types of pipettes are available, it is important to use only pipettes manufactured by reputable companies. Care and discretion should be used in selecting pipettes for clinical laboratory use, because their accuracy is one of the determining factors in producing accurate results.

Each manual pipette has at least one calibration or graduation mark on it, as does all volumetric glassware. A pipette is filled by using mechanical suction or an aspirator bulb. Mouth suction is never used. Strong acids, bases, solvents, or human specimens are much too potent or contaminated to risk pipetting them by mouth. Caustic liquids and some solvents are very dangerous; some destroy tissue immediately on contact. Some solvents have harmful vapors.

Pipettes are calibrated to deliver, or transfer, a specified volume from one vessel to another. Manual and automatic pipettes are available. Ergonomically correct pipettes are available on the market for conditions of frequent pipetting. For most general laboratory use, there are two main types of manual pipettes:

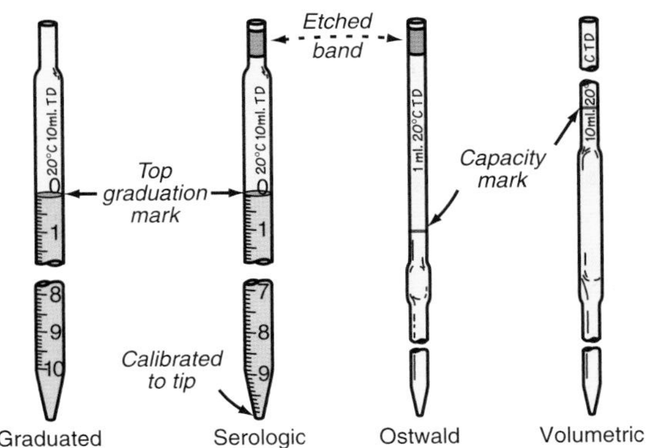

Fig. 6.2 Types of manual pipettes. *TD,* To deliver.

the volumetric (or transfer) pipette and the graduated (or measuring) pipette. They are classified according to whether they contain or deliver a specified amount; they may be called *to-contain pipettes* or *to-deliver pipettes.* A to-contain pipette is identified by the inscribed letters *TC* and a to-deliver pipette by the letters *TD.* The TD pipette is filled properly and allowed to drain completely into a receiving vessel. Portions of nonviscous samples are accurately measured by allowing the *volumetric pipette* to drain while it is held in the vertical position, using only the force of gravity. For most volumetric glassware, the temperature of calibration is usually 20° C, and this is inscribed on the pipette.

The opening (orifice) at the delivery tip of the pipette is of a certain size to allow a specified time for drainage when the pipette is held vertically. A pipette must be held vertically to ensure proper drainage. It will not drain as fast when held at a 45-degree angle.

Volumetric Pipettes. A volumetric, or transfer, pipette has been calibrated to deliver a fixed volume of liquid by drainage. These pipettes consist of a cylindrical bulb joined at both ends to narrow glass tubing. A calibration mark is etched around the upper suction tube, and the lower delivery tube is drawn out to a fine tip. Some important considerations concerning volumetric pipettes are that the calibration mark should not be too close to the top of the suction tube, the bulb should merge gradually into the lower delivery tube, and the delivery tip should have a gradual taper. To reduce drainage errors, the orifice should be of a size such that the outflow of the pipette is not too rapid. These pipettes should be made from a good-quality Kimax or Pyrex glass.

Volumetric pipettes are suitable for all accurate measurements of volumes of 1 mL or more and are calibrated to deliver the amount inscribed on them. This volume is measured from the calibration mark to the tip. A 5-mL volumetric pipette will deliver a single measured volume of 5 mL, and a 2-mL volumetric pipette will deliver 2 mL. The tolerance of volumetric pipettes increases with the capacity of the pipette. A 10-mL volumetric pipette will have a greater tolerance than a 2-mL pipette. The tolerance of a 5-mL volumetric pipette is 0.01 mL. When volumes of liquids are to be delivered with great accuracy, a volumetric pipette is used. Volumetric pipettes are used to measure standard solutions, unknown blood and plasma filtrates, serum, plasma, urine, cerebrospinal fluid, and some reagents.

Measurements with volumetric pipettes are done individually, and the volumes can be only whole milliliters, as determined by the pipette selected (such as 1, 2, 5, and 10 mL). To transfer 1 mL of a standard solution into a test tube volumetrically, a 1-mL volumetric pipette is used. To transfer 5 mL of the same solution, a 5-mL volumetric pipette is used. After a volumetric pipette drains, a drop remains inside the delivery tip. The specific volume the pipette is calibrated to deliver is dependent on the drop left in the pipette tip. Information inscribed on the pipette includes the temperature of calibration (usually 20° C), capacity, manufacturer, and use (TD). The technique involved in using volumetric pipettes correctly is very important, and a certain amount of skill is required (see Pipetting Technique Using Manual Pipettes).

Graduated Pipettes. Another way to deliver a particular amount of liquid is to deliver the amount of liquid contained between two calibration marks on a cylindrical tube or pipette. Such a pipette is called a *graduated pipette* or *measuring pipette.* It has several graduation, or calibration, marks (see Fig. 6.2). Many measurements in the laboratory do not require the precision of the volumetric pipette, so graduated pipettes are used when great accuracy is less critical. This does not mean that these pipettes may be used with less care than the volumetric pipettes. Graduated pipettes are used primarily in measuring reagents, but they are not calibrated with sufficient tolerance to use in measuring standard or control solutions, unknown specimens, or filtrates.

A graduated pipette is a straight piece of glass tubing with a tapered end and graduation marks on the stem, separating it into parts. Depending on the size used, graduated pipettes can be used to measure parts of a milliliter or many milliliters. These pipettes come in various sizes or capacities, including 0.1, 0.2, 1.0, 2.0, 5.0, 10, and 25 mL. If 4 mL of deionized water is to be measured into a test tube, a 5-mL graduated pipette would be the best choice. Graduated pipettes require draining between two marks; they introduce one more source of error compared with the volumetric pipettes, which have only one calibration mark. This makes measurements with the graduated pipette less precise. Because of this relatively poor precision, the graduated pipette is used when speed is more important than precision. It is used for measurements of reagents and is generally not considered accurate enough for measuring samples and standard solutions.

Two types of graduated pipettes are calibrated for delivery. A Mohr pipette is calibrated between two marks on the stem, and a serologic pipette has graduation marks down to the delivery tip. The serologic pipette has a larger orifice and therefore drains faster than the Mohr pipette.

The volume of the space between the last calibration mark and the delivery tip is not known in the Mohr pipette. In Mohr graduated pipettes, this space cannot be used for measuring fluids. Graduated pipettes are calibrated in much the same manner as volumetric pipettes, but they are not constructed to specifications that are as strict, and they have larger tolerances. The allowable tolerance for a 5-mL graduated pipette is 0.02 mL.

Serologic Pipettes. The serologic pipette is similar to the graduated pipette in appearance (see Fig. 6.2). The orifice, or tip opening, is larger in the serologic pipette than in other pipettes. The rate of the fall of liquid is much too fast for great accuracy or precision. Using the serologic pipette in chemistry would require impeding the flow of liquid from the delivery tip. The serologic pipette is graduated to the end of the delivery tip and has an etched band on the suction piece. It is therefore designed to be blown out mechanically. The serologic pipette is less precise than any of the pipettes discussed earlier. It is designed for use in serology, in which relative values are sought.

Specialized Pipettes

Micropipettes (To-Contain Pipettes). The micropipette, or to-contain pipette, when used properly, is one of the more precise pipettes used in the clinical laboratory. This type of pipette is calibrated to contain a specified amount of liquid. If a pipette contains only 0.1 mL and 0.1 mL of blood is needed for a laboratory determination, then none of the blood can be left inside the pipette. The entire contents of the pipette must be emptied. If this pipette is rinsed well with a diluting solution, all the blood or similar specimen will be removed from it. The correct way to use a TC pipette is to rinse it with a suitable diluent. Thus a TC pipette cannot be used properly unless the receiving vessel contains a diluent; that is, a TC pipette should not be used to deliver a specimen into an empty receiving vessel. Because all the liquid in a TC pipette is rinsed out and used, there is only one graduation mark.

Micropipettes are used when small amounts of blood or specimen are needed. Many procedures require only a small amount of blood, and a micropipette is used for this measurement. Because even a minute volume remaining in the pipette can cause a significant error in micromeasurement, most micropipettes are calibrated to contain the stated volume rather than to deliver it. They are generally available in small sizes from 1 to 500 mL.

Self-Filling Pipettes. A special disposable micropipette used in the hematology laboratory is a self-filling pipette accompanied by a polyethylene reagent reservoir. An example of this type of self-filling pipette is the BMP LeukoChek Test Kit for the microscopic counting of leukocytes and platelets in whole blood (see Chapter 11).

Capillary Pipettes. This inexpensive, disposable micropipette is made of capillary tubing with a calibration line marking a specified volume. The capillary micropipette is filled to the line by capillary action, and the measured liquid is delivered by positive pressure, as with a medicine dropper. These pipettes are usually calibrated TC and require rinsing to obtain the stated accuracy.

Pipetting

Care and discretion should be used in selecting pipettes for clinical laboratory use; their accuracy is one of the determining factors in the accuracy of the procedures done. As previously mentioned, several types of pipettes are used in the laboratory. Qualified personnel must understand their uses and gain experience in how to handle pipettes in clinical determinations. Practice is the key to success in the use of laboratory pipettes. To reiterate, the two categories of manual pipettes are to-contain (TC) and to-deliver (TD).

To-Contain Pipettes

The TC pipettes are calibrated to contain a specified amount of liquid but are not necessarily calibrated to deliver that exact amount. A small amount of fluid will cling to the inside wall of the TC pipette, and when used, these pipettes should be rinsed out with a diluting fluid to ensure that the entire contents have been emptied.

To-Deliver Pipettes

The TD pipettes are calibrated to deliver the amount of fluid designated on the pipette; this volume will flow out of the pipette by gravity when the pipette is held in a vertical position with its tip against the inside wall of the receiving vessel. A small amount of fluid will remain in the tip of the pipette; this amount is left in the tip because the calibrated portion has been delivered into the receiving vessel.

Blowout Pipettes

Another category of pipette is called *blowout.* The calibration of blowout pipettes is similar to that of TD pipettes, except that the drop remaining in the tip of the pipette must be "blown out" into the receiving vessel. If a pipette is to be blown out, an etched ring will be seen near the suction opening. A mechanical device or safety bulb must be used to blow out the entire contents of the pipette.

Pipetting Technique Using Manual Pipettes

It is important to develop a good technique for using pipettes (Fig. 6.3); only through practice can this be accomplished (Student Procedure Worksheet 6.1). With few exceptions, the same general steps apply to pipetting for all manual pipettes.

Laboratory accidents frequently result from improper pipetting techniques. The greatest potential hazard is pipetting performed by mouth instead of mechanical suction. Mouth pipetting is *never* acceptable in the clinical laboratory. Caustic reagents, contaminated specimens, and poisonous solutions are all pipetted at some point in the laboratory, and every precaution must be taken to ensure the safety of the person doing the work (see Chapter 2).

After the pipette has been filled above the top graduation mark, removed from the vessel, and held in a vertical position, the meniscus must be adjusted (Fig. 6.4). The meniscus is the curvature in the top surface of a liquid. The pipette should be held in such a way that the calibration mark is at eye level. The delivery tip is touched to the inside wall of the original vessel, not the liquid, and the meniscus of the liquid in the pipette is eased, or adjusted, down to the calibration mark.

When clear solutions are used, the bottom of the meniscus is read. For colored or viscous solutions, the top of the meniscus is read. All readings must be made with the eye at the level of the meniscus (see Fig. 6.4). Note that the pipette should be held steady with a finger of the opposite hand while the liquid is allowed to drain into a container.

Before the measured liquid in the pipette is allowed to drain into the receiving vessel, any liquid adhering to the outside of the pipette must be wiped off with a clean piece of gauze or tissue. If this is not done, any drops present on the outside of the pipette might drain into the receiving vessel along with the measured volume. This would make the volume greater than that specified, and an error would result.

Pipetting Technique Using Automatic Pipettes

Automatic Micropipettors. These automatic pipetting devices allow rapid, repetitive measurements and delivery of predetermined volumes of reagents or specimens. The most common type of micropipette used in many laboratories is one that is automatic or semiautomatic, called a *micropipettor.* These piston-operated devices allow repeated, accurate, reproducible delivery of specimens, reagents, and other liquids requiring measurement in small amounts. Many pipettors are continuously adjustable so that

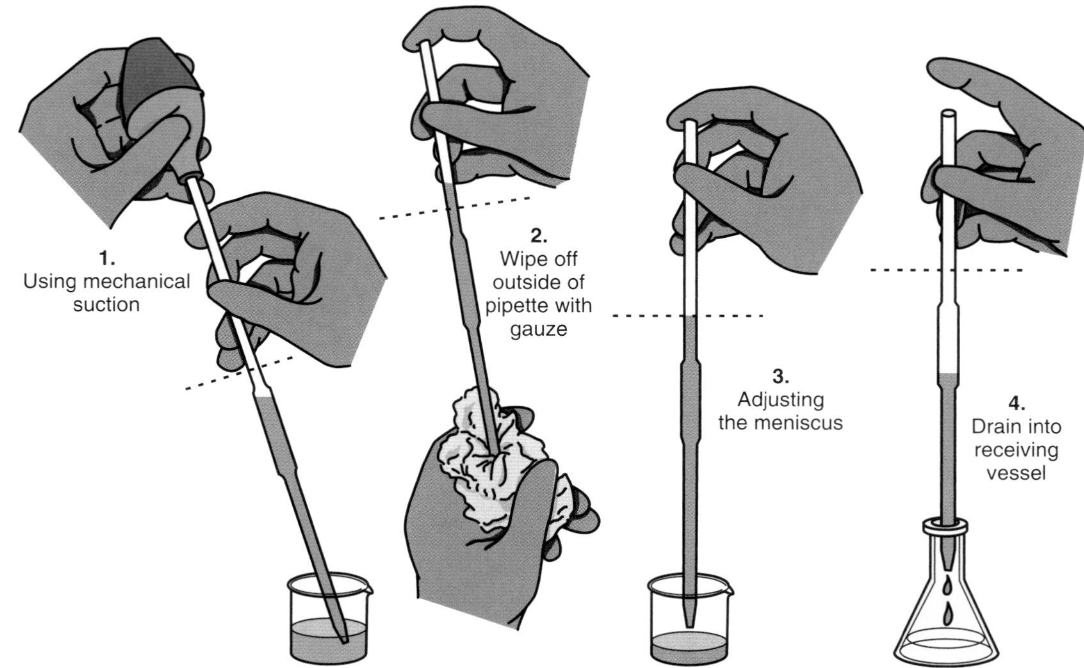

Fig. 6.3 Pipetting technique.

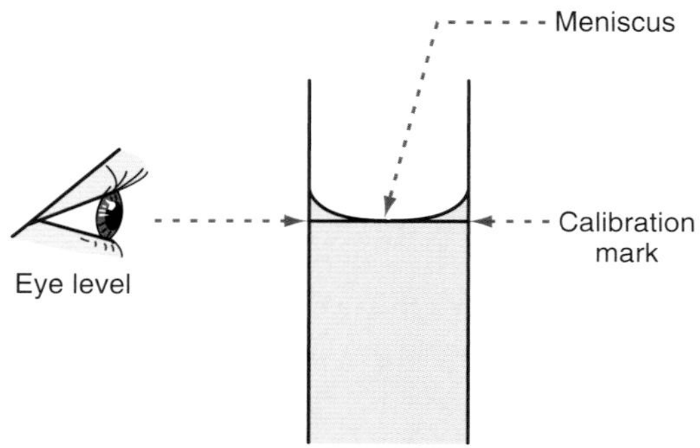

Fig. 6.4 Reading the meniscus.

variable volumes of liquids can be dispensed with the same device. Delivery volume is selected by adjusting the settings on the device. Different types or models are available and allow ranges of volume delivery, as from 0.5 to 500 mL. The calibration of these micropipettes should be checked periodically.

The piston (usually in the form of a thumb plunger) is depressed to a "stop" position on the pipetting device; the tip is placed in the liquid to be measured, and then slowly the plunger is allowed to rise back to the original position (Fig. 6.5). This will fill the tip with the desired volume of liquid. The tips are usually drawn along the inside wall of the vessel from which the measured volume is drawn so that any adhering liquid is removed from the end of the tip. These pipette tips are not usually wiped, as is done with the manual pipettes, because the plastic surface is considered nonwettable. The tip of the pipette device is then placed against the inside wall of the receiving vessel, and the plunger is depressed. When the manufacturer's directions for the device are followed, sample delivery volume is judged to be extremely accurate.

The pipette tips are usually made of disposable plastic, so no cleaning is necessary. Various types of tips are available. Some pipetting devices automatically eject the tip after use. These will also allow the user to insert a new tip and remove the used tip without touching it, minimizing infectious biohazard exposures.

Automatic and semiautomatic micropipettors are useful in many areas of laboratory work. Each of the different types must be carefully calibrated before use. The problems encountered with automatic pipetting depend largely on the nature of the solution to be pipetted. Some reagents cause more bubbles than others, and some are more viscous. Bubbles and viscous solutions can cause problems with measurement and delivery of samples and solutions.

Micropipettors contain or deliver from 1 to 500 mL. It is important to follow the manufacturer's instructions for the device being used because each may be slightly different (Student Procedure Worksheet 6.2).

Automatic Dispensers or Syringes. Many types of automatic dispensers or syringes are used in the laboratory for repetitive adding of multiple doses of the same reagent or diluent. These devices are used for measuring serial amounts of relatively small volumes of the same liquid. The volume to be dispensed is determined by the pipettor setting. Dispensers are available with a variety of volume settings. Some are available as syringes and others as bottle-top devices. Most of these dispensers can be cleaned by autoclaving.

Diluter-Dispensers. In automated instruments, diluter-dispensers are used to prepare a number of different samples for analysis. These devices pipette a selected aliquot of sample and diluent into the instrument or receiving vessel. These devices are mostly of the dual-piston type, one being used for the sample and the other for the diluent or reagent.

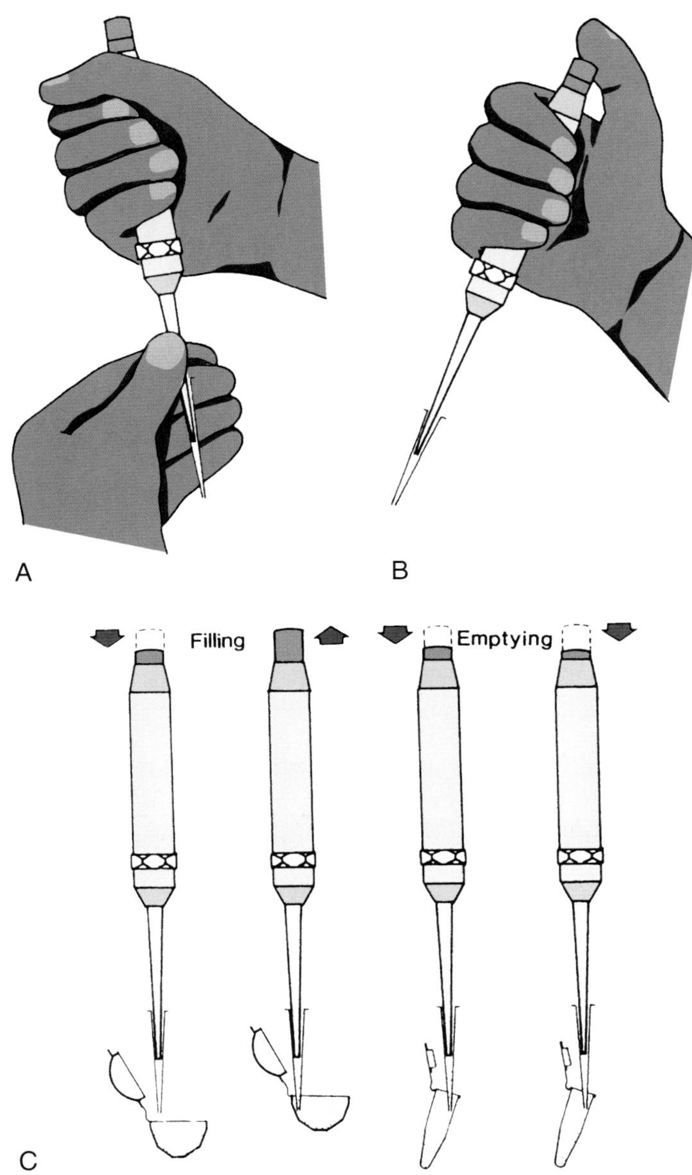

Fig. 6.5 **Steps in using piston-type automatic micropipette.** (A) Attaching proper tip size for range of pipette volume and twisting tip as it is pushed onto pipette to give an airtight, continuous seal. (B) Holding pipette before use. (C) Filling and emptying pipette tip. (From Kaplan LA, Pesce AJ: *Clinical chemistry: theory, analysis, correlation,* ed 5, St Louis, 2010, Elsevier/Mosby.)

Cleaning Laboratory Glassware and Plasticware

Many factors ensure accurate results in laboratory determinations, including the use of clean, unbroken glassware. There is no point in exercising care in obtaining specimens, handling the specimens, and making the laboratory determination if the laboratory ware used is not extremely clean. Plasticware must also be clean.

Since the widespread adoption of disposable glassware and plasticware, few pieces are cleaned for reuse. Only larger pieces of glassware (such as volumetric flasks, pipettes, and graduated cylinders) are usually cleaned. Various methods are used; general cleaning methods involve the use of a soap, detergent, or cleaning powder. In most laboratories, detergents are used. Laboratory ware that cannot be cleaned immediately after use should be rinsed with tap water and left to soak in a basin or pail of water to which a small amount of detergent has been added. If the dirty glassware has been soaking in a solution of the detergent water, the cleaning job will be much easier.

Glassware that is contaminated, as by use with patient specimens, must be decontaminated before it is washed. This can be done by presoaking in 5% bleach or by boiling, autoclaving, or some similar procedure. Most plasticware can be cleaned in the same manner as glassware and using ordinary glassware washing machines, but the use of any abrasive cleaning materials should be avoided.

Cleaning Pipettes

Nondisposable pipettes used in the laboratory are cleaned in a special way. Immediately after use, the pipettes should be placed in a special pipette container or cylinder containing water; the water should be high enough to cover the pipettes completely. Pipettes should be placed in the container carefully with the tip up to avoid breakage. When the pipettes are to be cleaned, they are removed from the cylinder and placed in another cylinder containing a cleaning solution. This cleaning solution can be a detergent or a commercial analytical cleaning product. The pipettes are allowed to soak in the cleaning solution for 30 minutes.

The next step involves thorough rinsing of the pipettes. This can be accomplished by hand, but more often an automatic pipette washer is used. The pipettes are rinsed with tap water, using the automatic washer, for 1 to 2 hours. They are then rinsed in deionized or distilled water two or three times and dried in a hot oven.

Glass Breakage

It is important in the clinical laboratory to check all glassware periodically to determine its condition. No broken or chipped glassware should be used; many laboratory accidents are caused this way. Serious cuts may result, and infections may develop.

Each time a laboratory procedure is carried out, the glassware used should be checked. Equipment such as beakers, pipettes, test tubes, and flasks should not have broken edges or cracks. To prevent breakage, glassware should be handled carefully, and personnel should avoid carrying too much glassware at one time in the laboratory.

LABORATORY BALANCES

General Use of Balances

In the traditional clinical laboratory, measurement of mass or weight was used in the preparation of some reagents and standard solutions. In many laboratories now, reagents, standard solutions, and control solutions are purchased ready to use, and the actual laboratory preparation of reagents and solutions is limited but some laboratories routinely prepare their own standard solutions.

Analytical Balance

The basic principle in the quantitative measurement of mass is to balance an unknown mass (the substance being weighed) with a known mass. The *electronic analytical balance* (Fig. 6.6) is a single-pan balance that uses an electromagnetic force to counterbalance the load placed on the pan. Electronic balances permit fast, accurate weighing with a high degree of resolution. These are easy to use and have replaced the traditional mechanically operated analytical balance in most clinical laboratories.

The analytical balance should be cleaned and adjusted at least once a year to ensure its continued accuracy and sensitivity. Its accuracy is what makes this instrument so essential in the clinical laboratory. The accuracy to which most analytical balances used in the clinical laboratory should weigh chemicals is usually 0.1 mg, or 0.0001 g. With the electronic balance, the weights are added by manipulating a series of dials.

Weighing errors will occur if the analytical balance is not properly positioned. The balance must be level; this is usually accomplished by adjusting the movable screws on the legs of

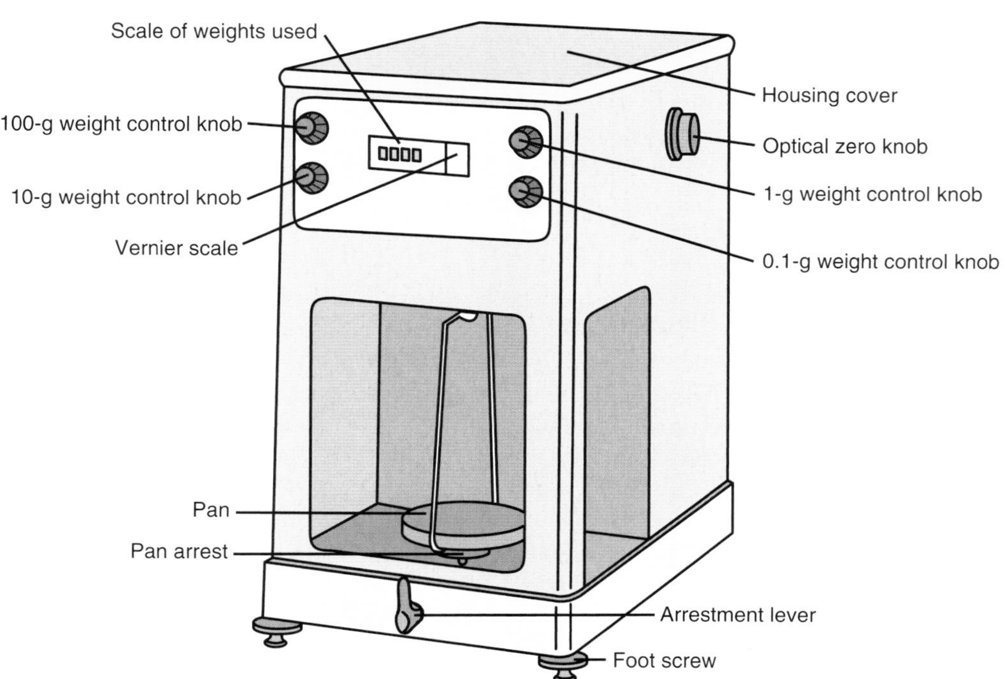

Fig. 6.6 Electronic analytical balance.

the balance. The firmness of support is also important. The bench or table on which the balance rests must be rigid and free from vibrations. Ideally, the analytical balance should be in an air-conditioned room. The temperature factor is most important. The balance should not be placed near hot objects (such as radiators, flames, stills, and electric ovens) or near cold objects and especially not near an open window. Sunlight or illumination from high-power lamps should be avoided in choosing a good location for the analytical balance.

The analytical balance is a delicate precision instrument that will not function properly if abused. The following general rules apply:

1. Set up the balance where it will be free from vibration.
2. Close the balance case before observing the reading; any air currents present will affect the weighing process.
3. Never weigh any chemical directly on the pan; a container of some type must be used for the chemical. Weigh an empty container first to establish the "tare" weight. This weight must be added to the desired weight of dry chemical.
4. On completion of weighing, clean up any chemical spilled on the pan or within the balance area.
5. Weighed materials should be transferred to labeled containers or made into solutions immediately.

Top-Loading Balance

A single-pan top-loading balance is one of the most common balances used in the laboratory (Student Procedure Worksheet 6.3). It is usually electronic and self-balancing. It is much faster and easier to use. A substance can be weighed in just a few seconds. Top-loading balances are used when the substance being weighed does not require as much analytical precision, as when reagents of a large volume are being prepared.

LABORATORY CENTRIFUGES

Centrifugation is used in the separation of a solid material from a liquid through the application of increased gravitational force by rapid rotation or spinning. It is also used in recovering solid materials from suspensions, as in the microscopic examination of urine. The solid material or sediment packed at the bottom of the centrifuge tube is sometimes called the **precipitate**, and the liquid or top portion is called the **supernatant**. Another important use for the centrifuge is in the separation of serum or plasma from cells in blood specimens. The suspended particles, solid material, or blood cells usually collect at the bottom of the centrifuge tube because the particles are heavier than the liquid. Occasionally, the particles are lighter than the liquid and will collect on the surface of the liquid when it is centrifuged. Centrifugation is employed in many areas of the clinical laboratory, including chemistry, urinalysis, hematology, and blood banking. Proper use of the centrifuge is important for anyone engaged in laboratory work.

Types of Centrifuges

Centrifuges facilitate the separation of particles in suspension by the application of centrifugal force. Several types of centrifuges are usually found in the same laboratory, each designed for special uses. The various types include table-model and floor-model centrifuges (some small and others very large), refrigerated centrifuges, ultracentrifuges, cytocentrifuges, and other centrifuges adapted for special procedures. Two traditional types of centrifuges are used in routine laboratory determinations: a conventional horizontal-head centrifuge with swinging buckets and a fixed angle–head centrifuge.

With the horizontal-head centrifuge, the cups holding the tubes of material to be centrifuged occupy a vertical position when the centrifuge is at rest but assume a horizontal position when the centrifuge revolves (Fig. 6.7). The horizontal-head, or swinging-bucket, centrifuge rotors hold the tubes being centrifuged in a vertical position when the centrifuge is at rest, but when the rotor is in motion, the tubes move and remain in a horizontal position. During the process of centrifugation, when the tube is in the horizontal position, the particles being centrifuged constantly move along the tube, and any sediment is distributed evenly against the bottom of the tube. When centrifugation is complete and the rotor is no longer turning, the surface of the sediment is flat, with the column of liquid resting above it.

For the fixed angle–head centrifuge, the cups are held in a rigid position at a fixed angle. This position makes the process of centrifuging more rapid than with the horizontal-head centrifuge. There is also less chance that the sediment will be disturbed when the centrifuge stops. During centrifugation, particles travel along the side of the tube to form a sediment that packs against the bottom and side of the tube. Fixed angle–head centrifuges are used when rapid centrifugation of solutions containing small particles is needed; an example is the microhematocrit centrifuge. The microhematocrit centrifuge used in many hematology laboratories for packing red blood cells attains a speed of about 10,000 to 15,000 rpm.

A cytocentrifuge uses a motor with very high torque and low inertia to spread monolayers of cells rapidly across a special slide for critical morphologic studies. This type of preparation can be used for blood, urine, body fluid, or any other liquid specimen that can be spread on a slide. An advantage of this technology is that only a small amount of sample is used, producing evenly distributed cells that can then be stained for microscopic study. The slide produced can be saved and examined at a later time, in contrast to "wet" preparations, which must be examined immediately.

Refrigerated centrifuges are available with internal refrigeration temperatures ranging from −15° C to −25° C during centrifugation. This permits centrifugation at higher speeds because the specimens are protected from the heat generated by the rotors of the centrifuge. The temperature of any refrigerated centrifuge should be checked regularly, and the thermometers should be checked periodically for accuracy.

Centrifuge Speed

Directions for use of a centrifuge are most frequently given in terms of speed, or revolutions per minute (rpm). The number of revolutions per minute and the centrifugal force generated are expressed as *relative centrifugal force (RCF)*. The number

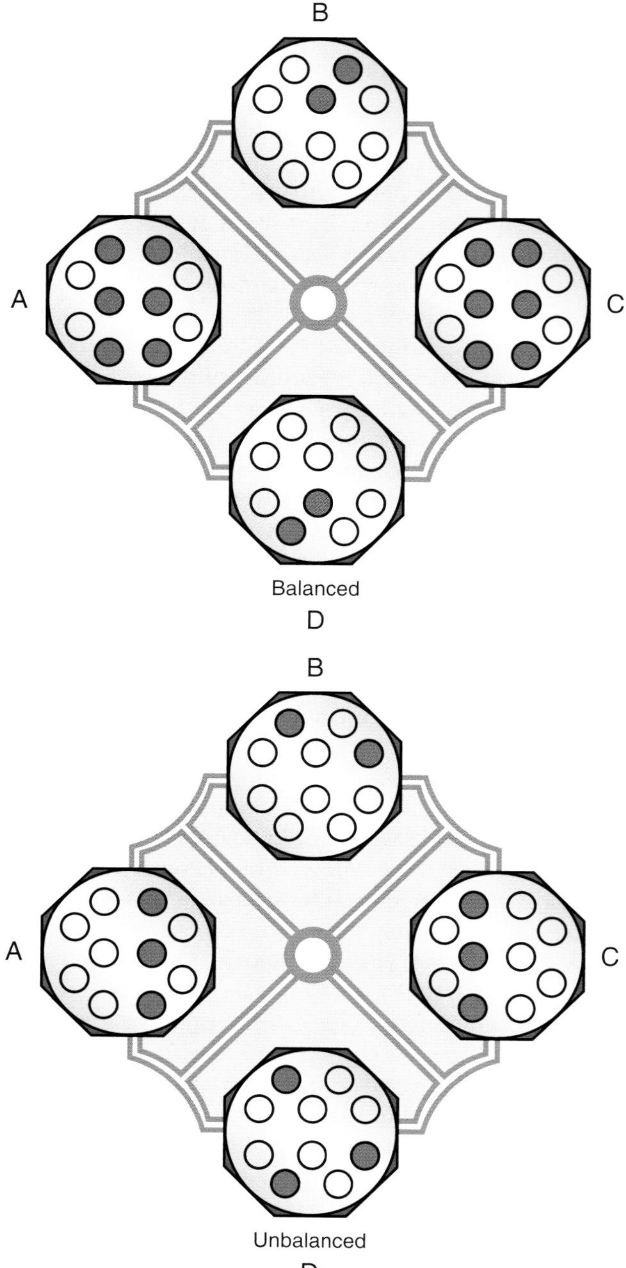

Fig. 6.7 Examples of balanced and unbalanced loads in a horizontal-head centrifuge. (A) Assuming that all tubes have been filled with an equal amount of liquid, this rotor load is balanced. Opposing bucket sets A-C and B-D are loaded with equal numbers of tubes and balanced across the center of rotation. Each bucket is also balanced with respect to its pivotal axis. (B) Even if all the tubes are filled equally, this rotor is improperly loaded. None of the bucket loads is balanced with respect to its pivotal axis. At operating speed, buckets A and C will not reach the horizontal position. Buckets B and D will pivot past the horizontal. Also note that the tube arrangement in the opposing buckets, B and D, is not symmetric across the center of rotation. (From *A centrifuge primer,* Palo Alto, CA, 1980, Spinco Division of Beckman Instruments.)

of revolutions per minute is related to the RCF by the following formula:

$$\mathrm{RCF} = 1.12 \times 10^{-5} \times r \times (\mathrm{rpm})^2$$

where *r* is the radius of the centrifuge expressed in centimeters. This is equal to the distance from the center of the centrifuge head to the bottom of the tube holder in the centrifuge bucket.

General laboratory centrifuges operate at speeds of up to 6000 rpm, generating RCF up to 7300 times the force of gravity (*g*). The top speed of most conventional centrifuges is about 3000 rpm. Conventional laboratory centrifuges of the horizontal type attain speeds of up to 3000 rpm, about 1700 *g*, without excessive heat production caused by friction between the head of the centrifuge and the air. Angle-head centrifuges produce less heat and may attain speeds of 7000 rpm (about 9000 *g*).

Ultracentrifuges are high-speed centrifuges generally used for research projects. For certain clinical uses, however, a small, air-driven ultracentrifuge is available that operates at 90,000 to 100,000 rpm and generates a maximum RCF of 178,000 *g*. Ultracentrifuges are often refrigerated.

A rheostat is used to set the desired speed; the setting on the rheostat dial does not necessarily correspond directly to revolutions per minute. The setting speeds on the rheostat can also change with variations in weight load and general aging of the centrifuge.

The College of American Pathologists (CAP) recommends that the number of revolutions per minute for a centrifuge used in chemistry laboratories be checked every 3 months. This periodic check can be performed most easily using a photoelectric or strobe tachometer. Timers and speed controls must also be checked periodically, with any corrections posted near the controls for the centrifuge.

Uses for Centrifuges

A primary use for centrifuges in clinical laboratories is to process blood specimens. Separation of cells or clotted blood from plasma or serum is achieved on an ongoing basis during the handling and processing of the many specimens needed for the various divisions of the clinical laboratory. The relative centrifugal force is not critical for the separation of serum from clot for most laboratory determinations. A force of at least 1000 *g* for 10 minutes will usually result in a good separation. When serum separator collection tubes are used that contain a silicone gel requiring displacement up the side of the tube, a greater centrifugal force is needed to displace this gel: 1000 to 1300 *g* for 10 minutes. An RCF of less than 1000 *g* may result in an incomplete displacement of the gel. It is always important to follow the manufacturer's directions when special collection tubes or serum separator devices are being used. These may require more narrowly defined conditions for centrifugation.

In the hematology laboratory, a tabletop version of the centrifuge has been specially adapted for determination of microhematocrit values. This centrifuge accelerates rapidly and can be stopped in seconds. Centrifugation is needed to prepare urinary sediment for microscopic examination. The urine specimen is centrifuged, the supernatant decanted, and the remaining sediment examined. Refrigerated centrifuges are used in the blood bank and for other temperature-sensitive laboratory procedures. Ultracentrifuges, which can generate *g* forces in the hundreds of thousands, are used in laboratories where tissue receptor assays and other assays requiring high-speed centrifugation are needed.

Technical Factors in Using Centrifuges

The most important rule to remember in using any centrifuge follows:

Always balance the tubes placed in the centrifuge.

To balance the centrifuge, in the centrifuge cup opposite the material to be centrifuged, a container of equivalent size and shape with an equal volume of liquid of the same specific gravity as the load must be placed (see Fig. 6.8 for examples of a properly balanced and an improperly balanced centrifuge). For most laboratory determinations, water may be placed in the balance load.

Tubes being centrifuged must be capped. Open tubes of blood should never be centrifuged because of the risk for aerosol spread of infection (see Chapter 2). Aerosols produced from the heat and vibration generated during the centrifugation process can increase the risk for infection to the laboratory personnel. Some evaporation of the sample can occur during centrifugation in uncapped specimen tubes.

Special centrifuge tubes can be used. These tubes are constructed to withstand the force exerted by the centrifuge. They have thicker glass walls or are made of a stronger, more resistant glass or plastic. Some of these tubes are conical, and some have round bottoms.

Before placing the centrifuge tubes in the cups or holders, check the cups to make certain the rubber cushions are in place. If some cushions are missing, the centrifuge will not be properly balanced. In addition, without the cushions, the tubes are more likely to break. When a tube breaks in the centrifuge cup, both the cup and the rubber cushion in the cup must be cleaned well to prevent further breakage resulting from the glass particles left behind.

Covers specially made for the centrifuge should be used, except in certain specified cases. Using the cover prevents possible danger from aerosol spread and from flying glass, should tubes break in the centrifuge. Keep the centrifuge cover closed at all times, even when not using the machine. In addition to posing danger from broken glass, using the centrifuge without the cover in place may cause the revolving parts of the centrifuge to vibrate, which causes excessive wear of the machine.

Do not try to stop the centrifuge with one's hands. It is generally best to let the machine stop by itself. A brake may be applied if the centrifuge is equipped with one. The brake should be used with caution because braking may cause some resuspension of the sediment. Many laboratories discourage use of the brake, except when it is evident that a tube or tubes have broken in the centrifuge.

Centrifuges should be checked, cleaned, and lubricated regularly to ensure proper operation. Centrifuges that are used routinely must be checked periodically with a photoelectric or strobe tachometer to comply with quality assurance guidelines set by CAP and others.[4]

Special Precautions for Centrifugation of Blood and Body Fluids

The laboratory centrifuge requires special precautions during handling of blood and body fluids.[5] These precautions include the following:

1. Place a biohazard label on the centrifuge.
2. Include centrifugation procedure and decontamination plan in laboratory standard operating procedures (SOPs).
3. After each use, check for possible spills or leaks.
4. If tube breakage occurs, turn centrifuge off immediately. Leave the lid closed for 30 minutes to reduce the risk for aerosols.
5. If tube breakage occurs, decontaminate centrifuge interior, safety cups or buckets, and rotors. The laboratory employee should wear proper gloves, remove debris, and dispose of it in a biohazard waste receptacle (glass needs to be disposed of in a rigid sharps container). Clean and disinfect centrifuge interior, rotors, safety cups, or buckets following the manufacturer's instructions.
6. If a spill of infectious materials transmitted by inhalation occurs in the centrifuge, hold your breath, close the centrifuge lid, turn off the centrifuge, and immediately leave the laboratory. Notify others to evacuate the laboratory, close the door, and post a biohazard spill sign at the laboratory door. Remove any contaminated protective clothing and place in a biohazard bag. Wash hands and any exposed skin surfaces with soap and water. Immediately report the incident to the laboratory supervisor.

LABORATORY REAGENT WATER

Laboratory reagent-grade water is water that is suitable for use in a specified procedure and does not interfere with the specificity, accuracy, and precision of an assay procedure. Process definitions alone, e.g., distilled or deionized water, do not adequately define required water quality. Laboratory water needs to have inorganic or organic impurities in the water removed before analysis.

Levels of Water Purity

A specialized category of purified water is the U.S. Pharmacopeial Convention (USP) water designation for drug production and analytical purposes, such as high-pressure liquid chromatography. The most updated information about chromatographic columns in USP can be found on the USP Chromatographic Columns website.

For most laboratory analysis, water specifications are described by the American Society for Testing and Materials (ASTM), International Organization for Standardization (ISO), and Clinical and Laboratory Standards Institute (CLSI). The ASTM uses the terminology type I, etc. In contrast, CLSI uses the designation clinical laboratory reagent water (CLRW) and designations such as special reagent water (SRW) and instrument feed water, neither of which is specifically defined and is intended to be determined on a local or application basis. ISO uses the term *grade* in place of *type*, with significant differences of criteria.

The three types of laboratory water recommended by the National Committee for Clinical Laboratory Standards Reagent Grade Water Specifications are organized as type I, type II, and type III[5] (Table 6.6).

Type I Reagent Water

Type I reagent water is the purest and should be used for procedures that require maximum water purity. Type I must be used for preparation of standard solutions, **buffers**, and controls, and in quantitative analytical procedures (especially

TABLE 6.6 Characteristics of the Three Grades of Reagent Water

Characteristic	Type I	Type II	Type III
Maximum colony count (CFU/mL)	10	1000	Not specified
pH	Not specified	Not specified	5.0–8.0
Silicate (mg/L SiO_2)	0.05	0.1	1.0

CFU, Colony-forming units; *SiO_2,* silicon dioxide.
Modified from National Committee for Clinical Laboratory Standards Reagent Grade Water Specifications, Laboratory Water: Its Importance and Applications. National Institutes of Health, Washington, DC, March 2013.

when nanogram or subnanogram measurements are required), electrophoresis, toxicology screening tests, and high-performance liquid chromatography. Type I water should be used immediately after it is produced; it cannot be stored.

Type II Reagent Water

For qualitative chemistry procedures and for most procedures done in hematology, immunology, microbiology, and other clinical test areas, type II reagent water is suitable. Type II water is used for general laboratory tests that do not require type I water.

Type III Reagent Water

Type III water can be used for some qualitative laboratory tests, such as those done in general urinalysis. Type III reagent water can be used as a water source for preparation of type I or type II water and for washing and rinsing laboratory glassware. Any glassware should be given a final rinse with either type I or type II water, depending on the intended use for the glassware.

Quality Control and Impurity Testing

Water must be monitored at regular intervals to evaluate the performance of the water purification system. Testing at periodic intervals should include the following:

- Microbial monitoring
- Resistivity
- pH
- Pyrogens
- Silica
- Organic contaminants

Several methods are available to test for water purity. With regard to the presence of inorganic ionized materials, as the purity of the water increases, the amount of dissolved ionized substances decreases, as does the ability of the water to conduct an electrical current. This principle is used in commercially available resistance test analyzers for water purity. As the ability of the water to conduct an electrical current decreases, the resistance increases. The presence of ionizable contaminants in distilled water or deionized water is most easily determined by measuring the conductance, or electrical resistance, of the water. This is the basis for having purity meters or conductivity warning lights on distillation and deionization apparatus.

Water of the highest purity will vary with the method of preparation and may be referred to as *nitrogen-free water, double-distilled water,* or *conductivity water,* depending on the actual method used. However, a measure of conductance does not consider the presence of nonionized substances (organic contaminants) such as dissolved gases. Especially important in the clinical laboratory is dissolved carbon dioxide (CO_2). To remove CO_2 from water, boil it immediately before use; it is often referred to as *gas-free water* or *CO_2-free water.* Such water may be necessary for the preparation of strongly alkaline solutions. Other potential water contaminants include substances dissolved from the storage container.

Accreditation or certification requirements for clinical laboratories, set up by state and federal agencies, have resulted in specific, well-defined criteria for water purity. The classification of and specifications for water purity are designed, for example, to enable laboratory personnel to specify the quality of the water needed for particular laboratory analyses and reagent preparation. Each test performed in the laboratory must be evaluated as to the type of water needed, to avoid potential interference with specificity, accuracy, and precision. It is well known, for example, that water contaminated with metal, when used in analyses of enzymes, can have a dramatic effect on the values obtained.

Storage of Reagent Water

It is important to store reagent water appropriately. Type I water must be used immediately after its production to prevent CO_2 from being absorbed into it. Types II and III water can be stored in borosilicate glass or polyethylene bottles but should be used as soon as possible to prevent contamination with airborne microbes. Containers should be tightly stoppered to prevent absorption of gases. It is also important to keep the delivery system for the water protected from chemical or microbiological contamination.

Purification of Water Process

The original source of water varies greatly with the health care facility. Water originating from rivers, lakes, springs, or wells contains a variety of inorganic, organic, and microbiological contaminants; no single purification system can remove them all. For this reason, a variety of methods in differing combinations are used to obtain the particular types of water used in a laboratory facility. Two general methods are employed to prepare water for laboratory use: deionization and distillation. Sometimes it is necessary to treat distilled water further with a deionization process to obtain the degree of water purity needed.

Distilled Water

In the process of distillation, water is boiled, and the resulting steam is cooled; condensed steam is distilled water. Many minerals are found in natural water, most often iron, magnesium, and calcium. Water from which these and other minerals have been removed by distillation is known as *distilled water.* The process of distillation also removes microbiological organisms, but volatile impurities such as CO_2, chlorine, and ammonia are not removed. Water that has been distilled meets the specifications for water types II and III.

Double-Distilled Water. Distilled or deionized water is not necessarily pure water. There may be contamination by dissolved gases, by nonvolatile substances carried over by steam in the distillation process, or by dissolved substances from storage containers. For example, in tests for nitrogen compounds (such as urea nitrogen, a common clinical chemistry determination), it is important to use ammonia-free (nitrogen-free) water. This may be specially purchased by the laboratory for such determinations or prepared in the laboratory by a specific method, double distillation, to remove the contaminating ammonia.

Deionized Water

In the process of deionization, water is passed through a resin column containing positively (+) and negatively (−) charged particles. These particles combine with ions present in the water to remove them; this water is known as *deionized water.* The only substances that will be removed in the process of deionization are those that can ionize. Organic substances and other substances that do not ionize are not removed. Further treatment with membrane filtration and activated charcoal is necessary to remove organic impurities, particulate matter, and microorganisms to produce type I water from deionized water.

Combinations of Deionization and Distillation

Water of higher purity is produced also by special distillation units in which the water is first deionized and then distilled, eliminating the need for double distillation. Other systems may first distill the water and then deionize it.

Reverse Osmosis

The process of reverse osmosis passes water under pressure through a semipermeable membrane made of cellulose acetate or other materials. This treatment removes approximately 90% of dissolved solids and 98% of organic impurities, insoluble matter, and microbiological organisms. Reverse osmosis does not remove dissolved gases and removes only about 10% of ionized particles.

Other Processes of Purification

Other water purification processes include ultrafiltration, ultraviolet oxidation and sterilization (used after other purification processes), and ozone water purification (used primarily in industrial settings). Filtration of water through semipermeable membranes will remove insoluble matter, pyrogens, and microorganisms if the pore size of the membrane is small enough. Adsorption by activated charcoal, clays, silicates, or metal oxides can remove organic matter. Type I water can be processed through a combination of deionization, filtration, and adsorption.

REAGENTS USED IN LABORATORY ASSAYS

Reagent Preparation

Instructions for preparing a reagent resemble a cooking recipe and specify what quantities of ingredients to mix together. The instructions identify the names of the chemicals needed, the number of grams or milligrams needed, and the total volume to which the particular reagent should be diluted. The solvent most often used for dilution is deionized or distilled water.

A *reagent* is defined as any substance used to produce a chemical reaction. In highly automated clinical laboratories, very few reagents are prepared by laboratory staff. In many cases, only water or buffer needs to be added to a prepackaged reagent. However, in some cases, clinical and research laboratories may need to prepare a reagent or solution for method validation or specialized analyses. In-house reagent preparation may be required because of reagent deterioration, supply and demand, or verified cost containment.

Grades of Chemicals

A chemical is a substance that occurs naturally or is obtained through a chemical process; it is used to produce a chemical effect or reaction. Chemicals are produced in various purities or grades. Analytical chemicals exist in varying grades of purity, as follows:

- Analytical reagent (AR) grade
- Chemically pure (CP) grade
- USP and *National Formulary* (NF) grade
- Technical or commercial grade

The label on the bottle and the supplier's catalog may give important information, such as the maximum limits of impurities or an actual analysis of the chemical. Directions for reagent preparation usually specify the grade and often state the particular brand of chemical.

Analytical Reagent Grade

The AR-grade chemicals are of a high degree of purity and are used often in the preparation of reagents in the clinical laboratory. The American Chemical Society (ACS) has developed specifications for many reagent-grade or AR-grade chemicals, and those that meet its standards are designated by the letters *ACS.*

Chemically Pure Grade

The CP-grade chemicals are sufficiently pure to be used in many analyses in the clinical laboratory. However, the CP designation does not reveal the limits of impurities that are tolerated. Therefore CP chemicals may not be acceptable for research and various clinical laboratory techniques unless they have been specifically analyzed for the desired procedure. It may be necessary to use CP grade when higher-purity biochemicals are not available.

USP and NF Grade

The USP-grade and NF-grade reagents meet the specifications published in the *U.S. Pharmacopeia* or the *National Formulary.* These reagents are generally less pure than CP-grade chemicals, because the tolerances specified are such that USP and NF chemicals are not injurious to health, rather than chemically pure.

Technical or Commercial Grade

The technical and commercial chemicals are used only for industrial purposes and are generally not used in the preparation of reagents for the clinical laboratory.

Hazardous Chemicals Communication Policies

Information and training regarding hazardous chemicals must be provided to all persons working with them in the clinical laboratory. Occupational Safety and Health Administration (OSHA) regulations ensure that all sites where hazardous chemicals are used comply with the necessary safety precautions. Any information about signs and symptoms associated with exposures to hazardous chemicals used in the laboratory must be communicated to all persons. Reference materials about the individual chemicals are provided by all chemical manufacturers and suppliers by means of the safety data sheet (SDS). This information accompanies the shipment of all hazardous chemicals and should be available in the laboratory for anyone to review. The SDS contains information about possible hazards, safe handling, storage, and disposal of the particular chemical it accompanies (see Chapter 2).

Storage of Chemicals

It is important that chemicals kept in the laboratory be stored properly. Chemicals that require refrigeration should be refrigerated immediately. Solids should be kept in a cool, dry place. Acids and bases should be stored separately in well-ventilated storage units. Flammable solvents (such as alcohol and chloroform) should be stored in specially constructed, well-ventilated storage units with appropriate labeling in accordance with OSHA regulations. Flammable solvents such as acetone and ether should always be stored in special safety cans or other appropriate storage devices and in approved storage units. Fuming and volatile chemicals such as solvents, strong acids, and strong bases should be opened, and reagent preparation resulting in fumes should be done only under a fume hood so that vapors will not escape into the room. Chemicals that absorb water should be weighed only after desiccation or drying in a hot oven; otherwise the weights will not be accurate.

It is essential that the label on a chemical be read for instructions about storage details. Most chemicals are stable at room temperature without desiccation. Some must be stored at refrigeration temperature, some must be frozen, and some that are light sensitive must be stored in brown bottles.

Reference Materials

Various organizations (such as CAP) supply certified clinical laboratory standards. The highest-grade or purest chemicals are available from NIST. Very few such compounds, standards, clinical type, are available to the clinical laboratory. Chemicals used to prepare standard solutions are the most highly purified types of chemicals available. This group includes primary, reference, and certified standards. Primary standards meet specifications set by the ACS Committee on ARs. Each lot of these chemicals is assayed, and the chemicals must be stable substances of definite composition.

Concentration of Solutions

Using solutions of the correct concentrations is of the greatest importance in attaining good results in the laboratory (see Chapter 7). Quantitative transfer, along with accurate initial measurement of a chemical, helps ensure that a solution will be of the correct concentration. The concentration of a solution may be expressed in different ways.

In the clinical chemistry laboratory, most measurements are concerned with the concentrations of substances in solutions. The solution is usually blood, serum, urine, cerebrospinal fluid, or other body fluid, and the substance to be measured is dissolved in the solution. Substances being measured in the analyses (whether organic or inorganic or of high or low molecular weight) are solutes. In comparison, the substance in which a solute is dissolved is called the solvent.

Buffers and pH

Buffers are weak acids or bases and their related salts that, as a result of their dissociation characteristics, minimize changes in the hydrogen ion concentration. Hydrogen ion concentration $[H^+]$ is often expressed as *pH.* The pH scale ranges from 0 to 16 and is a convenient way of expressing $[H^+]$. Measurement of the pH of blood and various body fluids (such as urine) is important in laboratory analyses.

A buffer's capacity to minimize changes in pH is related to the dissociation characteristics of the weak acid or base in the presence of its respective salt.

Transfer and Dilution of Chemicals for Reagents

In preparing any solution in the clinical laboratory, it is necessary to follow the practice known as *quantitative transfer* (Student Procedure Worksheet 6.4). It is essential that the entire amount of the weighed or measured substance be used in preparing the solution. In quantitative transfer, the entire amount of the measured substance is transferred from one vessel to another for dilution. The usual practice in preparing most laboratory reagents is to weigh the chemical in a beaker (or other suitable vessel, such as a disposable weighing boat) and quantitatively transfer the chemical to a volumetric flask for dilution with deionized or distilled water. The volumetric flask chosen must be the correct size; that is, it must hold the amount of solution desired for the total volume of the reagent being prepared.

The most common amount of solution prepared at one time is 1 L. If 1 L of reagent is needed, the measured chemical must be transferred quantitatively to a 1-L volumetric flask and diluted to the calibration mark with deionized water or the required solvent. The method of quantitative transfer requires great care and accuracy.

Dissolving the Chemical Into Solution

Several methods can be used to hasten the dissolution of solid materials. Heating usually increases the solubility of a chemical, and heat also causes the fluid to move (currents help in dissolving materials). Even mild heat, however, will decompose some chemicals, so heat must be used with caution. Agitation by a stirring rod or swirling by means of a mechanical shaker increases solubility by removing the saturated solution from contact with the chemical. Rapid addition of the solvent is another means of hastening the dissolution of solid materials. Some chemicals tend to cake and form aggregates as soon as the solvent is added. By adding the solvent quickly and keeping the solids in motion, aggregation may be prevented. Because the flask is calibrated at 20° C, the solution must be returned to room temperature before final adjustment is made.

Labeling the Reagent Container

Containers for storage of reagents (usually reagent bottles) should be labeled before the material is added. A reagent should never be placed in an unlabeled bottle or container. If an unlabeled container is found, the reagent in it must be discarded. Proper labeling of reagent bottles is of the greatest importance (see Chapter 2).

Checking a Reagent Before Use

After the prepared reagent is in the reagent bottle, it must be checked before it is put into actual use in any procedure. New lots or batches of reagents are generally run in parallel testing with existing reagents. Controls, standards, and calibrators are means of testing the new lot or batch with the existing reagent.

In addition, a reagent log should be kept to indicate date in use and date of expiration. This log should also note the lot numbers of controls. After the reagent has been checked, this is indicated on the label, and the solution can be used for laboratory testing.

Ready-Made Reagents

Many laboratories, especially those using large automated instruments, use ready-made reagents. The manufacturers of these instruments usually provide the necessary specific reagents for use with their instruments. These reagents must be handled with extreme care and always used according to the manufacturer's directions.

Immunoreagents

Special commercial reagent kits are often used for clinical immunology tests. A typical test kit will contain all necessary reagents, including standards, labeled antigen, and antibody plus any other associated reagents needed. The laboratory must maintain strict evaluation policies for these kits to ensure their reliability. The disadvantage of such kits is that the laboratory depends on the supplier to produce and maintain components, which must meet the necessary standards. Each new kit must be evaluated by the laboratory according to a strict protocol, and then a periodic monitoring program must be maintained to ensure the reliability of the results produced.

REFERENCES

1. National Institute of Standards and Technology, US Department of Commerce. NIST SP 330:2008 and NIST SP 811:2008. www.nist.gov.
2. ASTM Standard ASTM E288: *Laboratory testing standards*, West Conshohocken, Pa, 2012, ASTM International, https://doi.org/10.1520/C0033-03E01.
3. ASTM Standard ASTM E288.10: Standard specification for laboratory glass volumetric flasks, ASTM International, West Conshohocken, Pa. https://doi.org/10.1520/E0288-10. (Accessed May 29, 2013.)
4. Chemical safety: practices and procedures. Fred Hutchison Cancer Research Center. www.extranet.fhcrc.org.
5. ASTM D1193-06: *Standard specification for reagent water*, West Conshohocken, Pa, 2013, ASTM International, https://doi.org/10.1520/D1193-06R11 Accessed May 29, 2013.)

BIBLIOGRAPHY

Bishop ML, Fody EP, Schoeff L: *Clinical chemistry: techniques, principles, correlations*, ed 6, Philadelphia, 2010, Lippincott Williams & Wilkins.

Burtis CA, Ashwood ER, Bruns DE: *Tietz fundamentals of clinical chemistry*, ed 6, St Louis, 2008, Elsevier/Saunders.

Campbell JM, Campbell JB: *Laboratory mathematics: medical and biological applications*, ed 5, St Louis, 1997, Mosby.

Kaplan LA, Pesce AJ: *Clinical chemistry: theory, analysis, correlation*, ed 5, St Louis, 2010, Elsevier/Mosby.

U.S. Government: National Institutes of Health, National Committee for Clinical Laboratory Standards Reagent Grade Water Specifications, Laboratory Water: Its Importance and Applications. Washington, DC, March 2013.

REVIEW QUESTIONS (ANSWERS IN APPENDIX A)

Systems of Measurement

1. The metric system unit of volume is a:
   - **a.** Meter
   - **b.** Gram
   - **c.** Liter
   - **d.** Micron
2. The metric system unit of length is a:
   - **a.** Meter
   - **b.** Gram
   - **c.** Liter
   - **d.** Pound
3. The metric unit of mass is a:
   - **a.** Meter
   - **b.** Gram
   - **c.** Liter
   - **d.** Angstrom

International System (SI System)

4. Convert: 20° C = ___ ° F
   a. 25
   b. 53
   c. 68
   d. 86
5. Convert: 75° F = ___° C
   a. 15.5
   b. 21.0
   c. 23.8
   d. 32.6
6. The prefix milli- represents:
   a. 10^{-2}
   b. 10^{-3}
   c. 10^{-6}
   d. 10^{-9}
7. The prefix micro- represents:
   a. 10^{-2}
   b. 10^{-3}
   c. 10^{-6}
   d. 10^{-9}

Labware

8. The primary use of a 1-mL volumetric pipette is to:
   a. Prepare a reagent of specific total volume
   b. Measure an unknown serum sample
   c. Add a reagent to a reaction tube
   d. Measure an approximate amount of control specimen
9. The primary use of a 10-mL graduated pipette is to:
   a. Prepare a reagent of specific total volume
   b. Measure an unknown serum sample
   c. Add a reagent to a reaction tube
   d. Measure an approximate amount of control specimen
10. The primary use of a 100-mL volumetric flask is to:
    a. Prepare a reagent of specific total volume
    b. Measure an unknown serum sample
    c. Add a reagent to a reaction tube
    d. Measure an approximate amount of control specimen
11. An etched ring on a to-deliver (TD) pipette indicates:
    a. A small amount of fluid will remain in the tip of the pipette, and the fluid is left there.
    b. The drop remaining in the tip must be blown out.
    c. Either a or b.
    d. No significance.

Laboratory Balances

12. A top loading balance can be used appropriately when
    a. An increased degree of accuracy is weight is required.
    b. A substance being weighed does not require an extremely high degree of analytical precision.
    c. It is the only available balance in the laboratory.
    d. A small volume of reagent is being prepared.

Laboratory Centrifuges

13. A cytocentrifuge is used to spread:
    a. Liquid specimens evenly over a slide
    b. Monolayers of cells
    c. A large volume of specimen
    d. Both a and b

Laboratory Reagent Water

14. The purest type of reagent water is:
    a. Type I
    b. Type II
    c. Type III
    d. All are equal
15. Water from which minerals have been removed and that meets the specifications for type II and type III water is called:
    a. Distilled water
    b. Deionized water
    c. Reagent-grade water
    d. Charcoal-activated water

Reagents Used in Laboratory Assays

16. Grades of chemicals include all of the following *except:*
    a. Analytical reagent
    b. Chemically pure
    c. Commercial grade
    d. Industrial grade
17. Reference standards are chemicals whose purity has been ensured by the:
    a. National Institute of Standards and Technology
    b. Centers for Disease Control and Prevention
    c. Occupational Safety and Health Administration
    d. State licensing agencies
18. A solute is:
    a. The substance dissolved in the solution
    b. The substance that does the dissolving
    c. Always water
    d. Both b and c
19. A label for a reagent should bear:
    a. Name and concentration of reagent
    b. Date prepared and expiration date
    c. Initials of preparer
    d. All the above

Bonus Challenge Questions

20. You need to complete a chemistry procedure that involves diluting 1.5 mL of serum specimens to a 1:10 solution before performing testing. Which pipette is best suited for this task?
    a. Volumetric
    b. Serologic
    c. Micropipette
    d. Any of the above
21. You need to reconstitute quality control samples by adding 5 mL of deionized water to lyophilized material. Which pipette is best suited for this task?
    a. Volumetric
    b. Serologic
    c. Micropipette
    d. Any of the above

22. You need to perform some testing in the serology department. Which pipette is suitable for use in this department, but not for other tasks (such as pipetting small amounts of blood or specimen, measuring standard solution)?
    a. Volumetric
    b. Serologic
    c. Micropipette
    d. Erlenmeyer

Turgeon: Linné & Ringsrud's Clinical Laboratory Science, 8th Edition

STUDENT PROCEDURE WORKSHEET 6-1

Pipetting with Manual Pipettes

Read Chapter 6 in *Linné & Ringsrud's Clinical Laboratory Science: Concepts, Procedures, and Clinical Applications,* 8th edition, for a complete discussion of this topic.

Student Learning Outcomes

After reading Chapter 6, and at the completion of the laboratory exercise and review questions, the student will be able to:

- Correctly select and use various types of manual pipettes.
- Complete the end-of-procedure review questions with a grade of 80% or higher.

Supplies and Equipment

1. Volumetric pipettes (various sizes)
2. Graduated pipettes (various sizes)
3. Safety bulb
4. Gauze (or Kimwipes)
5. Distilled water

Instructions for the Procedure

Read the list of required equipment and supplies and the procedural steps. Follow the procedural steps in exact order.

SEQUENCE	PROCEDURAL STEP	INSTRUCTOR-OBSERVED ACCEPTABLE PERFORMANCE (CHECK IF ACCEPTABLE)
1	Assemble equipment and supplies.	
2	Wash your hands and put on gloves and eye protection as directed.	
3	Check the pipette to ascertain its correct size, being careful also to check for broken delivery or suction tips.	
4	Wearing protective gloves, hold the pipette lightly between the thumb and last three fingers, leaving the index finger free.	
5	Place the tip of the pipette well below the surface of the liquid to be pipetted.	
6	Using mechanical suction or an aspirator bulb, carefully draw the liquid up into the pipette until the level of liquid is well above the calibration mark.	
7	Quickly cover the suction opening at the top of the pipette with the index finger.	
8	Wipe the outside of the pipette dry with a piece of gauze or tissue to remove excess fluid.	
9	Hold the pipette in a vertical position, with the delivery tip against the inside of the original vessel. Carefully allow the liquid in the pipette to drain by gravity until the bottom of the meniscus is exactly at the calibration mark. (The meniscus is the concave or convex surface of a column of liquid as seen in a laboratory pipette.) To do this, do not entirely remove the index finger from the suction-hole end of the pipette; rather, by rolling the finger slightly over the opening, allow slow drainage to take place.	
10	While still holding the pipette in a vertical position, touch the tip of the pipette to the inside wall of the receiving vessel. Remove the index finger from the top of the pipette to permit free drainage. Remember to keep the pipette in a vertical position for correct drainage. In TD pipettes, a small amount of fluid will remain in the delivery tip.	
11	To be certain the drainage is as complete as possible, touch the delivery tip of the pipette to another area on the inside wall of the receiving vessel.	
12	Remove the pipette from the receiving vessel, and clean or discard appropriately.	
13	Discard used gauze and other contaminated supplies into a biohazard container.	
14	Clean equipment and return to proper storage.	
15	Clean work area with disinfectant solution.	
16	Remove gloves and discard into biohazard container.	
17	Wash hands using proper procedure.	

Procedural Evaluation

Student's Name ______________________________ Grade _________

Instructor's Signature ___________________________ Date ___________

Comments:

(Continued)

Turgeon: Linné & Ringsrud's Clinical Laboratory Science, 8th Edition

STUDENT PROCEDURE WORKSHEET 6-1

Pipetting with Manual Pipettes

Review Questions

Student's Name ______________________________ Date __________________

1. Describe the appearance of a volumetric pipette.

2. Describe the appearance of graduated pipette.

3. When would you select a volumetric pipette?

4. When would you select a graduated pipette?

Turgeon: Linné & Ringsrud's Clinical Laboratory Science, 8th Edition

STUDENT PROCEDURE WORKSHEET 6-2

Micropipetting

Read Chapter 6 in *Linné & Ringsrud's Clinical Laboratory Science: Concepts, Procedures, and Clinical Applications*, 8th edition, for a complete discussion of this topic.

Student Learning Outcomes

After reading Chapter 6, and at the completion of the laboratory exercise and review questions, the student will be able to:

- Use a micropipettor correctly.
- Complete the end-of-procedure review questions with a grade of 80% or higher.

Supplies and Equipment

1. Gloves
2. Deionized water
3. Pipettor
4. Pipettor tips
5. Gauze (or Kimwipes)
6. Beaker

Instructions for the Procedure

Read the list of required equipment and supplies and the procedural steps. Follow the procedural steps in exact order.

SEQUENCE	PROCEDURAL STEP	INSTRUCTOR-OBSERVED ACCEPTABLE PERFORMANCE (CHECK IF ACCEPTABLE)
NOTE: In general, the following steps apply for use of a micropipettor (see Fig. 6-5).		
1	Attach the proper tip to the pipettor, and set the delivery volume.	
2	Depress the piston to a stop position on the pipettor.	
3	Place the tip into the solution, and allow the piston to rise slowly back to its original position. (This fills the pipettor tip with the desired volume of solution.)	
4	Some tips are wiped with dry gauze at this step, and some are not wiped. Follow the manufacturer's directions.	
5	Place the tip on the wall of the receiving vessel and depress the piston, first to a stop position where the liquid is allowed to drain, then to a second stop position where the full dispensing of the liquid takes place.	
6	Some pipettors automatically eject the used tips, thus minimizing biohazard exposure. Dispose of the tip in the waste disposal receptacle.	

Procedural Evaluation

Student's Name ______________________ Grade ________

Instructor's Signature ______________________ Date ________

Comments:

(Continued)

Turgeon: Linné & Ringsrud's Clinical Laboratory Science, 8th Edition

STUDENT PROCEDURE WORKSHEET 6-2

Micropipetting

Review Questions

Student's Name ______________________________ Date ___________

1. What are some advantages to using a micropipettor?

2. What types of volume can be handled by a micropipettor?

Turgeon: Linné & Ringsrud's Clinical Laboratory Science, 8th Edition

STUDENT PROCEDURE WORKSHEET 6-3

Weighing with an Electronic Analytical Balance

Read Chapter 6 in *Linné & Ringsrud's Clinical Laboratory Science: Concepts, Procedures, and Clinical Applications,* 8th edition, for a complete discussion of this topic.

Student Learning Outcomes

After reading Chapter 6, and at the completion of the laboratory exercise and review questions, the student will be able to:

- Correctly weigh substances on an electronic analytical balance.
- Complete the end-of-procedure review questions with a grade of 80% or higher.

Supplies and Equipment

1. Electronic analytical balance (such as Mettler)
2. Disposable plastic weighing boat or weighing paper
3. Tweezers or tongs
4. Paper and pencil to record weights
5. Dry chemical (such as NaCl)
6. Gloves and lab coat
7. Antistatic brush
8. Distilled/deionized water
9. Standard set of weights
10. Gauze (or Kimwipes)

Instructions for the Procedure

Read the list of required equipment and supplies and the procedural steps. Follow the procedural steps in exact order.

SEQUENCE	PROCEDURAL STEP*	INSTRUCTOR-OBSERVED ACCEPTABLE PERFORMANCE (CHECK IF APPLICABLE)
1	Assemble equipment and supplies. Plug in the electronic balance. Open the side glass doors of the instrument, and clean weighing pan and base with the antistatic brush. A dry gauze square (or Kimwipe) dampened with distilled water can be used to remove any chemicals that may be stuck on the pan or floor base of the balance.	
2	Before turning on the instrument, be sure that the doors are closed. Analytical balances require a draft-free location on a solid bench that is free of vibrations. Some modern balances have built-in calibration masses to maintain accuracy. Older balances should be calibrated periodically with a standard mass. Turn on by pushing down on the gray bar and letting up quickly. Push again if the digital readout does not show 0.0000 g.	
3	Wash your hands and put on gloves and eye protection as directed.	
4	Before weighing, make certain the balance is properly leveled. Observe the spirit level (leveling bubble), and adjust the two rear balance feet that serve as leveling screws. **NOTE**: Do not lean on the bench while weighing.	
5	Turn on the balance by pressing the control bar. The display lights up for several seconds, then resets to 0.0000. Allow display to stabilize; (g) will appear after the numerical display.	
6	Using tweezers or tongs, place weighing boat or small, creased weighing paper on the balance pan. **NOTE**: Do not pick up tare containers with your bare hands, because your fingerprints add mass. Use gauze wipes or tongs to prevent this.	
7	Close the sliding glass doors. Wait for the green dot on the left to go out; this is the stability indicator light, indicating that the weight is stable. **NOTE**: Record the mass of the container, if you will need it later.	
8	Press the control bar to cancel out the weight of the container or paper *(tare weight)*. The display will again read 0.0000.	
9	Carefully add the substance to be weighed up to the desired mass. Do not attempt to reach a particular mass exactly.	
10	Before recording the mass, close the glass doors and wait until the stability detector lamp goes out. Record mass of solid.	

Turgeon: Linné & Ringsrud's Clinical Laboratory Science, 8th Edition

STUDENT PROCEDURE WORKSHEET 6-3

SEQUENCE	PROCEDURAL STEP*	INSTRUCTOR-OBSERVED ACCEPTABLE PERFORMANCE (CHECK IF APPLICABLE)
11	Use the antistatic brush provided to clean spills in the weighing chamber. Discard any disposable tare containers, weighing paper, or gauze pieces (or Kimwipes).	
12	Clean inside the instrument with the antistatic brush and a damp gauze wipe, if necessary. Return to proper storage, if not stored on the laboratory benchtop.	
13	Clean work area and wipe down benchtop with an appropriate solution.	

*Always check manufacturer directions for revisions to the procedure.

Procedural Evaluation

Student's Name ______________________________ Grade __________

Instructor's Signature ___________________________ Date ___________

Comments:

(Continued)

Turgeon: Linné & Ringsrud's Clinical Laboratory Science, 8th Edition

STUDENT PROCEDURE WORKSHEET 6-3

Weighing with an Electronic Balance

Review Questions

Student's Name ______________________________ Date____________

1. What is the purpose of the glass enclosure around a weighing pan of an electronic analytical balance?

2. How do you properly transfer objects or substances to a weighing pan?

3. What is the "tare" weight? What effect does it having on weighing an object?

Turgeon: Linné & Ringsrud's Clinical Laboratory Science, 8th Edition

STUDENT PROCEDURE WORKSHEET 6-4

Quantitative Transfer of Liquids

Read Chapter 6 in *Linné & Ringsrud's Clinical Laboratory Science: Concepts, Procedures, and Clinical Applications,* 8th edition, for a complete discussion of this topic.

Student Learning Outcomes
After reading Chapter 6, and at the completion of the laboratory exercise and review questions, the student will be able to:

- Correctly demonstrate techniques for quantitative transfer of liquids.
- Complete the end-of-procedure review questions with a grade of 80% or higher.

Supplies and Equipment

1. Volumetric flask (any size) with ground-glass stopper
2. Funnel
3. Beaker
4. Distilled/deionized water
5. Storage bottle with label
6. Waterproof pen

Instructions for the Procedure
Read the list of required equipment and supplies and the procedural steps. Follow the procedural steps in exact order.

SEQUENCE	PROCEDURAL STEP	INSTRUCTOR-OBSERVED ACCEPTABLE PERFORMANCE (CHECK IF APPLICABLE
1	Assemble equipment and supplies.	
2	Place a clean, dry funnel in the mouth of the volumetric flask.	
3	Carefully transfer the chemical in the measuring vessel (beaker) into the funnel.	
4	Wash the chemical into the flask with small amounts of deionized water or the required solvent for the reagent.	
5	Rinse the measuring vessel (beaker) three to five times with small portions of deionized water or the required solvent until all the chemical has been transferred from the vessel into the volumetric flask (add each rinsing to the flask).	
6	Rinse the funnel with deionized water or the required solvent, and remove the funnel from the volumetric flask.	
7	Dissolve the chemical in the flask by swirling or shaking it. Some chemicals are more difficult to dissolve than others. Dissolving the chemical occasionally becomes a problem and requires additional attention.	
8	Add deionized water or the required solvent to about 0.5 inch below the calibration line on the flask. Allow a few seconds for drainage of the fluid above the calibration line, and then carefully add deionized water or the required solvent to the calibration line (bottom of meniscus must be exactly on the calibration mark).	
9	Seal the flask with a ground-glass stopper, and mix well by inverting at least 20 times.	
10	Rinse a properly labeled reagent bottle with a small amount of the mixed reagent in the volumetric flask. Transfer the prepared reagent to the labeled reagent bottle for storage.	
11	Clean up work area, and place any unused supplies in storage.	
12	Wash hands using proper procedure.	

Procedural Evaluation

Student's Name ______________________________ Grade _________

Instructor's Signature ___________________________ Date ___________

Comments:

(Continued)

Turgeon: Linné & Ringsrud's Clinical Laboratory Science, 8th Edition

STUDENT PROCEDURE WORKSHEET 6-4

Quantitative Transfer of Liquids

Review Questions

Student's Name ______________________________ Date ______________

1. Does the solvent or the solute go into a volumetric flask first?

2. How do you transfer any remaining solute into a volumetric flask?

7

Laboratory Mathematics and Solution Preparation

http://evolve.elsevier.com/Turgeon/clinicallab/

CHAPTER OUTLINE

LEARNING OUTCOMES

Significant Figures
- Explain and apply the rules for rounding off numbers and using significant figures.

Exponents
- Describe the use of exponents and interpret exponents.

Density and Specific Gravity
- Define the terms *density* and *specific gravity.*

Expressions of Solution Concentration
- Prepare a percent solution.
- Define the terms molality, molarity, osmolality, and osmolarity.
- Calculate the osmolarity of given substances.

Proportions and Ratios
- Calculate proportions and ratios.

Concentrations of Solutions
- Calculate the requirements for solutions of a given volume and concentration.

Dilutions
- Describe the procedures for making a single dilution and a serial dilution.
- Calculate the amount of one solution needed to make a solution of a lesser concentration.
- Construct a table with the amount of serum and solvent for a 1:2, a 1:5, and a 1:10 serial dilution.

Review Questions
- Demonstrate comprehension of the chapter content by completing the end-of-chapter review questions with a grade of 80% or higher.

Note:
- indicates MLT and MLS core content

❖ indicates MLT (optional) and MLS advanced content

KEY TERMS

aliquot
density
dilution
gram-molecular weight
molality
molarity
osmolality
osmolarity
serial dilutions
significant figure
solute
solvent
specific gravity
standard solution
titer

Today's clinical laboratory requires a minimal amount of solution preparation and mathematical calculations. Most reagents are prepackaged for immediate use, and microprocessors perform various mathematical calculations. Calculations specific to hematology or clinical chemistry are discussed in discipline-specific chapters in Part II. In special circumstances, or more often in research laboratories, laboratory staff are required to calculate and prepare solutions for analytical assays or to calculate results.

SIGNIFICANT FIGURES

Using more digits than necessary to calculate and report the results of a laboratory determination has several disadvantages. It is important that the number used contain only the digits necessary for precision of the determination. Using more is misleading in that it ascribes more accuracy to the determination than is actually the case. There is also the danger of overlooking a decimal point and making an error in judging the magnitude of the answer. Digits in a number that are needed to express the precision of the measurement from which the number is derived are known as **significant figures**. A significant figure is known to be reasonably reliable. Judgment must be exercised in determining how many figures should be used. The following rules can assist in making such decisions:

1. Use the known accuracy of the method to determine the number of digits that are significant in the answer, and as a general rule, retain one more figure than this. For example, a urea nitrogen result was reported as 11.2 mg/dL. This would indicate that the result is accurate to the nearest tenth and that the exact value lies between 11.15 and 11.25. In reality, the accuracy of most urea nitrogen methods is ±10%, so the result reported as 11.2 mg/dL could actually vary from 10 to 12 mg/dL and should be reported as 11 mg/dL. In addition, if the decimal point were omitted or overlooked, the result could be taken as "112" mg/dL.
2. Take the accuracy of the least accurate measurement, or the measurement with the least number of significant figures, as the accuracy of the final result. In doing so, certain adjustments must be made in the addition and subtraction or multiplication and division of numerals. With addition or subtraction, for example, to add the following numerals:

   206.1
   7.56
   0.8764

   rewrite them as:

   206.1
   7.6
   0.9

In this example, the least accurate figure is accurate to one decimal place; this is therefore the determining factor. To determine the least accurate figure, use this rule: In a column of addition or subtraction in which the decimal points are placed one above the other, the number of significant figures in the final answer is determined by the first digit encountered going from left to right that terminates any one numeral.

In multiplication or division, using this example:

$$32.973 \div 4.3 =$$

the result should be reported as 7.7, following this rule:

The number of significant figures in the final product or quotient should not exceed the smallest number of significant figures in any one factor.

Rounding Off Numbers

Test results sometimes produce insignificant digits. It is then necessary to round off the numbers to a chosen number of significant value so as not to imply an accuracy of precision greater than the test is capable of delivering. Some general rules may be used in rounding off decimal values to the proper place. When the digit next to the last one to be retained is less than 5, the last digit should be left unchanged. When the digit next to the last one to be retained is greater than 5, the last digit is increased by 1. If the additional digit is 5, the last digit reported is changed to the nearest even number. Examples are as follows:

2.31463 g is rounded off to 2.3146 g.
5.34659 g is rounded off to 5.3466 g.
23.5 mg is rounded off to 24 mg.
24.5 mg is rounded off to 24 mg.

EXPONENTS

Exponents are used to indicate that a number must be multiplied by itself as many times as indicated by the exponent. The number to be multiplied by itself is called the *base*. Usually the exponent is written as a small superscript figure to the immediate right of the base figure; it is sometimes referred to as the *power* of the base. The exponent figure can have either a plus or a minus sign before it. The plus sign is usually implied and does not actually appear.

A positive exponent indicates the number of times the base is to be multiplied by itself. Examples of exponents with no sign or a plus sign (positive exponents) are:

$$10^2 = 10 \times 10 = 100$$
$$10^5 = 10 \times 10 \times 10 \times 10 \times 10 = 100{,}000$$
$$5^3 = 5 \times 5 \times 5 = 125$$

Clinical laboratory values in hematology cell counts are expressed exponentially. For example, the average of the reference range of the total erythrocyte count in an adult female is 4.8×10^{12}/L. The low end of the reference range of the total leukocyte count in an adult is 4.5×10^9/L.

A negative exponent indicates the number of times the reciprocal of the base is to be multiplied by itself. In other words, a negative exponent indicates a fraction. Examples of exponents with a minus sign (negative exponents) follow:

$$10^{-1} = \frac{1}{10} = 0.1$$
$$10^{-4} = \frac{1}{10} \times \frac{1}{10} \times \frac{1}{10} \times \frac{1}{10} = \frac{1}{10{,}000} = 0.0001$$

DENSITY AND SPECIFIC GRAVITY

Density is defined as the amount of matter per unit volume of a substance. All substances have this property, not solutions only. An example of the expression of density is the specific gravity of a substance.

Specific gravity can be used to determine the mass (weight) of solutions. It relates the weight of 1 mL of a solution and the weight of 1 mL of pure water at 4°C (1 g). Specific gravity is used in the clinical or research laboratory when preparing dilutions made from concentrated acids.

$$\text{Specific gravity} \times \text{Percent assay} = \text{Grams of compound/mL}$$

Example: Concentrated hydrochloric acid (HCl) has a specific gravity of 1.25 g/mL and an assay value of 38%. What is the amount of HCl/mL?

$$1.25\,\text{g/mL} \times 0.38 = 0.475\,\text{g of HCl/mL}$$

Once the number of grams (g) of HCl in the concentrated acid is known, further calculations can be performed to determine how many milliliters (mL) of the acid are needed to prepare various concentrations of HCl solutions.

EXPRESSIONS OF SOLUTION CONCENTRATION

Solutions are made up of a mixture of substances. Making up a solution usually involves two main parts: the substance that is being dissolved (the solute) and the substance into which the solute is being dissolved (the solvent). In working with solutions, it is necessary to know or be able to measure the relative amounts of the substance in solution, known as the *concentration of the solution.* Concentration is the amount of one substance relative to the amounts of the other substances in the solution (Student Worksheet 7.1).

Solution concentration is expressed in several ways. The most common methods used in clinical laboratories involve either weight per unit weight (w/w), also known as mass per unit mass (m/m); weight per unit volume (w/v), also known as mass per unit volume (m/v); or volume per unit volume (v/v). *Weight* is the term commonly used, although *mass* is really what is being measured. Mass is the amount of matter in something, and weight is the force of gravity on something. The most accurate measurement is weight per unit weight, because weight (or mass), unlike volume, does not vary with temperature. Probably the most common measurement is weight per unit volume. The least accurate measurement is volume per unit volume because of the changes in volume resulting from temperature changes. Volume per unit volume is used in preparing a liquid solution from another liquid substance.

Weight (Mass) per Unit Volume

The most common way of expressing concentration is by weight (mass) per unit volume (w/v). When weight (mass) per unit volume is used, the amount of solute (the substance that goes into solution) per volume of solution is expressed. Weight per unit volume is used most often when a solid chemical is diluted in a liquid. The usual way to express weight per unit volume is as grams per liter (g/L) or milligrams per milliliter (mg/mL). If a concentration of a certain solution is given as 10 g/L, it means there are 10 g of solute for every liter of solution. If a solution with a concentration of 10 mg/mL is desired, and if 100 mL of this solution is to be prepared, a proportion formula can be applied. Example:

$$\frac{10\,\text{mg}}{1\,\text{mL}} = \frac{x\,\text{mg}}{100\,\text{mL}} = 1000\,\text{mg (or 1 g)}.$$

One gram (1 g) of the desired solute is weighed and diluted to 100 mL.

A standard solution is usually expressed as milligrams per milliliter (mg/mL).

Volume per Unit Volume

Another way of expressing concentration is by volume per unit volume (v/v). Volume per unit volume is used to express concentration when a liquid chemical is diluted with another liquid. The concentration is expressed as the number of milliliters of liquid chemical per unit volume of solution. The usual way to express volume per unit volume is as milliliters per milliliter (mL/mL) or as milliliters per liter (mL/L). The number of milliliters of liquid chemical in 1 mL or 1 L of solution uses the volume per unit volume expression of concentration. If 10 mL of alcohol is diluted to 100 mL with water, the concentration is expressed as 10 mL/100 mL, or 10 mL/dL, or 0.1 mL/mL, or 100 mL/L. If a solution with a concentration of 0.5 mL/mL is desired, and 1 L is to be prepared, a proportion can again be used to solve the problem. An example follows:

$$\frac{0.5\,\text{mL}}{1\,\text{mL}} = \frac{x\,\text{mL}}{1000\,\text{mL}}$$
$$x = 500\,\text{mL}$$

Therefore 500 mL of the liquid chemical is measured accurately and diluted to 1000 mL (1 L). To express concentration in milliliters per liter, one needs to know how many milliliters of liquid chemical are in 1 L of the solution.

Any chemical (liquid or solid) can be made into a solution by diluting it with a solvent. The usual solvent is deionized or distilled water (see Laboratory Reagent Water, Chapter 6). If the desired chemical is a liquid, the amount needed is measured in milliliters or liters. On occasion, liquids are weighed, but the usual method is to measure their volume. If the desired chemical is a solid, the amount needed is weighed in grams or milligrams.

Percent

Another expression of concentration is the percent solution (%), although in the International System of Units (SI system) the preferred units are kilograms (or fractions thereof) per liter (w/v) or milliliters per liter (v/v). A description of the percent solution follows, because this expression of concentration is still used in some instances. *Percent* is defined as parts per hundred parts (the part can be any particular unit). Unless otherwise stated, a percent solution usually means grams or milliliters of solute per 100 mL of solution (g/100 mL or mL/100 mL). Recall that 100 mL is equal to 1 deciliter (dL). Percent solutions can be prepared using either liquid or solid chemicals. Percent solutions can be expressed either as weight per unit volume percent (w/v%) or as volume per unit volume percent (v/v%), depending on the state of the solute (chemical) used; that is, whether it is a solid or a liquid. When a solid chemical is dissolved in a liquid, *percent* means grams of solid in 100 mL of solution. If 10 g of sodium chloride (NaCl) is diluted to 100 mL with deionized water, the concentration is expressed as 10% (10 g/dL). If 2.5 g is diluted to 100 mL, the concentration is 2.5% (2.5 g/dL).

The following is an example of concentration expressed in percent: 10 grams of sodium hydroxide (NaOH) is diluted to 200 mL with water. What is the concentration in percent? A proportion can be set up to solve this problem, as follows:

$$\frac{10\,\text{g}}{200\,\text{mL}} = \frac{x\,\text{g}}{100\,\text{mL}}$$

x = 5% solution (preferably expressed as 5 g/dL)

Remember that the percent expression is based on how much solute is present in 100 mL (or 1 dL) of the solution.

Some concentrations of solutions are expressed as milligrams of solute in 100 mL of solution (mg%). When this method of expression is used, mg% is always specifically stated. If 25 mg of a chemical is diluted to 100 mL, the concentration in milligrams percent would be 25 mg% (preferably expressed as 25 mg/dL).

If a liquid chemical is used to prepare a percent solution, the concentration is expressed as volume per unit volume percent, or milliliters of solute per 100 mL of solution. If 10 mL of HCl is diluted to 100 mL with water, the concentration is 10% (preferably expressed as 10 mL/dL). If 10 mL of the same acid is diluted to 1 L (1000 mL), the concentration is 1% (preferably expressed as 1 mL/dL).

Molality

Molality is the number of moles of solute per kilogram of solvent. Because the density of water at 25°C is about 1 kilogram per liter, molality is approximately equal to molarity for dilute aqueous solutions at this temperature.

Example of Molality Calculation

What is the molality of a solution of 10 g NaOH in 500 g water?

Solution:

10 g NaOH/(40 g NaOH/1 mol NaOH) = 0.25 mol NaOH
500 g water × 1 kg/1000 g = 0.50 kg water
Molality = 0.25 mol/0.50 kg
Molality = 0.05 M/kg
Molality = 0.50 M

Molarity

The molarity of a solution is defined as the gram-molecular mass (or weight) of a compound per liter of solution. This is a weight-per-unit-volume method of expressing concentration. A basic formula follows:

$$\text{Molecular weight} \times \text{Molarity} = \text{Grams/liter}$$

Another way to define *molarity* is number of moles per liter (mol/L) of solution. A *mole* is the molecular weight of a compound in grams (1 mole = 1 gram-molecular weight). The number of moles of a compound equals the number of grams divided by the gram-molecular weight of that compound. One gram-molecular weight equals the sum of all atomic weights in a molecule of the compound, expressed in grams.

To determine the gram-molecular weight of a compound, the correct chemical formula must be known; then the sum of all the atomic weights in the compound can be found by consulting a periodic table of the elements or a chart with atomic masses of the elements.

Examples of Molarity Calculations

Sodium chloride has one sodium ion and one chloride ion; the correct formula is written as *NaCl.* The gram-molecular weight is derived by finding the sum of the atomic weights:

$$\begin{aligned} \text{Na} &= 23.0 \\ \text{Cl} &= 35.5 \\ \text{Gram molecular weight} &= 58.5 \end{aligned}$$

If the gram-molecular weight of NaCl is 58.5 g, a 1 molar (1 M) solution of NaCl would contain 58.5 g of NaCl per liter of solution, because molarity equals moles per liter, and 1 mol of NaCl equals 58.5 g.

For barium sulfate ($BaSO_4$), the gram-molecular weight equals 233 (the formula indicates that the compound has one barium, one sulfur, and four oxygen ions):

Because the gram-molecular weight is 233, a 1 M solution of $BaSO_4$ would contain 233 g of $BaSO_4$ per liter of solution.

The quantities of solutions needed will not always be in units of whole liters, and often fractions or multiples of a 1 M concentration will be desired. Parts of a molar solution are expressed as decimals. If a 1 M solution of NaCl contains 58.5 g of NaCl per liter of solution, a 0.5 M solution would contain one half of 58.5 g, or 29 g/L, and a 3 M solution would contain 3 times 58.5 g, or 175.5 g/L.

What is the molarity of a solution containing 30 g of NaCl per liter? Molarity equals the number of moles per liter, and the number of moles equals the grams divided by the gram-molecular weight.

Step 1: Find the gram-molecular weight of NaCl. It is 58.5 g (Na = 23 and Cl = 35.5).

Step 2: Find the moles per liter.

$$\frac{30\,\text{g/L}}{x} = \frac{58.5\,\text{g/L}}{1\,\text{mol}}$$

$$x = \frac{30\,\text{g/L} \times 1\,\text{mol}}{58.5\,\text{g/L}} = 0.513\,\text{mol NaCl}$$

Step 3: The number of moles per liter of solution equals the molarity; the solution in the example is therefore 0.513 M, rounded off to 0.5 M.

Equations might prove useful to some in working with molarity solutions, but all these equations can be derived by applying the commonsense proportion approach to molarity problems described later under Proportions and Ratios. Some equations are:

$$\text{Molarity} = \frac{\text{Moles of solute}}{\text{Liters of solution}}$$

$$\text{Molarity} = \frac{\text{Grams of solute}}{\text{Gram molecular weight}} \times \frac{1}{\text{Liters of solution}}$$

$$\text{Moles of solute} = \text{Molarity} \times \text{Liters of solution}$$

$$\text{Grams of solute} = \text{Molarity} \times \text{Gram molecular weight} \times \text{Liters of solution}$$

NOTE: These equations are all on the basis of 1 L of solution; if something other than 1 L is used, refer back to the 1-L basis (for example, 500 mL = 0.5 L; 2000 mL = 2 L).

Molarity does not provide a basis for direct comparison of strength for all solutions. For example, 1 L of 1 M NaOH will exactly neutralize 1 L of 1 M HCl, but it will neutralize only 0.5 L of 1 M sulfuric acid (H_2SO_4). It is therefore more convenient to choose a unit of concentration that will provide a basis for direct comparison of solution strengths. Such a unit is referred to as an *equivalent* (or equivalent weight or mass), and this term is used in describing normality.

Millimolarity

A milligram-molecular weight (the molecular weight expressed in milligrams) is a millimole (mmole). This is in contrast to the molarity described previously, which is the number of moles per liter. The following formulas compare the two:

$$\text{Molarity}\ (\textit{moles/liter}) = \frac{\text{g/L}}{\text{Molecular weight}}$$

$$\text{Millimoles/liter} = \frac{\text{mg/L}}{\text{Molecular weight}}$$

Osmolality and Osmolarity

Osmolality and osmolarity are units of solute concentration that are referred to in the analysis of body fluids. An osmole is related to *osmosis* and is used in reference to solutions where osmotic pressure is important, such as blood and urine.

Both osmolality and osmolarity are defined in terms of osmoles. An *osmole* is a unit of measurement that describes the number of moles of a compound that contribute to the osmotic pressure of a chemical solution.

Osmolality

Osmolality is defined as the number of osmoles of solute per kilogram of solvent. It is expressed in terms of osmol/kg or Osm/kg. In the clinical laboratory, osmolality is a more exact measurement of urine concentration than the urine specific gravity test. Urine osmolality is a measure of urine concentration based on the number of particles dissolved into the urine and is measured in milliosmols/kg. Serum osmolality is ordered primarily to investigate hyponatremia, or low sodium in the blood. Hyponatremia may be caused by sodium loss through the urine or by increased fluid in the bloodstream. Increased fluid may be caused by drinking excessive amounts of water, water retention, decreased ability of the kidneys to produce urine, or the presence of osmotically active agents such as glucose. Marathon runners can be affected by hyponatremia.

Osmolarity

Osmolarity is defined as the number of osmoles of solute per liter of solution. An osmole (osm) is the amount of a substance that will produce 1 mole (mol) of particles having osmotic activity. An osmole of any substance is equal to 1 gram-molecular weight (1 mol) of the substance divided by the number of particles formed by the dissociation of the molecules of the substance. For materials that do not ionize, 1 osm is equal to 1 mol. This gives an estimate of the osmotic activity of the solution—the relative number of particles dissolved in the solution. Osmolarity is an expression of weight per unit volume concentration.

For a solution of glucose, a substance that does not ionize or dissociate in aqueous solution, 1 osm of glucose is equal to 1 mol of glucose. For a solution of NaCl, which does ionize, 1 osm of NaCl is equal to 1 gram-molecular weight divided by the number of particles formed on ionization. NaCl completely ionizes in water to form one sodium ion (Na^+) and one chloride ion (Cl^-), or a total of two particles. The molecular weight of NaCl is 58.5. To calculate the osmolarity of NaCl, the following formula is used:

$$1\ \text{osm NaCl} = \frac{58.5}{2} = 29.25\ \text{g}$$

The osmolal gap is discussed in detail in Chapter 10, Introduction to Clinical Chemistry. The major contributors to the gap are glucose, Na^+, and blood urea nitrogen.

Titer

The term titer is used to express the concentration of antibody in serum. The difference between the concentration of antibody when a person is initially ill from an infection (such as infectious mononucleosis) and the concentration when convalescing from the same illness can be measured and expressed as the titer of antibody.

Proportions and Ratios

The use of proportions involves a commonsense approach to problem solving. Proportions are used to determine a quantity from a given ratio. A ratio is an amount of something compared with an amount of something else.

Ratios always describe a relative amount, and at least two values are always involved. For example, 5 g of something dissolved in 100 mL of something else can be expressed by the ratio 5:100 or by the decimal 0.05. Proportion is a means of saying that two ratios are equal. Thus the ratio 5:100 is equal, or proportional to, the ratio 1:20. This proportion can be expressed as 5:100 = 1:20. In the laboratory, proportions and ratios are useful when it is necessary to make more (or less) of the same thing. However, ratios and proportions can be used only when the concentration (or any other type of relationship) does not change.

The following is an example of a proportion or ratio problem: A formula calls for 5 g of NaCl in 1000 mL of solution. If only 500 mL of solution is needed, how much NaCl is required?

$$\frac{5\,\text{g}}{1000\,\text{mL}} = \frac{x\,\text{g}}{500\,\text{mL}}$$

$$x = \frac{5\,\text{g} \times 500\,\text{mL}}{1000\,\text{mL}}$$

$$x = 2.5\,\text{g NaCl}$$

In setting up ratio and proportion problems, the two ratios being compared must be written in the same order, and they must be in the same units. When specimens are diluted in various laboratory analyses, the ratio principle is applied (see later).

Concentrations of Solutions

To relate different concentrations of solutions that contain the same amount of substance (or solute), a basic relationship, or ratio, is used. The volume of one solution (V_1) times the concentration of that solution (C_1) equals the volume of the second solution (V_2) times the concentration of the second solution (C_2), as follows:

$$V_1 \times C_1 = V_2 \times C_2$$

If any three of the values are known, the fourth may be determined. This relationship shows that when a solution is diluted, the volume is increased as the concentration is decreased. The total amount of substance (or solute) remains unchanged. Several applications of this relationship are used in the clinical laboratory, such as dilution of specimens or preparation of weaker solutions from stronger solutions.

An example of making a less concentrated solution from a more concentrated solution follows. An NaOH solution is available that has a concentration of 10 g of NaOH per deciliter (dL) of solution (1 dL = 100 mL). To calculate the volume of the 10 g/dL NaOH solution required to prepare 1000 mL of 2 g/dL NaOH:

$$V_1 \times C_1 = V_2 \times C_2$$

$$x\,\text{mL} \times 10\,\text{g/dL} = 1000\,\text{mL} \times 2\,\text{g/dL}$$

$$x = \frac{2\,\text{g/dL} \times 1000\,\text{mL}}{10\,\text{g/dL}} = 200\,\text{mL}$$

$$10\,\text{g/dL} = 200\,\text{mL}$$

Note that this relationship is not a direct proportion but an inverse proportion. Because this is a proportion problem, it is important to remember that the concentrations and volumes on both sides of the equation must be expressed in the same units.

DILUTIONS

It is often necessary to make **dilutions** of specimens being analyzed or to make weaker solutions from stronger solutions in various laboratory procedures (Student Procedure Worksheet 7.2).

A laboratory professional must be capable of working with various dilution problems and *dilution factors.* In these problems, one must often be able to determine the concentration of material in each solution, the actual amount of material in each solution, and the total volume of each solution. All dilutions are a type of ratio. Dilution is an indication of relative concentration.

Diluting Specimens

In performing a laboratory assay, it may be necessary to dilute a specimen because of the high concentration of a constituent. The needed dilution will vary according to the procedure (see Use of Dilution Factors).

Dilution Factor

A dilution factor is used to correct for having used a diluted sample in a determination rather than the undiluted sample. The result (answer) using the dilution must be multiplied by the reciprocal of the dilution made.

For example, a dilution factor by which all determination answers are multiplied to give the concentration per 100 mL of sample (blood) may be calculated as follows:

1. Determine the volume of blood that is actually analyzed in the procedure. By use of a simple proportion, it is evident that 0.5 mL of blood diluted to 10 mL is equivalent to 1 mL of blood diluted to 20 mL.

$$\frac{0.5\,\text{mL blood}}{10\,\text{mL solution}} = \frac{1\,\text{mL blood}}{x\,\text{mL solution}}$$

$$x = \frac{1\,\text{mL blood} \times 10\,\text{mL}}{0.5\,\text{mL}} = 20\,\text{mL}$$

2. Using another simple proportion, the concentration of specimen (blood) in each milliliter of solution may be determined to be 0.05 mL of blood per milliliter of solution:

$$\frac{1\,\text{mL blood}}{20\,\text{mL solution}} = \frac{x\,\text{mL blood}}{1\,\text{mL solution}}$$

$$x = \frac{1\,\text{mL} \times 1\,\text{mL}}{20\,\text{mL}} = 0.05\,\text{mL}$$

3. Because 1 mL of the 1/20 dilution of blood is analyzed in the remaining steps of the procedure, 0.05 mL of blood is actually analyzed (1 mL of the dilution used × 0.05 mL/mL = 0.05 mL of blood analyzed).
4. To relate the concentration of the substance measured in the procedure to the concentration in 100 mL of blood (the units in which the result is to be expressed), another proportion may be used:

$$\frac{100\,\text{mL (volume of blood desired)}}{0.05\,\text{mL (volume of blood used)}} = \frac{\text{Concentration desired}}{\textit{Concentration}\text{ used or determined}}$$

$$\text{Concentration desired} = \frac{100\,\text{mL} \times \text{Concentration determined}}{0.05}$$

$$\text{Concentration desired} = 2000 \times \text{Value determined}$$

5. The concentration of the substance being measured in the volume of blood actually tested (0.05 mL) must be multiplied by 2000 to report the concentration per 100 mL of blood.

The preceding material may be summarized by the following statement and equations. In reporting results obtained from laboratory determinations, one must first quantify the amount of specimen actually analyzed in the procedure, then calculate the factor that will express the concentration in the desired terms of measurement. For the previous example:

$$\frac{0.5\ \text{mL (volume of blood used)}}{10\ \text{mL (volume of total dilution)}} = \frac{x\ \text{mL (volume of blood analyzed)}}{1\ \text{mL (volume of dilution used)}}$$

$$x = 0.05\ \text{mL (volume of blood actually analyzed)}$$

$$\frac{100\ \text{mL}\left(\begin{array}{c}\text{volume of blood required}\\ \text{for expression of result}\end{array}\right)}{0.05\ \text{mL (volume of blood actually analyzed)}} = 2000\ \text{(dilution factor)}$$

Single Dilutions

When the concentration of a particular substance in a specimen is too great to be accurately determined, or when there is less specimen available for analysis than the procedure requires, it may be necessary to dilute the original specimen or to further dilute the initial dilution (or filtrate). Such *single dilutions* can be expressed as 1/2, 1/5, or 1/10 dilutions. These dilutions refer to 1 unit of the original specimen diluted to a final volume of 2, 5, or 10 units, respectively. A dilution refers to the volume or number of parts of the substance to be diluted in the total volume, or parts, of the final solution. A dilution is an expression of concentration, not an expression of volume; it indicates the relative amount of substance in solution. Dilutions can be made singly or in series.

To calculate the concentration of a single dilution, multiply the original concentration by the dilution expressed as a fraction.

Calculation of the Concentration of a Single Dilution

A simple dilution uses the formula:

$$\frac{\text{Sample volume}}{\text{Sample volume} + \text{Diluent volume}}$$

or:

$$\frac{\text{Sample volume}}{\text{Total volume}}$$

A specimen contains 500 mg of substance per deciliter of blood. A 1/5 dilution of this specimen is prepared by volumetrically measuring 1 mL of the specimen and adding 4 mL of diluent. The concentration of substance in the dilution is:

$$500\ \text{mg/dL} \times {}^{1}/_{5} = 100\ \text{mg/dL}$$

Note that the concentration of the final solution (or dilution) is expressed in the same units as the original solution.

To obtain a dilution factor that can be applied to the answer to express it as a concentration per standard volume, proceed as follows. Rather than multiply by the dilution expressed as a fraction, multiply the determination value by the reciprocal of the dilution fraction. In the case of a 1/5 dilution, the dilution factor that would be applied to values obtained in the procedure would be 5, because the original specimen was five times more concentrated than the diluted specimen tested in the procedure.

Use of Dilution Factors

A 1/5 dilution of a specimen is prepared, and an aliquot (one of a number of equal parts) of the dilution is analyzed for a particular substance. The concentration of the substance in the aliquot is multiplied by 5 to determine its concentration in the original specimen. If the concentration of the dilution is 100 mg/dL, the concentration of the original specimen is:

$$100\ \text{mg/dL} \times 5\ \text{(dilution factor)} \doteq 500\ \text{mg/dL in blood}$$

Serial Dilutions

As mentioned previously, dilutions can be made singly or in series, in which case the original solution is further diluted. A general rule for calculating the concentrations of solutions obtained by dilution in series is to multiply the original concentration by the first dilution (expressed as a fraction), this by the second dilution, and so on until the desired concentration is known (Student Procedure Worksheet 7.2).

Several laboratory procedures, especially serologic tests, make use of a dilution series in which all dilutions, including or after the first one, are the same. Such dilutions are referred to as serial dilutions. A complete dilution series usually contains five or 10 tubes, although any single dilution may be made directly from an undiluted specimen or substance. In calculating the dilution or concentration of substance or serum in each tube of the dilution series, the rules previously discussed apply.

A five-tube twofold dilution may be prepared as follows (Fig. 7.1). A serum specimen is diluted 1/2 with buffer. A series of five tubes is prepared, in which each succeeding tube is rediluted 1/2. This is accomplished by placing 1 mL of diluent into each of four tubes (tubes 2–5). Tube 1 contains 1 mL of undiluted serum. Tube 2 contains 1 mL of undiluted serum plus 1 mL of diluent, resulting in a 1/2 dilution of serum. A 1-mL portion of the 1/2 dilution of serum is placed in tube 3, resulting in a 1/4 dilution of serum (${}^{1}/_{2} \times {}^{1}/_{2} = {}^{1}/_{4}$). A 1-mL portion of the 1/4 dilution from tube 3 is placed in tube 4, resulting in a 1/8 dilution (${}^{1}/_{4} \times {}^{1}/_{2} = {}^{1}/_{8}$). Finally, 1 mL of the 1/8 dilution from tube 4 is added to tube 5, resulting in a 1/16 dilution (${}^{1}/_{8} \times {}^{1}/_{2} = {}^{1}/_{16}$). One milliliter of the final dilution is discarded so that the volumes in all the tubes are equal. Note that each tube is diluted twice as much as the previous tube, and that the final volume in each tube is the same. The undiluted serum may also be given a dilution value: 1/1.

The concentration of serum in terms of milliliters in each tube is calculated by multiplying the previous concentration (mL) by the succeeding dilution. In the Fig. 7.1 example, tube 1 contains 1 mL of serum, tube 2 contains 1 mL × ${}^{1}/_{2}$ = 0.5

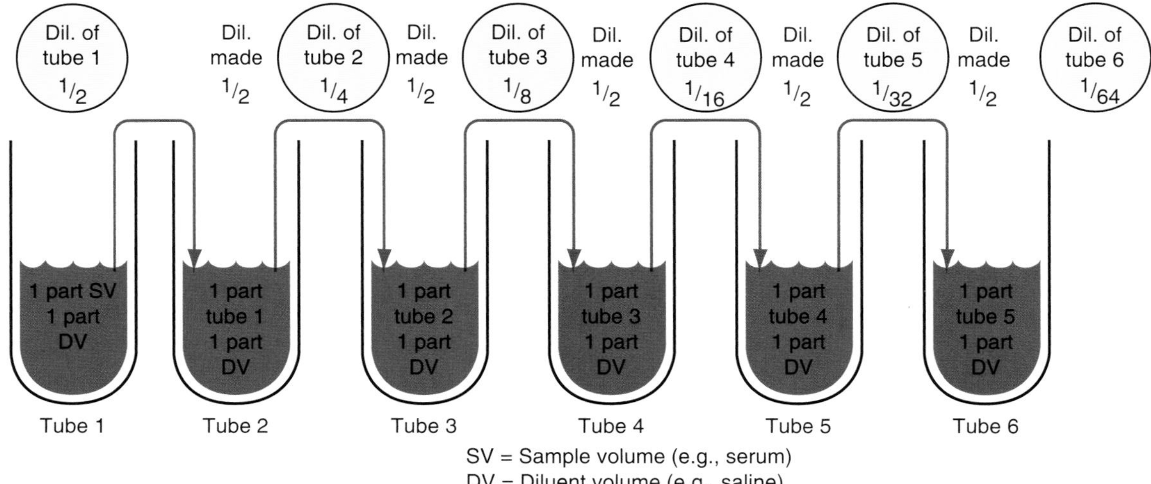

Fig. 7.1 Schematic of a twofold serial dilution. (From Doucette LJ: *Mathematics for the clinical laboratory*, ed 2, St Louis, 2011, Elsevier/Saunders.)

mL of serum, and tubes 3 to 5 contain 0.25, 0.125, and 0.06 mL of serum, respectively.

Other serial dilutions might be fivefold or tenfold; that is, each succeeding tube is diluted five or 10 times. A fivefold series would begin with 1 mL of serum in 4 mL of diluent and a total volume of 5 mL in each tube. A tenfold series would begin with 1 mL of serum in 9 mL of diluent and a total volume of 10 mL in each tube. Other systems might begin with a 1/2 dilution and then dilute five succeeding tubes 1/10. The dilutions in such a series would be 1/2, 1/20 $({}^{1}/{}_{2} \times {}^{1}/{}_{10} = {}^{1}/{}_{20})$, 1/200 $({}^{1}/{}_{20} \times {}^{1}/{}_{10} = {}^{1}/{}_{200})$, 1/2000, 1/20,000, and 1/200,000.

Calculation of the Concentration After a Series of Dilutions

A working solution is prepared from a stock solution (see next section). In that process, a stock solution with a concentration of 100 mg/dL is diluted 1/10 by volumetrically adding 1 mL of the solution to 9 mL of diluent. The diluted solution (intermediate solution) is further diluted 1/100 by volumetrically measuring 1 mL of intermediate solution and diluting to the mark in a 100-mL volumetric flask. The concentration of the final or working solution is:

$$100\ \text{mg/dL} \times {}^{1}/{}_{10} \times {}^{1}/{}_{100} = 0.1\ \text{mg/dL}$$

Standard Solutions

To determine the concentration of a substance in a specimen, there must be a basis of comparison. For analyses that result in a colored solution, a spectrophotometer is used to make this comparison. A standard solution is one that contains a known, exact amount of the substance being measured. It is prepared from high-quality reference material with measured, known amounts of a fixed and known chemical composition that can be obtained in a pure form. The standard solution is measured accurately and then treated in the testing procedure as if it were a specimen whose concentration is to be determined.

Standard solutions are purchased "ready made," already prepared from high-quality chemicals, or they can be prepared in the laboratory from high-quality chemicals that have been dried and stored in a desiccator. The standard chemical is weighed on the analytical balance and diluted volumetrically. This standard solution is usually most stable in a concentrated form, in which case it is usually referred to as a *stock standard.*

Working Standards

Working standards are prepared from the stock, and sometimes an intermediate form is prepared. The working standard (a more dilute form of the stock standard) is the one employed in the actual determination. Stock and working standards are usually stored in the refrigerator. The accuracy of a procedure is absolutely dependent on the standard solution used, so extreme care must be taken whenever these solutions are prepared or used in a clinical laboratory.

Standards Used in Spectrophotometry

To use the standard solution as a basis of comparison in quantitative analysis with the spectrophotometer, a series of calibrated cuvettes (or tubes) is prepared. Each cuvette contains a known, different amount of the standard solution. In this way, a series of cuvettes is available containing various known amounts of the standard. Standard cuvettes are carried through the same developmental steps as cuvettes containing specimens to be measured. This set of standard cuvettes is read in the spectrophotometer, and the galvanometer readings are recorded. These readings can be recorded in percent transmittance or in absorbance units. Standard solutions are also included in automated analytical methods.

Blank Solutions

For every procedure using the spectrophotometer, a blank solution must be included in the batch. A *blank solution* contains reagents used in the procedure, but it does not contain the substance to be measured. It is treated with the same reagents and processed along with the unknown specimens and the standards. The blank solution is set to read 100%T on the galvanometer viewing scale. In other words, the blank tube is set to transmit 100% of the light.

The other cuvettes in the same batch (such as unknown specimens and standards) transmit only a fraction of this light because they contain particles that absorb light (particles of the unknown substance), so only part of the 100% is transmitted. Using a blank solution corrects for any color that may be present because of the reagents used or an interaction between those reagents.

BIBLIOGRAPHY

Adams DS: *Lab math: a handbook of measurements, calculations and other quantitative skills for use at the bench,* Cold Spring Harbor, NY, 2003, Cold Spring Harbor Press.

Campbell JB, Campbell JM: *Laboratory mathematics: medical and biological applications,* ed 5, St Louis, 1997, Mosby.

Doucette LJ: *Basic mathematics for the health-related professions,* Philadelphia, 2000, Saunders.

Doucette LJ: *Mathematics for the clinical laboratory,* ed 2, St. Louis, 2011, Elsevier/Saunders.

Johnson CW, Timmons DL, Hall PE: *Essential lab math, concepts and applications for the chemical and clinical lab technician,* Clifton Park, NY, 2003, Thomson Delmar Learning.

Kaplan LA, Pesce AJ: *Clinical chemistry: theory, analysis, correlation,* ed 5, St Louis, 2010, Elsevier/Mosby.

REVIEW QUESTIONS (ANSWERS IN APPENDIX A)

Significant Figures

1. How would 6.32 be rounded off to one less decimal place?
   a. 6.32
   b. 6.4
   c. 7.0
   d. 6.3
2. How would 15.57 be rounded off to one less decimal place?
   a. 15.6
   b. 15.5
   c. 16.0
   d. 15.0
3. How would 25.96 be rounded off to one less decimal place?
   a. 26.0
   b. 25.9
   c. 25.6
   d. 26.96

Exponents

4. The exponent 10^{-2} represents:
   a. 100
   b. 1000
   c. 0.1
   d. 0.01

Density and Specific Gravity

5. A unique characteristic of specific gravity versus density is that specific gravity is:
   a. The amount of matter per unit volume of a substance
   b. That all substances have this property
   c. That it represents size of substance
   d. That it is applicable only to solutions

Expressions of Solution Concentration

6. Molarity is:
   a. The amount of one substance relative to the amounts of other substances in the solution
   b. Relative concentrations of the components of a mixture
   c. The gram-molecular mass (or weight) of a compound per liter of solution
   d. Expression of one amount relative to another amount
7. Three grams (3 g) of solute in 100 mL of solvent equals _____% (w/v).
   a. 0.3
   b. 3
   c. 30
   d. 300
8. Twenty grams (20 g) of solute dissolved in 1 L of solvent equals _____% (w/v).
   a. 0.2
   b. 2
   c. 20
   d. 200
9. If 6 mL of liquid is placed in a volumetric flask and the volume is brought to 100 mL total, the solution is what percent of liquid?
   a. 0.6%
   b. 6%
   c. 60%
   d. None of the above
10. How many grams of NaCl would be used to prepare 1000 mL of a 5% (w/v) solution of NaCl?
    a. 0.5 g
    b. 5 g
    c. 50 g
    d. 500 g
11. If there is 25 g of NaCl per liter of solution, what is the molarity?
    a. 0.25 M
    b. 0.43 M
    c. 0.50 M
    d. 1.00 M
12. How many grams of NaCl are needed to prepare 1000 mL of a 0.5 M solution of NaCl?
    a. 5 g
    b. 15 g
    c. 29 g
    d. 58.4 g

13. How much calcium chloride ($CaCl_2$) is needed to prepare 500 mL of a 0.5 M solution of $CaCl_2$?
    a. 27.8 g
    b. 40.0 g
    c. 57.8 g
    d. 115.6 g
14. What is the correct formula for calculating a percent (w/v) solution?
    a. Grams of solute/Volume of solution × 100
    b. Grams of solute × Volume of solvent × 100
    c. Volume of solvent/Grams of solute × 100
    d. Grams of solute × Volume of solvent/100
15. If a solution contains 20 g of solute dissolved in 0.5 L of water, what is the percentage of this solution?
    a. 2%
    b. 4%
    c. 6%
    d. 8%
16. How is a 25% w/w solution prepared?
    a. 0.25 g solute and 75 g solvent
    b. 2.5 g solute and 97.5 g solvent
    c. 25 g solute and 75 g solvent
    d. 75 g solute and 25 g solvent
17. How many milliliters (mL) of bleach in an original bottle are needed to prepare a 10% solution?
    a. 0.1 mL bleach and 100 mL water
    b. 1.0 mL bleach and 90 mL water
    c. 10 mL bleach and 90 mL water
    d. Bleach is already a 10% solution in the original bottle

Dilutions

18. Dilution is:
    a. The amount of one substance relative to the amounts of other substances in the solution
    b. Relative concentrations of the components of a mixture
    c. The gram-molecular mass (or weight) of a compound per liter of solution
    d. Expression of one amount relative to another amount
19. What is the dilution, if 1.0 mL of serum is added to 9.0 mL of diluent?
    a. 1/9
    b. 1/10
    c. 2/18
    d. 1:9
20. What volume of 25% alcohol is needed to prepare 500 mL of 15% alcohol?
    a. 30 mL
    b. 300 mL
    c. 350 mL
    d. 375 mL
21. A ratio is:
    a. The amount of one substance relative to the amounts of other substances in the solution
    b. Relative concentrations of the components of a mixture
    c. The gram-molecular mass (or weight) of a compound per liter of solution
    d. Expression of one amount relative to another amount
22. If only 25 mL of a 9% saline solution is available in the laboratory, how many mL of 5% saline solution can be prepared using all available saline solution?
    a. 4.5 mL
    b. 25.0 mL
    c. 45.0 mL
    d. 100 mL
23. Concentration is:
    a. The amount of one substance relative to the amounts of other substances in the solution
    b. Relative concentrations of the components of a mixture
    c. The gram-molecular mass (or weight) of a compound per liter of solution
    d. Expression of one amount relative to another amount
24. To prepare a 1/10 dilution, add _____ parts of serum to _____ parts distilled water.
    a. 1, 10
    b. 1, 9
    c. 0.5, 4.5
    d. Either b and c
25. If 0.1 mL of serum, 5 mL of reagent, and 4.9 mL of distilled water are mixed together, what is the dilution of the serum in the final solution?
    a. 1/5
    b. 1/10
    c. 1/50
    d. 1/100
26. If a glucose standard solution contains 10 mg/dL of glucose, a 1/10 dilution of this standard contains how much glucose?
    a. 0.01 mg/dL
    b. 0.1 mg/dL
    c. 1 mg/dL
    d. None of the above
27. What is the dilution factor if 4 mL of serum is added to 12 mL of diluent?
    a. 3
    b. 4
    c. 12
    d. 15
28. Serum is diluted with an equal amount of diluent (such as tube #1, 1/2 and tube #2, 1/2). What is the concentration in tube #2 if the original concentration was 100 mg/dL?
    a. 12.5 mg/dL
    b. 25.0 mg/dL
    c. 50.0 mg/dL
    d. 75.0 mg/dL
29. If a total of 125 mL of a 10% solution is diluted to 500 mL in a 500-mL volumetric flask, what is the concentration of the resulting new solution?
    a. 0.25%
    b. 2.5%
    c. 25%
    d. None of the above

Bonus Challenge Questions

30. You are asked to make a 1/2 dilution using 1.5 mL of serum. How much diluent do you need to use?
    a. 1.5 mL
    b. 3.0 mL
    c. 15 mL
    d. 30 mL
31. Which of the following "recipes" gives you a 1/5 dilution?
    a. 0.25 mL of serum + 4.75 mL of diluent
    b. 2 mL of serum + 18 mL of diluent
    c. 0.25 mL of serum + 1 mL of diluent
    d. 1.5 mL of serum + 13.5 mL of diluent
32. The dilution created by answer d. in Question #31 is:
    a. 1/20
    b. 1/10
    c. 1/100
    d. 1/1000
33. If you make a five-tube twofold dilution using 2 mL of serum, what is the concentration of serum in tube #4?
    a. 0.125 mL
    b. 0.25 mL
    c. 1 mL
    d. 2 mL

Turgeon: Linné & Ringsrud's Clinical Laboratory Science, 8th Edition

STUDENT PROCEDURE WORKSHEET 7-1

Preparing and Calculating Solution Concentrations

Read Chapter 7 in *Linné & Ringsrud's Clinical Laboratory Science: Concepts, Procedures, and Clinical Applications,* 8th edition, for a complete discussion of this topic.

Student Learning Outcomes

After reading Chapter 7, and at the completion of the laboratory exercise and review questions, the student will be able to:

- Calculate and mix solutions in the clinical laboratory.
- Complete the end-of-procedure practice problems with a grade of 80% or higher.

Equipment and Supplies

1. 0.85% normal saline in 100-mL beaker
2. Test tubes
3. Test tube rack
4. Marking pen
5. Graduated pipettes (1 mL)
6. Gauze (or Kimwipes)
7. Colored liquid imitation specimen
8. Lab coat, gloves, goggles, safety bulb

Instructions for the Procedure

Read the list of required equipment and supplies and the procedural steps. Follow the procedural steps in exact order.

SEQUENCE	PROCEDURAL STEP	INSTRUCTOR-OBSERVED ACCEPTABLE PERFORMANCE (CHECK IF ACCEPTABLE)
1	Collect and assemble the appropriate equipment and supplies.	
2	Label 10 test tubes (1-10).	
3	Check a 1-mL pipette to ascertain its correct size, being careful also to check for broken delivery or suction tips. a. Wearing protective gloves, hold the pipette lightly between the thumb and the last three fingers, leaving the index finger free. b. Place the tip of the pipette well below the surface of the saline to be pipetted. c. Using mechanical suction or an aspirator bulb, carefully draw the liquid up into the pipette until the level of liquid is well above the calibration mark. d. Quickly cover the suction opening at the top of the pipette with the index finger. e. Wipe the outside of the pipette dry with a piece of gauze (or Kimwipe) to remove excess fluid. f. Hold the pipette in a vertical position with the delivery tip against the inside of the original vessel. Carefully allow the liquid in the pipette to drain by gravity until the bottom of the meniscus is exactly at the calibration mark. To do this, do not entirely remove the index finger from the suction hole end of the pipette; rather, by rolling the finger slightly over the opening, allow slow drainage to take place. g. While still holding the pipette in a vertical position, touch the tip of the pipette to the inside wall of the receiving vessel. Remove the index finger from the top of the pipette to permit free drainage. Remember to keep the pipette in a vertical position for correct drainage. In TD (to-deliver) pipettes, a small amount of fluid will remain in the delivery tip. h. To be certain that the drainage is as complete as possible, touch the delivery tip of the pipette to another area on the inside wall of the test tube. i. Repeat this procedure to place 1 mL of saline into each of the 10 labeled tubes.	
4	Pipette 1 mL of imitation serum specimen into tube #1. Mix well by carefully moving the liquid up and down in the pipette.	
5	Repeat the step 3 instructions to begin transferring 1 mL of the mixture in tube #1 to tube #2. Repeat this procedure until you reach tube #10.	
6	Refer to pp. 175-176 to determine the concentrations in each tube.	

Procedural Evaluation

Student's Name ______________________________ Grade___________

Instructor's Signature ___________________________ Date___________

Comments:

Turgeon: Linné & Ringsrud's Clinical Laboratory Science, 8th Edition

STUDENT PROCEDURE WORKSHEET 7-2

Serial Dilutions

Read Chapter 7 in *Linné & Ringsrud's Clinical Laboratory Science: Concepts, Procedures, and Clinical Applications,* 8th edition, for a complete discussion of this topic.

Review Questions

Student's Name ______________________________ Date __________

1. Examine the table below.
What are the dilutions in tubes #2 through #6?

Tube	1	2	3	4	5	6
Saline (µL)	—	50	50	50	50	50
Serum (µL)	50	50	50 (1:2)	50 (1:4)	50 (1:8)	50 (1:16)
Mix and transfer to next tube	—	50	50	50	50	50
Final Dilution/titer	1:1					
IU/mL	200	100	25	12.5	6.25	3.175

2. How would you prepare a 1:10 dilution?

3. How would you prepare a 1:1000 dilution of a standard solution?

8

Basic and Contemporary Techniques in the Clinical Laboratory

http://evolve.elsevier.com/Turgeon/clinicallab/

CHAPTER OUTLINE

LEARNING OUTCOMES

Photometry

- Describe the basic principle of photometry.

Absorbance Spectrophotometry

- Describe the principle of absorbance spectrophotometry.
- Compare the observed colors of the visible spectrum and the corresponding wavelengths.
- Define Beer-Lambert law or Beer's law.

- Summarize the criteria for the preparation and use of a standard curve.
- Name the components and describe the functions of a spectrophotometer.
- Identify and describe the three quality control tests for spectrophotometers.

Reflectance Spectrophotometry
- Describe the principle of reflectance spectrophotometry.

Nephelometry
- Describe the principle, advantages, and disadvantages of nephelometry.

Flow (Cell) Cytometry
- Explain the principle of flow (cell) cytometry and its clinical application.

Immunoassays
- Describe the general characteristics of enzyme immunoassay.
- Identify and compare the three basic immunofluorescent labeling techniques.
- Critique the clinical applications of direct and indirect immunofluorescence assays.

Alternative Labeling Technologies
- Compare the six types of alternative labeling technologies.
- Describe the FISH technique.

Chemiluminescence
- Describe the process of chemiluminescence
- Name several medical uses of chemiluminescence.

Chromatography and Immunochromatography
- Describe the priniciples of lateral and vertical flow immunoassays.

Molecular Diagnostic Techniques
- Differentiate the steps in a polymerase chain reaction (PCR) amplification technique.
- Discuss the general concept of nucleic acid blotting.
- State the clinical applications of Western blotting techniques.

Electrochemical Methods
- Compare a pH electrode with an ion-selective electrode.
- Differentiate the steps in the electrophoresis technique.
- Compare immunoelectrophoresis and immunofixation electrophoresis.

Review Questions
- Demonstrate comprehension of the chapter content by completing the end-of-chapter review questions with a grade of 80% or higher.

Note:
- indicates MLT and MLS core content

❖ indicates MLT (optional) and MLS advanced content

KEY TERMS

absorbance
amplicon
Beer-Lambert (Beer's) law
chemiluminescence
chromatography
colorimeter
coulometry
electrophoresis
flow cytometry
immunoassay
immunofluorescence
ion-selective electrode (ISE)
molecular diagnostic techniques
nephelometry
photometry
polymerase chain reaction (PCR)
spectrometry
standard curve
turbidimetry
Western blot

In the clinical laboratory, there is a continual need for quantitative techniques of measurement. Instrumentation has become miniaturized, enabling the development of point-of-care devices. The methodologies used in technologically sophisticated automated analyzers are based on traditional approaches and technologies. General methods for common automated and manual assays in the chemistry laboratory include the use of photometry, spectrometry, ion-selective electrodes (ISEs), electrophoresis, nephelometry, and immunoassays. Molecular diagnostic techniques are becoming popular testing platforms in the clinical laboratory and for point-of-care testing (POCT).

Analytical techniques and instrumentation provide the foundation for all measurements made in a modern clinical laboratory. Most measurement techniques fall into one of the following four basic categories:

1. Spectrometry, including spectrophotometry, atomic absorption, and mass spectrophotometry
2. Luminescence, including fluorescence, chemiluminescence, and nephelometry
3. Electroanalytical methods, including immunoelectrophoresis (IEP) and immunofixation electrophoresis (IFE), potentiometry, and amperometry
4. Chromatography, including gas, liquid, and thin-layer techniques

PHOTOMETRY

Instruments that measure electromagnetic radiation have several concepts and components in common. One of the most frequently used techniques in the clinical laboratory is photometry or, specifically, absorbance or reflectance spectrophotometry. Photometry employs color and color variation to determine the concentrations of various substances. A photometric component is employed in many of the automated analyzers currently in use in the clinical laboratory, and any person performing clinical laboratory techniques should understand the principles of photometry.

Photometry is the measurement of the luminous intensity of light, or the amount of luminous light falling on a surface from a light source. Photometric instruments measure this intensity of light without consideration of wavelength. In contrast, spectrophotometry is the measurement of the intensity of light at selected wavelengths.

ABSORBANCE SPECTROPHOTOMETRY

In absorbance spectrophotometry, the concentration of an unknown sample is determined by measuring its absorption of light at a particular wavelength and comparing the result with that of a known standard solution measured at the same time and with the same wavelength. The intensity of the color is directly proportional to the concentration of the substance present.

The use of spectrophotometry, or colorimetry, as a means of quantitative measurement depends on primarily two factors: the color itself and the intensity of the color. Any substance to be measured by spectrophotometry must be either naturally colored or capable of being colored. An example of a substance that is colored to begin with is hemoglobin (determined by spectrophotometry in the hematology laboratory). Sugar, specifically glucose, is an example of a substance that is not colored to begin with but is capable of being colored by certain reagents and reactions. Sugar content can therefore be measured by spectrophotometry.

When spectrophotometry is used as a method for quantitative measurement, the unknown colored substance is compared with a similar substance of known strength (a standard solution). In absorbance spectrophotometry, the absorbance units or values for several different concentrations of a standard solution are determined by spectrophotometry and then plotted on graph paper. The resulting graph is known as a *standard calibration curve,* standard curve, or a Beer-Lambert (Beer's) law plot. Unknown specimens can then be read in the spectrophotometer, and their absorbance values can be used to determine their concentrations from the calibration curve.

The Nature of Light

To understand the use of absorbance spectrophotometry (and photometry in general), one must first understand the fundamentals of color. To understand color, one must also understand the nature of light and its effect on color as we see it. Light is a type of radiant energy, and it travels in the form of waves. The distance between waves is the wavelength of light. The term *light* is used to describe radiant energy with wavelengths visible to the human eye or wavelengths bordering on those visible to the human eye.

Electromagnetic radiation includes a spectrum of energy from short-wavelength, highly energetic gamma rays and x-rays on the left side of the spectrum to wavelengths of radio frequencies on the right side (Fig. 8.1). Visible light passes between these frequencies, with the color violet at the 400-nm wavelength and red at the 700-nm wavelength. As discussed next, these are the approximate limits of the visible spectrum.

The human eye responds to radiant energy, or light, with wavelengths between about 380 and 750 nm. A nanometer is 1×10^{-9} m. With modern photometric apparatus, shorter (ultraviolet [UV]) or longer (infrared) wavelengths can be measured. Modern instruments isolate a narrow wavelength range of the spectrum for measurements. Most instruments use filters (photometers) or prisms or gratings (spectrometers) to select or isolate a narrow range of the incident wavelength. The wavelength of light determines the color of the light seen by the human eye. Every color seen is light of a particular wavelength. A combination or mixture of light energy of different wavelengths is known as *daylight* or *white light.* When light is passed through a filter, a prism, or a diffraction grating, it can be broken into a spectrum of visible colors ranging from violet to red. The visible spectrum consists of the following range of colors: violet, blue, green, yellow, orange, and red. If white light is diffracted or partially absorbed by a filter or prism, it becomes visible as certain colors. The various portions of the spectrum may be identified by wavelengths ranging from 380 to 750 nm for the visible colors. Wavelengths below approximately 380 nm are UV, and those above 750 nm are infrared; these light waves are not visible to the human eye. Table 8.1 shows the wavelength ranges for the colors of the visible spectrum.

The color of light seen in the visible spectrum depends on the wavelength that is not absorbed. When light is not absorbed, it is transmitted. A colored solution has color because of its physical properties, which result in its absorbing certain wavelengths and transmitting others. When white light is passed through a solution, part of the light is absorbed, and the remaining light is

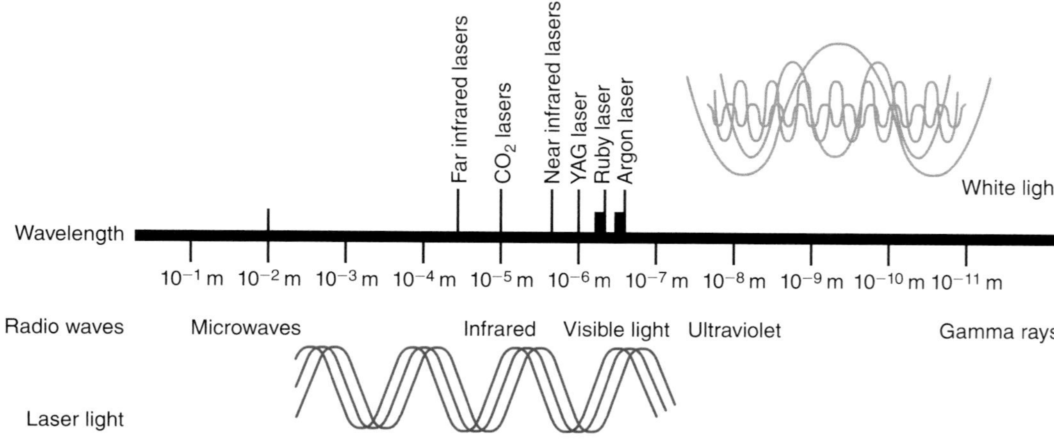

Fig. 8.1 The electromagnetic spectrum. *YAG,* Yttrium-aluminum-garnet. (From Turgeon ML: *Clinical hematology: theory and procedures,* ed 3, Philadelphia, 1999, Lippincott Williams & Wilkins.)

TABLE 8.1 Observed Colors of Visible Spectrum and Corresponding Wavelengths

Approximate Wavelength (nm)	Color Observed
<380	Not visible (ultraviolet light)
380–440	Violet
440–500	Blue
500–580	Green
580–600	Yellow
600–620	Orange
620–750	Red
>750	Not visible (infrared light)

transmitted. A rainbow is seen when there are droplets of moisture in the air that refract or filter certain rays of the sun and allow others to pass through. The colors of the rainbow range from red to violet—the visible spectrum.

Many compounds absorb UV or visible light. The following diagram shows a beam of monochromatic radiation of radiant power P_0, directed at a sample solution. Absorption takes place, and the beam of radiation leaving the sample has radiant power P.

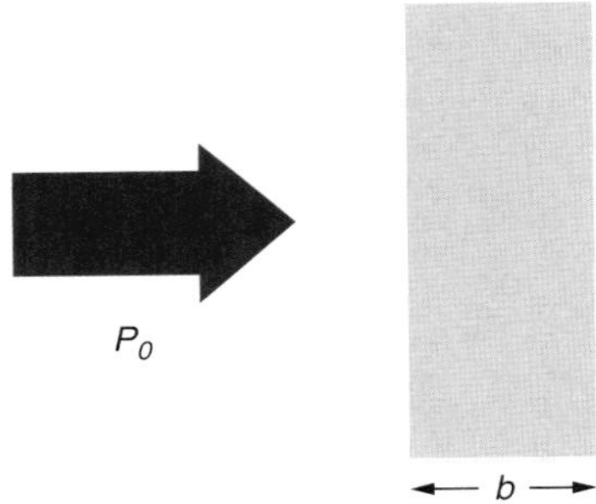

The amount of radiation absorbed may be measured in a number of ways:

Transmittance: $T = P/P_0$

% Transmittance: $\%T = 100\ T$

Absorbance:

$A = \log_{10} P_0/P$

$A = \log_{10} 1/T$

$A = \log_{10} 100/\%T$

$A = 2 - \log_{10} \%T$

The last equation, $A = 2 - \log_{10} \%T$, is worth remembering because it allows one to calculate absorbance easily from percentage transmittance data.

The relationship between absorbance and transmittance is illustrated by the following scale:

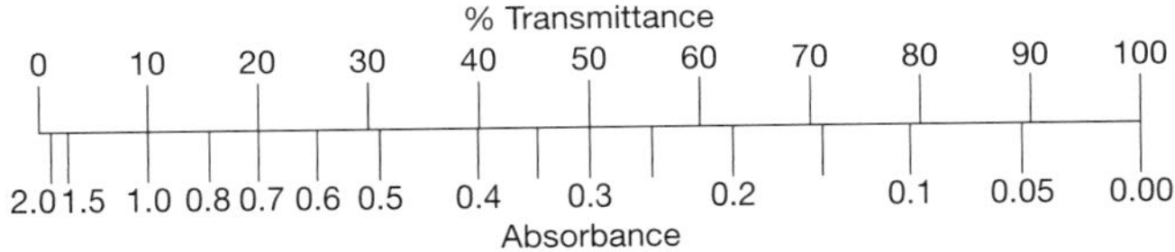

Therefore if all the light passes through a solution *without* any absorption, absorbance is zero, and percent transmittance is 100%. If all the light is absorbed, % transmittance is zero, and absorption is infinite.

Beer-Lambert (Beer's) Law

It is important to describe the Beer-Lambert law, or Beer's law, and explore its significance, because people who use this law often do not understand it, even though the equation representing the law is so straightforward, as follows:

$$A = \varepsilon bc$$

where:

A is absorbance (no units, because $A = \log_{10} P_0/P$).

ε is the molar absorptivity with units of L mol^{-1} cm^{-1}.

b is the path length of the sample; that is, the path length of the cuvette in which the sample is contained (we express this measurement in centimeters).

c is the concentration of the compound in solution, expressed in mol L^{-1}.

We prefer to express the law with this equation because absorbance is directly proportional to the other parameters, as long as the Beer's law is obeyed.

Absorbance and Transmittance of Light

Many solutions contain particles that absorb certain wavelengths and transmit others. Solutions appear to the human eye to have characteristic colors. The wavelength of light transmitted by the solution is recognized as color by the eye. A blue solution appears blue because particles in the solution absorb all the wavelengths except blue; the blue is the color transmitted and seen. A red solution appears red because all other wavelengths except red have been absorbed by the solution; the red wavelength passes through the solution.

Measurement by spectrophotometry is based on the reaction between the substance to be measured and a reagent, or chemical, used to produce color. The amount of color produced in a reaction between the substance to be measured and the reagent depends on the concentration of the substance. Therefore the intensity of the color is proportional to the concentration of the substance.

Beer's law states that the concentration of a substance is directly proportional to the amount of light absorbed or inversely proportional to the logarithm of the transmitted light. (*Percent transmittance* and *absorbance* are related photometric terms; see following discussion.) Beer's law is the basis for the use of photometry in quantitative measurement. If one saw a solution with a very intense red color, one would be correct in assuming that the solution had a high concentration of the substance that made it red. Another way of stating Beer's law is that any increase in the concentration of a color-producing substance will increase the amount of color seen.

As the Beer-Lambert law states, the depth at which the color is determined must be constant. The depth of the solution is regulated by the cuvette or container used to hold it. Increasing the depth of the solution through which the light must pass (by using a cuvette with a larger diameter) is the same as placing more particles between the light and the eye, thereby creating an apparent increase in the concentration, or intensity, of color.

Visible light is composed of wavelengths from 400 to 700 nm. When visible light passes through a colored solution, some wavelengths are transmitted and others are absorbed. You see the color of the transmitted wavelengths. For example, a red color results when a solution absorbs short wavelengths (green and blue) and transmits longer wavelengths (red). An absorbance spectrum (a plot of absorbance as a function of wavelength) is determined to select the optimal wavelength for analyzing a given compound. The optimal wavelength (A_{max}) for measuring absorbance is the wavelength that is most absorbed by the compound in question. This provides maximum sensitivity for measurements.

Expressions of Light Transmitted or Absorbed

There are two common methods of expressing the amount of light transmitted or light absorbed by a solution. (Another term for absorbed light is *optical density,* which is not generally used.) The units used to express the readings obtained by the electronic measuring device are either absorbance (A) units or percent transmittance (%T) units. Most spectrophotometers give readings in both units. Absorbance units are sometimes more difficult to read directly from the reading scale because it is divided logarithmically rather than in equal divisions (Fig. 8.2).

Absorbance is an expression of the amount of light absorbed by a solution. Absorbance values are directly proportional to the concentration of the solution and can be plotted on linear graph paper to give a straight line (Fig. 8.3A). Percent transmittance is the amount of light that passes through a colored solution compared with the amount of light that passes through a blank or standard solution. The blank solution contains all the reagents used in the procedure, but it does not contain the unknown substance being measured.

Percent transmittance varies from 0 to 100, with equal divisions on the viewing scale. As the concentration of the colored solution increases, the amount of light absorbed increases, and the percentage of light transmitted decreases. Transmitted light does not decrease in direct proportion to the concentration or color intensity of the solution being measured. Percent transmittance readings plotted against concentration will not give a straight line on linear graph paper (see Fig. 8.3B). A logarithmic relationship exists between percent transmittance and concentration, so when percent transmittance is plotted against concentration, semilogarithmic graph paper is used to obtain a straight line (see Fig. 8.3). Absorbance and percent transmittance are related in the following way:

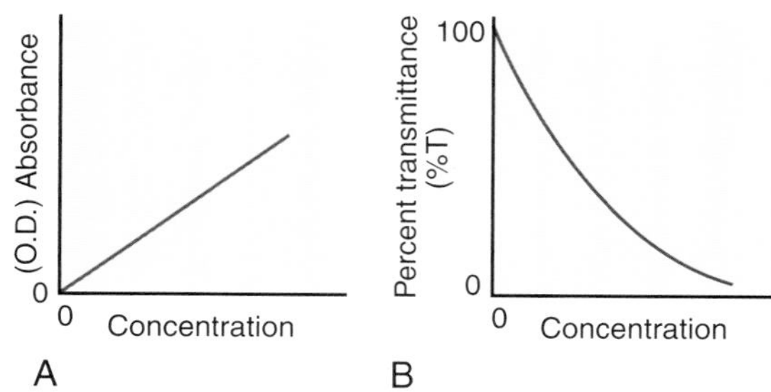

Fig. 8.3 Relationships of (A) absorbance and (B) percent transmittance to concentration when plotted using linear graph paper. (From Kaplan LA, Pesce AJ: *Clinical chemistry: theory, analysis, correlation,* ed 5, St Louis, 2010, Elsevier/Mosby.)

Absorbance = 2 minus the logarithm of the percent transmittance

or:

$$A = 2 - \log\%T$$

Therefore 2 is the logarithm of 100%T. A convenient conversion table for transmittance and absorbance is available in a standard chemistry reference book.

Preparation and Use of a Standard Curve

For our purposes, standard curves are defined as a graph with absorption (A) or %T plotted on the *y*-axis (vertical axis), and increasing concentrations of standard along the *x*-axis (horizontal axis). If Beer's law is followed, the resulting line representing absorbance versus concentration will be straight.

A standard curve is constructed after obtaining the %T/A readings from a number of solutions of known concentration (standards) used in a reaction or procedure. After the readings are obtained, each is plotted on semilogarithmic (%T) or linear (A) paper against the corresponding concentration. If the procedure follows Beer's law, the points plotted will generally lie such that a straight line can be drawn through them. The concentrations of controls and other unknowns (patient samples) can be determined by locating their %T/A readings on the line, then dropping down an imaginary line from that point to intersect the concentration axis.

Once a standard curve is developed for a particular test method on a particular spectrophotometer, it should be checked

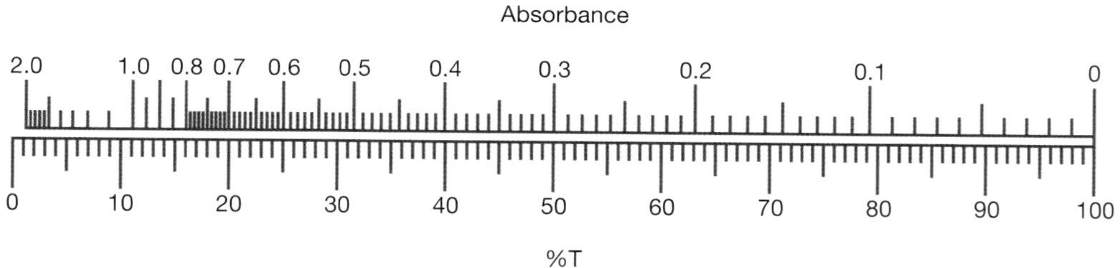

Fig. 8.2 Viewing scales showing divisions for reading percent transmittance versus absorbance. Absorbance is the measure of light stopped or absorbed. Percent transmittance is the measure of light transmitted through the solution. (From Campbell JB, Campbell JM: *Laboratory mathematics: medical and biological applications,* ed 5, St Louis, 1997, Mosby.)

periodically to determine that it is still good. A new curve should be constructed when there is a change in the following:

- Reagent lot numbers
- Methodology/procedure
- An instrument parameter (such as when a bulb is changed or the optics are cleaned)

Once the curve is drawn, a number of factors must be considered to determine its acceptability. The majority of the curve's points should be on or close to the line. Many reasons could explain why a point is not on the line. If the standards are formed from a series of dilutions, the accuracy of the dilutions must be suspect. Calculations of the dilutions and spectrophotometer errors are other possibilities. Whether the curve passes through the point of origin (the "0") varies with the procedure. If the Beer-Lambert law is followed and the procedure is linear at the lower concentrations, the curve's line generally goes through the zero.

Many laboratory tests require that the outcome of a carefully controlled chemical reaction be evaluated or read in a photometer (colorimeter or spectrophotometer). Because these instruments are capable only of measuring the amount of light allowed to pass through the cuvette, their readout devices display the percentage of light transmitted or the mathematically derived absorbance. One method of obtaining concentration from %T or absorbance is through the use of a standard curve.

In the current clinical laboratory, the preparation for the construction of a standard curve is not typically done manually. The steps formerly taken using graph paper to calculate the relationship between spectrophotometric readings for the standards and the unknowns have now been automated. However, sometimes in research laboratories or in the preparation of a new or special procedure, it may be necessary to prepare a standard curve manually. Moreover, to understand the concept of a standard curve and its function, one must also understand the principles behind constructing and using a standard curve (Student Procedure Worksheet 8.1).

Types of Graph Paper

Semilogarithmic (semilog) graph paper is used to plot %T readings from the photometer, because a logarithmic (log) relationship exists between percent and concentration, as previously described. The horizontal axis (x-axis) of semilog graph paper is a linear scale, and the vertical axis (y-axis) is a log scale (Fig. 8.4). Concentrations of the standard solutions are plotted on the horizontal axis. The transmittance or absorbance readings from the photometer are plotted along the vertical axis. When used, percent transmittance readings can be plotted directly on the log scale of the semilog graph paper (horizontal axis) because the concentration is proportional to the logarithm of the galvanometer reading. In this way, percent transmittance readings are converted to the appropriate numbers on the log scale. When percentages are plotted against concentrations on semilog graph paper, the proportional relationship is direct, and the necessary straight-line graph is obtained when the individual standard points are connected.

The criteria for a good standard curve are as follows:

- The line is straight.
- The line connects all points.
- The line goes through the origin, or intersect, of the two axes.

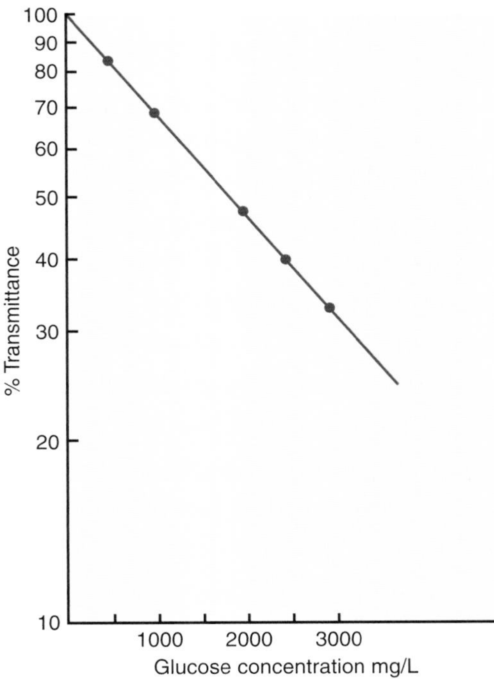

Fig. 8.4 Use of semilogarithmic graph paper showing percent transmittance plotted against concentration. (From Kaplan LA, Pesce AJ: *Clinical chemistry: theory, analysis, correlation,* ed 5, St Louis, 2010, Elsevier/Mosby.)

The origin of the graph paper is the point on the vertical and horizontal axes where there is 100%T and "0" concentration.

Linear graph paper can also be used to plot absorbance readings because absorbance of wavelengths of light is directly proportional to the concentration of the colored solution being read. This graph paper has linear scales on both the horizontal and the vertical axis. If linear graph paper is used to construct a standard curve, and only percent transmittance readings are available, these readings must first be converted to log values and the log values plotted on the vertical axis. Absorbance units can be plotted directly against the concentration on the linear graph paper to obtain a straight-line graph (Beer's law is followed). To eliminate the conversion of percent transmittance to absorbance when obtaining the necessary straight-line graph, the use of semilog graph paper is recommended.

Plotting a Standard Curve

When points are plotted on graph paper, whether they represent concentrations or galvanometer readings, care must be taken to note the intervals on the graph paper. Many errors result from carelessness in the initial plotting of points on the graph paper. Also, when a standard curve is prepared, the axes must be properly labeled, along with other information pertaining to the graph.

Sources of Error

The following is an abbreviated list of errors or problems encountered by students in the past. It is provided so you can be aware of pitfalls to avoid. Keep this list handy when preparing chemistry laboratory curves.

a. Bottom of y-axis did not start at 0.000.
b. Compressed y-axis or x-axis.

c. Uneven spacing of *y*-axis or *x*-axis.
d. Not labeling correctly/in the right place.
e. Drawing curve point-to-point.
f. Required information is missing/in the wrong place.
g. "Fat" pencil lines or double/smeared lines.
h. Making dots on curve's line for unknown's absorbance value.
i. Drawing dotted lines on graph representing how the concentration of unknown was determined.
j. Drawing circles around dots on the curve line.

Using a Standard Curve

Once the standard curve has been plotted, it is used to calculate the concentrations of any unknowns that were included in the same batch as the standards used to make the graph. Determining the concentration of a solution requires some way of comparing it with a solution of known concentration.

Fig. 8.5 shows a simplified example of the construction and use of a standard curve. In this example, three standard solutions are prepared with the following concentrations: standard 1 (S_1), 0.02 mg; standard 2 (S_2), 0.04 mg; and standard 3 (S_3), 0.06 mg. These concentrations are plotted on the linear (horizontal) scale of the semilogarithmic graph paper.

The three standard tubes are read in a photometer, giving the following readings in percent transmittance: $S_1 = 76\%T$, $S_2 = 58\%T$, and $S_3 = 45\%T$. The percent transmittance readings are plotted under their respective concentrations on the logarithmic (vertical) scale of the paper. The points are connected using a ruler. An undetermined substance gives a reading of 63%T. Using the graph in Fig. 8.5, the 63%T point on the vertical scale is found, followed horizontally to the graph line just drawn, and then followed vertically to the concentration scale. The degree of accuracy with which an unknown concentration can be read depends on the concentrations of the standards used. The accuracy of the unknown can be no greater than that of the standard solutions used. Standard solutions are usually weighed to the fourth decimal place. In this example, if the graph lines were present, the unknown concentration would be read as 0.0343 mg (the figure in the fourth decimal place is approximate).

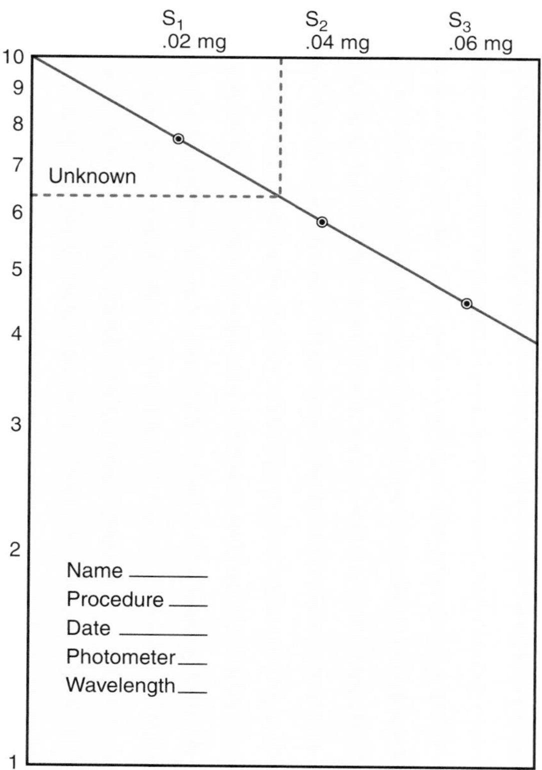

Fig. 8.5 Construction of a standard curve.

Rather than relying on a permanently established calibration curve, using standard solutions to standardize the analyses of each batch allows the clinical laboratory to produce more reliable results. It compensates for variables such as time, temperature, age of reagents, and condition of instruments. It is always best to use several different concentrations of the standard solution, not just one. To obtain reliable photometric information about the concentration of a substance, standard solutions must be used as the basis for comparison.

Instruments Used in Spectrophotometry

The instrument used to show the quantitative relationship between the colors of the undetermined solution and those of the standard solution is called a *spectrophotometer* or *colorimeter.* A spectrophotometer is used to measure the light transmitted by a solution to determine the concentration of the light-absorbing substance in the solution.

Most of the instruments used in photometry have some means of isolating a narrow wavelength, or range, of the color spectrum for measurements. Instruments using filters for this purpose are referred to as *filter photometers,* and those using prisms or diffraction gratings are called *spectrophotometers* or *photoelectric colorimeters.* Both types are used frequently in the clinical laboratory. Older colorimetric procedures used visual comparison of the color of an unknown with that of a standard. In general, visual colorimetry has been replaced by more specific and accurate photoelectric methods.

One current application of visual colorimetry employs various dry-reagent strip tests prevalent in many clinical chemistry tests (such as urinalysis). These strips can be read visually, although instruments are available that can read the developed color electronically.

Many types of spectrophotometers are in common use in the clinical laboratory (Fig. 8.6). The principle of most of these instruments is the same: The amount of light transmitted by the standard solution is compared with the amount of light transmitted by the solution of unknown concentration.

Photometers utilize an electronic device to compare the actual color intensities of the solutions measured. As the name implies, a spectrophotometer is really two instruments in a single case: a spectrometer, a device for producing light of a specific wavelength, the monochromator; and a photometer, a device for measuring light intensity. In the automated analyzing instruments used in many laboratories, a photometer is still a necessary component so that absorbance values for unknown and standard solutions can be determined. Some instruments contain a filter wheel that allows measurement of absorbance at any wavelength for which there is a filter on the wheel. Microprocessors control the location of the correct filter for the

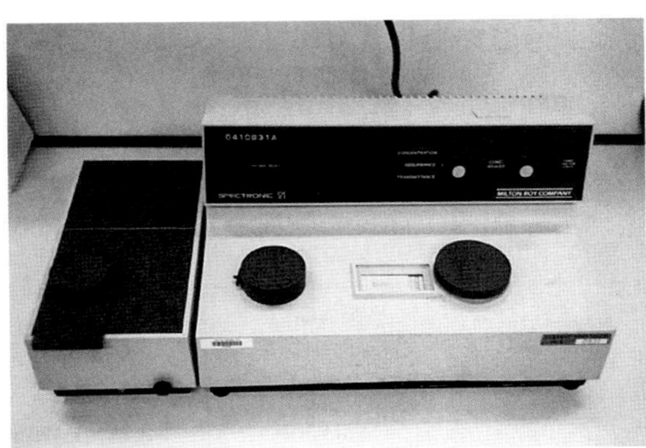

Fig. 8.6 Spectrophotometer. (From Rodak BF, Fritsma GA, Doig K: *Hematology: clinical principles and applications*, ed 3, St Louis, 2007, Elsevier/Saunders.)

particular analyte being measured. From the absorbance information, the computer microprocessor calculates the unknown concentration.

Parts Essential to All Spectrophotometers

The parts necessary to all spectrophotometers are a light source, a means to isolate light of a desired wavelength, fiber optics, cuvettes, a photodetector, a readout device, a recorder, and a microprocessor (Fig. 8.7).

Light Source

Each spectrophotometer must have a light source. This can be a light bulb constructed to give the optimum amount of light. The light source must be steady and constant; therefore use of a voltage regulator or an electronic power supply is recommended. The light source may be movable or stationary. The most common source of light for work in the visible or near-infrared region is the incandescent tungsten or tungsten-iodide lamp. Most emitted radiant energy is near-infrared. Often, a heat-absorbing filter is inserted between the lamp and sample to absorb the infrared radiation. The most common lamps for UV work are deuterium-discharge and mercury arc lamps.

Wavelength Isolator

Before the light from the light source reaches the sample of solution to be measured, the interfering wavelengths must be removed. A system of isolating a desired wavelength and excluding others is called a *monochromator;* the light is actually being reduced to a particular wavelength. Filters can be used to accomplish this. Some are very simple, composed of one or two pieces of colored glass. The more complicated filters are found in the better spectrophotometers. The filter must transmit a color the solution can absorb. A red filter transmits red, and a green filter transmits green. Filters are available to cover almost any point in the visible spectrum, and each filter has inscribed on it a number that indicates the wavelength of light that it transmits. For example, a filter inscribed with "540 nm" absorbs all light except that of wavelengths around 540 nm. Because the filter must transmit a color that the solution can absorb, for a red solution, the filter chosen should *not* be red (all colors except red are absorbed). The wavelength of light transmitted is therefore the important factor to consider in choosing the correct filter for a procedure.

Other means exist to provide light at the desired wavelength. One common instrument employs a diffraction grating with a special plate and slit to reduce the spectrum to the desired wavelength. The grating consists of a highly polished surface with numerous lines that break up white light into the spectrum. By moving the spectrum behind a slit (the light source must be movable), only one particular portion of the spectrum is allowed to pass through the narrow slit. The particular band of light, or wavelength, transmitted through the slit is indicated on a viewing scale on the machine. Certain wavelengths are more desirable than others for a particular color and procedure. The wavelength chosen is determined by running an absorption curve and selecting the correct wavelength after inspecting the curve obtained. Only when new methods are being developed is it necessary to run an absorption curve.

Cuvettes (Absorption Cells or Photometer Tubes)

Any light (of the wavelength selected) coming from the filter or diffraction grating will pass on to the solution in the cuvette. Glass cuvettes are relatively inexpensive and satisfactory, provided they are matched or calibrated. Calibrated cuvettes are tubes that have been optically matched so that the same solution in each will give the same reading on the photometer. In using calibrated cuvettes, the depth factor of Beer's law is kept constant. Depending on the concentration and thus the color of the solution, a certain amount of light will be absorbed by the solution. The light not absorbed by the solution is transmitted and passed on to an electronic measuring device. Alternatively, to eliminate the cuvette entirely, a flow-through apparatus can be used.

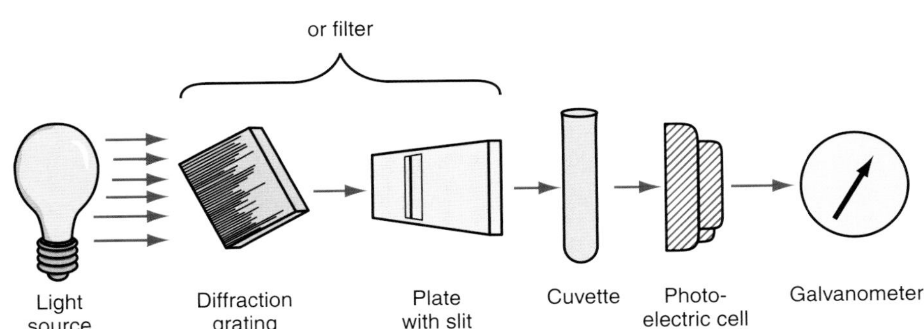

Fig. 8.7 Parts essential to all spectrophotometers.

Electronic Measuring Device

In the more common spectrophotometers, the electronic measuring device consists of a photoelectric cell and a galvanometer. The amount of light transmitted by the solution in the cuvette is measured by a photoelectric cell, a sensitive instrument producing electrons in proportion to the amount of light hitting it. The electrons are passed on to a galvanometer, where they are measured. The galvanometer records the amount of current (in the form of electrons) it receives from the photoelectric cell on a special viewing scale on the spectrophotometer. Results are reported in terms of percent transmittance (or in some cases, absorbance). The percent transmittance depends on the concentration of the solution and its depth. If the solution is very concentrated (the color appearing intense), less light will be transmitted than if it is dilute (pale). Therefore the reading on the galvanometer viewing scale will be lower for a more concentrated solution than for a dilute solution. This is the basis for the comparison of color intensity with the spectrophotometer.

Calibration of Cuvettes

If cuvettes are used, it is essential for their diameters to be uniform; that is, the depth of the cuvettes or tubes used in the spectrophotometer must be constant for Beer's law to apply. Precalibrated cuvettes must be checked before actual use in the laboratory. Calibrated cuvettes are optically matched so that the same solution in each will give the same percent transmittance reading on the galvanometer viewing scale.

For use in spectrophotometry, the cuvette is carefully checked to ensure that the solution in it gives the same reading as that in other calibrated cuvettes. To check cuvettes for uniformity, the same solution is read in many cuvettes. Readings are taken, and cuvettes that match within an established tolerance are used.

If new plain glass tubes are being calibrated for use as cuvettes, the tubes are rotated in the cuvette well to observe any variations in the reading seen with change of position in the well, because all tubes may not be perfectly round. The cuvette is etched at the point where the reading corresponds with the established tolerance for the absorption reading. Cuvettes that do not agree or do not correspond are not used for spectrophotometry. Different sizes of cuvettes can be used, depending on the spectrophotometer.

Care and Handling of Spectrophotometers

When a spectrophotometer is used, error caused by color in the reagents must be eliminated. Because color is so important, and because the color produced by the undetermined substance is the desired color, any color resulting from the reagents themselves or from interactions between the reagents could cause confusion and error. By using a blank solution, a correction can be made for any color resulting from the reagents used. The blank solution contains the same reagents as the unknown and standard tubes, with the exception of the substance being measured.

As with any expensive, delicate instrument, a spectrophotometer must be handled with care. The manufacturer supplies a manual of complete instructions on the care and use of a particular machine. Care should be taken not to spill reagents on the spectrophotometer. Spillage could damage the instrument, especially the photoelectric cell. Any reagents spilled must be wiped up immediately. Spectrophotometers with filters should not be operated without the filter in place; the unfiltered light from the light source may damage the photoelectric cell and the galvanometer. A spectrophotometer should be placed on a table with good support, where it will not be bumped or jarred (Student Procedure Worksheet 8.2).

Quality Control Tests for Spectrophotometers

Quality control testing for spectrophotometry consists of checking the following:

- Wavelength accuracy
- Stray light
- Linearity

Wavelength accuracy is ensured when the wavelength indicated on the control dial is the actual wavelength of light passed by the monochromator. This is checked with standard absorbing solution or with filters with maximum absorbance of known wavelength. Wavelength calibration can be tested by using a rare-earth glass filter (such as didymium) or a stable chromogen solution. Calibration at two wavelengths is necessary for instruments with diffraction gratings and at three wavelengths for instruments with prisms. Photoelectric accuracy can be checked by reading standard solutions of potassium dichromate or potassium nitrate. As an alternative, the National Bureau of Standards, now the National Institute of Standards and Technology, has sets of three neutral-density glass filters that have known absorbance at four wavelengths for each filter. These filters are not completely stable, however, and require periodic recalibration.

Stray light refers to any wavelengths outside the band transmitted by the monochromator. The most common causes of stray light are (1) reflections of light from scratches on optical surfaces or from dust particles anywhere in the light path and (2) higher-order spectra produced by diffraction gratings. Stray light is detected by using cutoff filters.

Linearity is demonstrated when a change in concentration results in a straight-line calibration curve, as discussed under Beer's law. Neutral-density filters to check linearity over a range of wavelengths are commercially available, as are sealed sets of various colors and concentrations.

REFLECTANCE SPECTROPHOTOMETRY

Reflectance spectrophotometry is another quantitative spectrophotometric technique; the light reflected from the surface of a colorimetric reaction is used to measure the amount of unknown colored product generated in the reaction. A beam of light is directed at a flat surface, and the amount of light reflected is measured in a reflectance spectrophotometer. A photodetector measures the amount of reflected light directed to it. This technology has been employed in automated instrumentation, including many of the handheld instruments for bedside testing and some of the smaller instruments used in physician offices and clinics.

Principle and Quality Control

Different surfaces have different optical properties. The optical properties of plastic strips or test paper are different from those of dry film. The use of a reflectance spectrophotometer requires the employment of a standard with the same specific surface optical properties as those of the surface used in the test system. The use of reflectance spectrophotometry provides the quantitative measurement of reactions on surfaces such as strips, cartridges, and dry film.

The amount of light reflected and then measured depends on the specific instrumentation employed. Variables include the angles at which the reflected light is measured and the area of the surface used for the measurement. Because this technology depends on products manufactured for use in the specific instrumentation, manufacturing processes (quality control considerations), and shipping and handling or storage problems can affect the resulting measurements.

Quality control for single-test instruments (using instrument-based systems) has been integrated into the device by the manufacturer. As long as the reagent packs or tabs have been properly stored and are used within the stated outdate, the manufacturer assures the user that calibration of the instrument will function automatically, that crucial quality control information has been encoded via the bar code on the unit packs, and that real-time processing is monitored. Use of the laboratory's usual quality control measures can be problematic for this technology because when single-test instrument-based systems are used, a new test system is created each time a new cartridge, pack, or strip is inserted into the instrument.

Parts of a Reflectance Spectrophotometer

The instrumentation necessary for a reflectance spectrophotometer is similar to that of a filter photometer, in which the filter serves to direct the selected wavelength for the methodology. A lamp generates light, which passes first through the filter and then a series of slits and is focused on the test surface (Fig. 8.8).

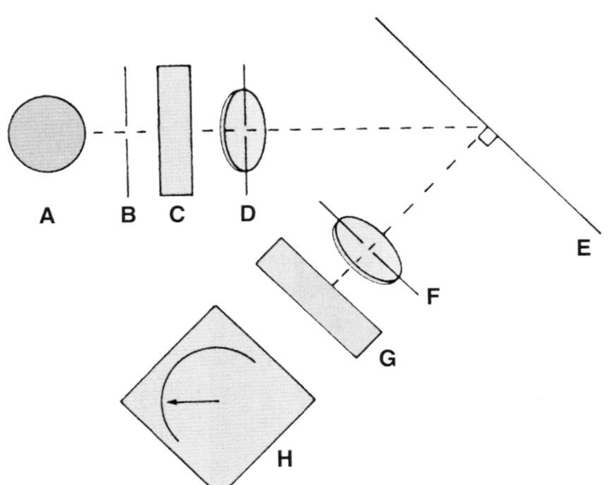

Fig. 8.8 Diagram of reflectance spectrophotometer. (A) Light source; (B) slit; (C) filter or wavelength selector; (D) lens or slit; (E) test surface; (F) lens or slit; (G) detector/photodetector device; (H) readout device. (From Kaplan LA, Pesce AJ: *Clinical chemistry: theory, analysis, correlation,* ed 5, St Louis, 2010, Elsevier/Mosby.)

As with a filter photometer, some light is absorbed by the filter; in the reflectance spectrophotometer, the remaining light is reflected. The light reflected is analogous to the light transmitted by the filter spectrophotometer. The reflected light then passes through a series of slits and lenses and on to the photodetector device, where the amount of light is measured and recorded as a signal. The signal is then converted to an appropriate readout.

Applications of Reflectance Spectrophotometry

Reflectance spectrophotometry can be used at the bedside or in handheld POCT devices; it is also used for home testing. Common POCT and self-testing instruments include those for quantitation of blood glucose (employing single-test methodology) in maintaining good diabetic control. The chemistry laboratory and therapeutic drug-monitoring analyzer systems also employ this technology (such as Vitros). In urinalysis testing, various instruments use dry-reagent reflectance spectrophotometry.

Fluorescence Spectrophotometry

On receiving UV radiation, the electrons of certain fluorescent substances absorb the radiation and become excited. After about 7 to 10 seconds, when the electron has returned to its ground state, this energy is released as a photon of light. When a molecule then absorbs this photon of radiant energy, the molecule has an increased level of energy, which it seeks to release because the energy of the molecule is now greater than that of its environment. When this excess energy is ejected as a photon, the result is fluorescence emission. Generally, this emitted light is in the visible part of the spectrum.

The intensity of the fluorescence is determined using a fluorometer, sometimes called a *spectrofluorometer* or *fluorescence spectrophotometer.* This measurement is governed by the same factors that affect the absorption of light (i.e., light path through the solution, concentration of the solution, wavelength of light being used) and also by the intensity of the UV exciting the substance. Only a few compounds can fluoresce, and in those that do, not all photons absorbed will be converted to fluorescent light. The list of fluorochromes is constantly changing, but common fluorochromes are fluorescein isothiocyanate (FITC, green) and phycoerythrin (PE, red).

NEPHELOMETRY

Light can be absorbed, reflected, scattered, or transmitted when it strikes a particle in a liquid. Nephelometry is the measurement of light that has been scattered. **Turbidimetry** is the measurement of loss of intensity of light transmitted through a solution as a result of the light's scattering (the solution becomes turbid). Turbidimetry will measure only light that is scattered, not absorbed or reflected by the particles in the suspension. Nephelometers are used to detect the amount of light scattered.

Nephelometry has become increasingly popular in diagnostic laboratories and depends on the light-scattering properties of antigen-antibody complexes (Fig. 8.9). The quantity of cloudiness or turbidity in a solution can be measured photometrically. When specific antigen-coated latex particles acting as reaction intensifiers are agglutinated by their corresponding antibody,

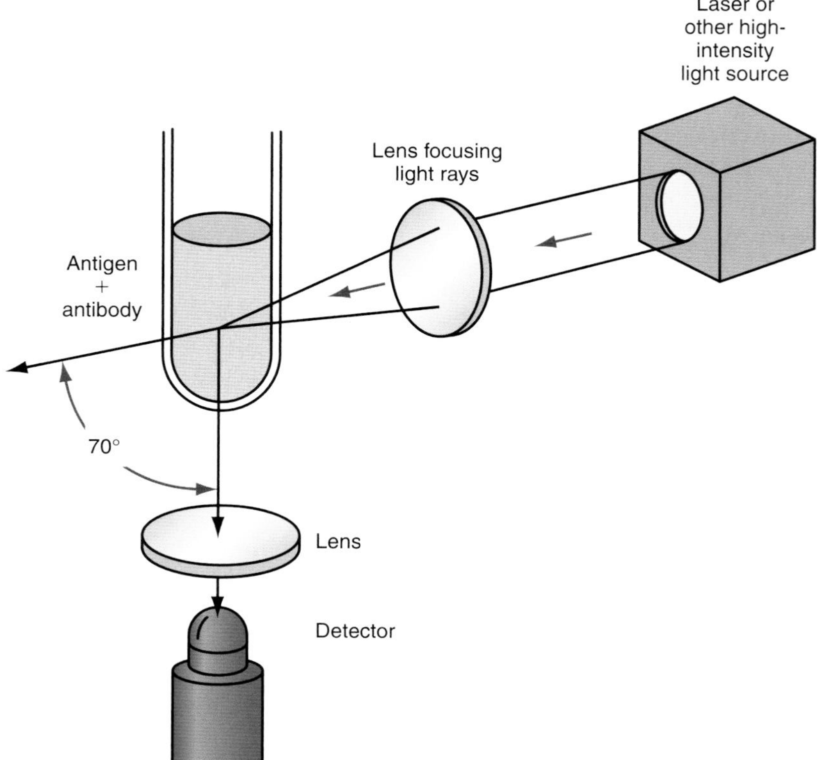

Fig. 8.9 Principle of nephelometry for the measurement of antigen-antibody reactions. Light rays are collected in a focusing lens and ultimately can be related to the antigen or antibody concentration in a sample. (From Turgeon ML: *Immunology and serology in laboratory medicine,* ed 5, St Louis, 2014, Elsevier/Mosby.)

the increased light scatter of a solution can be measured by nephelometry as the macromolecular complexes form. The use of polyethylene glycol enhances and stabilizes the precipitates, thus increasing the speed and sensitivity of the technique by controlling the particle size for optimal light angle deflection. The kinetics of this change can be determined when the photometric results are analyzed by computer.

Principles of Use

Formation of a macromolecular complex is a fundamental prerequisite for nephelometric protein quantitation. The procedure is based on the reaction between the protein being assayed and a specific antiserum. Protein in a patient specimen reacts with specific nephelometric antisera to human proteins and forms insoluble complexes. When light is passed through such a suspension, the resulting complexes of insoluble precipitants scatter incident light in solutions. The scattered light can be detected with a photodiode. The amount of scattered light is proportional to the number of insoluble complexes and can be quantitated by comparing the unknown patient values with standards of known protein concentration.

The relationship between the quantity of antigen and the measuring signal at a constant antibody concentration is given by the Heidelberger curve. If antibodies are present in excess, a proportional relationship exists between the antigen and the resulting signal. If the antigen overwhelms the quantity of antibody, the measured signal decreases.

By optimizing the reaction conditions, the typical antigen-antibody reactions as characterized by the Heidelberger curve are effectively shifted in the direction of high concentration. This ensures that these high concentrations will be measured on the ascending portion of the curve. At concentrations higher than the reference curve, the instrument will transmit an out-of-range warning.

Optical System and Measurement

In the nephelometric method, an infrared high-performance light-emitting diode is used as the light source. Because an entire solid angle is measured after convergence of this light through a lens system, an intense measuring signal is available when the primary beam is blocked off. In connection with the lens system, this produces a light beam of high collinearity with a wavelength of 840 nm. Light scattered in the forward direction in a solid angle to the primary beam ranges between 13 and 24 feet and is measured by a silicon photodiode with an integrated amplifier. The electrical signals generated are digitized, compared with reference curves, and converted into protein concentrations.

A fixed-time method of measurement is used routinely for precipitation reactions. Ten seconds after all reaction components have been mixed, an initial blank measurement with a cuvette is taken. Six minutes later a second measurement is taken, and after subtraction of the original 1-second blanking value, a final answer is calculated against the multiple-point or single-point calibration in the computerized program memory for the assay.

Advantages and Disadvantages

Nephelometry represents an automated system that is rapid, reproducible, relatively simple to operate, and very common in higher-volume laboratories. It has many applications in the immunology laboratory. Currently, instruments using a rate method and fixed-time approach are commercially available, with tests including C-reactive protein and rheumatoid factor.

Disadvantages include the high initial equipment cost. As for technical issues, interfering substances such as microbial contamination may cause protein denaturation and erroneous test results. Another potential complicating factor is that intrinsic specimen turbidity or lipemia may exceed the preset limits. In these cases, a clearing agent may be needed before an accurate assay can be performed.

FLOW (CELL) CYTOMETRY

Fundamentals of Laser Technology

In 1917 Einstein speculated that under certain conditions, atoms or molecules could absorb light or other radiation and then be stimulated to shed this gained energy. Since then, lasers have been developed with numerous medical and industrial applications.

The electromagnetic spectrum ranges from long radio waves to short, powerful gamma rays. Within this spectrum is a narrow band of visible or white light, composed of red, orange, yellow, green, blue, and violet light. Laser (*l*ight *a*mplification by *s*timulated *e*mission of *r*adiation) light ranges from the UV and infrared spectrum through all the colors of the rainbow. In contrast to other forms of radiation, laser light is concentrated. It is almost exclusively of one wavelength or color, and its parallel waves travel in one direction. Through the use of fluorescent dyes (such as FITC, green), laser light can occur in numerous wavelengths. Types of lasers include glass-filled tubes of helium and neon (most common); yttrium-aluminum-garnet (an imitation diamond), argon, and krypton.

Lasers sort the energy in atoms and molecules, concentrate it, and release it in powerful waves. In most lasers, a medium of gas, liquid, or crystal is energized by high-intensity light, an electrical discharge, or even nuclear radiation. When an atom extends beyond the orbits of its electrons, or when a molecule vibrates or changes its shape, it instantly snaps back, shedding energy in the form of a photon. The photon is the basic unit of all radiation. When a photon reaches an atom of the medium, the energy exchange stimulates the emission of another photon in the same wavelength and direction. This process continues until a cascade of growing energy sweeps through the medium.

Photons travel the length of the laser and bounce off mirrors. First a few and eventually countless photons synchronize themselves until an avalanche of light streaks between the mirrors. In some gas lasers, transparent disks (Brewster windows) are slanted at a precise angle that polarizes the laser's light. The photons, which are reflected back and forth, finally gain so much energy that they exit as a powerful beam. The power of lasers to pass on energy and information is rated in watts.

Principles of Flow Cytometry

Flow cytometry is based on staining cells in suspension with an appropriate fluorochrome, which may be an immunologic reagent, a dye that stains a specific component, or some other marker with specified reactivity. Fluorescent dyes used in flow cytometry must bind or react specifically with the cellular component of interest, such as reticulocytes, peroxidase enzyme, or deoxyribonucleic acid (DNA) content. Fluorescent dyes include acridine orange and PE.

Laser light is the most common light source used in flow cytometers because of its properties of intensity, stability, and monochromaticity. Argon is preferred for FITC labeling. Krypton is often used as a second laser in dual-analysis systems and serves as a better light source for compounds labeled by tetramethylrhodamine isothiocyanate and tetramethylcyclopropylrhodamine isothiocyanate.

The stained cells then pass through the laser beam in single file. The laser activates the dye, and the cell fluoresces. Although the fluorescence is emitted throughout a 360-degree circle, it is usually collected by optical sensors located 90 degrees relative to the laser beam. The fluorescence information is then transmitted to a computer. Flow cytometry performs fluorescence analysis on single cells at the general rate of 500 to 5000 cells per second.

Fig. 8.10 illustrates the parts of the laser flow cytometer. The computer is the heart of the instrument; it controls all decisions regarding data collection, analysis, and cell sorting. The major application of this technology is sorting the main cellular population into subpopulations, such as T lymphocytes and B lymphocytes, for further analysis.

IMMUNOASSAYS

Immunoassays utilize antigen-antibody reactions. When foreign material (called *antigens* or *immunogens*) is introduced into the body, protein molecules (called *antibodies*) are formed in response. For example, certain bacteria, when introduced into the body, elicit the production of specific antibodies. These antibodies combine specifically with the substance that stimulated the body to produce them initially, producing an antigen-antibody complex.

Antigens and antibodies are used as very specific reagents. In the laboratory, an antigen may be used as a reagent to detect the presence of antibodies in the serum of a patient. If the antibody is present, it shows that the person's body has responded previously to that specific antigen. This response can be elicited by exposure to a specific microorganism or by the presence of a drug or medication in the patient's serum. Antibodies are used to detect and measure an antigen (such as a drug or medication) present in the patient's serum.

Immunoassays can be divided into heterogeneous and homogeneous immunoassays.

- Heterogeneous immunoassays involve a solid phase (microwell, bead) and require washing steps to remove unbound antigens or antibodies. Heterogeneous immunoassays can have a competitive or noncompetitive format.
- Homogeneous immunoassays consist of only a liquid phase and do not require washing steps. Homogeneous

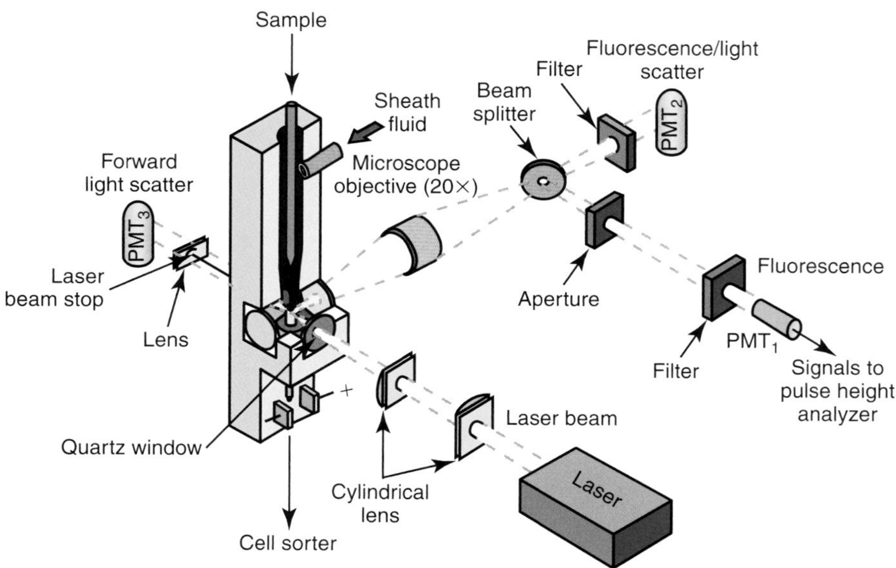

Fig. 8.10 Laser-flow cytometry. (Modified from Burtis CA, Ashwood ER, Bruns DB: *Tietz fundamentals of clinical chemistry,* ed 6, St Louis, 2008, Saunders.)

TABLE 8.2 Examples of Immunoassay Types

Type of Immunoassay	Antibody	Comments
Enzyme immunoassay	Enzyme-labeled antibody (such as horseradish peroxidase)	Competitive EIA Noncompetitive, such as direct EIA or indirect ELISA
Chemiluminescence	Chemiluminescent molecule–labeled antibody, such as isoluminol- or acridinium ester–labeled antibodies	
Electrochemiluminescence immunoassay	Electrochemiluminescent molecule–labeled antibody, such as ruthenium-labeled antibodies	
Fluoroimmunoassay	Fluorescent molecule–labeled antibody, such as europium-labeled antibodies or fluorescein-labeled antigens	Heterogeneous, such as time-resolved immunofluoroassay Homogeneous, such as fluorescence polarization immunoassay

EIA, Enzyme immunoassay; *ELISA,* enzyme-linked immunosorbent assay.

immunoassays are faster and easier to automate than heterogeneous immunoassays and have competitive formats.

The use of antigen-coated cells or particles in agglutination techniques may be considered the earliest method for labeling components in immunoassays. Applications of labels include enzyme immunoassays (EIAs), fluorescent substances, and chemiluminescence (Table 8.2).

Ideal characteristics of a label include the quality of being measurable by several methods, including visual inspection. The properties of a label used in an immunoassay determine the ways in which detection is possible. For example, coated latex particles can be detected by various methods: visual inspection, light scattering (nephelometry), and particle counting. The conversion of a colorless substrate into a colored product in EIA allows for two methods of detection: colorimetry and visual inspection.

Enzyme Immunoassay (EIA)

There are two general approaches to diagnosing diseases or conditions by immunoassay: testing for specific antigens or testing for antigen-specific antibodies. Some EIA procedures provide diagnostic information and measure antibodies to detect immune status (such as to detect either total antibody immunoglobulin [Ig]M or IgG). Enzyme-linked immunosorbent assay (ELISA), a type of EIA, is designed to detect antigens or antibodies by producing an enzyme-triggered color change.

The EIA method uses a nonisotopic label, compared to radioimmunoassay (RIA), which has the advantage of safety. EIA is usually an objective measurement that provides numeric results (Fig. 8.11). It uses the catalytic properties of enzymes to detect and quantitate immunologic reactions. An enzyme-labeled antibody or enzyme-labeled antigen conjugate is used in immunologic assays (Box 8.1). The enzyme with its substrate detects the presence and quantity of antigen or antibody in a patient specimen.

Various enzymes are used in EIA (see Table 8.2). Common enzyme labels include horseradish peroxidase, alkaline phosphatase, glucose-6-phosphate dehydrogenase, and beta-galactosidase. To be used in EIA, an enzyme must fulfill the following criteria:

- A high amount of stability
- Extreme specificity
- Absence from the antigen or antibody

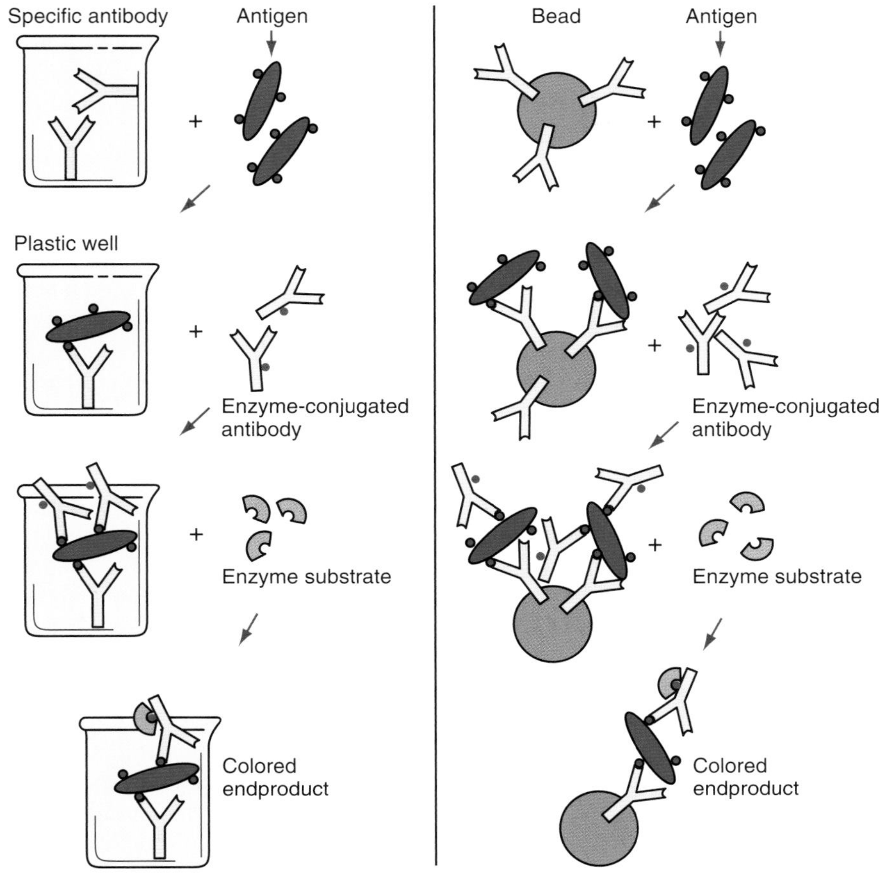

Fig. 8.11 Enzyme immunoassay. (From Forbes BA, Sahm DF, Weissfeld AS: *Bailey and Scott's diagnostic microbiology*, ed 12, St Louis, 2007, Mosby.)

- No alteration by inhibitor with the system

EIAs for Antigen Detection

When used for antigen detection (such as hepatitis B surface antigen), EIAs have four steps:

1. Antigen-specific antibody is attached to a solid-phase surface such as plastic beads.
2. Patient serum that may contain the antigen is added.
3. An enzyme-labeled antibody specific to the antigen (conjugate) is added next.
4. Chromogenic substrate is then added, which changes color in the presence of the enzyme. The amount of color that develops is proportional to the amount of antigen in the patient specimen.

BOX 8.1 Examples of Enzyme Immunoassays

Cytomegalovirus (IgG and IgM Ab)
Cytomegalovirus (Ag)
Hepatitis A (total Ab)
Hepatitis B (HB):
- Anti-HBs
- Anti-HBc
- Anti-HBe
- Anti-HBc (IgM)
- HBs Ag
- HBe Ag

Hepatitis delta virus (total Ab)
Hepatitis non-A, non-B
HIV Ab
HIV Ag
Rubella virus (IgG and IgM Ab)

Ab, Antibody; *Ag*, antigen; *HIV*, human immunodeficiency virus; *Ig*, immunoglobulin.

EIAs for Antibody Detection

Two major types of reaction formats are used in immunochemical assays:

- Competitive (limited reagent assays)
- Noncompetitive (excess reagent, two-site, and sandwich assays)

In a competitive assay, all reactants are added and mixed together either simultaneously or sequentially. In a simultaneous situation, the labeled antigen and unlabeled antigen compete to bind with antibody. In a *sequential* competitive reaction, unlabeled antigen is mixed with excess antibody, and binding is allowed to reach equilibrium. Labeled antigen is then added sequentially and allowed to equilibrate. After separation, the bound label is measured and used to calculate the unlabeled antigen concentration.

In noncompetitive assays, polyclonal or monoclonal antibodies are used. These assays are performed in either simultaneous or sequential modes. If a simultaneous mode is used, a high concentration of analyte saturates both the capture and the labeled antibodies. To avoid problems associated with high concentrations of antibody, such as chorionic gonadotropin, a sequential procedure is used. In a typical noncompetitive assay, the capture antibody initially is passively adsorbed or covalently bound to the surface of a solid phase. Then the antigen from the specimen is allowed to react and is captured by the solid-phase antibody. Other proteins then are washed away, and a labeled antibody (conjugate) is added that reacts with the bound antigen through a second and distinct antigen site, an epitope. After additional washings to remove the excess unbound labeled antibody, the bound label is measured, and its concentration or activity is directly proportional to the concentration of antigen.

Basic Immunofluorescence Labeling Techniques

Fluorescent labeling is another method of demonstrating the complexing of antigens and antibodies. Fluorescence techniques are extremely specific and sensitive. Antibodies may be conjugated to other markers in addition to fluorescent dyes; the use of these markers is called *colorimetric immunologic probe detection.* The use of enzyme-substrate marker systems has been expanded, and horseradish peroxidase can be used as a visual tag for the presence of antibody. These reagents have the advantage of requiring only a standard light microscope for analysis.

Fluorescent conjugates are used in the following basic methods:

1. Direct immunofluorescence assay
2. Inhibition immunofluorescence assay
3. Indirect immunofluorescence assay

Direct Immunofluorescence Assay

In the direct technique, a conjugated antibody is used to detect antigen-antibody reactions at a microscopic level (Fig. 8.12A). This technique can be applied to tissue sections or smears for microorganisms. Direct immunofluorescence assay can be used to detect nucleic acids in organisms such as cytomegalovirus (CMV), hepatitis B virus, Epstein-Barr virus, and *Chlamydia.*

When absorbing light of one wavelength, a fluorescent substance emits light of another (longer) wavelength. In fluorescent antibody microscopy (see Chapter 5), the incident or exciting light is often blue-green to UV. The light is provided by a high-pressure mercury arc lamp with a primary (such as blue-violet) filter between the lamp and the object that passes only fluorescein-exciting wavelengths. The color of the emitted light depends on the nature of the substance. Fluorescein gives off yellow-green light, and the rhodamines fluoresce in the red portion of the spectrum. The color observed in the fluorescence microscope depends on the secondary or barrier filter used in the eyepiece. A yellow filter absorbs the green fluorescence of fluorescein and transmits only yellow. Fluorescein fluoresces an intense apple-green color when excited.

Inhibition Immunofluorescence Assay

The inhibition immunofluorescence assay is a blocking test in which an antigen is first exposed to unlabeled antibody, then to labeled antibody, and finally is washed and examined. If the unlabeled and labeled antibodies are both homologous to the antigen, there should be no fluorescence. This result confirms the specificity of the fluorescent antibody technique. Antibody in an unknown serum can also be detected and identified by the inhibition test.

Indirect Immunofluorescence Assay

The indirect method is based on the fact that antibodies (immunoglobulins) not only react with homologous antigens, but also can act as antigens and react with antiimmunoglobulins (Fig. 8.12B). The serologic method most widely used for the detection of diverse antibodies is the indirect fluorescent antibody assay. Immunofluorescence is used extensively in the detection of autoantibodies and antibodies to tissue and cellular antigens. For example, antinuclear antibodies are frequently assayed by indirect fluorescence. By using tissue sections that contain a large number of antigens, it is possible to identify antibodies to several different antigens in a single test. The antigens are differentiated according to their various staining patterns.

Immunofluorescence can also be used to identify specific antigens on live cells in suspension (i.e., flow cytometry). When a live stained-cell suspension is put through a fluorescence-activated cell sorter, which measures fluorescence intensity, the cells are separated according to their particular fluorescent brightness. This technique permits isolation of various cell populations with different surface antigens (such as CD4+ and CD8+ lymphocytes).

In the indirect immunofluorescence assay, the antigen source (such as whole *Toxoplasma* microorganism or virus in infected tissue culture cells) to the specific antibody being tested is affixed to the surface of a microscope slide. The patient's serum is diluted and placed on the slide to cover the antigen source. If antibody is present in the serum, it will bind to its specific antigen. Unbound antibody is then removed by washing the slide. In the second phase of the procedure, antihuman globulin (directed specifically against IgM or IgG) conjugated to a fluorescent substance that will fluoresce when exposed to UV light is placed on the slide. This conjugated marker for human antibody

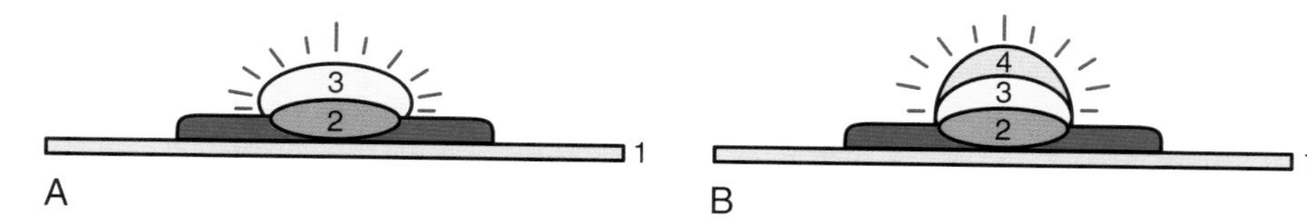

Fig. 8.12 Principles of direct and indirect fluorescence techniques. (A) Direct fluorescence. (B) Indirect fluorescence. *1,* Microscopic slide; *2,* cell (cytoplasm and nucleus); *3,* antiserum, conjugate in A and unconjugated in B; *4,* conjugated antiglobulin serum. (From Turgeon ML: *Immunology and serology in laboratory medicine,* ed 5, St Louis, 2014, Elsevier/Mosby.)

will bind to the antibody already bound to the antigen on the slide and serve as a marker for the antibody when viewed under a fluorescence microscope.

ALTERNATIVE LABELING TECHNOLOGIES

Time-Resolved Fluoroimmunoassay

Time-resolved assay means that the measurement of fluorescence should occur after a certain time frame to exclude background interference fluorescence. This form of immunoassay is heterogeneous with a direct format (sandwich assay) similar to that of direct ELISA.

Fluorescence Polarization Immunoassay

The fluorescence polarization immunoassay method is a homogeneous competitive fluoroimmunoassay. The polarization of the fluorescence from a fluorescein-antigen conjugate is determined by its rate of rotation during the lifetime of the excited state in solution.

Fluorescence In Situ Hybridization

Fluorescence in situ hybridization (FISH) uses fluorescent molecules to create brightly painted genes or chromosomes. FISH is a molecular cytogenetic technique that uses recombinant DNA technology. Probes, which are short sequences of single-strand DNA (ssDNA) that are complementary to the DNA sequences being examined, hybridize (bind) to the complementary DNA; because of the labeled fluorescent tags, the location of those sequences can be seen. Probes can be locus specific, centromeric repeat probes, or whole-chromosome probes. This protocol has potentially broad applications for clinical immunoassays and DNA hybridization analysis. FISH is both a labeling method and a molecular technique.

Signal Amplification Technology

Tyramide signal amplification (TSA) can be used in various fluorescence and colorimetric detection applications. TSA protocols are simple and require few changes to standard operating procedures. TSA provides a messenger RNA (mRNA) in situ hybridization protocol that is effective in detecting B cell clonality in plastic-embedded tissue specimens. Immunoglobulin light-chain mRNA molecules can be detected directly in paraffin-embedded tissue using fluorescein-labeled oligonucleotide probes. TSA amplification enables B cells to be detected in tissue sections without additional processing steps and specially prepared sections. Similar in situ hybridization technology can be used also for the detection of cytokines, such as interferon gamma (IFN-γ).

Magnetic Labeling Technology

Magnetic labeling technology is an application of the high-resolution magnetic recording technology developed for the computer disk drive industry. Increased density of microscopic, magnetically labeled biological samples (e.g., nucleic acid on a biochip) translates directly into reduced sample-processing times. Magnetic labeling can be applied to automated DNA sequences, DNA probe technology, and gel electrophoresis. Compared with other nonradioactive labeling systems, magnetic labels are inherently safe, instrumentation is less expensive, signals are almost permanent, and spatial resolution is increased.

In a magnetic label–based gel electrophoresis application sphere, DNA is analyzed. DNA is separated into bands using electrophoresis, and magnetic labels are bound to the DNA in each band. By applying and then removing a magnetic field, the magnetic domains in each label are oriented in the same direction, resulting in a net magnetic field near the bands in the direction of the applied field.

Radioimmunoassay

The infrequently used radioimmunoassay (RIA) method uses a radioactive label that can identify an immunocomponent at very low concentrations. In the 1960s researchers began to search for a substitute for the successful RIA method because of the inherent drawbacks of using radioactive isotopes as labels (such as radioactive waste and short shelf life). Today, chemiluminescent reactions have replaced most RIAs in the clinical laboratory. This relatively simple, cost-effective technology has sensitivity at least as good as that of RIA without the problems (such as disposal of radioactive waste).

CHEMILUMINESCENCE

Chemiluminescence is the emission of light by molecules in an excited state with a limited amount of emitted heat (luminescence) as the result of a chemical reaction.

Technical advances in methodologies, robotics, and computerization have led to expanded immunoassay automation. Newer systems are using chemiluminescent labels and substrates rather than older fluorescent labels and detection systems. Immunoassay systems have the potential to improve turnaround time with enhanced cost-effectiveness (Box 8.2).

Chemiluminescent assays are ultrasensitive and are widely used in automated immunoassays and DNA probe assay systems. Chemiluminescence has excellent sensitivity and dynamic range. It does not require sample radiation, and nonselective excitation and source instability are eliminated. Most chemiluminescent reagents and conjugates are stable and relatively nontoxic.

In immunoassays, chemiluminescent labels can be attached to an antigen or an antibody. Chemiluminescent labels are being used to detect proteins, viruses, oligonucleotides, and genomic nucleic acid sequences in immunoassays, DNA probe assays, DNA sequencing, and electrophoresis.

BOX 8.2 POTENTIAL BENEFITS OF IMMUNOASSAY AUTOMATION

- Ability to provide better service with less staff
- Savings on controls, duplicates, dilutions, and repeats
- Elimination of radioactive labels and associated regulations
- Better shelf life of reagents, with less disposal caused by outdating
- Better sample identification with bar-code labels and primary tube sampling
- Automation of sample delivery possible

Modified from Blick KE: Current trends in automation of immunoassays, *J Clin Ligand Assay* 22:6–12, 1999.

CHROMATOGRAPHY AND IMMUNOCHROMATOGRAPHY

The word *chromatography* comes from the Greek words *chromatos*, "color," and *graphein*, "to write." In chromatography, mixtures of solutes dissolved in a common solvent are separated from one another by a differential distribution of the solutes between two phases. The solvent, the first phase, is mobile and carries the mixture of solutes through the second phase. The second phase is a fixed or stationary phase. In variations in chromatographic techniques, the mobile phase ranges from liquids to gases and the stationary phase from sheets of cellulose paper to internally coated, fine capillary glass tubes. The varieties of chromatographic techniques as well as their applications to clinical assays have grown rapidly.

Types of Chromatographic Methods

The chromatographic method is used to separate the components of a given sample within a reasonable amount of time. The purpose of this separation technique is to detect or quantitate the particular component or group of components to be assayed in a pure form. By convention, the concentrations of solutes in a chromatographic system are plotted versus time or distance. The bands or zones of the various analytes separated in the technique are usually termed *peaks*.

Chromatographic methods are usually classified according to the physical state of the solute carrier phase. The two main categories of chromatography are gas chromatography, in which the solute phase is in a gaseous state, and liquid chromatography, in which the solute phase is a solution or liquid. The methods are further classified according to how the stationary-phase matrix is contained. For example, liquid chromatography is subdivided into flat and column methods. In flat chromatography, the stationary phase is supported on a flat sheet, such as cellulose paper (paper chromatography), or in a thin layer on a mechanical backing, such as glass or plastic (thin-layer chromatography). Column methods are classically liquid chromatography. Gas chromatography is done by a column method.

Lateral or Vertical Flow Immunoassays (Immunochromatography)

The lateral or vertical flow immunoassays, immunochromatography assay, is an extremely versatile and rapid method for visual detection of antigen in a blood sample on a test strip. The probes used in lateral or vertical flow assays are commonly based on gold nanoparticle antibody conjugates. Due to the optical properties of gold, a noble meta,l nanoparticles detection with the naked eye can be achieved with excellent sensitivity. The assay is simple to perform.

The basic technology that underlies lateral flow immunoassays was first described in the 1960s. The first real commercial application was an over-the -counter home pregnancy test launched in 1988. Since then, this technology has been employed to develop a wide and ever-growing range of assays. Strip assays are extremely versatile and are available for an extensive range of analytes from blood proteins to mycotoxins and from viral pathogens to bacterial toxins. A newly introduced test for Zika virus uses gold nanorods on paper to detect the virus within minutes. The test uses proteins attached to nanorods that change color when coming into contact with Zika-infected blood. In tests conducted from blood samples of four infected people and five uninfected people, the nanorod test could differentiate between the sample and no false-positives.

A typical lateral flow rapid test strip consist of the following components:

- Sample pad - an adsorbent pad onto which the test sample is applied.
- Conjugate or reagent pad – this contains antibodies specific to the target analyte conjugated to coloured particles (usually colloidal gold nanoparticles, or latex microspheres).
- Reaction membrane – typically a nitrocellulose or cellulose acetate membrane onto which anti-target analyte antibodies are immobilized in a line that crosses the membrane to act as a capture zone or test line (a control zone will also be present, containing antibodies specific for the conjugate antibodies).
- Wick or waste reservoir – a further absorbent pad designed to draw the sample across the reaction membrane by capillary action and collect it.

Sample pad – an adsorbent pad onto which the test sample is applied.

Conjugate or reagent pad – this contains antibodies specific to the target analyte conjugated to coloured particles (usually colloidal gold nanoparticles, or latex microspheres).

Reaction membrane – typically a nitrocellulose or cellulose acetate membrane onto which anti-target analyte antibodies are immobilized in a line that crosses the membrane to act as a capture zone or test line (a control zone will also be present, containing antibodies specific for the conjugate antibodies).

Wick or waste reservoir – a further absorbent pad designed to draw the sample across the reaction membrane by capillary action and collect it.

The components of the strip are usually fixed to an inert backing material and may be presented in a simple dipstick format or within a plastic casing with a sample port and reaction window showing the capture and control zones (see Fig. 8.13).

Vertical flow immunoassays rely on the same basic principles as common lateral flow immunoassay format with some modifications. The most apparent difference between the two methods being the vertical and lateral flow of fluid. Vertical flow technology has reduced assay time (<5 minutes), (See Table 8.3).

As with lateral flow, vertical flow immunoassays rely on the immobilization of a capture antibody on a reagent pad to which the sample of interest (with or without antigen to be detected) is applied. Detection of the bound antigen is subsequently achieved through the binding of an antigen specific antibody gold conjugate. This step completes a sandwich consisting of a capture antibody, an antigen and finally the gold conjugate and results in a direct and permanent visually detectable red coloured dot indicating the presence of the antigen.

MOLECULAR DIAGNOSTIC TECHNIQUES

Molecular testing is one of the fastest-growing diagnostic disciplines in the clinical laboratory. Since the complete human genome (sequence) became available in 2003, molecular testing has been expanded extensively. Clinical applications of molecular knowledge are being directly applied in cancer treatment

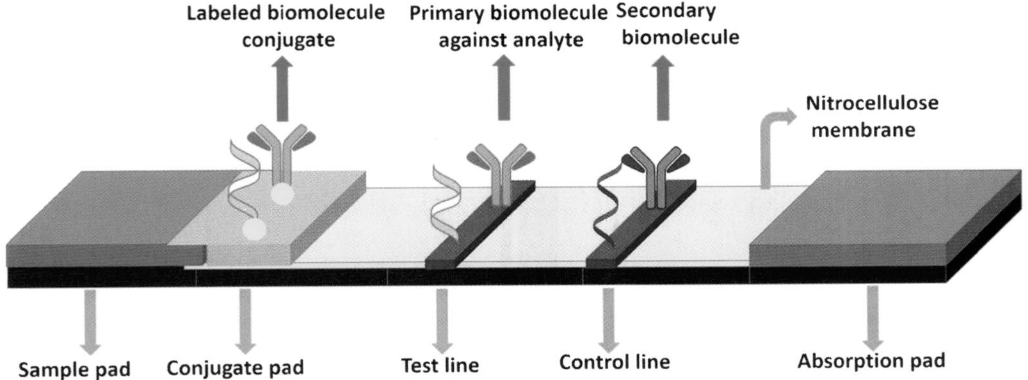

Fig. 8.13 Lateral flow immunoassay. Bahadır EB, Sezgintürk MK: Lateral flow assays: principles, designs and labels, *Trends Anal Chem* 82:286–306, 2016.

TABLE 8.3 Comparison of Lateral Flow and Vertical Flow Assay Methods

	Lateral Flow	Vertical Flow
Speed	Moderate	Fast
Ease of use	Easy	Easy
Readability or reliability of result after recommended reading time	Not recommended	Not applicable
Timed results	Requirement	No
Single window for sample and reagent	Yes	Yes
Hook effect[a]	Yes	No
Separation of sample and conjugate	No	Yes

[a]Using lateral flow, an undiluted specimen will overwhelm the internal color conjugate at the time of reaction before moving toward the reaction zone.
Modified from: Bahadır EB, Sezgintürk MK: Lateral flow assays: principles, designs and labels, *Trends Anal Chem* 82:286–306, 2016.

where personalized health care allows the tailoring of patient treatments based on the patient's genomic information. Table 8.4 presents specific molecular testing methods and their purpose. Molecular diagnostic testing and traditional serologic testing can complement each other in the establishment of infectious disease (Table 8.5).

Amplification Techniques in Molecular Biology

Polymerase chain reaction (PCR) is a molecular diagnostic technique that amplifies low levels of specific DNA sequences in a sample to higher quantities suitable for further analysis (Fig. 8.14). To use this technology, the target sequence to be amplified must be known. Typically, a target sequence ranges from 100 to 1000 base pairs in length. Two short DNA "primers" that are typically 16 to 20 base pairs long are used. Namely, the oligonucleotides (small portions of a single DNA strand) act as a template for the new DNA. These primer sequences are complementary to the 3-foot ends of the sequence to be amplified.

This enzymatic process is carried out in cycles. Each repeated cycle consists of the following:

- DNA denaturation: separation of the double DNA strands into two single strands through the use of heat.
- Primer annealing: recombination of the oligonucleotide primers with the single-strand original DNA.
- Extension of the primed DNA sequence: the enzyme DNA polymerase synthesizes new complementary strands by the extension of primers.

Each cycle theoretically doubles the amount of specific DNA sequence present and results in an exponential accumulation of the DNA fragment being amplified (amplicons). In general, this process is repeated approximately 30 times. At the end of 30 cycles, the reaction mixture should contain about 2^{30} molecules of the desired product. After cycling is completed, the amplification products can be examined in various ways. Typically the contents of the reaction vessel are subjected to gel electrophoresis. This allows visualization of the amplified gene segments (such as PCR products and bands) and a determination of their specificity. Additional product analysis by probe hybridization or direct DNA sequencing is often performed to verify further the authenticity of the amplicon.

The three important applications of PCR are as follows:

1. Amplification of DNA
2. Identification of a target sequence
3. Synthesis of a labeled antisense probe

Adaptations of the PCR technique have been developed. One adaptation uses nested primers and a two-step amplification process. PCR modifications include reverse transcriptase, multiplex, and real-time PCR.

Other Amplification Techniques

Strand Displacement Amplification. Strand displacement amplification is a fully automated method that amplifies target nucleic acid without the use of a thermocycler. A double-strand DNA (dsDNA) fragment is created and becomes the target for exponential amplification.

Transcription-Mediated Amplification. Transcription-mediated amplification (TMA), another isothermal assay, targets either DNA or ribonucleic acid (RNA) but generates RNA as its amplified product. This method is currently being used to detect microorganisms (such as *Mycobacterium tuberculosis*).

Nucleic Acid Sequence–Based Amplification. Nucleic acid sequence–based amplification is similar to TMA, but only RNA is targeted for amplification. Applications of this technique are detection and quantitation of human immunodeficiency virus (HIV) and detection of CMV.

TABLE 8.4 Molecular Testing Methods

Manufacturer	Test Name	Purpose of Testing
Abbott Molecular www.abbottmolecular.com	Abbott RealTime M2000 System	Automates PCR-based molecular diagnostic testing for infectious diseases
Avellino Laboratory USA www.avellinolab.com/us	Avellino-GENE Detection System (AGDS) Test	Detects gene mutation in corneal dystrophy
bioTheranostics www.biotheranostics.com	CancerTYPE ID	Differentiates expression of 92 genes to determine tumor site of origin in patient with metastatic cancer
	PRECIS Precision Medicine	Biomarker profiles for non–small cell lung cancer, colorectal cancer, breast cancer, gastric cancer, melanoma, and GIST
EKF Molecular Diagnostics www.ekfdiagnostics.com	PointMan DNA Enrichment Kits	Enriches rare mutated gene sequences in the *KRAS, BRAF,* and *EGFR* T90M sequence associated with melanoma, lung, and colorectal cancers
GenMark Diagnostics www.genmarkdx.com	eSensor Cystic Fibrosis Genotyping Test	Detects and identifies a cystic fibrosis panel of mutations and variants in the *CFTR* gene
	eSensor Respiratory Viral Panel	Detects 14 respiratory virus types and subtypes
Great Basin Corp www.gbscience.com	Portrait Benchtop Analyzer and Portrait Toxigenic *C. difficile* Assay	Detects toxigenic *Clostridia difficile*
Life Technologies www.lifetechnologies.com	Applied Biosystems 7500 Fast Dx Real-Time PCR Instrument	Detects and amplifies nucleic acid in real time and measures nucleic acid signals from reverse-transcribed RNA and converts them to comparative quantitative readouts using fluorescence detection of dual-labeled hydrolysis probes
	QuantStudio Dx Real-Time PCR Instrument	Performs fluorescence-based PCR to provide detection of FDA-cleared/approved nucleic acid sequences in human-derived specimens
Meridian Bioscience www.meridianbioscience.com	Illumigene Group A Streptococcus	Detects *Streptococcus pyogenes* in throat swab specimens
	Illumigene Mycoplasma	Detects *Mycoplasma*
Randox www.randox.com	STI Multiplex Array	Simultaneously detects 10 STIs from a single patient specimen
Roche Diagnostics www.mylabonline.com	Cobas HPV Test	Provides individual genotyping results for HPV 16 and 18, while simultaneously reporting 12 other high-risk HPV types as a pooled result
Siemens Healthcare Diagnostics usa.healthcare.siemens.com	Siemens Tissue Preparation System	Provides a process for isolation of high-quality nucleic acids from FFPE tissue samples
Thermo Fisher Scientific www.thermoscientific.com	ImmunoCAP Allergen Components	Reveals sensitization to unique proteins of the whole allergen test to help diagnose and optimize management

DNA, Deoxyribonucleic acid; *FDA,* U.S. Food and Drug Administration; *FFPE,* formalin-fixed paraffin-embedded; *GIST,* gastrointestinal stromal tumor; *HPV,* human papillomavirus; *PCR,* polymerase chain reaction; *RNA,* ribonucleic acid; *STI,* sexually transmitted infection.
Data from Tech guide, molecular testing, *Cl Lab Products* 43(8):20–26, 2013.

Ligase Chain Reaction Nucleic Acid Amplification. Oligonucleotide pairs hybridize to target sequences within the gene or the cryptic plasmid. The bound oligonucleotides are separated by a small gap at the target site. The enzyme DNA polymerase uses nucleotides in the ligase chain reaction (LCR) nucleic acid amplification reaction mixture to fill in this gap, creating a ligatable junction. Once the gap is filled, DNA ligase joins the oligonucleotide pairs to form a short, single-strand product that is complementary to the original target sequence. This product can itself serve as a target for hybridization and ligation of a second pair of oligonucleotides present in the LCR reaction mixture. Subsequent rounds of denaturation and ligation lead to the geometric accumulation of amplification product. The amplified products are detected by microparticle EIA.

Analysis of Amplification Products

Many of the revolutionary changes that have occurred in research in the biological sciences, particularly the Human Genome Project, can be attributed directly to the ability to manipulate DNA in defined ways. Molecular genetic testing focuses on the examination of nucleic acids (DNA or RNA) by special techniques to determine whether a specific nucleotide base sequence is present. Nucleic acid testing has expanded in various areas of the clinical laboratory, despite the higher costs associated with it. Clinical applications include genetic testing, hematopathology diagnosis and monitoring, and identification of infectious agents. The distinct advantages of molecular testing are as follows:

- Faster turnaround time
- Smaller sample volumes required
- Increased specificity and sensitivity

Conventional Analysis

DNA products resulting from PCR can be conventionally analyzed using agarose gel electrophoresis after ethidium bromide staining. This technique is simple to perform and is only an extra step after a PCR assay has been run.

Other Molecular Techniques

Other techniques are used to enhance both the sensitivity and the specificity of amplification techniques. Probe-based DNA detection systems have the advantage of providing sequence

TABLE 8.5 Relationship of Molecular and Serologic Testing for Infectious Disease

Polymerase Chain Reaction Result	IgM Result	IgG Result	Interpretation
Negative	Negative	Negative	No active or past infection
Positive	Positive	Positive	A recent primary infection with clinically detectable antibody evidence
Negative	Negative	Positive	Past infection with no current infection
Positive	Negative	Negative	Early primary infection with no clinically detected antibodies
Positive	Positive	Negative	Primary infection with clinically detectable levels of IgM
Positive	Negative	Positive	Past infection with clinically detectable titer as evidence
Negative	Positive	Negative	Contradictory results; retest by both methods, possibly a primary infection but has variations or mutations within its molecular target sequence
Negative	Positive	Positive	Contradictory results; retest by both methods with a substitution for an alternate target sequence

Brunstein JA: So happy together: integrating molecular and serological testing, *Med Lab Obs* 48(9):44–46, 2016.

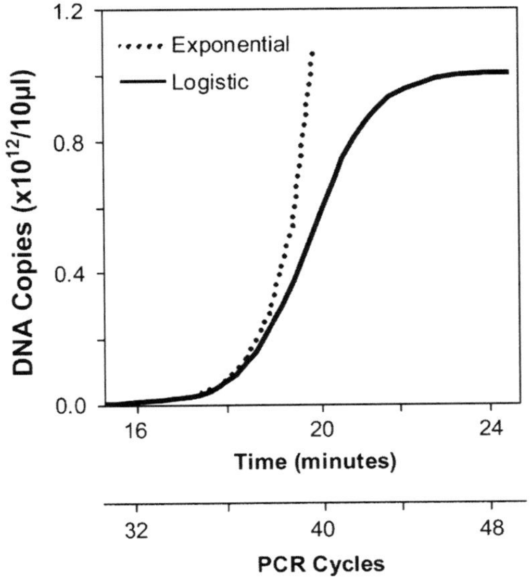

Fig. 8.14 Exponential and logistic curves for DNA amplified by polymerase chain reaction. (Modified with permission of the publisher from Wittwer CT, Kusukawa N: Real-time PCR. In Persing DH, Tenover FC, Versalovic J, et al, editors: *Molecular microbiology: diagnostic principles and practice,* Washington, DC, 2004, ASM Press, pp. 71–84, © 2004 ASM Press.)

specificity and decreased detection limits. Other techniques include hybridization protection assay, DNA EIA, automated DNA sequencing technology, single-strand conformational polymorphisms, and restriction fragment length polymorphism analysis. The selection of one technique over another is often based on a variety of factors (such as sensitivity and specificity profiles, cost, turnaround time, and local experience).

DNA Sequencing. The DNA sequencing method is considered to be the gold standard by which other molecular methods are compared. DNA sequencing displays the exact nucleotide or base sequence of a targeted fragment of DNA. The Sanger method, which uses a series of enzymatic reactions to produce segments of DNA complementary to the DNA being sequenced, is the most frequently used method for DNA sequencing. Automated sequencing techniques use primers with four different fluorescent labels.

The first step in sequencing a target is amplifying it in some way, either by cloning or in vitro amplification, usually PCR. Once the amplified DNA is purified from the clinical specimen (the target DNA), it is heat-denatured to separate the dsDNA into ssDNA.

The second step involves adding primers—short synthetic segments of ssDNA that contain a nucleotide sequence complementary to a short sequence of the target DNA—to the ssDNA. The patient's DNA serves as a template to copy. DNA polymerase catalyzes the addition of the appropriate nucleotides to the preexisting primer. DNA synthesis is terminated when the deoxynucleotide is embodied into a growing DNA chain.

Hybridization Techniques. Probe-hybridization assays involving the complementary pairing of a probe with a DNA or RNA strand derived from the patient specimen exist in many forms. The common feature of probe hybridization assays is the use of a labeled nucleic acid probe to examine a specimen for a specific homologous DNA or RNA sequence. The clinical probes are most often labeled with nonradioisotopic molecules such as digoxigenin, alkaline phosphatase, biotin, or a fluorescent compound. The detection systems are conjugate dependent and include chemiluminescent, fluorescent, and calorimetric methodologies.

Blotting Protocols

The Southern blot and Northern blot are used to detect DNA and RNA, respectively. These protocols share some procedural steps: electrophoretic separation of the patient's nucleic acid, transfer of nucleic acid fragments to a solid support (such as nitrocellulose or hybridization with a labeled probe of known nucleic acid sequence), and autoradiographic or colorimetric detection of the bands created by the probe–nucleic acid hybrid.

Western Blot

The Southern blot separates and identifies RNA fragments and proteins, and the Northern blot concentrates on isolating mRNA. In the Western blot technique, however, proteins are separated electrophoretically, transferred to membranes, and identified through the use of labeled antibodies specific for the protein of interest. The Western blot technique (Fig. 8.15) is used to detect antibodies to specific epitopes of electrophoretically separated subspecies of antigens. Electrophoresis of

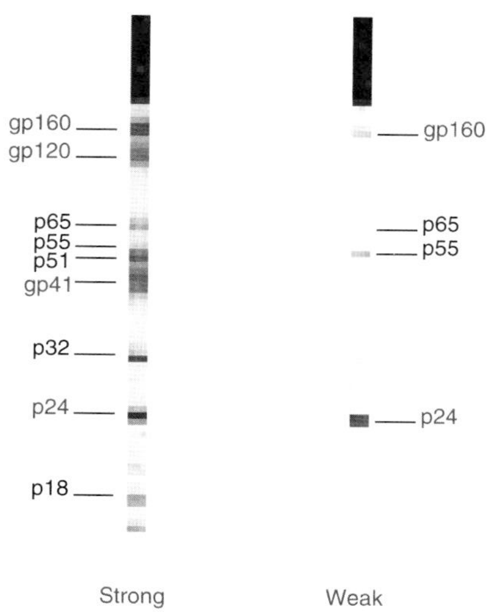

Fig. 8.15 Schematic of Western blotting. (From Burtis CA, Ashwood ER, Bruns DE: *Tietz textbook of clinical chemistry and molecular diagnostics,* ed 4, Philadelphia, 2006, Elsevier/Saunders.)

antigenic material yields separation of the antigenic components by molecular weight. Blotting the separated antigen to nitrocellulose, retaining the electrophoretic position, and causing it to react with the patient specimen will result in the binding of specific antibodies, if present, to each antigenic "band." Electrophoresis of known molecular weight standards allows for determining the molecular weight of each antigenic band to which antibodies may be produced. These antibodies are then detected using EIA reactions that characterize antibody specificity. Western blot is often used to confirm the specificity of antibodies detected by ELISA screening procedures.

Microarrays

Microarray (DNA chip) technology holds the promise of accelerating genetic analysis in much the same way that microprocessors have sped up computation. Microarrays are basically the product of bonding or direct synthesis of numerous specific DNA probes on a stationary, often silicon-based support. The chip may be tailored to particular disease processes. It is easily performed and readily automated. Microarrays are miniature gene fragments attached to glass chips. These chips are used to examine gene activity of thousands or tens of thousands of gene fragments and to identify genetic mutations, using a hybridization reaction between the sequences on the microarray and a fluorescent sample. After hybridization, the chips are scanned with high-speed fluorescence detectors, and the intensity of each spot is quantitated. The identity and amount of each sequence are revealed by the location and intensity of fluorescence displayed by each spot. Computers are used to analyze the data.

The applications of microarrays in clinical medicine include analysis of gene expression in malignancies (such as *BRCA1* mutations, tumor suppressor gene p53 mutations, genetic disease testing, and viral resistance mutation detection).

ELECTROCHEMICAL METHODS

When chemical energy is converted to an electrical current (a flow of electrons) in a galvanic cell, the term *electrochemistry* is used. Electrochemical reactions are characterized by a loss of electrons (oxidation) at the positive pole (anode) and a simultaneous gain of electrons (reduction) at the negative pole (cathode). The galvanic cell is made up of two parts called *half-cells,* each containing a metal in a solution of one of its salts. These methods involve the measurement of electrical signals associated with chemical systems that are within an electrochemical cell.

Electroanalytical chemistry uses electrochemistry for analysis purposes. In the clinical laboratory, electroanalytical methods are used to measure ions, drugs, hormones, metals, and gases. Methods are available for the rapid analysis of analytes present in relatively high concentrations in blood and urine, such as blood electrolytes (Na^+, K^+, Cl^-, HCO_3^-), and other analytes present in very low concentrations, such as heavy metals and drug metabolites. Three general electrochemical techniques are used in the clinical laboratory: potentiometric, voltammetric, and coulometric. This section discusses the electrochemical methods of potentiometry, coulometry, and electrophoresis.

Potentiometry

Potentiometry measures the potential of an electrode compared with the potential of another electrode. The method is based on the measurement of a voltage potential difference between two electrodes immersed in a solution under zero-current conditions. This difference in voltage between the two electrodes is usually measured on a pH or voltage meter. One electrode is called the *indicator electrode;* the other is the *reference electrode.* The reference electrode is an electrochemical half-cell that is used as a fixed reference for the cell potential measurements. One of the most common reference electrodes used for potentiometry is the silver or silver chloride electrode. The indicator electrode is the main component of potentiometric techniques. It is important that the indicator electrode be able to respond selectively to analyte species. The most common indicator electrode used in clinical chemistry is the ISE.

The use of ISEs is based on the measurement of a potential that develops across a selective membrane. The electrochemical cell response is based on an interaction between the membrane and the analyte being measured that alters the potential across the membrane. The specificity of the membrane interaction for the analyte determines the selectivity of the potential response to an analyte.

Electrodes and Ionic Concentration

Potentiometric methods of analysis involve the direct measurement of electrical potential caused by the activity of free ions. ISEs are designed to be sensitive toward individual ions. An ISE universally used in the clinical laboratory is the pH electrode. Specialized probes such as ISEs can measure concentrations of ionic species other than hydrogen ions [H^+], including fluoride, chloride, ammonia, sodium, potassium, calcium, sulfide, and nitrate ions.

An electrode is an electronic conductor in contact with an ionic conductor, the electrolyte. Passive (inert) electrodes act as electron donors or electron acceptors; active (participating) electrodes act as ion donors or ion acceptors. The electrode reaction is an electrochemical process in which charge transfer takes place at the interface between the electrode and the electrolyte.

By means of its potential, an indicator electrode shows the activity of an ion in a solution. The relationship between the potential and the activity is given by the Nernst equation (see later). The potential between an electrode and a solution cannot be directly measured; a reference electrode is needed. The reference electrode should have a known, or at least a constant, potential value under the prevailing experimental conditions.

The most essential component of a pH electrode is a special sensitive glass membrane that permits the passage of hydrogen ions but no other ionic species. When the electrode is immersed in a test solution containing hydrogen ions, the external ions diffuse through the membrane until equilibrium is reached between the external and internal concentrations. Thus there is a buildup of charge on the inside of the membrane that is proportional to the number of hydrogen ions in the external solution.

Because of the need for equilibrium conditions, there is minimal current flow. Therefore this potential difference between electrode and solution can be measured only relative to a separate and stable reference system that is also in contact with the test solution but that is unaffected by it. A sensitive, high-impedance millivolt meter or digital measuring system must be used to measure this potential difference accurately.

In fact, the potential difference developed across the membrane is directly proportional to the logarithm of the ionic concentration in the external solution. To determine the pH of an unknown solution, it is necessary only to measure the potential difference in two standard solutions of known pH, construct a straight-line calibration graph by plotting millivolts versus pH = (log [H^+]), then read off the unknown pH from the measured voltage.

To measure the electrode potential developed at the ion-selective membrane, the ISE/pH electrode must be immersed in the test solution together with a separate reference system, and the two must be connected by a millivolt measuring system. At equilibrium, the electrons added or removed from the solution by the ISE membrane (depending on whether it is cation or anion sensitive) are balanced by an equal and opposite charge at the reference interface. This causes a positive or negative deviation from the original stable reference voltage that is registered on the external measuring system.

The relationship between the ionic concentration (activity) and the electrode potential is expressed by the Nernst equation, as follows:

$$E\,cell = E^0 cell + (2.303RT/nF) \times \log(Q)$$

where:

E cell = cell potential under nonstandard conditions

E^0 cell = cell potential under standard conditions

2.303 = Conversion factor from natural to base-10 log

R = Gas constant (8.314 joules/degree/mole)

T = Absolute temperature

n = Number of moles of electrons exchanged in the electrochemical reaction (ol)

F = Faraday constant (96,500 coulombs)

Q = reaction quotient, which is the equilibrium expression with initial concentrations rather than equilibrium concentrations

Note that $2.303RT/nF$ is the slope of the line—from the straight-line plot of E versus log(A), which is the basis of ISE calibration graphs. This is an important diagnostic characteristic of the electrode; generally the slope drops lower as the electrode ages or is contaminated, and the lower the slope, the higher the errors on the sample measurements.

For practical use in measuring pH, it is usually not necessary for the operator to construct a calibration graph and to interpolate the results for unknown samples. Most pH electrodes are connected directly to a special pH meter, which performs the calibration automatically. This determines the slope mathematically and calculates the unknown pH value for immediate display on the meter.

These basic principles are exactly the same for all ISEs, so it would appear that all can be used as easily and rapidly as the pH electrode—simply by calibrating the equipment by measuring two known solutions, then immersing the electrodes in any test solution and reading the answer directly from a meter. Some other ions can be measured in this simple way, but this is not the case for most ions.

pH Electrodes and Meters

The pH measurement was originally used by the Danish biochemist Soren Sorensen to represent the hydrogen ion concentration, expressed in equivalents per liter, of an aqueous solution: pH = log[H^+]. In expressions of this type, enclosure of a chemical symbol within square brackets denotes that the concentration of the symbolized species is the quantity being considered.

The first commercially successful electronic pH meter was invented by Dr. Arnold Beckman in 1934. This instrument was the forerunner of modern electrochemical instrumentation and became an indispensable tool in analytical chemistry. Beginning in the 1950s, electrodes were also developed for other ions (such as F, Na^+, K^+, and Ag^+). The pH meter and ISE are now essential to scientific analysis, providing precise pH and concentration (ISE) measurements in handheld, bench-top, and high-performance meters for research, pharmaceutical, chemical, and environmental applications.

The term *pH* refers to the concentration of hydrogen ions ([H^+], also called *protons*) in a solution. For aqueous solutions, the scale ranges from 0 to 14, with pure water in the middle at 7. The more acid a solution, the lower is the pH reading (0–6.9), and alkaline solutions come in at the high end of the scale (7.1–14).

Paper test strips (such as urine dipsticks) are good for measuring approximate pH values, but chemical laboratories require more exact measurements. A pH meter is a boxy-looking instrument attached to a glass or plastic tube called a *probe*. Handheld pH meters have a probe directly attached to the instrument body. The probe has a glass bulb on one end and an electrical wire on the other. The wire sends data to the instrument when the glass bulb is dipped into a sample solution.

The pH meter measures [H^+] by sensing differences in the electrical charges inside and outside the probe. The glass bulb is made from silica (silicon dioxide) that contains added metal ions. Most of the oxygen atoms in the glass are surrounded by silicon and metal atoms. However, the oxygen atoms on the inside and outside surfaces of the bulb are not completely surrounded and can "grab" positively charged ions from the solution. When the bulb is dipped into an acid solution, H^+ ions bond with the outside surface of the glass bulb, forming electrically neutral Si–OH groups. The Si–O groups on the inside surface are in contact with a reference solution. The difference in electrical charge between the two surfaces creates an electrical potential, or voltage, and this causes an electrical current to flow through the wire at the other end of the probe.

Alkaline solutions have low $[H^+]$ and higher concentrations of negative ions such as OH. The excess negative charges are balanced with positively charged metal ions such as Na^+, and these positive ions hover close to the surface of the bulb rather than binding to the Si–O groups. This sets up a different sort of charge separation, and the resulting electrical signal registers a high pH.

Types of Meters

Analog Meters. The earliest type of pH meters were simple analog devices with a resolution of only 1 or 2 mV. The original meters were calibrated in millivolts, and the corresponding pH value was read from a calibration graph. Because pH electrodes are reasonably uniform and reproducible instruments, it is not necessary to have a unique calibration graph for each electrode. In this case the meters can be calibrated directly in pH units by the manufacturer and can simply be recalibrated each time they are used (to compensate for temperature changes or slight differences in electrode response) by immersing the electrode in just one pH buffer solution and adjusting the meter output to give the correct reading. This type of meter is simple and quick to use and is perfectly adequate for many pH measurements because it requires a modification of more than 5 mV to change the pH value by more than 0.1 pH units.

Simple precalibrated analog meters are not appropriate for ISE measurements.

Digital Meters. A major advance was made when digital meters were introduced with a resolution of 0.1 or even 0.01 mV. This enabled the analyst to measure and read the voltage with much greater accuracy and meant that the stability and reproducibility of the electrode response became the main limiting factors in determining the accuracy and precision.

Self-Calibrating, Direct-Reading Ion Meters. The next major advance occurred when microprocessors were introduced. These contained simple programs to calculate the slope and intercept from the calibration data, which were then used to calculate the sample concentration from the millivolt reading in the sample. The analyst can simply enter the concentrations of the standards and measure the millivolts, then immerse the electrodes in the sample and read the sample concentration directly from the meter. These meters are often confusing to operate, with small keypads and multifunction switches, and are not suitable for working in the nonlinear range of the electrodes, for using different slopes for different parts of the calibration range, or for measuring more than one ion at a time. It is often difficult for the analyst to assess the quality of the calibration or to detect errors in data entry, and it is still necessary for the results to be transferred manually to a permanent record.

Coulometry

Coulometry measures the amount of current passing between two electrodes in an electrochemical cell. The principle of coulometry involves the application of a constant current to generate a titrating agent; the time required to titrate a sample at constant current is measured and is related to the amount of analyte in the sample. The amount of current is directly proportional to the amount of substance produced or consumed by the electrode. Clinical applications of coulometry include the FreeStyle Connect blood glucose monitoring system (Abbott Labs) in the point-of-care setting (hospitals and medical clinics) and an older application for the measurement of chloride ions in serum, plasma, urine, and other body fluids.

Electrophoresis

Electrophoresis is the migration of charged solutes or particles in an electrical field. When charged particles are made to move, the variations in molecular structure can be seen because different molecules have different velocities in an electrical field. The assay using electrophoresis involves the movement of charged particles when an external electrical current is produced in a liquid environment.

The electrical field is applied to the solution through oppositely charged electrodes placed in the solution. Specific ions then travel through the solution toward the electrode of the opposite charge. Cations (positively charged particles) move toward the negatively charged electrode (cathode), and anions (negatively charged particles) move toward the positively charged electrode (anode) (Fig. 8.16).

Electrophoresis is a technique for separation and purification of ions, proteins, and other molecules of biochemical interest. It is used frequently in the clinical chemistry laboratory to separate serum proteins. The equipment needed for electrophoresis generally consists of a sample applicator; a solid medium (such as agar gel); a buffer system; an electrophoresis chamber,

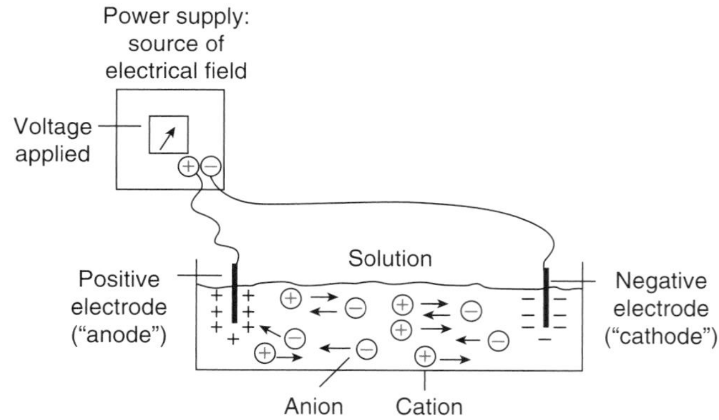

Fig. 8.16 Application of electrical field to solution of ions makes ions move. (From Kaplan LA, Pesce AJ: *Clinical chemistry: theory, analysis, correlation*, ed 5, St Louis, 2010, Elsevier/Mosby.)

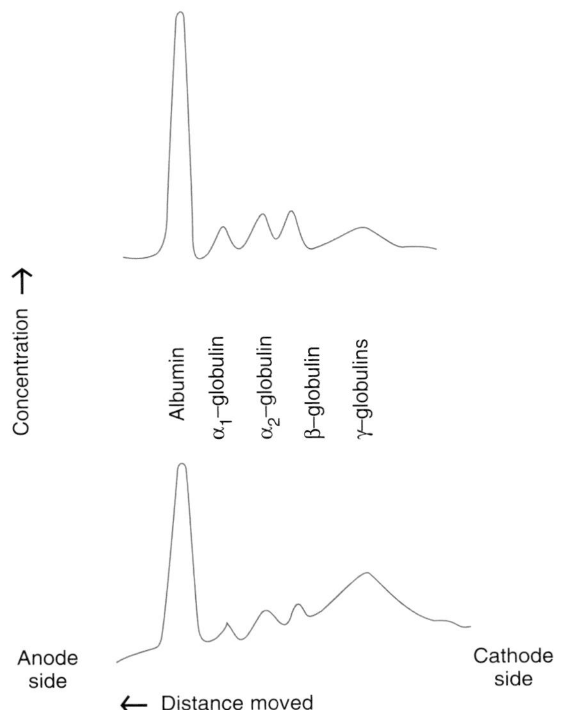

Fig. 8.17 Example of effect of disease (hepatic cirrhosis) on serum protein electrophoretic pattern. Upper profile, distribution characteristic of healthy people. (From Kaplan LA, Pesce AJ: *Clinical chemistry: theory, analysis, correlation,* ed 5, St Louis, 2010, Elsevier/Mosby.)

which houses the solid medium and the sample; electrodes and wicks; a timer; and a power supply. Additional supplies might be stains for proteins or other substances being assayed and reagents used to remove the stains and to transform the solid media into a stable carrier for further densitometry studies or for preservation needs, depending on the requirements of the laboratory.

Serum proteins, including immunoglobulins, are often separated by electrophoresis. Serum electrophoresis results in the separation of proteins into five fractions, using cellulose acetate as a support medium (Fig. 8.17). The immunologic applications of electrophoresis include identification of monoclonal proteins in serum or urine, IEP, and various blotting techniques.

Immunoelectrophoresis

IEP is an older method that has been largely replaced by IFE. IEP involves the electrophoresis of serum or urine followed by immunodiffusion. The size and position of precipitin bands provide the same type of information regarding equivalence or antibody excess as the double-immunodiffusion method. Proteins are differentiated not only by their electrophoretic mobility but also by their diffusion coefficient and antibody specificity.

IEP is a combination of the classic techniques of electrophoresis and double immunodiffusion and consists of two phases: electrophoresis and diffusion. In the first phase, serum is placed in an appropriate medium (such as cellulose acetate or agarose), then electrophoresed to separate its constituents according to electrophoretic mobilities: albumin and α_1-, α_2-, β-, and γ-globulin fractions. In the second phase, after electrophoresis, the fractions are allowed to act as antigens and interact with their corresponding antibodies. When a favorable antigen-to-antibody ratio exists (equivalence point), the antigen-antibody complex becomes visible as precipitin lines or bands. Diffusion is halted by rinsing the plate in 0.85% saline. Unbound protein is washed from the agarose with saline, and the antigen-antibody precipitin arcs are stained with a protein-sensitive stain.

Each line represents one specific protein. Proteins are thus differentiated not only by their electrophoretic mobility but also by their diffusion coefficient and antibody specificity. The antibody diffuses as a uniform band parallel to the antibody trough. If the proteins are homogeneous, the antigen diffuses in a circle, and the antigen-antibody precipitation line resembles a segment or arc of a circle. If the antigen is heterogeneous, the antigen-antibody line assumes an elliptical shape. One arc of precipitation forms for each constituent in the antigen mixture. This technique can be used to resolve the protein of normal serum into 25 to 40 distinct precipitation bands. The exact number depends on the strength and specificity of the antiserum used.

Normal Appearance of Precipitin Bands. Immunoprecipitation bands should be of normal curvature, symmetry, length, position, intensity, and distance from the antigen well and antibody trough. In normal serum, IgG, IgA, and IgM are present in sufficient concentrations of 10 mg/mL, 2 mg/mL, and 1 mg/mL, respectively, to produce precipitin lines. The normal concentrations of IgD and IgE are too low to be detected by IEP.

Clinical Applications. IEP is most frequently used to determine qualitatively the elevation or deficiency of specific classes of immunoglobulins. It is a reliable and accurate method for detecting both structural abnormalities and concentration changes in proteins. The most common application of IEP is in the diagnosis of a monoclonal gammopathy, a condition in which a single clone of plasma cells produces elevated levels of a single class and type of immunoglobulin. The most important application of IEP of urine is the demonstration of Bence Jones protein, a diagnostic sign of multiple myeloma.

Immunofixation Electrophoresis

IFE (Fig. 8.18), or simply *immunofixation,* has replaced IEP in the evaluation of monoclonal gammopathies because of its rapidity and ease of interpretation. IFE is a two-stage procedure using agarose gel protein electrophoresis in the first stage and immunoprecipitation in the second. The test specimen may be serum, urine, cerebrospinal fluid, or other body fluids. The primary use of IFE in clinical laboratories is for the characterization of monoclonal immunoglobulins.

Capillary Electrophoresis

In capillary electrophoresis, the classic separation techniques of zone electrophoresis, isotachophoresis, isoelectric focusing, and gel electrophoresis are performed in small-bore (10–100 μm) fused-silica capillary tubes from 20 to 200 cm in length. This method is efficient, sensitive, and rapid.

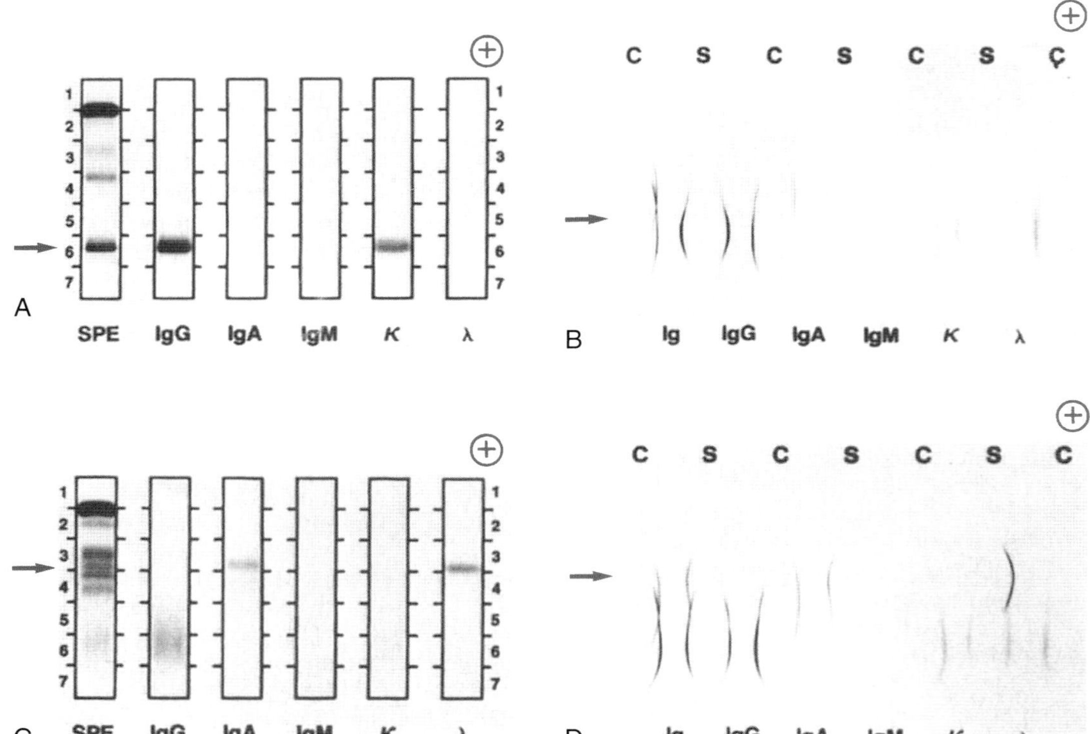

Fig. 8.18 Immunofixation electrophoresis. (From Burtis CA, Ashwood ER, Bruns DB: Tietz fundamentals of clinical chemistry, ed 6, St Louis, 2008, Saunders.)

BIBLIOGRAPHY

Abbott Laboratories: *Worldwide introduction of the new point-of-care glycemic control technology*, Paper presented at AACC Symposium, Orlando, Fla. 2005.

Astion ML, Wener MH, Hutchinson K: Autoantibody testing: The use of immunofluorescence and other assays, *Clin Lab News* (7):30–34, 2000.

Bahadır EB, Sezgintürk MK: Lateral flow assays: Principles, designs and labels, *Trends in Analytical Chemistry* 82:286–306, 2016.

Bakke AC: The principles of flow cytometry, *Lab Med* 32(4):207, 2001.

Bakker E: Is the DNA sequence the gold standard in genetic testing? Quality of molecular genetic tests assessed, *Clin Chem* 52:557–558, 2006.

Behring nephelometer system folder: Branchburg, NJ, 1987, Behring Diagnostics.

Bishop ML, Fody EP, Schoeff L: *Clinical chemistry: techniques, principles, correlations,* ed 6, Philadelphia, 2010, Lippincott Williams & Wilkins.

Blick KE: Current trends in automation of immunoassays, *J Clin Ligand Assay* 22(1):6, 1999.

Bruns DE, Ashwood ER, Burtis CA: *Fundamentals of molecular diagnostics,* St Louis, 2007, Elsevier/Saunders.

Brunstein J: A snapshot of the most common PCR application, *MLS Med Lab Obs* 49(3):44–45, 2017.

Brunstein J: Back to basics: nucleic acid amplification in the clinical lab, *MLS Med Lab Obs* 49(1):44–45, 2017.

Brunstein J: Molecular diagnostics: basic terms and principles, *MLO Med Lab Obs* 44(12):18–20, 2012.

Brunstein J: PCR: the basics of the polymerase chain reaction, *MLO Med Lab Obs* 45(4):32–35, 2013a.

Brunstein J: Endpoint PCR detection, *MLO Med Lab Obs* 45(5):38–40, 2013b.

Burtis CA, Ashwood ER, Bruns DE: *Tietz fundamentals of clinical chemistry,* ed 6, St Louis, 2008, Elsevier/Saunders.

Cook L: PCR then and now, *MLO Med Lab Obs* 48(11):46–48, 2016.

Estabrooks L: Gene sequencing in the clinical laboratory: benefits and dilemmas, *MLO Med Lab Obs* 44(10):28–30, 2012.

Forbes BA, Sahm DF, Weissfeld AS: *Bailey and Scott's diagnostic microbiology,* ed 12, St Louis, 2007, Elsevier/Mosby.

Giorda K: Assessing the suitability of NGS panels for clinical sequencing, *MLO Med Lab Obs* 49(4):36–37, 2017.

Helena Laboratories: Educational slide series. Protein electrophoresis and IFE and immunofixation for identification of monoclonal gammopathies. www.helena.com. Accessed November 2007.

Hyde A: Enzyme-linked immunosorbent assay (ELISA): an overview, Adv Med Lab Professionals: 13–16, *Oct* 9, 2006.

Jandreski MA: Chemiluminescence technology in immunoassays, *Lab Med* 29(9):555, 1998.

Kaplan LA, Pesce AJ: *Clinical chemistry: theory, analysis, correlation,* ed 5, St Louis, 2010, Elsevier/Mosby.

Killingsworth LM, Warren BM: *Immunofixation for the identification of monoclonal gammopathies,* Beaumont, Texas, 1986, Helena Laboratories.

Li SFY, Kricka LJ: Clinical analysis by microchip capillary electrophoresis, *Clin Chem* 52:42, 2006.

Mark HFL: Fluorescent in situ hybridization as an adjunct to conventional cytogenetics, *Ann Clin Lab Sci* 24(2):153–163, 1994.

Mathias PC, Turner EH, Scroggins SM: Applying Ancestry and Sex Computation as a Quality Control Tool in Targeted Next-Generation Sequencing, *Am J Clin Pathol* 145(3):308–315, 2016.
Raich T: The evolving role of technology in clinical microbiology, *MLO Med Lab Obs* 45(4):16–18, 2013.
Ritzmann EE: Immunoglobulin abnormalities. In Ritzman S, editor: *Serum protein abnormalities, diagnostic and clinical aspects*, Boston, 1976, Little, Brown.
Romain C, Lee C, Hu P: Digital PCR, *ASCLS Today* 27(3):10, 2013. 15.
Saunders CJ: Newborn Screening in the Age of Genomics: Innovation versus evidence, *Cl Lab News* 44(3):13–17, 2017.
Shankey TV: New applications of flow cytometry in the clinical lab, *MLO Med Lab Obs* 44(12):22–24, 2012.
Sun T: Immunofixation electrophoresis procedures. Protein abnormalities. In *Physiology of immunoglobulins diagnostic and clinical aspects*, New York, 1982, Alan R Liss. vol.1.
Turgeon ML: *Clinical hematology*, ed 6, Philadelphia, 2017, Lippincott Williams & Wilkins.
Turgeon ML: *Immunology and serology in laboratory medicine*, ed 6, St Louis, 2017, Elsevier/Mosby.
Wang Z, et al: In situ amplified chemiluminescent detection of DNA and immunoassay of IgG using special-shaped gold nanoparticles as label, *Clin Chem* 52:1958–1962, 2006.

REVIEW QUESTIONS (ANSWERS IN APPENDIX A)

Photometry

1. Photometry:
   a. Employs color to determine the concentrations of various substances
   b. Employs color variations to determine the concentrations of various substances
   c. Measures luminous intensity of light
   d. All the above

Absorbance Spectrophotometry

2. The function of the absorbance spectrophotometer is to measure the concentration of:
   a. Sodium or potassium in a body fluid or serum
   b. Glucose in blood by using dry-film technology
   c. Hemoglobin in a solution
   d. Dried blood on a filter paper

Reflectance Spectrophotometry

3. The function of the reflectance spectrophotometer is to measure the concentration of:
   a. Sodium or potassium in a body fluid or serum
   b. Glucose in blood by using dry-film technology
   c. Hemoglobin in a solution
   d. Dried blood on a filter paper
4. In the visible light spectrum, the color red is in what nanometer range?
   a. 380-440 nm
   b. 500-580 nm
   c. 600-620 nm
   d. 620-750 nm

   Questions 5 and 6: Fill in the blanks (use an answer only once) to complete the following statement correctly.

The Beer-Lambert (Beer's) law states that the concentration of a substance is:

5. ____ to the amount of light absorbed or
6. ____ to the logarithm of the transmitted light.
   a. Directly proportional
   b. Inversely proportional
   c. Not proportional
   d. Proportional to half of the concentration of a substance
7. A characteristic of absorbance is that it:
   a. Decreases as the concentration of a colored solution decreases
   b. Increases as the concentration of a colored solution increases
   c. Contains a known strength
   d. Detects amplicons
8. A characteristic of percent transmittance is that it:
   a. Decreases as the concentration of a colored solution decreases
   b. Increases as the concentration of a colored solution increases
   c. Contains a known strength
   d. Detects amplicons
9. A characteristic of a standard solution is that it:
   a. Decreases as the concentration of a colored solution decreases
   b. Increases as the concentration of a colored solution increases
   c. Contains a known strength
   d. Detects amplicons
10. Wavelength accuracy is:
    a. Checked with standard absorbing solution or filters
    b. Any wavelength outside of the band transmitted
    c. Demonstrated when a change in concentration results in a straight-line calibration curve
    d. Better at lower ranges of the visible spectrum
11. Stray light is:
    a. Checked with standard absorbing solution or filters
    b. Any wavelength outside of the band transmitted
    c. Demonstrated when a change in concentration results in a straight-line calibration curve
    d. Better at lower ranges of the visible spectrum
12. Reflectance spectrophotometry is used in:
    a. Point-of-care testing
    b. Some large chemical instruments
    c. Urinalysis automated instruments
    d. All the above

Nephelometry

13. Nephelometry measures the light scatter of:
    a. Ions
    b. Macromolecular complexes
    c. Antibodies
    d. Soluble antigens

Flow (Cell) Cytometry

14. *Laser* is an acronym for:
    a. Light amplification by stimulated emission of radiation
    b. Light augmentation by stimulated emission of radiation
    c. Light amplification of stimulated energy radiation
    d. Large-angle stimulated emission of radiation
15. All the following are descriptive characteristics of laser light *except:*
    a. Intensity
    b. Stability
    c. Polychromaticity
    d. Monochromaticity
16. A photon is a:
    a. Basic unit of light
    b. Basic unit of all radiation
    c. Component of an atom
    d. Component of laser light

Immunoassays

17. Which of the following statements correctly describes competitive immunoassay?
    a. A fixed amount of labeled antigen competes with unlabeled antigen from a patient specimen for a limited number of antibody-binding sites.
    b. The sample antigen binds to an antibody; a second antibody, labeled with a chemiluminescent label, binds to the antigen-antibody complex.
    c. Excess reagent; linear binding to one site.
    d. Capture antibody actively absorbed; antigen from specimen allowed to react.
18. Which of the following statements correctly describes sandwich immunoassay?
    a. A fixed amount of labeled antigen competes with unlabeled antigen from a patient specimen for a limited number of antibody-binding sites.
    b. The sample antigen binds to an antibody; a second antibody, labeled with a chemiluminescent label, binds to the antigen-antibody complex.
    c. It is a type of noncompetitive assay.
    d. Both b and c.
19. Which enzyme label is often used in immunoassay procedures?
    a. Acid phosphatase
    b. Horseradish peroxidase
    c. β-Galactose
    d. All the above
20. Enzyme immunoassay (EIA):
    a. Uses a nonisotopic label
    b. Uses antibody labeled with fluorescein isothiocyanate (FITC)
    c. Uses a colloidal particle consisting of a metal or an insoluble metal compound
    d. Is not a safe technique
21. Immunofluorescence technique:
    a. Uses a nonisotopic label
    b. Uses antibody labeled with fluorescein isothiocyanate (FITC)
    c. Uses a colloidal particle consisting of a metal or an insoluble metal compound
    d. Is not very sensitive or specific
22. Direct immunofluorescence assay:
    a. Is based on the fact that antibodies can act as antigens and react with antiimmunoglobulins
    b. Uses conjugated antibody to detect antigen-antibody reactions at a microscopic level
    c. Has antigen first exposed to unlabeled antibody, then labeled antibody
    d. Is not used for tissue sections or smears for microbiology
23. Inhibition immunofluorescence assay
    a. Is based on the fact that antibodies can act as antigens and react with antiimmunoglobulins
    b. Uses conjugated antibody to detect antigen-antibody reactions at a microscopic level
    c. Has antigen first exposed to unlabeled antibody, then labeled antibody
    d. Is based on the fact that if unlabeled and labeled antibodies are homologous to antigen, fluorescence is produced
24. Indirect immunofluorescence assay
    a. Is based on the fact that antibodies can act as antigens and react with antiimmunoglobulins
    b. Uses conjugated antibody to detect antigen-antibody reactions at a microscopic level
    c. Has antigen first exposed to unlabeled antibody, then labeled antibody
    d. Is rarely used to detect diverse antibodies

Questions 25 and 26: Fill in each blank with the letter that completes the following statement correctly.

Alternative Labeling Technologies

A fluorescent substance is one that while:

25. ______ light of one wavelength,
    a. Emitting
    b. Absorbing
    c. Generating bright
    d. Generating dull
26. ______ light of another (longer) wavelength.
    a. Emits
    b. Absorbs
    c. Reduces
    d. Increases
27. Which of the following is a characteristic of fluorescence in situ hybridization (FISH)?
    a. Semiconductor nanocrystals
    b. Method of tagging antibodies with superparamagnetic particles
    c. Technology based on two different 200-nm latex particles
    d. Molecular cytogenetic technique
28. Tyramide signal amplification (TSA) is of value in detecting:
    a. light chain mRNA molecules
    b. interferon gamma (IFN-γ)
    c. interleukin-4 (IL-4)
    d. All of the above

29. Magnetic labeling technology analyzes:
    a. RNA
    b. DNA
    c. radio waves
    d. light waves

Chemiluminescence

30. Newer automated systems use:
    a. Fluorescent labels and detection systems
    b. Electromagnetic systems
    c. Accelerated chemical reactions
    d. Luminescent labels and substrates
31. Chemiluminescence:
    a. Has excellent sensitivity and dynamic range
    b. Does not require sample radiation
    c. Uses unstable chemiluminescent reagents and conjugates
    d. Both a and b

Chromatography and Immunochromatography

32. In chromatography:
    a. Mixtures of solutes dissolved in a common solvent are separated from one another by a differential distribution of the solutes between two phases.
    b. Different molecules have different velocities in an electrical field.
    c. The amount of current passing between two electrodes in an electrochemical cell is measured.
    d. An oscillating current is applied to generate a titrating agent.
33. The element combined with an antibody to form a visible reaction in lateral flow immunoassays is:
    a. silver
    b. gold
    c. calcium
    d. magnesium

Molecular Diagnostic Techniques

34. PCR testing is useful in:
    a. Forensic testing
    b. Genetic testing
    c. Identification of the disease
    d. All the above
35. The traditional PCR technique:
    a. Extends the length of the genomic DNA
    b. Alters the original DNA nucleotide sequence
    c. Amplifies the target region of DNA
    d. Amplifies the target region of RNA
36. For the PCR reaction to take place, one must provide which of the following?
    a. Oligonucleotide primers
    b. Individual deoxynucleotides
    c. Thermostable DNA polymerase
    d. All the above
37. The enzyme reverse transcriptase converts:
    a. mRNA to cDNA
    b. tRNA to DNTP
    c. dsDNA to ssDNA
    d. Mitochondrial to nuclear DNA
38. DNA polymerase catalyzes:
    a. Primer annealing
    b. Primer extension
    c. Hybridization of DNA
    d. Hybridization of RNA
39. Which of the following is an application of Western blot immunoassay?
    a. Messenger RNA is studied.
    b. Called immunoblot, it is used to detect antibodies to subspecies of antigens.
    c. Single-strand DNA is studied.
    d. It involves isolating mRNA.

Electrochemical Methods

40. Which ion-selective electrode (ISE) is universally used in the clinical laboratory?
    a. pH electrode
    b. Fluoride electrode
    c. Chloride electrode
    d. Sodium electrode
41. An indicator electrode:
    a. Is the main component of potentiometric techniques
    b. Is an electrochemical half-cell that is used as a fixed reference for the cell potential measurements
    c. Does not show activity of an ion in solution
    d. Directly measures potential
42. A reference electrode:
    a. Is the main component of potentiometric techniques
    b. Is an electrochemical half-cell that is used as a fixed reference for the cell potential measurements
    c. Does not require a known or constant potential value
    d. Performs the same function as an indicator electrode
43. In coulometry:
    a. Mixtures of solutes dissolved in a common solvent are separated from one another by a differential distribution of the solutes between two phases.
    b. Different molecules have different velocities in an electrical field.
    c. The amount of current passing between two electrodes in an electrochemical cell is measured.
    d. An oscillating current is applied to generate a titrating agent.
44. In electrophoresis:
    a. Mixtures of solutes dissolved in a common solvent are separated from one another by a differential distribution of the solutes between two phases.
    b. Different molecules have different velocities in an electrical field.
    c. The amount of current passing between two electrodes in an electrochemical cell is measured.
    d. An oscillating current is applied to generate a titrating agent.
45. Using serum electrophoresis, protein can be separated into how many fractions?
    a. Three
    b. Four
    c. Five
    d. Six

46. Which of the following is the most common application of immunoelectrophoresis (IEP)?
    a. Identification of the absence of a normal serum protein
    b. Structural abnormalities of proteins
    c. Screening for circulating immune complexes
    d. Diagnosis of monoclonal gammopathies
47. Immunofixation electrophoresis is best used in the:
    a. Workup of a polyclonal gammopathy
    b. Workup of a monoclonal gammopathy
    c. Screening for circulating immune complexes
    d. Identification of hypercomplementemia
48. Immunoelectrophoresis involves:
    a. Separation of proteins based on the rate of migration of individual components in an electrical field
    b. Electrophoresis of serum or urine
    c. Double immunodiffusion following electrophoresis
    d. All the above
49. In immunoelectrophoresis (IEP), proteins are differentiated by:
    a. Electrophoresis
    b. Diffusion coefficient
    c. Antibody specificity
    d. All the above
50. The most important application of IEP of urine is:
    a. Diagnosis of monoclonal gammopathy
    b. Diagnosis of polyclonal gammopathy
    c. Diagnosis of autoimmune hemolysis
    d. Demonstration of Bence Jones (BJ) protein
51. Immunofixation electrophoresis (IFE) can test:
    a. Serum and urine
    b. Cerebrospinal fluid
    c. Whole blood
    d. Both a and b
52. The primary use of IFE is:
    a. Characterization of monoclonal immunoglobulins
    b. Characterization of polyclonal immunoglobulins
    c. Identification of monoclonal immunoglobulins
    d. Identification of polyclonal immunoglobulins

Chromatography

53. In chromatography:
    a. Mixtures of solutes dissolved in a common solvent are separated from one another by a differential distribution of the solutes between two phases.
    b. Different molecules have different velocities in an electrical field.
    c. The amount of current passing between two electrodes in an electrochemical cell is measured.
    d. An oscillating current is applied to generate titrating agent.

Bonus Challenge Questions 54 to 56: Answer each question below from the following choices:

54. You need to perform an immunofluorescence assay that has improved sensitivity, uses an unlabeled antibody to detect antigen, and is suitable for detecting a wide variety of antibodies. Which assay should you use?
    a. Direct immunofluorescence
    b. Inhibition immunofluorescence
    c. Indirect immunofluorescence
    d. Chemiluminescence
55. In which methodology does a negative reaction confirm specificity?
    a. Direct immunofluorescence
    b. Inhibition immunofluorescence
    c. Indirect immunofluorescence
    d. Chemiluminescence
56. In this procedure performed on a tissue sample, a specific nucleic acid is detected in an organism by an antibody directly tagged with a fluorochrome (the fluorescent dye). Which procedure is this?
    a. Direct immunofluorescence
    b. Inhibition immunofluorescence
    c. Indirect immunofluorescence
    d. Chemiluminescence

Turgeon: Linné & Ringsrud's Clinical Laboratory Science, 8th Edition

STUDENT PROCEDURE WORKSHEET 8-1

Using the Spectrophotometer

Read Chapter 8 in *Linné & Ringsrud's Clinical Laboratory Science: Concepts, Procedures, and Clinical Applications,* 8th edition, for a complete discussion of this topic.

Student Learning Outcomes

After reading Chapter 8, and at the completion of the laboratory exercise and review questions, the student will be able to:

- Operate a spectrophotometer.
- Correctly complete the end of procedure review questions with a grade of 80% or greater.

Equipment and Supplies

1. Spectrophotometer (Fischer Scientific Educational Spectrophotometer or similar equipment)
2. Cuvettes
3. Distilled H_2O
4. A colored solution, e.g. Biuret reagent or colored water.

Additonal solutions: various colored water solutions.

Optional solutions: various colors or concentrations of solutions

Instructions for the Procedure

Read the list of required equipment and supplies and the procedural steps. Follow the procedural steps in exact order.

SEQUENCE	PROCEDURAL STEP	INSTRUCTOR-OBSERVED ACCEPTABLE PERFORMANCE (CHECK IF ACCEPTABLE)
1	Plug in to warm up. Allow about 30 minutes for the spectrophotometer to warm up.	
2	With no cuvette in the chamber, a shutter cuts off all light from passing though the cuvette chamber. Under this condition, the instrument can be adjusted to read infinite absorbance (%T) by rotating the zero adjust knob. Do not touch this knob again during the rest of this procedure.	
3	Select the desired wavelength of light at which absorbance will be determined by rotating the wavelength selection knob until the desired wavelength is reached. A wavelength of 550 nm can be chosen to start the procedure.	
4	Fill the B (blank) cuvette with distilled water. Wipe the cuvette with a soft tissue and insert into the cuvette chamber. Align the mark on the cuvette to face you. *Optional:* Cover the cuvette chamber.	
5	Rotate the blank adjust knob (front right knob) to adjust absorbance to read zero.	
6	Remove the cuvette and place in a test tube rack. To have a matched set of cuvettes for reading, repeat step 4. The percent transmittance (%T) should remain at 100%T. If not, select another cuvette. Scratches on the cuvette can alter correct readings.	
7	Fill up another cuvette about three-fourths full with colored solution. Wipe the cuvette clean with a soft tissue and insert into the chamber, aligning mark to the front. Note that the scale for absorbance is the lower scale on the dial and should be read from right to left.	
8	For all readings of the dial, stand directly in front of the spectrophotometer. Record the %T or absorbance (OD) of the solution.	
9	To read additional specimens, you must reinsert the water blank cuvette and confirm that the spectrophotometer is still set at 100%T.	
10a	To locate the wavelength with the greatest absorption: After confirming that distilled water is 100%T, place the colored solution cuvette into the spectrophotometer. Rotate the absorbance dial until it displays the greatest absorbance. Begin at one end of the spectrum (for example, 400 nm) and increase the wavelength by 50 nm each time. Read absorbance and record. Once the wavelength of interest has been identified (see Table 1-A), repeat the process of reading and recording absorbance in smaller steps.	

(Continued)

Turgeon: Linné & Ringsrud's Clinical Laboratory Science, 8th Edition

STUDENT PROCEDURE WORKSHEET 8-1

SEQUENCE	PROCEDURAL STEP	INSTRUCTOR-OBSERVED ACCEPTABLE PERFORMANCE (CHECK IF ACCEPTABLE)
10b	NOTE: Sample color provides a good indication of what wavelength region to use. A yellow solution absorbs light in the 400- to 500-nm region. A red solution absorbs light between 500 and 600 nm, and blue solutions absorb light in the 600- to 700-nm range. A nanometer (nm) equals 10^{-9} meter.	
	When actually doing an assay with high and low concentration, check to be sure there is enough difference in absorbance between low and high analyte concentrations by measuring other standard solutions with expected low and high concentrations.	
11	Remove the final cuvette from the spectrophotometer, carefully rinse the cuvettes with distilled water. Store spectrophotometer cuvettes, keeping them separate from regular test tubes.	
12	If the instrument is stored on the benchtop, cover with a dust cover. Otherwise, unplug and place on a storage shelf.	

Procedural Evaluation

Student's Name ______________________ Grade ________

Instructor's Signature ______________________ Date ________

Comments:

TABLE 1-A

WAVELENGTH (nm)	ABSORBANCE
550	0.477
500	0.762
450	0.355
400	0.134

WAVELENGTH (nm)	ABSORBANCE
520	0.748
515	0.759
510	0.780
505	0.771
500	0.771
495	0.651
490	0.590

TABLE 1-B

WAVELENGTH	ABSORBANCE
512	0.769
511	0.773
510	0.780
509	0.787
508	0.781
507	0.764

Turgeon: Linné & Ringsrud's Clinical Laboratory Science, 8th Edition

STUDENT PROCEDURE WORKSHEET 8-1

Using the Spectrophotometer

Review Questions

1. What is the purpose of the distilled water blank?

2. What are the wavelength ranges for the colors-yellow, red and blue?

Turgeon: Linné & Ringsrud's Clinical Laboratory Science, 8th Edition

STUDENT PROCEDURE WORKSHEET 8-2

Preparing a Standard Curve

Read Chapter 8 in *Linné & Ringsrud's Clinical Laboratory Science: Concepts, Procedures, and Clinical Applications,* 8th edition, for a complete discussion of this topic.

Student Learning Outcomes

After reading Chapter 8 and at the completion of this laboratory exercise and review questions, a student will be able to:

- Prepare a standard curve with linear or semilog paper.
- Use a prepared curve to determine the concentrations for control and patient specimens.
- Correctly complete the end-of-procedure review questions with a grade of 80% or higher.

Equipment and Supplies

1. Linear graph paper
2. Semilog graph paper
3. Pencil or pen
4. Ruler
5. Various colored solutions
6. Cuvettes

Instructions for the Procedure

Read the list of required equipment and supplies and the procedural steps. Follow the procedural steps in exact order.

SEQUENCE	PROCEDURAL STEP	INSTRUCTOR-OBSERVED ACCEPTABLE PERFORMANCE (CHECK IF ACCEPTABLE)
1	Review an example of the preparation of standards for various concentrations to be used for manual preparation of a standard curve (see Results table below).	
2	Review the absorbance (OD) values obtained as the result of chemical analysis (see Results table below).	
Absorbance Method (Steps 3-5)		
3	Select a piece of regular linear graph paper. Use the *x*-axis (horizontal axis) for concentration. Determine the spacing between the grid lines by trial and error, depending on the usual concentrations for a specific procedure. The spaces between grid lines must consistently express units of concentrations. Use the *y*-axis (vertical axis) for absorbance (linear paper). The amount of spacing for absorbance readings is often determined through trial and error.	
4	Plot the points and draw the best straight line through the points beginning with bottom left corner lines as the anchor for the straight line.	
5	Once a standard curve has been prepared, the control and patient serum results can be read from the graph.	
Patient specimens	Determine the concentrations for each of the unknown (patient) specimens. Report results to instructor: Patient #1 0.150 Patient #2 0.444 Patient #3 0.230 Patient #4 0.600	

NOTE: To calculate a patient value rather from a graph, choose the stock standard dilution with the closest absorbance to the unknown patient specimen. Use the following formula:

$$\frac{\text{Absorbance (OD) of standard}}{\text{Concentration of standard}} = \frac{\text{Absorbance (OD) of unknown}}{\text{Concentration of unknown } (x)}$$

Example formula:

$$\frac{0.211}{100\text{ mg/dL}} = \frac{0.222}{x}$$

Patient value = 105 mg / dL

Turgeon: Linné & Ringsrud's Clinical Laboratory Science, 8th Edition

STUDENT PROCEDURE WORKSHEET 8-2

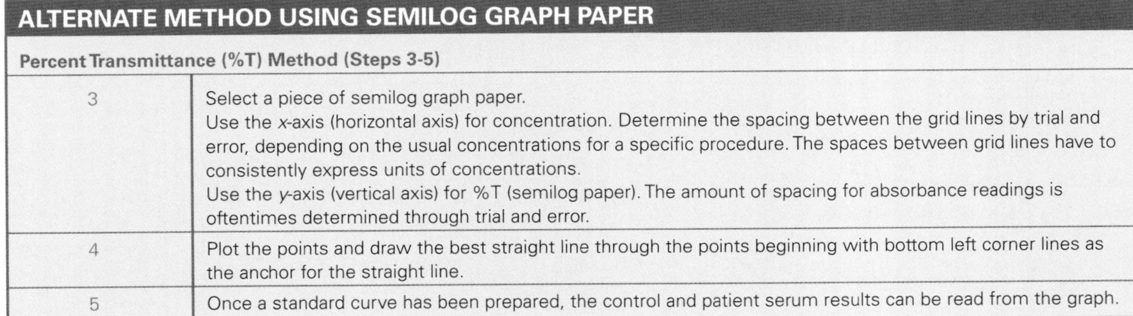

ALTERNATE METHOD USING SEMILOG GRAPH PAPER

Percent Transmittance (%T) Method (Steps 3-5)	
3	Select a piece of semilog graph paper. Use the *x*-axis (horizontal axis) for concentration. Determine the spacing between the grid lines by trial and error, depending on the usual concentrations for a specific procedure. The spaces between grid lines have to consistently express units of concentrations. Use the *y*-axis (vertical axis) for %T (semilog paper). The amount of spacing for absorbance readings is oftentimes determined through trial and error.
4	Plot the points and draw the best straight line through the points beginning with bottom left corner lines as the anchor for the straight line.
5	Once a standard curve has been prepared, the control and patient serum results can be read from the graph.

RESULTS FOR STANDARDS, CONTROLS, AND PATIENTS: ABSORBANCE AND PERCENT TRANSMITTANCE VALUES

CONCENTRATION OF STOCK STANDARD SOLUTION (mg/dL)	% TRANSMITTANCE	ABSORBANCE (OD)
0	100	0.000
25	89.5	0.480
50	75.5	0.100
100	61.5	0.211
200	40.0	0.398
500	25.0	0.900
1000	7.0	1.155

PATIENT RESULTS

Patient #1
Patient #2
Patient #3
Patient #4

Procedural Evaluation

Student's Name ______________________ Grade ________

Instructor's Signature ______________________ Date ________

Comments:

(Continued)

Turgeon: Linné & Ringsrud's Clinical Laboratory Science, 8th Edition

STUDENT PROCEDURE WORKSHEET 8-2

Preparing a Standard Curve

Review Questions

1. Make dilutions using a 20-mg/dL stock standard solution of uric acid. Complete the table to indicate preparation of various concentrations.

CONCENTRATION (mg/dL)	STOCK STANDARD (mL)	DISTILLED H_2O	TOTAL VOLUME OF DILUTION (mL)
0	0.0	5.0	5.0
2.5			5.0
5.0			5.0
7.5			5.0
10.0			5.0
12.5			5.0
20.0	5.0	0.0	5.0

2. Plot the following points on linear graph paper. Draw the best possible straight line. Submit your graph to your instructor.

STANDARD CONCENTRATION (mg/dL)	ABSORBANCE (OD)
0	0.000
25	0.054
50	0.100
100	0.206
200	0.407
500	0.900
1000	1.250

3. If the Control–Level I is 0.178 OD and Control–Level II is 0.457 OD, what are the values for each? Are they in or out of the published control reference levels?

4. Calculate the unknown patient concentrations of protein.

	PATIENT RESULTS ABSORBANCE	PATIENT RESULTS (mg/mL)
Patient #1	0.740	
Patient #2	0.433	
Patient #3	0.101	
Patient #4	0.399	
Patient #5	0.555	

9

Laboratory Testing: From Point of Care to Total Automation

http://evolve.elsevier.com/Turgeon/clinicallab/

CHAPTER OUTLINE

LEARNING OUTCOMES

Point-of-Care Testing
- Compare the major advantages and disadvantages of point-of-care testing (POCT).
- Identify the four categories of Clinical Laboratory Improvement Amendments (CLIA) test procedures.

Non–Instrument-Based Point-of-Care Testing
- Discuss non–instrument-based testing (such as pregnancy and fecal occult blood).

Handheld POCT Equipment
- Provide examples of handheld POCT devices.
- Identify at least six characteristics to consider when selecting a POCT instrument.

Emerging Patient-Centric Technologies
- Describe the challenges of POCT growth.

Overview of Informatics
- Compare the characteristics and functions of LIMS and LIS

Communication and Network Devices
- Compare local area network (LAN) and LIS communications.

Computer Applications
- Categorize examples of preanalytical, analytical, and postanalytical testing.

Overview of Automation
- Differentiate the major benefits of laboratory automation.
- Arrange and evaluate the five steps in automated analysis.

Case Study
❖ Analyze the patient history, clinical signs and symptoms, and laboratory data for the stated case studies, answer the related critical thinking questions, and conclude the most likely diagnosis.

Review Questions
- Demonstrate comprehension of the chapter content by completing the end-of-chapter review questions with a grade of 80% or higher.

Note:
- indicates MLT and MLS core content

❖ indicates MLT (optional) and MLS advanced content

KEY TERMS

autoverification
critical values
Delta checks
functionality
laboratory information management system (LIMS)
laboratory information system (LIS)
middleware
point-of-care testing (POCT)
provider-performed microscopy (PPM)
radio frequency identification device (RFID)
waived test

POINT-OF-CARE TESTING

For many years, the majority of laboratory testing was performed in a central laboratory. This was necessary because of the complexity of testing. With bar-code, network, and microcontroller technology, testing has emerged from the laboratory and is now taking place at the patient's bedside and at other nonlaboratory sites.

Point-of-care testing (POCT) or near-testing is defined as laboratory assays performed near the patient, wherever that may be. This type of off-site laboratory testing is also known as *near-patient testing* or *decentralized testing*. POCT offers the potential major advantage of reduced turnaround time of test results, which can improve patient management. The major drawback is cost. Other areas of concern include maintenance of quality control (QC) and quality assurance (QA) and proper integration of data (connectivity) into the patient's medical record.

The Importance of Decentralized Laboratory POCT Assays

Diagnostic laboratory tests are required to meet the health care needs of global populations. They are critical to the management of communicable and noncommunicable diseases, to the surveillance of emerging infectious threats such as the Ebola and Zika viruses, and to the safe and rational use of essential medicines, as identified by the World Health Organization (WHO). For each core of medical conditions, diagnostic tests considered essential for at least one of the following:
- Diagnosing the condition for which the medicine is indicated,
- Monitoring for medication efficacy, or
- Monitoring for medication toxicity.

The WHO has identified 147 essential laboratory tests (EDLs), which are sorted into 57 categories.[1] From this comprehensive inventory, 19 laboratory tests with the highest number of applications in essential medicine have been ranked (see Box 9.1). Some of the test categories have applications in more than one type of condition. Some of the tests deemed essential will probably be too expensive for resource-challenged countries to sustain. EDLs represent tests that should be reasonably available for people who need them, in the form of POCT or high-complexity reference laboratory tests.

BOX 9.1 Ranking of Selected Essential Diagnostics Laboratory (EDL) Tests[1,2]

1. Complete blood count
2. Liver enzymes
3. Renal function
4. Microscopy
5. Urinalysis
6. Nucleic acid testing (microbiology)
7. Electrolytes
8. Microbiology culture and sensitivity
9. Glucose
10. Antigen testing in microbiology
11. Serology
12. Human chorionic gonadotropin
13. Bacterial biochemical typing
14. Lipid panel
15. CD4+ lymphocyte count
16. Blood gases
17. Coagulation testing
18. Hemoglobin A_{1c}
19. Calcium

[1]Ranked by the number of drugs on the World Health Organization (WHO) List of Essential Medicines (2017) that satisfy the health care needs of the population and that are intended to be available at all times and at a price an individual and community can afford. 20th WHO Essential Medicines List (EML), World Health Organization (WHO), Geneva, Switzerland, March 2017.
[2]Schroeder LF, Guarner J, Elbireer A, et al.: Time for a model list of essential diagnostics, *N Engl J Med* 374(26):2511–2514, 2016.

Purpose and Cost

As the development of new POCT assays continues, it is important to assess the purpose of POCT versus traditional laboratory-based testing. Why is POCT being performed instead of routine laboratory testing? Advantages of POCT include the following:

- Patient convenience
- Smaller blood specimen required
- Faster turnaround time; testing performed near the patient
- Reduction of length of hospital stay
- Improved patient care management
- Easy-to-operate equipment

An appropriate POCT in the emergency department (ED), for example, may prevent the unnecessary admission of a patient into the hospital. Although POCT may appear to be beneficial, the downside of its low volume of tests may result in concerns about the proficiency of the testing personnel and may cause reagents and controls to outdate before reasonable usage, thus escalating costs. In determining the cost of a POCT program, one must look at the whole process of patient care rather than only at the cost of an individual POCT method versus the cost of the laboratory test method. Factors that should be assessed include the following[1]:

- Cost of training the testing personnel and maintenance of competency
- Labor associated with processing and analyzing the specimen
- Labor associated with maintaining the equipment
- Annual reagent, control, maintenance, and depreciation costs
- Costs of state licensing according to volume and test complexity
- Costs of proficiency programs for testing performed

Quality Control and Regulations

The use of instruments with stable calibration curves is important; a QC program should be available from the manufacturer. Data from the analyzing instruments should provide the necessary documentation of laboratory results. QC information can also be stored for confirmation of measurement validity. The instrument should be easy to use, and because staff members in many physician office laboratories have minimal or no laboratory training, limited training should be required for users of the instrument. The reagents, whether wet or dry, should be bar-coded, prepackaged, and stable for at least 6 months.

All sites performing laboratory testing are regulated under the Clinical Laboratory Improvement Amendments of 1988 (CLIA '88) and must be licensed to perform any testing they do. CLIA has granted deemed status to approved accreditation organizations and exempt states and allows these entities to accredit or license testing sites.[2] State and city governments may enact regulations, including those regarding qualifications of personnel performing the tests, which may be more, but not less, stringent than federal regulations.

Waived Testing

Diagnostic testing not performed within a traditional laboratory is called *waived testing* by TJC. CLIA '88 subjects all clinical laboratory testing to federal regulation and inspection. According to CLIA, test procedures are grouped into one of the following four categories: waived tests, moderately complex tests, highly complex tests, or provider-performed microscopy (PPM) tests (Table 9.1).

TABLE 9.1 CLIA Categories of Laboratory Testing

Category	Description
CLIA waived tests	Simple procedures with little chance of negative outcomes if performed inaccurately
CLIA moderately complex tests	More complex than waived tests but usually automated, such as blood counts and routine chemistries
CLIA highly complex tests	Usually are nonautomated or complicated tests requiring considerable judgment, such as microbiology or crossmatching of blood
CLIA PPM tests	Slide examinations of freshly collected body fluids

PPM, Provider-performed microscopy https://www.cms.gov.

A site performing only waived tests must have a Certificate of Waiver license from CLIA but will not be routinely inspected. The site must, however, adhere to manufacturers' instructions for performing the test. Good Laboratory Practice according to CLIA dictates appropriate-quality testing practices as outlined under the moderate- and high-complexity test requirements. These include the training of testing personnel, competency evaluation, and performance of QC. The Veterans Administration, College of American Pathologists (CAP), and The Joint Commission (TJC) do not recognize the waived category. These accreditation organizations have guidelines for waived testing and other POCT that must be met.[3]

Test complexity is determined by criteria that assess knowledge, training, reagent and material preparation, operational technique, QA/QC characteristics, maintenance and troubleshooting, and interpretation and judgment. Any over-the-counter test approved by the U.S. Food and Drug Administration (FDA) is automatically placed into the waived category. POCT falls within either the waived or the moderately complex category. However, the examination and interpretation associated with it, such as collecting and Gram-staining a specimen, can be classified as highly complex testing.

Evaluation of Quality

All laboratory testing must meet the same quality standards, regardless of where it is performed. Specific federal government regulatory requirements for waived testing include a Certificate of Waiver or application for a Certificate of Waiver, permission for inspections by the U.S. Department of Health and Human Services (HHS), evaluation of complaints by the public, and other requirements (42CFR 493.35 and 493.37). Waived testing must follow the manufacturer's instructions. Moderately complex POCT must meet the requirements listed for waived tests, plus instrument validation is required for each new instrument.[3]

Voluntary participation in QA programs can be another option. The Centers for Disease Control and Prevention invited providers to participate in a QA testing program for human immunodeficiency virus (HIV) that offers external performance evaluation for rapid tests. Ultimate responsibility and control of POCT reside with the CLIA-certified laboratory, which is

TABLE 9.2 Bedside Glucose Testing Systems

Vendor	Name of Instrument	Website
Abbott Diabetes Care	Precision Xceed Pro Blood Glucose and beta-Ketone Monitoring System	www.abbottdiabetescare.com
Arkray	Assure Platinum	www.arkayusa.com
	Assure 4	
HemoCue	Glucose 201 DM Analyzer	www.hemocue.com
	Glucose 201 Analyzer	
Medtronic Diabetes	iPro2 Professional CGM	www.medtronicdiabetes.com
Nova Biomedical	StatStrip Hospital Glucose Monitoring System	www.novabiomedical.com
Roche Diagnostics	Accu-Chek Inform II System	www.roche-diagnostics.us
	AccuData GTS	
	Accu-Chek Inform System	

Modified data from *CAP Today, March 2013*. Accessed October 14, 2018.

required to have a minimum of one credentialed laboratory staff member on-site who is responsible for each POCT program (such as glucose testing).

Written policies and procedures must be available for patient preparation, specimen collection and preservation, instrument calibration, QC and remedial actions, equipment performance evaluations, test performance, and results reporting and recording. The greatest source of error is preanalytical error, especially in the categories of patient identification and specimen collection.

Patient-Centric Laboratory Testing

An early example of decentralized health care is patient self-monitoring and managing of blood glucose levels using blood glucose meters or wearable continuous glucose monitors (Table 9.2). New technologies continue to expand the range of POCT.

A challenge for POCT growth is the current regulatory and CLIA '88 accreditation requirements, which were originally developed for the central laboratory, not for POCT in various settings. Hospital requirements for CLIA-waived devices are based on testing requirements developed for laboratory test systems. CLIA-waived self-testing does not require QA or proficiency testing, but in a hospital-based laboratory, both QA and proficiency testing are required.

In 2016, the FDA published the new final guidelines, "Blood Glucose Monitoring Test Systems for Prescription Point-of-Care Use" and "Self-Monitoring Blood Glucose Test Systems for Over-the-Counter Use." This was the first time that performance guidelines clearly differentiated the requirements for both types of CLIA-waived devices for professional or prescription use in a hospital or other professional care setting.

Personal Direct-to-Consumer Genetic Testing

The FDA approved marketing for 23andMe personal genome service genetic health risk (GHR) tests. These are the first direct-to-consumer tests that analyze DNA from a user's saliva to calculate genetic predisposition to 10 diseases or conditions (see Box 9.2). Risk associated with the tests includes false-positive and false-negative findings.

BOX 9.2 DNA Testing for Ten Conditions or Diseases with Genetic Predisposition

Alpha-1 antitrypsin deficiency
Celiac disease
Early-onset primary dystonia
Factor XI deficiency
Gaucher disease type 1
Glucose-6-phosphate dehydrogenase deficiency
Hereditary hemochromatosis
Hereditary thrombophilia
Late-onset Alzheimer disease
Parkinson disease

Food and Drug Administration, Release: FDA allows marketing of first direct-to-consumer tests that provide genetic risk information for certain conditions, www.fda.gov, April, 2017, updated March, 2018.

NON–INSTRUMENT-BASED POINT-OF-CARE TESTING

Ultralow-Cost Diagnostics

In resource-challenged countries, there is a widely recognized problem of insufficient laboratory testing capacity. In the absence of diagnostic tests, primary care providers are forced to relay on clinical symptoms that can often overlap between conditions. For example, children with malaria, bacterial sepsis or pneumonia may have indistinguishable symptoms. The problem of resolving inadequate laboratory testing must be addressed as a global healthcare delivery goal.

There is an additional urgent need for POCT diagnostic testing for sexually transmitted infections where the disease burden is the greatest. The acronym, ASSURED, has been developed to summarize the qualities desired in new POCT diagnostics. These qualities are: affordability, sensitivity, specificity, user-friendliness, rapidity, robustness, equipment-free, and the ability to deliver diagnostics to those who need them.[3]

The stability, size, and ease of use of the test are important, but the key is reducing costs (see Table 9.3). An example would be an inexpensive, user-friendly diagnostic platform for detecting the Zika virus. Ultimately, the development of such in-field

TABLE 9.3 Ultra-Low Cost Diagnostics

Name	Principle	Reference
The Paperfuge	A paper disc and strong rotates up to speeds of 125,000 rpm and can separate malaria parasites from red blood cells in 15 minutes.	https://www.who.int/features/factfiles/malaria/en/
The Foldscope	An optical microscope that can provide over 2,000x magnification. It is constructed from a flat sheet of papers, takes under 10 minutes to construct by following a series of folding steps.	https://www.kickstarter.com/
Multifunctional Lab-on-a-Chip	This 1 cent device is a combination of microfluidics, electronics, and inkjet printing technology which requires no clean room or trained personnel to create. It can separate cells based on their intrinsic electrical properties.	https://med.stanford.edu/
Cell-free, paper-based sensors for Zika for molecular diagnostics	This device is for strain-specific detection of Zika virus. After RNA amplification, blood droplets are applied to paper discs, which change color if Zika virus is present. The cost ranges from U.S. $ 0.10 to $1/test.	Rapid, Low-Cost Detection of Zika Virus Using Programmable Biomolecular Components. Pardee K, Green AA, Takahashi MK, et. al. Cell. 2016 May 19;165(5):1255–66. https://www.sciencedirect.com
A Paper-Based Biochip to Detect Whooping Cough	This is a 3D microfluidic point-of-care biochip which uses samples from nasal swabs to detect the presence o of the bacteria in under one hour. The device uses DNA amplification technology and has demonstrated a high sensitivity and specificity with results comparable to PCR.	https://www.cdc.gov/pertussis/countries/
Portable Zika Test	This device made from paper or plastic-based materials uses is the size of a tablet, uses saliva specimens to detect Zika in 15 minutes.	http://www.the-scientist.com https://www.acs.org/

testing for Zika and similar pathogens could help governments stay ahead of outbreaks and epidemics, curbing the spread of disease and lessening the burden on already challenged health care delivery systems.

Nonautomated POCT

POCT can be performed by nonautomated or automated methods. POCT may be done by manual rapid test methods such as those for pregnancy, occult blood, and infectious mononucleosis (Fig. 9.1). More rapid tests are being developed for the identification of infectious organisms (such as group A streptococcus and HIV) and cardiac markers (such as troponin). One example of an FDA-approved immunoassay for the detection of cardiac markers (free and complex troponins) in EDs, hospital settings, and point-of-care situations is Instant-View by Alfa Scientific Designs.

Most non–instrument-based tests apply the principles of competitive and noncompetitive immunoassay, enzymatic assay, or chemical reactions with a visually read endpoint. Tests for pregnancy (see procedure at http://evolve.elsevier.com/Turgeon/clinicallab), drugs of abuse, cardiac markers, and occult fecal blood (see Student Procedure Worksheet 9.1) are included in this category, and, tests using urine dipsticks or various microbial agents (such as the Rapid West Nile Virus IgM test by Spectral Diagnostics); testing for *Helicobacter pylori* (Fig. 9.2) is included. Manual entry of data into the medical record is the only mechanism available for non–instrument-based POCT systems.

The POCT assays usually test whole blood, although urine, feces, saliva, or throat swabs can also be tested. Rapid testing materials or kits are available in all of the diagnostic specialties

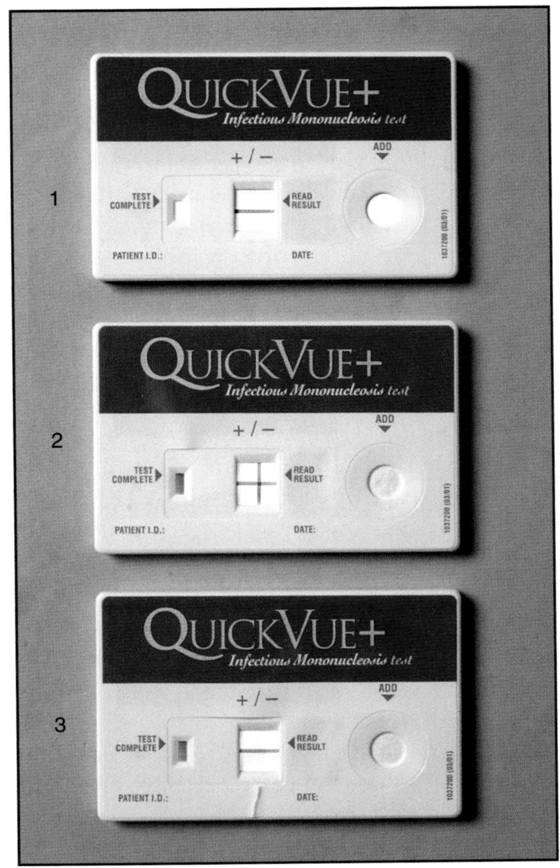

Fig. 9.1 Infectious mononucleosis test. (From Garrels M, Oatis CS: *Laboratory testing for ambulatory settings: a guide for health care professionals,* ed 2, Philadelphia, 2010, Saunders, Procedure 7–2D, p. 223.)

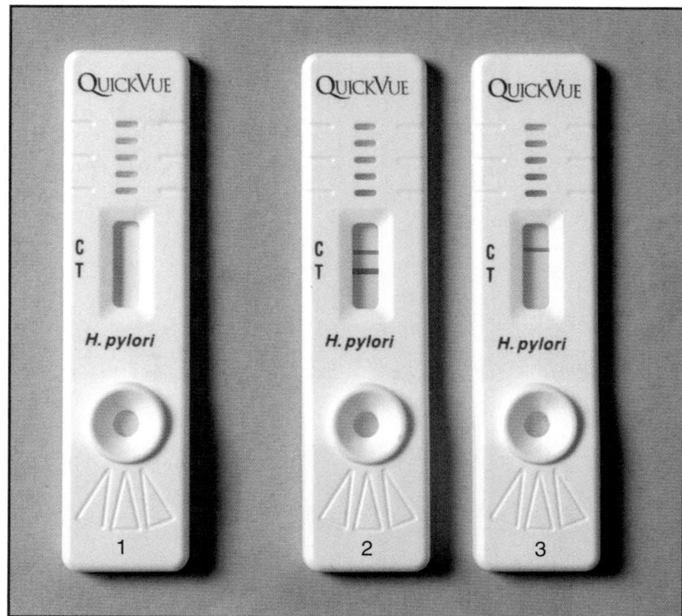

Fig. 9.2 *Helicobacter pylori* **test kit.** (From Garrels M, Oatis CS: *Laboratory testing for ambulatory settings: a guide for health care professionals*, ed 2, Philadelphia, 2010, Saunders, Procedure 7–3B, p. 224.)

of the clinical laboratory. An example of a recently CLIA-waived assay for HIV, which can test oral fluid plasma, and whole blood, is OraQuick Advance HIV-1/2 (www.oraquick.com). This rapid antibody test is a single-use qualitative immunoassay to detect antibodies to HIV types 1 (HIV-1) and 2 (HIV-2).

Pregnancy Tests

Pregnancy tests are designed to detect minute amounts of human chorionic gonadotropin (hCG), a glycoprotein hormone secreted by the trophoblast of the developing embryo that rapidly increases in the urine or serum during early stages of pregnancy. Many pregnancy test kits contain monoclonal antibody (mAb) directed against the beta subunit of the glycoprotein (β-hCG) to increase the specificity of the reaction.

Beta–Human Chorionic Gonadotropin

For the first 6 to 8 weeks after conception, β-hCG helps maintain the corpus luteum and stimulate the production of progesterone. In a normal pregnancy, detectable amounts of about 25 mIU/mL β-hCG are secreted 2 to 3 days (48–72 hours) after implantation, or approximately 8 to 10 days after conception or fertilization. Peak levels are reached approximately 2 to 3 months after the last menstrual period. Levels rise rapidly after conception. If a test is negative at this stage, the test should be repeated within 1 week. Most specimens will contain enough β-hCG for detection by the twelfth day after a missed period. Some test methods (such as enzyme-linked immunosorbent assay [ELISA]) use serum and detect increases in β-hCG much earlier, often within days of conception.

Specimen Collection

Most of the kits currently can be used for both serum and urine β-hCG but show better sensitivity with serum, because the concentration of β-hCG in serum is not subject to the wide variation found in urine β-hCG as a result of changes in urine concentration. Urine for the hCG assay (pregnancy test) must be collected at a suitable time after fertilization to allow the concentration of the hormone to rise to a significant detectable level. The first morning urine specimen is required because it contains the highest concentration of hormone. It should have a specific gravity of at least 1.015. The urine specimen is collected in a clean glass or plastic container. It may be refrigerated for up to 2 days or frozen at −20°C for at least 1 year. Thaw frozen samples by placing the frozen specimen in a water bath at 37°C, and then mix thoroughly before use. If turbidity or precipitation is present after thawing, filtering or centrifuging is recommended. Specimens containing blood, large amounts of protein, or excessive bacterial contamination should not be used. Do not refreeze.

Types of Pregnancy Tests

Immunologic pregnancy tests are done in one of several ways. Generally, these tests are easy to perform with blood or urine samples. A variety of commercial kits are available (Fig. 9.3).

Enzyme Immunoassays

Several ELISA tests are available as a result of mAb technology. In these tests, two types of mAb are used. One is a β-hCG–specific antibody bound to a membrane or other solid support medium. This can be a membrane in a tube or on a disk. The characteristics of nitrocellulose, nylon, or other membrane material can be used to enhance the speed and the sensitivity of ELISA reactions. An absorbent material below the membrane can help pull the liquid reactants through the membrane and help separate components that have not reacted from those that

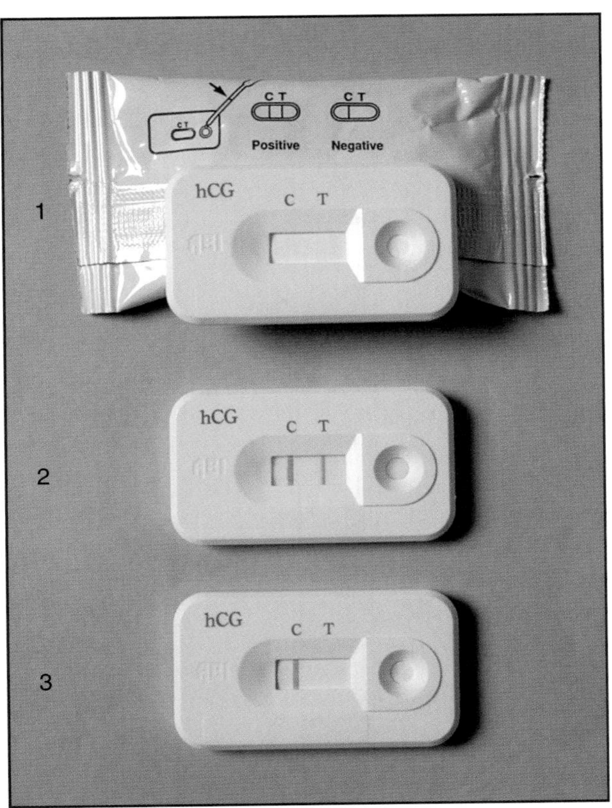

Fig. 9.3 Pregnancy testing. (From Garrels M, Oatis CS: *Laboratory testing for ambulatory settings: a guide for health care professionals,* ed 2, Philadelphia, 2010, Saunders, Procedure 7–1B, SureStep Pregnancy Test, p. 220.)

have formed antigen-antibody complexes and have bound to the membrane during the testing process. The washing steps are simplified in this way. When a specimen containing β-hCG is added (urine, plasma, serum, or whole blood can be used), the β-hCG molecules present are bound to the antibodies on the solid support membrane.

The second mAb is a β-hCG antibody that has been linked to a specific enzyme, alkaline phosphatase (ALP). This enzyme-linked antibody is added to the testing system and will bind to a different site on the β-hCG molecule, creating a sandwich of bound antibody–β-hCG–enzyme-labeled antibody. After an incubation period, any unbound enzyme-labeled antibody is washed free. A chromogenic substrate reagent is next added, which undergoes a specific color change in the presence of the ALP enzyme, indicating the presence of β-hCG. The color change is often to blue. Variations in these tests include the use of impregnated membranes and strips.

Test results should be reported as "β-hCG positive" or "β-hCG negative," not as "pregnancy positive" or "pregnancy negative," because of the possibility of a false-positive pregnancy test reaction. False-positive results are less common with the ELISA tests. ELISAs are very sensitive, giving positive reactions as early as 10 days after conception.

Fecal (Stool) Tests

There are three types of fecal (stool) tests: fecal occult blood, fecal immunochemical, and stool deoxyribonucleic acid (sDNA).

Fecal Occult Blood Test

For the fecal occult blood test (FOBT), tiny samples of stool are put on a special card or cloth and sent to a laboratory, which uses chemicals to find blood that cannot be seen with the naked eye. With some test kits, the chemicals can be added by the individual at home. FOBT tests are low cost and should be done every year after age 50.

Fecal Immunochemical Test

The fecal immunochemical test (FIT) may be easier to do at home than FOBT, with no drug or food restrictions and simpler collection of a stool sample, but it costs more. FIT also should be done every year after age 50.

Stool DNA Test

Instead of looking for blood in the stool, the sDNA test looks for abnormal DNA from cancer or polyp cells. Of the three tests, sDNA costs the most and should be done every 5 years after age 50.

Types of FOBT

There are two types of FOBT: chemical and immunologic.

Chemical Testing. For chemical testing, a solution containing the chemical guaiac and an oxidizing chemical is used. If blood is present in the sample of stool, the mixing of the solution with blood causes the guaiac to turn visibly blue. The blue color is caused by the interaction (promoted by the oxidizing agent) of the heme portion of the hemoglobin molecule, the oxygen-carrying molecule in red blood cells (RBCs), and the guaiac.

Immunologic Testing. A sample of stool is mixed with a solution that contains an antibody to globin, the protein part of the hemoglobin molecule. The antibody is combined with a small amount of gold. When the antibody-gold complex binds to the globin in stool, the antibody-gold-globin complex settles out of the solution as a visible line on the test strip.

Chemical versus Immunologic FOBT. In comparison with immunologic FOBT, chemical FOBT is inexpensive and easy, but it has the following disadvantages:

Substances in fruits and vegetables can mimic heme and cause chemical FOBTs to be falsely positive, that is, falsely abnormal. Therefore it is necessary to restrict certain fruits and vegetables before and during the collection of stool samples.

Unlike heme, which can travel intact from the stomach or small intestine and into the stool, globin is destroyed in the small intestine. As a result, a positive chemical FOBT can be caused by bleeding anywhere in the stomach or intestines, but a positive immunologic FOBT occurs only when there is bleeding into the colon.

Therefore it is necessary to restrict red meat containing hemoglobin before and during the collection of stool samples, or the heme from the ingested meat will cause a false-positive test.

Some drugs typically cause small amounts of bleeding into the stomach or small intestine. Moreover, vitamin C and a few other drugs can cause an abnormal chemical FOBT. Therefore these drugs must be stopped before and during the collection of samples.

The immunologic FOBT has additional advantages over the chemical test. First, the immunologic test is more sensitive for blood. This means that given the same amount of blood in the stool, the immunologic FOBT will more frequently be abnormal. In other words, it will more frequently detect cancers and precancerous polyps. Second, it is more specific for blood. That is, there will be fewer abnormal tests from interfering substances in the diet, and as a result, an abnormal immunologic test will more often be caused by cancer or a precancerous polyp. As a result, less follow-up testing (such as a colonoscopy) will be necessary to pursue a falsely abnormal FOBT.

Clinical Significance

Tests for hemoglobin in fecal specimens are often referred to as *tests for occult blood.* This is because hemoglobin may be present in the feces, as evidenced by positive chemical tests for blood, but may not be detected by the naked eye. In other words, occult blood is hidden blood and requires a chemical test for its detection. Occasionally, enough blood will be present in the feces to produce a tarry black or even bloody specimen. However, even bloody specimens should be tested chemically for occult blood. In such cases the outer portion is avoided, and the central portion of the formed stool is sampled. The detection of occult blood in feces is important in determining the cause of hypochromic anemias resulting from chronic loss of blood and in detecting ulcerative or neoplastic diseases of the gastrointestinal (GI) system. Blood in the feces may result from bleeding anywhere along the GI tract, from the mouth to the anus.

Tests for occult blood are especially useful for early detection and treatment of colorectal cancer. Such tests are useful because more than half of all cancers (excluding skin) are from the GI tract. Early detection results in good survival. Persons over age 50 should be screened annually for occult blood. They sample their own stool specimens for three consecutive collections, apply a thin film to the test slides, and mail or bring them to the laboratory for testing. Dietary considerations are important to avoid false-positive results, and special instructions are generally included with the test slides. It is now less common practice for the laboratory to receive the actual fecal specimen to be tested for occult blood.

Bleeding at any point in the GI system and representing as little as 2 mL of blood lost daily may be detected by the tests for occult blood. However, false-negative results occur for unknown reasons, possibly because of inhibitors in the feces.

Implications of both false-positive and false-negative tests are important clinically. Early diagnosis and treatment of serious disease might be missed with false-negative results, resulting in poor prognosis and death. Positive results are serious and require extensive further testing to determine the cause of bleeding or to rule out false-positive reactions. Further testing is both unpleasant for the patient and expensive.

Principle and Specificity

Numerous tests have been described for the detection of hemoglobin (or blood) in both urine and feces. Most of these tests are based on the same general principles and reaction. They all

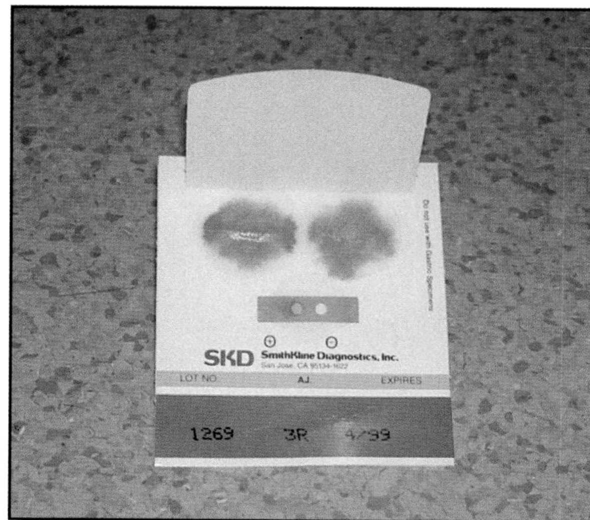

Fig. 9.4 Fecal occult blood test. (From Garrels M, Oatis CS: *Laboratory testing for ambulatory settings: a guide for health care professionals,* ed 2, Philadelphia, 2010, Saunders.)

make use of *peroxidase* activity in the heme portion of the hemoglobin molecule. As mentioned, most tests for occult blood in feces use *gum guaiac,* a phenolic compound that produces a blue color when oxidized. The tests require the presence of hydrogen peroxide (H_2O_2) or a suitable precursor. The peroxidase activity of the hemoglobin molecule results in the liberation of oxygen (O_2) from H_2O_2, and the released O_2 oxidizes gum guaiac to a blue oxidation product. The reaction (Fig. 9.4) is summarized as follows:

$$\text{Hemoglobin} + H_2O_2 \rightarrow \text{Oxygen}$$
(peroxidase activity)

$$\text{Oxygen} + \text{Reduced gum guaiac} \rightarrow$$
(colorless)

$$\text{Oxidized gum guaiac} + H_2O$$
(blue)

Interfering Substances and Dietary Considerations

Several interfering substances may give false-positive results for occult blood, including dietary substances with peroxidase activity, especially myoglobin and hemoglobin in red meat. Vegetable peroxidase, as found in horseradish, can also cause false-positive results. Several foods have been identified as causing erroneous reactions, including turnips, broccoli, bananas, black grapes, pears, plums, and melons. Cooking generally destroys these peroxidases, and therefore patients are generally instructed to eat only cooked foods. White blood cells (WBCs) and bacteria also have peroxidase activity that might result in false-positive reactions. Various drugs, including aspirin and aspirin-containing preparations and iron compounds, are known to increase GI bleeding, causing positive results. Vitamin C and other oxidants may give false-negative results.

Patients are generally instructed to eat no beef or lamb (including processed meats and liver) for 3 days before collecting the first specimen and to remain on this diet through the collection of three successive samples. They may eat well-cooked pork, poultry, and fish. They are also instructed to avoid raw fruits and vegetables, especially melons, radishes, turnips, and horseradish. Cooked fruits and vegetables are acceptable. Ingestion of high-fiber foods, such as whole-wheat bread, bran cereal, and popcorn, is encouraged. The ingestion of more than 250 mg/day of vitamin C is to be avoided because it may cause false-negative results. The mechanism of this interference is the same as for reagent strips used in urinalysis (UA). Aspirin and other nonsteroidal antiinflammatory drugs (NSAIDs) should be avoided for 7 days before and during the test period.

Guaiac Slide Test for Occult Blood

Various commercial tests have been developed to test for the presence of hemoglobin in feces. At least eight guaiac-based tests for occult blood are available commercially. The Hemoccult II (SmithKline Diagnostics), which seems to have the lowest rate of false-positive results, is described here (Student Procedure Worksheet 9.1). Other tests are similar. In all cases, the manufacturer's directions should be followed.

Hemoccult II is available as a slide test that contains filter paper uniformly impregnated with gum guaiac. The specimen is applied in a thin film in both of two boxes on the front side of the slide. This may be done by the patient or the laboratory. The specimen is applied with a wooden applicator, which is supplied with the test kit. The kit includes dietary information for the patient and instructions for collecting the specimen.

The American Cancer Society (ACS) recommends that for colorectal screening, two samples from three consecutive specimens be collected. Therefore test kits are usually supplied to patients in groups of three slides. The patient is instructed to allow the test slides to dry overnight, then return them to the physician or laboratory. The slides should be properly labeled. If the slides are to be mailed, they must be placed in an approved U.S. Postal Service mailing pouch (not a standard paper envelope).

When the slides are received in the laboratory, the specimen is tested on the back (opposite side) of the test slide. When the perforated window on the back of the slide is opened, two specimen windows plus positive and negative "performance monitor areas" (controls) are revealed. If the specimen is applied in the laboratory, it must air-dry before the developer solution is applied, to increase the sensitivity of the test. The developer solution is a stabilized mixture of H_2O_2 and denatured alcohol, which is supplied with the test. Only reagent supplied with the test slides can be used for color development. When the fecal specimen containing occult blood is applied to the guaiac-impregnated test paper, peroxidase in the specimen comes in contact with the guaiac. When the developing solution is then applied to the test paper, a reaction between the guaiac and peroxidase results in formation of a blue color.

The reaction requires that blood cells be hemolyzed for proper release of peroxidase. This usually takes place within the GI tract. If whole, undiluted blood is applied to the test paper, the RBCs may not hemolyze, and the reaction may be weak or atypical. The test is significantly more sensitive to the presence of occult blood if the specimen is allowed to dry on the slide before the developing solution is applied. The ACS recommends that slides be tested within 6 days of preparation and that the slides not be rehydrated. Also, a single positive smear should be considered a positive test result, even in the absence of dietary restriction.

HANDHELD POCT EQUIPMENT

Microprocessors in small and often handheld instruments provide automated, easy-to-perform testing with calibration and on-board QC (Tables 9.4A and B). Both handheld and small instruments may be used for testing (Fig. 9.5). Important characteristics of POCT devices are:

- Small blood sample
- Rapid turnaround time
- Easy portability with single-use disposable reagent cartridges or test strips
- Easy-to-perform protocol with one or two steps
- Accuracy and precision of results comparable to those with central laboratory analyzers
- Minimal QC tracking
- Storage at ambient temperature for reagents
- Bar-code technology for test packs, controls, and specimens
- Economical equipment cost and maintenance free
- Software for automatic calibration, system lockouts, and data management
- Hard copy or electronic data output that interfaces with a laboratory information system or other tracking software

One disadvantage of handheld POCT devices is the cost per test, which is more expensive than central laboratory testing. Errors from improper cleaning of devices between patients can produce a higher error rate for POCT than for central laboratory testing and can result in disease transmission to patients from the instruments. A challenge with waived tests is that testing is typically performed by nonlaboratory personnel. Training by laboratory professionals is essential to the accuracy of results.

Handheld or small analyzers are frequently located in intensive care units or surgery suites. Measurements taken can include glucose, blood coagulation studies such as prothrombin time (Fig. 9.6), and blood gases. Glucose testing with a portable analyzer is based on electrochemical measurement protocols that have been shown to be reliable but are affected by variability in blood hemoglobin level. Current technology uses reflectance photometry or biosensors. Optical sensing measures aggregate light from populations of targets. Some newer equipment uses non-optical sensing but it also relies on aggregate measurements of targets. The problem with aggregating measurements is that they are low in sensitivity. Sensitivity rapidly degrades as size is reduced into smaller forms. Nanopore, biological pores that are 2.5 nm in size, offer the promise of improved results from solid state nanopore sensing and measurement methods.[3]

Various forms of data output are used with POCT systems, including visual readings, display screen, printer, and various means of electronic transmission by Ethernet, infrared, and wireless radio signals such as Wi-Fi or Bluetooth.

TABLE 9.4A Examples of Handheld and Small Automated Point-of-Care Equipment for Blood Clinical Chemistry Specimen Testing

Chemistry Analysis	Assay Principle	Format	Representative Product or System (Manufacturer)
Glucose	Photometry: transmittance	Disposable individual microcuvette	HemoCue (www.hemocue.com)
Glucose	Potentiometry: electrochemistry	Biosensor strips: single test	Accu-Chek (Roche) (www.accu-chek.com)
Chemistry and drugs	Photometry: transmittance	Wet-reagent cartridges: single test	Vision (Abbott) (www.abbottdiagnostics.com)
Cardiac markers Creatine kinase-MB (CK-MB), myoglobin, and troponin I	Fluorometric enzyme immunoassay	Solid-phase radial partition immunoassay technology	Stratus CS (SCS; Dade Behring) (www.dadebehring.com)
Cardiac markers Creatine kinase-MB (CK-MB), myoglobin, and troponin I	Fluorescence immunoassay	Murine monoclonal and polyclonal antibodies against CK-MB, murine monoclonal and polyclonal antibodies against myoglobin, murine monoclonal and goat polyclonal antibodies against troponin I labeled with a fluorescent dye and immobilized on the solid phase, and stabilizers	Triage (Biosite) (www.biosite.com)
β-Type natriuretic peptide (BNP)	Fluorescence immunoassay	Murine monoclonal and polyclonal antibodies against BNP, labeled with a fluorescent dye and immobilized on the solid phase, and stabilizers	Triage BNP (Biosite) (www.biosite.com)
Blood gases and electrolytes	Electrochemical	Wet-reagent cartridges	i-STAT (Abbott) (www.abbottdiagnostics.com)
Hemoglobin A_{1c}	Coulometric biosensor technology	Test strip	Precision PCT (Abbott) (www.abbottdiagnostics.com)

TABLE 9.4B Examples of Point-of-Care Testing Blood Coagulation Analyzers

Assay	Method	Format	Representative Product or System (Manufacturer)
Prothrombin time with INR	Reflectance photometry	Test strip	Siemens https://usa.healthcare.siemens.com/point-of-care
Prothrombin time with INR	Reflectance photometry	Single-use cartridge	CoaguChek S (www.rochediagnostics.com)
Prothrombin time with INR, activated partial thromboplastin time, activated clotting time	Optical motion detection	Single-use tube containing an activator and a magnet	Hemochron Response 401/801[a] CoaguChek Pro (www.rochediagnostics.com)
Prothrombin time (PT)/INRatio Monitor	Platelet aggregation thromboelastography	Electrochemical test strip	HemoSense (www.hemosense.com)

INR, International normalized ratio.

[a]Three types of activator tubes are available. Equipment can perform thrombin time, heparin-neutralized thrombin time, high-dose thrombin time, fibrinogen, and protamine dose assay.

EMERGING PATIENT-CENTRIC TECHNOLOGIES

The Tricorder

The innovative product DxtER (pronounced "Dexter"), the 2017 winner of the Qualcomm Tricorder XPRIZE competition, is a prototype developed by Final Frontier Medical Devices. Modeled after the fictional medical tricorder from *Star Trek,* DxtER is a portable medical device designed to monitor health and diagnose illness from the comfort of home.

At the heart of DxtER is an artificially intelligent engine that learned to diagnose by integrating years of experience in clinical emergency medicine with data analysis from actual patients having a variety of medical conditions and outcomes. Included with DxtER is a collection of noninvasive sensors custom-designed to collect data on vital signs, body chemistry, and biological functions. The diagnostic engine synthesizes a patient's health data to make a quick and accurate assessment.

Technology Transfer

The National Aeronautics and Space Administration (NASA) needs compact, reliable, lightweight diagnostics for monitoring crew health on future space missions. A handful of current portable point-of-care devices provide generalized blood analysis but perform only a few tests at a time and rely on disposable components and diverse detection technologies to complete routine tests. None of these devices are suited for space travelers on extended missions.

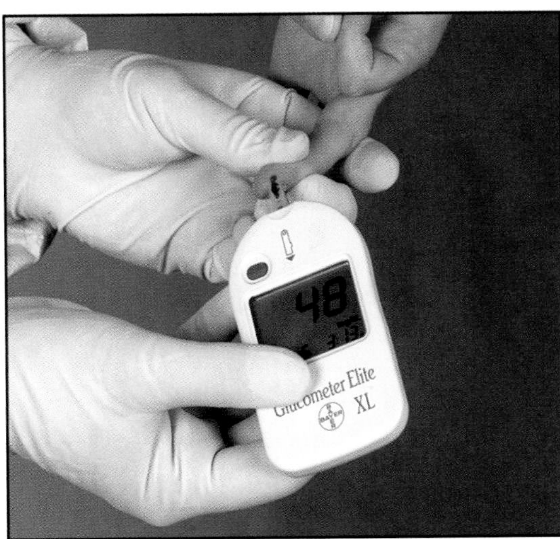

Fig. 9.5 Glucometer. (From Garrels M, Oatis CS: *Laboratory testing for ambulatory settings: a guide for health care professionals,* ed 2, Philadelphia, 2010, Saunders, Procedure 6–1B, p. 185.)

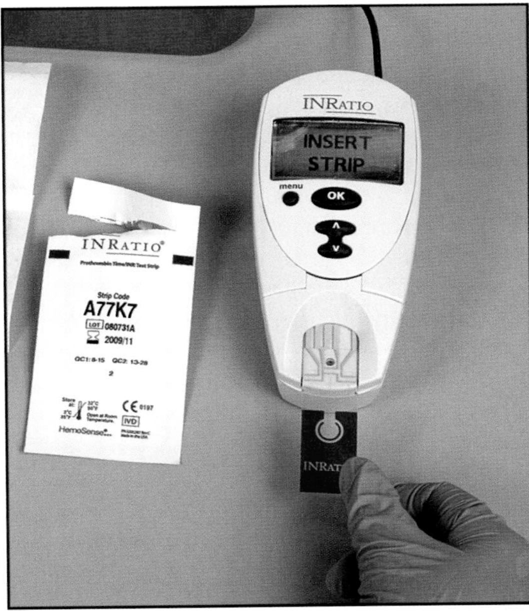

Fig. 9.6 Prothrombin time (PT) and international normalized ratio (INR). (From Garrels M, Oatis CS: *Laboratory testing for ambulatory settings: a guide for health care professionals,* ed 2, Philadelphia, 2010, Saunders, Procedure 5–6F, p. 158.)

In 2008, NASA's Glenn Research Center in Ohio and Johnson Space Center in Texas formed a technology transfer collaboration with the DNA Medicine Institute in Massachusetts. The goal of this collaboration is to seek innovative solutions to advance patient care and treat disease by drawing upon diverse and disparate fields including medicine, nanotechnology, genomics, biophysics, biochemistry, molecular biology, and advanced engineering. To date, this collaboration has produced a reusable microfluidic device that performs rapid, low-cost cell counts and measurements of electrolytes, proteins, and other biomarkers.

Microfluidics is the common thread that ties together many of the recent advancements in POCT. The microchannels associated with microfluidics are typically either etched or molded into glass, silicone, plastics, or paper and have certain qualities that can offer an advantage over traditional materials. Opko Diagnostics developed a microfluidics-based smartphone accessory that can test for HIV, syphilis, and hemoglobin. Cepheid's GeneXpert technology also employs microfluidics; a finger prick Ebola test runs on this system, and there are plans to develop finger prick HIV tests for GeneXpert Omni, a handheld molecular POCT instrument.

The reusable Handheld Electrolyte and Laboratory Technology for Humans (rHEALTH) sensor is a compact portable device that employs cutting-edge fluorescence detection optics, innovative microfluidics, and nanostrip reagents to perform 16 different tests in hematology, chemistry, or biomarker assays from a single drop of blood or bodily fluid. The limitations of testing a single drop of blood include significant variations among drops of blood collected from the same finger prick.

OVERVIEW OF INFORMATICS

Informatics software was traditionally divided into the sample-centric laboratory information management system (LIMS) and the patient-centric laboratory information system (LIS). Today there is no such thing as a "traditional" LIMS or LIS. The two systems have converged somewhat in functionality.

What Is LIMS?

A **LIMS** represents transmission of sample-centric information with the ultimate goal of providing accurate information in a timely manner to clinicians. LIMS is used because it can routinely integrate automation and data handling, provide uniform methodology with complete visibility, and lead to increased productivity and process integrity.

The essential requirements of an LIMS include secure login, flexibility to add-ons and software upgrades and, most importantly, data management. The number of laboratory tests has increased as a result of the development of new diagnostic assays and the increased use of automated, high-volume instruments and handheld devices. Because of the dramatic increase in the number of assays performed in the clinical laboratory and by POCT, and because these assays have produced so much analytical information, the ability to process this information efficiently and accurately has become essential.

LabWare of Wilmington, Delaware, is an example of an LIMS product with features to support clinical laboratory workflow, instrument interfacing, sampling, and aliquoting. This product allows for the addition of patient management features that enable the system to be patient-centric, while maintaining all sample management and tracking capabilities.

It is not possible to discuss LIMS without discussing automation. *Automation* describes an instrumental system that involves the mechanization of discrete processes and is "noninterventional" of self-regulating and self-timing. Many automated techniques make use of robotized units, as is typically seen in a QC

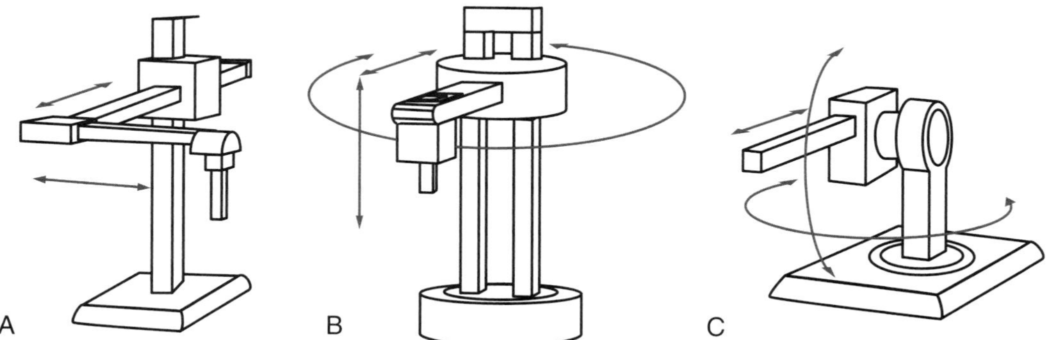

Fig. 9.7 Robotic arm performing sample handling. (From Burtis CA, Ashwood ER, Bruns DE: Tietz fundamentals of clinical chemistry, ed 6. Philadelphia, 2008, Saunders, Fig. 11.3, p. 181.)

BOX 9.3 Examples of Large Laboratory and Hospital Information Systems

Antek Healthware	www.antekhealthware.com
Cerner Corp.	www.cerner.com
Computer Service & Support (LIS Systems)	www.csslis.com
COVE Laboratory Software	www.covelab.com
Dawning Technologies	www.dawning.com
LabSoft	www.labsoftweb.com
Meditech	www.meditech.com
Orchard Software	www.orchardsoft.com
Psyche Systems Corporation	www.psychesystems.com
Sunquest Systems	www.sunquestinfo.com
Sysmex America	www.sysmex.com/usa/

Partial listing of information systems from *Medical Laboratory Observer*. Clinical Laboratory Reference 2009 to 2010, Laboratory Information Systems.

laboratory for procedures that are susceptible to gross method errors. *Robotics* describes the use of instrument management systems and the way in which information is handled. More recent revisions have produced *automated robotized systems* (Fig. 9.7) capable of handling multichannel information sources while running selected instruments.

Many LIMS vendors have developed systems for large and small clinical laboratories and off-site locations (Box 9.3). Every November, the CAP publishes a detailed survey of more than 35 LIMS (www.cap.org). Software products use process automation, robust interfaces, and rules-based technology to address regulatory issues, improve efficiency, reduce errors, and increase reimbursements.

What Is LIS?

The LIS is the tool for delivery of these laboratory data. The LIS is the integration of computers through a common database via various communication networks. When automated instruments are interfaced or point-of-care equipment is connected to an LIS, productivity improves and the risk for errors decreases because the data are delivered directly to a patient's record for physician review and to other departments, such as medical records and billing.

LIS can be applied to many laboratory-related preanalytical, analytical, and postanalytical functions: specimen processing, inventory control, QC, online monitoring, data entry on patient charts, and data interpretation. Advances in functionality of LIS with new technology are changing the approach to some fundamental laboratory tasks. LIS systems have incorporated more and more of what in the past would have been considered to be LIMS features. Some LIS systems now have full capability to manage the testing and samples that are taken as part of a patient's records. More LIS systems now allow those samples to be tracked for location and status of testing, and more LIS systems are now capable of importing data from instruments and other sources.

Technology-driven enhancements in LIS include the following[4]:

- QC storage and functionality
- Support of comprehensive analyzer interface, including calculations
- Tools to aid in compliance with regulations for laboratory procedures
- Capability to share data with third-party vendors
- Automated result report dissemination to support workflow models
- Rules-based logic for decision-making support

Various LISs on the market can be assessed (Student Procedure Worksheet 9.2). The Association for Pathology Informatics LIS toolkit can be used for assessment. This toolkit consists of a 6000-word white paper plus three appendices: (1) an 850-item list of simple functionality statements that a laboratory can use to specify the complex set of tasks an LIS should perform, each paired with a weighting measure from 1 to 4 to gauge importance for the laboratories; (2) a set of scenarios that a hospital can use as scripted demonstrations to elicit possible functionality gaps during live vendor displays; and (3) a list of the various categories that need to be considered when calculating the "total cost of ownership" of any specific LIS.

Input Devices

One of the most common peripheral input/output (I/O devices is the video display monitor. Monitors are usually cathode ray tube or liquid crystal display screens; important features include the diagonal dimension, the number of pixels (picture elements), resolution, and inclusion of a touch-sensitive surface. Touch screens allow interaction with the software application and CPU through a menu. Menus are lists of programs, functions, or other options offered by the system. A cursor is moved to the point on the list (such as a list of tests) that is the option of choice and placed on the test desired. The position of touch on the screen determines the choice. A stylus, the operator's finger, or a mouse can be used to interact with a touch-sensitive screen to indicate a menu choice.

Bar Codes

Computer technology is applied to phlebotomy through bar codes verifying both the patient and the ordered tests. One system, MediCopia (Lattice), indicates the tests, appropriate tubes, and quantity of tubes required for the patient and generates bar-coded laboratory labels for tube identification at the patient's bedside. This eliminates mislabeling because the only labels available are the ones printed for that particular patient. MediCopia automatically time-stamps operations, providing physicians with valuable information on when samples were drawn. All completed draws are sent via the handheld computer back to the LIS for reconciliation. MediCopia's integrated wireless radio technology allows the caregiver to receive "nonsweep" and "stat" test orders on the handheld unit without having to return to the docking station. Some software triggers the generation of specimen labels and prints those needed for the collection process. The patient demographic information will be printed on the labels (see Fig. 9.3), along with special accession numbers in some institutions. These accession numbers will be represented in the bar-coding format for each of the patient's specimen labels. Bar coding reduces errors in specimen handling and improves productivity. For the greatest benefit, specimen bar coding is also coordinated with the automated instruments used for testing, with the sampling done directly from the primary collection tube.

After collection, the specimen is sent to the laboratory for analysis. After testing is completed, a computerized system can be used for managing specimen storage and retrieval. An example of such a system is SpecTrack (Siemens Healthcare Diagnostics), an informatics software product enabling quick and easy storage and retrieval of specimens for the laboratory. Users can find the exact storage location of any specimen from all laboratories in their network, eliminating time-consuming searches in the refrigerator or cold room.

One-dimensional (1D) bar codes are linear and consist of a series of parallel lines of varying widths. The parallel lines encode data and are read by a laser optical device known as a *scanner* or *reader*. At present, bar-code labels are critical to laboratory operations where essential patient accessioning, clinical testing, or research functions occur. Bar-code readers may be used attached as input devices. They use either manually operated light pens or laser devices that read the bars on a label and convert these data to a sequence of numbers representing specific information (Fig. 9.8). This information can be patient identification, tests requested, or identification of a reagent for a test. Bar codes are being used on identification wristbands, allowing for better control of accuracy with patient identification, and on labels for specimen containers and test requests.

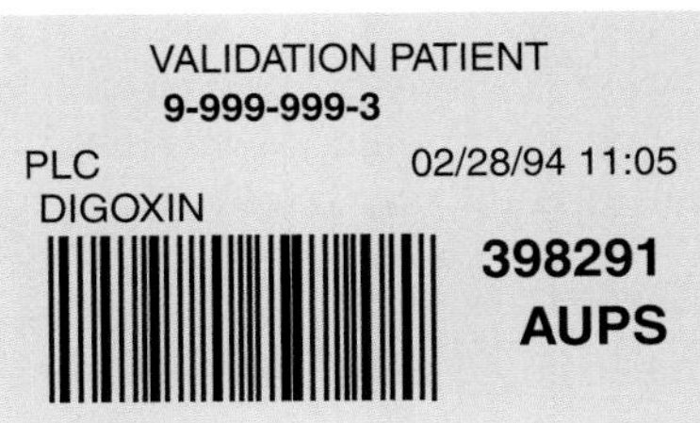

Fig. 9.8 Bar code.

The newest development in bar codes is the growing popularity of two-dimensional (2D) bar codes in the United States and Japan. A 2D bar code is nonlinear and consists of black-and-white "cells" or "modules" arranged in a matrix pattern—typically a square—which in turn encapsulates a "finder" pattern and a "reader" pattern. These 2D symbols are omnidirectionally scannable—upside down, backward or forward, and even diagonally.

A 2D bar code can store every bit of patient information in a tiny symbol that is 2 to 3 mm square, because 2D bar codes can store thousands of characters. The symbology of 2D bar codes is not as susceptible to printing defects or errors as traditional 1D bar codes. The coding pattern has a high level of redundancy, with the data dispersed in several locations throughout the symbology. This enables the bar code to be scanned correctly even if a portion of it has printed lightly or is missing altogether.

Specialized equipment is required to print 2D bar codes. The best printer for 2D labels is a direct thermal or thermal transfer printer. In addition, 2D bar codes cannot be read by a laser scanner but must be scanned by an image-based scanner employing a charge-coupled device or some other digital-camera sensor technology.[5]

Three-dimensional (3D) bar codes and QR codes are also being developed.

Radio Frequency Identification Devices

A radio frequency identification device (RFID) is an automatic identification method that involves storing and retrieving data using tags or transponders (such as those used for electronic toll collection on highways). Small RFID tags attached to products contain silicon chips and antennas that enable the tags to receive and respond to radio frequency queries from an RFID transceiver. Two kinds of RFID devices exist: passive and active. Active RFIDs provide real-time location for tracking and workflow improvement. RFID is being implemented in blood transfusion applications. RFID and bar codes can be viewed as complementing each other. The choice of technology will depend on the specific application.[6]

Output Devices

Output is any information a device generates as a result of its calculations or processing. The monitor, printers, and on-board instrument displays all can function as output devices. The computer directs the needed data from a storage device to the specific output device. An electronic chart or intermediate data may be displayed on a monitor. A printer is used for the production of hard copy and longer-lasting paper-printed records. Another specific output function of the printer is generating printed labels for specimen containers at the time of order entry for a test.

Data Storage Devices

An important LIS component is the data storage section. This contains all the necessary instructions and data needed to operate the computer system. Any short-term information, such as patient records and laboratory data, may also be stored temporarily in the memory. Massive storage devices are used for long-term memory. The CAP accreditation standards require that laboratories establish methods for communication of needed information to ensure prompt, reliable reporting of results and that they have appropriate data storage and retrieval capacity.[7]

Hard drives that are mass storage devices can be disks with a magnetic surface. Other forms of data storage are optical storage disks (such as CDs and DVDs), solid-state drives, or cloud storage.

Software

Software consists of the encoded instructions for the operation of a computer. Software programs that supply basic functions of the computer are called operating system (OS) programs, such as Microsoft Windows. Software programs are stored on various forms of media (such as hard drives) for operating the program and optical disks (CD/DVD-ROMs) or in cloud storage for distribution. Those that supply special functions for the users are called application programs (Apps).

Middleware

Middleware is computer software that connects software components or applications. Middleware sits "in the middle" between application software and large central computer systems that may be working on different OSs (Box 9.4).

BOX 9.4 Laboratory Information Systems and Middleware Vendors

Apex Healthware	www.apexhealthware.com
Aspyra	www.aspyra.com
Clinical Software Solutions	www.clin1.net
COVE Laboratory Software	www.covelab.com
Cerner	www.cerner.com/laboratory
CompuGroup Medical	www.cgmus.com
LigoLab Information Systems	www.ligolab.com
Orchard Software	www.orchardsoft.com
Psyche Systems	www.psychesystems.com
Sunquest Information Systems	www.sunquestinfo.com
Middleware Vendor	
Apex Healthcare	www.apexhardware.com
Beckman Coulter	www.beckmancoulter.com
COVE Laboratory Software	www.covelab.com
Dawning Technologies	www.dawning.com
Orchard Software	www.orchardsoft.com
Psyche Systems	www.psychesystems.com
Sysmex America	www.sysmex.com

Automation enhancements have emerged as the result of middleware. Middleware can boost workflow productivity and efficiency and can offer function otherwise not possible. It can be used to do the following:

- Process specimens from multiple locations
- Automate algorithms
- Initiate repeat testing
- Implement autoverification[8–10] and QC monitoring
- Detect patient misidentification errors
- Provide alerts for critical values

COMMUNICATION AND NETWORK DEVICES

For interaction with users, an LIS uses personal computers as workstations directly connected to the server for the LIS. Most laboratories connect workstations using routers to form a local area network (LAN) that can access the LIS server or the hospital information system (HIS). Not only can workstations be networked to the main server (LAN) to facilitate network communications, but software can also be configured to integrate wide area networks (WANs). A WAN connects multisite facilities into a single network.

In most health care venues, multiple software products are employed among the various departments. The exchange of information between the computer and the user is called *interfacing.* The use of an interface allows data from one or more systems to be automatically captured by the other systems. Interfacing is accomplished through several types of devices.

Most current systems use the Health Level 7 (HL7) standard for their interfaces. The goal in using this standard is to prevent misunderstandings between the computers by defining messages and their content. The HL7 standard is used primarily for financial and medical record information. It does not address many types of clinical information or other data, such as raw data from instrument interfaces.

For laboratory use, the interface specification should include what data will be transferred, where data will be transferred, when data will be transferred, and security and encryption considerations. Interfaces are important to the laboratory because they contribute to the overall effectiveness of the computer support of laboratory operations. It is critical to remember that interfaces pass patient information between computers without direct human intervention.

Interfacing of the workstation with the analytical testing instrument allows the test result to be entered directly into the computer information system or LIS and saves laboratory time. The test results data are transferred directly over a single wired or wireless interface. A unidirectional interface transmits or uploads results; a bidirectional interface allows for simultaneous transmission or downloading of information and for the reception of uploaded information from an instrument. An example is the LifeScan Accu-Chek, a bidirectional interface that patients and laboratories can use for the management of diabetes testing. Patients can both upload their test results from a point-of-care device and download information related to their care.

An LIS is often interfaced with other information systems, most often the HIS; interfacing allows electronic communication between two workstations. The HIS manages patient census information and demographics and systems for billing, and the more complex systems process and store patient medical information. The interfacing of the HIS and the laboratory workstation facilitates the exchange of test request orders, return of analytical results (the laboratory report), and charges for the tests ordered and reported. When the data are verified, nurses or physicians in the patient care areas can retrieve results through workstations, monitors, tablets, and printers.

This linking of hospital and laboratory workstations is not easy, and totally integrated systems require an institutional commitment to the process. A well-designed, easily accessible HIS-LIS database offers significant improvements in medical record keeping, patient care planning, budget planning, and general operations management tasks (Fig. 9.9).

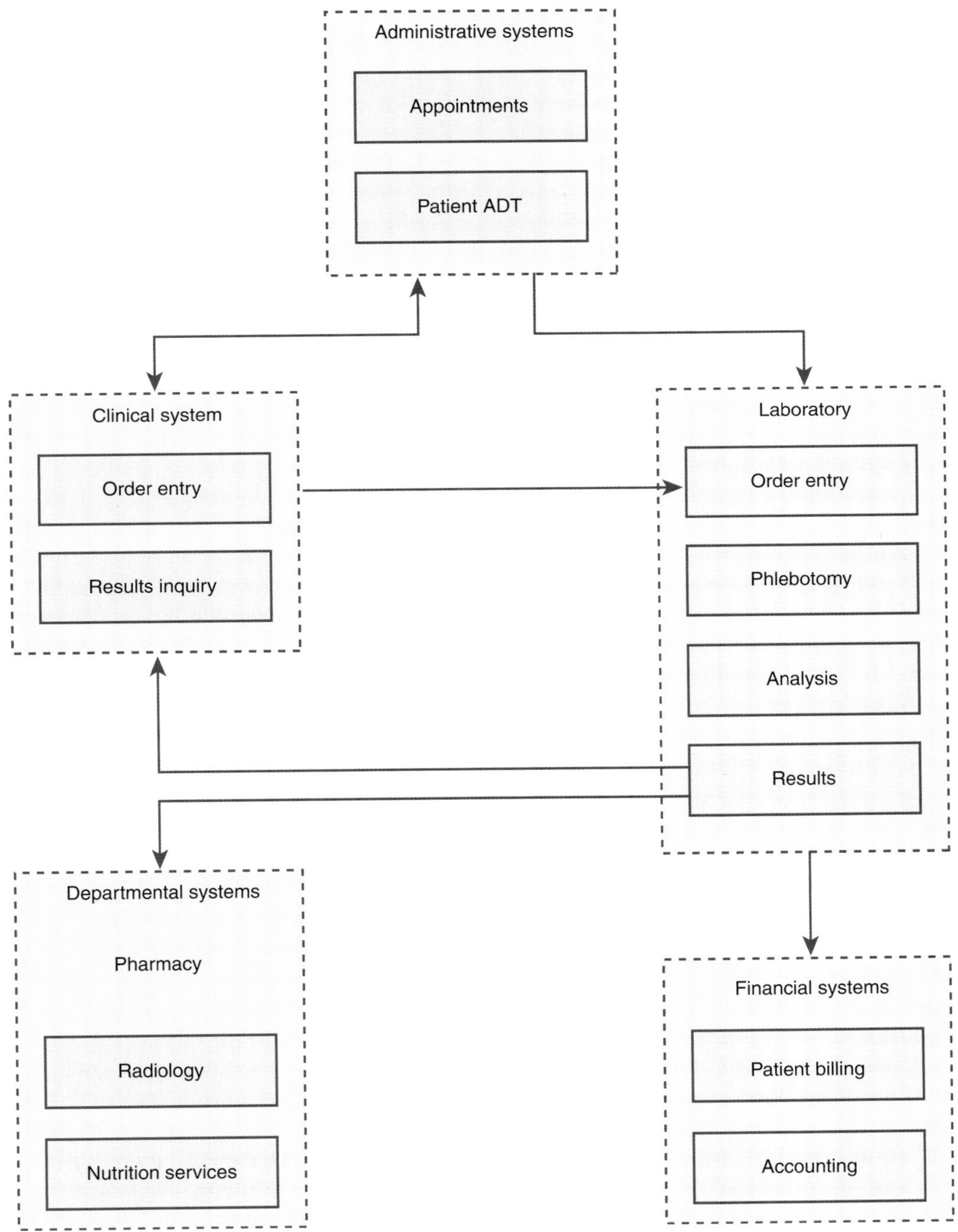

Fig. 9.9 **Interchange of information between systems.** (From Kaplan LA, Pesce AJ: *Clinical chemistry: theory, analysis, and correlation,* ed 5, St Louis, 2010, Mosby.)

Transmitting data is the primary productivity goal that any LIS system should achieve. Most systems are capable of network output of patient results to multiple locations. Many systems employ the Ethernet and Internet Wi-Fi to transmit information.

Future challenges for the clinical laboratory include interfacing and integration of information exchanged, handling of patient data through HL7 output, and validation of error-free software. Integration of information and connectivity needs continue to increase as POCT increases. Although the industry has developed many standards for information interchange, a multiplicity of information systems can still present a management and operational challenge. In addition, ensuring that the software supplied is error free and performs as specified is a crucial activity, both in the initial LIS implementation and in the installation of subsequent software releases. Most LIS vendors today utilize current Good Manufacturing Practices and are ISO 9000 certified. The laboratory should insist that its vendor follow the guidelines and procedures for software QA.

To guide the laboratory in future information technology, the Clinical and Laboratory Standards Institute (CLSI) has developed interrelated Laboratory Automation standards that address the design, compatibility, and integration of automated clinical laboratory systems worldwide and that include the following:

The Specimen Container/Specimen Carrier standard provides guidelines for designing and manufacturing specimen containers and carriers used for collecting and processing liquid samples, such as blood and urine, for clinical testing in laboratory automation systems.[11]

The Bar Codes for Specimen Container Identification standard provides specifications for using linear bar codes on specimen container tubes in the clinical laboratory and on laboratory automation systems.[12]

The Communications with Automated Clinical Laboratory Systems, Instruments, Devices, and Information Systems standard provides guidelines to facilitate the accurate and timely electronic exchange of data and information between the automated laboratory elements.[13]

The Systems Operational Requirements, Characteristics, and Information Elements standard describes the operational requirements, characteristics, and required information elements of clinical laboratory automation systems.[14]

The Electromechanical Interfaces standard provides guidance for developing a standard electromechanical interface between instruments and specimen-processing and specimen-handling devices used in automated laboratory testing procedures.[15]

Additional CLSI documents address various aspects of automation and informatics.[16–25] These guidelines are helpful as informational technology applications expand to include the following:

- *Providing primary care provider order entry.* The newest HISs access laboratory information and patient results through a laboratory web page. A newer postanalytical function of the LIS is retrieval of patient laboratory results by handheld devices. With password entry, primary care providers can order assays or retrieve results remotely.
- *Integrating total automation of laboratory systems.* New LISs and robotics are adapted for and integrated into total automated laboratory systems.
- *Monitoring the quality of laboratory results.* Use of automatic Westgard rules in QC analysis conveys appropriate warning to laboratory staff.
- *Interfacing of HIS and LIS.* The ability of the laboratory to retrieve data from medical records, including patient diagnosis, pharmacy data, and diagnostic imaging information, can contribute to overall quality of care.

COMPUTER APPLICATIONS

The application of the LIS has evolved from being exclusive to high-volume chemistry and hematology instrumentation to including all the other sections of the laboratory and off-site locations. General functions of the LIS can include patient identification, patient demographics, test ordering, specimen collection, specimen analysis, test results, and test interpretation. Coding systems for diagnosis, such as the CAP Systematized Nomenclature of Human and Veterinary Medicine, can also be managed by the LIS.

Most vendors separate the LIS into separate modules for various functions by department, such as specimen processing or high-volume hematology and chemistry testing. For example, a general laboratory system can fully automate clinical, financial, and managerial processes associated with the chemistry, hematology, coagulation, UA, immunology/serology, and toxicology sections of the clinical laboratory. Software can support all aspects of departmental workflow, including QC, instrument interfaces, result entry and review functions, autoverification, worksheets for the manual areas, and result inquiry. In addition, management report options are available to provide the laboratory manager with information necessary for the optimal operation of the laboratory.

The functions of LIS can be grouped into three categories: preanalytical, analytical, and postanalytical (Box 9.5).

Preanalytical (Preexamination) Functions

Using handheld technology reduces costs, improves workflow, and eliminates preventable medical errors. If data are collected and printed or transmitted directly, it is more efficient and accurate than manual recording.

Identifying and defining the patient in the computer system must take place before any testing is done. Most health care institutions assign a unique identification number to each patient and also enter other demographic information about the patient in the information database (such as name, gender, age or birth date, and referring or attending physician). These data are known as the *patient demographics.* This information is collected at admission to the facility and entered into the HIS. The information is then transferred electronically from the HIS to the LIS.

BOX 9.5 Examples of Laboratory Information System Functionality

Preanalytical (Preexamination)

Reduction of manual tasks, such as test ordering and specimen accessioning
Specimen labels
Specimen tracking between workstations
Centrifugation and cap removal
Error reduction, such as in correct specimen identification
Validation, such as the right assay being performed on the right tube type
Specimen integrity, such as correct volume of specimen and absence of interference from hemolysis or lipemia

Analytical (Examination)

Automated results entry
Manual results entry
Quality control
Validation of results
Output data processing
Network to laboratory automation systems

Postanalytical (Postexamination)

Archive of patient cumulative reports
Archive of specimens, such as frozen storage
Disposal of individual tubes
Workload recording
Billing
Network to other systems

Test ordering, or order entry, is an important first step in use of the LIS. Specific data are needed during the order entry process: a patient number and a patient name, name of ordering physician(s), name of physician(s) to receive the report, test request time and date, time the specimen was or will be collected, name of person entering the request, tests to be performed, priority of the test request (such as "stat" or routine), and any other specimen comments pertaining to the request.

Orders can be received most efficiently by the LIS through a network with the HIS. The laboratory can also receive a paper copy of the tests requested—the test request form or requisition from which laboratory personnel enter the test request into the LIS. The same data are needed on the paper form as are needed on the electronic order. The computer will generate collection lists, work lists, or logs with patient demographics and any necessary collection or analysis information. For example, work lists generated may include a loading list for a particular analyzer. The LIS has numerous checks and balances built into it as a part of the order entry process.

Analytical (Examination) Functions

An automated analyzer must link each specimen to its specific test request. This is best done automatically through the use of bar codes on the specimen label but can be done manually by the laboratory staff, who can link the sample at the instrument to the specimen number in the computer.

Molecular and Genetic Data

Molecular testing, including cytogenetics and molecular detection, is being supported by information systems today. The software development cycle continues, and linkage of databases of relevant genetic information is in progress. Currently, modules exist that can support karyotype results entry and fluorescence in situ hybridization data. Flow cytometry and cytogenetics are supported by vendors such as Millennium Helix (Cerner), where a unique karyotype editor that promotes compliance with ISCN and pairing karyotypes into easily searchable and coded concepts has been developed. Cerner's Clinical Bioinformatics Ontology (CBO) standardizes molecular findings to promote extensive analytical capabilities. The CBO has almost 12,000 unique concepts. This promotes the comparison of results between patients, which supports family member comparisons.

The Millennium Helix also provides context-sensitive links to Online Mendelian Inheritance in Man, a database of information and references about human genes and genetic disorders, and to the National Center for Biotechnology Information (NCBI). Established in 1988 as a national resource for molecular biology information, NCBI creates public databases, conducts research in computational biology, develops software tools for analyzing genome data, and disseminates biomedical information—all for the better understanding of molecular processes affecting human health and disease.

Another company offering modality-specific modules for cytogenetics, flow cytometry, and molecular testing is SCC Soft Computer. The cytogenetics module interfaces with flow cytometry instruments. Functionality includes data capture and scatterplot images.

Autoverification

Any results generated must be verified (approved or reviewed) by the laboratory staff before the data are released to the patient report. *Autoverification* is a process whereby computer-based algorithms automatically perform actions on a defined subset of laboratory results without the need for manual intervention.[8–10] Useful data for autoverification can include the display of "flags" signifying results that are outside the reference range values, the presence of critical values or panic values (possible life-threatening values), values out of the technical range for the analyzer, or results that fail other checks and balances built into the system.

Autoverification can be of three types: rules-based systems, neural networks, and pattern recognition. *Rules-based systems* are the most traditional. *Pattern recognition* is the most complex of the systems. *Neural networks* are midway between the two other types. The type of system selected depends on an analysis of how many tests the laboratory offers, the expected turnaround time, and the complexity of test results. Rules-based systems are the most common and the easiest to implement. Many newer automated instruments include autoverification systems. In a simple laboratory operation such as a satellite laboratory, the systems are inexpensive.

Autoverification of Clinical Laboratory Results (CLSI Approved Guideline AUTO 10-A) provides a general outline that allows each laboratory to design, implement, validate, and customize rules for autoverification based on the needs of its patient population.

QA procedures, including the use of QC solutions, are part of the analytical functions of the analyzer and its interfaced computer. CLIA '88 regulations require documentation of all QC data associated with any test results reported.

Postanalytical (Postexamination) Functions

The end product of the work done by the clinical laboratory consists of the testing results produced by the particular methodology used, which are provided in the laboratory report. The data can be electronically transmitted to printers, computer terminals, or handheld pager terminals, giving rapid access to the test information for the user.

Laboratory Report

An important use for the laboratory computer is to provide a comprehensive laboratory report that complies with Health Insurance Portability and Accountability Act regulations and contains all the test information generated by the various laboratories that have performed analyses for a single patient. A paper report is still required by most accreditation agencies and by current medical practice. CLIA '88 regulations require that every LIS has the capacity to print or reprint reports easily when needed. The format of the report should be such that the test results are clear and unambiguous. Many questions need answering to establish or rule out a particular diagnosis, and the report should facilitate this process. The report should indicate any abnormality with a flag.

If an abnormal result is reported, the clinician needs to evaluate the results. Questions that should be considered include the following: What is the predictive value of the test for the disease in question? Is the result meaningful? What other factors could produce the result? What should be done next?

If the diagnosis has already been made, the information on the report form can be used for other purposes, such as managing the patient's treatment plan. The physician must know the result of the most recent laboratory test, what clinically significant changes have occurred since the last test (through the retrieval of current and historical data), whether changes in therapy are indicated, and when the test should be performed next. This information constitutes an interpretive report.

An interpretive report form should give information about the range of reference values, should flag any abnormal values, and provide these data in a readily accessible format to support laboratories in the interpretation of clinical results in specific diagnostic areas, such as cerebrospinal fluid testing, urine assessment, and protein profiling. Besides the graphical presentation of patient results and the calculation of formulas, this program provides suggestions for the clinical interpretation of specific protein results.

In the reporting of results, Delta checks of current and previous patient results and flagging of abnormal and questionable results are being integrated into LIS operation. The International Consensus Group for Hematology Review[26] has guidelines that define the delta limit for a particular test as the amount by which the most recent automated analyzer patient test result may differ from a previous test result. Delta limits should be established for each laboratory by taking into account physiologic considerations and the characteristics of the automated analyzer used in that laboratory. Delta pass occurs when the result of the most recent automated analyzer patient test result does not differ by more than the delta limit from the previous patient test result; delta fail is when the result of the most recent patient test result differs by more than the predefined delta limit from the patient's previous test result.

Critical Patient Results

Critical patient results must be communicated immediately. The traditional way is by phone contact with the primary care provider. With automated LIS, it is essential to achieve electronic line of sight from the test order to the receipt and acknowledgment of the critical result by the appropriate health care professional. An automated process that supports critical result reporting with a manual call center backup system creates error-proof critical laboratory assay communication and improves the quality of patient care and laboratory staff productivity.

In addition, CLIA '88 has led to major changes in clinical laboratory data storage requirements. Records of test requests and results must be retained in a conveniently retrievable manner for 10 years for anatomic pathology and cytology results, 5 years for blood bank and immunohematology (human leukocyte antigen typing) results, and 2 years for all other results.

Voluntary accreditation agencies (such as CAP and TJC) often act as initial reviewers for compliance with federal and state regulations. These requirements for data processing include reporting procedures for documenting and validating software, documenting software and hardware maintenance, and communicating standard operating procedures. CAP laboratory inspection checklists have added requirements for review of computerized verification of results, security, and privacy procedures.

OVERVIEW OF AUTOMATION

Automated systems complete the process for sample-handling systems such as centrifuging and aliquoting and deliver the sample directly to the instruments for analysis. Aging of the population and development of more laboratory assays have resulted in an increasing number of laboratory tests done every year. It is estimated that clinical laboratories generate up to 80% of the information physicians rely on to make crucial treatment decisions.[27]

In addition, patients and physicians, especially ED staff, expect that accurate test results will be available quickly. The expectation of fast turnaround time has affected the development of both central laboratory equipment and POCT instruments. Major advances in clinical laboratory testing include miniaturization of test equipment and linking patients, specimens, and automated instruments of all sizes to robotics and information technology systems. With an impending shortage of skilled laboratory staff and economic forces creating more intense competition, clinical laboratories see automation as a key to survival.

Benefits of Automation

The major benefits of laboratory automation follow:

- Reduction of medical errors
- Reduced specimen sample volume
- Increased accuracy and precision (reduced coefficient of variation)
- Improved safety for laboratory staff (such as stopper removal or piercing)
- Faster turnaround time of results
- Partially alleviating the impending shortage of skilled laboratory staff

According to a U.S. Institute of Medicine report, medical errors in the United States may contribute to up to 98,000 deaths and more than 1 million injuries each year.[28] New TJC guidelines highlight the importance of proper identification of patient samples; a mistake in labeling or misidentification can lead to critical medical errors such as transfusion of blood products or medication to the wrong patient. The report identified several critical errors concerning laboratory processes, including delay in diagnosis.

Patient safety benefits from automation include workflow standardization for more precise, consistently reliable test results and improved test turnaround time for faster diagnosis and better patient care. Automated specimen processing and testing also improve safety for laboratory technologists. Because technologists are now handling blood samples less frequently, their exposure to pathogens and sharps injuries is reduced dramatically.

In addition to alleviating the impending shortage of laboratory staff, automation can produce a more dynamic and robust laboratory. Clinical laboratory professionals can spend more time on difficult cases while automated instruments handle routine work.

Process of Automation

As mentioned, CLSI has developed interrelated standards addressing the design, compatibility, and integration of automated clinical laboratory systems worldwide. Automation can be applied to any or all of the steps used to perform a manual assay. Automated systems include the following:

- Some type of device for sampling the patient's specimen or other samples to be tested (such as blanks, controls, and standard solutions)
- A mechanism to add the specimen to reagents in the proper sequence
- Incubation modules when needed for the specific reaction
- A measuring device (such as photometric technology) to quantitate the extent of the reaction
- A recording mechanism to provide the final reading or permanent record of the analytical result

Most analyzers are capable of processing a variety of specimens. To increase efficiency, it is generally advisable to perform as many steps as possible without manual intervention. Full automation reduces the possibility of human errors that arise from repetitive and boring manipulations done by laboratory staff, such as pipetting errors in routine procedures.

Steps in Automated Analysis

The major steps designed by manufacturers to mimic manual techniques are as follows:

- Specimen collection and processing
- Specimen and reagent measurement and delivery
- Chemical reaction phase
- Measurement phase
- Signal processing and data handling

Specimen Collection and Processing

The specimen must be collected properly, labeled, and transported to the laboratory for analysis. Specimen handling and processing are vital steps in the total analytical process. To eliminate problems associated with manually handling specimens, systems have been developed to automate this process. Automation of specimen preparation steps can include the use of bar-coded labels on samples, which allow electronic identification of the samples and of the tests requested. Bar coding can identify a sample and the reagents or analyses needed and relay this information to the automated analyzer. This can prevent clerical errors that could result in improperly entering patient data for analysis. In addition, bar coding allows for automated specimen storage and retrieval.

If whole blood is used, specimen preparation time is eliminated. Whole blood may also be applied manually or by automated techniques to dry-reagent cartridges or test strips containing reagents for visual observations or instrument readings of a quantitative change.

Specimen and Reagent Measurement and Delivery

Automated instruments combine reagents and a measured amount of specimen in a prescribed manner to yield a specific final concentration. This combination of predetermined amounts of reagent and sample is termed *proportioning*. It is important that reagents be introduced to the sample in the proper amounts and in specific sequences for the analysis to be carried through correctly.

The most common configuration for specimen testing with large automated equipment is the random-access analyzer. Random-access analysis assays are performed on a collection of specimens sequentially, with each specimen analyzed for a different selection of tests. Assays are selected through the use of different containers of liquid reagents, reagent packs, or reagent tables, depending on the analyzer. The random-access analyzer does all the selected determinations on a patient sample before it goes on to the next sample. These analyzers can process different assay combinations for individual specimens. The microprocessor enables the analyzer to perform up to 30 determinations. The selected tests are ordered from the menu, and the testing is begun with the unordered tests left undone. A sampling device begins the process by measuring the exact amount of sample into the required cells. The microprocessor controls the addition of the necessary diluents and reagents to each cell. After the proper reacting period, the microprocessor begins the spectrophotometric measurements of the various cells, the reaction results are calculated, control values are checked, and the results are reported. Some analyzers of this type have a circular configuration utilizing an analytical turntable device for the various cells. Other random-access analyzers have a parallel configuration.

Chemical Reaction Phase

Reagents may be classified as liquid or dry systems for use with automated analyzers. Reagent handling varies according to instrument capabilities and methodologies. Special test packets may be inserted into an instrument. The Vitros analyzer uses slides to contain the entire reagent chemistry system. Multiple layers on the slide are backed by a clear polyester support. The coating is sandwiched in a plastic mount.

The chemical reaction phase consists of mixing, separation, incubation, and reaction time. In continuous-flow analyzers, when the sample probe rises from the cup, air is aspirated for a specified time to produce a bubble between the sample and reagent plugs of liquid. In most discrete analyzers, the chemical reactants are held in individual moving containers that are either reusable or disposable. These reaction containers also function as cuvettes for optical analysis (such as Siemen's ADVIA), or the reactants may be placed in a stationary reaction chamber in which a flow-through process or reaction mixture occurs before and after the optical reading. In continuous-flow systems, flow-through cuvettes are used and optical readings taken during the flow of reactant fluids.

In automated analyzers, incubation is simply a waiting period in which the test mixture is allowed time to react. This is done at a specified, constant temperature controlled by the analyzer.

Measurement Phase

Traditionally, automated chemistry analyzers have relied on photometers and spectrophotometry for measurement of absorbance (see Chapter 8). Alternative measurement methods include nephelometry, chemiluminescence, enzyme immunoassay, and ion-selective electrodes.

To ensure the accuracy of results obtained with automated systems, there must be frequent standardization of methods. Once the standardization has been done, a well-designed automated system maintains or reproduces the prescribed conditions with great precision. Frequent standardization and running of control specimens are essential to ensure this accuracy and precision. CLIA '88 mandated regulations in the use of control specimens for certain tests. For laboratories doing moderately complex or highly complex testing using automated analyzers, a minimum of two control specimens (negative or normal and positive or increased) must be run once every 8 hours of operation or once per shift when patient specimens are being run.

Signal Processing and Data Handling

The simplest method of reading results is visual instrument readout using light-emitting diodes or a monitor. Results can be converted to hard copy, or the readout can be transmitted electronically with verified results.

Most data management devices are computer-based modules with manufacturers' proprietary software that interfaces with one or more analyzers and the host LIS. These software programs offer automated QC data management, with storage and evaluation of QC results against the laboratory's predefined acceptable limits. Every LIS has the capability for data autoverification, the process in which the computer performs the initial review and verification of test results. Data that fall within a set of predefined parameters or rules established by the laboratory are automatically verified in the LIS and the patient's files. The LIS may transmit results directly to a server or wireless pager. Laboratory staff must review all the data that fall outside the set of parameters or rules.

Automated Analyzers

Many different analyzers continue to be manufactured for use in the central clinical laboratory and for off-site testing. The choice of instrument depends on several factors: the volume of determinations done in the laboratory, type of data profile to be generated, level of staffing, initial cost of the instrument, its maintenance and operation costs, and time required for each analysis.

Automated instruments have been designed to perform the most frequently ordered tests. Versatility and flexibility are often just as important as high volume and speed of testing, but automation is also desirable for less frequently ordered tests.

In the case of large-volume hospital and reference laboratories, a completely automated laboratory system may be used. Each automated instrument can operate separately or integrated with other laboratory instruments. Instruments can be linked into a single continuous operation that can include robotic specimen processing.

Initially, highly automated systems were introduced in larger-volume clinical chemistry and hematology laboratories. Today, automation and semiautomation exist in other clinical laboratory sections including UA, blood bank, and microbiology. Applicable information related to automation or semiautomation for each clinical specialty is included in specific clinical chapters (Chapters 10–17).

CASE STUDY

CASE STUDY 9.1

A 25-year-old woman comes to the clinic for pregnancy testing. She reports that her last menstrual period was 30 days ago. A random urine specimen is collected for testing. The result for this test is reported as negative. The physical examination indicates that the woman is pregnant.

Multiple-Choice Questions

1. What is a possible reason for the false-negative test result?
   a. The specific gravity was greater than 1.015.
   b. The lack of agglutination seen on the test slide was interpreted as a negative test result.
   c. The concentration of hCG present in the specimen is too low to be detected.
   d. The patient had ingested an excessive amount of aspirin.
2. If conception is estimated to have taken place about 2 weeks before her visit to the clinic, and if this is an average pregnancy, what would be the normal average serum hCG concentration at the time of this patient's visit?
   a. 25 mIU/mL
   b. 50 mIU/mL
   c. 500 mIU/mL
   d. 30,000 mIU/mL
3. If this patient was not pregnant, a reason for a false-positive result could be:
   a. A urine specific gravity of less than 1.015
   b. Treatment for infertility with an hCG injection
   c. Conducting the assay at 1 week of gestation
   d. Use of a random urine specimen

Answers are in Appendix A.

Critical Thinking Group Discussion Questions

1. What are the factors in performing an accurate pregnancy test?
2. What are possible causes of a false-negative pregnancy test?

Answers published on EVOLVE Instructor website.

REFERENCES

1. World Health Organization (WHO), 20th WHO Essential Medicines List (EML), Geneva, Switzerland, March 2017.
2. US Department of Health and Human Services, Health Care Financing Administration: Clinical laboratory improvement amendments of 1988, *Fed Regist* 60(78), 1995. Final rules with comment period.
3. Heller D: Nanopore technology offers a way forward for point-of-care diagnostics, Med Lab Obs 50(2): 22–24, 2018.
4. Kasoff J: Advances in LIS functionality, *Adv Med Lab Professionals* 20(16):16–19, 2008.
5. Hattie M: *Bar coding: labs go 2D*, September 2009, www.mlo-online.com.
6. Smith TJ: Barcode: meet your match, Adv Med Lab Professionals 18:12–13, *Dec* 4, 2006.
7. College of American Pathologists: Accreditation standards. www.cap.org (Accessed 13.06.13.).
8. Winsten D: Molecular, genetic data and the LIS, *Adv Med Lab Professionals* 20(15):22–25, 2008.
9. Lehman C, Burgnener R, Munoz O: Autoverification and laboratory quality, *Crit Values* 2(4):24–27, 2009.
10. Graham KJ: Lab limelight: autoverification, *Adv Med Lab Professionals* 19(1):22, 2007.
11. Clinical and Laboratory Standards Institute: Autoverification of clinical laboratory test results approved standard 2006, Wayne, Pa, AUTO 10.
12. Clinical and Laboratory Standards Institute: Laboratory automation: specimen container/specimen carrier: approved standard, 2ed 2000, Wayne, Pa, AUTO 01.
13. Clinical and Laboratory Standards Institute: Laboratory automation: bar codes for specimen container identification: approved standard 2006, Wayne, Pa, AUTO 02.
14. Clinical and Laboratory Standards Institute: Laboratory automation: communications with automated clinical laboratory systems, instruments, devices, and information systems2nd ed 2009, Wayne, Pa, AUTO 03.
15. Clinical and Laboratory Standards Institute: Laboratory automation: systems operational requirements, characteristics, and information elements: approved standard 2001, Wayne, Pa, AUTO 04.
16. Clinical and Laboratory Standards Institute: Laboratory automation: electromechanical interfaces: approved standard 2001, Wayne, Pa, AUTO 05.
17. Clinical and Laboratory Standards Institute: Laboratory automation: data content for specimen identification: approved standard 2004, Wayne, Pa, AUTO 07.
18. Clinical and Laboratory Standards Institute: Protocols to validate laboratory information systems: proposed guideline 2006, Wayne, Pa, AUTO 08.
19. Clinical and Laboratory Standards Institute: Remote access to clinical laboratory diagnostic devices via the Internet: proposed standard 2006, Wayne, Pa, AUTO 09.
20. Clinical and Laboratory Standards Institute: Laboratory instruments and data management systems: design of software user interfaces and end-user software systems validation, operation, and monitoring ed 2 2003, Wayne, Pa, 2003, AUTO 13.
21. Clinical and Laboratory Standards Institute: Standard Specification for low-level protocol to transfer messages between clinical laboratory instruments and computer systems 2008, Wayne, Pa, LIS 01.
22. Clinical and Laboratory Standards Institute: Specification for transferring information between clinical laboratory instruments and information systems: approved standarded 2 2004, Wayne, Pa, LIS 02.
23. Clinical and Laboratory Standards Institute: Standard guide for selection of a clinical laboratory information management system 2003, Wayne, Pa, LIS 03-A.
24. Clinical and Laboratory Standards Institute: Standard guide for documentation of clinical laboratory computer systems 2003, Wayne, Pa, LIS 04.
25. Clinical and Laboratory Standards Institute: Standard Specification for transferring information between clinical instruments and independent computer systems, 2ed, 2004, Wayne, Pa, LIS 05.
26. International Society for Laboratory Hematology: Consensus Guidelines, www.islh.org, accessed July 6, 2014.
27. Beckman-Coulter Conference: Lab automation, Calif, 2003, Palm Springs.
28. US Institute of Medicine: To err is human, Washington, DC, 1999, US Government Printing Office.

BIBLIOGRAPHY

Altinier S, Mion M, Cappelletti A, et al: Rapid measurement of cardiac markers on Stratus CS, *Clin Chem* 46:991, 2000.

Bartholow TL, Parwant AV, Becich MJ: A blueprint for laboratory information systems: lab data architecture of the future, *Critical Values* 4(2):25–28, 2011.

Bickers J: A wireless environmental monitoring system for the clinical laboratory, *MLO Med Lab Obs* 45(5):60–61, 2013.

Bond MM, Richards-Kortum RR: Drop-to-drop variation in the cellular components of fingerprick blood: implications for point-of-care diagnostic development, *Am J Clin Pathol* 144(6):885–894, 2015.

Brown SM: *Bioinformatics: a biologist's guide to biocomputing and the Internet,* New York, 2000, Eaton.

Burtis CA, Ashwood ER, Bruns DE: *Tietz fundamentals of clinical chemistry,* ed 6, St Louis, 2008, Elsevier/Saunders.

Clark JL, Rao LV: Retrospective analysis of point-of-care and laboratory-based hemoglobin A1c testing, *JALM* 1(5):502–509, 2017.

Clinical Lab Products: Whole Blood Rapid Pregnancy Test Certified for Over-the-Counter Sales in Europe, clpmag.com 40(4), June, 2018.

DuBois JA: *Advances in POCT technologies outpace regulatory and accreditation requirements, MLO Med Lab Obs 49(2): 42-45,* 2017.

Esmon A, Ruckstuhl V: Clinical lab heating and cooling equipment: critical to new innovations, *MLO Med Lab Obs* 45(5):56–58, 2013.

Felciano RM: Looking ahead: the future bioinformatics of genetic testing and precision medicine, *MLO* 49(5):40–41, 2017.

Futrell K: The EHR-LIS nexus, *MLO Med Lab Obs* 45(5):42–44, 2013.

Gonnelli G: Planning for laboratory automation, *MLO* 49(8):40, 2017.

Jefferson R: LIS selection guide: research your unique requirements before purchasing or upgrading your LIS, *Adv Med Lab Professionals* 14(13):14, 2002.

Jefferson R: POL connectivity: LIS to reference lab and beyond, *Adv Med Lab Professionals* 15(4):13, 2003.

Joint Commission on Accreditation of Healthcare Organizations: *Comprehensive accreditation manual for laboratory and point-of-care testing, Oak Brook Terrace, Ill, 2005,* Department of Communications Laboratory Accreditation, 2005–2006, Program.

Kaplan LA, Pesce AJ: *Clinical chemistry: theory, analysis, and correlation,* ed 5, St Louis, 2010, Elsevier/Mosby.

Katz B, Marques MB: Point-of-care testing in oral anticoagulation: what is the point? *MLO Med Lab Obs* 36:30–35, 2004.

Lyle J: The final frontier in software testing automation, *MLO* 49(8):48–49, 2017.

McMahan J: HIPAA and the Lab Information System Act will have direct effect on use of LIS, *Adv Med Lab Professionals* 14(3):8, 2002.

McMahan J: Primer on LIS interfaces, *Adv Med Lab Professionals* 14(20):8, 2002.

McMahan J: Necessary evils of information technology, *Adv Med Lab Professionals* 17(9):14, 2005.

Menhardt W: The future state of informatics and the clinical lab, *MLO* 49(5):38–41, 2017.

Murray P: How did your lab do with POCT? *MLO Med Lab Obs* 49(2):40, 2017.

Nolen JDL: Riding the waves of lab automation, *MLO* 49(8):38, 2017.

Paxton A: Toolkit lets labs make the case for the right LIS, *CAP Today* 27(8):1, 2013. 28–34.

Sarker DK: *Quality systems and control for pharmaceuticals,* West Sussex, England, 2008, Wiley.

Schroeder LF, Guarner J, Elbireer A, et al: Time for a Model List of Essential Diagnostics, *N Engl J Med* 374(26):2511–2514, 2016.

Smith T: Making IT work: relieving the IS headache, *Adv Med Lab Professionals* 14(2):24, 2002.

Turgeon ML: *Immunology and serology in laboratory medicine,* ed 6, St Louis, 2018, Elsevier/Mosby.

University of South Florida, https://www.usfhealthonline.com/resources/key-concepts/what-is-health-informatics/, 2018

U.S. Department of Health and Human Services (HHS): Standards for privacy of individually identifiable health information, 45 CFR Parts 160 and 164, Washington, DC, 2003, HHS.

U.S. Food and Drug Administration (FDA): FDA releases two final guidance documents on blood glucose monitors: *Cl Lab News* 42(12):20, 2016.

Verne B: *Size up this critical medical laboratory automation*, July 2005. www.mlo-online.com.

Wray B, Denton J: Achieving automation process improvement through innovative barcoding strategies, *MLO* 49(8):47, 2017.

REVIEW QUESTIONS (ANSWERS IN APPENDIX A)

Point-of-Care Testing

1. A major advantage of POCT is:
   a. Faster turnaround time
   b. Lower cost
   c. Ease of use
   d. Both a and b
2. POCTS assays are usually in which CLIA category?
   a. Waived
   b. Provider-performed microscopy
   c. Moderately complex
   d. Highly complex
3. Over-the-counter test kits are in which CLIA category?
   a. Waived
   b. Provider-performed microscopy
   c. Moderately complex
   d. Highly complex
4. An early example of decentralized health care is:
   a. Patient self-monitoring of blood glucose
   b. INR coagulation testing
   c. Electrolyte testing
   d. Hemoglobin determination
5. An early commercial example of direct consumer genetic testing is:
   a. 23andMe
   b. Full metabolic laboratory panel
   c. Hemoglobin alterations
   d. Cholesterol assay

Non–Instrument-Based Point-of-Care Testing

6. What is the concentration at which most sensitive current laboratory assays can give a positive serum hCG result?
   a. 25 mIU/mL
   b. 50 mIU/mL
   c. 100 mIU/mL
   d. 100,000 mIU/mL

7. The most specific assays for human chorionic gonadotropin (hCG) use antibody reagents against which subunit of hCG?
   a. Alpha
   b. Beta
   c. Gamma
   d. Chorionic

Handheld POCT Equipment

8. An important characteristic to be considered when selecting a POCT instrument is:
   a. Rapid turnaround time
   b. Easy-to-perform protocol
   c. Refrigerated storage of reagents
   d. Both a and b

Emerging Patient-Centric Technologies

9. The tricorder is modeled after:
   a. *Star Trek* ideas
   b. original cell counters
   c. flow cell principles
   d. digital imaging

Overview of Informatics

10. What is the ultimate goal of the laboratory?
    a. Perform more tests.
    b. Hire less staff.
    c. Quickly produce results.
    d. Produce accurate information in a timely manner.
11. Computer technology can be used for:
    a. Specimen processing
    b. Inventory control
    c. Ordering tests
    d. All the above
12. The function of a CPU is:
    a. Short-term memory
    b. Executes software instructions
    c. Exchange of information
    d. A printer
13. The function of an interface is:
    a. Short-term memory
    b. Executes software instructions
    c. Exchange of information
    d. Bar-code reader

Communication and Network Devices

14. The laboratory can have directly connected computers that can access the hospital record system by:
    a. Use of routers
    b. Forming an LAN
    c. Using a WAN
    d. Both a and b

Computer Applications

15. An example of laboratory information system functionality is:
    a. Specimen tracking
    b. Quality control
    c. Archive patient cumulative reports
    d. All the above
16. Future challenges for laboratory automation standards include all of the following *except:*
    a. Design of laboratory specimen containers
    b. Design of bar codes for specimen identification
    c. Developing uniform collection devices
    d. Developing a standard electromechanical interface

Overview of Automation

17. The major benefit(s) of laboratory automation is (are):
    a. Reduction in medical errors.
    b. Improved safety for laboratory staff.
    c. Faster turnaround time.
    d. All the above.
18. Steps in automation designed to mimic manual techniques include:
    a. Pipetting of specimen
    b. Pipetting of reagents
    c. Measurement of chemical reactions
    d. All the above

Bonus Challenge *Questions 19 and 20:* Answer the questions based on the following laboratory situation.

Amanda is working within the chemistry department and is reviewing results before she releases them to be sent to the patient charts. All testing within the chemistry department is performed on an automated analyzer. She notices that John Smith has an abnormally high bilirubin result that is flagged as a delta check failure (a result that does not match previously filed results), and all his liver function tests are abnormal. On a sample tested that morning, Mr. Smith's bilirubin level was normal, as were all his liver function tests.

Amanda begins troubleshooting the current test result, taking note of the five steps of automated analysis. She first looks at Mr. Smith's current sample and notices there are two bar-code labels, one placed over the top of the other, on the test tube.

19. What do you think is the most likely cause of this problem?
    a. Specimen collection and processing error
    b. Chemical reaction phase error
    c. Measurement phase error
    d. Signal processing and data handling error

Later on in the day, Amanda is again reviewing results before releasing them, and she notices an error message on Amy Brown's test results: "Short Sample Detected." No results are available for Ms. Brown's chemistry profile, but other patients on the machine before and after this sample had no issues with the test results. Amanda begins troubleshooting the problem.

20. What do you think is the most likely cause of this error?
    a. Specimen collection and processing error
    b. Specimen and reagent measurement and delivery
    c. Measurement phase error
    d. Signal processing and data handling error

Turgeon: Linné & Ringsrud's Clinical Laboratory Science, 8th Edition

STUDENT PROCEDURE WORKSHEET 9.1

Fecal Occult Blood Testing

Read Chapter 9 in *Linné & Ringsrud's Clinical Laboratory Science: Concepts, Procedures, and Clinical Applications,* 8th edition, for a complete discussion of this procedure.

Student Learning Outcome

After reading Chapter 9, and at the completion of the laboratory exercise and review questions, the student will be able to:

- Explain the fecal occult blood procedure: purpose, specimen, collection, and test results.
- Correctly complete the end-of-procedure review questions with a grade of 80% or higher.

Hemoccult II SENSA[elite] Method

Principle

This procedure is based on the oxidation of guaiac, a natural resin, by H_2O_2 to a blue-colored compound if heme is present in a fecal specimen. The heme portion of hemoglobin has peroxidase activity, which catalyzes the oxidation of α-guaiaconic acid (active component of the guaiac paper) by H_2O_2 (active component of the developer) to form a highly conjugated, blue quinine compound.

Specimen

Patient Preparation and Instructions

- *General:* Patients may ingest pork, chicken, turkey, and fish; fruits and vegetables; high-fiber foods; and acetaminophen.
- *Avoid 7 days before specimen collection and during specimen collection:* No more than one adult aspirin (325 mg) a day; no other NSAIDs (such as ibuprofen).
- *Avoid 3 days before specimen collection:* No red meat (such as beef, lamb, and liver); no more than 250 mg vitamin C a day from supplements, citrus fruits, and juices. An average orange contains approximately 70 to 75 mg vitamin C; 100% of recommended daily allowance of vitamin C is 60 mg.

Specimen Collection

- The patient should write his or her name and the physician's name on the front of the test card. Fill in Day 1 collection date. Open Day 1 flap.
- Patients should be advised to place plastic wrap on the toilet seat and to defecate onto the plastic. Obtain a small stool sample with provided applicator stick. Apply thin smear in box A. Reuse applicator stick to obtain a second sample from a different part of the stool specimen. Apply thin smear in box B. Discard specimen and supplies. Close flap. Store test card in the patient kit envelope. Let dry. Do not store smeared test card in any moisture-proof material (such as plastic bag).
- Repeat the previous steps for Day 2 and Day 3.
- Insert completed and overnight air-dried test card into enclosed U.S. Postal Service–approved mailing pouch. Peel tape from flap. Fold flap over. Press firmly to seal.
- Deliver or mail sealed mailing pouch to the physician or laboratory within 10 days of Day 1 collection date.

Equipment and Supplies

1. Hemoccult II SENSA[elite] slides (test cards)
2. Hemoccult II SENSA[elite] developer. Stabilized mixture of less then 4.2% hydrogen peroxide, 80% denatured ethyl alcohol, and enhancer in an aqueous solution; consult material safety data sheet (MSDS) for additional information. Do not use in eyes; avoid contact with skin.

   NOTE: Store test cards and developer at controlled room temperature (15 °C to 30 °C) in original packaging. Do not refrigerate or freeze. Protect from heat and light. Do not store with volatile chemicals such as ammonia, bleach, bromine, iodine, and household cleaners.

   - When stored as recommended, the slides and developer will remain stable until the expiration dates that appear on each slide and developer bottle.
3. Applicator sticks
4. Patient screening kit with dispensing envelopes and patient instructions
5. Flushable collection tissue or plastic wrap
6. Mailing pouches (for return of test cards)
7. Hemoccult II SENSA[elite] product instructions

Instructions for the Procedure

Read the list of required equipment and supplies and the procedural steps. Follow the procedural steps in exact order.

SEQUENCE	PROCEDURAL STEP	INSTRUCTOR-OBSERVED ACCEPTABLE PERFORMANCE (CHECK IF ACCEPTABLE)
1	Wash your hands and put on gloves and eye protection as directed.	
2	Assemble kit materials and supplies.	
3	If fecal (stool) specimen has been applied to the two paper guaiac squares, begin testing in a fume hood or biosafety cabinet.	
4	**Color development** (performed in laboratory) Turn the slide over and open the perforated flap to expose the backs of boxes A and B and the performance monitor (control) area.	
5	Apply 2 drops of the developer (hydrogen peroxide) directly over each smear (boxes A and B) and start the timer for 60 seconds.	
6	Read the results at the appropriate time.	
7	Observe the slide for any blue color at the edge of the smear. This is a positive result.	

Turgeon: Linné & Ringsrud's Clinical Laboratory Science, 8th Edition

STUDENT PROCEDURE WORKSHEET 9.1

SEQUENCE	PROCEDURAL STEP	INSTRUCTOR-OBSERVED ACCEPTABLE PERFORMANCE (CHECK IF ACCEPTABLE)
8	**Quality control (QC)** The positive and negative "performance monitor area," an internal control, is located under the sample area. Perform QC step by applying 1 drop of developer between the positive and negative performance areas. Read the results at the appropriate time: Positive = blue color Negative = no blue color (colorless) If these results are not obtained, repeat the QC step with a new slide. NOTE: Develop on slide performance monitor areas (controls): Apply 1 drop only of peroxide solution between the positive and negative performance areas. Always test the specimen and read and interpret the results before developing the controls. A blue color from the positive control might spread into the specimen and cause confusion or a false-positive reaction. Read the results within 10 seconds. A blue color will appear in the positive performance monitor area and no color in the negative performance monitor area if the slides and developer are reacting according to product specifications.	
9	Record the patient and quality control results.	
10	Discard used lancets in a sharps container and discard gauze and other contaminated supplies into a biohazard container.	
11	Clean equipment and return to proper storage.	
12	Clean work area with disinfectant solution.	
13	Remove gloves and discard into biohazard container.	
14	Wash hands using proper procedure.	

NOTE: Always check manufacturer directions for revisions to the procedure.

Reporting Results

Any trace of blue color is positive, whether the intensity of color development is weak or strong. Reagent paper that has turned blue or blue-green before use should be discarded. If discolored test paper has been used by the patient, the test should be repeated if there is any question in interpretation.

False-Positive Results

Substances that can cause false-positive test results:

- Red meat (beef, lamb, liver)
- Aspirin (>325 mg/day) and other NSAIDs (such as ibuprofen and naproxen)
- Corticosteroids, phenylbutazone, reserpine, anticoagulants, antimetabolites, and cancer chemotherapeutic drugs
- Alcohol in excess
- Application of antiseptic preparations containing iodine (such as povidone-iodine mixture)

False-Negative Results

Substances that can cause false-negative results:

- Ascorbic acid (vitamin C) in excess of 250 mg/day
- Excessive amounts of vitamin C–enriched foods, citrus fruits, and juices
- Iron supplements that contain quantities of vitamin C in excess of 250 mg/day

Limitations

Bowel lesions may not bleed at all or may bleed intermittently. Blood, if present, may not be distributed uniformly in the specimen. Consequently, a test result may be negative even when disease is present.

Clinical Applications

The Hemoccult II SENSA^{elite} is a rapid qualitative method for detecting fecal occult blood, which may be indicative of gastrointestinal disease. It is recommended for professional use as a diagnostic aid during routine physical examinations; to monitor hospital patients for gastrointestinal bleeding (such as iron deficiency anemia in recuperating from surgery); to follow patients with peptic ulcer, ulcerative colitis, and other conditions; and in screening programs of asymptomatic patients for colorectal cancer.

Procedural Evaluation

Student's Name ______________________________ Grade _________

Instructor's Signature ___________________________ Date ___________

Comments:

Turgeon: Linné & Ringsrud's Clinical Laboratory Science, 8th Edition

STUDENT PROCEDURE WORKSHEET 9.1

Fecal Occult Blood Testing

Review Questions

1. Describe proper patient specimen collection procedures.

2. What are possible sources of error for a false-positive result?

3. What are possible sources of error for a false-negative result?

Turgeon: Linné & Ringsrud's Clinical Laboratory Science, 8th Edition

STUDENT PROCEDURE WORKSHEET 9.2

Student Assignment*[1]

Choosing an LIS system or equipment for your laboratory[2]

Read Chapter 9 in *Linné & Ringsrud's Clinical Laboratory Science: Concepts, Procedures, and Clinical Applications,* 8th edition, for a complete discussion of this activity.

Student Learning Outcomes

After reading Chapter 9, and at the completion of this laboratory exercise and review questions, the student will be able to:

- List important features considered when selecting an LIS.
- Utilize recent *CAP Today* Product Guides to compare features of current LISs.
- Describe and compare the features of two LIS systems assigned by the instructor.

SEQUENCE	PROCEDURAL STEP
1	Locate the most recent College of American Pathologists publication, *CAP Today,* at www.captodayonline.com. Click on the "Product Guides" tab.
2	Select at least ten comparative characteristics related to the two assigned LISs.
3	Set up a table with three columns labeled: Characteristic, System #1, and System #2
4	Enter the data for each system in the respective column.
5	Compare at least five characteristics that you think are the most appropriate for the two systems using a narrative essay style.
6	Submit a written summary (minimum of 150 words) to your instructor for grading.

[1]Special thanks to Professor Joan Radtke, Rush University, Department of Medical Laboratory Science, Chicago.
[2]This assignment can be applied to any automated instrument.

10

Introduction to the Principles and Practice of Clinical Chemistry

http://evolve.elsevier.com/Turgeon

CHAPTER OUTLINE

LEARNING OUTCOMES

Glucose and glucose metabolism

- Differentiate various aspects of the normal physiology of glucose metabolism, including glycogenesis, gluconeogenesis, lipogenesis, and glycolysis.

Diabetes

- Compare and contrast the pathophysiology of types 1 and 2 diabetes, and gestational diabetes.
- Describe the symptoms of diabetes.
- Compare the diagnostic criteria for types 1 and 2 diabetes, and gestational diabetes mellitus.
- Compare the conditions of hyperglycemia and hypoglycemia.
- Describe the collection procedures and various types of blood specimens for glucose analysis.
- Compare point-of-care testing to traditional testing methods for glucose.
- Describe the methods for qualitative and semiquantitative determination of glucose.
- ❖ Explain the significance of glycosylated hemoglobin in the management of diabetes.

Electrolytes

- Identify and describe the function of sodium, potassium, calcium, and magnesium in blood and body fluids.
- Discuss the causes and results of electrolyte imbalances.
- Compare osmolality and osmolarity.
- ❖ Assess osmolality and osmolal gap and apply them to clinical situations.
- ❖ Calculate an anion gap and apply it to clinical situations.

Acid-base balance and blood gases

- ❖ Explain the role and alterations of acid-base balance and blood gases in the body.

Renal function

- Compare and contrast renal function assays.
- ❖ Describe the clinical applications of creatinine clearance, estimated glomerular filtration rate, cystatin C, and beta-2 microglobulin testing.
- ❖ Explain the chemical aspects of blood urea nitrogen and the normal reference range.
- ❖ Compare the eGFR and the GFR.

Uric acid

- Interpret the clinical significance of uric acid analysis.

Lipids

- Define the terms lipemia, BNP, saturated and unsaturated fats, and atherosclerosis.
- Assess the biochemical and physiologic characteristics of cholesterol, triglycerides, and lipoprotein.

Cardiovascular Disease

- List significant risk factors in the assessment of cardiovascular disease.

- Compare various systems for assessing cardiovascular disease risk assessment.
- Compare and contrast at least three cardiac markers of acute myocardial infarction.

Liver and pancreatic testing

- Name liver and pancreatic assays and explain their clinical significance.
- Describe the physiology of bilirubin formation and associated abnormal conditions.

❖ Differentiate between various forms of bilirubin, and understand the clinical significance of various forms.

Hormone assays

- Compare and contrast thyroid hormone assays and describe the clinical applications.

Tumor markers

❖ Identify various tumor markers and at least one use.

Therapeutic drug monitoring

- Describe therapeutic drug assays.

Drugs of abuse

❖ Identify drugs of abuse.

Automation in Clinical Chemistry

- Compare the chemical method principles used in various chemistry and immunochemistry analyzers.

Case Studies

❖ Analyze the patient history, clinical signs and symptoms, and laboratory data for the stated case studies, answer the related critical thinking questions, and conclude the most likely diagnosis.

Review Questions

- Demonstrate comprehension of the chapter content by completing the end-of-chapter review questions with a grade of 80% or higher.

Note:

- indicates MLT and MLS core content

❖ indicates MLT (optional) and MLS advanced content

KEY TERMS

anion gap
bilirubin
glomerular filtration rate (GFR)
gluconeogenesis
glycogenesis
glycogenolysis
glycolysis
glycosuria
hemoglobin A_{1c} (Hb A_{1c})
hyperglycemia
hyperkalemia
hypoglycemia
hypokalemia
jaundice
lipogenesis
lipoproteins
polyuria
postprandial
triglycerides
tumor-specific markers
uremia

Chemistry is an area in which changes continue to occur because of the introduction of new methodologies and increasingly sophisticated instrumentation. This chapter describes selected classic manual methods and analytical approaches currently in common use. An understanding of both classic and current methods is helpful in mastering the basics of manual testing and automated testing. Groups of major clinical applications are discussed.

GLUCOSE AND GLUCOSE METABOLISM

One of the most frequently performed determinations in the clinical chemistry laboratory is blood glucose. *Glucose* is a simple sugar, or monosaccharide, derived from the breakdown of dietary carbohydrates (Fig. 10.1). Intestinal absorption of carbohydrates occurs in the small intestine, where monosaccharides, the single-sugar units of carbohydrates, are absorbed. Nonglucose monosaccharides, including galactose and fructose, are converted to glucose by the liver.

At any given time, the blood glucose level is under the control of a number of hormones. Insulin, a hormone secreted by the pancreas after a meal, responds to high glucose levels, promoting glucose entry into cells (Fig. 10.2). Glucose may also be converted, under the action of insulin, to protein and fat (lipogenesis), with the latter stored as fat (adipose) tissue. Most body cells have limited glycogen stores, but the liver and skeletal muscles store larger amounts of glycogen. Glycogen constitutes 10% of the total weight of the liver.

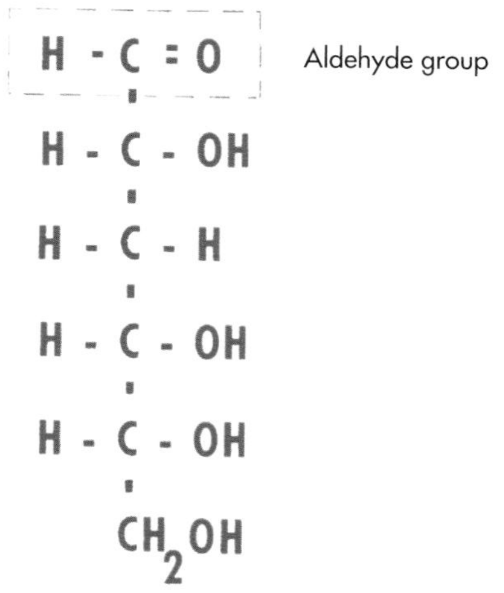

H - C = O   Aldehyde group
H - C - OH
H - C - H
H - C - OH
H - C - OH
CH_2OH

Fig. 10.1 Glucose molecule.

Depending on the needs of the cell, glucose may undergo anaerobic and aerobic metabolism to yield energy as adenosine triphosphate (ATP). Gluconeogenesis, the formation of glucose from lactate or amino acids, is stimulated by the hormones glucagon, cortisol, and thyroxine (T_4). Alternatively, glucose may be biochemically converted to and stored as glycogen (glycogenesis).

Glucose is the primary source of energy for most body cells. Insulin regulates the concentration of blood glucose by promoting its entry into the cell, which is followed by a number of

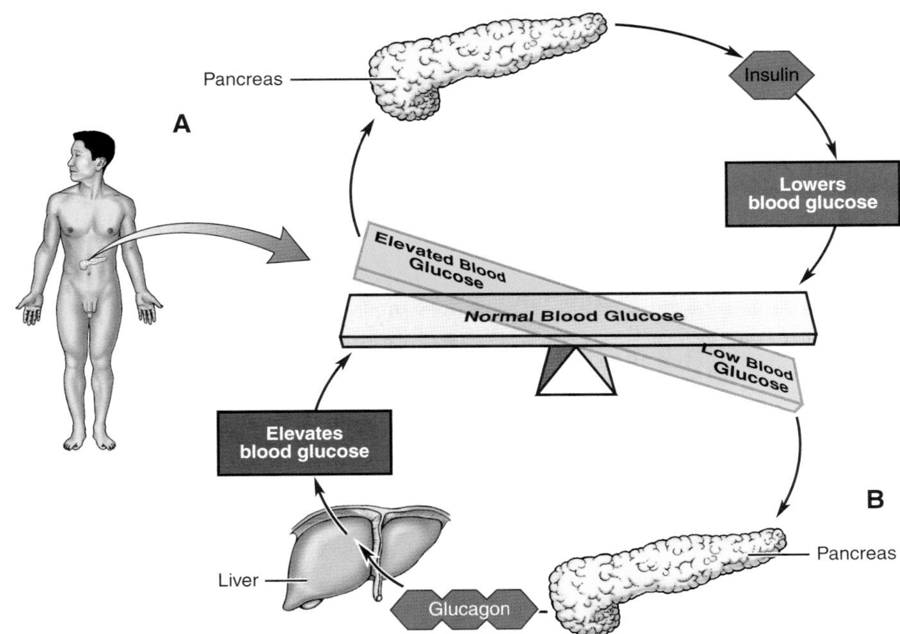

Fig. 10.2 Glucose balance. Homeostatic balancing of glucose levels. (A) When glucose level is too high, insulin lowers it to normal. (B) When glucose level is too low, glucagon raises it to normal. (From Herlihy M: *The human body in health and illness,* ed 2, Philadelphia, 2003, Saunders.)

possible metabolic fates: glycolysis, glycogenesis, lipogenesis, and protein synthesis. Several hormones have the effect of maintaining the blood glucose concentration during the fasting state. These hormones have varied cellular effects, but all oppose the action of insulin by raising the blood glucose level. Glucagon, secreted by the alpha (α) cells of the pancreas, is the major hormone that opposes the action of insulin, increasing blood glucose by stimulating the breakdown of glycogen (glycogenolysis) by the liver. A number of other hormones, some secondary to pituitary hormone release, also promote glycogenolysis, the degradation of glycogen to form glucose.

The normal reference range for fasting blood glucose is less than 100 mg/dL. Plasma glucose level increases rapidly after a carbohydrate-rich meal, returning to normal 1½ to 2 hours after eating (postprandial level). Many diseases alter normal glucose metabolism. The most frequent cause of an increase in blood glucose, or hyperglycemia, is diabetes.

Hypoglycemia, defined as a blood glucose level less than 50 mg/dL, may have severe consequences. One cause of hypoglycemia in diabetic patients is an excessive dose of insulin. The body secretes a number of hormones that increase blood glucose levels, but only insulin lowers blood sugar.

DIABETES

The incidence of diabetes is rising. The U.S. Centers for Disease Control and Prevention (CDC)[1] and the American Diabetes Association (ADA)[2] estimate that 8.3% of the population of the United States now have diabetes. Currently, 18.8 million persons have been diagnosed with diabetes, and 7 million are estimated to have the disease but are undiagnosed. There are considerable racial and ethnic differences in diabetes, with the highest rates for non-Hispanic blacks, Hispanics, and Asian Americans compared with whites. Diabetes-associated complications remain the leading cause of mortality related to heart disease or stroke and are associated with long-term damage, including failure of organs such as the eyes and kidneys.

The classification of diabetes includes the following four clinical classes:

- Type 1 diabetes (results from β-cell destruction, usually leading to absolute insulin deficiency)
- Type 2 diabetes (results from a progressive insulin secretory defect with insulin resistance)
- Gestational diabetes mellitus (GDM), diagnosed during pregnancy
- Other specific types of diabetes from other causes, such as genetic defects in β-cell function; genetic defects in insulin action; diseases of exocrine pancreas such as cystic fibrosis (CF); and chemically or drug-induced diabetes, such as occurs during treatment of acquired immunodeficiency syndrome or after organ transplantation

Type 1 Diabetes

Type 1 diabetes, or insulin-dependent diabetes, is usually diagnosed in children and young adults, and was previously called *juvenile diabetes.* The genetic marker, human leukocyte antigen class II genes on chromosome 6p21, is associated with both type 1 diabetes and celiac disease. Celiac disease is increasing in patients with type 1 diabetes and occurs with greater frequency than in the general population.

Type 1 diabetes results from the lack of insulin caused by cell-mediated autoimmune destruction of insulin-secreting pancreatic beta (β) cells. The autoimmune process leading to type 1 diabetes begins years before manifestation of clinical signs and symptoms. An estimated 80% to 90% reduction in the number of β cells is required to induce symptomatic type 1 diabetes. Children have a more rapid rate of islet cell destruction than adults. Circulating antibodies can be demonstrated in the serum of individuals with type 1 diabetes. Indicators of autoimmune destruction of the pancreas include islet cell antibodies and insulin antibodies.

The breakdown of fat (lipolysis) from adipose tissue to supply energy in diabetes can be life- threatening. Increased lipolysis results in increased concentrations of ketone bodies, which can lead to ketoacidosis, particularly in type 1 diabetic patients with absolute insulin deficiency. The result may be a dangerous decrease in blood pH or acidosis.

Type 2 Diabetes

Adults

The prevalence of type 2 diabetes has more than doubled since 1996 (Fig. 10.3). The incidence of type 2 diabetes, or non–insulin-dependent diabetes, is usually associated with occurrence later in life and with a gradual onset, usually after 40 years of age. However, more children and adolescents are being diagnosed with type 2 diabetes as well.

Type 2 diabetes is characterized by insulin resistance and progressive hyperglycemia. Type 2 diabetic patients can develop complications similar to those noted in type 1 diabetes, but ketoacidosis is less likely to occur. Type 2 diabetes is also associated with the development of atherosclerosis and with an increased risk for coronary artery disease (CAD) and cerebrovascular accident (stroke).

Higher fasting plasma glucose concentrations within the normoglycemic range constitute an independent risk factor for type 2 diabetes among young men. Such levels, along with body mass index (BMI) and triglyceride levels, may help identify apparently healthy men at increased risk for developing type 2 diabetes.[3]

Children and Adolescents

Testing for type 2 diabetes should be considered in children age 18 years or younger who are overweight. A BMI above the 85th percentile for age and gender, above the 85th percentile weight for height, or greater than 120% of ideal weight for height are risk factors. In addition to the BMI risk factor, two or more of any of the following risk factors put children at risk for developing type 2 diabetes:

- Family history of type 2 diabetes in first- or second-degree relative
- Race/ethnicity (Native/Indian American, African American, Latino, Asian American, Pacific Islander)
- Signs of insulin resistance or conditions associated with insulin resistance such as acanthosis nigricans, hypertension, dyslipidemia, polycystic ovary syndrome, or small-for-gestational-age birth weight
- Maternal history of diabetes or GDM during child's gestation

Children and adolescents should begin being tested at the age of 10 years or at onset of puberty (if it occurs at age <10), and should be done every 3 years after that.

Symptoms of Diabetes

The primary symptoms of diabetes are excessive urination (polyuria), abnormally high blood glucose (hyperglycemia) and urine glucose (glycosuria), excessive thirst (polydipsia), constant hunger (polyphagia), and sudden weight loss. During acute episodes of the disease, excessive blood ketones (ketonemia) and urinary ketones (ketonuria) may be detected.

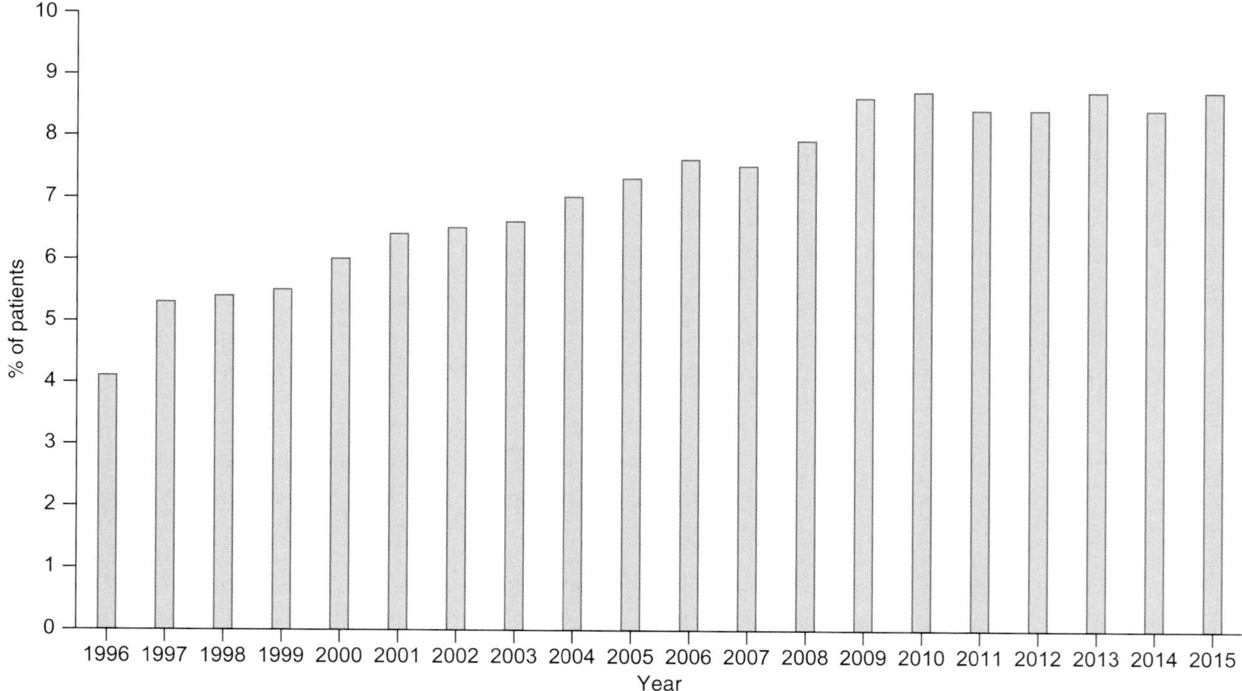

Fig. 10.3 Type 2 Diabetes. Long-term Trends in Diabetes, April 2017, CDC's Division of Diabetes Translation. U.S. Diabetes Surveillance System, http://www.cdc.gov/diabetes/data, accessed Oct. 1, 2018.

These symptoms are all caused by the body's inability to metabolize glucose and the resulting consequences of high glucose levels.

Glucosuria is a consequence of hyperglycemia. The amount of glucose reabsorbed by the kidneys is equivalent to the amount entering the filtration system. The reabsorption increases with an increase in glucose concentration up to approximately 11 mmol/L (198 mg/dL). At this threshold, the system becomes saturated and the maximal reabsorption rate, the glucose transport maximum (Tm_G), is reached. No more glucose can be absorbed, and the kidneys begin excreting it in the urine. This is the beginning of glycosuria. The actual renal threshold is not a single point but a curve, where excretion begins to occur at plasma glucose levels of ~10 mmol/L (180 mg/dL), then increasing more gradually rather than abruptly. As the reabsorption approaches the Tm_G, it trails off and becomes parallel to the glucose concentration threshold. The actual diagnosis of diabetes is established by determining blood glucose levels (Table 10.1).

Gestational Diabetes Mellitus

GDM is defined as glucose intolerance that is first recognized during pregnancy. Based on the 2013 ADA diagnostic criteria for GDM,[2] it is estimated that gestational diabetes affects 18% of pregnancies.

Diabetes in pregnancy needs to be recognized (Table 10.2). The hypothesis for the development of gestational diabetes supports the belief that placental hormones block the action of a mother's insulin in her body. This is called *insulin resistance.* Insulin resistance makes it difficult for the mother's body to use insulin, and she may need up to three times as much insulin. GDM occurs when a mother develops hyperglycemia.

Gestational diabetes affects the mother in late pregnancy, after the fetus has been formed but while the baby is growing.

TABLE 10.1 Diagnosis of Diabetes and Increased Risk (Prediabetes)*

	AMERICAN DIABETES ASSOCIATION GOAL FOR:		
Diabetes Test	**Normal**	**Diagnosis of Diabetes**	**Increased Risk (Prediabetes)/ Impaired Fasting Glucose**
HbA_{1c}	Less than 5.7%	6.5% or higher	5.7%–6.4%
Fasting plasma glucose	Less than 100 mg/dL	126 mg/dL or higher	100–125 mg/dL
2-hour plasma glucose (OGTT)	Less than 140 mg/dL mg/dL	200 mg/dL or higher	140–199 mg/dL
Random plasma glucose		Greater than or equal to 200 mg/dL	

HbA_{1c}, Hemoglobin A_{1c}; *OGTT,* oral glucose tolerance test.
Reference: American Diabetes Association: Standards of Medical Care in Diabetes—2018 Abridged for Primary Care Providers, *Clinical Diabetes* 2018 Jan; 36(1):14–37.

TABLE 10.2 Gestational Diabetes Mellitus Screening and Care*

GDM Screening	Results
Screen for GDM at 24–28 weeks using a 75-g dose of glucose for OGTT.	Fasting: ≥92 mg/dL (5.1 mmol/L) 1 hour: ≥180 mg/dL (10.0 mmol/L) 2 hour: ≥153 mg/dL (8.5 mmol/L)
Screen women with GDM for persistent diabetes 6–12 weeks postpartum using OGTT and nonpregnancy diagnostic criteria.	
Continue to screen women with history of GDM for diabetes or prediabetes at least every 3 years.	
Women with GDM history and prediabetes should receive lifestyle interventions or metformin for diabetes prevention.	

Preconception Care	Risks
Maintain HbA_{1c} levels as close to below 7.0% as possible before attempting conception.	
Provide preconception counseling starting at puberty for all women of childbearing potential.	
Evaluate and treat (if necessary) in women contemplating pregnancy.	Diabetic retinopathy Nephropathy Neuropathy Cardiovascular disease
Evaluate, consider risk/benefit profile of medications being used for treatment of diabetes and associated conditions before conception.	Statins, ACEIs, ARBs, and most noninsulin therapies are contraindicated or not recommended in pregnancy.

ACEI, Angiotensin-converting enzyme inhibitor; *ARB,* angiotensin receptor blocker; *GDM,* gestational diabetes mellitus; *HbA_{1c},* hemoglobin A_{1c}; *OGTT,* oral glucose tolerance test.
*Pregnant women not known to have diabetes.
Modified from American Diabetes Association: Position statement: Diagnosis and classification of diabetes mellitus, *Diabetes Care* 37:S81–S90, 2014

Therefore GDM does not cause the types of birth defects sometimes seen in babies whose mothers had diabetes before pregnancy. However, untreated or poorly controlled GDM can harm an unborn baby. When GDM exists, a pregnant woman's pancreas works overtime to produce insulin, but the insulin does not lower the blood glucose levels. Although insulin does not cross the placenta, glucose and other nutrients do. Thus extra blood glucose goes through the placenta, resulting in high blood glucose levels in the unborn baby as well. This causes the fetal pancreas to make extra insulin to react the blood glucose. Because the baby is receiving more energy than it needs to grow and develop, the extra energy is stored as fat. This can produce a "fat" infant with health problems of his or her own, including damage to the shoulders during birth. Because of the extra insulin made by the pancreas, the newborn may have very low blood glucose levels at birth and is also at higher risk for breathing problems. An infant with excess insulin becomes a child who is at risk for obesity and an adult at risk for type 2 diabetes.

Other Causes of Hyperglycemia

In some cases, high blood glucose values are caused by conditions other than diabetes. Hyperglycemia can be secondary to traumatic brain injury; febrile disease; certain liver diseases; and overactivity of the adrenal, pituitary, or thyroid gland. Often, hyperglycemic patients exhibit impaired glucose tolerance when the fasting glucose or 2-hour postprandial glucose level is elevated above normal.

Stress-induced hyperglycemia is a condition encountered in nondiabetic persons and diabetic patients, and is common in patients with severe illness. It is standard procedure for hospitalized patients in intensive care to have their blood glucose levels monitored frequently. Maintenance of the blood sugar at close to normal limits, referred to as *tight glycemic control,* is accomplished by infusion of intravenous (IV) insulin. Bedside testing for blood glucose has made this possible. This procedure has been shown to reduce morbidity significantly, including renal dysfunction, and mortality in critically ill patients with stress-induced hyperglycemia.[4]

Hypoglycemia

Hypoglycemia is a blood glucose concentration below the fasting value, with a transient decline in blood sugar 1½ to 2 hours after a meal. Glycogen storage disease, associated with impaired breakdown of stored glycogen in the liver, causes hypoglycemia. Other causes of low blood glucose include islet cell hyperplasia and insulinoma. Both these conditions result in an increased concentration of insulin in the blood, hyperinsulinemia. A decrease in blood glucose is life-threatening because the brain and cardiac cells depend on glucose in the blood and interstitial fluids.

Hypoglycemia can lead to nausea and vomiting, muscle spasms, unconsciousness, and death. The most common causes of hypoglycemia in neonates are prematurity, maternal diabetes, GDM, and maternal toxemia. These conditions are usually transient. If the onset of hypoglycemia is in early infancy, it is usually less transitory and may be caused by an inborn error of metabolism or ketotic hypoglycemia, a type of hypoglycemia that usually develops after fasting or a febrile illness.

Diagnosis of Diabetes

In the past, diabetes was diagnosed based on the measurement of glucose on either fasting plasma glucose or 2-hour plasma glucose level in the oral glucose (75 g) tolerance test (OGTT). In 2013 ADA Clinical Practice Guidelines recommended the use of glycated hemoglobin (**hemoglobin A_{1c} [HbA_{1c}]**) to diagnose diabetes.

Traditionally, the diagnosis of diabetes type 1 and type 2 was made on the basis of an elevated fasting glucose level. The ADA proposes that fasting plasma glucose be measured in all asymptomatic patients age 45 and older and that screening be considered at a younger age in those at increased risk for diabetes. The former gold standard of the 3- to-5-hour OGTT is currently not recommended by the ADA or the International Expert Committee. Both organizations continue to recommend use of the 2-hour oral glucose challenge test, especially in women with GDM. Current recommendations from the National Diabetes Data Group are that the OGTT be performed after 3 days on a diet containing a minimum of 150 g of carbohydrates per day. The following day, after an overnight fast, 75 g of glucose is given in water (H_2O). Five blood specimens are usually collected, one before glucose administration and then every 30 minutes up to 2 hours after glucose ingestion. ADA and International Expert Committee set the diagnostic criteria for abnormal glucose tolerance, a blood glucose level of 200 mg/dL or greater at 2 hours, as diagnostic of diabetes, and set a level of 140 to 199 mg/dL as impaired glucose tolerance. About one-third of patients who develop diabetes may not exhibit impaired glucose tolerance.

A fasting glucose concentration of 126 mg/dL or greater on more than one occasion is considered diagnostic of diabetes. In the absence of clinical symptoms, a glucose level between 100 and 125 mg/dL indicates an increased risk for diabetes (prediabetes) and is called *impaired fasting glucose.*

Glycemic Biomarker: Hemoglobin A_{1c}

Measurement of glycated proteins, primarily glycosylated HbA_{1c}, has been widely used for routine long-term monitoring of glucose. HbA_{1c} is now recommended by the ADA for diagnosis and for monitoring purposes every 3 months, but it does have some limitations. Therefore use of other glycated protein biomarkers is necessary.

Hemoglobin A is formed when glucose binds to an amino group that is part of the HbA protein. The reaction occurs at the N-terminal valine of the hemoglobin beta chains (see Chapter 11, Fig. 11.6). Formation of HbA_{1c} is nonenzymatic and occurs over the life span (average 120 days) of the red blood cell (RBC). Because RBCs are freely permeable to blood glucose, the amount of total HbA_{1c} is related to the time-averaged glucose concentration over the 120 days before the measurement. According to the American Diabetes Association, 2018[5] the accepted adult values of HbA_{1c} are

Normal	Less than 5.7%
Prediabetic	5.7%–6.4%
Diabetic	6.5% or higher

HbA_{1c} testing should be performed at least twice a year if patients are meeting treatment goals and have stable glycemic control. For patients whose therapy has changed or who are not meeting glycemic goals, HbA_{1c} testing should be conducted quarterly.

Common automated chemistry analyzers can use an enzymatic assay such as Diazyme A_{1c} (Hitachi 7170). Glycosylated hemoglobin methods also include electrophoresis, ion exchange chromatography, and high-performance liquid chromatography (HPLC).

Emerging Glycemic Biomarkers

In addition to hemoglobin, other proteins in the blood can also be glycated. Fructose amine and glycoalbumin can be used as an estimation of glucose control.

Glycated albumin (GA) is based on the half-life of serum albumin, rather than on the average blood glucose concentration, over a shorter time frame than the 2- to 3-month review associated with HbA_{1c} methods. The glycated serum protein (GSP)/GA ratio profiles the patient's glucose control over the

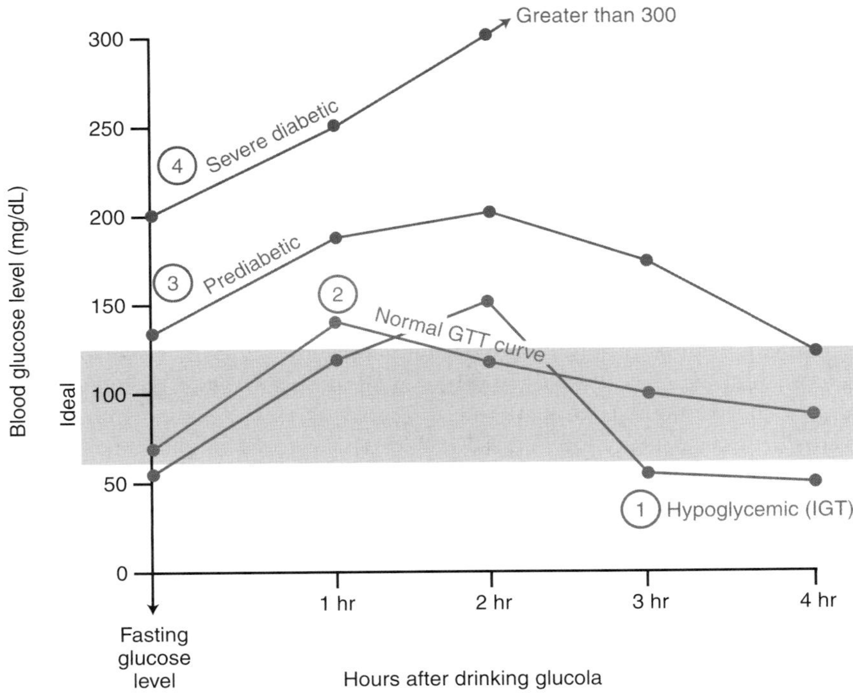

Fig. 10.4 Glucose curve. Comparative patterns of glucose tolerance testing (GTT) results. Compare the blood glucose levels for each condition during the initial fasting test, then the subsequent levels for each hourly test after consumption of the glucose drink. *IGT,* Impaired glucose tolerance. (From Garrels M, Oatis CS: *Laboratory testing for ambulatory settings: a guide for health care professionals,* Philadelphia, 2006, Saunders.)

preceding 2 to 3 weeks and is a more rapid evaluation of the effectiveness of diet, exercise, and medication adjustments. Specific advantages of GSP/GA include efficient monitoring of patients receiving hemodialysis or peritoneal dialysis and of those with GDM, hemolytic anemia, or blood loss.[6]

Collection of Blood Specimens for Glucose

Capillary Blood Specimens

An advantage of using whole blood is the convenience of measuring glucose directly with capillary blood, as for infants in mass screening programs for the detection of diabetes, and as in the home monitoring done by many diabetic patients. Capillary blood must be thought of as essentially arterial rather than venous. In the fasting state, the arterial (capillary) blood glucose concentration is 5 mg/dL higher than the venous concentration.

Venous Blood Specimens

Whole blood, plasma, or serum from a fasting patient can be used for a glucose assay. An evacuated (gray-top) tube containing the preservative *sodium fluoride* is often used for the collection of blood for glucose testing. Fluoride inhibits glucose metabolism by the cells in the sample, allowing for an accurate glucose determination if a number of hours will elapse before analysis. Glycolysis decreases serum glucose by approximately 5% to 7% per hour (5–10 mg/dL) in normal, uncentrifuged coagulated blood at room temperature.[7]

Use of serum or plasma separator gel tubes, processed as quickly as possible (within 30 minutes), is another method of collection.

Types of Blood Specimens

Because the amount of glucose in the blood increases after a meal, it is important that assays to monitor glucose metabolism be done on fasting blood specimens or on specimens drawn 2 hours after a meal (2-hour postprandial). A random sample of blood is of limited value for a glucose determination. The term *fasting* means that the patient has had no food or drink for 8 to 12 hours. A strict fast is necessary, including no coffee, tea, or other caffeinated drink, and no drugs that might affect the blood glucose level. Patients also should avoid emotional disturbances that might cause liberation of glucose into the blood.

For nonpregnant women, the fasting serum or plasma glucose concentration should normally be less than 110 mg/dL, and the postprandial value should be less than 126 mg/dL.

In the detection and treatment of diabetes, it is sometimes necessary to have more information than can be obtained from testing only the fasting specimen for glucose. Patients with mild or diet-controlled diabetes may have fasting serum or plasma glucose levels within the normal range, but they may be unable to produce sufficient insulin for prompt metabolism of ingested carbohydrates. As a result, the serum or plasma glucose rises to abnormally high levels, and the return to normal levels is delayed. Such a pattern will be noted with an OGTT (Fig. 10.4).

Other Body Fluids

Glucose testing may be requested on other body fluids, such as cerebrospinal fluid (CSF) and urine. CSF should be analyzed for glucose immediately because contamination with bacteria will quickly reduce the level of glucose. If a delay in measurement is unavoidable, the specimen should be centrifuged and stored at 4°C or −20°C.[8]

In a 24-hour collection of urine, glucose may be stabilized by the addition of a preservative. Urine specimens should be stored at 4°C during collection because they can lose up to 40% of the glucose concentration after 24 hours at room temperature.

Point-of-Care Testing for Glucose

Many patients regularly monitor their own blood glucose concentrations to reduce their risk for developing diabetic complications. Advances in capillary blood glucose meters have made it possible for almost all diabetic patients to test themselves with these easy-to-use instruments. However, blood glucose meters, as consumer products, do differ from traditional laboratory methods for measuring glucose. Manufacturers of point-of-care instruments must balance accuracy with many other factors to ensure that these meters perform properly in the hands of patients Table 10.3).

Specimens used for patient point-of-care testing (POCT) are generally capillary blood obtained by finger puncture. Products using reagent test strips for monitoring blood glucose include OneTouch (LifeScan), Accu-Chek Easy (Boehringer Mannheim), and Glucometer Elite (Bayer). The strips used for these tests are impregnated with the enzyme glucose oxidase. Glucose present in the blood is converted to gluconic acid and hydrogen peroxide (H_2O_2) by the glucose oxidase used to catalyze the reaction. A second enzyme, peroxidase, is also present on the strip. The peroxidase uses the H_2O_2 formed in the first reaction to oxidize an indicator also present on the strip to give a detectable color change. The color change can be read on a reflectance meter, where the result (in mg/dL) is visualized. The results of capillary whole blood are converted to plasma glucose values by the instrument.

TABLE 10.3 Glucose Point-of-Care Testing Meters versus Laboratory Instruments

Laboratory Instruments	POCT Glucose Meter
No hematocrit effect by analysis of serum or plasma	Hematocrit effect mitigated by measurement or algorithms
Can cost >$10,000	Costs <$100
Maintenance costs >$1000 per year	No maintenance required
Trained laboratory personnel perform test	Patient performs test
Calibration many times each day	No user calibration
Controlled environment	Variables include temperature and altitude
Controls tested frequently	Control solution use limited
Large piece of equipment, sensitive to vibrations and shock	Small, portable, resistant to vibrations and shock
≥5-mL specimen	≤1-μL specimen
≥60-second throughput	≤10-second throughput
±4% to ±10% inaccuracy	Inaccuracy generally ≥2 × reference method (laboratory instrument)

POCT, Point-of-care testing.
From Malone B: Blood glucose meters, glucose analysis: laboratory instruments versus points-of-care meters, *Adv Med Clin Laboratory News* 36(5):3, 2010.

Various other methods of testing are used in POCT meters (Table 10.4). Another product, HemoCue Glucose, uses transmittance photometry and single-test cartridges. The cartridge is inserted into a microcuvette that draws up 5 mL into the photometer, where the analysis takes place and the result is displayed. The reaction is based on the glucose dehydrogenase method. The cartridge/microcuvette is the unique part to this system; it is a self-filling, disposable cuvette and serves as a pipette, test tube, and measuring vessel. The reagent is contained in the tip of the microcuvette, where the chemical reaction takes place. Another new blood glucose and β-ketone point-of-care monitoring system is manufactured by Abbott.

Another new blood glucose and β-ketone point-of-care monitoring system is manufactured by Abbott.

The majority of point-of-care-testing and training are overseen by the laboratory, but nonlaboratory personnel perform the testing. It is important that users of these bedside or home-monitoring methodologies be fully instructed in and informed about their proper use. The instruments must be calibrated with either control solutions of glucose of a known concentration or with a calibration strip or cartridge supplied with each lot of test strips or cartridges. The procedure supplied by the manufacturer must always be followed when any of these products is used.

Methods for Qualitative and Semiquantitative Determination of Glucose

Qualitative laboratory testing provides a semiquantitative estimation of the amount of glucose present in a specimen such as urine. Glucose methods once relied on the reducing ability of glucose as demonstrated by the classic Benedict's reaction. A reducing sugar, such as glucose, converts cupric ions (Cu^{2+}) in alkaline solution to Cu^{+} ions, producing a color change. This reaction is the basis for Clinitest tablets, which react with urinary reducing substances, but the test detects reducing sugars that are not specifically glucose. Urine dipstick methods for glucose determination use test strips impregnated with enzyme reagent (see Chapter 13).

TABLE 10.4 Comparative Point-of-Care Testing Principles

Manufacturer	Instrument Series	Operational Type/Reagent Type	Test Principle
Abbott Point of Care	Piccolo Xpress	Discrete/self-contained single-use cartridges-packages-slides	Photometry, enzymatic
		Disk loaded directly into instrument	
		Benchtop	
	i-STAT-1 analyzer	Self-contained single-use cartridges-packages-slides	Potentiometry, amperometric, conductometric
		Handheld	

Methods for Quantitative Determination of Glucose

The most common quantitative methods for glucose determination use the enzymes glucose oxidase and hexokinase.

Glucose Oxidase

Glucose oxidase catalyzes the oxidation of β-D-glucose to gluconic acid by utilizing molecular oxygen as an electron acceptor with simultaneous production of hydrogen peroxide. The enzyme is specific for β-D-glucose, the form of glucose in the blood. In some methods, the amount of H_2O_2 produced or oxygen consumed is measured by an electrode. In other methods, a second enzyme, peroxidase, catalyzes the oxidation of a chromogen to a colored product. In this case the color formed is proportional to the amount of glucose present. When peroxidase is used in these procedures, the test is subject to interference from reducing agents such as ascorbic acid, which react with H_2O_2, resulting in falsely low results.

Glucose oxidase reaction.

$$\beta\text{-D-glucose } H_2O \xrightarrow{\text{glucoseoxidase}} \text{D-gluconic acid} + H_2O_2$$

$$2H_2O_2 + 4\text{ Aminopyrine} + 1,7\text{-Dehydroxynapthylene} \xrightarrow{\text{peroxidase}} \text{A red dye} + H_2O$$

The glucose oxidase procedure has been adapted to a wide range of automated instruments. Vitros Clinical Chemistry Analyzers (Johnson & Johnson) employ dry chemical reagents in either strip or film form. In these instruments, the oxidation of an indicator dye is used to form a colored compound that results from the action of H_2O_2 and peroxidase. The specimen is deposited on the Vitros Clinical Chemistry Slide and is evenly distributed by the spreading layer. H_2O and any nonprotein components, including glucose, move to the underlying reagent layer. After a fixed incubation period, the reflectance density of the red dye formed in the reaction is measured by the spectrophotometer through the transparent polyester support. The result is obtained in about 5 minutes.

Glucose oxidase methods can be used to measure glucose in CSF. These methods should not be used for urine unless the urine is pretreated, because urine contains a high concentration of substances that interfere with the peroxidase reaction.

Hexokinase

The hexokinase method is the one used most often in automated chemistry analyzers. Hexokinase methods are less subject to interference than the glucose oxidase–peroxidase methods. In this enzymatic method glucose is converted to glucose-6-phosphate (G-6-P) by hexokinase in the presence of ATP, a phosphate donor. Glucose-6-phosphate dehydrogenase then converts the G-6-P to gluconate-6-P in the presence of NADP+. As the NADP+is reduced to NADPH during this reaction, the resulting increase in absorbance at 340 nm (secondary wavelength = 700 nm) is measured.

Hexokinase Reaction.

$$\text{Glucose} + \text{ATP} \xrightarrow{\text{hexokinase}} \text{Glucose-6-phosphate} + \text{ADP} + H^+$$

$$\text{Glucose-6-phosphate} + \text{NADP} \xrightarrow[\text{dehydrogenase}]{\text{glucose-6-phosphate}} \text{6-Phosphogluconate} + \text{NADPH} + H^+$$

This is an endpoint reaction that is specific for glucose and is proportional to the amount of glucose present in the original specimen. Although other hexoses (six-carbon sugars) can also react in the hexokinase procedure, they are not normally encountered in the blood. If plasma is to be used with this procedure, fluoride, heparin, oxalate, and ethylenediaminetetraacetic acid (EDTA) are acceptable anticoagulants.

The hexokinase method is also an excellent test to determine glucose in urine and other biological fluids. This method has been proposed as a basis-of-reference method because of its accuracy and precision.

Glucose Reference Values

Reference values[9] for the individual glucose methods can vary significantly. Each laboratory must determine and evaluate the reference range for its particular facility.

There is no significant difference in serum or plasma glucose concentration between males and females or between races. In normal CSF, the glucose concentration is about two-thirds of the plasma level. It is important to measure the blood glucose concentration simultaneously when CSF glucose is tested so that the CSF glucose results can be evaluated appropriately. There is normally no detectable glucose in urine.

In the asymptomatic child or adolescent screened because of a high risk for diabetes, a test with fasting plasma glucose (FPG) ≥126 mg/dL (7 mmol/L), 2-h PG ≥200 mg/dL (11.1 mmol/L), or A1C ≥6.5% should be repeated on a separate day to confirm the diagnosis.

Diabetes in Children and Adolescents

Criteria for the diagnosis of diabetes

FPG ≥126 mg/dL (7.0 mmol/L). Fasting is defined as no caloric intake for at least 8 h.*

OR

2-h PG ≥200 mg/dL (11.1 mmol/L) during an OGTT. The test should be performed as described by the WHO, using a glucose load containing the equivalent of 1.75 g/kg up to a maximum of 75 g anhydrous glucose dissolved in water.*

OR

A1C ≥6.5% (48 mmol/mol). The test should be performed in a laboratory using a method that is NGSP certified[†] and standardized to the DCCT assay.*

OR

In a patient with classic symptoms of hyperglycemia or hyperglycemic crisis, a random PG ≥200 mg/dL (11.1 mmol/L).

Chiang JL, Maahs DM, Garvey KC, et.al.:, Reference Type 1 Diabetes in Children and Adolescents: A Position Statement by the American Diabetes Association Diabetes Care 2018 Sep; 41(9): 2026–2044.

Laboratory Tests for Diabetic Management

In addition to blood glucose or HbA_{1c}, two other tests are used to manage diabetic patients, for ketones and microalbumin.

Ketone Bodies

During carbohydrate deprivation caused by decreased carbohydrate utilization such as occurs during diabetes starvation, fasting, or prolonged vomiting, blood levels of ketones derived from lipid breakdown increase to meet energy needs. The three ketone bodies are:

- Acetone (2%)
- Acetoacetic acid (20%)
- 3-β-Hydroxybutyric acid (78%)

Ketonemia refers to the accumulation of ketones in blood, and *ketonuria* refers to accumulation of ketones in urine. Measurement of ketones is recommended for patients with type 1 diabetes during acute illness, and in other conditions including stress, pregnancy, and extremely elevated blood glucose levels, or if signs of ketoacidosis are present.

A common method for screening for ketones uses sodium nitroprusside in the urine reagent strip test and Acetest tablets. Sodium nitroprusside reacts with acetoacetic acid in an alkaline pH to form a purple color. An enzymatic method employed by some automated instruments uses the enzyme β-hydroxybutyrate dehydrogenase to detect either β-hydroxybutyric acid or acetoacetic acid, depending on the pH of the solution used.

Microalbumin

Diabetes causes progressive changes in renal tissue, resulting in diabetic nephropathy. This complication develops over many years. An early sign of degeneration is an increase in urinary albumin. Microalbuminuria is a powerful predictor for the future development of diabetic nephropathy.

The use of a random spot collection for the measurement of a microalbumin/creatinine ratio is the preferred method. Microalbuminuria is confirmed when two specimens collected within a 6-month period are elevated. Chemistry and immunoassay integrated analyzers, such as ci8200 (Abbott Laboratories), perform microalbumin analysis. POCT for microalbuminuria screening also is available (such as HemoCue Urine Albumin System).

ELECTROLYTES

Electrolytes are substances that form or exist as ions or charged particles when dissolved in H_2O. Electrolytes facilitate many crucial functions in the body such as fluid volume, osmotic pressure, myocardial cell contractibility, neuromuscular cell excitability, and acid-base balance. Electrolytes are either negatively charged anions or positively charged cations. Cations move toward the cathode and anions toward the anode in an electrical field. Electrolytes include sodium (Na^+), potassium (K^+), calcium (Ca^{2+}), magnesium (Mg^{2+}), chloride (Cl^-), bicarbonate (HCO_3^-), sulfate (SO_4^{2-}), and phosphate (PO_4^{2-}).

The chief positively charged constituents (cations) are Na^+ and K^+. The chief negatively charged constituents (anions) are Cl^- and HCO_3^-. Because Na^+, K^+, Cl^-, and HCO_3^- represent the major electrolytes, they are most likely to show variation when an electrolyte problem exists. These four electrolytes are discussed together because changes in the concentration of one are almost always accompanied by changes in the concentration of one or more of the others.

Water-based body fluid can be divided into two major compartments: intracellular fluid (ICF) and extracellular fluid (ECF). ICF is located within the cell membrane and contains primarily potassium ions and phosphate ions. The ECF is found outside of cell membranes and can be divided into interstitial fluid (fluid between and around the cells) and intravascular fluid (blood plasma). ECF contains primarily sodium ions and chloride ions. Although electrolytes are found throughout the body, their concentrations or activities vary from one body compartment to another. Assays are usually done on plasma or serum.

It is essential that the positively charged particles balance, or electrically neutralize, the negatively charged particles. The kidneys and lungs are the organs that exert the most control over electrolyte concentration. If the body is unable to maintain normal control over acceptable concentrations of electrolytes, either by excretion or conservation, an electrolyte imbalance occurs. Having an abnormal concentration of one or more of the electrolyte constituents is extremely harmful to the patient and can be fatal because most of the body's essential metabolic processes are affected by or dependent on electrolyte balance.

Sodium

Na^+ is the major cation, or positively charged particle, and is found in the highest concentration in ECF. It is significant in maintaining water distribution, plasma volume, and osmotic pressure. Na^+ is associated with the levels of Cl^- and HCO_3^- ions and has a major role in maintaining the acid-base balance of the body cells and excitation of nerve and muscle cells.

A low serum Na^+ level is called *hyponatremia*. Low Na^+ levels are found in a variety of conditions, including severe polyuria, metabolic acidosis, Addison disease, diarrhea, and some renal tubular diseases. A high level of Na^+ is called *hypernatremia*. Clinical conditions resulting in excess body Na^+ include cardiac failure (congestive heart failure), liver disease (ascites), and renal disease (nephritic syndrome). An increased Na^+ level is found in Cushing syndrome (in which there is hyperactivity of the adrenal cortex and an excess production of hormones), severe dehydration caused by primary H_2O loss, certain types of brain injury, diabetic coma after therapy with insulin, and after excess treatment with Na^+ salts. The kidneys can conserve or excrete large concentrations of Na^+ depending on the Na^+ concentration of the ECFs and the blood volume.

Osmolality

Osmolality is based on the number of dissolved particles in a solution. Osmolality measures the total concentration of all the ions and molecules present in serum or urine. Na^+, glucose, and urea are major contributors to the total osmolality of serum (Boxes 10.1 and 10.2). The reference range of osmolality for adults is 275 to 295 mOsm/kg. In contrast, in the calculation of the osmolal gap (Box 10.3)—the difference between the calculated osmolality and the measured osmolality—elevation in the gap is usually caused by factors other than Na^+, glucose, or blood urea nitrogen. Clinically, the presence of ketones or alcohol in the plasma can elevate the osmolal gap. The average osmolal gap is 0 to 10 mOsm/kg H_2O.

BOX 10.1 Osmolality of Plasma

$$\text{Osmolality}(\text{osmol/kg } H_2O) = 1.86(Na^+) + \frac{(\text{glucose})}{18} + \frac{\text{BUN}}{2.8}$$

note:

- 1.86 = Used because each sodium ion is balanced by an anion, but dissociation is not perfect.
- 18 = Molecular weight of glucose is 180; factor of 18 converts mg/dL to mmol/L. This is the unit used to express osmolality.
- 2.8 = Represents the molecular weight of blood urea nitrogen (BUN), which is 28; therefore 2.8 is used.

BOX 10.2 Case Study of Plasma Osmolality

A 40-year-old woman suffering from vomiting and diarrhea had the following laboratory values: Na^+ 145 mmol/L, glucose 750 mg/dL, blood urea nitrogen (BUN) 25 mg/dL.

$$\text{Osmolality}(\text{osmol/kg } H_2O) = 1.86(Na^+) + \frac{(\text{glucose})}{18} + \frac{\text{BUN}}{2.8}$$

Calculation:

$$\begin{aligned}\text{Osmolality}(\text{osmol/kg } H_2O) &= 1.86(145) + \frac{750}{18} + \frac{25}{2.8} \\ &= 270 + 41.7 + 8.9 \\ &= 321 \text{ mOsm/kg } H_2O\end{aligned}$$

BOX 10.3 Case Study of Osmolal Gap

The patient is a 22-year-old intoxicated man with Na^+ 142 mmol/L, glucose 105 mg/dL, and blood urea nitrogen (BUN) 12 mg/dL. His measured plasma osmolality is 320 mOsm/kg. His calculated osmolality is 274 mOsm/kg. What is the osmolal gap measurement in this patient?

$$\begin{aligned}\text{Osmolal gap} &= \text{Calculated osmolality} - \text{Measured plasma osmolality} \\ &= 320 - 274 \text{ mOsm/kg} \\ &= 46 \text{ mOsm/kg}\end{aligned}$$

Average reference range of osmolal gap = 0 to 10 mOsm/kg H_2O

Osmolality is important because it is the condition to which the hypothalamus responds. If a calculated osmolality is elevated above the reference range, the patient has dehydration. The regulation of osmolality affects the Na^+ concentration in plasma mainly because Na^+ and associated anions account for approximately 90% of the osmotic activity in plasma.

Regulation of Plasma Na^+

The following three processes are important to the regulation of plasma Na^+ concentration:

- Intake of H_2O in response to thirst, which is stimulated or suppressed by plasma osmolality
- Excretion of H_2O, which is influenced primarily by antidiuretic hormone (ADH) released in response to changes in either blood volume or osmolality
- Regulation of blood volume, which affects Na^+ excretion through aldosterone, angiotensin II, and atrial natriuretic peptide

Potassium

K^+ is the major intracellular cation with 98% of K^+ located in the ICF (see Special Considerations for Specimens). K^+ has an important influence on the muscle activity of the heart. In addition, K^+ is important in cellular metabolism in the regulation of protein and glycogen synthesis.

The ratio of intracellular to extracellular K^+ concentration results in a voltage difference across the cell membrane when the cell is at rest (resting membrane potential), which makes K^+ a major determinant of resting membrane potential and thus is essential for neuromuscular cell excitability. The overall difference between a cell's resting membrane potential and the cell's threshold potential initiates an action potential and nerve impulse. An elevated K^+ decreases the resting membrane potential compared with low plasma K^+ concentration, which increases the resting membrane potential. Alterations in cell excitability cause muscle weakness, paralysis, or arrhythmia.

Hypokalemia (abnormally low K^+ levels) can result from prolonged diarrhea or vomiting, or from inadequate intake of dietary K^+. Even in conditions of K^+ deficiency, the kidney continues to excrete K^+. The body has no effective mechanism to protect itself from excessive loss of K^+, so a regular daily intake of K^+ is essential.

An elevated K^+ level in serum is called *hyperkalemia*. Because K^+ is excreted primarily by the kidney, the level becomes elevated in kidney dysfunction or urinary obstruction. As with Na^+, K^+ is influenced by the presence of the adrenocortical hormones and is associated with acid-base balance. In renal tubular acidosis, there is increased retention of K^+ in the serum. One important purpose of renal dialysis is the removal of accumulated K^+ from the plasma. Potassium levels greater than 10.0 mEq/L (10.0 mmol/L) are usually associated with death as a result of vascular collapse of the heart.

Sodium and Potassium in Body Fluids

Urinary Na^+ excretion varies with dietary intake, but for individuals on an average diet containing 8 to 15 g/day, a range of 40 to 220 mmol/day is typical. Diurnal variation exists in Na^+ excretion, with reduced levels at night.

After K^+ is absorbed by the gastrointestinal tract, it is rapidly distributed, with most excreted by the kidneys. K^+ filtered through the glomeruli is reabsorbed almost completely in the proximal tubules and then secreted in the distal tubules in exchange for Na^+ under the influence of aldosterone.

Factors that regulate distal tubular secretion of K^+ include the following:

- Na^+ and K^+ intake
- H_2O flow rate in the distal tubules
- Plasma level of mineralocorticoids
- Acid-base balance

Renal regulation of K^+ excretion is influenced by renal tubular acidosis and by metabolic and respiratory acidosis and alkalosis. Retention of K^+ is present in patients with chronic renal failure.

The Na^+ concentration of CSF is 138 to 150 mmol/L. Mean fecal Na^+ excretion generally is considered to be less than 10 mmol/day. In cases of severe diarrhea, fecal loss of K^+ may be as much as 60 mmol/day. CSF values for K^+ are approximately 70% of plasma values. Urinary excretion of K^+ varies with dietary intake but typically ranges from 25 to 125 mmol/day.

Chloride

Cl^- is found in serum, plasma, CSF, tissue fluid, and urine. Physiologically, only the concentration of Cl^- in the ECF is important.

The chief extracellular anions are Cl^- and HCO_3^-, and there is a reciprocal relationship between them: A decrease in the amount of one produces an increase in the amount of the other. The Cl^- ion is the most important anion of the ECFs in the body. It is the major anion that counterbalances the major cation, Na^+. This means that the sum of all the cations equals the sum of all the anions.

In the blood, two-thirds of Cl^- is found in the plasma and one-third in the RBCs. Because of the difference in Cl^- concentration between the RBCs and the plasma, the test for Cl^- is routinely performed on plasma (or serum) and not on whole blood.

Cl^- has an important role in two main functions in the body: (1) determining the osmotic pressure, which controls the distribution of H_2O among cells, plasma, and interstitial fluid; and (2) maintaining electrical neutrality.

Cl^- plays an important role in the buffering action when carbon dioxide (CO_2) exchange takes place in the RBCs. This activity is known as the *chloride shift*. When blood is oxygenated, Cl^- travels from the RBCs to the plasma, and at the same time, HCO_3^- leaves the plasma and enters the RBCs. An example of the Cl^- shift in the laboratory is the replacement action that occurs when a specimen for a Cl^- determination is allowed to stand for a time before the cells and plasma are separated. When whole blood comes into contact with air, CO_2 (and thus HCO_3^-) escapes from the blood. While CO_2 leaves the plasma, Cl^- diffuses (or shifts) out of the RBCs to replace HCO_3^-, which is reentering the cell to maintain equilibrium. The contact between whole blood and air has the effect of lowering the plasma CO_2 and raising the plasma Cl^-. Specimens of whole blood left in contact with air can produce falsely high plasma or serum Cl^- values. The cells must be removed from the plasma by centrifugation as quickly as possible. Once separated from the cells, the serum or plasma has a very stable Cl^- concentration.

Another important function of Cl^- is to regulate the fluid content of the body and its influence on the kidney. The kidney maintains the electrolyte concentration of the plasma within very narrow limits. Renal function is set to regulate the composition of the ECF first and the volume second. Consequently, if the body loses salt (Na^+ Cl^-), H_2O is lost.

High serum or plasma Cl^- values are seen in dehydration and conditions that cause decreased renal blood flow, such as congestive heart failure. Excessive treatment with or dietary intake of Cl^- also results in high serum levels. Low serum or plasma Cl^- values may be seen when salt is lost, such as in chronic pyelonephritis. A low Cl^- value may also be seen in metabolic acidotic conditions that are caused by excessive production or diminished excretion of acids, such as diabetic acidosis and renal failure. Prolonged vomiting from any cause may ultimately result in a decrease in serum and body Cl^- levels.

Bicarbonate

HCO_3^-, after Cl^-, is the other major extracellular anion in body fluids. While the blood perfuses the lungs, CO_2 and H_2O are formed. During the metabolic processes, carbonic acid (H_2CO_3) dissociates and forms HCO_3^-. This is a reversible reaction, and depending on body tissue requirements, HCO_3^- may be reconverted to H_2CO_3, followed by the formation of H_2O and CO_2. The reactions are:

$$CO_2(\text{gas}) \leftrightarrow CO_2(\text{dissolved}) + H_2O \leftrightarrow H_2CO_3 \leftrightarrow H^+ + HCO_3^-$$

HCO_3^- is filtered by the kidney, but little or no HCO_3^- is found in the urine. The proximal tubules reabsorb 85% of HCO_3^-, and the remaining 15% is reabsorbed by the distal tubules. HCO_3^- is most often measured with other combined forms of CO_2 (CO_2, HCO_3^-, carbamino groups) as total CO_2. Because about 90% of all the CO_2 in serum is in the form of HCO_3^-, this combined form approximates the actual HCO_3^- concentration very closely. Total CO_2 is the total of H_2CO_3, dissolved CO_2 gas, and HCO_3^-. Assay methods for HCO_3^- are actually a measure of total CO_2.

Along with pH and CO_2 pressure (P_{CO_2}) determinations, the total CO_2 concentration is a useful measurement in evaluating acid-base disorders. The HCO_3^- or CO_2 value in itself is not as significant as the value in the context of the other electrolytes assayed. Assays for total CO_2 are performed by using a P_{CO_2} electrode to measure the rate of released CO_2 being formed.

Anion Gap

The calculation of the mathematical difference between the anions (Cl^- and HCO_3^-) and the cations (Na^+ and K^+) is known as the **anion gap** (Box 10.4). If Cl^- and HCO_3^- are summed and subtracted from the sum of Na^+ and K^+ concentrations, the difference should be less than 16 mmol/L, with a range of 10 to 20 mmol/L. If the anion gap exceeds 16 mmol/L, this is usually an indication of increased concentrations of the unmeasured anions (PO_4^{3-}, SO_4^{2-}, protein ions). Increased anion gaps can also result from ketotic states, lactic acidosis, salicylate and methanol ingestion, **uremia**, or increased plasma proteins. Decreased anion gaps of less than 10 mmol/L can result from either an increase in unmeasured cations (Ca^{2+}, Mg^{2+}) or a decrease in the unmeasured anions.

The anion gap is also useful as a quality control measure for electrolyte results. If an increased anion gap is found for electrolytes in a healthy person, one or more of the test results may be erroneous, and the tests should be repeated.

Special Considerations for Specimens

Plasma can be assayed for electrolyte concentration after use of lithium or sodium heparin as the anticoagulant, except in testing

BOX 10.4

Anion Gap (AG)

$$AG = (Na^+) - ([Cl^-] + [HCO_3^-]) \text{ Reference range } 8-16\text{ mmol/L}$$

or:

$$([Na^+] + [K^+]) - ([Cl^-] + [HCO_3^-]) \text{ Reference range } 10-20\text{ mmol/L}$$

Reference: Langman L, Bechtel LK, Holstege: Clinical Toxicology in Burtis CA, Bruns DE, Tietz Fund. of Cl Chem and Molecular Diagnostics, Elsevier, 2015.

for Na^+, in which case sodium heparin cannot be used. Electrolyte testing can also be done on serum. Capillary samples can be collected into microcontainers or capillary tubes. Centrifugation should be done using the unopened primary collection tubes, and the plasma or serum should be separated from the RBCs promptly. Each assay has specific requirements and technical factors relating to the specimen collection and handling.

Sodium

Lithium heparinized plasma, serum, urine, and other body fluids are suitable specimens. Sodium heparin should not be used, as already noted, because the presence of Na^+ will interfere with the assay for Na^+. Cells must be separated from serum or plasma as soon as possible.

Na^+ is stable in serum for at least 1 week at room or refrigerator temperature, or it can be frozen for up to 1 year. Na^+ can be measured in 24-hour urine specimens and in CSF.

Potassium

Lithium or sodium heparin is the preferred anticoagulant for plasma specimens; an anticoagulant containing K^+ cannot be used. Serum can also be tested. The collection of blood for K^+ studies requires special attention and technique. Because the concentration of K^+ in the RBC is about 20 times that in serum or plasma, hemolysis must be avoided. The following technical errors can contribute to elevated K^+:

- Recentrifugation of specimens in gel tubes
- Inadequate centrifugation
- Centrifuging blood specimen tubes with the stoppers removed
- Pouring blood from one tube to another
- Delayed centrifugation
- Refrigerating a specimen before K^+ analysis
- Improper venipuncture technique such as IV fluid contamination

To avoid a shift of K^+ from the RBCs to the plasma or serum, it is important to separate the cells from the plasma or serum within 3 hours of collection. When blood is collected for a K^+ test, the patient should not open and close the fist before venipuncture; this muscle action can increase plasma K^+ levels by 10% to 20%. K^+ levels in plasma are about 0.1 to 0.2 mmol/L lower than those in serum because of the release of K^+ from ruptured platelets during the coagulation process.

K^+ in serum promptly separated from the blood clot is stable for at least 1 week at room or refrigerator temperature. Specimens may be frozen for up to 1 year. K^+ levels in urine vary with dietary intake and are measured in a 24-hour collection.

Chloride

The anticoagulant used most frequently for Cl^- is lithium or sodium heparin. Serum separator gel tubes are also often used for specimens in Cl^- testing. Cl^- is assayed in serum, plasma, urine, or sweat, and in other body fluids. Moderate hemolysis does not significantly affect Cl^- concentration in the serum.

Bicarbonate

Lithium- or sodium-heparinized plasma or serum may be used for the HCO_3^- assay. Arterial blood is generally collected. The pH and HCO_3^- concentrations are most accurately determined immediately when the tube is opened and as quickly as possible after collection and centrifugation of the unopened tube. A specimen to be assayed for total CO_2 must be handled anaerobically to minimize losses of CO_2 and HCO_3^- (converted to CO_2) into the atmosphere. A falsely low total CO_2 would result if this loss had occurred. In the laboratory, the specimen can be protected by placing a stopper on the container.

Methods for Quantitative Measurement

Four electrolytes—Na^+, K^+, Cl^-, and HCO_3^-—are generally grouped together for testing, called an *electrolyte profile.*

Sodium and Potassium

Ion-selective electrode (ISE) potentiometry uses a glass ion exchange membrane for Na^+ assay and a valinomycin neutral-carrier membrane for K^+ assay and has been incorporated into many automated chemistry analyzers. ISE methods measure the activity of an ion in the H_2O-volume fraction in which it is dissolved. Generally, two types of ISE measurements are made on biological samples: direct and indirect. Direct measurements are becoming more common. Direct measurement is done on undiluted samples; indirect measurement requires prediluted samples for measurement of ion activity. Lipemia and protein cause a false decrease in indirect ISE measurements because they occupy plasma volume.

The Vitros Clinical Chemistry Analyzer uses the ISE method. This instrument uses a dry multilayered slide with a self-contained analytical element coated on a polyester support. Each slide contains a pair of ISEs; one is used as a reference electrode and the other as a measuring electrode. Depending on which slide electrode is selected, the instrument can assay Na^+ or K^+. Another ISE is also available for Cl^- assay using this same instrument. In this method, 10 mL of specimen and reference standard is applied to the appropriate Vitros Clinical Chemistry Slide, and the slide is introduced into the instrument. An electrometer in the instrument measures the potential difference between the two half-cells of the reference and the sample, and the result is calculated.

Chloride

The most common methods for Cl^- assays use ISE-based technology. The sensing element is usually silver–silver Cl^- or silver sulfide.

Another common method for Cl^- assay employs a quantitative displacement of thiocyanate by Cl^- from mercuric thiocyanate and formation of a red ferric thiocyanate complex. The amount of the colored compound, as measured with a spectrophotometer, is proportional to the concentration of Cl^- present in the specimen. In this method, Cl^- first combines with free mercury ions to form a colorless compound, then displaces any thiocyanate from mercuric thiocyanate. The free thiocyanate ions react with iron to produce the red-colored end product.

Sweat Chloride. The Cl^- content of sweat is useful in diagnosing Cystic Fibrosis (CF), a disease of the exocrine glands. Traditional analysis involves collection of a sweat sample from forearm stimulation with the use of pilocarpine nitrate in a process referred to as *iontophoresis.* Cl^- concentration can then be measured directly with the use of ISEs. Newer molecular diagnostic analysis is available.

Affected infants usually have concentrations of sweat Cl^- greater than 60 mmol/L; affected adults have concentrations greater than 70 mmol/L (reference values average about 40 mmol/L). In 98% of patients with CF, the secretion of Cl^- in sweat is two to five times that of normal. The Cl^- content of normal sweat varies with age.

Bicarbonate

The routine HCO_3^- (determined as total CO_2) assay is automated. The first step in automated methods in general is the acidification of the sample to convert the various forms of HCO_3^- present to gaseous CO_2. To keep automated methods in control, another important consideration for HCO_3^- assays is the need to include several standard solutions with the assay of the unknowns.

Other Electrolytes

Calcium

Ca^{2+} is essential for myocardial contraction. A decreased level of ionized Ca^{2+} impairs cardiac function and produces irregular muscle spasms (tetany). Three hormones—parathyroid hormone (PTH), vitamin D, and calcitonin—regulate serum Ca^{2+}.

Most Ca^{2+} in the body is part of bone. Only 1% is in the blood and in other ECFs. Ca^{2+} in blood exists as free Ca^{2+} ions or ionized Ca^{2+} (45%), or is bound to protein or anions.

Calcium has many important functions in the body, including bone mineralization, muscle contraction and excitability, blood hemostasis, plasma membrane stability, and as a second messenger in enzyme activation.

Most of the body's calcium is crystallized in the skeleton. The remainder of calcium exists in three forms: ionized; bonded with the anions bicarbonate, lactate, phosphate, or citrate; or bound to plasma proteins (predominating albumin).

Imbalances of Ca^{2+} are often expressed as neuromuscular symptoms. If a patient has *hypocalcemia,* neuromuscular irritability and cardiac irregularities are primary symptoms. Hypocalcemia is frequently due to chronic renal failure. Mild *hypercalcemia* often has asymptomatic results. Hypercalcemia is caused by primary hyperparathyroidism or malignancy involving PTH-related protein-producing tumors.

Ionized calcium (Ca^{2+}) represents about 50% of plasma and is the only physiologically active form. Forty percent of Ca^{2+} is bound to proteins. Most laboratories can analyze both total Ca^{2+} and ionized Ca^{2+}. Ionized Ca^{2+} is a more reliable indicator of disorders because total calcium measurements can be altered by changes in the concentrations of anions and plasma proteins caused by surgery or serious illness. The preferred specimen for total Ca^{2+} determinations is serum. It is important that a serum specimen for ionized Ca^{2+} remain *uncapped* until immediately before analysis, because loss of CO_2 produces an increase in pH and altered protein binding.

Magnesium

Mg^{2+} is the second most abundant intracellular cation in the body. Most of the total body Mg^{2+} is found in bone. Less than 1% is present in the plasma. Two-thirds of Mg^{2+} present in serum is free or ionized. Mg^{2+} has many functions in the body and is an essential cofactor of more than 300 enzymes. Measurement of Mg^{2+} is useful in cardiovascular, metabolic, and neuromuscular disorders. Serum levels are useful in determining acute changes in the ion.

Hypomagnesemia is most frequently observed in hospitalized patients in intensive care units or in patients receiving diuretics or digitalis therapy. Hypomagnesemia is rare in nonhospitalized patients. Symptoms do not usually occur until serum Mg^{2+} levels fall below 0.5 mmol/L. Manifestations of hypomagnesemia most often involve the cardiovascular and neuromuscular systems. Metabolic conditions such as hyponatremia, hypokalemia, hypocalcemia, or hypophosphatemia, or psychiatric symptoms such as depression, agitation, or psychosis can also occur.

Hypermagnesemia is seen less frequently than hypomagnesemia. Severe elevations of Mg^{2+} level usually result from decreased renal function and an intake of commonly prescribed Mg^{2+}-containing medications such as antacids.

Nonhemolyzed serum or lithium heparin plasma may be analyzed. Hemolysis must be avoided because the concentration of Mg^{2+} inside an erythrocyte is 10 times greater than in the ECF. Citrate and EDTA anticoagulants are unacceptable because they will bind with Mg^{2+}.

The three most common methods for measuring total serum Mg^{2+} are colorimetric: calmagite, formazan dye, and methylthymol blue. One limitation in the measurement of total Mg^{2+} concentrations in serum is that approximately 25% of Mg^{2+} is protein bound. Total Mg^{2+} may not reflect the physiologically active, free ionized Mg^{2+}. Because Mg^{2+} is primarily an intracellular ion, serum concentrations will not necessarily reflect the status of intracellular Mg^{2+}. As much as a 20% depletion of tissue or cellular Mg^{2+} may not be reflected in the serum Mg^{2+} concentrations.

Reference Values

Reference values[7,9] are generally instrument specific. Manufacturers' manuals must be consulted for specific reference values for a particular instrument and specimen type.

Analyte	Specimen	Reference Range	Type of Patient	Comments
Sodium	Serum or Plasma	136-145 mmol/L	Infancy-Adult	
	24 hr. Urine	40-220 mmol/24 hr	Adult male	On average diet
		27-287 mmol/24 hr	Adult female	On average diet
	CSF	70% of value determined simultaneously for plasma or serum Na		
	Sweat	40-40 mmol/L		>70 mmol/L suggests Cystic Fibrosis
Potassium	Serum	3.5-5.1 mmol/L	Adults	
		3.7-5.9 mmol/L	Newborns	
	Plasma	3.5-4.5 mmol/L	Adult Male	On average diet
		3.4-4.4 mmol/L	Adult Female	On average diet
	Urine	25-125 mmol/24 hr	Adult	On average diet

Continued

Chloride	Serum or Plasma	98-107 mmol/L	Adult	
	Serum or Plasma	Upper limit 110 mmol/L	Full term and premature infants	
	Urine	10-250 mmol/L	Adult	Varies with diet
	CSF	118-132 mmol/L		
	Sweat	5-35 mmol/L	Adult	30-70 mmol/L marginal result > 60 mmol/L for 98% of patients with Cystic Fibrosis
Bicarbonate	Serum	22-29 mmol/L	Adult	Newborn infants have lower values
Calcium (total)	Arterial blood	21-28 mmol/L	Adult	
	Serum or Plasma	2.15-2.57 mmol/L	Adult	Alternate reference
		2.15-2.65 mmol/L	Children	range 8.6-10.3 mg/dL
Calcium (ionized or free)	Serum or Plasma	1.15-1.33 mmol/L	Adult	Alternate reference
		1.20-1.48 mmol/L	Neonates	range 4.6-5.3 mg/dL (adults) Children slightly higher reference values Alternate reference range 4.8-5.9 mg/dL
Magnesium	Serum	1.7-2.4 mmol/L	Adults	
		1.5-2.2 mmol/L	Newborns	
		0.45-0.60 mmol/L (free)		
	Urine	12-291 mg/24hr		

Reference: McMillen, GA, Burtis CA, Bruns DE, Tietz Fund. of Cl Chem and Molecular Diagnostics, Chap 50, Table 50-1, Information for the Clinical Laboratory, ed 7, Elsevier, 2015.

ACID-BASE BALANCE AND BLOOD GASES

Many abnormal conditions are accompanied by disturbances of acid-base balance and electrolyte composition. These changes are usually apparent in the acid-base pattern and in the anion-cation composition of ECF such as blood plasma.

A description of acid-base balance involves an accounting of the carbonic (H_2CO_3, HCO_3^-, CO_3^{2-}, CO_2) and noncarbonic acids and conjugate bases in terms of input (intake plus metabolic production) and output (excretion plus metabolic conversion) over a given time interval. The acid-base status of the body fluids typically is assessed by measurements of total CO_2, plasma pH, and P_{CO_2}, because the HCO_3^- system is the most important buffering system of the plasma.[7]

The normal hydrogen ion concentration [H^+] in extracellular body fluid ranges from pH 7.34 to pH 7.44. Through mechanisms that involve the lungs and kidneys, the body controls and excretes H^+ to maintain pH homeostasis. The buffer systems present in all body fluids are the body's first line of defense against extreme changes in H^+. All buffers consist of a weak acid, such as H_2CO_3, and its salt or conjugate base, such as HCO_3^-, for the HCO_3^- buffer system. Other buffers include the PO_4^{3-} buffer system.

The role of the lungs and kidneys in maintaining pH is depicted with the Henderson-Hasselbalch equation. The numerator (HCO_3^-) denotes kidney functions, and the denominator (P_{CO_2}) denotes lung function.

$$pH = pK' + \log \frac{cCHO_3^-}{\alpha \times P_{CO_2}}$$

Note:
$cHCO_3$ = total concentration of CO_2 minus concentration of dissolved CO_2, including a small amount of dissolved carbonic acid.
α = solubility coefficient of CO_2.
P_{CO_2} = partial pressure of oxygen.

This equation can also be written as:

$$pH = 6.1 + (cHCO_3^- / cdCO_2)$$

Note:
6.1 = pK for carbonic acid/bicarbonate system.
$cHCO_3$ = total concentration of CO_2 minus concentration of dissolved CO_2, including a small amount of dissolved carbonic acid.
$cdCO_2$ = concentration of dissolved CO_2 including a small amount of dissolved carbonic acid.

The average normal ratio of the concentrations of HCO_3^- and dissolved CO_2 in plasma is 25 (mmol)/1.25 (mmol/L) = 20/1. Any change in the concentration of either HCO_3^- or dissolved CO_2 is accompanied by a change in pH. The change in the ratio can occur because of a change in either the numerator (renal component) or the denominator (respiratory component).

Clinical terms are used to describe the acid-base status of a patient. *Acidemia* is defined as an arterial blood pH of less than 7.35, and *alkalemia* is defined as an arterial blood pH of greater than 7.45. The terms *acidosis* and *alkalosis* refer to pathologic states that lead to acidemia or alkalemia. If an acid-base disorder is caused by ventilatory (lung) dysfunction, it is called *respiratory*. If the renal or metabolic system is involved, it is called *metabolic*. Acid-base disorders are traditionally classified as follows:

- Metabolic acidosis
- Metabolic alkalosis
- Respiratory acidosis
- Respiratory alkalosis

Metabolic acidosis is detected by decreased plasma HCO_3^-. HCO_3^- is lost in the buffering of excess acid. Causes of metabolic acidosis include the following:

1. Production of organic acids that exceed the rate of elimination, as in diabetic acidosis
2. Reduced excretion of acids (H^+), with an accumulation of acid that consumes HCO_3^-, as in renal failure
3. Excessive loss of HCO_3^-, as with increased renal excretion or excessive loss of duodenal fluid, as occurs in severe diarrhea

Metabolic alkalosis occurs when excess base is added to the system, base elimination is decreased, or acid-rich fluids are lost. Conditions leading to metabolic alkalosis are numerous and include prolonged vomiting, upper duodenal obstruction, or Cushing syndrome.

Respiratory acidosis is a condition of decreased elimination of CO_2. Causes of decreased elimination include chronic obstructive pulmonary disease, which is the most common cause, drugs such as narcotics and barbiturates, infections of the central nervous system such as meningitis or encephalitis, coma caused by intracranial hemorrhage, and sleep apnea.

Respiratory alkalosis is a condition caused by increased rate or depth of respiration, or both; it produces excess elimination of acid through the respiratory system. Factors contributing to the cause of respiratory alkalosis include anxiety or hysteria, febrile states, and asthma.

If a patient has a straightforward acid-base disorder, laboratory results are classic (Table 10.5). However, most cases of acid-base imbalance deviate from being a simple disorder because of compensatory responses by the respiratory and renal systems attempting to correct the imbalance in this dynamic situation.

RENAL FUNCTION

Kidney disease affects at least 8 million Americans. More people die annually from kidney failure than from colon cancer, breast cancer, or prostate cancer. Chronic kidney disease or kidney failure significantly increases a patient's risk for cardiovascular disease (CVD).

A variety of laboratory assays can be performed to support a diagnosis of renal disease or dysfunction (Box 10.5) and (Table 10.6). The reference values of the glomerular filtration rate (GFR) varies by gender and age. For example, a 17–24-year-old male normal value ranges from 93–131 compared to an 80+-year-old female with a rate of 48–85.

Nitrogen (N) exists in the body in many forms, mostly in components of complex substances. Nitrogen-containing substances are classified into two main groups: protein nitrogen (protein substances containing nitrogen) and nonprotein nitrogen (NPN). Urea is the major NPN constituent and accounts for more than 75% of the total NPN excreted by the body; other NPNs, in order of their quantitative importance, are amino acids, uric acid, creatinine, creatine, and ammonia.

TABLE 10.5 Classification and Characteristics of Simple Acid-Base Disorders

	Primary Change	Compensatory Response
Metabolic		
Acidosis	↓ $cHCO_3^-$	↓ Pco_2
Alkalosis	↑ $cHCO_3^-$	↑ Pco_2
Respiratory		
Acidosis	↑ Pco_2	↑ $cHCO_3^-$
Alkalosis	↓ Pco_2	↓ $cHCO_3^-$

$cHCO_3^-$, Cytoplasmic bicarbonate; *Pco_2*, partial pressure of carbon dioxide.

Modified from Burtis CA, Ashwood ER, Bruns DE: *Tietz fundamentals of clinical chemistry*, ed 6, St Louis, 2008, Elsevier/Saunders, p. 668.

BOX 10.5 Renal Function Panel

Assay	Type of Specimen
Albumin	Serum or plasma
Calcium	Serum or plasma
Carbon dioxide	Serum or plasma
Creatinine	Serum or plasma
Chloride	Serum or plasma
Glucose	Serum or plasma
Phosphorus, inorganic	Serum or plasma
Potassium	Serum or plasma
Sodium	Serum or plasma
Urea nitrogen	Serum or plasma

From www.aruplab.com, September, 2018.

TABLE 10.6 Laboratory Assay Characteristics of Reduced Kidney Function or Damage[7,9]

Assay	Reference Interval	Comments
Reduced glomerular filtration rate (GFR)	< mL/min/1.73m² Age and gender dependent*	Monitor renal function with test results of serum creatinine reference intervals.
Albumin	3.9-24.4 mg/dL	≥ 30 mg/24 hrs is diagnostic of albuminuria
Albumin-creatinine ratio, urine	51-80 yrs Male 800-2100 mg/dL Female 500-1400 mg/dL	Reference value varies with age. Peak is at >50 years old. Detect early kidney disease in those with diabetes or other risk factors (e.g., hypertension).
Urinary sediment	Various abnormalities	Tubular disorders
Electrolytes	Na=136-145 mmol/L K=3.5-5.1 mmol/L Cl=98-107 mmol/L HCO_3^- = 22-29 mmol/L	Adult values
Alpha-1 microglobulin (urine)	0.0-1.2 mg/dL	Aids in diagnosis of proximal tubule injury and/or impaired proximal tubular function. May indicate renal involvement in patients with urinary tract infections or diabetes mellitus.
Alpha-2 macroglobulin urine	131-293 mg/dL	May be used as a marker of membrane permeability in serum and fluids; may be used as a screening test of renal function. May be used as a marker of membrane permeability in urine or as an indirect marker for liver fibrosis.

Continued

TABLE 10.6 Laboratory Assay Characteristics of Reduced Kidney Function or Damage[7,9]—cont'd

Assay	Reference Interval	Comments
Beta-2 microglobulin	0-300 μg/L	May indicate renal involvement in patients with diabetic nephropathy, cadmium toxicity, or progressing idiopathic membranous nephropathy. Evaluate renal tubular damage. Monitor exposure to mercury and cadmium.
Cystatin C	Representative value 18 yrs and older 0.5-1.0 mg/L	May be a maker of renal disease but the assay lacks specificity. Reference value varies with age.
Creatinine	00.62-1.10 mg/dL male 00.45-0.75 mg/dL female	Values are age dependent
Microalbumin/ creatinine ratio		Useful in monitoring diabetic nephropathy in insulin-dependent diabetes mellitus

*GFR reference ranges, Burtis CA, Bruns DE: Tietz fundamentals of clinical chemistry, Table 50–1 ed 7, St Louis, 2015, Elsevier/Saunders, p. 965.
Modified from Burtis CA, Bruns DE: Tietz fundamentals of clinical chemistry, Table 50-1 ed 7, St Louis, 2015, Elsevier/Saunders, p. 981

Normally, more than 90% of the urea is excreted through the kidneys. Urea nitrogen, uric acid, and creatinine occur in increased levels as a consequence of decreased renal function. Most laboratories perform serum urea nitrogen measurements in conjunction with creatinine tests when tests for renal function are needed, because as combined assays they are more specific indicators of renal function disorders. The usefulness of the serum urea nitrogen test alone in determining kidney function is limited because of variable blood levels as the result of nonrenal factors. It is common practice to calculate a urea nitrogen/creatinine ratio:

$$\frac{\text{Serum urea nitrogen(mg/dL)}}{\text{Serum creatinine(mg/dL)}}$$

The normal ratio for a person on a normal diet is between 12 and 20. Significantly lower ratios indicate acute tubular necrosis, low protein intake, starvation, or severe liver disease. High ratios with normal creatinine values indicate tissue breakdown, prerenal azotemia, or high protein intake. High ratios with increased creatinine may indicate a postrenal obstruction or prerenal azotemia associated with a renal disease.

Urea/Urea Nitrogen

Urea (urea nitrogen) is the chief component of the NPN material in the blood; it is distributed throughout the body H_2O, and it is equal in concentration in the ICF and ECF. Gross alterations in NPN usually reflect a change in the concentration of urea. The liver is the sole site of urea formation. While protein breaks down (for example, while amino acids undergo deamination), *ammonia* is formed in increased amounts. This potentially toxic substance is removed in the liver, where the ammonia combines with other amino acids and is converted to urea by enzymes present in the liver. Urea is a waste product of protein metabolism, which is normally removed from the blood in the kidneys. The amount of urea in the blood is determined by the amount of dietary protein and by the kidney's ability to excrete urea. If the kidney is impaired, urea is not removed from the blood and accumulates in the blood. An increased concentration of serum or plasma urea may indicate a flaw in the filtering system of the kidneys.

Assays for urea/urea nitrogen and creatinine are performed concurrently because creatinine is considered to be a better single test for kidney function than urea nitrogen alone.

Clinical Significance

The assay for urea is only a rough estimate of renal function and will not show any significant level of increased concentration until the glomerular filtration rate (GFR) is decreased by at least 50%. A more reliable single index of renal function is the test for serum creatinine (S_{CR}). Contrary to urea concentration, creatinine concentration is relatively independent of protein intake (from the diet), degree of hydration, and protein metabolism.

The amount of urea in the blood is determined by the dietary protein and the kidney's ability to excrete urea. If the kidney is impaired, the urea is not removed from the blood, and while it accumulates, the urea level increases. The urea concentration is influenced also by diet; people who are undernourished or who are on low-protein diets may have urea levels that are not accurate indications of kidney function. Because the concentration of urea is directly related to protein metabolism, the protein content of the diet will affect the amount of urea in the blood. The ability of the kidneys to remove urea from the blood will also affect the urea content. Urea concentration is influenced primarily by the protein intake. In the normal kidney, urea is removed from the blood and excreted in the urine. If kidney function is impaired, urea will not be removed from the blood, resulting in a high urea concentration in the blood. Considerable deterioration must usually be present before the urea level rises above the reference range.

The condition of abnormally high urea nitrogen in the blood is called *uremia*. A significant increase in the plasma concentrations of urea and creatinine, in kidney insufficiency, is known as *azotemia*. Decreased levels are usually not clinically significant unless liver damage is suspected. During pregnancy, urea levels lower than normal are often seen. Azotemia can result from prerenal, renal, or postrenal causes:

- Prerenal azotemia is the result of poor perfusion of the kidneys and therefore diminished glomerular filtration. The kidneys are otherwise normal in their functioning capabilities. Poor perfusion can result from dehydration, shock, diminished blood volume, or congestive heart failure. Another cause of prerenal azotemia is increased protein breakdown, as in fever, stress, or severe burns.
- Renal azotemia is caused primarily by diminished glomerular filtration as a consequence of acute or chronic renal disease. Such diseases include acute glomerulonephritis, chronic glomerulonephritis, polycystic kidney disease, and nephrosclerosis.

- Postrenal azotemia is usually the result of any type of obstruction in which urea is reabsorbed into the circulation. Obstruction can be caused by stones, an enlarged prostate gland, or tumors.

Specimens

Urea may be determined directly from serum, heparinized (sodium or lithium heparin) plasma, urine, or other biological specimens. Anticoagulants containing fluoride (gray-top evacuated tubes) will also interfere with methods using urease because fluoride inhibits the urease reaction. Urea can be lost through bacterial action, so the specimen should be analyzed within a few hours after collection or should be preserved by refrigeration. Refrigeration at 4°C to 8°C preserves the urea without measurable change for up to 72 hours.

Urine urea is particularly susceptible to bacterial action, so in addition to refrigerating the urine specimen at 4°C to 8°C, maintaining the pH at less than 4 can help reduce the loss of urea.

Methods for Quantitative Determination

The oldest method for urea assay is the addition of the enzyme urease to whole blood, serum, or plasma. During incubation with urease, urea is converted to ammonium carbonate ($[NH_4]_2CO_3$) by the urease. The ammonia in the $(NH_4)_2CO_3$ is analyzed in one of several ways. One classic manual method, devised by Gentzkow,[10] measures the amount of $(NH_4)_2CO_3$ formed by having it react with Nessler's solution.

The most common automated methods in use today are indirect methods based on a preliminary hydrolysis step in which the urea present is converted to ammonia by the enzyme urease. The measurement of ammonia differs according to specific instrumentation. In one commonly used analyzer, an enzymatic measurement of the ammonia formed is accomplished by an indicator reaction using glutamate dehydrogenase (GLDH) to oxidize nicotinamide adenine dinucleotide (NADH) to NAD^+. The disappearance of NADPH is measured at 340 nm. It is a very specific, rapid test for urea. The reaction follows:

$$\text{Urea} + H_2O \xleftarrow{\text{urease}} (NH_4)_2CO_3$$

$$NH_4{}^+ + \alpha - \text{Ketoglutaric acid} + \text{NADH} \xrightarrow{\text{GLDH}} \text{ADP} + H^+ + NAD^+ + \text{Glutamic acid}$$

The kidneys and lungs are the organs that exert the most control over electrolyte concentration.

Potentiometric methods using an ammonia ISE are available. Urea may be measured by condensation with diacetyl monoxime in the presence of strong acid and an oxidizing agent to form a yellow diazine derivative. Iron (III) and thiosemicarbazide are added to the reaction mixture to stabilize the color.

Urea Nitrogen, Serum:	
Adult	6–20 mg/dL (2.1–7.1 mmol urea/L)
>60 yr	8–23 mg/dL (2.9–8.2 mmol urea/L)
Infant/child	5–18 mg/dL (1.8–6.4 mmol urea/L)
Urea Nitrogen, Urine:	
12–20 g/24 h (428–714 mmol urea/24 h)	

Modified from Burtis CA, Bruns DE: Tietz fundamentals of clinical chemistry, Table 50-1 ed 7, St Louis, 2015, Elsevier/Saunders, p. 965.

Reference Values

Values in parentheses are in SI units.[7]

Creatinine

Creatinine in the blood results from the spontaneous formation of creatinine from creatine and creatine phosphate. Its formation and release into the body fluids occur at a constant rate and have a direct relationship to muscle mass. Therefore creatinine concentration varies with age and gender. The clearance of creatinine from the plasma by the kidney is measured as an indicator of the GFR. Serum or plasma specimens are preferred over whole blood because considerable noncreatinine chromogens are present in RBCs, which can cause falsely elevated creatinine assay results.

Specimens

Serum, heparinized plasma, or diluted urine can be assayed for creatinine. Ammonium heparinized plasma should not be used for methods that measure ammonia production to quantify creatinine. Usually, urine is diluted 1:100 or 1:200. Creatinine is stable in serum or plasma for up to 1 week if the specimen has been refrigerated. It is important to separate the cells promptly to prevent hemolysis and to minimize ammonia production. Hemolysis causes falsely elevated creatinine values.

Methods for Quantitative Determination

Most methods for creatinine employ the Jaffe reaction,[11] the oldest clinical chemistry method still in use. Creatinine reacts with alkaline picrate to form an orange-red solution that is measured in the spectrophotometer. To improve the specificity of the reaction and to eliminate interference from the many noncreatinine substances in blood that can also react with the alkaline picrate solution and yield falsely elevated values, an acidification step is added. These noncreatinine Jaffe-reacting chromogens include proteins, glucose, ascorbic acid, and pyruvate. The color from true creatinine is less resistant to acidification than the color from the noncreatinine substances. The difference between the two colors is measured photometrically.

Kinetic alkaline picrate methods and enzymatic creatinine methods are often used in automated analyzers. Kinetic methods have reduced some of the interferences caused by noncreatinine chromogens. A kinetic Jaffe method measures the rate of color change, with the interference by slower-reacting chromogens minimized. Another approach to the analysis of creatinine is the measurement of the color formed when creatinine reacts with 3,5-dinitrobenzoate. This method has been successfully adapted to a reagent strip, but the color is less stable than that of the classic Jaffe chromogen assay.

Enzymatic methods, such as creatinine aminohydrolase (creatinine deaminase) or creatininase (creatinine amidohydrolase), make the reaction more specific and more sensitive for creatinine than the colorimetric methods.

Reference Values

Values in parentheses are in SI units.[9]

Creatinine, Serum, or Plasma (Jaffe kinetic or enzymatic method):	
Adult men	0.62–1.10 mg/dL (55–96 μmol/L)
Adult women	0.45–0.75 mg/dL (40–66 μmol/L)
Creatinine, Urine: Jaffe, Manual	
Adult men	14–26 mg/kg/24 h (124–230 μmol/kg/24 h)
Adult women	11–20 mg/kg/24 h (97–177 μmol/kg/24 h)
Creatinine excretion decreases with age	
Creatinine Clearance: See GFR	

Modified from Burtis CA, Bruns DE: Tietz fundamentals of clinical chemistry,Table 50-1 ed 7, St Louis, 2015, Elsevier/Saunders, p. 965.

Clinical Significance

Creatinine in the blood results from creatine originating in the muscles of the body. Creatinine is freely filtered by the glomeruli of the kidney, with a small percentage secreted by the renal tubules, but it is not reabsorbed under normal circumstances. There is a relatively constant excretion of creatinine in the urine that parallels creatinine production. In renal disease, the creatinine excretion is impaired, as reflected by increased creatinine in the blood.

The serum creatinine, S_{CR} concentration is relatively constant and is somewhat higher in males than in females. The constancy of concentration and excretion makes creatinine a good measure of renal function, especially of glomerular filtration. The concentration of creatinine is not affected by dietary intake, degree of dehydration in the body, or protein metabolism, which makes the assay a more reliable single screening index of renal function than the urea assay.

A useful index relates creatinine excretion to muscle mass or lean body weight, taking into consideration variables in individual body sizes. This index is known as the *creatinine clearance (C_{CR})*.

Creatinine Clearance. C_{CR} is defined as milliliters of plasma cleared of creatinine by the kidneys per minute. The result is normalized to a standard person's surface area by using the height and weight of the patient. C_{CR} is an indirect method used to assess the glomerular filtration functioning capabilities of the kidneys.

To perform this test for C_{CR}, timed specimens of both blood and urine must be collected. All voided urine must be carefully collected for 24 hours. The urine specimen is preserved by refrigeration as successive additions are made to the total collection. Blood is collected at about 12 hours into the urine collection period. Creatinine is measured in the blood (serum or plasma) and in the timed urine specimen (24 hours). The C_{CR} is calculated as follows:

$$U/P \times V \times 1.73/A = \text{Plasma Cleared(mL)/min}$$

where *U* is the urine creatinine concentration (mg/dL), *P* is the plasma creatinine concentration (mg/dL), *V* is the volume in milliliters of urine excreted per minute, *A* is the patient's body surface area in square meters, and 1.73 is the standard body surface area in square meters. A nomogram is used to find the patient's body surface area. Most automated analyzers have calculating capabilities for this value if the specific patient height and weight data are entered into the system.

Estimated Glomerular Filtration Rate

The estimated glomerular filtration rate (eGFR) is used to screen for and detect early kidney damage, to help diagnose chronic kidney disease, and to monitor kidney status. This assay is a calculation based on the results of an S_{CR} test, along with other variables such as age, sex, and race (e.g., African American, non–African American), depending on the equation used. The calculation for eGFR is intended to be used when kidney function and creatinine production are stable.

The creatinine clearance, C_{CR} test also provides an estimate of kidney function and of the actual GFR. However, in addition to the S_{CR}, this test requires a timed urine collection (24 hours) for urine creatinine measurement to compare blood and urine creatinine concentrations and to calculate the clearance.

The amount of the substance filtered from the blood (plasma concentration, or *Px*) by the kidneys should equal the amount excreted in the urine (urine concentration, or *Ux*). *V* is the urine flow. The equation for calculation follows:

$$\text{GFR} \times \text{Px} = \text{Ux} \times \text{V}$$

Inulin has historically been the gold standard for measurement of GFR. The best method for directly determining the GFR is an "inulin clearance." It involves introducing a fluid containing the marker molecule inulin (*not* insulin) by IV infusion and then collecting timed urines over a period of hours. The urine volumes are measured, and the inulin in each sample is measured to allow determination of the GFR. An alternative to inulin clearance is the measurement of radiolabeled substances such as iothalamate. The determination of GFR with these compounds is rarely done because of cost and inconvenience to the patient.

Prediction Equations

The National Kidney Disease Education Program and National Kidney Foundation recommend that laboratories use prediction equations to estimate GFR from S_{CR} for patients with chronic kidney disease and for patients at risk for developing chronic kidney disease. Some groups advocate the use of the Cockcroft-Gault Modification of Diet in Renal Disease (MDRD) Study equation as a prediction equation. The MDRD equation is considered to be more accurate because it factors in ethnicity, age, and gender. The MDRD equation has gained widespread use for the estimation of creatinine clearance C_{CR} because of its enhanced accuracy in the estimation of GFR.

$$C_{CR}(\text{mL/min}) = \frac{(140 - \text{Age}) \times \text{Weight}}{72 \times S_{CR}} \times (0.85 \text{ if female})$$

The Cockcroft-Gault formula is used for medical decision-making.[12] The importance of an acc[12] the GFR, as provided by this equation, is exemplified by the following uses of GFR:

1. Detect the onset of renal insufficiency.
2. Adjust drug dosages for drugs excreted by the kidney.
3. Evaluate therapies instituted for patients with chronic renal disease.
4. Document eligibility for Medicare reimbursement in end-stage renal disease.

5. Accrue points for patients awaiting cadaveric kidney transplants.

Abbreviated MDRD Equation

$$GFR(mL/min/1.73m^2) = 186 \times S_{CR}^{-1.154} \times Age^{-0.203}$$

C_{CR} values decrease approximately 6.5 mL/min/1.73 m^2 per decade.

Cystatin C

Cystatin C has been identified as a marker superior to S_{CR} for GFR assessment. Cystatin is a low-molecular-weight part of the cystatin superfamily of cysteine proteinase inhibitors that is thought to be a potentially more reliable marker for GFR. A significant advantage of cystatin is that it is present in constant amounts in all body cells and is not influenced by muscle mass. Cystatin C can be measured by either particle-enhanced turbidimetry or particle-enhanced nephelometry. Both immunoassay methods produce rapid and precise measurements.

GFR is inversely proportional to cystatin C concentration: If GFR is elevated, cystatin C concentration is decreased, and vice versa.

Reference Value

A common reference interval for cystatin C in women and men was calculated to be 0.54 to 1.21 mg/L (median 0.85 mg/L, range 0.42–1.39 mg/L).[13]

Clinical Significance

This novel serum marker of the GFR is a critical measure of normal kidney function. Cystatin C is at least as good as S_{CR} for detecting renal dysfunction.

Creatine

Creatine is synthesized primarily in the liver and then transported to other tissue, such as muscle, where it serves as a high-energy source to drive metabolic reactions. Creatine phosphate loses phosphoric acid and creatine loses H_2O to form creatinine, which passes into the plasma. Creatine can increase the performance of athletes in activities that require quick bursts of energy, such as sprinting, and can help athletes to recover faster after expending bursts of energy.

Clinical Significance

Elevated levels of creatine are found in muscular diseases or with injury such as muscular dystrophy or trauma. Creatine testing is rarely performed.

URIC ACID

Uric acid is the final breakdown product of purine nucleoside metabolism. Three major disease states associated with elevated plasma uric acid are gout, increased catabolism of nucleic acids, and renal disease. Both renal damage and increased nuclear catabolism resulting from chemotherapy contribute to increased serum uric acid levels.

Uric acid can be measured in heparinized plasma, serum, or urine. Serum should be removed from cells as quickly as possible to prevent dilution by intracellular contents. Diet can affect uric acid concentrations. Uric acid is stable in plasma or serum after RBCs have been removed. Serum samples may be stored refrigerated for 3 to 5 days.[14]

Methods of analysis for uric acid include enzymatic methods such as uricase, chemical methods such as phosphotungstic acid (PTA), and HPLC. The PTA method is based on the development of a blue reaction as PTA is reduced by urate in alkaline medium. The color is read at 650 to 700 nm. HPLC using ion exchange or reversed-phase columns is employed to separate and quantify uric acid.

Uricase is a reaction measured in either the kinetic or the equilibrium mode. The decrease of absorbance while urate is converted has been measured at wavelengths varying from 282 to 292 nm. Most current enzymatic assays for uric acid in serum involve a peroxidase system coupled with one of several oxygen acceptors to produce a chromogen:

$$\text{Uric acid} \xrightarrow{\text{uricase}} \text{Allantoin} + H_2O_2 + CO_2$$

Reference Values[9]

Uric Acid (uricase method):	
Adult, female, serum	0.15–0.35 mmol/L
Adult, male	0.21–0.42 mmol/L
Child	2.0–3.5 mg/dL
Urine, 24 hour (average diet)	250–750 mg/day

Modified from Burtis CA, Bruns DE: Tietz fundamentals of clinical chemistry, Table 50-1 ed 7, St Louis, 2015, Elsevier/Saunders, p. 981.

Clinical Significance

Plasma levels of uric acid are variable and higher in males than in females. Plasma urate is completely filterable, and both proximal tubular resorption and distal tubular secretion occur. With advanced chronic renal failure, the plasma uric acid level progressively increases.[14] With progressive renal failure, uric acid is retained. Uric acid concentration in the blood increases in advanced chronic renal failure, but this rarely results in classic gout. Uric acid is elevated in about 40% of patients with essential hypertension. Uric acid levels may also be elevated by thiazide diuretics, leading to gout in some cases.[15]

LIPIDS

Lipids are a class of biochemical compounds. The major plasma lipids, including cholesterol (or total cholesterol [TC]) and the triglycerides, do not circulate freely in solution in plasma but are bound to proteins and transported as macromolecular complexes called *lipoproteins.*

Lipids play an important role in many metabolic processes. They act as:

- Hormone or hormone precursors
- Energy storage and metabolic fuels

- Structural and functional components in cell membranes
- Insulation to allow conduction of nerve impulses or heat loss

Lipids are important because a clear relationship has been demonstrated between plasma lipids and lipoproteins and atherosclerosis. Atherosclerosis, a condition of deposition of plaques in the blood vessels, has been proven to lead to CAD. A lipid profile is useful in the evaluation of risk status for coronary heart disease (CHD).[16,17] Recently, lipid and lipoprotein profiles have been suggested for children 9 to 11 years old and again at 17 to 19 years.[18]

Cholesterol

Cholesterol is found in animal fats. Only a portion of the body's cholesterol is derived from dietary intake; about 70% of the daily production of cholesterol comes from the liver. Although increases in cholesterol have been implicated in increased atherosclerotic diseases, cholesterol is also an essential component for normal biological functions. It serves as an essential structural component of animal cell membranes and subcellular particles and as a precursor of bile acids and all steroid hormones, including sex and adrenal hormones.

Measurement of Cholesterol Specimen

A serum specimen collected in a serum separator evacuated tube from a patient who has been fasting for 12 to 15 hours is the preferred lipid-testing specimen. If a serum separator collection tube is not used, serum for analysis must be separated from RBCs to prevent an exchange of cholesterol between RBC membranes and the serum or plasma. If analysis must be delayed, the serum can be refrigerated at 4°C for several days.

Total Cholesterol

In routine laboratories, the most common methodology used to determine cholesterol is by enzymatic assay. In most automated methods, the enzyme cholesterol esterase hydrolyzes cholesterol esters to free cholesterol. The free cholesterol produced, along with free cholesterol that was initially present in the sample, is then oxidized in a reaction catalyzed by cholesterol oxidase. The H_2O_2 formed oxidizes various compounds to form a colored product that is measured photometrically; the magnitude of the colored compound formed is proportional to the amount of cholesterol present in the sample. Some interference factors are noted with lipemic samples when direct methods are used.

Familial Lecithin Cholesterol Acyltransferase Deficiency

Familial lecithin cholesterol acyltransferase deficiency is a rare disorder inherited as a recessive trait. It is characterized by lack of the enzyme that normally esterifies cholesterol in the plasma. The disorder is manifested by marked hypercholesterolemia and hyperphospholipidemia (free cholesterol and lecithin), together with hypertriglyceridemia.

Renal and liver failure, anemia, and lens opacities are common in familial lecithin cholesterol acyltransferase deficiency. Treatment with a fat-restricted diet reduces the concentration of lipoprotein complexes in plasma and may help prevent kidney damage. Kidney transplantation has been successful for renal failure.

Triglycerides

The fat found in food is composed mainly of triglycerides. A very small proportion of the lipids, about 1% to 2%, includes cholesterol and other fats. Lipids constitute 95% of tissue storage fat and are transported to and from body tissues in lipoprotein complexes.

Triglycerides are digested by the action of pancreatic and intestinal lipases. After absorption, triglycerides are resynthesized in the intestinal epithelial cells and combined with cholesterol and apolipoprotein B48 to form chylomicrons. Chylomicrons give serum its characteristic milky appearance (lipemia) when blood is drawn after a meal.

Measurement of Triglycerides

The appearance of the plasma or serum can be observed and noted after a minimum 12-hour fast. If the plasma is clear, the triglyceride level is probably less than 200 mg/dL. When the plasma appears hazy or turbid, the triglyceride level has increased to greater than 300 mg/dL, and if the specimen appears opaque and milky (lipemic, from chylomicrons), the triglyceride level is probably greater than 600 mg/dL.

Triglyceride methods are usually enzymatic. In most automated enzymatic methods, hydrolysis of the triglyceride present in the sample is usually achieved by lipase (triacylglycerol acylhydrolase). The resulting glycerol produced is assayed by various coupled-enzyme methods. The presence of free glycerol in the samples can interfere with the analysis; assays adjust for this positive interference. Reagents must be carefully checked in automated methodologies because some reagents have a short period of stability after reconstitution.

Secondary Hypertriglyceridemia

The most common forms of hypertriglyceridemia seen in clinical practice are those secondary to alcohol and drug consumption and those associated with disorders such as chronic, severe, uncontrolled diabetes mellitus.

Lipoproteins

Lipids are transported in the plasma to various body tissues by lipoproteins. **Lipoproteins** are particles with triglycerides and cholesterol esters in their core and phospholipids and free cholesterol near the surface. Lipoproteins also contain one or more specific proteins, apolipoproteins, located on the surface of the particle.

The major lipoprotein classes—chylomicron, very-low-density (pre-β) lipoprotein (VLDL), low-density (β-) lipoprotein (LDL), and high-density (α-) lipoprotein (HDL)—although closely interrelated, are usually classified in terms of physicochemical properties. Based on differences in their hydrated densities, lipoproteins can be separated by ultracentrifugation into the following:

- Chylomicrons
- VLDLs
- Intermediate-density lipoproteins

- LDLs, which carry about 70% of total plasma cholesterol
- HDLs, including HDL2 and HDL3 groups.

In a fasting state, most plasma triglycerides are present in VLDLs. In a nonfasting state, chylomicrons appear transiently and contribute significantly to the total plasma triglyceride levels.

Apolipoprotein E (apo E) is present on plasma lipoproteins, including chylomicrons, VLDLs, and HDLs. Apo E plays an important role in lipoprotein metabolism as the ligand for lipoprotein receptors. Apo E may also be involved in nerve regeneration, the immune response, and the differentiation of nerve and muscle cells.

Clinical Significance

The major plasma lipids of interest are total cholesterol (TC) and the triglycerides. When an elevation of these plasma lipids is observed, the condition is called *hyperlipidemia.*

For patients without clinical evidence of coronary or other atherosclerotic vascular disease, the National Cholesterol Education Program (NCEP) recommends health screening, including measurement of TC and HDL cholesterol, at least once every 5 years.

This evaluation should include fasting levels of TC, triglyceride, and HDL. LDL is then calculated by applying the following formula:

$$\text{LDL cholesterol} = \frac{\text{TC} - \text{HDL cholesterol} - \text{triglycerides}}{5}$$

This formula is valid only when triglyceride is <400 mg/dL.

The NCEP recommends that treatment decisions be based on the calculated level of LDL. For patients with an elevated LDL who have fewer than two risk factors in addition to elevated LDL and who do not have clinical evidence of atherosclerotic disease, the goal of treatment is an LDL level less than 160 mg/dL. For those who have at least two other risk factors, the goal of treatment is an LDL level less than 130 mg/dL. When LDL levels remain higher than 160 mg/dL despite dietary measures, and the patient has two or more risk factors (in addition to high LDL), or when LDL levels remain higher than 190 mg/dL even without added risk factors, the addition of drug treatment should be considered.

For those with CAD, peripheral vascular disease, or cerebrovascular disease, the goal of treatment is an LDL less than 100 mg/dL.

All patients with clinical evidence of coronary or other atherosclerotic disease should be evaluated with a fasting blood sample for measurement of TC, triglyceride, and HDL. LDL is calculated.

In contrast to plasma TC, it is unclear whether plasma triglycerides are independent risk variables. A triglyceride level of less than 150 mg/dL is considered normal, 150 to 199 mg/dL is borderline high, and 200-499 mg/dL is high. Hypertriglyceridemia has been associated with diabetes, hyperuricemia, and pancreatitis.

Secondary Elevations of Low-Density Lipoproteins

In North America and Europe, dietary cholesterol and saturated fats are the most common causes of mild to moderate elevations of LDL. Hypercholesterolemia is common in biliary cirrhosis, as is a marked increase in the serum phospholipids and an elevated free cholesterol/cholesterol ester ratio (>0.2).

Hypercholesterolemia resulting from increased LDL levels may be associated with the following disorders:

- Endocrinopathies such as hypothyroidism and diabetes mellitus; hypercholesterolemia usually reversed by hormone therapy
- Hypoproteinemias, as in nephrotic syndrome
- Metabolic aberrations, such as acute porphyria
- Dietary excesses with cholesterol-rich foods, producing elevated LDL levels
- Menopause without estrogen replacement therapy
- Secondary to increased HDL levels in postmenopausal women or in younger women who take oral contraceptives or hormone replacement therapy, which contains primarily estrogen

Reference Values

Healthy Blood Cholesterol

Demographic	Total Cholesterol	Non-HDL	LDL	HDL
Age 19 or younger	Less than 170 mg/dL	Less than 120 mg/dL	Less than 100 mg/dL	More than 45mg/dL
Men age 20 or older	125-200 mg/dL	Less than 130 mg/dL	Less than 100 mg/dL	40 mg/dL or higher
Women age 20 or older	125 to 200 mg/dL	Less than 130 mg/dL	Less than 100 mg/dL	50 mg/dL or higher

National Heart, Lung, and Blood Institute, https://nhlbi.nih.gov, accessed 10.10.18.

Interpretive Data

Men older than 45 and women older than 55 or premature menopause without estrogen replacement therapy:

+1 Family history of premature CHD
+1 Current smoker
+1 Hypertension
+1 Diabetes mellitus
+1 Low HDL cholesterol: 39 mg/dL or less
−1 High HDL cholesterol: 60 mg/dL or greater

LDL cholesterol (measured), therapeutic goal:

- 100 mg/dL or less if CHD is present
- 129 mg/dL or less if no CHD and two or more risk factors
- 159 mg/dL or less if no CHD

CARDIOVASCULAR DISEASE

Recent laboratory studies[15] have shown that a cholesterol efflux capacity of HDL assay is a better predictor of CVD than HDL cholesterol. A major disadvantage of this assay is that the cholesterol efflux capacity measurement is not a simple procedure and involves radioisotope-labeled cholesterol and cultured macrophages. Another related method, a cell-free assay, has been developed to evaluate the capacity of HDL to accept additional cholesterol. It is called cholesterol uptake capacity. This assay uses fluorescently labeled cholesterol and an antiapolipoprotein A1 antibody. This assay offers a potential new assay for the assessment of CVD.

Risk factors for CVD include:

- Age
- Gender
- Race
- Total cholesterol
- HDL cholesterol
- Blood pressure
- Diabetic diagnosis
- Smoking history

Risk factors were originally established by the Framingham Heart Study. The Third Report of the Expert Panel on Detection, Evaluation, and Treatment of High Blood Cholesterol in Adults (Adult Treatment Panel III, or ATP III) has presented the NCEP[16] updated recommendations (Table 10.7) on cholesterol testing and management. ATP III, based on the previous ATP I and ATP II studies with LDL, continues to be identified as the primary target of cholesterol-lowering therapy. New features of ATP III include:

- Use of the lipoprotein profile as the first test for high cholesterol
- A new level at which low HDL becomes a major heart disease risk factor
- A new set of "Therapeutic Lifestyle Changes" to improve cholesterol levels
- Aggressive treatment of persons who are at relatively high risk for CHD because of multiple risk factors
- An increased focus on a cluster of heart disease risk factors known as "metabolic syndrome"
- Increased attention to the treatment of high triglycerides

In 2013 a new assessment of cardiovascular risk algorithm[17] was introduced by the American College of Cardiology (ACC)/American Heart Association (AHA) (http://circ.ahajournals.org). This model assesses the 10-year risk for heart disease or stroke.

Originally, the evidence and recommendations in the guidelines focused on the large proportion of the adult white male population without clinical signs or symptoms of advanced symptomatic CVD (ASCVD), who merit evaluation for the primary prevention of ASCVD. The guidelines did not apply to those with clinically manifest ASCVD, who require secondary prevention approaches, or to highly selected patient subgroups, such as patients with symptoms suggestive of CVD who require diagnostic strategies rather than risk assessment. In addition, these recommendations were not developed for use in specific subgroups of asymptomatic individuals at unusually high risk, such as those with genetically determined extreme values of traditional risk factors (e.g., patients with familial hypercholesterolemia).

Newer assessment strategies offer the major advantages of estimating CVD risk for more segments of the population, including women, and of providing risk estimates specific to African Americans. Promoting lifetime risk estimation may represent an additional step forward in supporting lifestyle behavior changes.

Serial Sampling for Cardiac Markers

After the onset of symptoms of a myocardial infarction (MI), such as chest pain, there is a time window during which the cardiac markers released from myocardial tissue have elevated values in blood. Although the pattern varies somewhat among individuals, a typical pattern is defined for each marker (Fig. 10.5). Some studies have recommended sampling a sequence of blood specimens collected on admission and at 2 to 4 hours, 6 to 8 hours, and 12 hours after MI is suspected. The European Society of Cardiology and ACC consensus report stressed the importance of serial sampling for cardiac markers, recommending sampling on presentation, at 6 to 9 hours, and again at 12 to 24 hours if earlier specimens were negative and clinical suspicion of MI is high.[19] POCT or central laboratory testing must be available 24 hours a day.

TABLE 10.7 Coronary Heart Disease Risk Factors

Factor	Options Studied/Acceptable Range of Values	Factors or Optimal Values
M *or* F	M *or* F	M = higher risk
Age (yr)	20–79	82% of CHD deaths are patients age 65 or older
Hereditary*	All races and ethnicities	African American, Mexican Americans, American Indians, Native Hawaiians and some Asian Americans = higher risk
Total cholesterol	130–200 mg/dL	<180 mg/dL
HDL cholesterol	20–100 mg/dL	50 mg/dL
BP	90–200 mm Hg	110 mm Hg
Treatment for high BP	Y *or* N	N
Diabetes	Y *or* N	N
Smoker	Y *or* N	N

BP, Blood pressure; *CHD,* coronary heart disease; *F,* female; *HDL,* high-density lipoprotein; *M,* male; *N,* no; *Y,* yes; *yr,* years.
*Children of parents with heart disease are more likely to develop heart disease.
Reference: Third Report of the Expert Panel on Detection, Evaluation, and Treatment of High Blood Cholesterol in Adults (Adult Treatment Panel III, or ATP III) presents the National Cholesterol Education Program (NCEP) updated recommendations on cholesterol testing and management. Updated November 2013. https://www.lipid.org

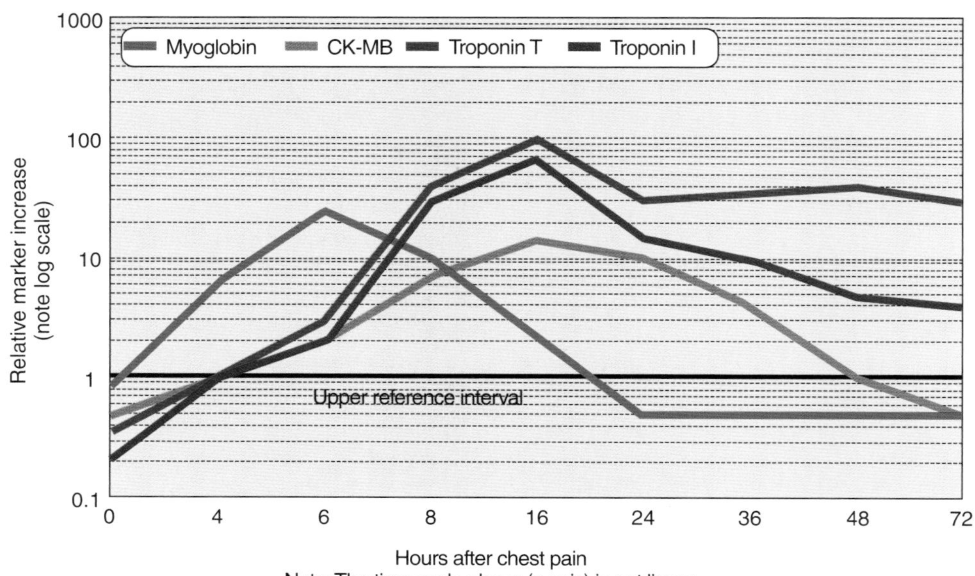

Fig. 10.5 Relative marker increase after myocardial infarction. Markers are expressed as multiples of the upper limit of the reference interval. Therefore the relative increase varies depending on the normal reference interval used. The time scale (*x*-axis) is not linear. (Modified from Wu A: *Cardiac markers,* Totowa, NJ, 1998, Humana Press.)

Before the introduction of current cardiac markers, physicians used total creatine kinase (CK) and lactate dehydrogenase (LDH) isoenzymes to diagnose and assess myocardial damage. Not only have these markers been eliminated, but the traditional standard of laboratory diagnosis of acute MI, the myoglobin (MB) isoform of CK (CK-MB), is also requested less frequently.

More than two decades ago, monoclonal antibody–based assays for cardiac-specific troponin T (cTn) and cTn I isoforms were introduced as cardiac markers. The universal definition of MI includes the typical rise or fall of cTns, with at least one value above the 99th percentile of a healthy reference population. This finding must be accompanied by at least one of the following clinical factors: presence of ischemic symptoms, electrocardiographic changes, or imaging evidence of loss of viable myocardium or a new wall motion abnormality.[20]

The current marker assay combination for diagnosis of acute MI and myocardial injury follows:

- MB
- Troponins
- CK isoenzyme (CK-MB)

Myoglobin

A heme protein found in striated skeletal and cardiac muscles, MB is an early marker of injury to muscle tissue. A rise in MB concentration is detectable in blood as early as 1 to 3 hours after the onset of MI symptoms and can be used to rule out the diagnosis in the 2- to 6-hour period after the onset of symptoms. The disadvantage of MB is that it is not cardiac specific. It can be increased in trauma, diseases of the skeletal muscle, and renal failure. MB concentrations for adult men range from 30 to 90 ng/dL; women typically demonstrate concentrations of less than 50 ng/mL.

MB can be measured by latex agglutination, enzyme-linked immunosorbent assay, immunonephelometry, and fluoroimmunoassay. A spot test using immunochromatography is also available.

Troponins

Cardiac troponin is currently acknowledged as the gold standard of cardiac biomarkers. Troponin is a complex of three proteins that bind to the thin filaments of striated cardiac or skeletal muscle and regulate muscle contraction. The complex consists of:

- Troponin T (TnT)
- Troponin I (TnI)
- Troponin C (TnC)

The largest portion of TnI released into the blood circulation after damage to myocardial tissue is in the form of a complex with cardiac-specific TnC (cTnC). Troponins remain elevated in blood for 4 to 10 days after MI and thus are valuable for late-presenting patients.

In 2017, the Food and Drug Administration approved the next-generation troponin assay, Roche's TnT Gen 5 Stat. This highly sensitive troponin has created concerns that the more elevated results will occur due to structural heart disease or other types of nonischemic etiologies that exist in critically ill patients, but not necessarily myocardial infarction.

Creatine Kinase Myoglobin

CK-MB can become elevated after tissue injury. An increased ratio of MB_2/MB_1 is sensitive for early diagnosis of myocardial cell death. CK-MB is relatively cardiospecific because of excellent sensitivity within 4 to 6 hours after onset of symptoms in MI patients.

Homocysteine

Homocysteine is an amino acid in the blood. Epidemiologic studies have shown that too much homocysteine in the blood, hyperhomocysteinemia, can be caused by folate, vitamin B_6, and vitamin B_{12} deficiencies. Hyperhomocysteinemia is related to a higher risk for CHD, stroke, and peripheral vascular disease.

Homocysteine may have an effect on atherosclerosis by damaging the inner lining of arteries and promoting blood clots. A direct causal link has not been established, but findings suggest that laboratory testing for plasma homocysteine levels can improve the assessment of cardiovascular risk. It may be particularly useful in patients who have a personal or family history of CVD but who do not have the well-established risk factors (smoking, high blood cholesterol, high blood pressure).

C-Reactive Protein

Cardiovascular disease is now considered a process with a low-level inflammatory component. C-reactive protein (CRP) is an inflammation-sensitive protein that can be measured by immunoassays (see Chapter 16). It is being used as an indicator of risk for CVD.

CRP appears to be one of the most sensitive acute-phase indicators of inflammation in certain populations of patients, especially middle-aged and older healthy individuals. There are two forms of this test: (1) monitoring the "traditional" inflammatory processes and (2) performing the highly sensitive CRP (hsCRP), also referred to as *cardioCRP*. The hsCRP detects the same protein as the traditional CRP but can detect small changes down to 0.3 mg/dL. The AHA and CDC cardiovascular risk stratification guidelines state that patients with hsCRP levels below 1 mg/L are at low risk, whereas 1 to 3 mg/L is average risk, and greater than 3 mg/L is defined as high risk. A single hsCRP value at one point in time is statistically of little to no value when assessing cardiovascular risk. In cases of elevated hsCRP levels, a patient should be tested again 2 weeks after the first assay to determine whether the level remains elevated. Patients with high CRP values cannot benefit from the hsCRP because elevated CRP masks the smaller changes. If a value is greater than 10 mg/L, it is important to search for an infection or inflammation.

Natriuretic Peptides

B-type natriuretic peptide (BNP), formerly known as *brain natriuretic peptide*, is used to differentiate dyspnea caused by heart failure from pulmonary disease. The heart is the major source of circulating BNP and releases this polypeptide in response to both ventricle volume expansion and pressure overload. As such, BNP is used as a diagnostic tool for heart failure.

Miscellaneous Markers

As with CRP, fibrinogen is an acute-phase protein produced in response to inflammation. Including measurement of fibrinogen in screening for cardiovascular risk may be valuable in identifying patients who need aggressive heart disease prevention strategies.

The D-dimer is the end product of the ongoing process of thrombus formation and dissolution that occurs at the site of active plaques in acute coronary syndrome (ACS). It can be used for early detection of myocardial cell damage, but it is not specific and can be detected in other conditions in which plaque forms.

Microalbuminuria is an independent risk factor for CVD in patients with diabetes or hypertension (see earlier discussion).

Although many potential biomarkers of cardiac ischemia have been proposed (Box 10.6), these emerging markers have added little value to diagnosis and risk stratification. There is a continuum from vascular inflammation to myocardial dysfunction, along with associated biomarkers, with each stage of ACS. The following biochemical profile markers are associated with the various stages of ACS:

- Proinflammatory cytokines
- Plaque destabilization
- Plaque rupture
- Acute-phase reactants such as CRP
- Ischemia
- Necrosis such as cTnT and CTnI
- Myocardial dysfunction such as BNP and nucleotidase–proBNP

The search continues for the next superstar cardiac biomarker to identify a circulating blood abnormality before a cardiac event such as MI occurs.[21]

BOX 10.6 Examples of Biomarkers in Heart Failure

- Adhesion molecules
- CD40 ligand
- Choline
- C-reactive protein (CRP)
- Cytokines
- Fatty acid–binding protein
- Glycogen phosphorylase-BB
- Ischemia-modified albumin
- Isopentanes
- Monocyte chemotactic protein
- Myoglobin
- Natriuretic peptides
- Oxidized low-density lipoprotein (LDL)
- Phospholipase A_2
- Placental growth factor
- Pregnancy-associated plasma protein A
- Serum amyloid
- Unbound free fatty acids

From Apple FS: Cardiac ischemia, *Clin Laboratory News* 35(9):9, 2009.

LIVER AND PANCREATIC TESTING

To assess liver disease, laboratory assays are best used in groups as a battery of tests (Table 10.8). If abnormal, biochemical tests of liver function suggest a category of liver disease, as follows:

- Hepatocellular damage
- Cholestasis
- Excretory function
- Biosynthetic function

TABLE 10.8 Laboratory Assays to Assess Liver Disease

Category	Laboratory Assay	Comments
Assays of the protein synthesis function of the liver	Total protein, albumin, and globulins (calculated) albumin/globulin ratio (calculated)	Altered albumin to globulin ratio in liver disease
	Coagulation factors	All factors produced in liver Factors II, VII, IX, and X are vitamin-K sensitive (i.e., require adequate quantities of vitamin K for production); PT is collective measure of factors II, V, VII, and X Elevated PT unresponsive to vitamin K supplementation suggests poor liver functionality
Hepatocellular disease or damage	Aspartate transaminase (AST)	Found in numerous tissues including liver, cardiac muscle, skeletal muscle, kidneys, brain, and pancreas.
	Alanine transaminase (ALT)	Found primarily in liver; considered best laboratory test for liver injury.
	γ-glutamyltransferase (GGT)	Very sensitive to small liver insults (for example, alcohol consumption); may be elevated in hepatocellular disease
Liver excretory function	Total bilirubin,	Heme product from catalysis and conjugation with glucuronic acid
	Direct bilirubin,	Three fractions: conjugated, unconjugated, and delta bilirubin (albumin bound)
	Indirect bilirubin (calculated)	Causes jaundice when concentrations < 1.5 mg/dL
	Urine bilirubin	Performed qualitatively using urine dipstick
Hepatic dysfunction	Blood ammonia	Liver converts ammonia to urea. Significant liver dysfunction results in elevated serum ammonia. Poor correlation exists between ammonia level and degree of liver disease.
Hepatobiliary disease	5′-Nucleotidase;	Very sensitive and specific for hepatobiliary disease
Cholestasis	Alkaline phosphatase (ALP)	Usually increased during periods of growth (such as in children and teenagers) and during pregnancy

PT, prothrombin time.
Modified from Burtis CA, Bruns DE: Tietz fundamentals of clinical chemistry, Table 37-6, ed 7, St Louis, 2015, Elsevier/Saunders, p. 721.

Ammonia

Ammonia arises from the breakdown of amino acids, and high concentrations are neurotoxic. Clinical conditions in which blood ammonia levels are useful include hepatic failure, Reye syndrome, and inherited deficiencies of urea cycle enzymes. Liver disease is the most common cause of abnormal ammonia metabolism. Ammonia is used to monitor the progress of disease severity.

Careful specimen handling is extremely important for plasma ammonia assays. Whole-blood ammonia concentration rises rapidly after specimen collection because of in vitro amino acid breakdown. Heparin and EDTA are suitable anticoagulants. Samples should be centrifuged at 0°C to 4°C within 20 minutes of collection and the plasma or serum removed. Specimens should be assayed as soon as possible or frozen.

Methods of measurement include ISEs, which measure the change in pH of a solution of ammonium Cl^- as ammonia diffuses across a semipermeable membrane, and an enzymatic assay using GLDH.

Ammonia Reference Values[22]

0–1 day old	64–107 μmol/L
2–14 days old	56–92 μmol/L
15 days to 17 years old	21–50 μmol/L
18 years and older	0–27 μmol/L

Clinical Significance

Significant hyperammonemia during childhood can be observed with urea cycle defects, many of the organic acidemias, transient hyperammonemia of the newborn, and fatty acid oxidation defects. In these cases, ammonia levels are greatly elevated and frequently exceed 1000 μmol/L. Hyperammonemia can also be seen in conditions associated with liver dysfunction or renal failure, but ammonia levels in these cases of liver disease rarely exceed 500 μmol/L. Mild transient hyperammonemia is relatively common in newborns, can reach levels that are twice normal, and is usually asymptomatic.

Bilirubin

A frequently used assay for assessing liver excretory function is the measurement of serum bilirubin concentration. **Bilirubin** is derived from the iron-containing heme portion of hemoglobin, which is released from the breakdown of RBCs. Bilirubin complexed to albumin, called *unconjugated bilirubin,* is transported to the liver, where it is processed into conjugated bilirubin by the liver cells. In this form, bilirubin enters the bile fluid for transport to the small intestine. In the small intestine, most of the conjugated bilirubin is converted to urobilinogens (see Chapter 13). At least four bilirubin fractions can be separated and identified by liquid chromatography, the least understood being the delta fraction (B delta), which apparently is covalently bound to albumin.

Clinical Significance

Jaundice. Jaundice, or icterus, the yellow discoloration of plasma, skin, and mucous membranes, is caused by the abnormal metabolism, accumulation, or retention of bilirubin. There are three types of jaundice: prehepatic, hepatic, and posthepatic.

Increased hemolysis of RBCs, as occurs in hemolytic anemia, can result in prehepatic jaundice. Hepatitis and cirrhosis of the liver can result in hepatic jaundice. Obstruction of the biliary tract caused by strictures, neoplasms, or stones can also result in jaundice.

The clinical finding of jaundice is nonspecific and can result from a variety of disorders. Specific disorders involving bilirubin metabolism represent specific defects in the way the liver processes the bilirubin. These can be transport defects, impairment in the conjugation step in the liver itself (hepatic function), or a defect in the excretory function of transporting the conjugated bilirubin from the liver cells into bile fluid.

Neonatal Jaundice. Elevations in serum bilirubin occur in some infants, especially premature babies in the first few days of life. This is an example of physiologic jaundice and may involve a deficiency of the enzyme that transfers glucuronate groups onto bilirubin or may signal liver immaturity. Some infants lack glucuronosyltransferase, the enzyme necessary for conjugation of bilirubin glucuronide, which results in a rapid buildup of unconjugated bilirubin. The unconjugated bilirubin readily passes into the brain and nerve cells and is deposited in the nuclei of these cells. This condition is called *kernicterus* and can result in cell damage leading to mental impairment or death.

Neonatal jaundice can persist until glucuronosyltransferase is produced by the liver of the newborn, usually within 3 to 5 days. All newborns have serum unconjugated bilirubin values greater than the reference values in a healthy adult, and 50% of newborns will be clinically jaundiced during the first few days of life.

Normal, healthy, full-term neonates can have unconjugated bilirubin values up to 4 to 5 mg/dL, and values may be as high as 10 mg/dL in a small percentage of newborns. These elevated values usually decrease to normal levels in 7 to 10 days. If toxic levels do occur, exceeding 20 to 25 mg/dL, treatment must be rapidly initiated. Infants with physiologic jaundice can be treated with phototherapy.

Specimens

Bilirubin analyses may be done on serum or plasma, although serum is preferred. The blood should be drawn when the patient is in a fasting state to avoid alimentary lipemia, which can result in falsely increased bilirubin values because of the turbidity of the specimen. Exposure of serum to heat and light results in oxidation of bilirubin. For this reason, specimens for bilirubin assays must be protected from the light. The procedure should be carried out as soon as possible, at least within 2 or 3 hours after the blood has clotted. Specimens can be stored in the dark in a refrigerator for up to 1 week or in the freezer for 3 months without significant loss of bilirubin.

Methods for Quantitative Determination of Bilirubin

Most assays for serum bilirubin are based on a diazo reaction. In this procedure, bilirubin reacts with diazotized sulfanilic acid to form azobilirubin, which has a red-purple color. This basic reaction was modified by the addition of alcohol, usually methanol, which accelerates the reaction of unconjugated bilirubin, called *indirect bilirubin*. The reacting substance, in the absence of alcohol, is the direct fraction of bilirubin, or conjugated bilirubin. Total bilirubin is the combination of conjugated and unconjugated bilirubin.

Many procedures involve a modification of the original Malloy-Evelyn technique, which uses a diazo reaction with methanol added.[23] Another common procedure is the Jendrassik-Grof modification, which is carried out in an alkaline solution.[24] Both the Malloy-Evelyn and the Jendrassik-Grof modifications have been automated and are currently used to perform bilirubin assays.

Automated Bilirubin Assays

In the Vitros Clinical Chemistry Analyzers, bilirubin is separated from the protein matrix by means of thin-film technology. Dry reagents are within the multilayered slides, and the reaction occurs within the layers while the serum passes through them. Total bilirubin is determined by diazotization after unconjugated bilirubin and conjugated bilirubin have been dissociated from albumin. The bilirubin diffuses into a polymer layer that complexes with the bilirubin. The reaction is monitored with a reflectance spectrophotometer. This method provides for the measurement of direct bilirubin.

Reference Values[9]

Total Serum Bilirubin, Adult:
0–2.0 mg/dL 0–34 µmol/L

Direct (conjugated) Serum Bilirubin:
0–3.4 µmol/L

Total Serum Bilirubin, Infants:

Age	Premature	Full Term
Cord	<2.0 mg/dL	<2.0 mg/dL
0–1 day	<8.0 mg/dL	2.0–6.0 mg/dL
1–2 days	<12.0 mg/dL	6.0–10.0 mg/dL
3–5 days	<8.0 mg/dL	<8.0 mg/dL

Enzymes

Tests for several serum enzymes are used in the differential diagnosis of liver disease. These tests include alkaline phosphatase (ALP), γ-glutamyltransferase (GGT), LDH, aspartate transaminase (AST) and alanine transaminase (ALT), and 5′ nucleotidase. Bile acids, triglycerides, cholesterol, serum proteins, coagulation proteins, and urea and ammonia assays are also used in the diagnosis of liver disease.

Aspartate Transaminase and Alanine Transaminase

These transaminase enzymes catalyze the conversion of aspartate and alanine to oxaloacetate and pyruvate, respectively. The highest level of ALT, also called *alanine aminotransferase,* is found primarily in the liver. AST, also called *aspartate aminotransferase,* is found in the liver, heart, kidney, and muscle tissue. Acute destruction of tissue in any of these areas with damage at the cellular level results in rapid release of the enzymes into the serum. ALT and AST are elevated at the onset of viral jaundice and in chronic active hepatitis. With the onset of acute liver necrosis, both enzymes also are increased, but the increase in ALT is higher.

γ-Glutamyltransferase

GGT normally has its highest concentration in the renal tissue, but it is also generally elevated in liver disease. Serum GGT is usually elevated earlier than the other liver enzymes in diseases such as acute cholecystitis, acute pancreatitis, acute and subacute liver necrosis, and neoplasms of sites where liver metastases are present. Increased GGT levels are found in the blood when there is obstruction to bile flow, or cholestasis. Elevation of GGT is seen in chronic alcoholism.

Alkaline Phosphatase

ALP can be present in many tissues. It is generally localized in the membranes of cells. The highest activity of ALP is found in the liver, bone, intestine, kidney, and placenta. The enzyme appears to facilitate the transfer of metabolites across cell membranes and is associated with lipid transport and the calcification process in bone synthesis. Increased blood levels are found when cholestasis or bone degeneration is present.

Proteins

Hypoproteinemia is a condition involving a total protein level less than the reference interval. It can be caused by an excessive loss of protein in the urine in renal disease, leakage into the gastrointestinal tract in inflammatory conditions, loss of blood, and severe burns. A dietary deficiency and intestinal malabsorption may be other causes. Decreased protein synthesis is observed in liver disease. Hyperproteinemia is not seen as often as hypoproteinemia. Dehydration is an example of a condition that would contribute to an increased level of total serum protein.

Albumin is the major protein synthesized by the liver and present in the circulating blood. When the liver has been chronically damaged (such as with cirrhosis), the albumin level may be low (hypoalbuminemia). Malnutrition can also cause a low albumin level, with no associated liver disease.

Serum is the most frequently analyzed specimen for total protein or protein fractions, including albumin and globulin (Student Procedure Worksheet 10.1). The reference interval for total protein is 6.5 to 8.3 g/dL for ambulatory adults. The reference range for albumin is 3.5 to 5.5 g/dL.

The classic colorimetric method for the measurement of total protein and albumin is the Biuret method. In this reaction, Cu^{2+} complexes with the groups involved in the peptide bond. In an alkaline medium and in the presence of at least two peptide bonds, a violet-colored chelate is formed. Biuret reagent also contains Na^+–K^+ tartrate, which complexes with Cu^{2+} to prevent their precipitation in the alkaline solution, and K^+ iodide, which acts as an antioxidant. The test solution is measured photometrically; the darker the solution, the higher the concentration of protein. A handheld refractometer can also be used.

Dye-binding methods can also be used to measure total proteins and are the most frequently used methods for determining albumin. This methodology is based on the ability of most proteins in serum to bind to dyes such as bromophenol blue. Coomassie brilliant blue 250 bound to protein is used in a spectrophotometric method, but dye-binding methods are frequently used to stain protein bands after electrophoresis.

In normal healthy individuals, the various plasma proteins are present in delicately balanced concentrations, with a normal ratio of albumin to globulin (A/G ratio) of 2:1. A reversal in this ratio can be observed in disease of the kidney and liver. Chronic infections also produce a decrease in the albumin concentration.

Serum Protein Electrophoresis

Electrophoresis separates proteins on the basis of their electrical charge densities (Fig. 10.6). The direction of movement depends on whether the charge is positive or negative; cations (positive net charge) migrate to the cathode (negative terminal), and anions (negative net charge) migrate to the anode (positive terminal) (Fig. 10.7). The speed of the migration depends on the degree of ionization of the protein at the pH of the buffer solution. In addition to the charge density, the velocity of movement also depends on the electrical field strength, size and shape of the molecule, temperature, and characteristics of the buffer.

Cellulose acetate is the support medium typically used. Proteins can be separated into five distinct protein zones, which constitute many individual proteins:

- Albumin
- Alpha-1 (α_1-) globulin
- Alpha-2 (α_2-) globulin
- Beta (β-) globulins
- Gamma (γ-) globulins

This method of analysis is useful for evaluation of patients who have abnormal liver function tests, because it allows a direct quantification of multiple serum proteins.

By modifying the standard electrophoretic technique, high-resolution protein electrophoresis, the five major fractions can be separated further (see Chapter 8). The technique is usually performed with an agarose gel support medium.

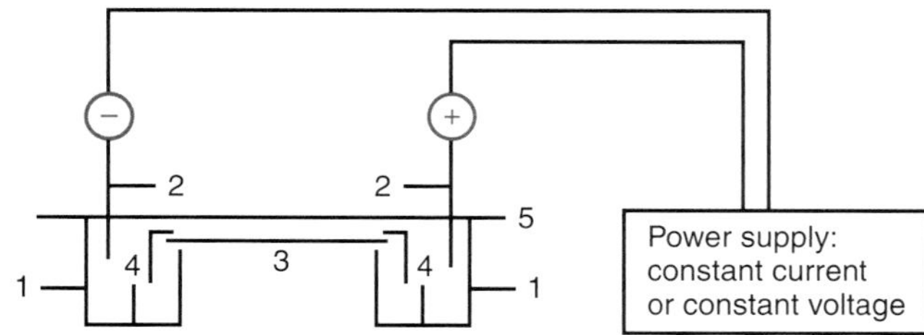

Fig. 10.6 Typical electrophoresis apparatus. Schematic diagram shows two buffer boxes with baffle plates; *1,* electrodes; *2,* electrophoretic support; *3,* wicks; *4,* cover; *5,* power supply. (From Burtis CA, Ashwood ER, Bruns DE: *Tietz fundamentals of clinical chemistry,* ed 6, St Louis, 2008, Elsevier/Saunders.)

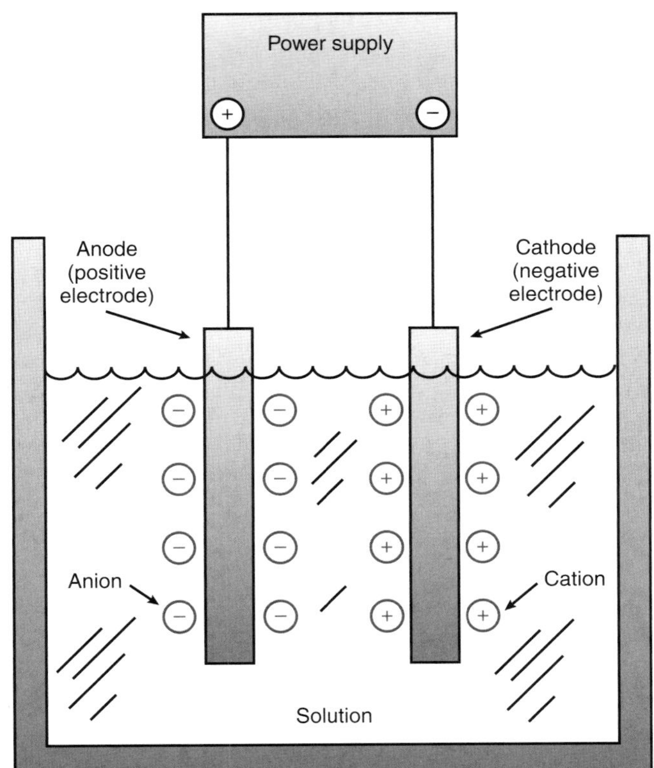

Fig. 10.7 Movement of cations and anions in an electrical field. (From Burtis CA, Ashwood ER, Bruns DE: *Tietz fundamentals of clinical chemistry*, ed 6, St Louis, 2008, Elsevier/Saunders.)

Zone	Serum Proteins	Found in Zones
1	Prealbumin zone	Prealbumin
2	Albumin zone	Albumin
3	Albumin-α_1 interzone	1.1.1.1 α-Lipoprotein, alpha fetoprotein (AFP)
4	α_1 zone	1.1.1.2 α_1-Antitrypsin, α_1-acid-glycoprotein
5	α_1-α_2 interzone	1.1.1.3 Gc-globulin, inter-α-trypsin inhibitor, α_1-antichymotrypsin
6	α_2 zone	α_2-Macroglobulin, haptoglobin
7	α_2-β_1 interzone	Cold insoluble globulin, hemoglobin
8	β_1 zone	Transferrin
9	β_2-β_1 interzone	β-Lipoprotein
10	β_2 zone	C3
11	γ_1 zone	IgA (fibrinogen), IgM (monoclonal Igs, light chains)
12	γ_2 zone	IgM (C-reactive protein), IgM monoclonal Igs, light chains

The most significant finding from an electrophoretic pattern is monoclonal immunoglobulin (Ig) disease. A spike in the α, β, or α_2 indicates a need for further consideration of a monoclonal disorder. A deficiency of IgG suggests an immunodeficiency disorder or nephrotic syndrome.

Proteins in Other Body Fluids

Urine and CSF are the body fluids most frequently analyzed for protein concentration. Increases in protein in the urine result from either glomerular or tubular dysfunction. Abnormally increased total CSF proteins may be found in conditions where there is an increased permeability of the capillary endothelial barrier through which ultrafiltration occurs, such as meningitis, multiple sclerosis, or cerebral infarction. The degree of permeability can be evaluated by measuring the CSF albumin and comparing it with the serum albumin. Diagnosis of specific disorders frequently requires measurement of individual protein fractions.

Coagulation: Prothrombin Time

Another measure of hepatic synthetic function is the prothrombin time (PT). The serum proteins are associated with the incorporation of vitamin K metabolites into a protein that allows normal coagulation (clotting of blood). If a patient has a prolonged PT, liver disease may be present, but a prolonged PT is not a specific test for liver disease. Diseases such as malnutrition, in which decreased vitamin K ingestion is present, may result in prolonged PT.

Pancreatic Function

The pancreas is a large gland involved in the digestive process and a gland that produces insulin and glucagon. Both of these hormones are involved in carbohydrate metabolism. Other than trauma, three diseases cause most cases of pancreatic disease:

- Cystic fibrosis (CF)
- Pancreatitis
- Pancreatic carcinoma

CF is an inherited autosomal recessive disorder that causes the small and large ducts and the acini (grapelike clusters lining the ducts) to dilate and change into small cysts filled with mucus. This eventually results in pancreatic secretions not reaching the digestive tract, possibly leading to an obstruction. The Cl^- content of sweat is useful in diagnosing CF, a disease of the exocrine glands. Affected infants usually have concentrations of sweat Cl^- greater than 60 mmol/L; adult values are typically greater than 70 mmol/L (reference values average about 49 mmol/L). In 98% of CF patients, the secretion of Cl^- in sweat is two to five times that of normal. The determination of increased Cl^- in sweat and an increase of other electrolytes is useful in the diagnosis of CF. The Cl^- content of normal sweat varies with age. To collect the sample, the patient is induced to sweat, and the sweat can be measured directly by use of ISEs.

Pancreatitis, inflammation of the pancreas, is caused by autodigestion of the pancreas from reflux of bile or duodenal contents into the pancreatic duct. It may be acute, chronic, or relapsing and recurrent. Pancreatic carcinoma is the fifth most common form of fatal cancer in the United States.

Laboratory assays of pancreatic function include assays for the enzymes amylase and lipase. In addition, assessment of extrahepatic obstruction (such as bilirubin) and endocrine-related tests (such as glucose) can reflect changes in the endocrine cells of the pancreas. Stool specimens can also be analyzed for excess fat and for the enzymes trypsin and chymotrypsin.

Amylase is an enzyme that catalyzes the breakdown of starch and glycogen. The islet cells of the pancreas and salivary glands are the major tissue of serum amylase. Amylase is the major digestive enzyme of starches. The clinical significance of serum and urine amylase is in the diagnosis of acute pancreatitis. Amylase begins to increase in concentration in the blood 2 to 12 hours after onset of an attack and peaks at 24 hours.

Lipase is an enzyme that hydrolyzes the ester linkage of fats to produce alcohols and fatty acids. Lipase is found primarily in the pancreas. Clinical assays of serum lipase are limited almost exclusively to the diagnosis of acute pancreatitis.

HORMONE ASSAYS

A *hormone* is defined as a chemical substance produced by a specialized gland in one part of the body and carried to a distant target organ where a regulatory response is elicited. Hormones may also be secreted by nonglandular tissues in more than one site and transported by mechanisms other than the blood circulation. A frequently performed hormone assay is measurement of thyroid hormone.

Thyroid

The thyroid is one of the largest endocrine glands in the body. This hormone-producing gland is found in the front at the base of the neck. The trace mineral iodine is essential for the production of thyroid hormones. In some parts of the world, iodine deficiency is common, but the addition of iodine to table salt has virtually eliminated this problem in the United States. In areas of the world where iodine is lacking in the diet, the thyroid gland can be considerably enlarged, resulting in the development of a goiter. The thyroid gland is sensitive to the effects of various radioactive isotopes of iodine produced by nuclear fission. In the event of large releases of such material into the environment, such as occurred during the Chernobyl disaster, the uptake of radioactive iodine isotopes by the thyroid can result in an increase in thyroid cancer in children. Theoretically, the selective uptake of radioactive isotopes of iodine can be blocked by saturating the uptake mechanism with a large surplus of nonradioactive iodine taken in the form of K^+ iodide tablets.

The thyroid secretes hormones, principally T_4 and triiodothyronine (T_3). The amount of thyroid hormone secreted from the gland is about 90% T_4 and about 10% T_3. The function of thyroid hormones is to control metabolism (the rate at which the body uses fats and carbohydrates), help control body temperature, influence heart rate, and help regulate the production of protein. The rate at which T_4 and T_3 are released is controlled by the pituitary gland and the hypothalamus. The hypothalamus signals the pituitary gland to make the hormone thyroid-stimulating hormone (TSH). The pituitary gland then releases TSH; the concentration of TSH depends on how much T_4 and T_3 are in the blood. The thyroid gland also regulates its production of hormones based on the amount of TSH it receives.

Calcitonin is another hormone produced by the thyroid gland. It participates in regulating the amount of Ca^{2+} in the blood and in maintaining Ca^{2+} homeostasis.

Hypothyroidism

The thyroid's hormone secretion process usually works well, but it sometimes fails to produce enough hormones, a condition called *hypothyroidism*. The autoimmune disease referred to as *Hashimoto thyroiditis* is the most common cause of hypothyroidism. Exogenous factors that contribute to hypothyroidism are radiation therapy, thyroidectomy, or medications such as lithium.

Some women develop hypothyroidism during or after pregnancy, a condition known as *postpartum hypothyroidism*. If untreated during pregnancy, hypothyroidism increases the risk for miscarriage, premature delivery, and preeclampsia. It can also adversely affect the developing fetus and can cause fetal death or a low IQ (endemic cretinism) in liveborn infants.

Women are five to eight times more likely than men to develop hypothyroidism. Women 40 to 60 years old are more likely to experience hypothyroidism. Although hypothyroidism most often affects middle-aged women, anyone can develop hypothyroidism, including infants and teenagers.

Hyperthyroidism

In hyperthyroidism, a condition resulting from an overactive thyroid, too much T_4 is produced. Graves disease, an autoimmune disorder in which antibodies produced by the immune system stimulate the thyroid to produce too much T_4, is the most common cause of hyperthyroidism. Hyperthyroidism can significantly accelerate the body's metabolism, causing sudden weight loss, a rapid or irregular heartbeat, sweating, and nervousness or irritability. Table 10.9 compares the features of hypothyroidism and hyperthyroidism.

Laboratory Diagnosis

A wide variety of laboratory assays are available for thyroid disease testing (Table 10.10). If hypothyroidism is suspected, initial evaluation should include TSH, free T_4, and thyroid antibodies. Some common medicines can interfere with assay results (Table 10.11).

TUMOR MARKERS

In tumor immunology, a fundamental tenet is that when a normal cell is transformed into a malignant cell, it develops unique antigens not normally present on the mature normal cell. A tumor marker such as a hormone or enzyme is a substance present in or produced by a tumor itself, or produced by the host in response to a tumor, which can be used to differentiate a tumor from normal tissue or to determine the presence of a tumor. Nonneoplastic conditions can also exhibit tumor marker

TABLE 10.9 Comparison of Hypothyroidism and Hyperthyroidism

Diagnosis	Thyroid-Stimulating Hormone	Free Thyroxine
Hypothyroidism	Increased	Decreased
Hyperthyroidism	Decreased	Increased

TABLE 10.10 Thyroid Laboratory Assays

Assay Name	Recommended Use
TSH	Initial screening test for suspected hypothyroidism and hyperthyroidism. TSH falls and may be less than the lower adult reference limit in 20% of pregnancies. Most reliable marker of thyroid function when illness is suspected.
Thyroxine, free (free T_4)*	Reference intervals for free T_4 have not been well established in pregnant patients; some advocate use of total T_4 in place of free T_4 during pregnancy. In 2% of pregnancies, T_4 is supranormal at about 10–12 weeks, because hCG is at its peak and TSH is at its nadir.
Thyroid antibodies	Detect antibodies for diagnosing autoimmune disease. Test includes thyroid peroxidase and thyroglobulin antibodies.
Thyroxine	Some advocate using total T_4 in place of free T_4 during pregnancy.
Thyroid-stimulating immunoglobulin	Detects thyroid antibodies for diagnosing autoimmune disease (Graves disease).
TPO antibody	Detects antibodies for diagnosing autoimmune disease.
TRAb	Detects antibodies for diagnosing autoimmune disease.
Thyroglobulin antibody	Detects antibodies for diagnosing autoimmune disease. Test is part of thyroid antibody panel.

hCG, Human chorionic gonadotropin; *TPO,* thyroid peroxidase; *TRAb,* thyroid-stimulating hormone receptor antibody; *TSH,* thyroid-stimulating hormone.
*Serum is the preferred specimen used in the measurement of T_4, but plasma ethylenediaminetetraacetic acid or heparin is also used. Storage of serum specimens at room temperature up to 7 days results in no significant loss of T_4.
Modified from Burtis CA, Bruns DE: Tietz fundamentals of clinical chemistry, Table 50-1 ed 7, St Louis, 2015, Elsevier/Saunders, p. 965.

activity. Some tumor markers are used to screen for cancer, but markers are used more often to monitor recurrence of cancer or to determine the degree of tumor burden in the patient. To be of any practical use, the tumor marker must be able to reveal the presence of the tumor while it is still susceptible to destructive treatment by surgical or other means. Tumor markers can be measured quantitatively in tissues and body fluids using biochemical, immunochemical, or molecular tests.

Tumor markers play an especially important role in the diagnosis and monitoring of patients with prostate, breast, and bladder cancers. At Memorial Sloan-Kettering Cancer Center in New York, the three tumor markers with the most remarkable increase in volume of testing are carcinoembryonic antigen (CEA), prostate-specific antigen (PSA), and cancer antigen (CA) 15-3.

Older, well-established markers include ALP and collagen-type markers in bone cancer, Igs in myeloma, catecholamines and their derivatives in neuroblastoma and pheochromocytoma, and serotonin metabolites in carcinoid. In addition, there are many breast tissue prognostic markers, including hormone receptors, cathepsin D, HER/neu oncogenes, and plasminogen receptors and inhibitors. The list of U.S. Food and Drug Administration–approved tumor markers continues to grow. Multiple marker combinations may also be useful in the management of some types of cancer.

Specific Markers

Tumor-specific markers[24] include the following:

- Alpha fetoprotein (AFP)
- Beta subunit of human chorionic gonadotropin (β-hCG)
- CA 15-3/CA27.29
- CA 19-9
- CA-125
- Carcinoembryonic antigen (CEA)
- Prostate-specific antigen (PSA)
- Miscellaneous hormone markers

Alpha Fetoprotein

AFP is normally synthesized by the fetal liver and yolk sac. AFP is secreted in the serum in nanogram to milligram quantities in hepatocarcinoma, endodermal sinus tumors, nonseminomatous testicular cancer, teratocarcinoma of the testis or ovary, and malignant tumors of the mediastinum and sacrococcyx. In addition, a small percentage of patients with gastric and pancreatic cancer with liver metastasis may have elevated AFP levels. Both AFP and β-hCG should be quantitated initially in all patients with teratocarcinoma, because one or both markers may be secreted in 85% of patients (see Chapter 16). The concentration of AFP may be elevated also in nonneoplastic conditions such as hepatitis and CF.

TABLE 10.11 Examples of Drugs That May Alter Thyroid Function Assays

Drug	TSH	T_3		T_4		Mechanism
		Total	Free	Total	Free	
Androgens	Normal	Reduced	Normal	Reduced	Normal	Reduced TBG synthesis
Aspirin	Normal	Increased	Normal	Increased	Normal	Reduced TBG binding
Estrogens	Normal	Increased	Normal	Increased	Normal	Increased TBG synthesis
Lithium	Increased	Reduced	Reduced	Reduced	Reduced	T_3 and T_4 release inhibition
Neuroleptic	Normal	Increased	Normal	Increased	Normal	Increased TBG synthesis

T_3, Triiodothyronine; *T_4,* thyroxine; *TBG,* thyroxine-binding globulin; *TSH,* thyroid-stimulating hormone.
Modified from Dominguez LJ, Bevilacqua M, Dibella G, et al: Diagnosing and managing thyroid disease in the nursing home, *J Am Med Dir Assoc* 9:11, 2008.

AFP is a very reliable marker for following a patient's response to chemotherapy and radiation therapy. Levels should be obtained every 2 to 4 weeks (metabolic half-life in vivo is 4 days).

Beta Subunit of Human Chorionic Gonadotropin

The ectopic protein β-hCG is a sensitive tumor marker with a metabolic half-life in vivo of 16 hours. A serum level of β-hCG greater than 1 ng/mL strongly suggests pregnancy or a malignant tumor, such as endodermal sinus tumor, teratocarcinoma, choriocarcinoma, molar pregnancy, testicular embryonal carcinoma, or oat cell carcinoma of the lung.

CA15-3/CA 27.29

The two main purposes of the CA 15-3/CA27.29 assay are: 1. to monitor disease progression and/or response to therapy in patients with metastatic breast cancer, and to detect cancer recurrence in patients treated previously for stages II or III breast cancer who are clinically free of the disease. It is not recommended as an assay for breast cancer screening. Patients with confirmed breast carcinoma frequently have CA 15-3 values in the same range as healthy individuals but patients with other conditions, including liver disease, some inflammatory conditions, and other carcinomas. A change in the CA 15-3/CA27.29 concentration is more predictive than the absolute concentration. Changes in tumor burden are reflected by changes in the tumor marker concentration.

CA 19-9

Levels of CA 19-9 are elevated in patients with pancreatic, hepatobiliary, colorectal, gastric, hepatocellular, pancreatic, and breast cancers. Its main use is as a marker for colorectal and pancreatic carcinoma.

CA 125

The CA 125 marker is elevated in carcinomas and benign disease of various organs, including pelvic inflammatory disease and endometriosis, but it is most useful in ovarian and endometrial carcinomas.

Carcinoembryonic Antigen (CEA)

CEA plasma levels greater than 12 ng/mL are strongly correlated with malignancy. Elevated neoplastic states frequently associated with an increased CEA level are endodermally derived gastrointestinal neoplasms and neck and breast carcinomas. Also, 20% of smokers and 7% of former smokers have elevated CEA levels.

CEA is used clinically to monitor tumor progress in patients who have diagnosed cancer with a high blood CEA level. If treatment leads to a decline to normal levels (<2.5 ng/mL), an increase in CEA may indicate cancer recurrence. A persistent elevation is indicative of residual disease or poor therapeutic response. In patients who have undergone colon cancer resection surgery, the rate of clearance of CEA levels usually returns to normal within 1 month but may take as long as 4 months. Blood specimens should be obtained 2 to 4 weeks apart to detect a trend.

Prostate-Specific Antigen (PSA)

Prostate cancer is the second leading cause of cancer death among American men. PSA is a marker specific for prostate tissue. Routine PSA screening is highly controversial as a marker in the diagnosis of prostate cancer. However, PSA screening may reduce prostate cancer mortality risk but is associated with false-positive results, biopsy complications, and overdiagnosis. Blood levels of PSA are increased when normal glandular structure is disrupted by benign or malignant tumor inflammation. Serum PSA is directly proportional to tumor volume, with a greater increase per unit volume of cancer compared with benign hyperplasia.

In 2018, an updated study on PSA screening recommendations was published in the Journal of the American Medical Association[25] that is consistent with the guidelines of the American Urologic Association (AUA).[26] This recommendation is that men from 55 to 69 years of age should make individual decisions with their clinicians about being screened for prostate cancer. Screening offers a small potential benefit of reducing the chance of death from prostate cancer in some men. However, if the concentration of PSA begins to accelerate over a period of months, it becomes important to follow the acceleration, which may warrant further radiological follow up and biopsy. Patients need to balance benefits and harms of treatment options. In addition, the new draft advises that men older than 70 years of age should not be screened because the potential benefits of screening do not outweigh the harms.

According to the AUA, routine PSA screening in asymptomatic men can lead to psychological harm and biopsy-related complications. Negative outcomes associated with prostate cancer screening include the detection of cancers that otherwise would have remained undetected without screening (overdiagnosis), subsequent treatment of these cancers (overtreatment), and the associated side effects from a treatment that does not improve survival. The AUA discourages the use of PSA screening for early diagnosis of prostate cancer in older men, especially those who have associated comorbidities that limit life expectancy to 10 to 15 years or less, for whom diagnosis and treatment are unlikely to improve health outcomes.

PSA level determination appears to be useful for monitoring progression and response to treatment among patients with prostate cancer. Accurate pretreatment staging using PSA assay is crucial in prostate cancer management. Serum PSA levels correlate with the risk for extraprostatic extension, seminal vesicle invasion, and lymph node involvement. Patients with serum PSA levels of less than 10.0 ng/mL are more likely to respond to local therapy.

Miscellaneous Enzyme Markers

LDH is elevated in a wide variety of malignancies and other medical disorders. The level of LDH has been shown to correlate to tumor mass in solid tumors, so it can be used to monitor progression of these tumors.

Neuron-specific enolase has been detected in neuroblastoma, pheochromocytoma, oat cell carcinomas, medullary thyroid and C cell parathyroid carcinomas, and other neural crest–derived cancers.

Placental ALP can be detected during pregnancy. It is also associated with the neoplastic conditions of seminoma and ovarian cancer.

Miscellaneous Hormone Markers

Elevated or inappropriate serum levels of hormones can function as tumor markers. Adrenocorticotropic hormone (ACTH, corticotropin), calcitonin, and catecholamines may be secreted by differentiated tumors of endocrine organs and squamous cell lung tumors. Oat cell carcinomas may produce β-hCG, ADH, serotonin, calcitonin, PTH (parathormone), and ACTH. These hormones can be used to follow a patient's response to therapy.

In addition, some breast cancers demonstrate progesterone and estradiol (estrogen) receptors, which are strongly correlated with a positive response to antihormone therapy. Patients with neuroblastomas and pheochromocytomas secrete catecholamine metabolites that can be detected in the urine. Neuroblastomas also release neuron-specific enolase and ferritin; these markers can be used for diagnosis and prognosis.

Breast, Ovarian, and Cervical Cancer Markers

For more than a decade, cancer antigens have been used to monitor therapy and evaluate recurrence of cancer. Estrogen and progesterone receptors are universally accepted as both prognostic markers and therapeutic choice indicators. A relatively new approach has been the use of the oncogene HER_2/neu as a prognostic indicator and a marker related to the choice of therapy. This has been particularly useful since the introduction of Herceptin as a chemotherapeutic agent that targets the HER_2/neu receptor. Breast cancer patients who express HER_2/neu in their cancers have a poor prognosis with shorter disease-free and overall survival than patients who do not express the oncogene. HER_2/neu in serum may be used to detect early recurrence, and elevated serum levels of HER_2/neu correlate with the presence of metastatic disease and suggest a poor prognosis. Combining HER_2/neu serum measurements with other markers such as CEA or CA 15-3 may improve the sensitivity of detection of recurrence.

THERAPEUTIC DRUG MONITORING

Therapeutic drug monitoring (TDM) is the process by which the concentration of a chemical substance administered therapeutically or diagnostically is measured. TDM is of value for only a limited number of drugs. For it to be clinically worthwhile, the following criteria should be met:

1. An established relationship between plasma drug concentration and therapeutic response or toxicity
2. A poor relationship between plasma concentration and drug dosage
3. A good clinical indication for the assay (such as no response to treatment, suspected noncompliance, signs of toxicity)
4. Appropriately timed peak–trough specimens with proper patient information
5. An adequate amount of clinical information to allow the interpretation of laboratory assay results

Peak and Trough

For many drugs, a relationship exists between the drug concentration in plasma and the clinical effects of the drug. Any concentration larger than the minimum may be toxic, but a minimum concentration is needed to achieve the desired pharmacologic effect. The therapeutic range of a drug is a concentration somewhere in the middle of the concentration–response curve.

Initially, a greater proportion of drug is absorbed than is distributed, metabolized, and eliminated; this is the peak concentration. Most drugs are administered in a series of doses. Depending on the drug half-life in the normal population sample, this time ranges from less than 1 day to more than 3 months. For drugs with a long half-life compared with the dosing interval, drug accumulation can be dramatic (i.e., drug concentrations after the first dose are much lower than drug concentrations at steady state). The goal of therapy is to have the drug accumulate until a steady state is achieved, or equal drug input and output occurs. In general, a blood specimen should *not* be taken until "steady state" has been achieved, or approximately five times the drug's half-life. The peak concentration and trough concentration, or minimum steady-state concentration, oscillate after each dose within a certain range. The goal is to achieve the therapeutic range.

Drugs in various categories can be monitored and include the following:

- Aminoglycoside antibiotics, such as gentamicin
- Glycopeptide antibiotics, such as vancomycin
- Anticonvulsant (antiepileptic) drugs, such as carbamazepine, phenytoin, ethosuximide, phenobarbitone, and valproic acid
- Cardioactive drugs, such as digoxin
- Respiratory stimulants, such as theophylline
- Tricyclic antidepressants, such as amitriptyline, clomipramine, desipramine, dothiepin, imipramine, and nortriptyline
- Selective serotonin receptor inhibitor antidepressants such as fluoxetine
- Mood stabilizers, especially lithium citrate

It is important to record the exact time and date of the specimen in relation to the last dose of the drug (Table 10.12), with a note of all other drugs prescribed. Effective and safe therapeutic plasma concentrations of drugs vary.

DRUGS OF ABUSE

Assessment of drugs of abuse or overdose can occur with prescription, over-the-counter, or illicit drugs. Testing for drugs of abuse can be performed by various methods. Rapid POCT is simple and of immediate value to a primary care provider. Drugs of abuse include alcohol, marijuana, cocaine, benzodiazepines, barbiturates, opiates, and amphetamines.

AUTOMATION IN CLINICAL CHEMISTRY

Clinical Chemistry and Immunochemistry Analyzers

The earliest automated testing occurred in clinical chemistry. Manufacturers continue to develop new assays for low-volume testing (Table 10.13) and high-volume testing (Table 10.14) using clinical chemistry analyzers. Many of the methods replicate standard manual reactions. Unique methods such as chemiluminescence have been developed for immunoassays performed by automated analyzers (Table 10.15).

TABLE 10.12 Target and Toxic Ranges for Therapeutic Drug Monitoring[9]

Drug	Target Range	Toxic Level
Amitriptyline (+ nortriptyline)	8-200 ng/mL	>300 ng/mL
Caffeine		>20 μg/mL
Carbamazepine	4-12 μg/mL	>15 μg/mL
Desipramine	100-300 ng/mL	>300 ng/mL
Digoxin	≥ ng/mL12 hrs after dose in heart failure	>3.0 ng/mL
Ethosuximide	40-100 μg/mL	>150 μg/mL
Fluoxetine (+ norfluoxetine)	120-500 ng/mL	>1000 ng/mL
Gabapentin	2-20 μg/mL	>12 μg/mL
Imipramine (+ desipramine)	175-300 ng/mL	>300 ng/mL
Lamotrigine	2.5-15 μg/mL	μg/mL
Nortriptyline	70-170 ng/mL	>300 ng/mL
Phenobarbitone	10-40 μg/mL	Coma, with reflexes (65-117 μg/mL) Coma, without reflexes (>100 μg/mL
Phenytoin	10-20 μg/mL	>20 μg/mL
Theophylline, adults†	Bronchodilator 8-20 μg/mL	>20 μg/mL
Theophylline, neonates‡	6-13 μg/mL	
Valproic acid§	50-100 μg/mL	>100 μg/mL
Vigabatrin	0.8-36	

†Theophylline used to treat asthma in adults.
‡Theophylline used to treat neonatal apnea.
§For valproic acid, there is no established target range. If the predose concentration is greater than 100 mg/L with no clear therapeutic effect, further increases in dose are unlikely to be beneficial.
Modified from Burtis CA, Bruns DE: Tietz fundamentals of clinical chemistry, Table 50-2, ed 7, St Louis, 2015, Elsevier/Saunders, pp. 983-990.

TABLE 10.13 Summary of Features of Representative Chemistry Analyzers for Low-Volume Laboratories

Manufacturer	Instrument Series	Operational Type/Reagent Type	Test Principle
Abbott Point of Care	Piccolo Xpress	Discrete/self-contained single-use cartridges-packages-slides Disc loaded directly into instrument Benchtop	Photometry, enzymatic
	i-STAT-1 analyzer	Self-contained single-use cartridges-packages-slides Handheld	Potentiometry, amperometric, conductometric
Alfa Wassermann Diagnostic Technologies	ACE Alera Clinical Chemistry System	Benchtop	Photometry, potentiometry (ISE), homogeneous EIA, turbidimetry
AMS Diagnostics	LIASYS	Batch, random access, discrete, continuous random access Benchtop	Photometry, potentiometry (ISE), turbidimetry
Awareness Technology	ChemWell-T	Batch, random access, discrete, continuous random access/open reagent system Benchtop	Photometry
Beckman Coulter	AU480 Clinical System	Continuous random access/open reagent system Floor standing	Photometry, potentiometry (ISE), homogeneous EIA, turbidimetry, latex agglutination
Carolina Liquid Chemistries	BioLis	Batch, random access, continuous random access/open reagent system Benchtop	Photometry, potentiometry
ELITech Clinical Systems	Selectra ProM Chemistry Systems	Continuous random access, discrete/random access, batch/self-contained multiuse cartridges-packages-slides Benchtop	Photometry, potentiometry, /turbidimetric homogeneous EIA

Continued

TABLE 10.13 Summary of Features of Representative Chemistry Analyzers for Low-Volume Laboratories—cont'd

Manufacturer	Instrument Series	Operational Type/Reagent Type	Test Principle
Horiba Medical	Pentra C200	Continuous random access, discrete, random access, batch/self-contained single-use cartridges-packages–open reagent system Benchtop	Photometry, potentiometry (ISE), turbidimetric
Medica	Easy RA	Batch, random access, discrete, continuous random access, batch/self-contained multiuse cartridges-packages-slides Benchtop	Photometry, potentiometry, turbidimetric immunoassay, EIA
MedTest DX	Poly Chem	Batch, random access/open reagent system Benchtop	Photometry, turbidimetry, potentiometry (ISE)
Nova Biomedical	Stat Profile pHOx Ultra	Discrete/self-contained multiuse cartridges Benchtop	Potentiometry (ISE), optical, reflectance
Randox Laboratories	RX Daytona	Random access/self-contained multiuse cartridges-packages-slides Benchtop	Photometry, potentiometry (ISE), latex-enhanced immunoturbidimetry
Roche Diagnostics	Cobas c311	Continuous random access/self-contained multiuse cassettes Floor standing	Photometry, potentiometry
SDI Biomed	SDI CA 480 Clinical Chemistry System	Random access/self-contained single-use cartridges-packages-slides Benchtop	Photometry, potentiometry, selected methodologies
Siemens	Dimension EXL	Batch, random access/continuous random access/self-contained multiuse cartridges Floor standing	Photometry, potentiometry, turbidimetry, other
Vital Diagnostics	Eon 100 Automated Chemistry Analyzer	Random access, continuous random access/self-contained multiuse cartridges-packages-slides Benchtop	Photometry, potentiometry,

EIA, Enzyme immunoassay; *ISE,* ion-selective electrode.
Data from College of American Pathologists: Chemistry analyzers for low-volume laboratories, *CAP Today* 27(8):35–47, 2013.

TABLE 10.14 Summary of Features of Representative Large-Volume Clinical Chemistry Analyzers

Manufacturer	Instrument Series	Type	Test Principle
Abbott (www.abbott.com)	Architect c8000	Random access	Photometry, potentiometry*
Beckman Coulter (www.beckmancoulter.com)	Synchron Series	Random access	Photometry, potentiometry, various types of turbidimetry, enzyme immunoassay
Ortho Clinical Diagnostics (www.orthoclinical.com)	Vitros Series	Random access	Potentiometry, colorimetry
Roche (www.roche-diagnostics.us)	Integra Cobra	Random access discrete	Photometry, potentiometry
Siemens Diagnostics Healthcare System (www.medical.siemens.com)	ADVIA	Random access batch	Photometry, potentiometry, turbidimetry

*Potentiometry: ion-selective electrode and electrochemiluminescence.

TABLE 10.15 Summary of Features of Representative Immunochemistry Analyzers

Manufacturer	Instrument Series	Test Principle	Type	Test Menus
Abbott	AxSYM	Chemiluminescence	Random access	Hormones, tumor markers, cardiac markers, toxicology, fertility/pregnancy, hepatitis markers, TDM
Beckman Coulter	ACCESS	Chemiluminescence	Random access	Hormones, tumor markers, cardiac markers, anemia profile, some TDM, infectious disease markers
BioMerieux	VITAS	Enzyme Linked Fluorescent Assay (ELFA)	Batch	Hormones, some TDM, infectious disease markers, D-dimer assay
Roche	ELECSYS	Electrochemiluminescence	Random access	Hormones, tumor markers, cardiac markers, anemia profile, hepatitis markers
Siemens Diagnostics Healthcare Systems	ADVIA Centaur	Chemiluminescence	Random access	Hormones, tumor markers, cardiac markers, TDM, anemia profile

TDM, Therapeutic drug monitoring.

CASE STUDIES

CASE STUDY 10.1

A 35-year-old man (height 67 inches, weight 73.3 kg) with known chronic renal disease for 6 months has blood drawn for S_{CR} and urea tests. Urine is collected for a 24-hour quantitative creatinine test; the total volume of urine collected is 1139 mL. The following laboratory results are obtained for the testing done:
Urine creatinine: 56 mg/dL
Serum creatinine: 9.6 mg/dL
Serum urea: 75 mg/dL

Multiple-Choice Questions

Answers are in Appendix A.

1. Given these data, what is this patient's standardized creatinine clearance?
   a. 4.3 mL/min
   b. 4.6 mL/min
   c. 5.8 mL/min
   d. 6.2 mL/min
2. A newer measurement of kidney function is:
   a. Ultrasound
   b. Urine microscopy
   c. Erythropoietin assay
   d. GFR

Critical Thinking Group Discussion Questions

1. What does an elevated serum BUN suggest?
2. What does an elevated creatinine suggest?
3. What is the clinical significance of the GFR and the urea nitrogen/creatinine ratio?

Note: Narrative answers published on EVOLVE instructor site.

CASE STUDY 10.2

As part of a lipid-screening profile, the following results were obtained for a blood specimen drawn from a 30-year-old woman immediately after she had eaten breakfast:
Triglycerides: 300 mg/dL
Cholesterol: 180 mg/dL

Multiple-Choice Question

Answer is in Appendix A.

1. Which of the following would be a reasonable explanation for these results?
   a. The results fall within the reference values for the two tests; they are not affected by the recent meal.
   b. The cholesterol is normal, but the triglyceride test is elevated; retest using a 12-hour fasting specimen, because the triglyceride test may be affected by the recent meal.
   c. The results are elevated for the two tests; retest for both using a 12-hour fasting specimen, because both the cholesterol and the triglyceride test may be affected by the recent meal.
   d. The results for both tests are below the normal reference values despite the recent meal.

Critical Thinking Group Discussion Questions

1. What other laboratory assays would be of value?
2. Discuss the chances that this patient will develop atherosclerosis.

Note: Narrative answers published on EVOLVE instructor site.

CASE STUDY 10.3

An adult male patient with jaundice complains of fatigue. He has a decreased blood hemoglobin level, RBC microhematocrit, and a total serum bilirubin value of 7.5 mg/dL, most of which represents unconjugated bilirubin. His liver enzyme tests are within the normal reference ranges.

Multiple-Choice Questions

Answers are in Appendix A.

1. The total bilirubin value is:
   a. Below the normal reference range
   b. Within the normal reference range
   c. Slightly above the normal reference range
   d. Extremely elevated above the reference range
2. The most likely disease process for this patient is:
   a. Gallstone obstructing the common bile duct
   b. Hemolytic anemia in which his red blood cells are being destroyed
   c. Infectious (viral) hepatitis
   d. Cirrhosis of the liver

Critical Thinking Group Discussion Questions

1. What laboratory assays could be performed to rule out viral hepatitis?
2. What are possible causes for this patient's jaundice?

Note: Narrative answers published on EVOLVE instructor site.

CASE STUDY 10.4

An 8-year-old boy comes to see his family physician with his mother. He has been urinating excessively and has also been drinking an excessive quantity of H_2O. He recently recovered from a viral upper respiratory infection, he has lost some weight since his last visit to the clinic 6 months ago, and he has a slight fever (100°F). Laboratory tests are ordered, fasting blood is drawn for testing, and a urinalysis is done. The following laboratory results are reported:
Serum creatinine: 0.8 mg/dL
Serum glucose: 180 mg/dL
White blood count: 15 × 10^9/L
Hemoglobin: 14.0 g/dL

Urinalysis

Specific gravity: 1.025
Glucose: 1000 mg/dL

Continued

CASE STUDY 10.4—cont'd

Ketones: Moderate
Protein, nitrite, blood: Negative
Sediment: No abnormal findings

Multiple-Choice Questions

Answers are in Appendix A.

1. The presence of ketones in the patient's urine is evidence of:
   a. Starvation
   b. Diabetic ketoacidosis
   c. Elevated glucose in the urine
   d. A protein imbalance
2. On the basis of the case history and the laboratory findings, what is a likely diagnosis of this patient's disease?
   a. Diabetes mellitus
   b. Hyperthyroidism
   c. Acute glomerulonephritis
   d. Recurring upper respiratory infection

Critical Thinking Group Discussion Questions

1. Does this patient have any evidence of renal disease?
2. Why does the patient have glucose in his urine?

Note: Narrative answers published on EVOLVE instructor site.

CASE STUDY 10.5

A 40-year-old woman with nausea, vomiting, and jaundice is seen in the clinic. Laboratory tests are ordered on blood and urine. The following laboratory results are reported:
Hemoglobin: Normal
White blood cell count: Normal

Serum Bilirubin

Total: 6.5 mg/dL
Conjugated (direct): 5.0 mg/dL

Serum Enzymes

Alanine transaminase (ALT): 300 U/L (normal: 0–45 U/L)
Alkaline phosphatase (ALP): 180 U/L (normal: 0–150 U/L)

Urine

Appearance: Dark brown
Urobilinogen: Normal/decreased
Bilirubin: Positive

Multiple-Choice Questions

Answers are in Appendix A.

1. The total bilirubin value is:
   a. Below the normal reference range
   b. Within the normal reference range
   c. Slightly above the normal reference range
   d. Extremely elevated above the reference range
2. These results can best be interpreted as representing which of the following?
   a. Unconjugated hyperbilirubinemia, probably from hemolysis
   b. Unconjugated hyperbilirubinemia, probably from an injury to the liver cells
   c. Conjugated hyperbilirubinemia, probably from biliary tract disease
   d. Conjugated hyperbilirubinemia, probably from obstruction (such as gallstones)

Critical Thinking Group Discussion Questions

1. Discuss the possible causes of jaundice in this patient.
2. Where in the bilirubin pathway is the system overloaded or altered?

Note: Narrative answers published on EVOLVE instructor site.

CASE STUDY 10.6

A 35-year-old man is admitted to the emergency department with chest pain; past history reveals other episodes of this same pain but of a shorter duration. Inquiry into his personal habits reveals that he is a cigarette smoker and that he follows a modified low-fat diet and engages in some regular exercise. His father died of ischemic heart disease at age 45, and other members of his family have had lipid-related disorders. Fasting blood is drawn for chemistry and hematology tests and urine collected for examination. Laboratory results are:
Hemoglobin: 15.0 g/dL
White blood cell count: Mildly elevated
Serum glucose: 120 mg/dL
Serum triglycerides: 300 mg/dL
Serum LDL cholesterol: 150 mg/dL
Serum total cholesterol: 275 mg/dL

Serum Enzymes

Aspartate aminotransferase (AST): 60 U/L (normal: 0–45 U/L)
γ-Glutamyltransferase (GGT): 70 U/L (normal: 0–45 U/L)
Alkaline phosphatase (ALP): 180 U/L (normal: 0–150 U/L)

Urinalysis

Normal findings

Multiple-Choice Questions

Answers are in Appendix A.

1. Which factor in the patient's history and laboratory findings is considered to be a positive risk factor for development of life-threatening coronary heart disease in this patient?
   a. High HDL cholesterol level
   b. Low triglyceride level
   c. Family history
   d. Strenuous exercise
2. Behavior change should immediately focus on which of the risk factors noted in this patient?
   a. Lowering the LDL cholesterol
   b. Lowering the total cholesterol
   c. Giving up smoking cigarettes
   d. Engaging in a more strenuous exercise program

Critical Thinking Group Discussion Questions

1. Which patient issues should be addressed to lower this patient's risk for a myocardial infarction?
2. What other laboratory tests would be of value?

Note: Narrative answers published on EVOLVE instructor site.

CASE STUDY 10.7

A 60-year-old man with a history of alcoholism is seen in an urgent care clinic; he complains of extreme pain in his upper abdomen. He has been experiencing pain on and off for the past 10 days. Now he is yellow (jaundiced) and feels extremely ill. He also mentions that his stool specimens have lost their normal color and look like clay. Blood is drawn for testing and urine collected for urinalysis. The following urinalysis results were obtained:

Physical Appearance
Color: Brown (yellow-brown)
Transparency: Clear

Chemical Screening
pH: 6.5
Specific gravity: 1.020
Protein (reagent strip): Negative
Blood: Negative
Nitrite: Negative
Leukocyte esterase: Negative
Glucose: Negative
Ketones: Negative
Bilirubin: Large
Urobilinogen: Normal

Microscopic Examination
Red blood cells: 0 to 2/hpf
White blood cells: 0 to 2/hpf

Multiple-Choice Questions
Answers are in Appendix A.

1. The abnormal urine color is caused by which of the following?
   a. Bilirubin
   b. Free bilirubin
   c. Unconjugated bilirubin
   d. Urobilinogen
2. The lack of color in the feces is caused by an absence of which of the following?
   a. Bilirubin glucuronide
   b. Free bilirubin
   c. Unconjugated bilirubin
   d. Urobilinogen
3. This patient's jaundice is the result of the presence of which of the following?
   a. Bilirubin glucuronide
   b. Unconjugated bilirubin
   c. Urobilinogen
   d. More than one of the above

Critical Thinking Group Discussion Questions

1. Based on the patient's history and the urinalysis results, what is the biological cause of this patient's jaundice?
2. How is this patient's physiology disrupted to produce abnormal laboratory results?

Note: Narrative answers published on EVOLVE instructor site.

REFERENCES

1. US Department of Health and Human Services, Centers for Disease Control and Prevention: *National diabetes fact sheet,* 2011.
2. American Diabetes Association: Position statement: diagnosis and classification of diabetes mellitus, *Diabetes Care* 37:S81–S90, 2014.
3. Tirosh A, et al: Normal fasting plasma glucose levels and type 2 diabetes in young men, *N Engl J Med* 353:14, 2005.
4. Krinsley JD: Effect of an intensive glucose management protocol in the mortality of critically ill adult patients, *Mayo Clin Proc* 79:9992, 2004.
5. American Diabetes Association: Standards of Medical Care in Diabetes–2018 Abridged for Primary Care Providers, *Clinical Diabetes* 36(1):14–37, 2018.
6. Gupta MK: Glycemic biomarkers as tools for diagnosis and monitoring of diabetes, *MLO Med Lab Obs* 45(3):8–14, 2013.
7. Burtis CA, Ashwood ER, editors: *Tietz fundamentals of clinical chemistry*, 4 ed., Philadelphia, 1996, Saunders.
8. Clinical Laboratory Buyers Guide and Annual Report: Clinical laboratory reference, 2005–2006, *Adv Admin Lab* 14(12), 2005.
9. Burtis CA, Bruns DE: *Tietz fundamentals of clinical chemistry,* Table 50-1, 50-2, ed 7, St Louis, 2015, Elsevier/Saunders.
10. Gentzkow CJ: Accurate method for determination of blood urea nitrogen by direct nesslerization, *J Biol Chem* 143:531, 1942.
11. Jaffe M: Uber den Niederschlag welchen Pikrinsaure in normalen Harn erzeugt und uber eine neue Reaktion des Kreatininins, *Z Physiol Chem* 10:391, 1886.
12. Levey AS, Bosch JP, Lewis JB, et al: A more accurate method to estimate glomerular filtration rate from serum creatinine: a new prediction equation, *Ann Intern Med* 130:461, 1999.
13. Erlandsen EJ, Randers E, Kristensen JH: Reference intervals for serum cystatin C and serum creatinine in adults, *Clin Chem Lab Med* 36:393–397, 1998.
14. Bishop ML, Fody EP: *Clinical chemistry: principles, procedures, correlations,* ed 5, Philadelphia, 2018, Lippincott Williams & Wilkins p 484230.
15. Harada A, Toh R, Murakami K, et al: Cholesterol Uptake Capacity: A new Measure of HDL Functionality for Coronary Risk, *J of Applied Laboratory Medicine* 1(6), 2015.
16. Third Report of the Expert Panel on Detection, evaluation, and treatment of high blood cholesterol in adults (adult treatment panel III), the National Cholesterol Education Program (NCEP) updated recommendations, https://www.lipid.org/practicetools/guidelines/national, accessed Oct, 2018.
17. Goff DC, Lloyd-Jones DM, Bennett G, et al: 2013 ACC/AHA Guideline on the Assessment of Cardiovascular Risk, *Circulation* 129(25 suppl 2):S49–S73, June, 2014.
18. Rollins G: Universal lipid screening in children, *Clin Lab News* 38(3):1–4, 2012.
19. Myocardial infarction redefined: a consensus document of the Joint European Society of Cardiology/American College of Cardiology Committee for the Redefinition of Myocardial Infarction, *J Am Coll Cardiol* 36(3):959, 2000.
20. Thomas S, Kavsak P, Devereaux PJ: Cardiac troponin, *Clin Lab News* 39(4):8–10, 2013.
21. Rollins G: A look at emerging cardiac biomarkers, *Clin Lab News* 38(1):3–5, 2012.
22. Tolman KG, Raj R: Liver function. In Burtis CA, Ashwood ER, editors: *Tietz textbook of clinical chemistry*, 3 ed., Philadelphia, 1999, Saunders.
23. Malloy HT, Evelyn KA: The determination of bilirubin with the photoelectric colorimeter, *J Biol Chem* 119:481, 1937.

24. National Cancer Institute: Tumor Markers, https://www.cancer.gov, accessed Sept. 28, 2018.
25. Fenton JJ, Weyrich MS, Durbin S: Evidence Summary: Other Supporting Document for Prostate Cancer: Screening, *JAMA* 319 (18):1914–1931, 2018.
26. Am. Urological Association: Early Detection of Prostate Cancer Published 2013; Reviewed and Validity Confirmed 2018, www.auanet.org, accessed Oct. 1, 2018.

BIBLIOGRAPHY

American Proficiency Institute-2015: APIC 153882151-CME/CMLE Electrolytes, Am Soc of Clin Path, Clinical Laboratory, www.ascp.org, accessed May, 2017.

Atkinson MA, Maclaren JK: The pathogenesis of insulin-dependent diabetes mellitus, *N Engl J Med* 331(21):1428, 1994.

Chloupkova M: Hemoglobin A_{1c}: new approach to the diagnosis of diabetes mellitus, *ASCLS Today* 27(3):6–7, 2013.

Clinical and Laboratory Standards Institute: *Standardization of sodium and potassium ion-selective electrode systems to the flame photometric reference method: approved standard,* ed 2, 2000. Wayne, Pa, reaffirmed June 2003, C29-A2.

Clinical and Laboratory Standards Institute: *Sweat testing: sample collection and quantitative analysis: approved guideline,* ed 2, 2000. Wayne, Pa, C34-A2.

Clinical and Laboratory Standards Institute: *Point-of-care blood glucose testing in acute and chronic care facilities: approved guideline,* ed 2, 2002. Wayne, Pa, C30-A2.

Clinical and Laboratory Standards Institute: *Glucose testing in settings without laboratory support: approved guideline,* ed 2, 2005. Wayne, Pa, AST4-A2.

Elefano EC, et al: *Analytical evaluation of $HgbA_{1c}$, microalbumin, CRP, and RF on Architect ci8200 integrated system and workflow computer simulation. Abstract 24. Pushing the Technology Envelope II: an Exploration of the Future of Clinical Laboratory Testing,* Baltimore, 2005, Oak Ridge Conference.

Faix JD, Thienpont LM: Thyroid stimulating hormone, *Clin Lab News* 39(5):8–10, 2013.

Foreback C: Diabetes epidemic, *Clin Lab Products* 42(11):8–10, 2012.

Harada A, Toh R, Murakami K, et al: Cholesterol Uptake Capacity: A new Measure of HDL Functionality for Coronary Risk, *J of Applied Laboratory Medicine* 1(6), 2017.

Larson TS: Lab estimation of GFR, *Clin Lab News* 30(6):8, 2004.

Miller WG: Glomerular filtration rate, *Clin Lab News* 37(12):10–12, 2011.

Milojkovic R: A heightened awareness: hemoglobin variants and HbA_{1c}, *MLO Med Lab Obs* 45(5):50–54, 2013.

Poudel RR: Renal glucose handling in diabetes and sodium glucose cotransporter 2 inhibition, *Indian J Endocrinol Metab* 17(4):588–593, 2013.

Rezendes DA, Faix JD: The role of the clinical laboratory in the new approach to diabetes, *Clin Lab News* 23(7):1, 1997.

Robinson K, Kongable GL: Lactate in critical illness: implications for monitoring, *US Respir Dis* 6:3–6, 2010.

Sandoval Y, Erfan Ayubi: Prognostic Value of High-Sensitivity Cardiac Troponin T Compared with Risk Scores in Stable Cardiovascular Disease: Methodological Issues The American Journal of Medicine, 130(10):1358–1365, 2017.

Tracey RP: C-reactive protein and cardiovascular disease, *Clin Lab News* 24(8):14, 1998.

White A, Foley KF: *Lab Q*, No. 1508 Clin Chem, Am Soc of Clin Path. In *Clinical Laboratory*, www.ascp.org, accessed May, 2015.

Woeste S: Diagnosing prostate cancer, *Lab Med* 36(7):399, 2005.

REVIEW QUESTIONS (ANSWERS IN APPENDIX A)

Note:
❖ indicates MLT (optional) & MLS advanced content

Glucose and Glucose Metabolism

1. One of the major hormones that controls high glucose levels after a meal is:
   - **a.** Insulin
   - **b.** Thyroxine
   - **c.** Glucagon
   - **d.** Lipase
2. In a person with normal glucose metabolism, the blood glucose level usually increases rapidly after carbohydrates are ingested but returns to a normal level after:
   - **a.** 30 minutes
   - **b.** 45 minutes
   - **c.** 60 minutes
   - **d.** 120 minutes
3. Which of the following organs uses glucose from digested carbohydrates and stores it as glycogen for later use as a source of immediate energy by the muscles?
   - **a.** Kidneys
   - **b.** Liver
   - **c.** Pancreas
   - **d.** Thyroid

Diabetes

4. In a person with impaired glucose metabolism, such as in type 1 diabetes, what is true about the blood glucose level?
   - **a.** It increases rapidly after carbohydrates are ingested but returns to a normal level after 120 minutes.
   - **b.** It increases rapidly after carbohydrates are ingested and stays greatly elevated even after 120 minutes.
   - **c.** It does not increase after carbohydrates are ingested and stays at a low level until the next meal.
   - **d.** It increases rapidly after carbohydrates are ingested but returns to a normal level after 30 minutes.
5. Which of the following is not a classic symptom of type 1 diabetes?
   - **a.** Polyuria
   - **b.** Polydipsia
   - **c.** Polyphagia
   - **d.** Proteinuria

6. Which of the following statements is true about type 1 diabetes?
   a. It is associated with an insufficient amount of insulin secreted by the pancreas.
   b. It is associated with inefficient activity of the insulin secreted by the pancreas.
   c. It is a more frequent type of diabetes than the non–insulin-dependent diabetes (type 2).
   d. Good control of this disease will eliminate complications in the future.
7. What can be the result of uncontrolled elevated blood glucose?
   a. Coma from insulin shock
   b. Diabetic coma
   c. Ketones in the urine
   d. Both b and c
8. Gestational diabetes can occur during pregnancy in some women. Which of the following can occur for a significant number of these women?
   a. Can develop type 1 diabetes at a later date
   b. Can develop type 2 diabetes at a later date
   c. Continue to manifest signs of diabetes after delivery
   d. No effect
9. The level of glycosylated hemoglobin in a diabetic patient reflects which of the following?
   a. Blood glucose concentration at the time blood was collected
   b. Average blood glucose concentration over the past week
   c. Average blood glucose concentration over the past 2 to 3 months (life span of a red cell)
   d. More than one of the above

Electrolytes

10. A sweat chloride result of 50 mmol/L is obtained for an adult patient who has a history of respiratory problems. What would be the best interpretation of these results, based on known reference values?
    a. Normal sweat chloride, not consistent with cystic fibrosis
    b. Marginally elevated results, borderline for cystic fibrosis
    c. Elevated results, diagnostic of cystic fibrosis
    d. Normal sweat chloride, consistent with cystic fibrosis
11. Which of the following electrolytes is the chief cation in the plasma, is found in the highest concentration in the extravascular fluid, and has the main function of maintaining osmotic pressure?
    a. Potassium
    b. Sodium
    c. Calcium
    d. Magnesium
12. Analysis of a serum specimen gives a potassium result of 6.0 mmol/L. Before the result is reported to the physician, what additional step should be taken?
    a. The serum should be observed for hemolysis; hemolysis of the red cells will shift potassium from the cells into the serum, resulting in a falsely elevated potassium value.
    b. The serum should be observed for evidence of jaundice; jaundiced serum will result in a falsely elevated potassium value.
    c. The test should be run again on the same specimen.
    d. Nothing needs to be done; simply report the result.

❖ 13. The anion gap can be increased in patients with:
    a. Lactic acidosis
    b. Toxin ingestion
    c. Uremia
    d. More than one of the above

❖ 14. Calculation of the anion gap is useful for quality control for:
    a. Calcium
    b. Tests in the electrolyte profile (sodium, potassium, chloride, and bicarbonate)
    c. Phosphorus
    d. Magnesium

Acid-Base Balance and Blood Gases

❖ 15. Ninety percent of the carbon dioxide present in the blood is in the form of:
    a. Bicarbonate ions
    b. Carbonate
    c. Dissolved CO_2
    d. Carbonic acid

❖ Questions 16 to 19: Match the following acid-base disorders with the corresponding laboratory findings (a–d).

16. ___ Metabolic acidosis
17. ___ Metabolic alkalosis
18. ___ Respiratory acidosis
19. ___ Respiratory alkalosis

Key: $cHCO_3^-$, Cytoplasmic bicarbonate; Pco_2, partial pressure of carbon dioxide.

a. $\downarrow cHCO_3^-$
b. $\uparrow cHCO_3^-$
c. $\uparrow Pco_2$
d. $\downarrow Pco_2$

Renal Function

20. Nitrogen is excreted principally in the form of:
    a. Creatinine
    b. Creatine
    c. Uric acid
    d. Urea
21. The main waste product of protein metabolism is:
    a. Creatinine
    b. Creatine
    c. Uric acid
    d. Urea
22. The protein content of the diet will affect primarily the test results for:
    a. Creatinine
    b. Creatine
    c. Uric acid
    d. Urea or urea nitrogen

23. Creatinine concentration in the blood has a direct relationship to:
 a. Muscle mass
 b. Dietary protein intake
 c. Age and gender
 d. More than one of the above
24. In the Jaffe reaction, a red-orange chromogen is formed when creatinine reacts with:
 a. Picric acid
 b. Biuret reagent
 c. Diacetyl monoxime
 d. Both a and b
25. Creatinine clearance is used to assess the:
 a. Glomerular filtration capabilities of the kidneys
 b. Tubular secretion of creatinine
 c. Dietary intake of protein
 d. Glomerular and tubular mass
26. Expected creatinine clearance for a patient with chronic renal disease would be:
 a. Very low; renal glomerular filtration is functioning normally.
 b. Normal; renal glomerular filtration is functioning normally.
 c. Very high; renal glomerular filtration is not functioning normally.
 d. Very low; renal glomerular filtration is not functioning normally.
27. A serum creatinine result of 6.6 mg/dL is most likely to be found in conjunction with which of the following other laboratory results?
 a. Urea, 15 mg/dL
 b. Urea, 85 mg/dL
 c. Urea nitrogen, 10 mg/dL
 d. Urea nitrogen/creatinine ratio, 15
28. Microalbumin is useful in:
 a. Monitoring diabetic nephropathy in Type I diabetes
 b. Monitoring renal function
 c. Detecting urinary tract infections
 d. Detecting membrane permeability in serum and fluids
29. Testing blood from a patient with acute glomerulonephritis would most likely result in which of the following laboratory findings?
 a. Decreased creatinine
 b. Decreased urea
 c. Increased glucose
 d. Increased creatinine

Uric Acid

30. Uric acid is the final breakdown product of which type of metabolism?
 a. Urea
 b. Glucose
 c. Purine
 d. Bilirubin

Lipids

31. Which of the following lipid results would be expected to be falsely elevated in a blood specimen drawn from a nonfasting patient?
 a. Total cholesterol
 b. Triglycerides
 c. HDL cholesterol
 d. More than one of the above
32. Blood is collected from a patient who has been fasting since 3 a.m.; the collection time is 7 a.m. Which of the following tests would not give a valid test result?
 a. Cholesterol
 b. Triglycerides
 c. Total bilirubin
 d. Either A or B
33. Which of the following laboratory values is considered healthy for a 19 year old?
 a. HDL cholesterol 45 mg/dL or greater
 b. HDL cholesterol 39 mg/dL or less
 c. LDL cholesterol 129 mg/dL or less
 d. Total cholesterol 199 mg/dL or less
34. Noting the appearance of plasma or serum can give important preliminary findings about lipid levels in the blood when it is collected from a fasting patient. When the specimen appears opaque and milky (lipemic), what is the approximate expected level of triglycerides in the sample?
 a. Within the normal range; test is unaffected by meals.
 b. From 200 to 300 mg/dL.
 c. Greater than 600 mg/dL.
 d. No preliminary findings can be made from observation of the serum.
35. When a hyperlipidemic condition exists for a sufficient time, it may be associated with the development of which of the following conditions?
 a. Obesity
 b. Diabetes mellitus
 c. Atherosclerosis
 d. Viral hepatitis
36. In what major organ of the body is the majority of the body's cholesterol synthesized?
 a. Heart
 b. Pancreas
 c. Gallbladder
 d. Liver
37. What is the cutoff for a healthy LDL cholesterol concentration for a female 20 years or older?
 a. <100 mg/dL
 b. <160 mg/dL
 c. <200 mg/dL
 d. <300 mg/dL

Cardiovascular Disease

38. Which of the following is considered a primary risk factor for the development of coronary heart disease later in life?
    a. Cigarette smoking
    b. Stress
    c. Diabetes mellitus
    d. Lack of exercise
39. Which of the following is considered a secondary risk factor for the development of coronary heart disease later in life?
    a. Cigarette smoking
    b. Increased HDL cholesterol
    c. Decreased HDL cholesterol
    d. Obesity
40. In the analysis of cardiac markers, which marker increases first?
    a. Myoglobin
    b. CK-MB fraction
    c. Troponin T
    d. Troponin I
41. Which cardiac marker persists at the highest concentration for the longest length of time?
    a. Myoglobin
    b. CK-MB fraction
    c. Troponin T
    d. Troponin I

Liver and Pancreatic Testing

42. Which of the following enzymes is found primarily in the liver?
    a. Aspartate transaminase
    b. Alkaline phosphatase
    c. Alanine transaminase
    d. γ-Glutamyltransferase
43. Elevated concentrations of serum amylase and lipase are often seen in:
    a. Acid reflux disease
    b. Gallstones
    c. Acute pancreatitis
    d. Acute pharyngitis
44. What is the classic symptom or manifestation of liver disease?
    a. Hemolysis of red cells
    b. Jaundice
    c. Kernicterus
    d. Formation of gallstones

❖ 45. In an adult, if total bilirubin value is 3.1 mg/dL and conjugated bilirubin is 1.1 mg/dL, what is the unconjugated bilirubin value?
    a. 2.0 mg/dL
    b. 4.2 mg/dL
    c. 1.0 mg/dL
    d. 3.4 mg/dL

❖ 46. A rapid buildup of unconjugated bilirubin in a newborn can result in kernicterus, which is an accumulation of bilirubin in the:
    a. Heart tissue
    b. Liver cells
    c. Brain tissue
    d. Kidney tissue

❖ 47. Impairment of conjugation of bilirubin by the liver cells is:
    a. Prehepatic jaundice
    b. Hepatic jaundice
    c. Posthepatic jaundice
    d. None of these phases

❖ 48. Transport defects involving release of the bilirubin bound to plasma albumin to the liver cell for conjugation with glucuronide is:
    a. Prehepatic jaundice
    b. Hepatic jaundice
    c. Posthepatic jaundice
    d. None of these phases

❖ 49. Defect in transporting the conjugated bilirubin out of the liver cells and into the bile fluid is:
    a. Prehepatic jaundice
    b. Hepatic jaundice
    c. Posthepatic jaundice
    d. None of these phases

❖ 50. In which of the following conditions resulting in jaundice is there an increase in both conjugated and unconjugated bilirubin?
    a. Hemolysis of red cells
    b. Viral hepatitis
    c. Obstruction from gallstones
    d. Constriction of biliary tract from neoplasm

❖ 51. In which of the following conditions resulting in jaundice is there an increase primarily in unconjugated bilirubin?
    a. Increased hemolysis of red cells
    b. Viral hepatitis
    c. Biliary obstruction
    d. Cirrhosis of the liver

52. In a premature newborn, a deficiency of what enzyme can affect the conjugation of bilirubin glucuronide in the liver?
    a. Glucuronosyltransferase
    b. Aspartate transaminase
    c. Alanine transaminase
    d. γ-Glutamyltransferase

Hormone Assays

❖ 53. Hormones secreted by the thyroid include:
    a. Thyroxine
    b. Triiodothyronine
    c. Insulin
    d. Both a and b

Tumor Markers

❖ 54. Tumor markers include:
    a. Carcinoembryonic antigen (CEA)
    b. Alpha fetoprotein
    c. Beta subunit of human chorionic gonadotropin
    d. All the above

Therapeutic Drug Monitoring

❖ **55.** In therapeutic drug monitoring assays, it is extremely important to test the specimen:
a. Exactly 8 hours after the drug is ingested
b. At the established peak and/or trough intervals
c. For competing antibodies to the drug
d. Before the establishment of a steady state

Drugs of Abuse

❖ **56.** Drugs of abuse include:
a. Acetaminophen
b. Salicylic acid
c. Amphetamines
d. Antibiotics

Challenge Questions

The following patient results were obtained:

Assay	Result
pH	7.6
Pco_2	20 mm Hg
Po_2	128 mm Hg
HCO_3^-	15 mmol/L
Na^+	138 mmol/L
K^+	3.9 mmol/L
Cl^-	107 mmol/L
Tco_2	24 mmol/L

❖ **57.** The blood pH is:
a. Alkaline
b. Acidic
c. Very acidic
d. Neutral

❖ **58.** The most likely condition is:
a. Blood specimen is not delivered on ice promptly to the laboratory.
b. Blood specimen contained air bubbles.
c. Patient is in a state of partially compensated metabolic alkalosis.
d. Patient is in a state of partially compensated respiratory alkalosis.

Automation in Clinical Chemistry

❖ **59.** A unique assay method developed for automated immunoassay that does not replicate standard manual reactions is:
a. Chemiluminescence
b. Photometry
c. Ion-selective electrode
d. Colorimetry

Turgeon: Linné & Ringsrud's Clinical Laboratory Science, 8th Edition

STUDENT PROCEDURE WORKSHEET 10-1

Calculating Total Protein Concentration

Student Learning Outcomes

See Chapter 10 of *Linné & Ringsrud's Clinical Laboratory Science: Concepts, Procedures, and Clinical Applications*, 8th edition, for a complete discussion of this procedure. After reading Chapter 10, and at the completion of this laboratory exercise and review questions, the student will be able to:

- Describe specimen requirements including length and temperature of storage.
- Explain how to calculate a patient's total protein based on the absorbance of the specimen and a known serum albumin standard.
- Complete the end-of-procedure review questions with a grade of 80% or higher.

Principle

For the assay of total protein using Biuret reagent, the color formed in the reaction is proportional to the protein concentration and is measured in a spectrophotometer at 540 nm (520-560 nm).

Specimen

A nonhemolyzed serum specimen is preferred, although plasma from whole blood collected in heparin is suitable. Total protein samples may be stored for at least 7 days at room temperature (18 °C-25 °C) and for at least 1 month at 4 °C.

Equipment, Supplies, and Reagents (Manual Procedure)

1. Total protein reagent (Biuret method). Ready for use with human plasma or serum. Store at 2 °C-25 °C until the expiration date stated on bottle (Thermo Scientific/Fisher Scientific, Cat. No. TR 34021).
2. Total protein standard (bovine serum albumin 5.0 mg/mL)
3. Pipettes and gauze (or Kimwipes)
4. Timer
5. Spectrophotometer and cuvettes
6. Test tubes, wax pencil, test tube rack, Parafilm

Quality Control

Normal and abnormal controls with known values must be tested with patient tests.

Reference Range

6.0-8.3 g/dL

Clinical Significance

Total protein values are increased in dehydration, multiple myeloma, and chronic liver diseases. Decreased levels are found in renal disease and terminal liver failure.

Procedure Notes

Indications of reagent deterioration include turbidity, control values not in reported assay ranges, and absorbance (OD) at 540 nm > 0.200.

Instructions for the Procedure

Read the list of required equipment, supplies, and reagents and the procedural steps. Follow the procedural steps in exact order.

SEQUENCE	PROCEDURAL STEP	INSTRUCTOR-OBSERVED ACCEPTABLE PERFORMANCE (CHECK IF ACCEPTABLE)
1	Don gloves and gown. Turn on spectrophotometer to warm up. Set the instrument to 540 nm.	
2	Label test tubes for patients and controls. Include a reagent blank test tube.	
3	Pipette 250 µL of Biuret reagent to each of the respectively labeled test tubes.	
4	Pipette 5 µL of serum to each of the respectively labeled test tubes.	
5	Cover each tube and mix gently by inverting. Allow to stand for 10 minutes.	
6	Set the spectrophotometer to 100%T or 0 O.D. absorbance with the Biuret reagent blank.	
7	Decant a portion of each specimen-Biuret mixture to fill a cuvette about three-fourths full. Read and record each value.	
8	Calculate or *(optional)* read the concentrations from a standard curve.	

(Continued)

Turgeon: Linné & Ringsrud's Clinical Laboratory Science, 8th Edition

STUDENT PROCEDURE WORKSHEET 10-1

Calculations

Total protein = Absorbance of unknown/Absorbance of TP standard × Standard value
Example: Absorbance of standard = 0.319; Absorbance of unknown = 0.396
Value of standard = 5.0 g/dL
Total protein = 0.396/0.319 × 5.0 = 6.21 g/dL

Protein Standard Curve

TEST TUBE DILUTIONS	ML OF BOVINE STANDARD ALBUMIN (5 mg/ml)	ML OF UNKNOWN	ML OF H_2O	PROTEIN CONCENTRATION (mg)
1	0.0	—	2.0	0
2	0.1	—	1.9	0.5
3	0.3	—	1.7	1.5
4	0.5	—	1.5	2.5
5	0.7	—	1.3	3.5
6	1.0	—	1.0	5.0
7	—	1.0	1.0	Unknown
8	—	1.0	1.0	Unknown

1. Pipette 3.0 mL of Biuret reagent to each of the test tubes. Mix.
2. Allow to stand for 10 min.
3. Transfer the content of each test to fill a cuvette three-fourths full.
4. Set spectrophotometer at 100%T/0 Absorbance at 540 nm.
5. Read and record the absorbance (OD) of each test tube.
6. Plot the standard curve on conventional graph paper. *x*-axis = mg of protein, *y*-axis = absorbance (OD) of each tube. Draw the best possible straight line on the graph paper with 0.0 as the beginning of the line. Locate the absorbance of the unknown specimen, and locate where this value intercepts the straight line. Read straight down from the point where an imaginary line intersects the protein concentration. This is the protein value of the unknown.

Results

TEST TUBE DILUTIONS	ABSORBANCE (OD)	PROTEIN CONCENTRATION (mg)
1		0.0
2		0.5
3		1.5
4		2.5
5		3.5
6		5.0

Results of Unknown Specimens

SPECIMEN IDENTIFICATION	RESULTS

(Continued)

Turgeon: Linné & Ringsrud's Clinical Laboratory Science, 8th Edition

STUDENT PROCEDURE WORKSHEET 10-1

Calculating Total Protein Concentration

Review Questions

1. If the Biuret reagent was allowed to stand for 1 hour, what would be the effect on the accuracy of the test?

2. What clinical conditions can cause an increase in serum total protein?

3. State the equation for calculating a patient's total protein value based on using a known total protein standard.

4. What is the normal range for creatinine clearance for this patient?

Procedural Evaluation

Student's Name ______________________ Grade________

Instructor's Signature ______________________ Date________

Comments:

11

An Introduction to the Principles and Practice of Clinical Hematology

http://evolve.elsevier.com/Turgeon/clinicallab

CHAPTER CONTENTS

LEARNING OUTCOMES

Hematopoiesis: Overall Blood Cell Maturation and Function
- Differentiate the stages of hematopoiesis.

Erythrocytes
- Distinguish the cellular characteristics in the formation of erythrocytes.
- Describe hemoglobin synthesis and normal and abnormal types of hemoglobin.
- Explain the difference between normal hemoglobin and abnormal hemoglobin S.

Leukocytes
- Distinguish the cellular characteristics in the formation of leukocytes.
- Identify the types of mature leukocytes found in circulating blood, and describe the characteristics of each.

Lymphocyte maturation and function
- Describe the process of maturation and functional differences between subsets of lymphocytes.
- Compare and calculate, if needed, the total, relative, and absolute counts of lymphocytes and other peripheral blood leukocytes.

Thrombocytes
- Distinguish the cellular characteristics in the formation of thrombocytes.

Clinical Hematology Procedures
- Discuss the mode and applications for the three types of anticoagulants used for hematology assays.
- Assess at least three types of unsuitable blood specimens and the effect of each on test results.
- Compare the effects of isotonic, hypotonic, and hypertonic solutions on blood cells.
- Hemoglobin
- Microhematocrit
- Describe the procedure for counting and calculating erythrocytes, leukocytes, and platelets.
- Calculate a corrected white cell count.
- Automated cell-counting methods

Additional Hematology Procedures
- Describe the calculations and applications of a reticulocyte count.
- Describe the application of the erythrocyte sedimentation rate (ESR).
- Describe the principle of the microhematocrit determination.

Red Blood Cell Indices
- Calculate red blood cell indices of mean corpuscular volume (MCV), mean corpuscular hemoglobin (MCH), and mean corpuscular hemoglobin concentration (MCHC).
- Explain the formula and application of the red cell distribution width (RDW).

Microscopic Examination of the Peripheral Blood Film
- Identify and describe the morphologic alterations of size, shape, color, inclusions, and abnormal distribution patterns in erythrocytes.
- Compare the three categories of anemia, based on morphology.
- Identify and describe leukocyte alterations.

Case Studies

❖ Analyze the patient history, clinical signs and symptoms, and laboratory data for the stated case studies, answer the related critical thinking questions, and conclude the most likely diagnosis.

Review Questions

❖ Demonstrate comprehension of the chapter content by completing the end-of-chapter review questions with a grade of 80% or higher.

Note:
- indicates MLT and MLS core content

❖ indicates MLT (optional) and MLS advanced content

KEY TERMS

erythrocytes
hematopoiesis
hemoglobin (Hb)
hemoglobinopathies
leukocytes
lymphocytes
monocytes
mononuclear phagocytic system
oxyhemoglobin (HbO_2)
phagocytosis
platelets (thrombocytes)
reduced hemoglobin
reticulocytes
segmented neutrophils
supravital stains

HEMATOPOIESIS: OVERALL BLOOD CELL MATURATION AND FUNCTION

The total volume of blood in an average adult is about 6 L, or 7% to 8% of the body weight. About 45% of this amount is composed of red blood cells (RBCs; erythrocytes), white blood cells (WBCs; leukocytes), and platelets (thrombocytes); the remaining 55% is the liquid fraction, plasma. The formed elements of whole blood are suspended in plasma. Approximately 90% of the composition of plasma is water; the remaining 10% consists of soluble biochemicals, including proteins, carbohydrates, vitamins, hormones, enzymes, lipids, salts, and trace metals.

Blood cell production, or hematopoiesis (Fig. 11.1), begins in embryonic development. In the embryo, self-renewing hematopoietic stem cells develop initially in the primitive yolk sac and then migrate to the fetal liver. Beginning in the fetal liver and later in bone marrow, these pluripotential CD34+, hematopoietic stem cells give rise to the earliest myeloid and lymphoid progenitors. Less than 1% of the marrow consists of stem cells. They have the ability to repopulate the bone marrow after injury or lethal radiation, which is the basis of bone marrow transplantation.

Until age 5 years, the marrow in all the bones is red and cellular, and actively produces cells. Between 5 and 7 years of age, the long bones become inactive, and fat cells appear to replace the active marrow. Through the maturing years, red marrow in the other bones is gradually displaced by fat cells and transformed into yellow marrow. After age 18 to 20 years, red marrow remains only in the vertebrae, ribs, sternum, skull, and partially in the femur and humerus.

Blood cell differentiation and maturation occur primarily in bone marrow, where the environment is well organized and complex. Mature cells must migrate across the sinusoidal

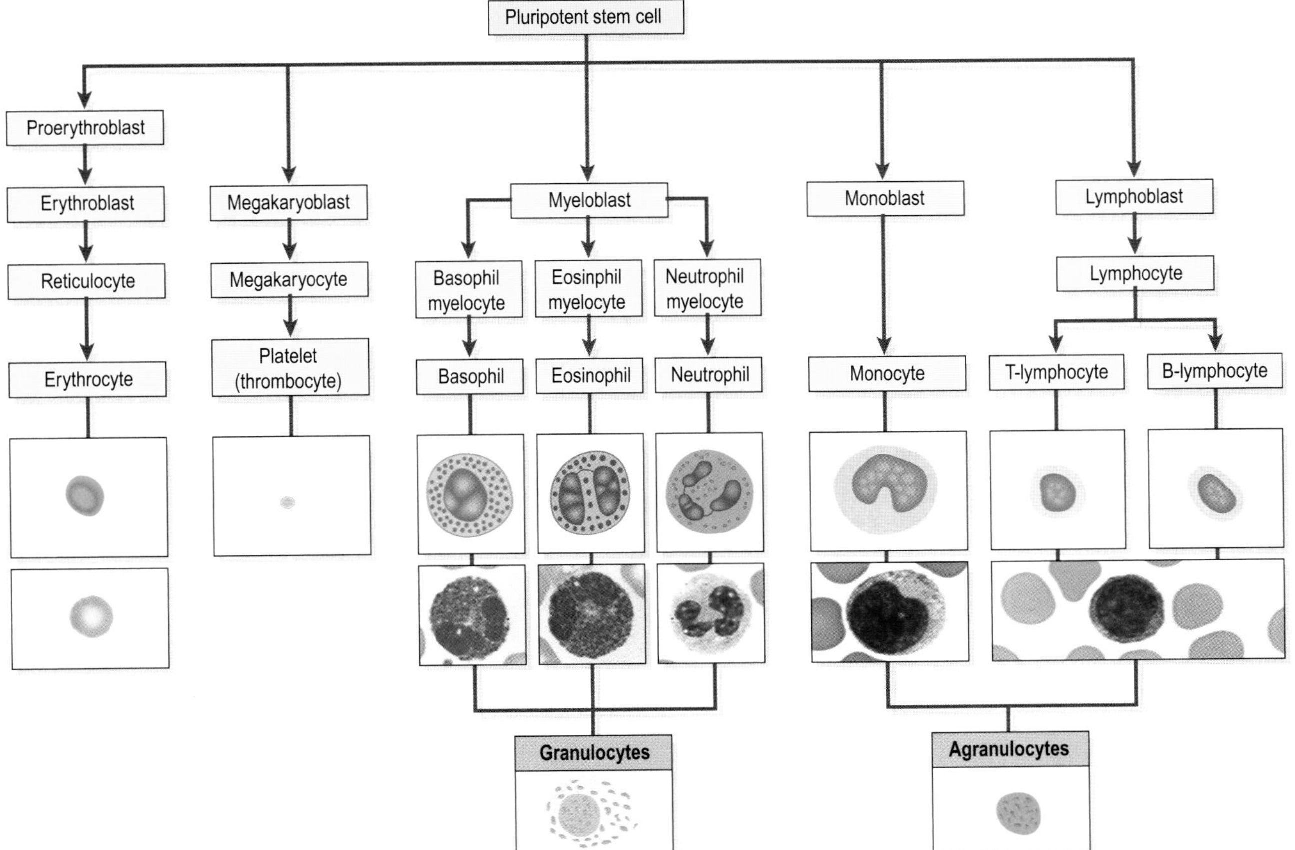

Fig. 11.1 Diagram of hematopoiesis. (From Waugh A, Grant A: Ross and Wilson anatomy and physiology in health and illness, ed. 12, p. 64)

endothelia of the marrow capillaries to enter the peripheral circulation. The endothelial membrane allows passage of the more deformable mature cells and holds back the immature cells, which are more rigid and less motile. Pathologic processes can facilitate the release of more immature cells by affecting the cellular composition of the sinusoidal endothelia.

Myeloid progenitors differentiate into colony-forming cells of the erythroid and myeloid lineages. Erythrocytes, platelets, neutrophils, monocytes and macrophages, eosinophils, basophils, and mast cells (tissues) all mature from the common myeloid progenitor cell.

Lymphoid progenitors give rise to natural killer cells, T lymphocytes, and B lymphocytes. B lymphocytes (B cells) differentiate further in the bone marrow and further still on encountering an antigen. T lymphocytes (T cells) differentiate and acquire antigen specificity, principally in the thymus and, in some cases, other lymphoid organs. If productive gene rearrangement does not occur as the result of antigen exposure, the lymphocytes will die. T cells develop in the thymus and extrathymic tissues from a lymphoid precursor. Lymphocytes circulate in the peripheral blood and lymphatic tissues and through secondary lymphoid organs such as the lymph nodes and spleen. B cells develop from lymphoid progenitors in the bone marrow and at sites at which the B cell encounters antigen, such as secondary lymphoid organs.[1]

All stages in the maturation process are gradual, and it is often impossible to identify an exact stage with certainty. The most immature forms of all cell types appear very similar morphologically, and their identification is often based on surrounding cell types in various stages of development.

ERYTHROCYTES

Erythrocyte Function and Maturation

The main function of the RBC is to carry oxygen to the cells of the body. Oxygen is transported in a chemical combination with hemoglobin (Hb). The concentration of Hb in the blood is a measure of its capacity to carry oxygen, on which all cells are absolutely dependent for energy and therefore life. In the tissues, oxygen is exchanged for carbon dioxide, which is carried to the lungs for excretion in exchange for oxygen. To combine with and transport oxygen, the Hb molecule must have a certain combination of heme (which contains iron) and globin. Deficiencies in the presence or metabolism of these substances will result in a decrease in Hb- and oxygen-carrying capacity.

RBCs gradually progress from one stage to another, steadily decreasing in size. The mature RBC is about 7 to 8 μm in diameter. The RBC begins as a nucleated cell within the bone marrow. As the cell matures in the bone marrow, its diameter decreases, and the nucleus becomes denser and smaller, and is finally released from the cell (extruded). The mature RBC is often described as a biconcave disk that lacks a nucleus. During maturation, the concentration of Hb increases in the cell. This is seen as a progressive change in color of the cytoplasm from blue to orange on a Wright-stained blood film. The whole sequence of maturation from an early cell precursor to a circulating RBC takes 3 to 5 days (Table 11.1).

RBCs (erythrocytes) are normally produced in the bone marrow, except in early fetal development. RBC maturation exists in six stages of development. Different systems of naming (nomenclature) have been used to describe these RBC developmental stages. The stages of maturation (Fig. 11.2) from the youngest to the mature cell are (1) rubriblast (pronormoblast), (2) prorubricyte (basophilic normoblast), (3) rubricyte (polychromatophilic normoblast), (4) metarubricyte (orthochromic normoblast), (5) reticulocyte (polychromatic erythrocyte), and (6) mature erythrocyte (Fig. 11.3).

The earliest rubriblast appears morphologically similar to other blasts such as myeloblasts or lymphoblasts, but cells of the erythrocyte series tend to stain more intensely blue than blast cells related to other cell lines. The intensity of the blue

TABLE 11.1 Erythrocyte Development

Nomenclature Rubriblastic	Alternate Nomenclature Normoblastic	Percent in Bone Marrow	Hours in Bone Marrow	Overall Size	N/C Ratio	Nucleus	Cytoplasm
Rubriblast	Pronormoblast	1	12	12–20	8:1	Round to oval shape with 1 or 2 nucleoli; chromatin has fine clumps	Intensely blue
Prorubricyte	Basophilic normoblast	1–4	20	10–15	6:1	Some chromatin clumping, no (or 1) nucleoli	Deeper, richer blue than blast
Rubricyte	Polychromatic normoblast	10–20	30	10–12	4:1	No nucleoli, clumpy chromatin	Murky gray-blue
Metarubricyte	Orthochromic normoblast	5–10	48	8–10	1:2	Nucleus is almost or completely pyknotic; incapable of DNA synthesis	Pink-orange; slightly bluish hue
Reticulocyte	Reticulocyte	1	48–72	8–10	—	No nucleus	Bluish hue
Reticulocyte*	Reticulocyte	—	24–48	8–8.5	—	No nucleus	—

N/C, Nuclear/cytoplasmic; *DNA*, deoxyribonucleic acid.
*Note circulating peripheral blood.

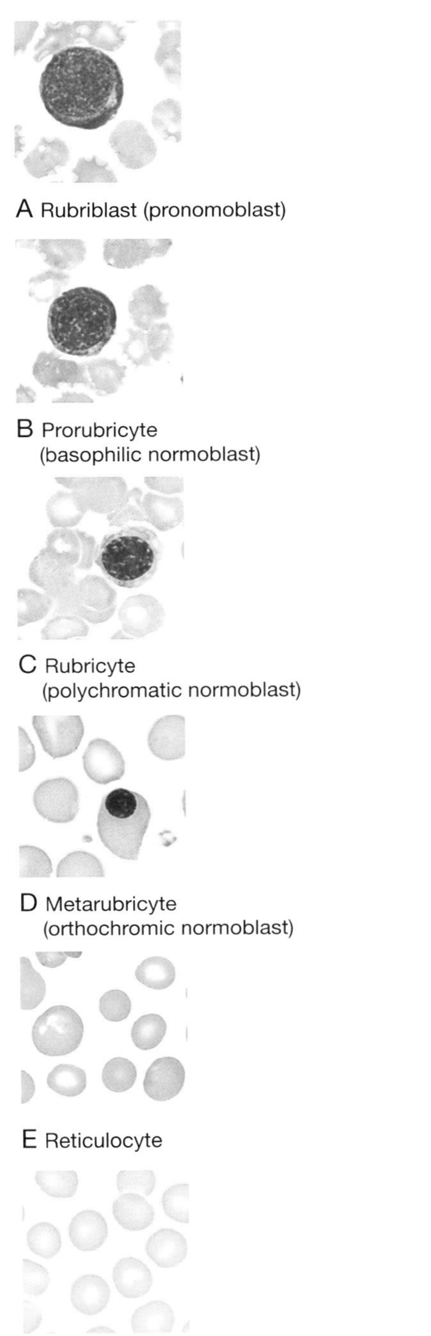

Fig. 11.2 Maturation of red blood cells series. (A) Rubriblast (pronormoblast); (B) prorubricyte (basophilic normoblast); (C) rubricyte (polychromatophilic normoblast); (D) metarubricyte (orthochromic normoblast); reticulocyte (diffusely basophilic erythrocyte); (E) polychromatic erythrocyte; (F) mature erythrocyte. (Turgeon M: *Clinical hematology,* ed 5, Philadelphia, 2011, Lippincott Williams & Wilkins, Fig. 5.2, p. 94.)

color results from the combination of Hb and ribonucleic acid (RNA) in the cytoplasm. The stages are described in terms of the staining reaction of the cytoplasm as it gains in Hb concentration: basophilic cytoplasm is blue, polychromatophilic cytoplasm shows shades of blue and gray as Hb increases, and orthochromic cytoplasm is orange-red.

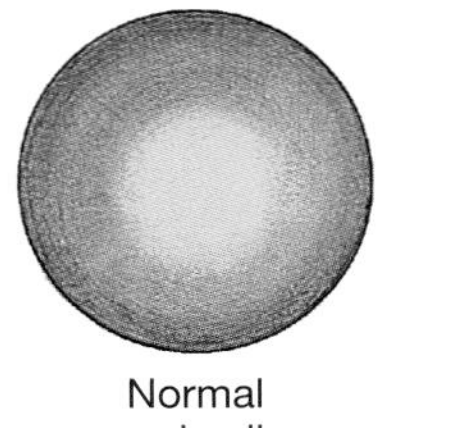

Fig. 11.3 Normal red blood cell.

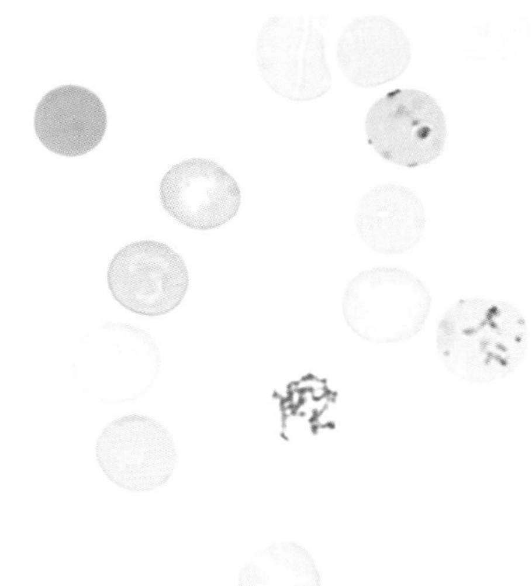

Fig. 11.4 Reticulocytes stained with new methylene blue. (From Carr JH, Rodak BF: *Clinical hematology atlas,* ed 3, St Louis, 2009, Saunders.)

The nucleus is generally round and in the center of the cell. In the early stages, the chromatin is fine and lacelike. As the cell matures and the nucleus becomes smaller, the chromatin becomes coarse and more condensed. Finally, the nucleus degenerates into clumps or a solid pyknotic mass, which is eventually released (or extruded) from the cell. At the same time, the color of the nucleus changes from purplish red to dark blue. When the nucleus is extruded, it is phagocytosed and digested by marrow macrophages.

After a few days in the bone marrow as reticulocytes, the RBCs squeeze through an opening in the endothelial lining of the marrow cavity and enter the peripheral circulatory system. *Reticulocytes* become fully mature in 1 or 2 days in the circulating blood, and all RNA disappears. Normally, about 1% of the circulating RBCs are reticulocytes (Fig. 11.4). The number of reticulocytes (percentage) in the peripheral blood is an indication of the degree of RBC production by the bone marrow. A reticulocyte is about the same size as, or slightly larger than, a mature RBC. Reticulocytes differ morphologically from mature RBCs because they contain a fine basophilic reticulum or network of RNA, a cytoplasmic remnant that decreases as the cell matures. With Wright stain, reticulocytes appear pink-gray or pale purple; they have a slight bluish tinge. This polychromasia or polychromatophilia (many colors) represents the presence of

TABLE 11.2 Red Blood Cell Counts, Hematocrit, and Hemoglobin

Adult Reference Values[1]

Red blood cell count	Male	4.5–5.9 × 10^{12}/L
	Female	4.5–5.1 × 10^{12}/L
Hematocrit	Male	41.5%–50.4%
	Female	35.9%–44.6%
Hemoglobin	Male	14.0–17.5 g/dL
	Female	12.3–15.3 g/dL

Pediatric Reference Values[2]

	Age	Mean	2 SD Range
Red blood cell count	Birth (cord blood)	4.7 × 10^{12}/L	3.9–5.5 × 10^{12}/L
	1 to 3 days of age	5.3 × 10^{12}/L	4.0–6.6 × 10^{12}/L
	3–6 months	3.8 × 10^{12}/L	3.1–4.5 × 10^{12}/L
	6–12 years	4.6 × 10^{12}/L	4.0–5.2 × 10^{12}/L
	12–18 years		
	Male	4.9 × 10^{12}/L	4.5–5.3 × 10^{12}/L
	Female	4.6 × 10^{12}/L	4.1–5.1 × 10^{12}/L
Hematocrit	Birth (cord blood)	51%	42%–60%
	1 to 3 days of age	56%	45%–67%
	3–6 months	35%	29%–41%
	6–12 years	40%	35%–45%
	12–18 years		
	Male	43%	36%–50%
	Female	41%	37%–45%
Hemoglobin	Birth (cord blood)	16.5 g/dL	13.5–19.5 g/dL
	1 to 3 days of age	18.5 g/dL	14.5–22.5 g/dL
	3–6 months	11.5 g/dL	9.5–13.5 g/dL
	6–12 years	13.5 g/dL	11.5–15.5 g/dL
	12–18 years		
	Male	14.5 g/dL	13.0–16.0 g/dL
	Female	14.0 g/dL	12.0–16.0 g/dL

[1]McPherson, P: *Henry's clinical diagnosis and management by laboratory methods,* ed 22, St Louis, Elsevier, 2011, Table A 5.9, p. 1502.
[2]Greer JP, et al: *Wintrobe's clinical hematology,* Vol. 2, ed 12, Lippincott Williams & Wilkins, 2009, Table B.2, p. 2584.
SD, standard deviation.

RNA within the cell. With special supravital stains, such as brilliant cresyl blue or new methylene blue, the basophilic reticulum of RNA appears as blue strands or dotlike structures.

RBCs have a total life span of about 120 days, and the bone marrow releases new cells into the circulatory system every day. The concentration of RBCs and the measurement of the packed volume of RBCs (microhematocrit) are important laboratory measurements for the detection of anemia or overproduction of RBCs (Table 11.2). Worn-out RBCs are removed from the blood circulation by the mononuclear phagocytic system, which is composed of connective tissue cells that carry on phagocytosis, a process in which a cell engulfs and digests foreign material. These cells are located in the blood sinusoids (tiny blood vessels) in the liver, spleen, and bone marrow, and in the lining of the lymph channels in the lymph nodes.

Many cellular components of worn-out RBCs are reusable, including iron (from the *heme* portion of the Hb molecule) and protein (from the *globin* portion of the Hb molecule) (see Fig. 11.5). The remaining heme portion of the Hb molecule (with iron removed) is converted to bilirubin, concentrated in the bile, and eliminated from the body in feces and, to a much smaller extent, in urine, as urobilin and urobilinogen.

Dubin-Johnson syndrome is an inherited, relapsing, benign disorder of bilirubin metabolism. This rare autosomal recessive condition is characterized by conjugated hyperbilirubinemia with normal liver transaminases, a unique pattern of urinary excretion of heme metabolites (coproporphyrins), and the deposition of a pigment that gives the liver a characteristic black color. Rotor syndrome, also called Rotor type hyperbilirubinemia, is a rare, relatively benign autosomal recessive bilirubin disorder. It is a distinct disease, yet it is similar to Dubin-Johnson syndrome because both diseases cause an increase in conjugated bilirubin. In addition, Crigler-Najjar syndrome is a rare genetic disorder characterized by an inability to properly convert and clear bilirubin from the body.

Fig. 11.6 shows a schematic representation of the RBC formation and destruction process. Erythrocytes can be broken down by both extravascular (Fig. 11.7) and intravascular metabolism (Fig. 11.8).

Hemoglobin Synthesis, Structure, and Function

Hb synthesis is a complex process, starting in the bone marrow with the production of the erythrocytes. The heme (iron-containing) portion of the molecule combines with globin (the protein portion) and forms an activated form of Hb that is ready to transport oxygen. Each Hb molecule consists of four heme groups and a globin moiety, which is composed of four polypeptide chains.

Heme

Heme is itself a complex molecule. It is made up of a series of tetrapyrrole rings, terminating in protoporphyrin, with a central iron (see Fig. 11.5A). Because the *heme* molecule is a porphyrin, a group of diseases called the *porphyrias* result from certain disorders of heme synthesis. Normally, heme is excreted from the body as bilirubin, which is eventually converted to the various bile salts and pigments. Iron is normally removed and retained by the mononuclear phagocytic system, stored, and reused in the production of new Hb.

Globin

The globin portion of the Hb molecule is a protein substance that consists of four chains of amino acids (polypeptides). Each of the four globin chains is attached to a heme portion to form a single Hb molecule (see Fig. 11.5B).

Hemoglobin Function

Iron is essential for the primary function of the Hb molecule: carrying oxygen to the tissues. If iron is lacking, anemia results because Hb is not formed in sufficient quantity. When reduced hemoglobin is exposed to oxygen at increased pressure, oxygen is taken up at the iron atom until each molecule of Hb has bound four oxygen molecules, with one molecule at each iron atom. This is not a true oxidation-reduction (redox) reaction, so the Hb molecule carrying oxygen is said to be oxygenated. The molecule fully saturated with oxygen (four oxygen molecules per Hb

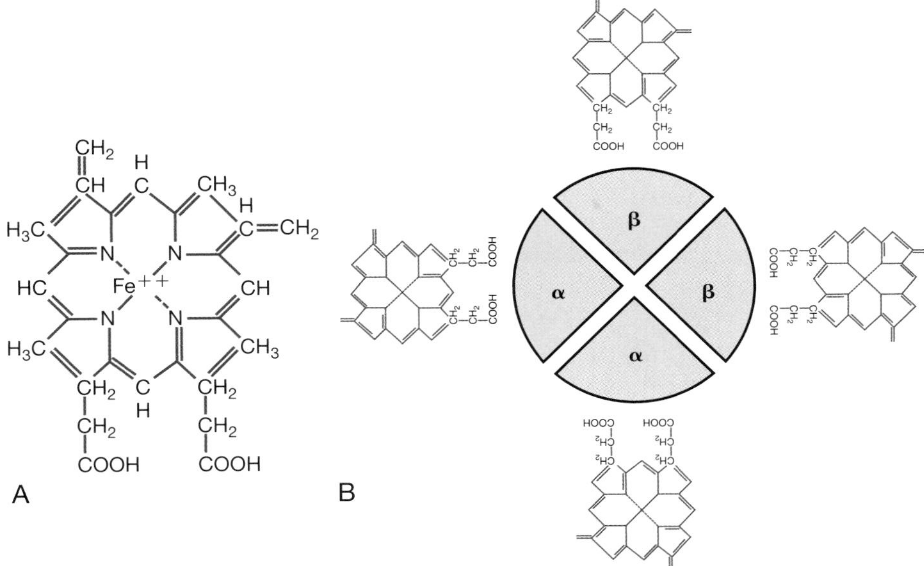

Fig. 11.5 Hemoglobin molecules. (A) The heme moiety consists of one protoporphyrin ring (four pyrrole rings that are joined to each other) with a single iron atom (Fe^{2+}). A complete hemoglobin molecule consists of four heme molecules. (B) Normal adult hemoglobin (hemoglobin A) consists of four heme groups and four globin chains: two alpha chains and two beta chains.

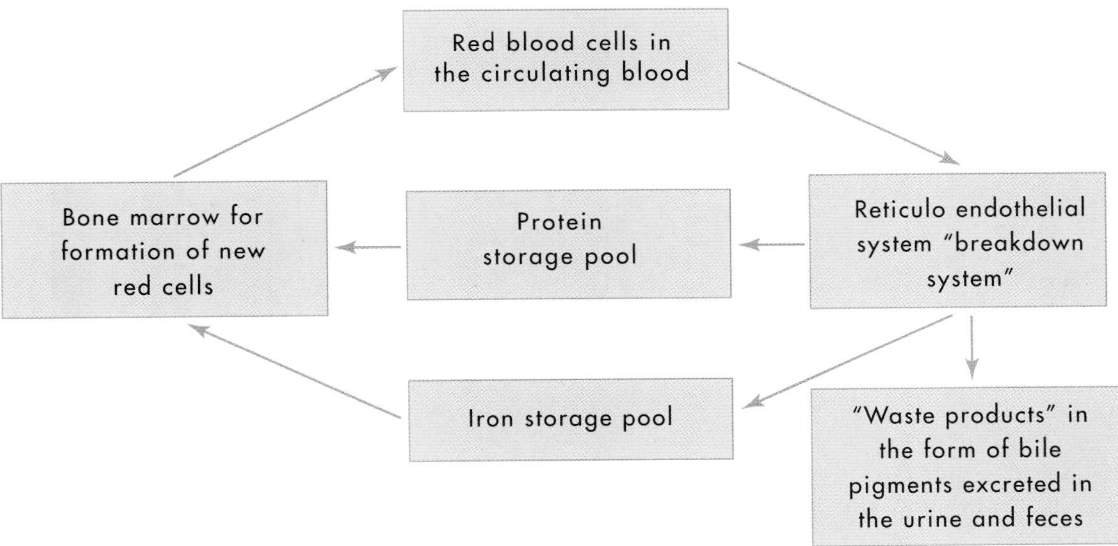

Fig. 11.6 Red blood cell formation and destruction process.

molecule) is called oxyhemoglobin (HbO_2). It contains 1.34 mL of oxygen per gram of Hb. HbO_2 carries oxygen from the lungs to the tissues of the body. Hb returning to the lungs with carbon dioxide from the tissues is known as *reduced hemoglobin.*

Hemoglobin Variants

Different structural forms of Hb may occur in the RBCs. These Hb variants differ in the content and sequence of amino acids in the globin chains. The alpha (α) chain is composed of 141 amino acids in a specific sequence, and the beta (β) chain contains 146 amino acids of a specific sequence. Other polypeptide globin chains that may be encountered include gamma (γ), delta (δ), and possibly epsilon (ε).

Normal Adult Hemoglobins: A and A_2

The principal adult Hb (HbA) contains two α and two β globin chains. In another form of adult Hb, HbA_2, the α chains are paired with two δ polypeptide chains. The δ chains are related to β chains, but 10 amino acids have been substituted. These are the major normal forms of HbA. Other genetically determined forms of Hb may be demonstrated by means of electrophoresis.

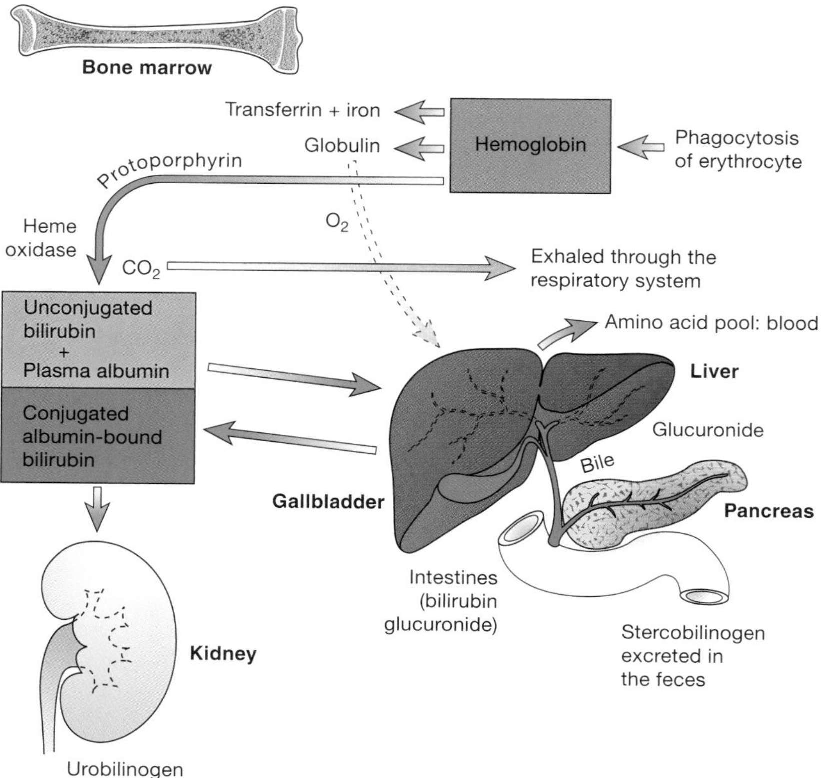

Fig. 11.7 Extravascular metabolism. (From Turgeon M: *Clinical hematology,* ed 5, Philadelphia, 2011, Lippincott Williams & Wilkins.)

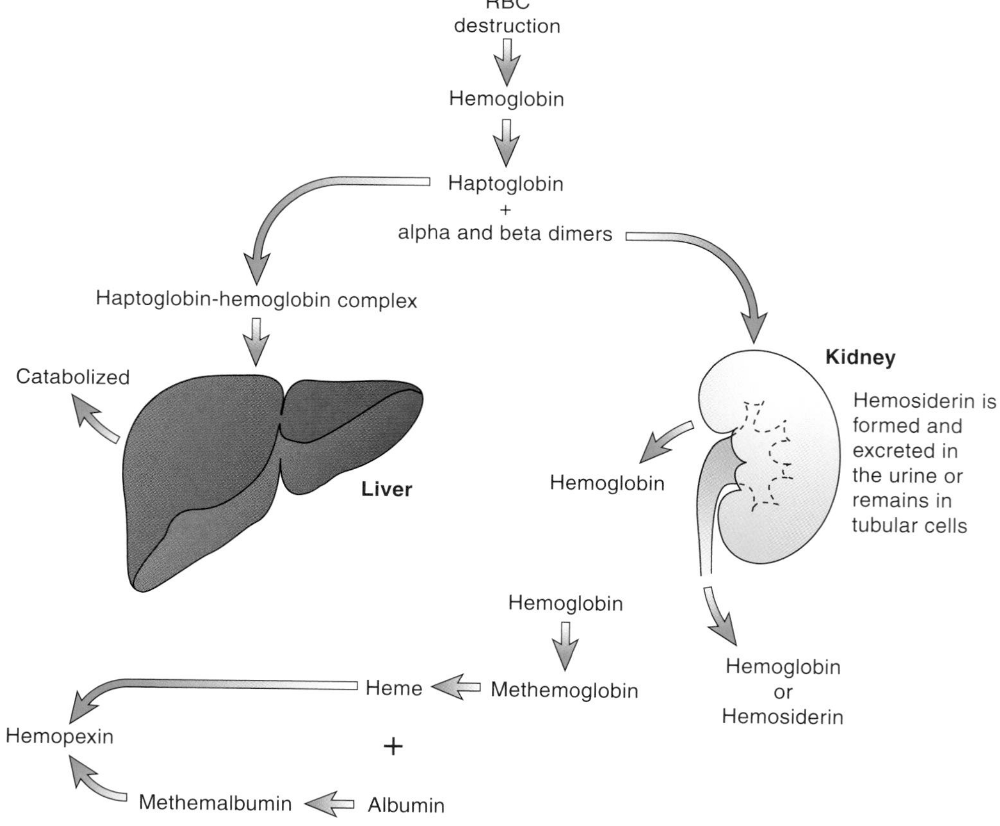

Fig. 11.8 Intravascular metabolism. (From Turgeon M: *Clinical hematology,* ed 5, Philadelphia, 2011, Lippincott Williams & Wilkins.)

Many abnormal forms of Hb lead to clinical illness because they interfere with the blood's oxygen-carrying capacity.

The combination of HbA and HbA_2 should normally make up 95% of the Hb in an adult, with fetal Hb (HbF) making up 5% or less.

Hemoglobin F

HbF is the major form found during intrauterine life and at birth. In HbF, the two α globin chains are paired with two γ chains. HbA is formed in small amounts by the fetus and rapidly increases after birth.

Abnormal Hemoglobin Variants

Disorders in which structurally abnormal Hb is considered to play an important role pathologically are called hemoglobinopathies. In some hemoglobinopathies, all the Hb is in one abnormal form. In other types, two abnormal forms may be present, or some normal forms and some abnormal forms may be present. The structurally abnormal Hbs usually consist of polypeptide chains with a normal number of amino acids, but with a single amino acid substitution. These substitutions are under genetic control, and the hemoglobinopathies may either be inherited or the result of genetic mutations. In clinically significant disease, either the α or the β chain may be affected; however, most of the hemoglobinopathies are the result of β-chain abnormalities.

The four clinically important abnormal Hbs are HbS, HbC, HbD, and HbE. These are all genetic disorders that affect the protein portion of the Hb molecule by altering the structure of the polypeptide chain. These abnormal Hbs and the normal forms can be distinguished from one another by various methods, including high-performance liquid chromatography and electrophoresis.

Hemoglobin S. The most common abnormal Hb is HbS. It is responsible for the genetic disorder called *sickle cell anemia* (Fig. 11.9 and Fig. 11.10), which is found predominantly in the black population. It is *also known as sickle cell disease (HbSS).* Sickle cell trait is acquired genetically as well.

HbS has an amino acid substitution in the β chain, where valine is substituted for glutamic acid at the sixth position in the normal β chain (Fig. 11.11). It causes "sickling" of the RBCs under conditions of reduced oxygen concentration.

Hemoglobin C. HbC results from an amino acid substitution of lysine for glutamic acid on the sixth position of the β chain. It may be inherited in combination with HbS and may occur in a homozygous or heterozygous state. The RBCs may appear as target cells when HbC is present; less frequently, crystals of precipitated HbC may be seen in the RBCs.

Hemoglobin Derivatives

Circulating blood carries a composite of derivatives of Hb. Most of the Hb in circulating blood is HbO_2 and reduced Hb. Other Hb derivatives found in normal circulating blood include carboxyhemoglobin (HbCO; Hb combined with carbon monoxide [CO]); methemoglobin, or hemoglobin (Hi), which is oxidized

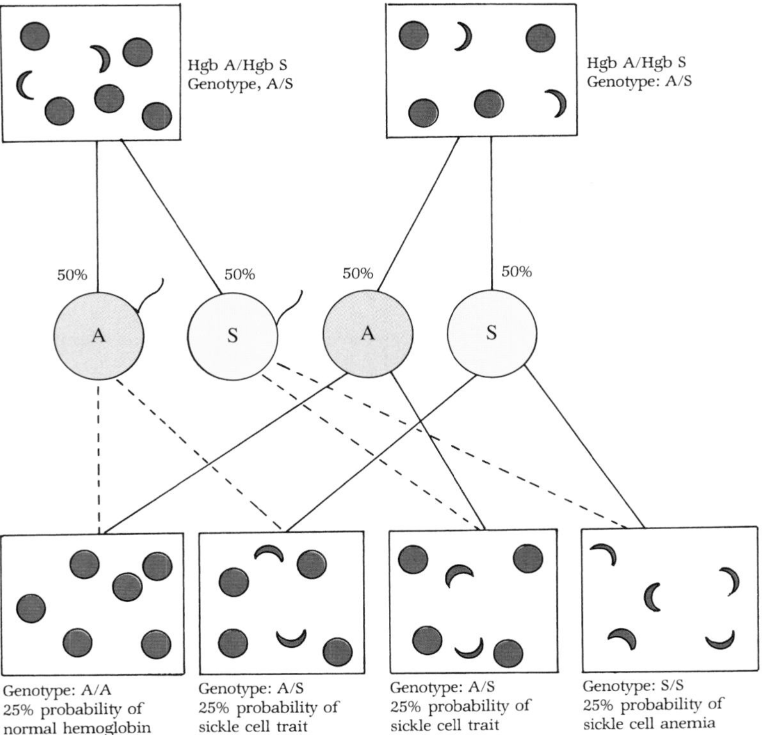

Fig. 11.9 Hemoglobin S genetics. Sickle cell trait and anemia. When two persons with sickle cell trait (genotype: A/S) produce offspring, the expected genotypic ratio is 1:2:1, or a 25% chance of offspring with a normal hemoglobin (A/A), a 50% chance of offspring with sickle cell train (A/S), and a 25% chance of offspring with sickle cell anemia (S/S). *Hgb,* Hemoglobin. (From Turgeon M: *Clinical hematology,* ed 5, Philadelphia, 2011, Lippincott Williams & Wilkins, Fig. 3.11, p. 62.)

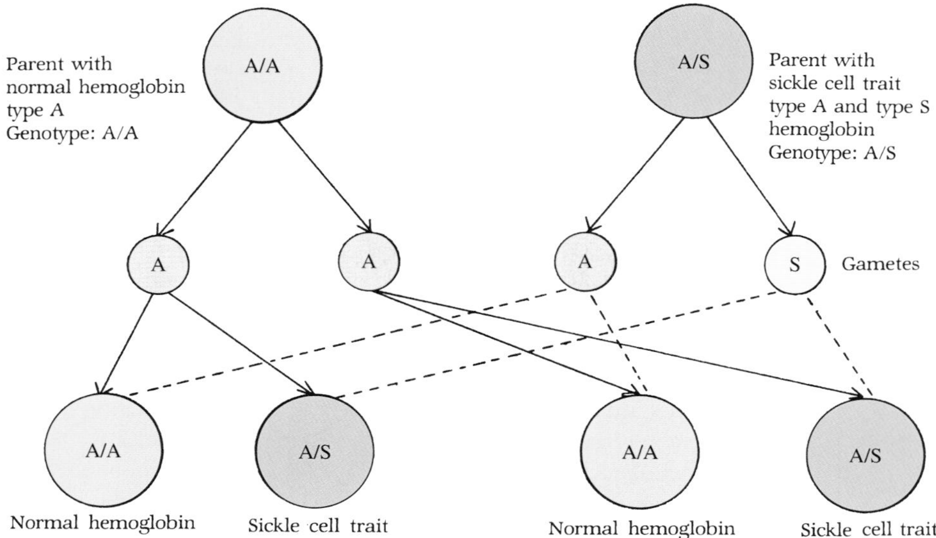

Fig. 11.10 Inheritance of hemoglobin S. Offspring probabilities are 50% normal hemoglobin A/A and 50% hemoglobin A/S (sickle cell trait). (From Turgeon M: *Clinical hematology*, ed 5, Philadelphia, 2011, Lippincott Williams & Wilkins, Fig. 3.13, p. 63.)

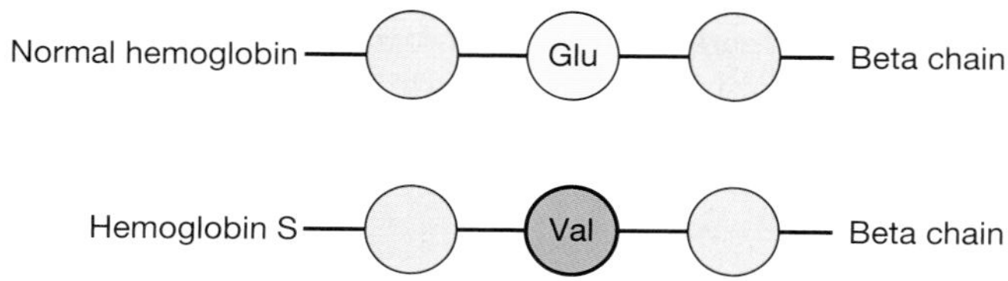

Fig. 11.11 Hemoglobin S amino acid sequence. Hemoglobin S differs from hemoglobin A by one amino acid that resides on the beta chain of the hemoglobin molecule. On this chain, valine (Val) is substituted for glutamic acid (Glu) at the sixth position of the chain. (From Turgeon M: *Clinical hematology*, ed 5, Philadelphia, 2011, Lippincott Williams & Wilkins, Fig. 3.12, p. 62.)

Hb; and minor amounts of other derivatives. When iron in the Hb molecule is converted from the 2+ to the ferric 3+ state, it can combine with other substances besides oxygen and is no longer capable of oxygen transport. When sufficient quantities of these Hb derivatives are present in circulating blood, hypoxia (lack of oxygen) or cyanosis (bluish discoloration of skin and mucous membranes) will be seen clinically.

Oxyhemoglobin and Reduced Hemoglobin

HbO_2 and reduced Hb are the major forms of circulating Hb. The main function of Hb is to transport oxygen from the lungs, where oxygen tension is high, to the tissues, where it is low. At the increased oxygen tension (100 mm Hg) in the lungs, Hb is oxygenated by the reversible association of an oxygen molecule at each iron atom, forming HbO_2. At the reduced oxygen tension of the tissues (down to 20 mm Hg), oxygen is dissociated from the iron in each heme group and replaced by carbon dioxide. This is called *reduced hemoglobin.* This is not an oxidation-reduction reaction, because iron is in the ferrous state in both HbO_2 and Hb.

Carboxyhemoglobin

The Hb molecule has a much greater affinity for CO than for oxygen and will readily combine with CO if it is present in even a low concentration. The affinity of CO for Hb is 200 times greater than the affinity of oxygen. HbCO cannot bind to and carry oxygen and will result in CO poisoning even at relatively low CO concentrations. The formation of HbCO is reversible, and if CO is removed, the Hb will once again combine with oxygen. Clinically, with sufficient HbCO levels, the skin will turn bright cherry red; at high levels (>50% to 70% of total Hb), the individual can be asphyxiated. HbCO is normally found in small amounts, especially in the blood of smokers, where concentrations range from 1% to 10% of circulating Hb.

Methemoglobin

Methemoglobin, also referred to as *hemiglobin* (Hi), is a Hb derivative in which the iron has been oxidized from the ferrous to the ferric state and therefore is incapable of combining reversibly with oxygen. The formation of methemoglobin is usually an acquired condition resulting from the presence of certain chemicals or drugs, and it is reversible. An inherited methemoglobinemia may result from a structurally abnormal globin chain or an RBC enzyme defect. Up to 1.5% of circulating Hb is normally methemoglobin.

The formation of methemoglobin is used as an intermediary in the cyanmethemoglobin (or hemiglobincyanide [HiCN]) method for the quantitation of whole-blood Hb.

Hemiglobincyanide (Cyanmethemoglobin)

To measure total Hb concentration in blood, it is necessary to prepare a stable derivative containing all the Hb forms that are present. All forms of circulating Hb are readily converted to HiCN, except for sulfhemoglobin, which is rarely present in significant amounts. For this reason, the HiCN, or cyanmethemoglobin, method is standard for the determination of Hb.

Sulfhemoglobin

Another abnormal Hb derivative is sulfhemoglobin. The formation of sulfhemoglobin is irreversible, and it remains in the RBC for the cell's entire 120-day life span. Its exact nature is unclear, but sulfhemoglobulin is thought to be formed by the action of some drugs and chemicals, such as sulfonamides. Although sulfhemoglobin is incapable of transporting oxygen and cannot be converted back to normally functioning Hb, it rarely exceeds 10% of the total Hb. This is not a life-threatening level, although sulfhemoglobinemia may be seen clinically as cyanosis.

Variations in Hemoglobin Concentrations

The reference (or normal) values for Hb in peripheral blood vary with the age and gender of the individual (see Table 11.2). Altitude also affects the Hb measurement in that the normal Hb concentration is higher at high altitudes than at sea level.

At 1 to 2 days of age, hemoglobin concentration is normally 14.5 to 22.5 g/dL. It decreases to 9.5 to 13.5 g/dL by about 3 to 6 months of age. By 6 years of age, a normal hemoglobin value is 11.5 g/dL to 15.5 g/dL. Adult values range from 12 to 16 g/dL in women and 13.5 to 17.5 g/dL in men. There may be a slight decrease in hemoglobin level after 50 years of age.

When the Hb value is below normal, the patient is said to be *anemic*. Anemia is a common condition and frequently is a complication of other diseases (see Erythrocyte Alterations). In this condition, circulating erythrocytes may be deficient in number, in total Hb content per unit of blood volume, or both. A decrease in Hb can result from bleeding conditions in which the patient loses erythrocytes. An increase in Hb, usually caused by an increase in the number of erythrocytes (erythrocytosis), is seen in polycythemia and newborn infants.

LEUKOCYTES

Formed elements of the blood go through a series of developmental stages. Normally, only mature cells are seen in the peripheral blood circulation (Fig. 11.12). Immature cells may appear in the peripheral blood in certain disease states. Each cell type has a normal life span and function (see Tables 11.2 through 11.5).

Granulocyte Maturation and Function

Neutrophils normally mature in the bone marrow (Fig. 11.13) in the following stages, from the youngest to the most mature: myeloblast, promyelocyte, myelocyte, metamyelocyte, band, and segmented neutrophils. These maturation stages are similar for all granulocytes (Table 11.3).

Cells of the neutrophil series are generally round with smooth margins or edges. As the cells mature, they become progressively smaller (Fig. 11.14). Most immature cells have cytoplasm that stains dark blue and becomes light pink as the cells mature. As the cells mature from the myeloblast to the

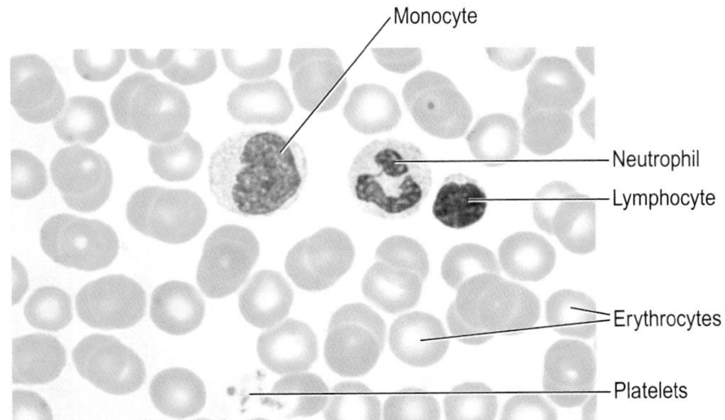

Fig. 11.12 A blood smear showing erythrocytes, a monocyte, a neutrophil, a lymphocyte, and a platelet. (From Waugh A, Grant A: Ross and Wilson anatomy and physiology in health and illness, ed. 12, p. 63.)

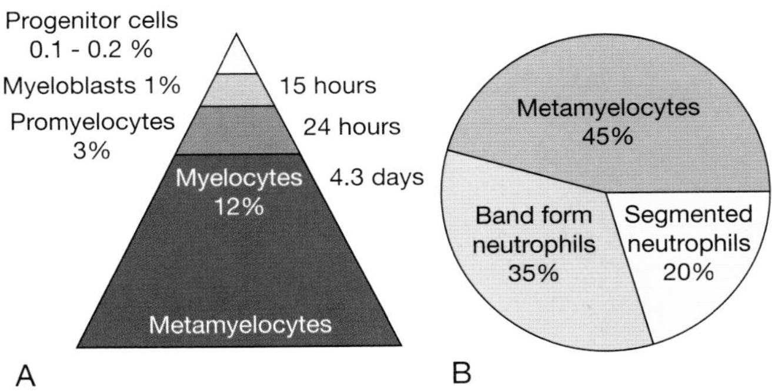

Fig. 11.13 Bone marrow compartments: differentiation of granulocytes. (A) Proliferative; (B) maturation/storage. (From Turgeon M: *Clinical hematology,* ed 5, Philadelphia, 2011, Lippincott Williams & Wilkins, Fig. 14.1, p. 236.)

promyelocyte stage, nonspecific granules that stain blue to reddish purple appear in the cytoplasm. Eventually, these nonspecific granules are replaced by specific neutrophilic granules.

Nuclear changes also occur as the cells mature. In the myeloblast, the nucleus is round or oval and very large in proportion to the rest of the cell. As the cell matures, the nucleus decreases in relative size and begins to contort or form lobes. At the same time, the nuclear chromatin changes from a fine, delicate pattern to the more clumped pattern characteristic of the mature cell. The staining of the nucleus also changes from reddish purple to bluish purple as the cell matures. Nucleoli may be apparent in the early forms but gradually disappear as the chromatin thickens and the cell matures.

The term *shift to the left* refers to the release into the peripheral blood of immature cell forms normally present only in bone marrow.

Neutrophils exist in the peripheral blood for about 10 hours after they are released from the marrow. During this time, they move back and forth between the general blood circulation and the walls of the blood vessels, where they accumulate. They also leave the blood and enter the tissues, where they carry out their primary functions. In the tissues, neutrophils are used to fight bacterial infections and are then destroyed or eliminated from

TABLE 11.3 Granulocytic Leukocyte Development

Nomenclature	Overall Size (mM)	N/C Ratio	Nuclear Characteristics	Cytoplasmic Characteristics
Myeloblast	10–18	4:1	Oval or round shape, 1 to 5 nucleoli	Auer rods can be present, no granules
Promyelocyte	14–20	3:1	Oval or round shape, 1 to 5 nucleoli	Heavy granulation
Myelocyte	12–18	2:1–1:1	Oval or indented	Specific blue-pink granules
Metamyelocyte	10–18	1:1	Indented	Specific blue-pink granules
Band	10–16	1:1	Elongated, curved	Specific blue-pink granules
Segmented neutrophil	10–16	1:1	Distinct lobes	Specific blue-pink granules
Mature basophil	10–16	1:1	Distinct lobes	Blue-black granules
Mature eosinophil	10–16	1:1	Distinct lobes	Orange granules

N/C, nuclear/cytoplasmic.

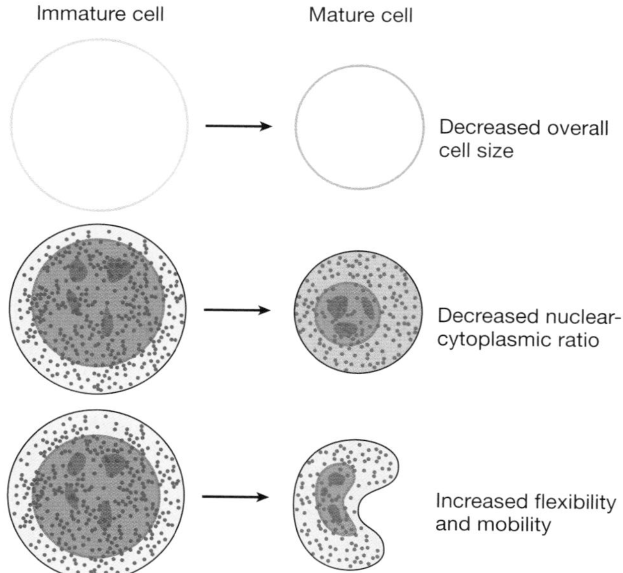

Fig. 11.14 Comparative maturational characteristics. As cells mature, they are able to move through the sinusoids of the bone marrow because of a decreased overall cell size, a decreased nuclear cytoplasmic ratio, and increased flexibility and mobility. (From Turgeon M: *Clinical hematology*, ed 5, Philadelphia, 2011, Lippincott Williams & Wilkins, Fig. 14.2, p. 236.)

the body by the excretory system (intestinal tract, urine, lungs, or saliva).

Metabolically, neutrophils are very active and can carry out both anaerobic and aerobic glycolysis. The neutrophilic granules contain several digestive enzymes that are able to destroy many types of bacteria. The cells are capable of random locomotion and can be directed to an area of infection by the process of chemotaxis. Once in the tissues, the neutrophils destroy bacteria by engulfing them and releasing digestive enzymes into the phagocytic vacuole thus formed.

The first recognizable precursor of eosinophils is the eosinophil myelocyte. Culture studies show that there is a separate eosinophilic-committed progenitor cell (colony-forming unit, eosinophil). Eosinophil myeloblasts cannot be recognized microscopically from the neutrophilic myeloblast. Eosinophils exist in the peripheral blood for less than 8 hours after release from the marrow and have a short survival time in the tissues.

The function of eosinophils is not completely understood. They do leave the peripheral blood when adrenocorticosteroid hormones increase and proliferate in response to immunologic stimuli. Eosinophils are capable of locomotion and phagocytosis, and respond to foreign proteins. They are active in allergic reactions and certain parasitic infections, especially those involving parasitic invasion of the tissues.

Basophils occur in very low numbers (mean 0.6 %) in normal peripheral blood. The first recognizable basophilic cell type is the basophil myelocyte, which contains basophilic granules. Their life span in blood is similar to that of neutrophils and eosinophils, and they are capable of sluggish locomotion. The granules contain histamine, heparin or a heparinlike substance, and peroxidase. The rapid release of mediators from immunoglobulin E (IgE)–primed basophils and mast cells activated by exposure to parasite-associated antigens is thought to contribute significantly to the local inflammation associated with IgE-dependent immune responses to parasites. If the same events are triggered by antigens from pollen, food, drugs, or insect venom, the result is a disorder of immediate hypersensitivity (see Chapter 16).

Normal Leukocyte Morphology

Five types of WBCs are normally encountered in peripheral blood: neutrophils (segmented and band), eosinophils, basophils, monocytes, and lymphocytes (Fig. 11.15A–E and Fig. 11.16). To identify leukocyte morphology, the cells should be examined for the following features:

- Nuclear chromatin pattern
- Nuclear shape
- Size and number of nucleoli, when present
- Cytoplasmic inclusions
- Nuclear/cytoplasmic (N/C) ratio

When a blood film is stained with Wright (a Romanowsky) stain and examined with the microscope, the majority of the cells seen will be RBCs, which appear as small, rounded, pink, or reddish-orange bodies. Scattered among the red-staining cells are the less numerous leukocytes.

The leukocytes are larger and more complex in appearance than the RBCs. They consist of a nucleus surrounded by cytoplasm. Usually the nucleus is centrally located and is a prominent purple-staining body. It can be round or oval (as in the lymphocyte) or lobulated (as in the neutrophil and eosinophil). The cytoplasm, which gives the cell its shape, stains a variety of

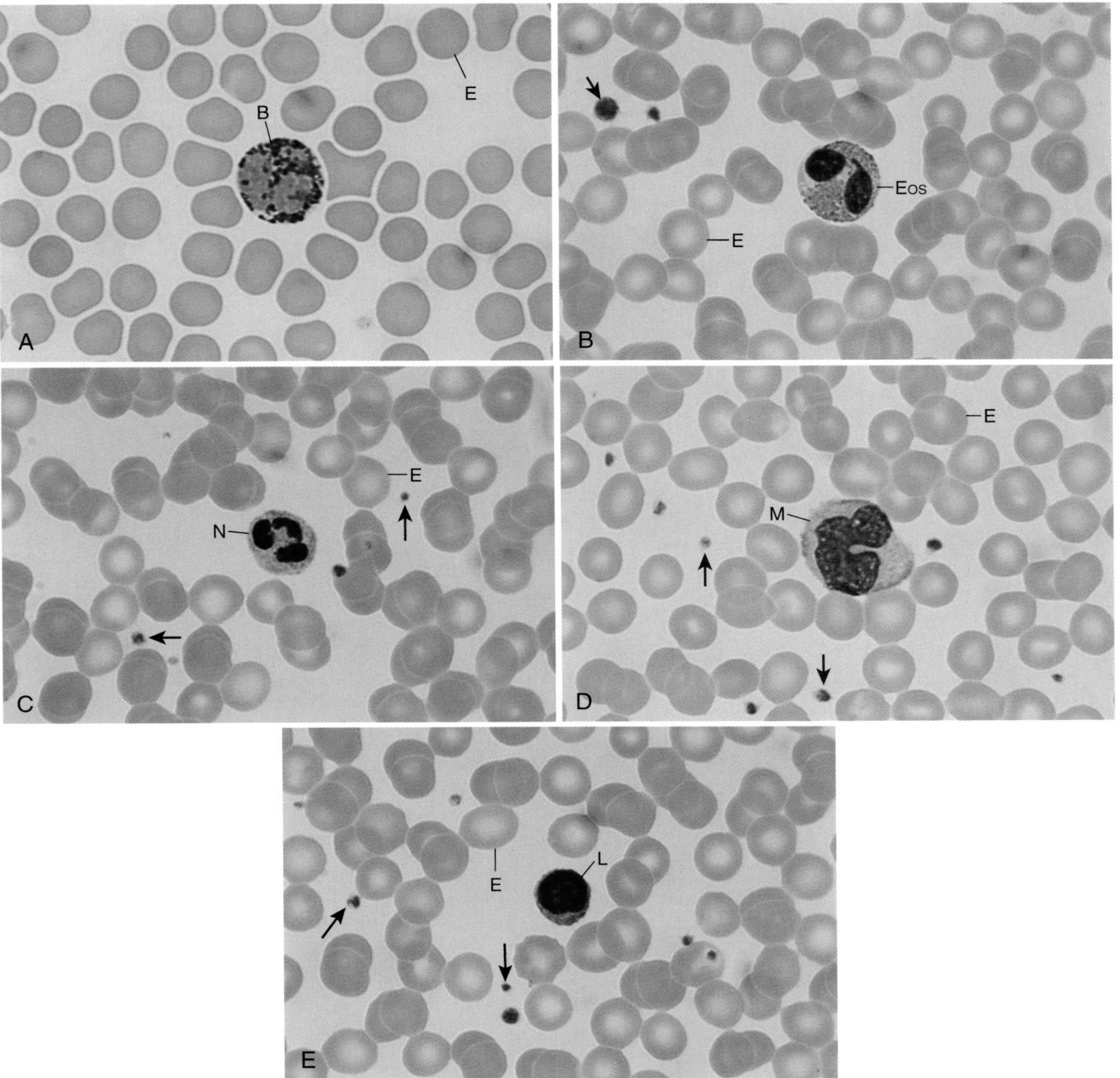

Fig. 11.15 (A) Blood (smear) showing basophil (×1325); E, erythrocyte; B, basophil. (B) Blood (smear showing eosinophil) (×1325); E, erythrocyte; eos, eosinophil; *arrow,* platelet. (C) Blood (smear showing neutrophil) (×1325); E, erythrocyte; *arrows,* platetets; N, neutrophil. (D) Blood (smear showing monocyte) (×1325); E, erythrocyte; M, monocyte; *arrows,* platelets. (E) Blood (smear showing lymphocyte) (×1325); E, erythrocyte; *arrows,* platelets; L, lymphocyte. (From Gartner LP, Hiatt JL: *Color textbook of histology,* ed 2, Burlington, 2001, Elsevier.)

colors, depending on its contents. The size of the cell, the shape and size of the nucleus, and the staining reactions of the nucleus and the cytoplasm aid in the identification of leukocytes.

Leukocytes are categorized as granulocytes and nongranulocytes (lymphocytes), and 100 cells are identified in the leukocyte differential procedure (Table 11.4). Granulocytes are leukocytes that come from the myeloid series of cell development. As mature cells, neutrophils, eosinophils, and basophils contain specific granulation in their cytoplasm. Monocytes are classified as myeloid cells that contain nonspecific granulation. Lymphocytes are cells derived from the lymphoid series of cell development. They are nongranulocytes that may contain nonspecific granulation.

Segmented Neutrophils

The most numerous of the granulocytes are polymorphonuclear neutrophil leukocytes, or segmented neutrophil leukocytes. Neutrophils make up about 59% of the leukocytes in peripheral blood, with a range of 35% to 71%. Infants and children have fewer neutrophils and more lymphocytes.

Neutrophils are generally round cells, varying in diameter from 10 to 15 μm. The nucleus forms a relatively small part

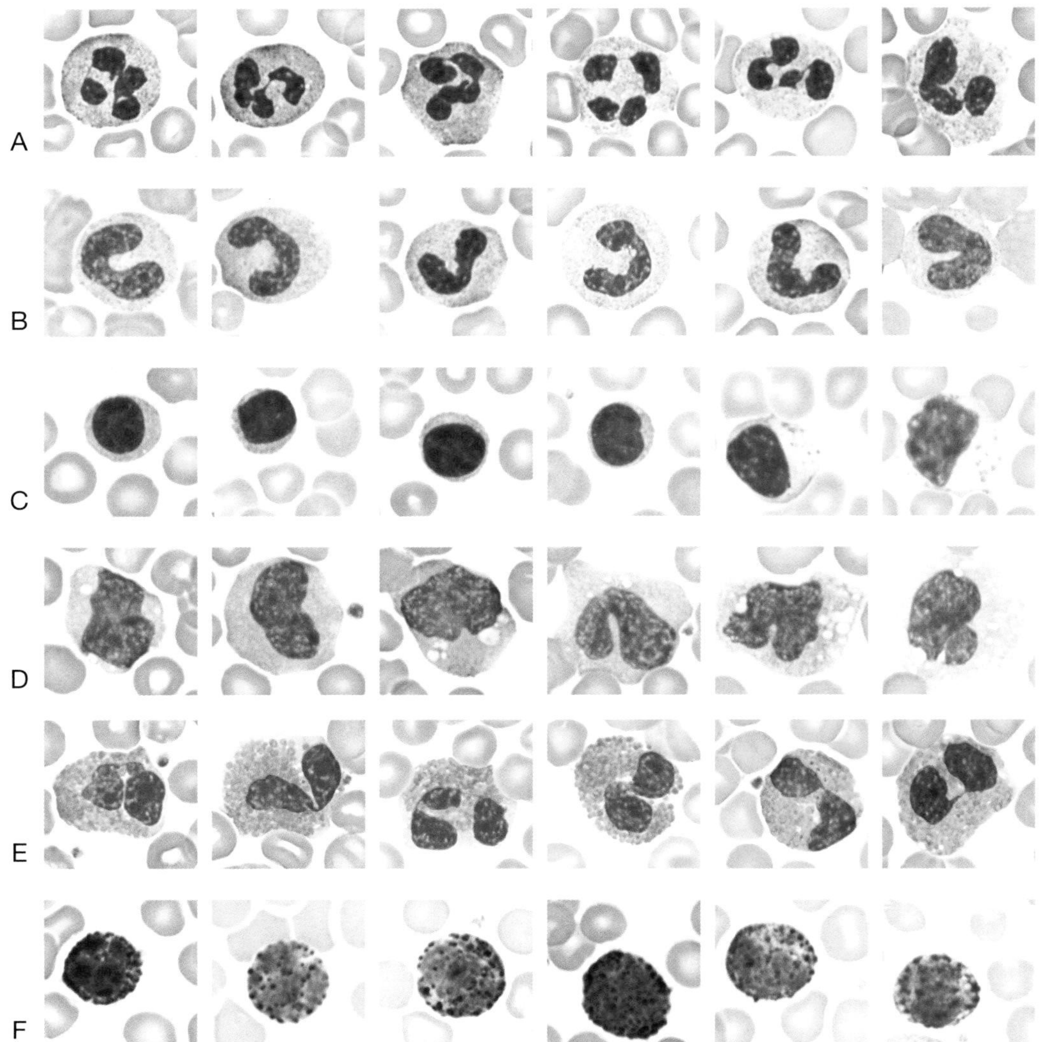

Fig. 11.16 Normal leukocytes. (A) Polymorphonuclear neutrophils; (B) band neutrophils; (C) lymphocytes; (D) monocytes; (E) eosinophils; and (F) basophils. (From Carr JH, Rodak BF: *Clinical hematology atlas,* ed 3, St Louis, 2009, Saunders.)

TABLE 11.4 Comparison of Normal Leukocytes in Peripheral Blood

Nomenclature	Nuclear Shape	Chromatin	Cytoplasmic Color	Granules	Average Percentage
Segmented neutrophil	Lobulated	Very clumped	Pink	Many, pinkish blue	56%
Band neutrophil	Curved	Moderately clumped	Blue, pink	Many, pinkish blue	3%
Lymphocyte	Round	Smooth	Light blue	Few red (azurophilic)	34%
Monocyte	Indented, folded, or twisted	Lacelike	Gray	Fine, dusty blue	4%
Eosinophil	Lobulated	Very clumped	Granulated	Many, orange	2%–3%
Basophil	Lobulated	Very clumped	Granulated	Many, dark blue	0.6%

of the cell. The nucleus can assume various shapes, but it is usually lobular. That is, the nucleus is usually constricted, forming a series of lobes connected by narrow strands or filaments of chromatin; it may have two to five lobes. The nuclear chromatin is coarse and clumped and stains deep purple. These irregular chromatin masses are distinct and distinguishable from the lighter-purple parachromatin. The nuclear membrane is distinct, and no nucleoli are visible. The N/C ratio is 1:3. The abundant cytoplasm is colorless or faintly pink and contains a large number of very small, often indiscrete, lilac-specific neutrophilic granules distributed irregularly throughout it. A variable number of nonspecific azurophilic granules may be present.

Band Neutrophils

The band neutrophil is a younger form of the mature neutrophil. Laboratories differ in the reporting of band neutrophils.

Some classify and report band and segmented neutrophils separately; others report total neutrophils. Normal adults generally have about 3% band neutrophils in their peripheral blood. An obvious increase of band neutrophils should be reported.

Morphologically, band neutrophils resemble segmented cells, except for the shape of the nucleus. In band neutrophils the nucleus may be rod- or band-shaped, when distinct lobes have not yet formed, or it may have begun to form lobes. In the latter case, the lobes are connected by wide strips or bands rather than by narrow threads or filaments, as in segmented neutrophils. The differentiation between band and segmented neutrophils may be difficult; if there is doubt, the cell should be classified as "segmented."

Generally, an increased WBC count (leukocytosis) results from an increase in the absolute number of neutrophils present in the blood; in this case, it is called neutrophilia. Neutrophilia is found in acute infections (especially bacterial infections); metabolic, chemical, and drug intoxications; acute hemorrhage; postoperative states; certain noninflammatory conditions, such as coronary thrombosis; malignant neoplasms; and after acute hemolytic episodes. Neutrophilia is usually accompanied by a shift to the left, or an increase in the number of immature cells, and by toxic changes in the cytoplasm. An increase in the number of band forms, which may be accompanied by the presence of more immature neutrophils, is significant. Toxic changes in the neutrophil cytoplasm are indicated by the presence of deeply stained basophilic (or toxic) granules, pale-blue Döhle bodies, and vacuolization, or pyknosis. The cell size may be increased or decreased.

Recent research[2] has determined that the absolute neutrophil count (ANC), immature neutrophil count (INC), and immature-to-total neutrophil ratio (ITR) are better indicators of invasive meningococcal *(Neisseria meningitides)* infection than the total WBC or total (absolute) neutrophil count alone (see Reporting Leukocyte Results). In pediatric cases where the child is febrile, it is recommended that the ANC, INC, and ITR be considered, rather than just the total WBC or ANC. About one-third of febrile children with meningococcal infection had completely normal total WBC counts. If the ANC is generated by an automated differential count, it can be falsely reassuring in 37% of patients in whom ANC is normal or only mildly abnormal. This ANC error results from exclusion of bands or other immature neutrophils in the ANC calculation.

Neutropenia is a reduction of the ANC. Severe neutropenia has been called *agranulocytosis*. The risk for infection is considerably increased as the neutrophil count falls below about $1 \times 10^9/L$. For this reason, neutrophil counts are important in the care of patients who are undergoing chemotherapy or who have other conditions in which the bone marrow is suppressed.

Eosinophils

Eosinophils are granulocytes and generally make up about 3% of the circulating leukocytes. They are slightly larger than neutrophils, usually 12 to 16 μm in diameter. The nucleus occupies a relatively small part of the cell. The nucleus is usually bilobed, and occasionally three lobes are seen. The nuclear structure is similar to that of the neutrophil, but the lobes are plumper and the chromatin often stains lighter purple than in the neutrophil. The nuclear membrane is distinct, and no nucleoli are visible. The cytoplasm is usually colorless, but it may be faintly basophilic. It is crowded with spherical acidophilic granules, which stain red-orange with eosin and are larger and more distinct than neutrophilic granules. The granules are evenly distributed throughout the cytoplasm but are rarely seen overlying the nucleus. They are hard, firm bodies that are not easily damaged; they remain intact when pressed into the nucleus or even when the whole cell is damaged and the cell membrane is broken. Eosinophilic granules are also highly refractive, a feature that is often a valuable distinguishing characteristic.

Eosinophilia, an increase above normal in the number of eosinophils, is associated with a wide variety of conditions, but especially with allergic reactions, drug reactions, certain skin disorders, parasitic infestations, collagen vascular diseases, Hodgkin disease, and myeloproliferative diseases. Eosinopenia, or decreased number of eosinophils, is seen with hyperadrenalism.

Basophils

Basophils, which are also granulocytes, normally constitute an average of 0.6% of the total circulating leukocytes. They are about the same size as neutrophils, 10 to 14 μm in diameter, but their nuclei usually occupy a relatively greater proportion of the cell. The nucleus is often extremely irregular in shape, varying from a lobular form to a form showing indentations that are not deep enough to divide it into definite lobes. The nuclear pattern is indistinct; there appears to be a mixture of chromatin and parachromatin, and this mixture stains purple or blue and shows little structure. The nuclear membrane is fairly distinct, and no nucleoli are visible. The cytoplasm is usually colorless; it contains a variable number of deeply stained, coarse, round, or angular basophilic granules. The granules (metachromatic) stain deep purple or black; occasionally a few smaller, brownish granules may be present. They may overlie and obscure the nucleus. Because the granules are soluble in water, occasionally a few or even most of them may be dissolved during the staining procedure. When this occurs, the cell will contain vacuoles in place of granules, and the cytoplasm may appear grayish or brownish in their vicinity. The cytoplasm of a mature basophil is colorless. An immature basophil has a pale-blue cytoplasm and can be seen in myelogenous leukemias.

Basophilia, an increase in the number of basophils, can be observed in chronic myelogenous leukemia (CML). It is also seen in allergic reactions, myeloid metaplasia, and polycythemia vera. The basophil number may increase temporarily after irradiation, and basophilia may be present in chronic hemolytic anemia and after splenectomy.

Tissue basophils, also called mast cells, are similar but not identical to basophilic granulocytes. They are larger and differ somewhat in their chemical makeup and function.

Monocyte Maturation and Function

Monocytes, as with granulocytes, are produced mainly in the bone marrow. However, new research demonstrates that adult tissue macrophages originate during embryonic development and not from circulating monocytes.

TABLE 11.5 Monocytic Leukocyte Development

Nomenclature	Overall Size (mm)	N/C Ratio	Nuclear Characteristics	Cytoplasmic Characteristics
Monoblast	12–20	4:1	Oval or folded shape; 1, 2, or more nucleoli	Vacuoles variable, irregularly shaped
Promonocyte	12–20	3:1–2:1	Elongated, folded, 0 to 2 nucleoli	Blue-gray, abundant, vacuoles variable
Mature monocyte	12–18	2:1–1:1	Horseshoe-shaped, folded, lacelike chromatin	Vacuoles common, blue-gray, abundant

N/C, nuclear/cytoplasmic.

The stages of development are myelomonoblast, promonocyte, and monocyte (Table 11.5). The myelomonoblast looks very similar to the myeloblast or the lymphoblast, and it may be impossible to distinguish myelomonoblasts morphologically on films prepared with Wright stain. In such cases, the term *blast* is used. It may be necessary to classify the type of blast present on the basis of other cell types in the area.

Monocytes remain in the peripheral blood for hours to days after leaving the bone marrow, depending on the reference cited. They are very motile phagocytic cells, but unlike neutrophils, monocytes do not die after they engage in phagocytic activity. Instead, after 1 to 3 days in the peripheral blood, monocytes move into the body tissues and are transformed into macrophages; they may remain for months, depending on location. Macrophages are thought to be derived from both monocytes and histiocytic cells.

In addition to phagocytosing bacteria, macrophages interact with lymphocytes in the synthesis of antibodies. Macrophages process and present antigens to T cells.

The mononuclear phagocytes (monocytes and macrophages) are important in the defense against microorganisms, including mycobacteria, fungi, bacteria, protozoa, and viruses. They play a role in immune response, phagocytic defense, and the inflammatory response. They also secrete cytokines, remove senescent blood cells, and have antitumor activity.

Monocytes

Monocytes, like granulocytes, are derived from the myeloid cell line. They make up about 4% to 6% of normal circulating leukocytes, ranging from 2% to 10% depending on the laboratory or author. Monocytes are the largest of the normal leukocytes, usually larger than neutrophils, measuring from 12 to 22 µm in diameter.

The nucleus is fairly large; it may be round, oval, indented, lobular, notched, or rarely even segmented, but most frequently it is indented or horseshoe shaped. The nuclear chromatin stains light purple and is delicate or lacy. Chromatin and parachromatin are sharply segregated, and the chromatin is distributed in a linear arrangement of delicate strands, which gives the nucleus a stringy appearance. (Occasionally the nuclear pattern resembles that of a lymphocyte, and the cytoplasmic differences must be relied on for identification.) The nuclear membrane is delicate but not distinct, and nucleoli usually are not seen.

The cytoplasm is abundant and stains gray or gray-blue. It may contain numerous small, poorly defined granules, resulting in a "ground-glass" appearance, and is often vacuolated. Extremely fine and abundant azurophilic granules are present; this granulation is called *azure dust* and is seen only in monocytes. The granules vary in color from light pink to bright purplish- red. In addition, phagocytized particles may be seen in the cytoplasm.

LYMPHOCYTE MATURATION AND FUNCTION

The lymphatic system consists of a network of vessels throughout most of the body tissues. The smaller vessels unite to form larger and larger vessels, which finally come together in two main trunks, the right lymphatic duct and the thoracic duct. The ducts empty into the circulatory system through veins in the neck. Lymph nodes are located all along the lymphatic vessels, and the lymph (fluid within the system) circulates through the nodes as it progresses through the lymphatic system. Many of the lymphocytes are formed in the lymph nodes and circulate back and forth between the blood, the organs, and the lymphatic tissues. Functionally, there are two types of lymphocytes: T cells, or T lymphocytes, and B cells, or B lymphocytes.

T cells arise in the thymus from fetal liver or bone marrow precursors that seed the thymus during embryonic development. These CD34+ progenitor cells develop in the thymic cortex. B lymphocytes are derived from hematopoietic stem cells by a complex series of differentiation events that occur in the fetal liver and, in adult life, in the bone marrow. B-lymphocyte differentiation is complex and proceeds through both an antigen-independent and an antigen-dependent state, culminating in the generation of mature, end-stage, nonmotile cells called *plasma cells.* Some activated B cells differentiate into memory B cells, which are long-lived cells that circulate in the blood.

The stages of lymphoid development are lymphoblast, prolymphocyte, and mature lymphocyte (Table 11.6). Lymphocytes will differentiate into T lymphocytes or B lymphocytes, but this distinction is not determined in a leukocyte differential count.

Lymphocytes act to direct the immune response system of the body. Maturation of lymphocytes in the bone marrow or thymus results in cells that are immunocompetent. The cells are able to respond to antigenic challenges by directing the immune responses of the host defense. They migrate to various sites in the body to await antigenic stimulus and activation. Only when immunologic studies are performed can these cells be identified as belonging to specific subsets of lymphocytes. As lymphocytes mature, their identity and function are specified by the antigenic structures on their external membrane surface.

T lymphocytes mature in the thymus, an organ found in the anterior mediastinum, and function in cell-mediated immune responses such as delayed hypersensitivity, graft-versus-host reactions, and allograft rejection. T cells make up the majority

TABLE 11.6 Lymphocyte Development

Nomenclature	Overall Size (mm)	N/C Ratio	Nuclear Characteristics	Cytoplasmic Characteristics
Lymphoblast	15–20	4:1	Round or oval, one or two nucleoli	Medium blue
Prolymphocyte	15–18	4:1 to 3:1	Oval, slightly indented	Medium blue; may have few azurophilic granules
Mature lymphocyte	Small: 6–9 Large: 17–20	Small: 4:1–3:1 Large: 2:1	Round or oval	Light blue; few azurophilic granules may be present

N/C, nuclear/cytoplasmic.

of the lymphocytes circulating in the peripheral blood. In the periphery of the thymus, they further differentiate into multiple different T cell subpopulations with different functions, including cytotoxicity and the secretion of soluble factors, termed *cytokines.* Many different cytokines have been identified, including 25 interleukin molecules and more than 40 chemokines; their functions include growth promotion, differentiation, chemotaxis, and cell stimulation.

B lymphocytes most likely mature in the bone marrow and function primarily in antibody production or the formation of Igs. B cells constitute about 10% to 30% of the blood lymphocytes. Memory B cells may live for years, but mature B cells that are not activated live for only days. B lymphocytes undergo blast transformation into plasma cells with appropriate antigen stimulation.

Lymphocytes

Lymphocytes make up about 34% of the leukocytes in the normal adult. Infants and children normally have more lymphocytes and fewer neutrophils than adults, a reversed differential. Lymphocytes fall into two general groups: small (approximately 7–10 μm) and large (up to 20 μm). Most normal lymphocytes are small.

When observed microscopically, lymphocytes are described based on their size and cytoplasmic granularity. Small lymphocytes are found in the greatest numbers. The small lymphocyte is composed chiefly of nucleus and is the type of lymphocyte predominating in normal adult blood. It is about the same size as a normocytic RBC and is a useful size marker during examination of the peripheral blood film, especially in cases of megaloblastic anemia, in which all cell forms other than lymphocytes are increased in diameter. The nucleus is round or slightly notched, and the nuclear chromatin is in the form of coarse, dense, deeply staining blocks. There is relatively little parachromatin, and it is not very distinct. Almost the entire nucleus stains deep purple. The nuclear membrane is heavy and distinct, and nucleoli are not usually seen. The cytoplasm appears in the form of a narrow band that stains pale blue with few, if any, red (azure) granules.

The large lymphocyte shows a further increase in the size of the nucleus and an increase in the relative amount of cytoplasm. The nucleus contains more parachromatin and thus stains more lightly than the nuclei of the smaller forms. The chromatin is still present in clumps, without distinct outlines because of the blending of chromatin and parachromatin. The nuclear membrane is distinct, and nucleoli usually are not seen. The cytoplasm in this form can be abundant, and azure granules are frequently seen. The cytoplasm color varies from colorless to a clear light or medium blue. The cytoplasm of the large granular lymphocyte can be deeply basophilic. Mature lymphocytes include different subsets of highly specialized lymphocytes. Morphologically, B and T lymphocytes appear identical on a Wright-stained blood film.

After antigenic stimulation, small lymphocytes can undergo transformation. These transformed cells appear large (15–25 μm) on Wright-stained films, with a relatively large amount of deep-blue cytoplasm, and are called *large granular lymphocytes.* The large nucleus has a reticular appearance, with uniform chromatin and prominent nucleoli. Such cells have various names, including *reactive, atypical, variant,* and *reticular lymphocytes.*

Nucleoli are rarely seen in lymphocytes of normal blood, but they may be seen in cells that have been crushed during the spreading of the film. Blood lymphocytes may contain nucleoli, but they are normally obscured by the coarse nuclear chromatin.

It is sometimes difficult to distinguish between nucleated RBCs and small lymphocytes. The staining reaction of the parachromatin of the two cells is an important diagnostic criterion; the parachromatin of the lymphocyte is pale blue or violet, and that of the nucleated RBC is pinkish blue. The N/C ratio is much higher in lymphocytes than in nucleated red cells.

Lymphocytosis, an increase in the number of lymphocytes, is associated with viral infections. It is characteristic of certain acute infections such as infectious mononucleosis; pertussis, mumps, and rubella; and German measles; and of chronic infections such as tuberculosis, brucellosis, and infectious hepatitis. The changes seen in these diseases have been referred to as *reactive* or *atypical changes* and are particularly associated with infectious mononucleosis. The cells are called *reactive lymphocytes* because the increased amount and apparent activity of the cytoplasm indicate that it may be reacting to some sort of stimulus. These cells can be referred to as *variant forms.*

Plasma Cells

The plasma cell is rarely seen alongside the five types of mature WBCs that normally appear in the peripheral blood. A greater concentration of plasma cells can be seen in the bone marrow. Plasma cells are large with a round or oval nucleus that is usually in an eccentric position. The chromatin consists of deeply stained, heavy masses that may be arranged in a radial pattern. The cytoplasm is strongly basophilic. There may be a pale, clear zone in the cytoplasm to one side of the nucleus, referred to as a *hof.* Immature forms may occasionally be seen. Plasma cells function in the synthesis of Igs. They may be found in the peripheral blood of patients with measles, chickenpox, or scarlet fever, and in the malignant conditions of multiple myeloma and plasmacytic leukemia.

Reporting Leukocyte Results (Total, Relative, and Absolute Counts)

The total, relative, and absolute WBC counts, both neutrophils and lymphocytes, are important data (Table 11.7). The total amount of leukocytes in the circulating blood varies by age. Fluctuations of the total leukocyte count can be seen as the result of the circadian rhythm.

The differential leukocyte counts of numbers and types of leukocytes are traditionally reported in percent numbers; cells are identified when examining and counting 100 WBCs in a systematic manner. These results are reported in relative numbers, or percentages.

The alternative method is to report the differentials in terms of absolute numbers. Using this method, the numbers and types of cells counted are reported in number of cells $\times$ 10^9/L. Increases or decreases of individual cell lines are reported individually, along with the total WBC count. The absolute count provides a much more accurate measure of the actual numbers of cell types present in the peripheral blood. The absolute cell count by cell type is obtained by multiplying the relative number of WBCs (in decimal units) by the total WBC count per liter.

For example, if a patient's WBC count is 7.0 $\times$ 10^9/L and 70% neutrophils are identified in the leukocyte differential, the relative neutrophil count is 70%. The ANC is:

$$0.70 \times (7.0 \times 10^9/\text{L} = 4.9 \times 10^9 \text{ neutrophils/L}(4900/\mu\text{L})$$

TABLE 11.7 Total, Relative Percentage, and Absolute Leukocyte Reference Values

Pediatric WBC Count (×10^9/L)[1]		
Age	**Mean**	**Range**
At birth	18.1 × 10^9/L	9.0–30.0 × 10^9/L
1 day (capillary blood)	18.9 × 10^9/L	9.4–34.0 × 10^9/L
6 months	11.9 × 10^9/L	6.0–17.5 × 10^9/L
10 years	8.1 × 10^9/L	4.5–13.5 × 10^9/L
21 years	7.4 × 10^9/L	4.5–11.0 × 10^9/L
Pediatric Relative Percentage Reference Values		
Birth	Neutrophils	61%
	Lymphocytes	31%
1 year	Neutrophils	31%
	Lymphocytes	61%
10 years	Neutrophils	54%
	Lymphocytes	38%
Adult WBC Count (×10^9/L)[2]		
4.4–11.3 × 10^9/L		
Adult Relative Percentage Reference Values		
Neutrophils		
Band		3%
Segmented		56%
Eosinophils		2.7%
Basophils		0.3%
Lymphocytes		34%
Monocytes		4%
Absolute Cell Counts (Adults)[2]		
PMNs		1.8–7.8 × 10^9/L
Band neutrophils		0–0.7 × 10^9/L
Lymphocytes		1.0–4.8 × 10^9/L

PMN, Polymorphonuclear; *WBC,* white blood cell.
[1]Greer JP, et al: *Wintrobe's clinical hematology,* vol 2, ed 12, Philadelphia, 2009, Lippincott Williams & Wilkins, Tables B.2 and B.4, pp. 2584–2585.
[2]McPherson RA, Pincus MR: *Henry's clinical diagnosis and management by laboratory methods,* ed 22, St Louis, 2011, Elsevier, Table A 5.9, p. 1502.

THROMBOCYTES

Another formed element of the circulating blood is the platelet, or thrombocyte.

Platelet (Thrombocyte) Maturation and Function

Platelets are produced in the bone marrow by cells called *megakaryocytes,* which are large and multinucleated. Platelets do not have a nucleus and are not actually cells; they are portions of cytoplasm pinched off from megakaryocytes and released into the bloodstream (Table 11.8).

Mature platelets are small, colorless bodies 1.5 to 4 μm in diameter. Platelets are generally round or ovoid, although they may have projections called *pseudopods.* Platelets have a colorless to pale-blue background substance containing centrally located, purplish-red granules.

In the bloodstream, platelets are an essential part of the blood-clotting mechanism. They act to maintain the structure or integrity of the endothelial cells lining the vascular system by plugging any gaps in the lining. They also function in the clotting process by (1) acting as plugs around the opening of a wound and (2) releasing certain factors necessary for the formation of a blood clot.

Reference Values

Platelet Reference Range.
$150 - 450 \times 10^9/\text{L}$

CLINICAL HEMATOLOGY PROCEDURES

Laboratory tests performed in the hematology laboratory include the following:

- Counting the number or concentration of cells
- Determining the relative distribution of various types of cells
- Measuring biochemical abnormalities of the blood

Several hematologic tests are basic to the initial evaluation and follow-up of a patient. The complete blood count (CBC) forms the foundation procedure performed in hematology. The CBC consists of the measurement of Hb, hematocrit (Hct), RBC count with morphology, WBC count with differential, and platelet estimate. The RBC indices of mean corpuscular volume (MCV),

TABLE 11.8 Development of Platelets

Nomenclature	Overall Size (mm)	N/C Ratio	Nuclear Characteristics	Cytoplasmic Characteristics
Megakaryocyte	30–160	1:1–1:12	Lobulated	Pinkish blue, abundant
Platelet	2–4	—	Anuclear	Light-blue fragments

N/C, nuclear/cytoplasmic.

mean corpuscular hemoglobin (MCH), and MCH concentration (MCHC) are now a standard part of a routine automated CBC.

Anticoagulants

Various types of anticoagulants are commonly used in the hematology laboratory: dipotassium (K_2) ethylenediaminetetraacetic acid (EDTA), tripotassium (K_3) EDTA, heparin, and sodium citrate. Each of the anticoagulant types prevents the coagulation of whole blood in a specific manner. The proper proportion of anticoagulant to whole blood is important to avoid the introduction of errors into test results. The specific type of anticoagulant needed for a procedure should be stated in the laboratory procedure manual.

EDTA

K_2 EDTA and K_3 EDTA are found in lavender-top evacuated tubes. EDTA is used in concentrations of 1.5 mg per 1 mL of whole blood. The mode of action of this anticoagulant is that it removes ionized calcium through the process of *chelation*. This process forms an insoluble calcium salt that prevents blood coagulation. EDTA is the most frequently used anticoagulant in hematology for the CBC or any of its component tests (Hb, packed cell volume or microhematocrit, total leukocyte count and leukocyte differential count, platelet count, and the erythrocyte sedimentation rate [ESR]).

The proper ratio of EDTA to whole blood is important because some test results will be altered if the ratio is incorrect. Excessive EDTA produces shrinkage of erythrocytes, thus affecting tests such as the manually performed packed cell volume (microhematocrit).

Blood cells in an anticoagulated specimen undergo degenerative changes over time. If a blood specimen is collected in EDTA and kept at room temperature, CBC results can remain relatively unchanged for a few days, but over time, significant changes in the relative and absolute numbers of neutrophils and lymphocytes will occur. In just one day, changes can be observed microscopically. These changes include chromatin degradation, cytoplasmic fragmentation in WBCs, and RBC deformations. For this reason, it is recommended that peripheral blood smears be prepared within 2 to 3 hours, preferably within 1 hour, after blood specimen collection.

Heparin

Heparin is used as an in vitro and in vivo anticoagulant. It is found in green-top evacuated tubes. The heparin concentration is 14 to 17 U/mL. Heparin acts as an antithrombin, or substance that inactivates the blood-clotting factor thrombin. This inactivation of thrombin is caused by the complexing of heparin with the antithrombin III molecule, catalyzing the inhibition of thrombin. The in vitro formation of fibrin in heparinized plasma opposes the anticoagulation action of heparin and can result in the subsequent formation of fibrin in the plasma. Heparin is the preferred anticoagulant for the osmotic fragility test and is used to coat "micro" (capillary blood) collection tubes. Heparin is an inappropriate anticoagulant for many hematologic tests, including Wright-stained blood smears, because the smear will stain too blue.

Sodium Citrate

Sodium citrate in the concentration of a 3.2% solution, found in a blue-top evacuated tube, has been adopted as the appropriate concentration by the International Council for Standardization in Haematology (ICSH) and the International Society on Thrombosis and Haemostasis. It also appears in the College of American Pathologists revised checklist section for hematology and coagulation as the appropriate concentration.

Sodium citrate removes calcium from the coagulation system by precipitating it into an unusable form. Sodium citrate is effective as an anticoagulant because of its mild calcium-chelating properties. This anticoagulant is used for the traditional Westergren ESR (see section Determination, under Erythrocyte Sedimentation Rate). The correct ratio of one part anticoagulant to nine parts of whole blood in blood collection tubes is critical. An excess of anticoagulant can alter the expected dilution of blood and produce errors in the results.

Processing and Testing the Specimen

After the blood specimen has been collected from the patient, it must be transported to the laboratory for analysis. Assuming that the specimen was properly labeled when it was drawn and that it has been handled properly, it is examined in the laboratory as quickly as possible to prevent deterioration. Laboratory tests are done on fresh specimens whenever possible. WBC counts, microhematocrit, platelet counts, and sedimentation rates can be determined up to 24 hours after blood is collected in EDTA if refrigerated at 4°C.

Immediately after the blood has been properly drawn and placed in the tube containing the anticoagulant, it should be gently mixed by inversion 5 to 10 times. This is necessary to ensure thorough contact with the anticoagulant. Clotted specimens are absolutely unacceptable for most tests done in the hematology laboratory, especially cell counts. If there is even a tiny clot in a specimen, the cell count will be grossly inaccurate. To comply with Standard Precautions, gloves must be worn during all laboratory handling and testing using blood specimens. All samples are to be considered as potentially infectious, and the proper use of barrier-protective apparel and devices is essential.

When a preserved specimen is allowed to stand for a time, the components will settle into three distinct layers (Fig. 11.17):

1. Top layer: plasma
2. Middle layer: buffy coat, a grayish-white cellular layer composed of WBCs and platelets
3. Bottom layer: RBCs

Some hematologic procedures are based on the ability of the blood specimen to settle into layers when it has been preserved by use of an anticoagulant. Immediately before a test is performed on a blood specimen, the blood sample must be mixed by repeated gentle inversion at least 15 times. This can be accomplished by hand or with a mechanical tube inverter. If the blood sample has stood for a few minutes, it should be mixed again.

Appearance of Specimens

When the blood specimen has been properly drawn and processed, plasma will have a light-yellow or straw color. Occasionally, the plasma may have an altered color resulting from a disease process or from improper collection or handling of the specimen.

Hemolysis

The breakup or rupturing of RBCs, hemolysis, can produce red-colored plasma. Hemolysis is one of the changes resulting from alterations in osmotic pressure in the solution surrounding the red cells. Hemolysis can occur when the membrane surrounding the RBCs has been mechanically ruptured either in vivo, as the result of a disease process, or in vitro, as the result of difficult collection or poor handling.

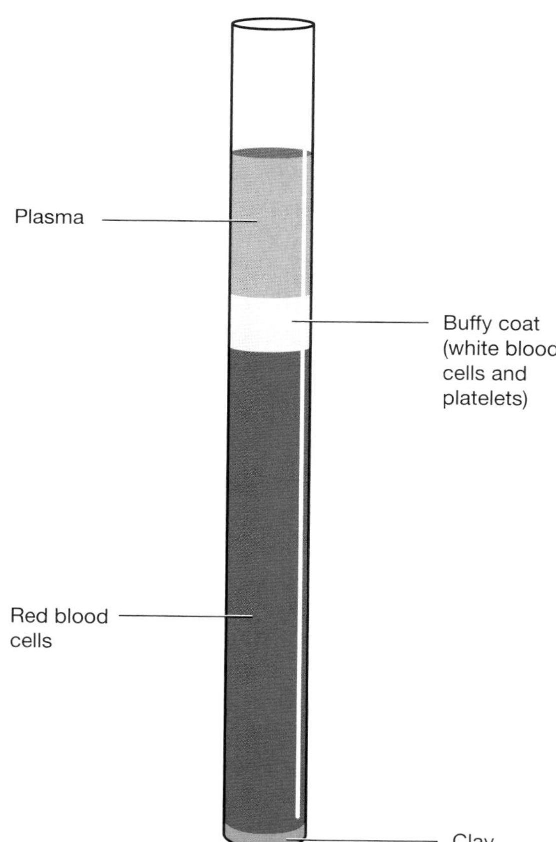

Fig. 11.17 Layers of normal blood. (Modified from Rodak BF, Fritsma GA, Doig K: *Hematology: clinical principles and applications,* ed 3, St Louis, 2007, Saunders.)

Unsuitable Hematologic Specimens

Two types of blood samples are unsuitable for hematology tests: clotted samples and hemolyzed samples. Clotted specimens are unsuitable for cell counts because the cells trapped in the clot are not counted. A cell count on a clotted sample will be falsely low. In hemolyzed specimens, the RBCs are no longer intact and will yield a falsely decreased RBC count and packed RBC results. The release of Hb and other constituents from intact RBCs elevates potassium ions (K^+) in the specimen. This will produce inaccurate chemistry results for K^+ and have an effect on other assays, such as Hb. Although hemolyzed specimens are generally considered unacceptable for testing, in certain cases of intravascular hemolysis, hemolysis is a clinically significant finding and not cause for rejection of the specimen for testing.

Homeostasis

All the fluid and cellular elements that make up the blood are in a constant state of exchange. The overall effect is a state of equilibrium in which the supply is equal to the demand for normal body function. This state of equilibrium is termed homeostasis, and various tests done on blood measure the overall state of homeostasis within the body. Many of the constituents of plasma (or serum, if the blood is allowed to clot) are measured in the clinical chemistry laboratory (see Chapter 10).

Osmosis and Osmotic Pressure

The principle of osmotic pressure and osmosis is important whenever a solution or diluent is used as part of a hematologic procedure. In simple terms, osmosis is the passage of a solvent through a membrane from a dilute solution into a more concentrated one. The difference in concentration between the solutions on either side of the membrane causes the phenomenon called osmotic pressure. If the concentrations of these solutions are the same, there will be no pressure (Fig. 11.18).

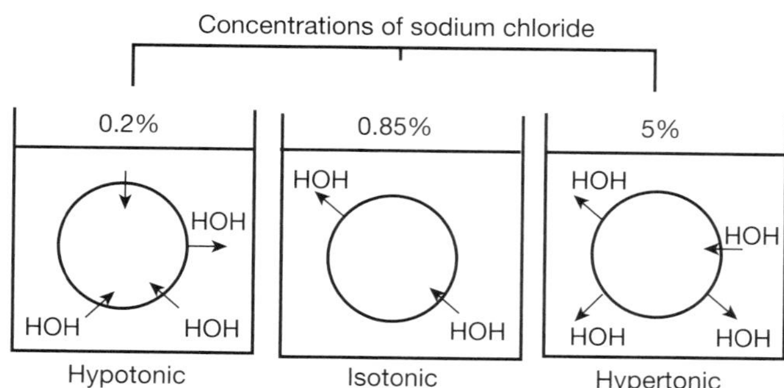

Fig. 11.18 Osmosis. A comparison of erythrocytes in three concentrations of sodium chloride solution demonstrates the net movement of water molecules into and out of the cell. If the net movement of water into the cell is in excess, the cell will lyse. If the net movement of water out of the cell is in excess, the cell will crenate. (From Turgeon M: *Clinical hematology,* ed 1, p. 40, Fig 2.2.)

Isotonic, Hypotonic, and Hypertonic Solutions

When the concentration is the same in the diluent solution as it is inside the RBC, the diluent is called an isotonic solution. If the diluent is less concentrated than the inside of the RBC, the solution is called hypotonic. From the definition of osmosis, it can be seen that in the case of a hypotonic (dilute) solution, the passage of diluent will be from outside the RBC into the RBC, causing the cell to swell and eventually to rupture, or hemolyze.

If the solution outside the RBC is more concentrated than that inside it, the outside solution is called *hypertonic*. In the case of a hypertonic solution, the osmosis of the solvent is from the inside of the red cell to the surrounding solution. When this happens, the RBC will shrink from loss of liquid and will become crenated.

When in plasma, the RBCs are in an isotonic solution. For this reason, any diluent used to dilute blood for hematology tests must have the same ionic concentration as plasma. When a solution has the same concentration or is isotonic with plasma, it is called a physiologic solution. One common physiologic solution is isotonic saline solution, a 0.85-g/dL solution of sodium chloride. If RBCs are placed in an isotonic saline solution, their size is preserved. Hypotonic and hypertonic solutions are unsatisfactory as diluents for hematologic studies.

Hemoglobin Measurement in the Laboratory

The determination of hemoglobin can be performed separately or as part of a routine CBC. Although the meaning of the CBC will vary somewhat from institution to institution, the measurement of hemoglobin is standard and is part of the automated instrumentation that includes cells counts and a calculated Hct.

Hemiglobincyanide (Cyanmethemoglobin) Method

The HiCN, or cyanmethemoglobin, method uses a modified Drabkin reagent that contains potassium cyanide; potassium ferricyanide; dihydrogen potassium phosphate, which shortens the conversion time to 3 minutes; and a nonionic detergent that minimizes turbidity and enhances RBC lysis. When the cyanmethemoglobin reagent is mixed with the blood specimen, the stable pigment HiCN is formed and can be measured quantitatively in a spectrophotometer.

Automated Hemoglobinometry

Various automated and semiautomated techniques measure Hb and determine the WBC count, RBC count, Hct, and RBC indices. Hb determinations done by an automated instrument generally use the traditional cyanmethemoglobin method. The sample is lysed by using the detergent-modified Drabkin reagent, and light absorbance is measured at 540 nm.

Specimens

The test for Hb can be done on free-flowing capillary blood obtained from a finger puncture or on venous blood preserved with an anticoagulant. The anticoagulant of choice for hematologic studies, including Hb determinations, is EDTA. The Hb content of blood remains unchanged for several days when the blood is properly anticoagulated and refrigerated at 4°C.

Point-of-Care Hemoglobin Assay

Single-analyte systems are available and are waived under the Clinical Laboratory Improvement Amendments of 1988 (CLIA '88).

The HemoCue method is an example of a single-purpose, self-contained instrument that measures Hb only and is waived under CLIA '88. It gives a reliable quantitative value and can be performed within 45 seconds. The instrument uses a microcuvette that serves as a sampling device, a test tube, and a measuring device. It automatically measures precisely 10 μL of blood from a capillary puncture or from a tube of anticoagulated blood collected by venipuncture. The microcuvette does not require mixing or dispensing of reagents. It contains an exact quantity of a dry reagent that yields a reaction when contact is made with the measured blood sample. Once the blood is sampled, the microcuvette is placed into the HemoCue photometer, and the Hb concentration is displayed in g/dL.

Principle: Hemoglobin Determination: Hemocue Method. This point-of-care testing assay for Hb is based on a modified azide-methemoglobin reaction. Erythrocyte membranes are disintegrated by sodium deoxycholate, releasing the Hb from the cells. Sodium nitrite converts the Hb iron from the ferrous to the ferric state to form methemoglobin, which then combines with azide to form azide-methemoglobin. The concentration of azide-methemoglobin is measured optically to determine the Hb concentration in the patient's blood (see procedure at http://evolve.elsevier.com/Turgeon/clinicallab).

The mean Hb level for the black population of both genders and all ages is reported to be 0.5 to 1.0 g/dL below the mean for the comparable white population.

Hematocrit (Packed Cell Volume)

The Hct, or packed cell volume, is a macroscopic observation of volume of the packed RBCs in a sample of whole blood, if measured by manual technique (Fig. 11.19). The manual procedure is relatively simple and reliable. An Hct is used in evaluating and classifying the various types of anemias according to RBC indices.

When whole blood is centrifuged, the heavier particles fall to the bottom of the tube, and the lighter particles settle on top of the heavier cells. The Hct is the percentage of RBCs in a volume of whole blood. Hct is expressed as units of percent or as a ratio in the International System of Units (SI) system.

When the Hct result is read, it is important to take the reading at the top of the RBC layer, particularly when there is an extremely elevated WBC or platelet count. The buffy coat should not be included in the measurement of RBC volume for the Hct result. Automated hematology instruments give a calculated Hct value and generally have replaced the manual methods.

A quick quality control check in healthy patients (normochromic, normocytic) is done by comparing the Hb with the Hct results (in % units), using the following formula:

$$\text{Hgb} \times 3 = \text{Hct} \pm 3$$

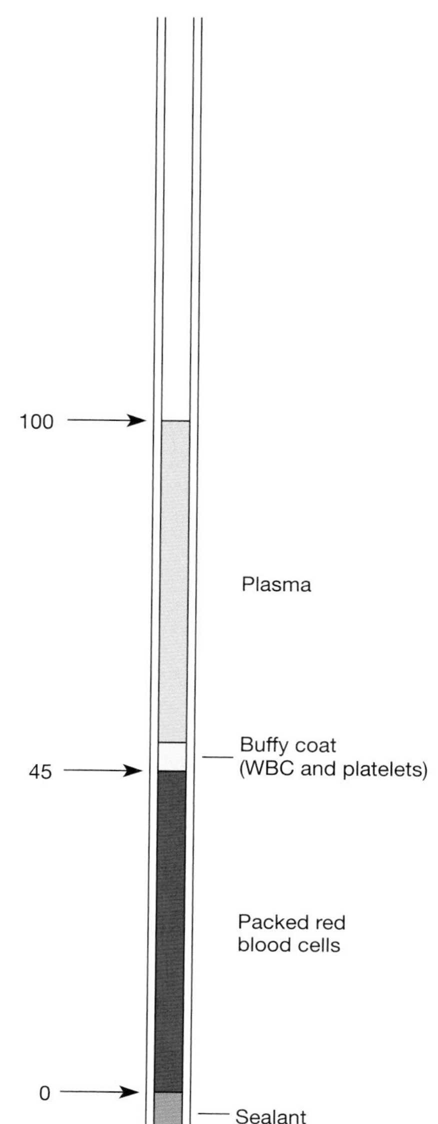

Fig. 11.19 Microhematocrit tube.

Methods for Measurement

The spun microhematocrit method can be done with either free-flowing capillary blood from a skin puncture or EDTA-anticoagulated venous blood (Student Procedure Worksheet 11.1). Only a very small amount of blood is needed. The test uses a high-speed centrifuge with a relatively short centrifugation time.

An automated Hct result is obtained when multiparameter instruments are used. This result is computed from individual red cell volumes (MCV) and the red cell count and is not affected by the trapped plasma that is left in the RBC column for the manual methods. Hct value obtained with the automated instruments is slightly lower than the value obtained by the centrifugation methods.

Specimens

Again, for the spun microhematocrit method, either venous blood anticoagulated with EDTA or free-flowing capillary blood may be used. With capillary blood, microhematocrit tubes coated with heparin are used. With venous blood, plain uncoated microhematocrit tubes must be used. Blood that has been properly anticoagulated with EDTA is used for automated analysis.

Capillary Tubes for Microhematocrit

Special nongraduated capillary tubes are used. These tubes are 1 mm in diameter and 7 cm long. They can be purchased lined with dried heparin for use with capillary blood or plain (without heparin) for use with previously anticoagulated venous blood. Some type of seal is needed for one end of the tube before it can be centrifuged. A special sealing compound (similar to modeling clay) can be used for this purpose. Also available are tubes with a self-sealing plug and a multilayered Mylar wrap; these ensure safer blood handling by preventing both breakage during collection and centrifugation and the resulting contamination of the sealant.

Blood Cell Counts

Counting the various cells found in blood is a fundamental procedure in the hematology laboratory. In modern laboratories, most cell counts are performed with automated equipment, but body fluids (see Chapter 14) may be analyzed by automated or manual methods. Electronic counting devices avoid human error, which is significant in manual cell counts, and are statistically more accurate because of sampling; these devices count many more cells than can be counted manually.

The procedures in this chapter are presented in a format consistent with the guidelines set forth by the Clinical and Laboratory Standards Institute (CLSI),[3] as follows:

1. Procedure title and specific method
2. Test principle, including type of reaction and clinical reasons for the test
3. Specimen collection and preparation
4. Equipment, supplies, and reagents
5. Calibration of a standard curve
6. Quality control
7. Procedure
8. Calculations
9. Reporting results (normal values)
10. Procedure notes, including sources of error, clinical applications, and limitations of the procedure
11. References

Units Reported

Because there are a great number of cells per unit volume of blood, it is necessary to dilute the blood before attempting to count the cells. Methods for counting cells are designed to obtain the number of cells in 1 L of whole blood; this is the SI unit of measurement of volume recommended by the ICSH.

The enumerated constituents are reported in units per liter of blood; the number of cells actually counted (platelets, RBCs, WBCs) must be converted to the number present per liter of blood. Previously, cells were counted and reported as the number of cells per cubic millimeter (mm^3). This was a convenient unit of measurement because cells were counted in a hemocytometer, an accurately ruled chamber or device where cells were counted in areas of square millimeters, and results were converted to number per cubic millimeter. One cubic millimeter is essentially equal to one microliter. This is summarized as follows:

$$1\ mm^3 = 1\ \mu L = 1/10^{-6} L$$

Therefore:

$$1 \times 10^6\ \mu L = 1\ L$$

Specimens

Free-flowing capillary blood obtained from a skin puncture (see Chapter 4) or venous blood preserved with an anticoagulant may be used. The anticoagulant of choice is EDTA.

Before any blood sample is used, it must be checked to ensure that it has been preserved with the proper anticoagulant, that it has been properly labeled, and that its appearance indicates a good collection technique was used. Each sample should be checked for hemolysis and small clots, known as *fibrin clots,* as soon as it is received. Clotted blood or samples with fibrin clots are unacceptable for cell counts. Standard Precautions must always be used when any blood specimen is handled.

Diluents Used

White Cell Counts. For leukocytes to be counted, the diluting fluid must destroy the more numerous RBCs so that WBCs may be counted more readily. (WBCs need not be eliminated when RBCs are being counted.) The principle of osmotic pressure is again employed, but in a different way. A lysing agent hemolyzes the RBCs; it converts the Hb released from red cells into acid hematin, which gives the resulting solution a brown color. The intensity of the brown color is directly related to the amount of Hb present in the RBCs.

Counting Red and White Blood Cells

The RBC (erythrocyte) and WBC (leukocyte) counts are basic procedures performed by automated instruments. Although generally replaced by automated cell counts, manual leukocyte counts may still be done in special circumstances such as when a whole blood cell count is extremely low (see http://evolve.elsevier.com/Turgeon/clinicallab), or in cerebrospinal fluid or synovial fluid (see Chapter 14).

Clinical Significance of Cell Counts

Red Blood Cell Counts. *Anemia* is a term generally applied to a decrease in the number of RBCs. There are many types of anemias (see later discussion). Anemia can be caused by excessive blood loss or blood destruction (hemolytic anemia). Anemias caused by decreased blood cell or Hb formation include pernicious anemia (PA), bone marrow failure anemia, and iron deficiency anemia. Polycythemia is a condition in which the number of erythrocytes is increased.

White Blood Cell Counts. The normal WBC count varies with age and gender (see Table 11.7).

An increase in the WBC (leukocyte) count above the normal upper limit is termed *leukocytosis.* A decrease below the normal lower limit is termed *leukopenia.* Leukopenia may occur with certain viral infections, with typhoid fever and malaria, after radiation therapy, after the administration of certain drugs, and in PA. Leukocytosis may occur in many acute infections (especially bacterial infections), in severe malaria, after hemorrhage, during pregnancy, postoperatively, in some forms of anemia, in some carcinomas, and in leukemia.

Leukemia is characterized by uncontrolled proliferation of one or more of the various hematopoietic cells and is associated with many changes in the circulating cells of the blood. Blood films prepared from patients with leukemia should be examined only by a qualified person—a pathologist or an experienced clinical laboratory scientist. There are two main classifications of leukemia, *lymphocytic* and *myelocytic,* according to the predominant type of leukocyte seen. Leukemias are further divided into the subclassifications acute and chronic. In the *acute* condition, the disease progresses rapidly, and morphologic changes are marked. In the *chronic* condition, the changes are neither as rapid nor as marked.

As mentioned earlier, the WBC count is used to indicate the presence of infection and to follow the progress of certain diseases. It may be elevated in acute bacterial infections, appendicitis, pregnancy, hemolytic disease of the newborn, uremia, and ulcers. It may be decreased in hepatitis, rheumatoid arthritis, cirrhosis of the liver, and systemic lupus erythematosus. A child's leukocyte count usually shows a much greater variation during disease than an adult's count. An individual's leukocyte count is subject to some variation during a normal day, being slightly higher in the afternoon than in the morning. There is also an increase in the WBC count after strenuous exercise, emotional stress, and anxiety.

Platelet Counts

Platelets, or thrombocytes, function in blood coagulation and are therefore associated with the bleeding and clotting, or *hemostatic,* mechanism of the body. Platelets are formed in the bone marrow from megakaryocytes. They are difficult to count accurately for several reasons: Platelets are small and difficult to discern, and they have an adhesive character and become attached to surfaces or to particles of debris in the diluting fluid. They disintegrate easily and are difficult to distinguish from debris. Because of their sticky nature, platelets clump easily and tend to adhere to other platelets in clumps. The clumping tendency of platelets is decreased if EDTA is used as an anticoagulant.

Specimens

Capillary blood from a finger puncture can be used, but venous blood generally gives more satisfactory results. Platelet counts on capillary blood are generally lower than those on venous blood because of immediate platelet clumping at the puncture site. Again, EDTA is the anticoagulant of choice for platelet counts because it lessens the tendency for platelet clumping.

Methods Used to Count Platelets

Most platelet counts are performed using automated instruments. The quantitative platelet count is correlated with a semiquantitative estimate from a stained peripheral blood smear. If the instrument count and the blood smear do not match, a manual platelet count is performed (see procedure at http://evolve.elsevier.com/Turgeon/clinicallab). This rare situation typically happens when the platelet count is very low and the patient has a moderate number of schistocytes.

Clinical Significance of Platelet Count

Platelet Reference Range.

$150 - 450 \times 10^9/L$

A count lower than normal may be associated with a generalized bleeding tendency and a prolonged bleeding time. A count higher than normal may be associated with a tendency toward thrombosis. There are several diseases in which a high or low platelet count can result.

Thrombocytopenia, or a decrease in platelets, is found in thrombocytopenic purpura, in some infectious diseases, in some acute leukemias, in some anemias (aplastic and pernicious), and when the patient is undergoing radiation treatment or chemotherapy.

Thrombocytosis, or an increase in platelets, can be found in rheumatic fever, in asphyxiation, after surgical treatment, after splenectomy, with acute blood loss, and with some types of chemotherapy used in the treatment of leukemia.

Automated Hematology Instrument Technology

Automated analyzers now form the backbone of clinical hematology laboratories both large and small. Smaller analyzers are commonly used in STAT labs, freestanding clinics, physicians' offices, and small hospital laboratories. Larger and more complex systems are used in larger clinical and research laboratories.

The degree of instrumental sophistication is frequently described by the number of parameters that the instrument generates. The term *parameter* is a statistical term that refers to any numerical value that describes an entire population. Parameter should be clearly distinguished from the term *sample,* which is a subset of a population.

Smaller hematology instruments measure erythrocytes (RBCs), leukocytes (WBCs), and platelets. Entry-level hematology instruments generate eight measured or calculated parameters: WBC, RBC, Hb, Hct; red blood cell indices: MCV, MCH, and MCHC; and platelets.

Various types of automation (Table 11.9) use different ways to count RBCs and WBCs, to differentiate leukocytes, and to calculate other cellular components (e.g., MCH and MCHC). Hemoglobin is measured by the traditional cyanmethemoglobin flow-cell method at 525 and 546 nm, depending on the instrument manufacturer.

Computerized systems generally flag high or low patient results. These systems are automated from sample aspiration through result printout. Additional basic parameters include erythrocyte morphology information expressed as red blood cell distribution width (RDW), mean platelet volume (MPV), or leukocyte histogram differential. The expression of other calculated output varies depending on the manufacturer.

Models and features of instrumentation change rapidly. The reader is advised to refer to the respective manufacturers' websites for any current updates.

TABLE 11.9 Examples of Automated Hematology Instrument Manufacturers

Manufacturer	Address	Series
Abbott Diagnostics	www.abbott.com	Cell-Dyn
Beckman Coulter	www.beckmancoulter.com	Coulter HmX, LH, and AcT diff family
Cella Vision	www.cellavision.com	DM
Horiba ABX Diagnostics	www.abx.com	Pentra
Siemens Healthcare Diagnostics	www.medical.siemens.com	ADVIA
Sysmex	www.sysemx.com	XE

Principles of Cell Counting

Most automated cell counters can be classified as one of two types: those using electrical resistance and those using optical methods with focused laser beams, in which cells cause a change in the deflection of a beam of light. In cell counters using optical methods, deflections are converted to measurable pulses by a photomultiplier tube. In electrical resistance cell counters, blood cells passing through an aperture through which a current is flowing cause a change in electrical resistance that is counted as voltage pulses. The voltage pulses are amplified and can be displayed on an oscilloscope screen. Each spike indicates a cell. Both types of instruments count thousands of cells in a few seconds, and both increase the precision of cell counts compared with manual methods.

Hemoglobin Measurement

Hemoglobin is measured by the traditional cyanmethemoglobin flow-cell method at 525 and 546 nm, depending on the instrument manufacturer. Many instruments also count immature erythrocytes (reticulocytes). Because models and features of instrumentation change rapidly, the reader is advised to refer to the respective manufacturer's website.

Automated Cell-Counting Methods

Instruments for cell counting and automated differential analysis (Table 11.10) are now routinely found in most laboratories. Because automated instruments count a much larger numbers of cells than manual counting methods, there is greater precision. Thousands of particles pass through the instrument's aperture in a few seconds. Smaller analyzers are commonly used in STAT and lower-volume hematology laboratories. Larger and more complex systems are used in larger clinical and research

TABLE 11.10 Examples of Automated Hematology Technology

Manufacturer	Series	Measurement Technology
Abbott Diagnostics www.abbott.com	Cell-Dyn	WBC and differential
	Sapphire	Four-angle optical multiangle polarized scatter separation (MAPSS) plus three-color fluorescent flow cytometry, multiple scatterplot analysis
		Nucleated RBCs
		Four-angle optical MAPSS plus red fluorescence; no extra reagent, no reflex testing requirement; multiple scatterplot analysis
		Platelets
		Dual-angle optical analysis, no extra reagent, no reflex testing requirement
	Ruby	Reticulocytes
		Patented RNA fluorescent flow cytometry, random and continuous access
		Monoclonal
		Immuno T-Cell (CD3/4/8) reagent; Immuno Plt (CD61) assay
		MAPSS laser technology for WBC enumeration and identification using four angles of light scatter on up to 10,000 cells per dilution
		Red blood cell and platelet counts are performed using optical laser light scatter analysis
		WBC and differential four-angle optical MAPSS, multiple scatterplot analysis
		Platelets dual-angle optical analysis, no extra reagent, no reflex testing requirement
	Cell-Dyn Emerald 22	Reticulocytes: new methylene blue NCCLS method, supravital staining technique
		Electrical impedance for WBC, RBC, and platelet counting
		Absorption spectrophotometry for hemoglobin
	Cell-Dyn Emerald	Uni-Flow technology for WBC classification
		Electrical impedance for WBC, RBC, and platelet counting
		Absorption spectrophotometry for hemoglobin
Beckman Coulter www.beckmancoulter.com		1.1 AcT 5diff CP (Cap Pierce), AcT diff2, AcT diff analyzer, LH 750 hematology analyzer, LH 780 hematology analyzer, UniCel DxH Slidemaker Stainer, cellular analysis system
		ClearLLab Reagents (T1, T2, T3, B1, B2 and M) are the first FDA-approved flow cytometry tests designed to help detect a variety of leukemias and lymphomas
Horiba ABX Diagnostics www.abx.com		Pentra Nexus, ABX Pentra DX-DF 120, ABX Pentra 120, ABX Pentra XL 80, Pentra XLR, Pentra ABX 60, Yumizen
Siemens Healthcare Diagnostics www.medical.siemens.com		ADVIA
		CBC results: WBC, RBC, HGB, HCT, MCV, MCH, MCHC, CHCM, RDW, HDW, CH, CHDW, PLT
		Differential results (absolute and %) Neut, Lymph, Mono, Eos, Baso, LUC (large unstained cells)
		Platelet results: PLT, MPV, PDW, PCT
		Reticulocyte results: (absolute and %) Retic, MCVr, CHCMr, RDWr, HDWr, CHr, CHDWr
		CSF assay results optional
		Morphology results (user-definable)
		WBC left shift, atypical lymph, blasts, immature granulocytes, myeloperoxidase deficiency
		RBD and PLT NRBC, ANISO, MICRO, MACRO, HC VAR, HYPO, HYPER, RBC fragments, RBC ghosts, platelet clumps, large platelets
Sysmex www.sysemx.com	Sysmex XN Series	• Slidemaker-stainer (SP50), Body fluid model, PLT-F (fluorescent platelet) discrete testing channel, reticulocyte channel
	Sysmex XL Series	• Low-WBC application (standard) improves reliability of analysis. Provides a 6-part differential (including immature granulocytes) on every sample aiding in the assessment of sepsis and other hematologic disorders
		• CBC with 5-part WBC differential (NEUT+ LYMPH+MONO+EO+BASO)
	Sysmex XS Series	• 3-part diff analyzers CBC with 8 parameters, including a 3-part WBC differential with an absolute neutrophil count
		• Alifax erythrocyte sedimentation rate
CellaVision www.cellavision.com	DM96 DM1200 DM9600	CellaVision
		Neural network technology
		Peripheral blood application WBC Differential; delivers pre-classification into 17 cell types
		Advanced RBC application
		Result parameters RBC precharacterization: automated pre-characterization of polychromatic cells, hypochromic cells, anisocytosis, microcytes, macrocytes, poikilocytosis, target cells, schistocytes, helmet cells, sickle cells, spherocytes elliptocytes, ovalocytes, teardrop cells, stomatocytes, acanthocytes, echinocytes, Howell-Jolly bodies, Pappenheimer bodies, basophilic stippling and parasites
		Body fluid application WBC Differential; delivers pre-classification into 5 cell types

laboratories. Significant innovations include automated front-end (preanalytical [preexamination]) instrumentation and robotics, and total work cells linked by a track or conveyor.

The instrument's degree of sophistication is frequently described by the number of parameters that the instrument generates. Parameter is a statistical term that refers to any numeric value that describes an entire population. Currently, the term *data point* is also used to refer to a measured output.

The cellular elements of the blood (erythrocytes, leukocytes, and platelets) can be counted based on one of two classic methods:

- Electrical impedance
- Optical detection

Electrical Impedance Principle

In the basic Coulter counter, cells passing through an aperture through which a current is flowing cause changes in electrical resistance that are counted as voltage pulses (Fig. 11.20). A reduced-pressure system operated by a vacuum unit draws the suspension through the aperture into a system of tubing following a column of mercury. The Coulter system is based on the principle that cells are poor electrical conductors compared with a saline diluent that is a good conductor.

A current flows through the aperture between the internal and external electrodes. Each cell that passes through the aperture displaces an equal volume of conductive solution, increasing the electrical resistance and creating a voltage pulse, because its resistance is much greater than that of the conductive solution. The pulses are counted. If two or more cells enter the aperture at the same time, they will be counted as one cell. This produces a *coincidence error.*

Optical Detection Principle

In the optical or hydrodynamic focusing method of cell counting and cell sizing, laser light is used. A diluted blood specimen passes in a steady stream through which a beam of laser light is focused. As each cell passes through the sensing zone of the flow cell, it scatters the focused light. Scattered light is detected by a photodetector and converted into an electrical pulse. The number of pulses generated is directly proportional to the number of cells passing through the sensing zone in a specific period. The instrument accomplishing this task is known as a flow cytometer.

Light is scattered at angles proportional to the structural features of a cell as it passes through the light beam (Fig. 11.21). Most laser systems use light sensors that detect forward scatter of the beam (180 degrees from the light source) and right-angle (90 degree) scatter. Forward scatter is correlated with cell volume or density, analogous to the impedance counting of the Coulter instruments. Right-angle deflection depends on cellular contents, mainly the granularity of the cell cytoplasm. Photodetectors convert the light signals to electrical impulses that are processed by a computer. Both intrinsic and extrinsic properties of cells can be analyzed by flow cytometry. Intrinsic properties include forward and right-angle light scatter, which correlate with size and granularity of a cell, respectively. In contrast, extrinsic properties rely on the binding of various probes to the cells. A fluorochrome dye can be employed in the cell suspension to enhance the cell identification. This dye can directly stain or tag certain cell components, such as a granule or an enzyme. The dye can be attached to an immunologic component, such as an antibody to a lymphocyte surface antigen. Different wavelengths of light excite different types of fluorochrome dyes, enabling particular tagged cells to be counted separately.

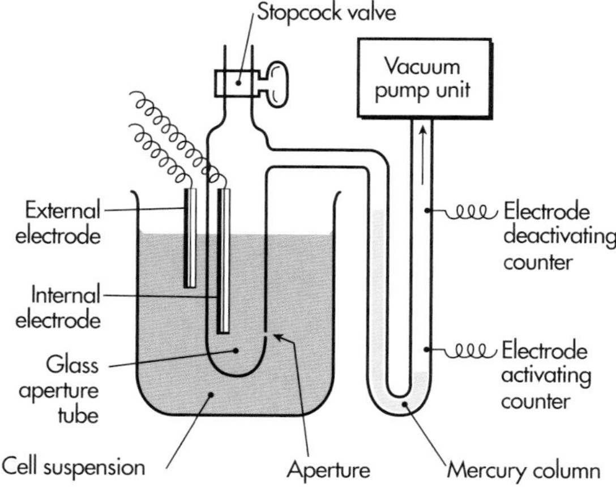

Fig. 11.20 Schematic diagram of a cell counter based on counting voltage pulse (Coulter principle). Cells flow through an aperture that separates two compartments. Electrical potential between electrodes changes as cells pass. Number of impulses translates to cell count, and pulse amplitude depends on cell volume that displaces conductive fluid.

Histograms

A histogram or graphic representation of output provides information about erythrocyte, leukocyte, and platelet frequency and cellular identification. The display of data includes cell counts, RBC indices, and WBC differentials (Fig. 11.22). Characteristics can be used to differentiate the various types of WBCs and to produce scatter plots with a five-part differential.

Erythrocyte Histogram

The erythrocyte histogram reflects the native size of erythrocytes or any other particles in the erythrocyte size range. In a homogeneous cell population, the curve assumes a symmetric bell-shaped or Gaussian distribution. A wide or more flattened curve is seen when the standard deviation (SD) from the mean is increased.

Red Cell Distribution Width

A new parameter, the red cell distribution width (RDW), expresses the coefficient of variation of the erythrocyte volume distribution. It is calculated directly from the histogram. A portion of the curve at the extreme ends is excluded from the computation to eliminate clumps of platelets, large platelets, or electrical interference on the left side of the curve. The portion of the right side of the curve that is excluded represents grouped or clumped erythrocytes.

The RDW is calculated by dividing the SD by the mean of the red cell size distribution:

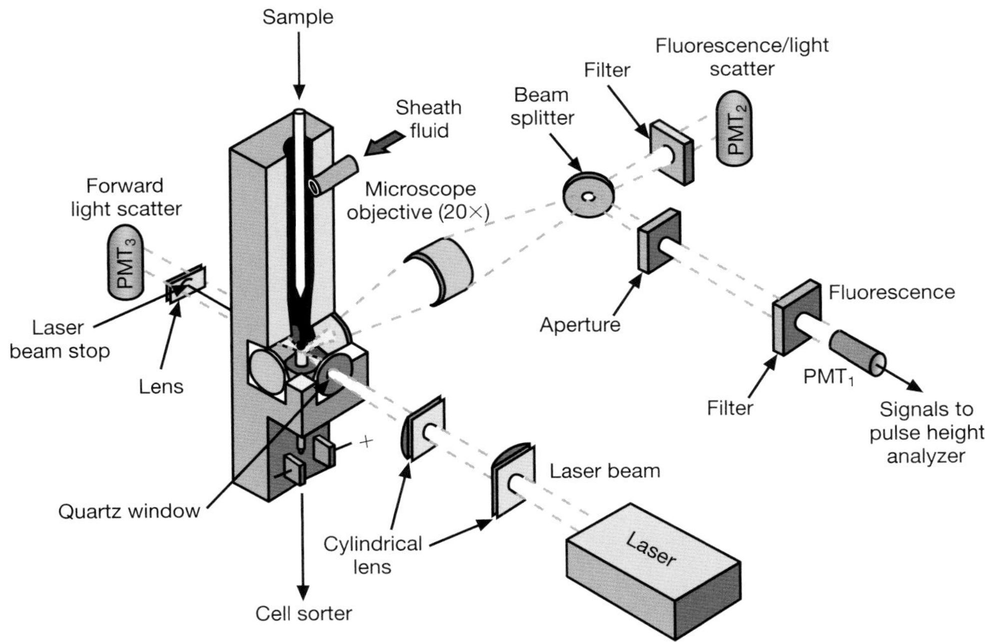

Fig. 11.21 Schematic diagram of a flow cytometer. (From Burtis CA, Ashwood ER, Bruns DE: *Tietz fundamentals of clinical chemistry,* ed 6, St Louis, 2008, Saunders.)

$$\text{RDW } (\%) = \frac{\text{Standard deviation (SD) of MCV}}{\text{Mean MCV}} \times 100$$

The RDW is expressed numerically as the coefficient of variation percentage.

RDW Reference Range.
11.5% to 14.5%

The RDW is increased above the normal limits in iron deficiency, vitamin B_{12} deficiency, and folic acid deficiency. In the hemoglobinopathies, the RDW is increased in proportion to the degree of anemia that accompanies the Hb disorder.

Examples of Automated Hematology Technology

The Abbott Cell-Dyn series uses multiangle polarized scatter separation flow cytometry with hydrodynamic focusing of the cell stream (see Chapter 8). It features dual leukocyte counting methods. The leukocyte differential is accomplished by light scatter with 0, 90, 10, and 90 (depolarized) degrees, and nuclear optical count is accomplished by light scatter at 0 and 10 degrees. Erythrocytes and platelets are counted by light scatter at 0 and 10 degrees. A unique feature is cyanide-free hemoglobinometry. One system (Cell-Dyn 4000) features three independent measurements and focused flow impedance. Multidimensional light scatter and fluorescence detection are used as well.

The Siemens Diagnostics Healthcare System's ADVIA series uses Unifluidics, a darkfield optical method. Dual leukocyte methods of peroxidase staining and basophil lobularity are used. Erythrocytes and platelets are counted by flow cytometry. Hemoglobin has dual readings and colorimetric or cyanmethemoglobin and corpuscular hemoglobin mean concentration.

The Beckman Coulter Z1 series uses electrical impedance to measure the volume of the cells by direct current (DC). Radio frequency (RF) or conductivity is used to gather information related to cell size and internal structure. Scatter or laser light is used to obtain information about cellular granularity and cell surface structure. Opacity is monitored to delineate internal structure, including nuclear size, density, and N/C ratio. A 3D analysis is the output.

Sysmex systems analyze erythrocytes and platelets by hydrodynamic focusing, DC, and automatic discrimination (Fig. 11.23). The leukocyte count is analyzed by the DC detection method and automatic discrimination. A five-part differential is produced for leukocytes by a differential detector channel (analyzed by RF and DC). A differential scattergram and an immature myeloid information scattergram are produced.

Automated Leukocyte Differentiation

Many of the multiparameter hematology analyzers provide differentiation of leukocytes as three-cell or five-cell differentials in a histogram. The histogram differentiates lymphocytes, mononuclear cells, and granulocytes. Mononuclear cells include blasts or other immature cells, such as promyelocytes and myelocytes, and monocytes; however, in a normal specimen, monocytes represent the mononuclear cells.

In an environment of cost containment and shortage of laboratory personnel, together with more and more sophisticated instrumentation, the CBC often uses an automated rather than a manual leukocyte differential. Automated differentials can provide an in-depth amount of information because many thousands of cells are analyzed rapidly.

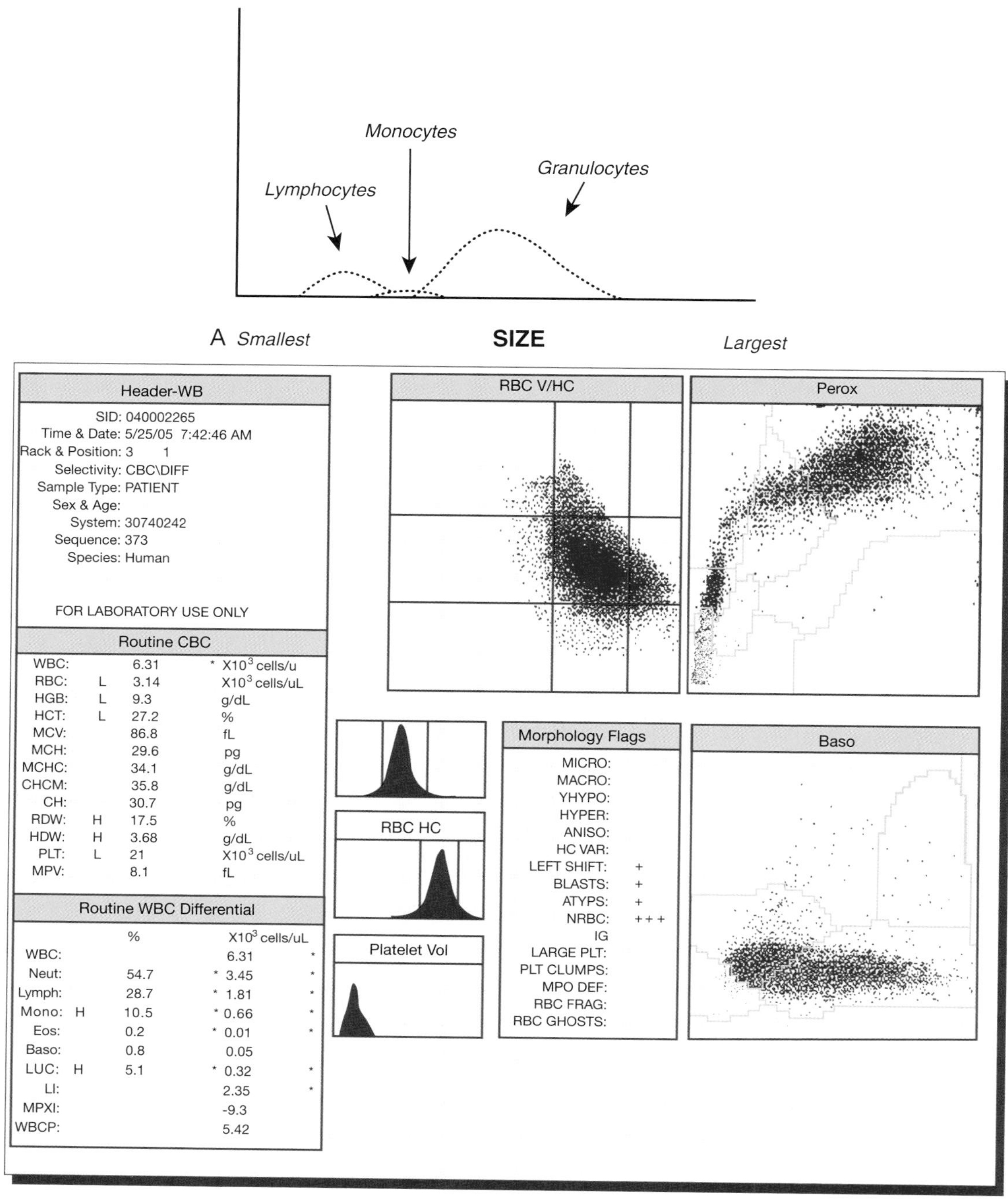

Fig. 11.22 (A) Normal Coulter complete blood count (CBC) readout. (B) Abnormal Coulter CBC readout. (Panel B is from Rodak BF, Fritsma GA, Keohane EM: *Hematology: clinical principles and applications,* ed 4, St Louis, 2012, Saunders.)

Leukocytes can be differentiated by various methods. Analysis can be by:

1. Impedance-related conductivity
2. Light-scattering measurements of cell volume
3. Automated continuous-flow systems that use cytochemical and light-scattering measurements
4. Automated computer image analysis of a blood film prepared by an instrument
5. Digital microscopy using neural network systems (Fig. 11.24)

Size-referenced leukocyte histograms display the classification of leukocytes according to size after lysis. It does not display the native cell size. The lytic reagent causes a cytochemical reaction. As a result of the reaction, the cytoplasm collapses around the nucleus, producing differential shrinkage. As a result, the histogram of leukocyte subpopulations reflects the sorting of these cells by their relative size, which is related primarily to their nuclear size.

Although the Coulter principle uses a size-distributed histogram of leukocytes, other technologies are available for

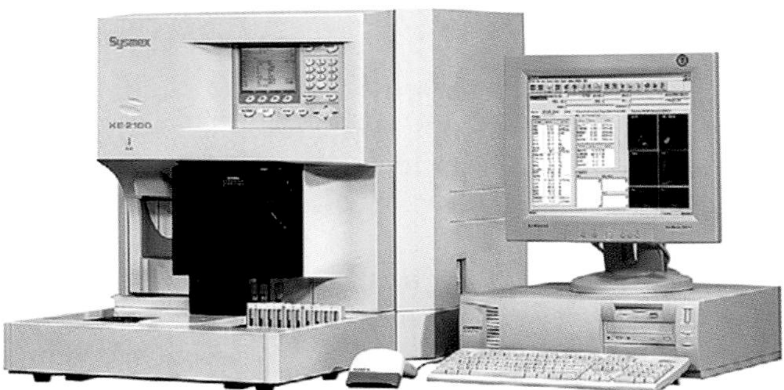

Fig. 11.23 Hematology Automation; Sysmex XE-2100. (Courtesy Sysmex Inc., Mundelein, IL.)

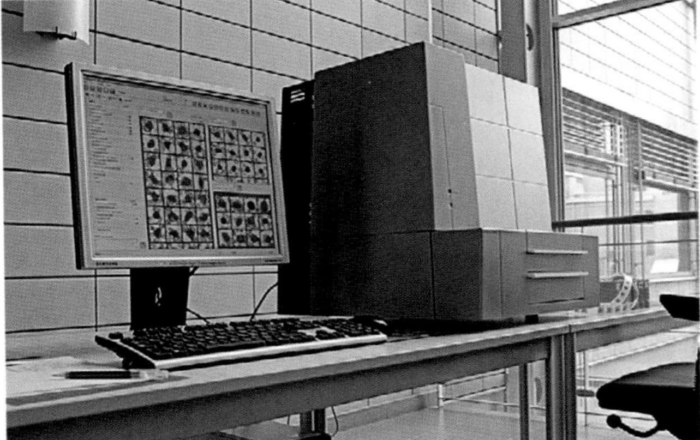

Fig. 11.24 Hematology CellaVision DM96. (Courtesy CellaVision Inc., Jupiter, FL.)

differentiating leukocytes, including the CellaVision digital microscope system or immunophenotyping using flow cytometry (see Chapter 8).

Platelet Histograms

Platelet counting and sizing in both the electrical impedance and optical systems reflect the native cell size. In the electrical impedance method, counting and sizing take place in the RBC aperture. In the optical system, forward light scatter pattern discrimination between erythrocytes and platelets in the flow cell determines the platelet count and frequency distribution.

Mean Platelet Volume Calculation. The MPV is a measure of the average volume of platelets in a sample. It is derived from the same data as the platelet count. The volume increases while the platelet count decreases. Because of this inverse relationship, the MPV and the platelet count must be considered together.

Platelet Distribution Width. The platelet distribution width (PDW) is a measure of the uniformity of platelet size in a blood specimen. This parameter serves as a validity check and monitors false results. A normal PDW is less than 20%.

New Automation Technology. Technology continues to deliver new automation capabilities in hematology. For example, automated reticulocyte counting was a leading-edge technology a few years ago but is a routinely measured parameter in many clinical laboratories today. Some of the latest instruments prepare and stain peripheral blood smears and automatically correct for leukocyte (WBC) interference.

Newly developed instrumental capabilities continue to be developed. Some of the innovations include

- Quantitation of nucleated erythrocyte (NRBC) counts
- Enumeration of immature granulocytes (IGs)
- Quantitation of CD4 lymphocytes by random access
- Analysis for CD34, CD38, and CD61 cell markers
- Measurement of reticulocyte hemoglobin
- Enumeration of hematopoietic progenitor cells (HPCs)
- Identification of RBC abnormal sizes and shapes

A hybrid version of cell image analysis is the Sysmex® Cell Image Analysis Portfolio, which combines the Sysmex DI-60 and CellaVision DM series analyzers. The DM9600 or 1200 analyzer locates blood cells on a prepared slide, preclassifies the white blood cells, precharacterizes parts of the RBC morphology, and provides functionality for platelet estimation.

Quality Control

All automated methods require the use of quality assurance measures (see Chapter 3), including quality control materials to ensure that the instrument is functioning correctly and that valid results are reported.

ADDITIONAL HEMATOLOGY PROCEDURES

The procedures discussed so far are usually part of a CBC. Two additional tests, the reticulocyte count and the ESR, are frequently performed in the hematology laboratory.

Reticulocyte Counts

Reticulocytes are young erythrocytes that have matured enough to have lost their nuclei but not their cytoplasmic RNA. They do not have the full amount of Hb. The number of reticulocytes is a measure of the regeneration or production of RBCs. Using the reticulocyte count and the immature RBC fraction is a means of establishing that a bone marrow/stem cell transplant is successful. Reticulocytes appear in a Wright-stained blood film as polychromatophilic RBCs because of the basophilic cytoplasmic remnant of the immature erythrocyte RNA. See Procedure[4] on http://evolve.elsevier.com/Turgeon/clinicallab).

Normal Erythropoiesis and Reticulocytes

In the circulating blood, 0.5% to 2.5% of the RBCs are usually reticulocytes. This is based on an average RBC life span of 120 days, with replacement of approximately 1% of the adult circulating erythrocytes each day. A reticulocyte count above this level, reticulocytosis, is a clinical indication that the body is attempting to meet an increased need for RBCs. An increase in reticulocytes is observed when RBCs are being hemolyzed in the body. Increased reticulocyte counts and polychromasia are characteristic of a hemolytic condition subsequent to blood loss, treatment of anemia, or other causes. The demand for RBCs may be so great in some patients that nucleated erythrocytes are prematurely released from the bone marrow.

Clinical Uses for Reticulocyte Counts

The reticulocyte count is used to follow therapeutic measures for anemias in which the patient is deficient in, or lacking, one of the substances essential for manufacturing RBCs. When the deficiency has been diagnosed, therapy is begun. This consists of supplying the body the missing essential substances and waiting for it to react by increasing erythrocyte production. New RBCs will be released rapidly into the circulating blood, many before they are fully matured, in response to therapy. The corresponding increase in the reticulocyte count indicates a favorable response to therapy.

The response to therapy in iron deficiency anemia (treated with iron) and PA (treated with vitamin B_{12}) is followed by reticulocyte counts. While the total RBC count and the Hb concentration reach normal levels, erythrocyte regeneration slows to the normal rate, allowing more time for maturation of the RBCs in the bone marrow. This is indicated by the presence of fewer reticulocytes in the circulating blood.

Reference Values

Reticulocytes	
Adults	0.5%–2.5%
Newborn	2.5%–6.0%

Erythrocyte Sedimentation Rate

If blood is prevented from clotting (by using blood collected in citrate anticoagulant) and allowed to settle, sedimentation of the erythrocytes will occur. The rate at which the RBCs fall is known as the erythrocyte sedimentation rate, or ESR. This rate depends on three main factors:

1. Number and size of erythrocyte particles
2. Plasma factors
3. Certain technical and mechanical factors

The most important factor determining the rate of fall of the RBCs is the size of the falling particle: The larger the particle, the faster it falls. The size of the falling particles depends on the formation of RBC *rouleaux,* which in turn depends on the presence of certain factors in the plasma. In normal blood, RBCs tend to remain separate from one another because they are negatively charged (zeta potential) and tend to repel each other. In many pathologic conditions, the phenomenon of rouleaux is caused by alteration of the erythrocyte surface charge by plasma proteins.

The protein that is most often involved is fibrinogen, although increases in gamma globulins or abnormal proteins also produce this effect. With increased concentrations of large molecules in the plasma, there is a greater tendency for erythrocytes to pile up in rouleaux formation.

Determination

There are two manual methods[1] for performing an ESR: the traditional Westergren method and the modified Westergren method. The traditional Westergren method requires blood anticoagulated with sodium citrate[1]; the modified Westergren method requires EDTA anticoagulant. Newer automated ESRs tend to use EDTA anticoagulated blood.[5] EDTA is considered to introduce less dilutional error than citrate. Some laboratories may offer both methods as options. The reference range for ESR varies with age, gender, and the specific methodology used. See Procedure http://evolve.elsevier.com/Turgeon/clinicallab).

A newer method for performance of the ESR right from EDTA tubes is being manufactured by Streck (streck.com). This system, Cube 30 Touch or Mini-Cube, produces results in approximately 20 minutes.

Clinical Significance

The ESR is a nonspecific screening test for inflammatory activity. It is a measure of the presence and severity of pathologic processes. In the vast majority of infections, there is at least some increase in the ESR; chorea and undulant fever are two exceptions. The ESR also increases in most cases of acute myocardial infarction and other inflammatory conditions. While patients recover, the ESR slowly returns to normal. The ESR may still be increased long after other clinical manifestations have disappeared, showing that the defense mechanisms of the body continue to be more active than normal.

Changes in the number and shape of erythrocytes also affect the ESR. In anemia the ESR is increased, more so in megaloblastic than iron deficiency anemias. The rate of sedimentation is inhibited by variations in RBC shape, including spherocytes, acanthocytes, and sickle cell formation.

Increased numbers of erythrocytes, as seen in patients with polycythemia and failure of the right side of the heart, tend to cause a marked slowing of sedimentation (decreased ESR). When the Hct is greater than 48% to 50%, sedimentation is greatly slowed regardless of any factors present that might otherwise accelerate it.

A decrease in the ESR will result when the plasma fibrinogen level is decreased, as in patients with severe liver disease. The ESR is not increased in viral diseases, such as infectious mononucleosis and acute hepatitis, probably because fibrinogen production is not increased in these diseases, despite a pronounced inflammatory reaction. The ESR is also not usually increased in chronic degenerative joint disease, but it is increased in inflammatory joint disease.

Reference Values

Younger Than 50 Years	
Male	0–10 mm/hr
Female	0–13 mm/hr
Older Than 50 Years	
Male	0–15 mm/hr
Female	0–20 mm/hr

RED BLOOD CELL INDICES

In the classification of anemias, quantitative measurements of the average size, Hb content, and Hb concentration of RBCs are especially useful (see Erythrocyte Alterations). These can be calculated from red cell count, Hb concentration, and Hct. The indices are the MCV, the MCH, and the MCHC.

The MCV represents the volume or size of the average RBC, the MCH represents the weight of Hb in the average RBC, and the MCHC represents the Hb concentration or color of the average RBC. A derived measurement determined electronically is the RDW, a measurement of the degree of variability in RBC size (see earlier discussion). Determination of these indices has become routine with the use of automated multiparameter instruments. These instruments measure the Hb, MCV, and RBC count, then automatically calculate the Hct, MCH, and MCHC.

When the indices are calculated from manually determined values for Hb, Hct, and RBC count, the greatest inaccuracy results from errors associated with the RBC count. Electronically counting the number of RBCs significantly reduces this error. Indices calculated by electronic methods have been found to be more accurate. It is important to verify all indices against observations of stained blood films. When the RBC indices are used in conjunction with an examination of the stained blood film, a clear picture of RBC morphology is obtained.

Because an RBC is very small and the amount of Hb in a single cell is minute, the units in which the RBCs are measured and recorded are micrometers (μm) and picograms (pg). With automated hematology instrumentation, reporting the red cell indices is routine, and the data are considered highly reliable. RBC indices are calculated from the following hematology data (with abbreviations) in units as indicated:

Test Name	Abbreviation	Units
Hematocrit	Hct	%
Packed cell volume	PCV	L/L
Red blood cell count	RBC	$\times 10^{12}$/L
Hemoglobin	Hb	g/dL

Mean Corpuscular Volume

The MCV is the average volume of an RBC in femtoliters (fL). One fL = 10^{-15} L = one cubic micrometer (μm^3). The MCV is calculated manually by dividing the volume of packed RBCs (Hct) by the number of RBCs, using the formula:

$$\text{MCV(fL)} = \frac{\text{Hct} \times 1}{\text{RBC}}$$

The factor 10 is introduced to convert the Hct reading (in %) from volume of packed RBCs per 100 mL to volume per liter. Example: If the Hct is 45% and the RBC count is 5 × 10^{12} cells per liter:

$$\text{MCV} = \frac{45 \times 10}{5} = 90\ \text{fL}$$

MCV ADULT REFERENCE VALUE[1]
80 to 96 fL

The MCV indicates whether the RBCs will appear small (microcytic), normal (normocytic), or large (macrocytic). If the MCV is less than 80 fL, the RBCs will be microcytic. If it is greater than 100 fL, the RBCs will be macrocytic. If it is within the normal range, the RBCs will be normocytic. In some macrocytic anemias, such as PA, the MCV may be as high as 150 fL. In microcytic anemia with marked iron deficiency, it may be 60 to 70 fL. The chief source of error in the MCV is the considerable error in the manual RBC count, if used.

With automated cell counters and electronically calculated indices, the MCV is measured directly, and the Hct is calculated from MCV and RBC count (Hct = MCV × RBC). The MCV is now considered the most reliable automated index and is probably the most effective discriminant for the classification of anemias. Previously, the MCHC was the most reliable index because it was calculated from the two manual measurements that could be done most accurately, Hct and Hb.

Mean Corpuscular Hemoglobin

The MCH is the content (weight) of Hb in the average RBC. It is measured in picograms. One picogram (pg) = 10^{-12} g = 1 micromicrogram (μμg). The MCH is obtained by dividing the Hb by the red cell count. A simple formula can be used to calculate this value:

$$\text{MCH(pg)} = \frac{\text{Hb} \times 10}{\text{RBC}}$$

The factor 10 is used to convert the Hb from grams per deciliter to grams per liter.

Example: if the Hb is 15 g/dL and the RBC is 5 × 10^{12} cells per liter:

$$\text{MCH} = \frac{15 \times 10}{5} = 30\ \text{pg}$$

MCH ADULT REFERENCE VALUE[1]
27 to 33 pg

MCH should always correlate with the MCV and the MCHC. MCH may be as high as 50 pg in macrocytic anemias or as low as 20 pg or less in hypochromic microcytic anemias.

The chief source of MCH error is the RBC count, if done manually. However, when the red cell count is determined by electronic cell counters, the MCH is a reliable index.

Mean Corpuscular Hemoglobin Concentration

The MCHC is the average Hb concentration in a given volume of packed RBCs. It is expressed as grams per deciliter. MCHC may be calculated from the MCV and the MCH or from the Hb and Hct values by using the following formula:

$$\text{MCHC (g/dL)} = \frac{\text{MCH}}{\text{MCV}} \times 100$$

or

$$\text{MCHC (g/dL)} = \frac{\text{Hb}}{\text{Hct}} \times 100$$

Example: If the Hb concentration is 15 g/dL and the Hct is 45%:

$$\text{MCHC} = \frac{15}{45} \times 100 = 33.3\ g/dL$$

If a packed cell volume of 0.45 is used in the previous example:

$$\text{MCHC} = \frac{15}{0.45} = 33.3\ \text{g/dL}$$

MCHC ADULT REFERENCE RANGE[1]
33 to 36 g/dL

Values below 32 g/dL indicate hypochromasia. An MCHC above 40 g/dL would indicate malfunctioning of the instrument. An impossibly high MCHC (>40 g/dL) also could indicate the presence of cold agglutinins in the specimen. An MCHC of 37 g/dL is near the upper limits for Hb solubility and near the physiologic upper limits for the MCHC. The MCHC typically increases only in spherocytosis. In other anemias, it is decreased or normal. In true hypochromic anemias, Hb concentration is reduced, and values as low as 20 to 25 g/dL may be seen.

Summary of Red Blood Cell Indices Reference Values

Mean corpuscular volume (MCV): range 80–96.1 fL
Mean corpuscular hemoglobin (MCH): range 27.5–33.2 pg
Mean corpuscular hemoglobin concentration (MCHC): range 33.4–35.5 g/dL

Red Blood Cell Distribution Width

The RDW is a measurement of the degree of anisocytosis present, or the degree of variability in RBC size, in a blood sample. This measurement is derived by the automated multiparameter instruments that can directly measure the MCV. If anisocytosis is present on the peripheral blood film, and the variation in RBC size is prominent, there is an increase in SD of the MCV from the mean.

In Coulter instruments such as Coulter Counter model S-Plus, a red cell histogram is plotted, and the RDW (%) is defined as the coefficient of variation of the MCV:

$$\text{RDW}(\%) = \frac{\text{Standard deviation (SD) of MCV}}{\text{Mean MCV}} \times 100$$

Red Blood Cell Distribution Width Adult Reference Range[1]
11.5% to 14.5%
Varies with the type of instrument used.

Accuracy and Precaution

The entire range of disorders seen in hematology includes hereditary, immunologic, nutritional, metabolic, traumatic, and inflammatory conditions. Many disorders, either primarily hematologic in nature or, more frequently, hematologic manifestations secondary to other diseases, can produce abnormalities of the red cells, white cells, and platelets. Additional laboratory assays can assist in detection of the primary cause of hematologic abnormalities. Physicians depend on laboratory results, in combination with the clinical history and physical examination, to determine the state of health or disease of a patient.

Any manual RBC count, Hct, or Hb concentration used in the calculations must be accurate. It is also essential to check the appearance of the RBCs in a well-stained blood film against the calculated indices. The calculations must agree with the appearance of RBCs in the blood film. For example, a corresponding decrease in Hb color intensity should be observed on the blood film when there is a low MCHC (increase in amount of central pallor in RBCs), but often it is difficult to recognize hypochromasia under these circumstances. The MCHC is often below 30 g/dL before hypochromasia is observed on the blood film.

MICROSCOPIC EXAMINATION OF THE PERIPHERAL BLOOD FILM

Microscopic examination of the peripheral blood is done by preparing (Student Procedure Worksheet 11.2), staining (Student Procedure Worksheet 11.3), and examining a thin smear of blood on a slide (Student Procedure Worksheet 11.4). With the use of automatic counting devices that determine Hb, Hct, RBC, WBC, and platelet counts, together with MCV, MCH, MCHC, RDW, WBC differential, and histograms, there is a tendency to place less emphasis on the routine examination of the peripheral blood film.

Traditionally, the microscopic examination of the peripheral blood film has been used to study the morphology of RBCs (erythrocytes), WBCs (leukocytes), and platelets. The percentage of each leukocyte cell type present in a peripheral blood film can be determined by direct microscopic observation, the WBC (leukocyte) differential. An additional examination of the bone marrow may be necessary in certain cases, but this is not a routine procedure. Platelets are also routinely assessed in clinical hematologic studies by observing their number and morphology in the peripheral blood film.

Sources of Blood for the Blood Film

Fresh blood from a finger or heel puncture can be used for morphologic examination of the white and red cells. CLSI has deleted the use of the big toe as a site for collecting peripheral blood because of the lack of documentation supporting or discouraging blood collection from this site.[1]

The finger must not be squeezed excessively to obtain the drop of blood, and it must not be touched with the slide. Only the drop of blood should touch the slide. Any oils or moisture from the finger will lead to a poorly prepared film.

Most of the work in the hematology laboratory is done on venous blood. EDTA is the anticoagulant of choice because it preserves the morphologic features of WBCs and RBCs and gives a more even distribution of platelets. If blood is collected in EDTA for morphologic studies, the film should be prepared as soon as possible, certainly within 2 hours.

Microscopic Examination of the Blood Film

Morphologic changes in the RBCs and WBCs seen on the stained blood film aid in diagnosis. Certain diseases produce characteristic alterations of RBCs, WBCs, and platelets, in addition to other clinical signs.

Accurate examination of the blood film depends on proper use of the microscope (see Chapter 5). A blood film is first examined with the low-power (10×) objective, with the slide being moved by the mechanical stage to position different areas into the field of view. The proper area for examination is where the RBCs are barely touching or overlapping each other.

Scattered among the RBCs, which appear as small, round, reddish-orange bodies, are the less numerous WBCs, which are larger and more complex in appearance than the RBCs. The WBCs consist of nuclei surrounded by cytoplasm. The nuclei stain purple, and the cytoplasms stain different colors depending on their contents.

Low-power objective (10×) examination includes:

1. Evaluation of the overall quality of the blood film smear preparation and staining
2. Estimate of the RBC and WBC counts
3. Scanning the blood film for abnormal cells and clumps of platelets

1. Evaluate the Quality of the Blood Film

   The film should be thin enough that the red and white cells are clearly separated. The space between the cells should be clear. There should be no precipitated dye. The red and white cells should be properly stained, and there should be no large accumulation of WBCs at the feather edge of the blood film. If the blood film does not meet these criteria, it should not be examined further; a new film must be made.

2. Estimate the Red and White Cell Counts

   A rough estimate of the RBC count as increased, decreased, or normal can be made by noting the number of cells and the space between them. Normally, fewer and fewer intercellular spaces will be seen as the observer moves into the thicker portion of the blood film. In the optimal counting area, there should be no agglutination (clumping) or rouleaux formation (cells stacked like coins). The optimal counting area is generally two to three microscope fields in from the feather edge.

   To find the optimal counting area, focus on the feather edge and then begin moving into the body of the blood film. At the very thin edge of the film, about one or two microscope fields into the body of the blood film, the RBCs flatten out, appear completely filled with Hb (showing no area of central pallor), and are generally distorted and show a cobblestone appearance. In the thick end of the film, the morphologic characteristics of all cell types are difficult to distinguish, and the RBCs show an apparent rouleaux formation.

   The number of WBCs is estimated in the optimal counting area of the film. With the low-power (10×) objective and the usual 10× eyepiece (a total magnification of 100×), five leukocytes in one low-power field are equal to approximately 1000 cells per microliter, or the number of cells per low-power field times 200 equals the number of cells per microliter. In other words, five WBCs in one low-power field are equal to a WBC count of approximately 1×10^9/L; thus the number of WBCs per low-power field divided by 5 is equal to the number of cells $\times 10^9$ per liter. As a general observation, approximately 20 to 30 WBCs per field are equivalent to a WBC count of approximately 5×10^9/L. Under the same magnification, 40 to 60 WBCs per field are equivalent to a WBC count of approximately 10×10^9/L.

3. Scan the Blood Film for Abnormal Cells and Clumps of Platelets

   The slide should also be examined under low power for the presence of immature or abnormal cells. With experience, the cells may be recognizable under low power; however, they are positively identified under oil immersion. If very few such abnormal cells are present, they may be overlooked if the slide is examined under oil immersion alone, in which the examination area is much smaller. Such abnormal cells should be sought especially in the feather edge and along the sides of the slide.

   The optimal counting area, sides, and feather edge should also be scanned for clumps of platelets. Clumps of platelets should not be seen normally; however, when the platelet count is increased, they may be found along the sides and in the feather edge.

High-Dry Objective (43×). The high-dry (43×) objective is not suitable for examination of blood films, because important morphologic changes cannot be seen at this magnification.

Oil-Immersion Objective (100×). With the low-power objective, in one area of the film the RBCs are just touching and are not overlapping or piled on top of one another. When this area has been found, the oil-immersion (100×) objective should be used next (Fig. 11.25).

To change to the oil-immersion lens, the low-power objective is moved out of position, and a drop of immersion oil is placed on the selected area of the blood film. The oil-immersion lens is moved into the oil while the viewer looks at it from the side. The oil must be in direct contact with the lens. If necessary, it can be focused with the fine adjustment. If the slide has been placed

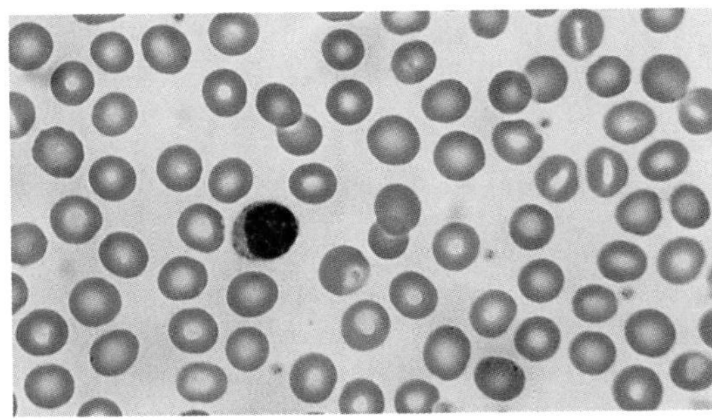

Fig. 11.25 Stained peripheral blood smear demonstrating appropriate area in which to perform white blood cell differential and morphology assessment and platelet estimate. Entire field would contain 200 to 250 red blood cells (×1000). (From Carr JH, Rodak BF: *Clinical hematology atlas,* ed 3, St Louis, 2009, Saunders.)

upside down on the microscope stage, it will be impossible to bring the blood cells into focus. More light will be needed with the oil-immersion lens. It can be obtained by repositioning the condenser (which should be all the way up for maximum resolution under oil immersion), opening the iris diaphragm, and increasing the intensity of the light source.

Under the oil-immersion objective, RBCs appear as round, unstructured bodies containing no nuclei, granules, or discrete material. The red color is darker at the edge of the cell than in the center. This variation is caused by the biconcave shape of the red cell, which contains less pigment (Hb) in its thinner center. With oil immersion, most RBCs in a normal blood film are about the same size, averaging 7.2 μm in diameter. A normal RBC is uniformly round on a dry film, although variations in shape can be produced by poor spreading technique in the preparation of the blood film.

Oil-immersion examination (100 × objective) includes:

1. Examination of the erythrocytes for alterations and variations in morphology
2. Estimation of platelet count and evaluation of morphologic changes
3. Differential count of the leukocytes
4. Examination of the leukocytes for morphologic alterations

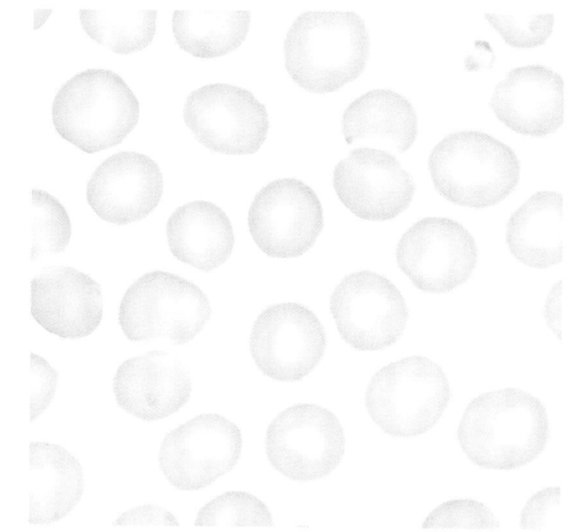

Fig. 11.26 Normal red blood cells (erythrocytes). (From Carr JH, Rodak BF: *Clinical hematology atlas,* ed 3, St Louis, 2009, Saunders.)

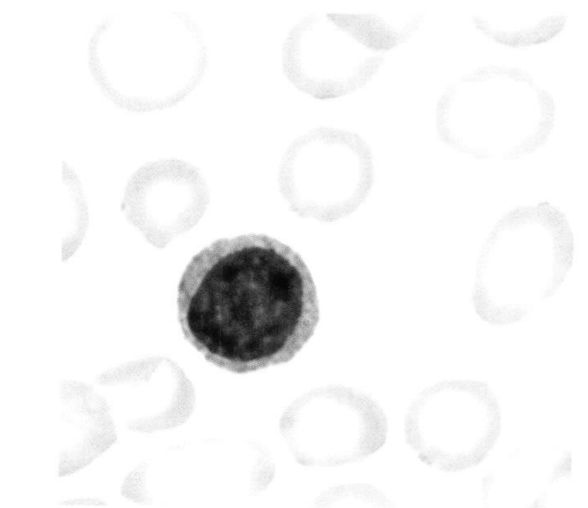

Fig. 11.27 Hypochromic red blood cells. (From Carr JH, Rodak BF: *Clinical hematology atlas,* ed 3, St Louis, 2009, Saunders.)

Erythrocyte Alterations

Examine the erythrocytes for alterations and variations in morphologic features. The normal RBC is a nonnucleated, biconcave disk containing Hb. Most RBCs measure 7.2 to 7.9 μm on a stained blood film. The normal RBC is approximately 2 μm thick. The mean volume, calculated from the Hct and the RBC count, is 87 fL. In estimating the diameters of WBCs or other structures, it is often advantageous to use the RBC as an approximate 7-μm reference.

When RBCs are examined morphologically, the following characteristics must be observed and noted:

1. Variations in color or staining reaction
2. Variations in size (anisocytosis)
3. Variations in shape (poikilocytosis)
4. Variations in structure and inclusions
5. Presence of artifacts and abnormal distribution patterns
6. Presence of nucleated red cells

Various terms are used to describe changes in the RBC size, shape, and staining reaction. The degree of the observed RBC alteration is noted as slight, moderate, or marked. The morphologic alterations of erythrocytes listed are further described as follows:

1. Variations in Color or Staining Reaction

The normal RBC appears as a disk with a rim of Hb and a clear central area, referred to as *central pallor*. The area of central pallor is normally less than one-third the RBC's diameter, although there is some variation within the film. The amount of color in the cell (the staining reaction) and the corresponding amount of central pallor reflect the amount of Hb in the cell. Normal RBCs are pink. RBCs with a normal amount of color are referred to as *normochromic* or, less frequently, *orthochromatic*. Normochromic, normocytic RBCs are shown in Fig. 11.26.

RBCs that are very pale and show an increased area of central pallor (making up more than one-third that of the cell) are termed *hypochromic* (Fig. 11.27). Hypochromia is the result of a decrease in the Hb content of the cell and is often accompanied by a decrease in cell size. This is seen as a decreased MCV, or *microcytosis*, as evidenced by low MCH and MCHC values. The cells tend to flatten out on the blood film and may appear normal in size. Such RBCs are particularly characteristic of iron deficiency anemias.

An increase in RBC color, hyperchromia, cannot exist, because normal RBCs are filled with Hb and cannot be oversaturated, or the cell membrane would burst. However, certain RBCs appear to have an increased Hb content. For example, cells that are larger than normal (macrocytes) are also thicker, and therefore the color intensity appears greater on the blood film. Another abnormally shaped erythrocyte, the spherocyte, which is a round cell without a depression in the center, also appears hyperchromic because it is thicker and stains equally throughout the cell.

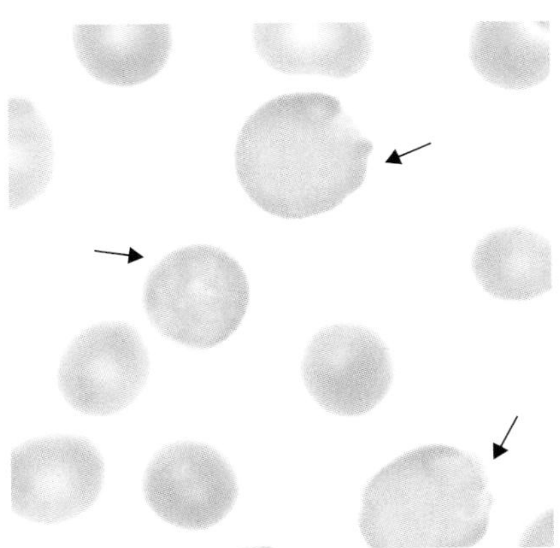

Fig. 11.28 Polychromatic red cells. (From Carr JH, Rodak BF: *Clinical hematology atlas*, ed 3, St Louis, 2009, Saunders.)

Variation in staining color (pinkish blue) is called *polychromatophilia* or polychromasia. Polychromasia refers to RBCs that show a faint blue or blue-orange color with Wright stain (Fig. 11.28). This is a mixed staining reaction, because both blue RNA and red Hb are present. Polychromic cells are young cells that have just extruded their nuclei and stain diffusely basophilic because of the presence of small numbers of ribosomes (or cytoplasmic RNA). When such cells enter the bloodstream, they lack 20% of their final Hb content and retain the ribosomes for Hb synthesis. Polychromatophilic RBCs are generally larger than mature cells. With supravital dyes, such as new methylene blue, the RNA reticulum stains blue, and the cells are called reticulocytes. The degree of polychromasia (or an increased reticulocyte count) is an indication of increased erythrocyte formation by the marrow and is characteristically seen in the various hemolytic anemias.

2. Alterations in Size

Anisocytosis is a general term indicating increased variation in the size of RBCs in the blood film. The degree of anisocytosis is reflected by the RDW. Examples of anisocytosis include microcytosis and macrocytosis (Fig. 11.29).

Microcytes are small RBCs, less than 6.5 μm in diameter, with an MCV less than 78 fL (Fig. 11.30). They are often associated with hypochromasia, but their decreased size may not be appreciated on the blood film because they tend to flatten out. Microcytosis is characteristic of iron deficiency anemia, thalassemia, lead poisoning, sideroblastic anemia, idiopathic pulmonary hemosiderosis, and anemias of chronic diseases.

Macrocytes are large RBCs (Fig. 11.31). They have a mean cell diameter greater than 9 μm or an MCV greater than 100 fL. They should be differentiated from polychromatophilic erythrocytes, which are also large. Macrocytes are characteristic of the megaloblastic anemias of folic acid or vitamin B_{12} deficiency.

3. Alterations in Shape

When an RBC is not being subjected to external deforming processes, its normal shape is that of a smooth biconcave disk. One term used to describe a red cell with a normal shape is discocyte (Fig. 11.32).

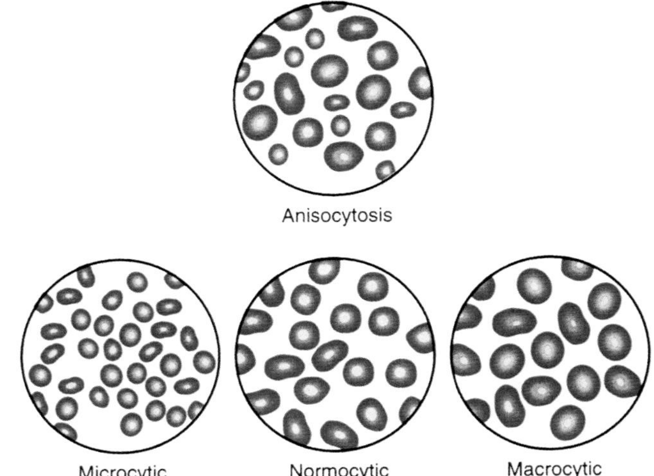

Fig. 11.29 Variation in erythrocyte size. (From Turgeon M: *Clinical hematology,* ed 5, Philadelphia, 2011, Lippincott Williams & Wilkins, Fig. 6.2.)

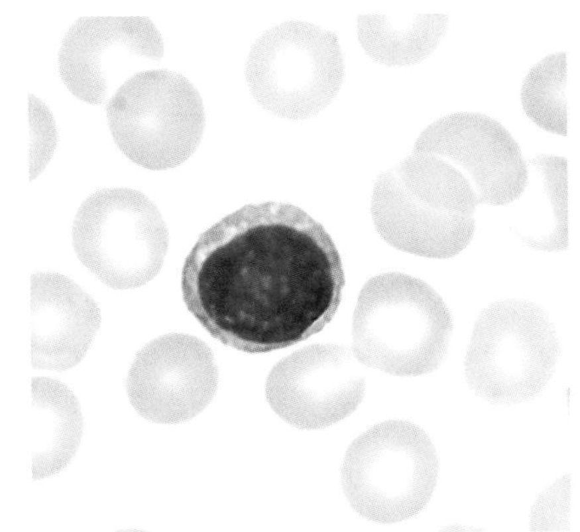

Fig. 11.30 Microcytosis. (From Carr JH, Rodak BF: *Clinical hematology atlas,* ed 3, St Louis, 2009, Saunders.)

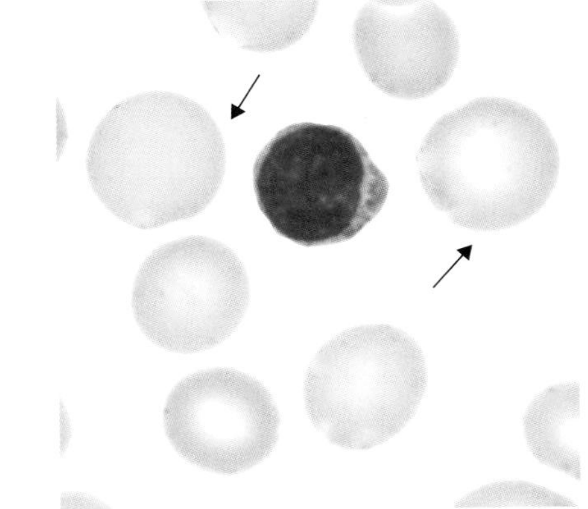

Fig. 11.31 Macrocytosis (macrocytes, *arrows*). (From Carr JH, Rodak BF: *Clinical hematology atlas,* ed 3, St Louis, 2009, Saunders.)

The general term for a variation in the shape of a normal discocyte is poikilocytosis. Some abnormal RBC shapes have specific names (Fig. 11.32A–K). Variations in shapes are found in a variety of anemias and hemolytic states, and a particular shape may or may not indicate a specific type of disease.

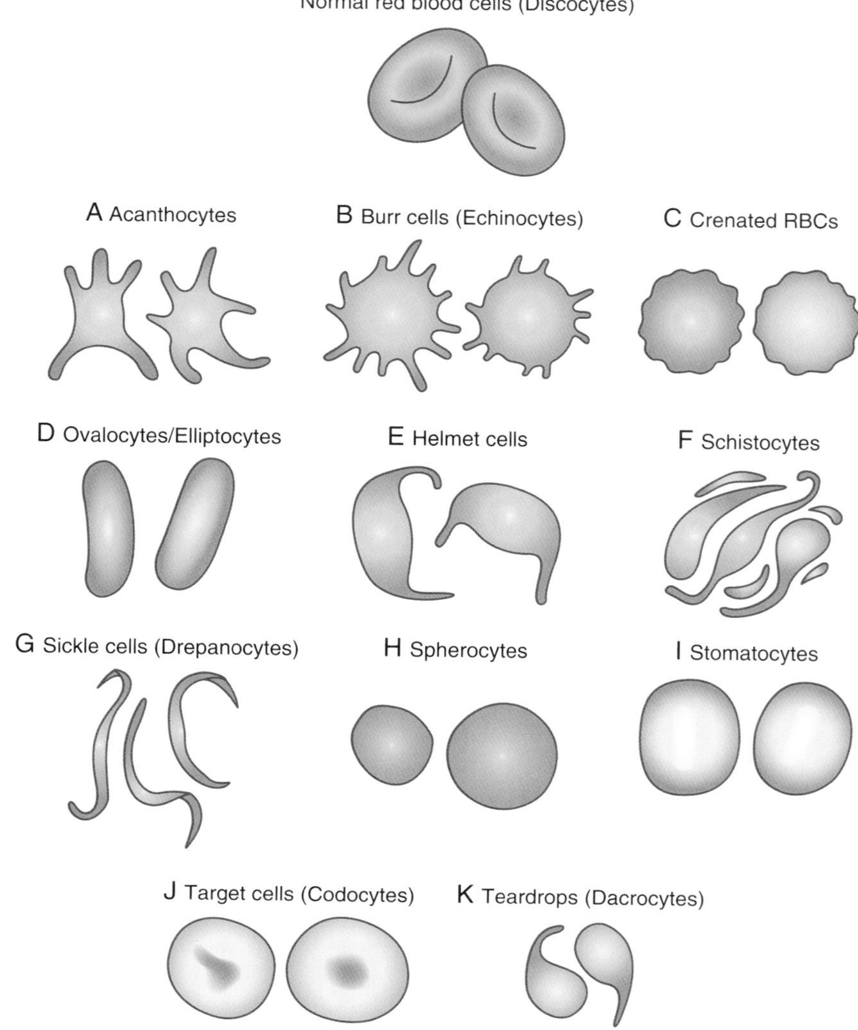

Fig. 11.32 Variations in red blood cell (RBC) shape. Normal red blood cells (discocytes): A, acanthocytes; B, burr cells; C, crenated RBCs; D, ovalocytes/elliptocytes; E, helmet cells; F, schistocytes; G, sickle cells; H, spherocytes; I, stomatocytes; J, target cells; K, teardrops. (Adapted from Turgeon M: *Clinical hematology,* ed 5, Philadelphia, 2011, Lippincott Williams & Wilkins.)

Examples of poikilocytosis include:

- Acanthocytes
- Blister cells
- Burr cells
- Crenated RBCs
- Helmet cells
- Ovalocytes and elliptocytes
- Schistocytes
- Sickle cells
- Spherocytes
- Stomatocytes

1. Target cells
2. Teardrops

Acanthocyte (Thorn, Spike Cell, Spur Cell). Acanthocytes are similar to echinocytes, but their spiny projections are irregularly distributed around the cell membrane (Fig. 11.32A). They are not artifacts and cannot revert to normal cells. Acanthocytes are related to and may occur with schistocytes and represent serious pathologic conditions.

Blister Cell (Marginal Achromatic). Blister cells are RBCs with a clear bubble surrounded by a thin layer of RBC membrane at the periphery of a cell.

Burr Cell (Echinocyte). Burr cells, or echinocytes, are RBCs with spicular, or spiny, projections regularly distributed around the cell membrane (Fig. 11.32B). They can usually revert back to normal cells.

Crenated. Crenated RBCs (Fig. 11.32C) resemble echinocytes with scalloped edges distributed evenly around the cell membrane. These crenated cells are an artifact resulting from incorrect preparation of the blood film, usually failure to dry it adequately.

Elliptocyte and Ovalocyte. Elliptocytes and ovalocytes are oval, or egg shaped, showing varying degrees of elliptical shaping from slightly oval to almost a cylindrical form (Fig. 11.32D).

Large elliptocytes, called *macro-ovalocytes,* are characteristic of megaloblastic anemias. Because of their increased size and thickness, these cells may not show an area of central pallor on the blood film. More elongated forms may occur in a variety of conditions, the most striking and least pathologic being hereditary elliptocytosis.

Helmet Cell. Helmet cells (Fig. 11.32E) are small triangular cells with one or two pointed ends that resemble a helmet.

Schistocyte (Fragmented Cell). Schistocytes have a variety of names and forms, depending on the remaining structure after the cell is physically fragmented (Fig. 11.32F). *Schistocytosis* is a very serious pathologic condition. It may be the result of mechanical fracture of cells while they pass through the circulatory system, as on filaments of fibrin resulting from disseminated intravascular coagulation or on artificial heart valves. Schistocytes are also seen in patients with severe burns. The fragmentation may also be the result of toxic or metabolic injury, as seen with certain malignancies. Schistocytes are characteristic of microangiopathic hemolytic anemias, and their presence is a danger signal requiring immediate action by the physician.

Sickle Cell (Drepanocyte). Sickle cells are typically narrow and shaped like a sickle with two pointed ends (Fig. 11.32G). They may also vary from crescent shaped to bipolar spiculated forms to cells with long, irregular spicules. Sickle cells are the result of a genetic condition in which abnormal HbS is present in a homozygous state in RBCs. Sickling of red cells is enhanced by lack of oxygen. Sickle cells may be found in HbSS or when HbSC or HbS β-thalassemia is present. Sickle cells are not found in sickle trait alone such as HbAS.

Spherocyte. Spherocytes are RBCs that are not biconcave; instead, they appear round or spherical because of the loss of a portion of the cell membrane (Fig. 11.32H). As a result, they are small cells, usually less than 6 μm in diameter, and are often called *microspherocytes.* They appear hyperchromic, staining a uniform intense orange-red because of the lack of central pallor, a result of the round shape. Spherocytes are characteristic of certain hemolytic anemias, both hereditary (hereditary spherocytosis) and acquired, such as drug induced. They also are associated with the presence of polychromasia and an increased reticulocyte count.

Stomatocyte. Stomatocytes show a slitlike or mouthlike, rather than round, area of central pallor on the blood film (Fig. 11.32I). They are not biconcave but bowl shaped, or concave on only one side. They are often found in chronic liver disease.

Target Cell (Codocyte). Target cells resemble targets, showing a peripheral ring of Hb, an area of pallor or clearing, and a central area of Hb (Fig. 11.32J). The codocyte circulates as a bell-shaped cell but takes on the target shape when dried on a slide for morphologic examination. Target cells represent another membrane defect; they have excessive cell membrane in relation to the amount of Hb. They are seen in a variety of clinical conditions, especially in various Hb abnormalities and in chronic liver disease.

Teardrop Cell (Dacryocyte). These pear-shaped or teardrop-shaped RBCs have an elongated point or tail at one end (Fig. 11.32K). They may be the result of the cell squeezing and subsequently fracturing while it passes through the spleen.

4. Red Cell Inclusions

Several inclusions are also seen under certain conditions. Artifacts can appear as inclusions. Examples include:

- Basophilic stippling
- Siderocytes
- Howell-Jolly bodies
- Cabot rings
- Parasitized RBCs
- Platelet on top of erythrocyte
- Punched-out RBCs

Basophilic Stippling. The presence of dark-blue granules evenly distributed throughout the RBC is called *basophilic stippling* (Fig. 11.33). The stippling may be very fine and dotlike, or coarse and larger. The stippled cell may resemble the polychromatophilic erythrocyte, but these are actual granules, not merely an overall blueness. Stippling does not exist in the circulating RBC but results from precipitation of ribosomes and RNA in the staining process. However, the stippling is not an artifact in the clinical sense because it may indicate abnormal erythrocyte formation in the marrow, as in thalassemia minor, megaloblastic anemia, and lead poisoning.

Siderocyte (Pappenheimer Body). Siderocytes contain small, dense, blue-purple granules of free iron uncombined with Hb (Fig. 11.34). Usually, only one or two of these granules are present in a cell, and they are located in the cell periphery. Siderocytes may be confused with Howell-Jolly bodies and can be distinguished and seen better with a specific stain for iron, such as Prussian blue. When siderocytes, or siderosomes, are Wright-stained, they are sometimes called *Pappenheimer bodies.* They are rarely seen in peripheral blood, except after removal of the spleen.

Howell-Jolly Bodies. Howell-Jolly bodies are round, densely staining purple granules that stain similar to dense nuclear chromatin (Fig. 11.35). Usually, only one or two such bodies are seen

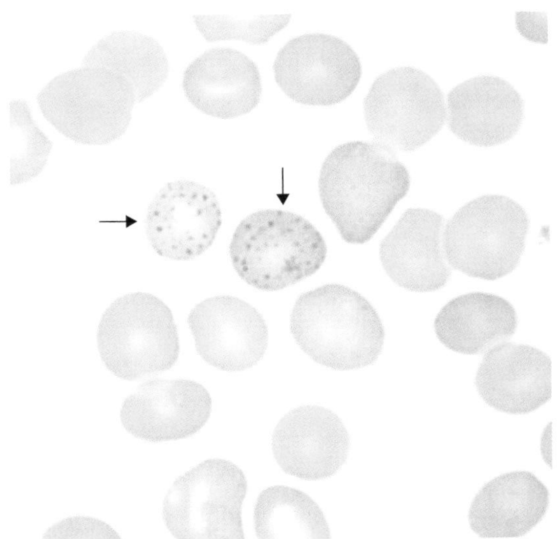

Fig. 11.33 Basophilic stippling in cell *(arrows).* (From Carr JH, Rodak BF: Clinical hematology atlas, ed 3, St Louis, 2009, Saunders.)

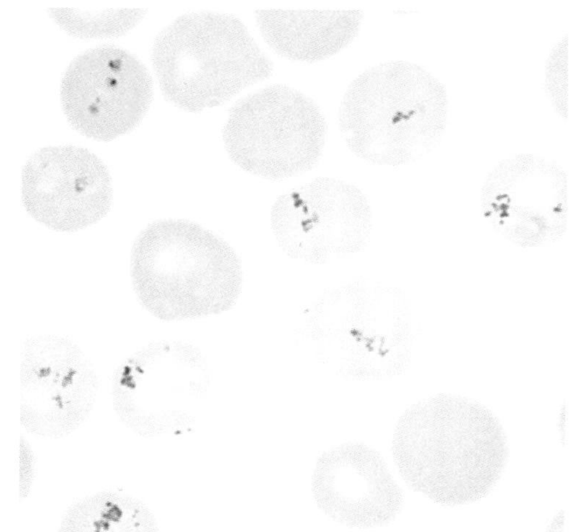

Fig. 11.34 Siderotic granules (iron stain). (From Carr JH, Rodak BF: *Clinical hematology atlas,* ed 3, St Louis, 2009, Saunders.)

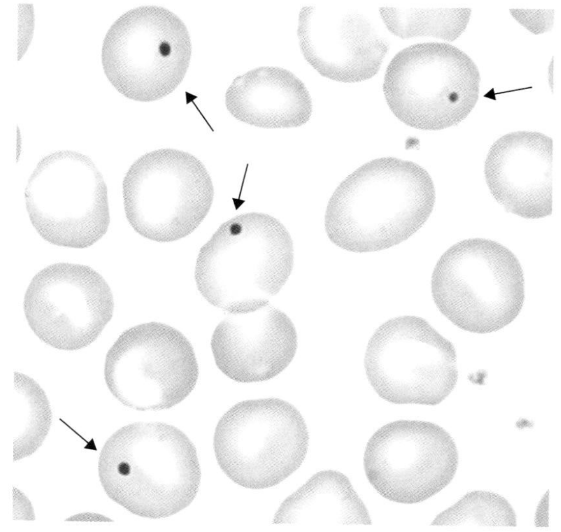

Fig. 11.35 Howell-Jolly bodies shown in cells *(arrows).* (From Carr JH, Rodak BF: *Clinical hematology atlas,* ed 3, St Louis, 2009, Saunders.)

in the RBCs. They are eccentrically located in the RBC and less than 1 μm in diameter. Howell-Jolly bodies are remnants of the erythrocyte nucleus and thus are DNA. Under normal conditions, they are derived from nuclear fragmentation (karyorrhexis) or incomplete expulsion of the nucleus in the later stages of RBC maturation, and they are thought to be aberrant chromosomes in certain abnormal conditions. These nuclear remnants are normally removed from the reticulocytes in the peripheral blood by a pitting process while they pass through the spleen. Therefore they are seen in peripheral blood after removal of the spleen and in cases of abnormal erythrocyte formation, such as megaloblastic anemias and some hemolytic anemias.

Cabot Rings. The threadlike red-violet strands known as *Cabot rings* occur in ring, twisted, or figure-8 shapes in reticulocytes and are rare. Their origin is unknown, but they are thought to result from abnormal erythrocyte formation during mitosis and can be seen in megaloblastic anemias and lead poisoning.

Parasitized Red Cell (Malarial). In patients with malaria, various stages of the malaria parasites may be seen in the erythrocytes (Fig. 11.36). Depending on the species of malaria organism present, the parasites may be confused with Cabot rings, basophilic stippling, or platelets lying on top of RBCs.

Platelet on Top of Erythrocyte. When a platelet rests on top of RBCs in the blood film, it may be confused with inclusions, especially the trophozoite stage of malaria organisms (Fig. 11.37). In such cases, the overlying platelets should be compared with those in the surrounding field. If the platelet is on top of the RBC, neither the platelet nor the RBC can be focused in the same plane, because the platelet is not in the RBC.

Punched-Out Red Cells. Erythrocytes with a punched-out appearance rather than a normal area of central pallor are also

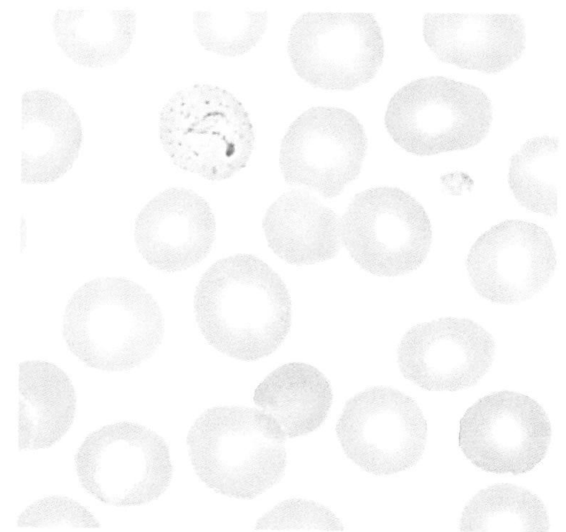

Fig. 11.36 Parasitized red cells (malarial). (From Carr JH, Rodak BF: *Clinical hematology atlas,* ed 3, St Louis, 2009, Saunders.)

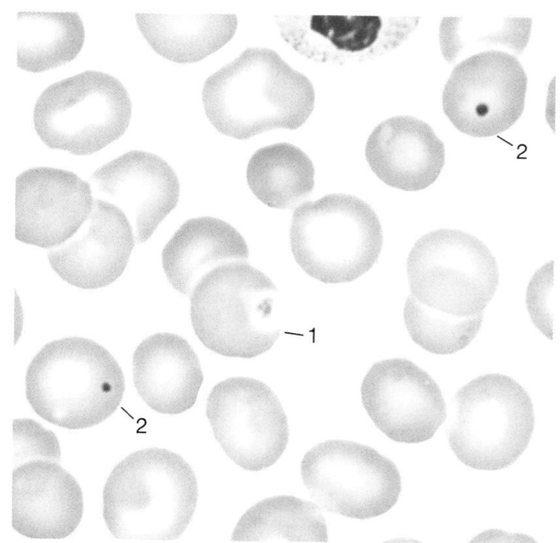

Fig. 11.37 Platelets on red blood cell (1) and Howell-Jolly bodies (2). (From Carr JH, Rodak BF: *Clinical hematology atlas,* ed 3, St Louis, 2009, Saunders.)

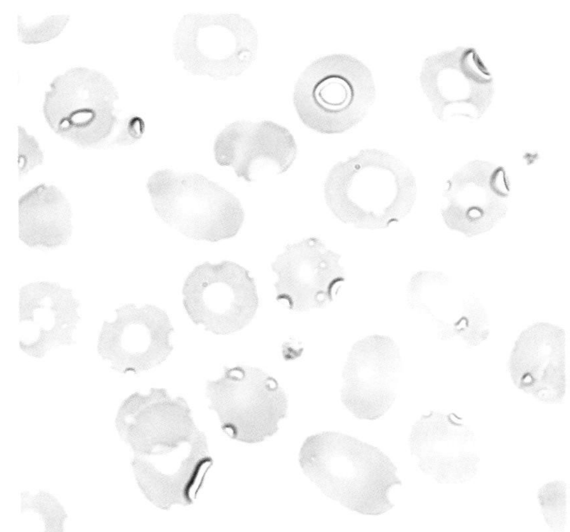

Fig. 11.38 Drying artifact in red cells showing punched-out appearance. (From Carr JH, Rodak BF: *Clinical hematology atlas,* ed 3, St Louis, 2009, Saunders.)

drying artifacts (Fig. 11.38). These should not be confused with hypochromic RBCs. The remaining cell shows a normal staining reaction with this artifact.

5. Abnormal Red Cell Distribution

Abnormal red cell distribution includes rouleaux formation and agglutination.

Rouleaux Formation. Rouleaux represents an abnormal distribution pattern of RBCs, which stick together or become aligned in aggregates that look like stacks of coins (Fig. 11.39). This arrangement is a typical artifact in the thick area of blood films. It is clinically significant when found in the normal examination area and is associated with elevated plasma fibrinogen or globulin, with a corresponding increase in ESR, such as with multiple myeloma.

Agglutination. Agglutination—irregular or amorphous clumping of RBCs in the blood film—represents another alteration in erythrocyte distribution. Clinically, this may be caused by the presence of a cold agglutinin (antibody) in the patient's serum and may indicate an autoimmune hemolytic state or anemia.

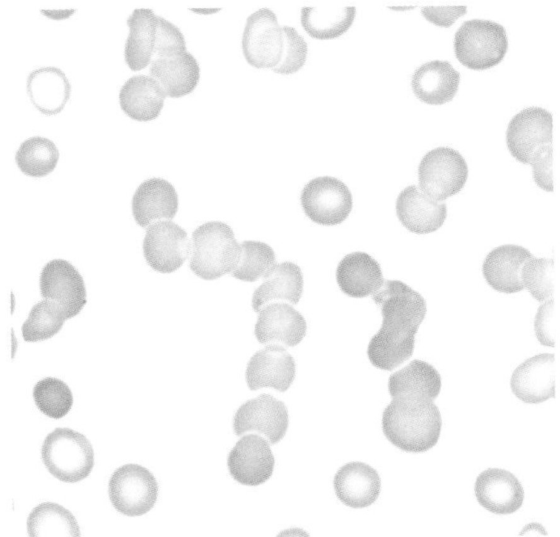

Fig. 11.39 Rouleaux formation, an abnormal distribution pattern. (From Carr JH, Rodak BF: *Clinical hematology atlas,* ed 3, St Louis, 2009, Saunders.)

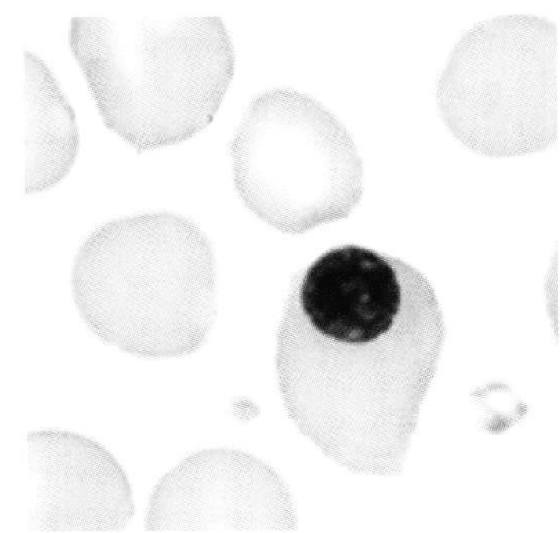

Fig. 11.40 Nucleated red cell (orthochromic normoblast). (From Carr JH, Rodak BF: *Clinical hematology atlas,* ed 3, St Louis, 2009, Saunders.)

6. Presence of Nucleated Red Cells

When nucleated metarubricytes (normoblasts) are seen on the blood film (Fig. 11.40), the number of these cells per 100 WBCs is reported. It is necessary to correct the total WBC count when nucleated RBCs are present (see formula for correction).

Platelet Estimation

Estimate the platelet count and evaluate for morphologic changes. The blood film is examined with the oil-immersion objective to estimate the number of platelets and to detect morphologic alterations. The platelet count is estimated as adequate, decreased, or increased.

Platelets generally vary from 2 to 5 μm in diameter. They are ovoid structures with a colorless to pale-blue background containing centrally located, reddish to violet granules. Platelets are not cells but portions of cytoplasm pinched off from megakaryocytes (giant cells of the bone marrow). Platelets are often increased in size when the blood is being actively regenerated; their size is also a function of age, with younger cells generally being larger. Bizarre forms are also noted after splenectomy and in myelofibrosis, hemorrhagic thrombocytosis, and polycythemia vera. Giant platelets are characteristic of platelet disorders associated with thrombocytopenia and the megaloblastic anemias.

Normally, 6 to 20 platelets should be seen in each oil-immersion field, representing a normal platelet count of 150 to 450 $\times$ 10^9/L. A rough estimate of the platelet count can be made by letting each platelet seen in an oil-immersion field equal approximately 20 $\times$ 10^9/L. The difference in normal values is probably a result of the use of specimens from different sources. The lower value is more consistent with capillary blood, where some of the platelets are used in the clotting mechanism, and the higher value is consistent with anticoagulated venous blood. Estimate the platelet count as adequate, decreased, or increased and report as follows:

a. Report the platelet estimate as adequate if 6 to 20 platelets are seen per oil-immersion field. Several fields should be checked, and the platelets may be estimated while the WBC differential is being done.

b. Report the platelets as decreased if the average number of platelets is less than 6, unless the blood film was prepared on capillary blood. In the latter case, 3 to 5 platelets per oil-immersion field is normal. Before reporting as decreased, scan the slide for clumps of platelets with the low-power objective, especially at the feather edge. If the blood film is well made (without aggregates at the feather edge) and platelets can be found only with great difficulty, the platelet count is below 20×10^9/L, and the estimate should be reported as decreased. In addition, the tube of blood should be rechecked for the presence of clots, because platelets would be used in the clots and the blood film value artificially decreased.
c. Report the platelets as increased if there are more than 20 platelets per oil-immersion field. If many masses of platelets are present at the feather edge, and if platelets in the body of the film are sufficiently abundant to attract the attention of the observer, it is reasonable to assume that the platelet count is increased.
d. Observe the platelet morphology. Report the presence of large, bizarre, or atypical forms. This may be done while the leukocyte differential is performed.

Perform the Differential Count of White Cells

The differential count consists of identifying and counting a minimum of 100 WBCs. After the RBCs and platelets have been examined, the WBCs are classified and counted in the optimal counting area of the blood film under oil immersion.

In certain situations, it may be necessary to count more or fewer than 100 cells. If the relative numbers of specific types of WBCs differ greatly from the accepted normal values, it is advisable to count 200 cells or more before recording percentages. Specifically, 200 cells should be counted if more than 5% of the cells are eosinophils, if more than 2% are basophils, if more than 10% are monocytes, or if the percentage of lymphocytes is greater than 50%. If the differential for an adult with a normal WBC count shows fewer than 15 or more than 40 lymphocytes, an additional 100 cells should be counted on another blood film to rule out distribution errors.

In cases of leukopenia, if the WBC count is less than 1×10^9/L, only 50 cells need to be counted in the leukocyte differential. When such changes are made, the percentages of the different cell types must be calculated, and the number of cells actually counted in the differential must be noted on the report form, for example, "3% basophils, 200 cells counted." Occasionally, the absolute number of cells of each type is of interest, although values are usually reported as percentages. To calculate the absolute value, multiply the percentage of each cell type, expressed as a decimal, by the total WBC count.

Examine the Leukocytes for Morphologic Alterations

All WBCs in the circulating blood should be mature. The presence of immature WBCs in the blood is considered abnormal. Immature WBCs may be differentiated from mature cells by size; by the appearance of intracellular structures such as granules; by changes in nucleoli, chromatin, or nucleus; and by staining properties.

There is a progressive decrease in cell size with maturity, with the nucleus becoming smaller and the N/C ratio decreasing. In granulocytes, granules appear with maturity. In immature WBCs the nucleus is round; with age it becomes lobular or indented. Chromatin is fine and lacy in the young cell and eventually becomes coarse and clumped. Nucleoli may be present in young cells and absent in the mature forms. The cytoplasm is basophilic (stains blue) in young granulocytes and eventually turns pink with maturity. The young nucleus stains reddish violet and becomes strongly basophilic with maturity. The granules in the cytoplasm assume specific staining qualities with increasing cell maturity.

Certain evidence of cell function is observed that is characteristic of specific developmental stages of the WBCs. Examples are the presence of nucleoli, which indicate a young cell; mitotic figures, which indicate a young cell; cytoplasmic inclusions, which are characteristic of a mature cell; and phagocytosis, seen in mature cells (see Granulocyte Alterations).

When the WBCs are being classified and counted, any morphologic alterations or abnormalities should be noted. A WBC cannot be skipped simply because it cannot be identified. Experience is necessary for morphologic studies of WBCs, especially when an immature or abnormal cell is seen. Persons with limited training in hematology should not attempt to identify abnormal WBCs. Persons with limited training should be able to identify and classify normal WBCs, but should be encouraged to seek assistance when a questionable cell is seen.

Types of Anemias

Clinically, alterations in erythrocyte morphology are associated with many diseases and especially with anemia. Anemia is not a specific disease, but a condition in which there is a decrease in the oxygen-carrying capacity of the blood and therefore in the amount of oxygen reaching the tissues and organs. Its causes are many and varied, and the type of anemia present and its underlying cause must be determined before treatment can be effectively undertaken. It may or may not be the result of a disorder of the blood or blood-forming tissues.

Clinically, all patients with anemia have similar symptoms or complaints, regardless of the cause of the anemia. The severity generally depends on the Hb concentration of the blood, because most symptoms result from the decreased oxygen-carrying capacity. The primary complaints are fatigue and shortness of breath. Other common complaints are faintness, dizziness, heart palpitation, and headache.

Once the existence of anemia has been demonstrated, usually on the basis of the blood Hb concentration, the underlying cause must be determined. In addition, the case history, physical examination, and various laboratory procedures, including the appearance of the RBCs on the peripheral blood film, are helpful in establishing the diagnosis.

Anemias can be classified according to either the appearance of the RBCs (morphologic classification) or the physiologic cause of the anemia (etiologic or pathogenic classification) (Table 11.11). Morphologically, anemias are generally classified as follows:

TABLE 11.11 Etiologic Classification of Anemias

Type	Example
Blood Loss	
Acute	Trauma
Chronic	Colon cancer
Impaired Production	
Aplastic anemia	Radiation exposure
Iron deficiency anemia	Excessive menstrual bleeding
Sideroblastic anemia	Faulty iron utilization
Anemia of chronic diseases	Cancer
Megaloblastic anemia	Pernicious anemia
Hemolytic Anemia	
Inherited defects	Hereditary spherocytosis
Acquired disorders	Hemolytic disease of the newborn
Hemolytic-hemoglobin disorders	Sickle cell anemia, thalassemias

1. Normochromic-normocytic
2. Macrocytic
3. Hypochromic-microcytic

Normochromic-Normocytic Anemias

Normochromic-normocytic anemias are characterized by normal-appearing RBCs on the peripheral blood film and RBC indices within the reference range. The cells produced by the marrow are normal, but the number of cells in circulation is reduced for a variety of reasons, including acute blood loss. Conditions resulting in increased plasma volume, such as overhydration, will also result in normochromic-normocytic anemia. If the bone marrow is suppressed (hypoplastic), as seen in cases of aplastic anemia, the RBCs that remain are normal, although the number is decreased. Suppressed marrow results in a deficiency of the myeloid series, which is seen as decreased leukocyte and platelet counts. If the marrow is infiltrated with a neoplasm or malignancy, such as leukemia or multiple myeloma, the remaining RBCs appear normal but are decreased in number. In certain hemolytic diseases and chronic kidney and liver diseases, the erythrocytes appear normal but also are reduced in number.

Macrocytic Anemias

Macrocytic anemias are represented primarily by the megaloblastic anemias resulting from vitamin B_{12} or folic acid deficiency, or both. The deficiency may be nutritional or may result from a malabsorption syndrome such as PA, in which the patient is unable to absorb vitamin B_{12}. In either case, the deficiency leads to a nuclear maturation defect and megaloblastic anemia. The marrow shows certain changes in the myeloid series, including the erythrocytes, granulocytes, and megakaryocytes (platelets). Megaloblastic changes are characterized by larger cells having a more open chromatin pattern in the nucleus and by the presence of larger, hypersegmented mature neutrophils in the peripheral blood. The enlarged RBCs (macrocytes) have MCV values of 120 to 140 fL. Actual hyperchromasia is impossible, but the RBCs appear to contain more Hb because of their increased size and therefore thickness. Although the anemia may be severe, the RBC count is decreased more than the Hb concentration, because the cells that are present are large and almost completely filled with Hb. Other changes seen in the blood film include anisocytosis (erythrocytes varying in size), poikilocytosis (erythrocytes varying in shape), and Howell-Jolly bodies.

Nutritional deficiency of vitamin B_{12} is relatively rare, but nutritional deficiency of folic acid is fairly common. It may be found in chronic alcoholism or other conditions in which the diet is not well balanced. Folate deficiency is observed also when the requirement is increased, as in pregnancy, infancy, certain hemolytic anemias, and hyperthyroidism. Celiac disease, tropical sprue, certain drugs, contraceptives, and liver disease may lead to malabsorption and megaloblastic anemia.

Megaloblastic erythrocytes have an abnormal developmental sequence. Although it is similar to the sequence of maturation in normoblasts, megaloblasts are larger. As they develop, cells of the megaloblastic sequence have a more open or immature chromatin pattern in the nucleus, referred to as *asynchronous maturation* or *dyssynchronous development* of the nucleus and cytoplasm. In megaloblastic anemia, these changes are not limited to the erythrocyte series; all types of cells normally produced in the bone marrow are similarly affected, as evidenced by large, hypersegmented neutrophils. Lymphocytes are unaffected, and a small lymphocyte is a useful visual size marker.

Hypochromic-Microcytic Anemias

Hypochromic-microcytic anemias can be the most common types encountered, with iron deficiency anemia being the type most frequently seen. Iron deficiency is not a simple classification, because there are several possible causes of this clinical condition. In simplified terms, iron deficiency anemia may result from the following:

- Decreased iron intake (either from inadequate diet or impaired absorption) (Fig. 11.41)
- Increased iron loss (generally from chronic bleeding from a variety of causes)
- An error of iron metabolism (sideroblastic anemias)
- Increased iron requirements in infancy, pregnancy, and lactation

The cause of the anemia must be determined (Fig. 11.42) to treat it. If it results from a dietary deficiency of iron, a relatively simple and effective treatment is to administer iron, usually orally as ferrous sulfate tablets. However, if it is caused by another condition, the administration of iron will be ineffective and may do harm either in itself, such as in the anemias of chronic disorders or thalassemias, in which iron overload is a possibility, or because it delays the use of appropriate therapy.

If the iron deficiency anemia results from chronic bleeding, the cause of the bleeding must be determined. The bleeding is most often gastrointestinal, although women with excessive menstrual flow often develop iron deficiency anemia. Gastrointestinal bleeding leading to iron deficiency anemia may result from such causes as ulcer, carcinoma or other neoplasms, hemorrhoids, hookworm, or even the ingestion of salicylate (usually as aspirin). The treatment is different for each of these causes.

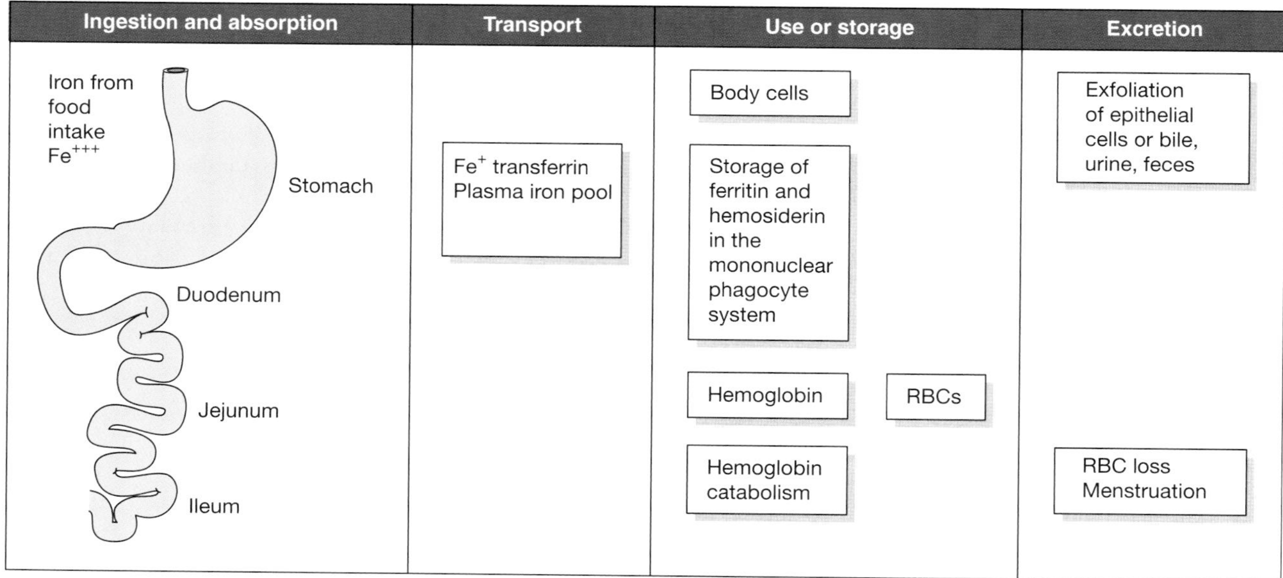

Fig. 11.41 Iron physiology. (From Turgeon M: *Clinical hematology,* ed 5, Philadelphia, 2011, Lippincott Williams & Wilkins.)

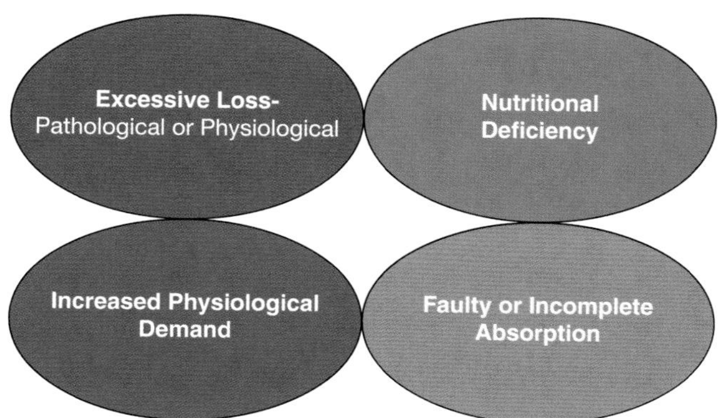

Fig. 11.42 Factors in iron deficiency. (From Turgeon M: *Clinical hematology,* ed 5, Philadelphia, 2011, Lippincott Williams & Wilkins.)

All iron deficiency anemias produce similar changes in erythrocyte morphology. The RBCs are smaller than normal (microcytic), and MCV is decreased. Unfortunately, the decreased size is not always as apparent on the blood film as it is in the MCV value. In iron deficiency anemia, the amount of Hb within each RBC is significantly decreased; such cells are hypochromic (deficient in color). This appears in the RBC volume, which is primarily a function of Hb, but may not be evident on the slide because the hypochromic RBC spreads out or flattens and may appear to be of normal size or even larger than normal. The hypochromic cell is extremely pale, showing only a thin rim of color with a significantly increased area of central pallor, which occupies more than one-third of the cell. The decreased Hb per RBC is measured in the laboratory as decreased MCH and MCHC. Other changes characteristic of iron deficiency anemia include anisocytosis and poikilocytosis, which vary in degree with the severity of the disease and are reflected by an increased RDW. Other tests that may be useful in the investigation of iron deficiency anemias include examination of the stool for occult blood, determination of serum iron and total iron-binding capacity, radiographic study of the gastrointestinal tract, and, rarely, bone marrow examination.

Another group of anemias, which demonstrate mild to severe microcytosis and hypochromia, consists of disorders in the synthesis of globin, a component of the Hb molecule. These are the thalassemias, a group of inherited disorders of Hb synthesis. Microcytosis, hypochromasia, and basophilic stippling are general observations. Anisocytosis, poikilocytosis, and target cells may be present and decreased osmotic fragility. Actual differentiation of α and β forms of thalassemia require additional laboratory testing.

Hypochromic-microcytic anemias also include those resulting from disorders of porphyrin and heme synthesis. As a result, the Hb molecule is malformed. The sideroblastic anemias are a heterogeneous group of disorders that have in common increased storage of iron, especially in the mononuclear phagocytic system. The bone marrow in these conditions shows sideroblasts, nucleated RBCs with granules of iron that can be demonstrated with Prussian blue stain. The granules occur characteristically in a full or partial ring around the nucleus. Besides microcytosis and hypochromasia, the peripheral blood from these patients shows siderocytes, nonnucleated RBCs with granules of iron. Because the body is already overloaded with iron that is not being used appropriately, iron therapy in these anemias would be harmful to the patient.

A number of chemicals cause sideroblastic anemias by inhibiting heme synthesis. Lead poisoning produces an anemia that is characteristically mildly microcytic and hypochromic and is often characterized by basophilic stippling of the RBCs. It is most often seen in children who have ingested lead paint chips and may be seen in adults with industrial exposure to lead.

Hemolytic Anemias

One problem with a morphologic classification of anemias is that it does not deal conveniently with a broad etiologic class of anemias, the hemolytic anemias. These are sometimes classified as normochromic-normocytic based on calculated indices. However, RDW is greatly increased in hemolytic anemia because of anisocytosis and poikilocytosis, unlike in the other normochromic-normocytic anemias. In addition, because of the increased number of young RBCs (reticulocytes), which are larger than mature cells, MCV is increased in hemolytic anemia, although not as much as for the megaloblastic anemias.

The hemolytic anemias are generally classified as congenital or acquired. They are characterized by increased destruction or hemolysis of RBCs from a variety of causes, accompanied by increased erythrocyte production by the bone marrow. This is seen as polychromasia and even nucleated forms of RBCs on Wright-stained blood films and as increased reticulocyte counts. Anisocytosis and poikilocytosis with increased RDW are characteristic of hemolytic anemias in general. An inherited form of spherocytic anemia, hereditary spherocytosis, results from an inherited erythrocyte abnormality and is characterized by spherocytes in the peripheral blood. This condition is indistinguishable morphologically from certain acquired disorders that result in spherocytic anemia. In such cases, a useful laboratory test is the direct antiglobulin test (DAT), formerly called the *Coombs test.*

The DAT is used to detect RBCs that have been coated with antibodies. This is one of the most useful procedures for distinguishing immune from nonimmune mechanisms that can underlie hemolytic anemias. When RBCs are precoated with an antibody, the DAT usually will be positive unless the amount of antibody on the cell membrane is too small. Erythrocytes can become sensitized when an autoimmune process is in effect. In this type of disorder, antibodies are produced by the patient's own immune system and react with specific antigens on the patient's own RBCs. These anemias can be temperature induced or drug induced.

Other changes of shape (poikilocytosis) are characteristic of certain hemolytic anemias. Elliptocytes are characteristic of hereditary elliptocytosis, an erythrocyte membrane disorder. Sickle cells are characteristic of sickle cell anemia, an inherited Hb abnormality. Schistocytes, or fragmented cells, are characteristic of the microangiopathic hemolytic anemias and may be produced by mechanical fragmentation resulting from an intravascular pathologic condition or intravascular coagulation.

Leukocyte Alterations

Quantitative changes in leukocytes are measured by the WBC count, the actual number of leukocytes in a certain volume of blood. Again, a WBC count above normal is called *leukocytosis;* a count below normal is called *leukopenia.* There can also be increases or decreases in number of any of the five WBC types enumerated collectively in the WBC count, and such changes are measured by the white cell differential. Quantitative changes in any of the cell types are described by the following terms: *neutrophilia* (increase) or *neutropenia* (decrease), *eosinophilia* or *eosinopenia, basophilia* or *basopenia, lymphocytosis* or *lymphopenia,* and *monocytosis* or *monocytopenia.*

In addition, these increases or decreases may be relative or absolute. If the change is *absolute,* the particular cell type shows a numeric increase or decrease from its normal concentration in the blood. If it is *relative,* there is an alteration (either high or low) of the percentage of the particular cell type, as determined in the leukocyte differential, whereas the numerical concentration is within normal values. Finally, there may be both an absolute and a relative change when both the percentage and the numeric values are above or below normal.

The term *shift to the left* refers to the presence of younger or more immature granulocytic (usually neutrophilic) cell forms than are normally found in the peripheral blood.

Granulocyte Alterations

Most alterations in leukocyte morphology can be classified as (1) toxic or reactive changes, (2) anomalous changes, or (3) leukemic or other malignant changes.

Toxic Changes and Granulocyte Alterations

Toxic changes are seen in neutrophils and are generally associated with a bacterial infection or a toxic reaction. Changes in the cytoplasm are seen on a blood film as toxic granulation, vacuolization, or the presence of Döhle bodies.

Döhle Bodies. Döhle bodies are round or oval, small, clear, light-blue–staining areas found in the neutrophil cytoplasm. They are remnants of cytoplasmic RNA from an earlier stage of neutrophil development and are often seen together with toxic granulation in infections, in burns, after administration of toxic agents, and in pregnancy.

Toxic Granulation. Toxic granules are deeply staining basophilic or blue-black, larger-than-normal granules found in the cytoplasm of neutrophils, bands, and metamyelocytes (Fig. 11.43). They resemble the primary granules seen in the promyelocyte, an early developmental stage of the neutrophil.

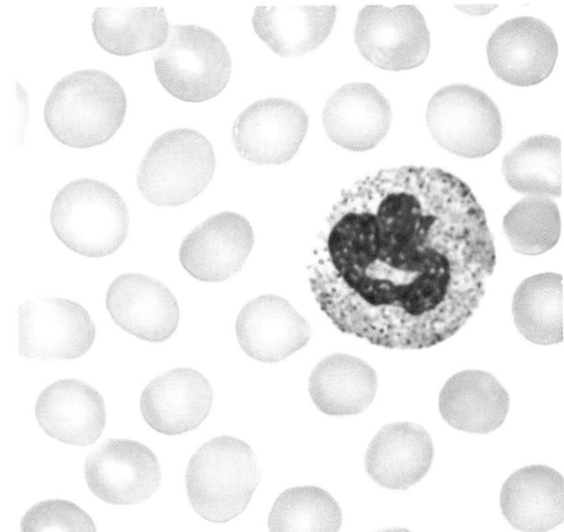

Fig. 11.43 Polymorphonuclear toxic granulation. (From Carr JH, Rodak BF: *Clinical hematology atlas,* ed 3, St Louis, 2009, Saunders.)

Their presence is associated with acute bacterial infections, drug poisoning, and burns.

Toxic Vacuolization. Vacuoles are also signs of toxic change and imply the occurrence of phagocytosis. Sites of digestion of phagocytized material are seen as vacuoles in the cytoplasm of neutrophils and bands, and vacuoles are often found in association with toxic granulation.

Granulocyte Nuclear Alterations

Auer Rods (Bodies). Auer rods or bodies are slender rod-shaped or needle-shaped bodies found in the cytoplasm; they stain reddish purple, similar to azurophilic granules (Fig. 11.44), and are composed of lysosomal material and fused primary granules. Auer rods can be observed in the cytoplasms of myeloblasts or monoblasts, and are considered diagnostic in distinguishing myeloblastic from lymphoblastic leukemias.

Barr Bodies. A Barr body is a small knob attached to or projecting from a lobe of the neutrophil nucleus and consisting of the same nuclear chromatin or substance. It is often referred to as the *sex chromatin* or *sex chromosome* because it is seen in some neutrophils of normal females and is thought to be an inactivated X chromosome.

Hypersegmentation of Nucleus. Neutrophils that are hypersegmented contain six or more lobes in their nuclei. They are characteristic of the megaloblastic anemias of vitamin B_{12} and folic acid deficiency and have been called PA neutrophils. The megaloblastic neutrophil is larger than a normal-sized neutrophil.

Anomalous Changes

An *anomaly* is a "deviation from the rule" or an irregularity. Hematologic deviations from normal may be congenital or acquired.

Pelger-Huët Anomaly. Pelger-Huët anomaly is seen as a failure of the granulocyte nucleus to segment or form lobes normally (hyposegmentation). The neutrophil nuclei are band shaped or at most have two lobes. In addition, the chromatin is quite coarsely clumped. This is a benign anomaly that can be inherited or acquired. In its acquired form, it is known as pseudo–Pelger-Huët anomaly.

Chédiak-Higashi Anomaly. In Chédiak-Higashi anomaly, large amorphous granules are observed in the neutrophil cytoplasm; granules are also seen in the lymphocyte and monocyte cytoplasm. This syndrome is inherited and rare, and patients have been treated with bone marrow transplantation.

May-Hegglin Anomaly. May-Hegglin anomaly is inherited, and most patients have no clinical symptoms. Blue inclusion bodies similar to Döhle bodies are present in neutrophils but are usually larger and have more sharply defined borders. Platelets may be decreased in number, but some giant forms can be present.

Alder-Reilly Anomaly. Alder-Reilly anomaly is inherited and often associated with mucopolysaccharidoses. Heavy, dark, azurophilic granulation is observed in neutrophils, eosinophils, basophils, and sometimes lymphocytes and monocytes.

Lymphocyte Alterations

Variant Lymphocytes (Reactive or Atypical Lymphocytes)

Reactive, atypical, or variant lymphocytes (Fig. 11.45) are associated with viral infections such as infectious mononucleosis. In general, the cytoplasm increases in amount and appears to be reacting to a stimulus. The cytoplasm tends to become more intensely blue in color (cytoplasmic basophilia). The basophilia tends to be localized, either *peripherally,* with an increased blue color around the outer edge of the cell, or *radially,* with areas of blueness radiating from the more central nucleus to the outer edges of the cell like spokes of a wheel. The reactive cell may also show increases or decreases in cytoplasmic volume. Cells with increased cytoplasmic volume, when observed on films prepared with Wright stain, tend to show indentations by adjacent structures, especially RBCs. The cytoplasm appears to be flowing around and almost engulfing such structures. The cells also tend to have an increased number of nonspecific azurophilic granules in the cytoplasm.

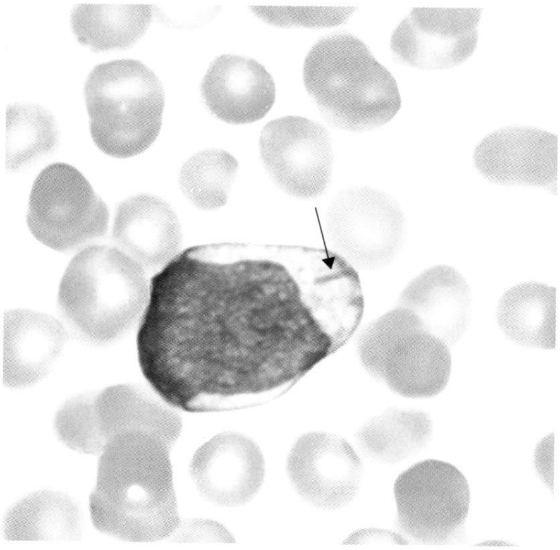

Fig. 11.44 Auer rod *(arrow)* in myeloblast. (From Carr JH, Rodak BF: *Clinical hematology atlas,* ed 3, St Louis, 2009, Saunders.)

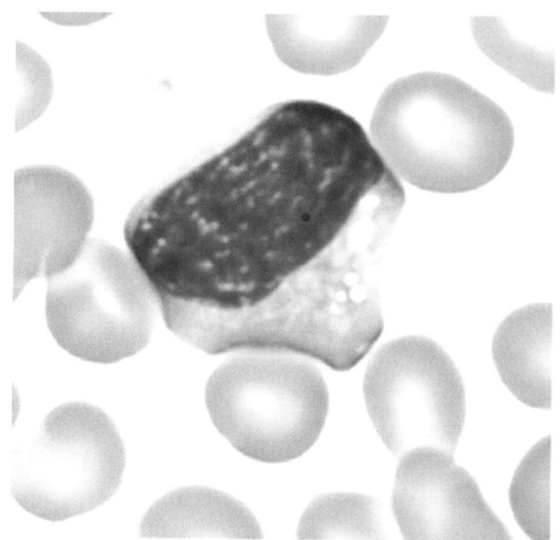

Fig. 11.45 Reactive lymphocyte. (From Carr JH, Rodak BF: *Clinical hematology atlas,* ed 3, St Louis, 2009, Saunders.)

Reactive or atypical lymphocytes also show nuclear changes. There is generally a sharper separation of chromatin and parachromatin. The nucleus may become loose and delicate, resembling an earlier developmental stage. In other cases, the nucleus becomes oval or kidney shaped with heavy clumps of deeply stained chromatin and resemble plasma cells. The reactive lymphocyte may resemble the lymphoblast, and it may be necessary to rule out leukemia.

Smudge or basket cells are damaged WBCs. Smudge cells are cellular fragments consisting of battered or frayed nuclei with no cytoplasm. Smudge cells are not counted as part of the WBC differential. Smudge cells are not significant unless present in large numbers. They may be associated with chronic lymphocytic leukemia (CLL).

Malignant or Leukemic Changes

The hematologic malignancies include a large and varied group of diseases. The leukemias may be classified as follows:

1. Acute myelogenous leukemia (AML), also known as acute nonlymphoblastic leukemia
2. Chronic myeloproliferative disorders, including CML
3. Acute lymphoblastic leukemia (ALL)
4. Chronic lymphoproliferative disorders, including CLL and lymphomas

Most leukemias exist as an abnormal, uncontrolled proliferation of one or more of the various hematopoietic cells that progressively displace normal cellular elements. In the case of CLL, the abnormality is a condition of lymphocyte accumulation in the blood and organs caused by a defect in apoptosis.

Classification

Leukemias are classified morphologically as *lymphocytic* (or lymphoid) and *myelogenous* (or myeloid). The youngest cell forms, or blasts, common to these leukemias are the lymphoblast and the myeloblast, respectively. It may be impossible to distinguish between the two types of blasts morphologically. The presence of Auer rods (rods or granules of lysosomal material, an azurophilic substance) in the cytoplasm is characteristically diagnostic of the myeloblast. However, Auer rods are not seen in all cases of myelogenous leukemia. Other considerations in the differentiation of myeloblasts and lymphoblasts are the N/C ratio, the number of nucleoli, and the nuclear chromatin pattern, but these differences are often inconclusive and may be misleading. If more mature cells are present, they may aid in the morphologic identification.

Leukemias can be classified as acute or chronic on the basis of clinical course (prognosis) and the number of blasts present. Acute leukemias usually occur with sudden onset.

The patient usually has anemia that increases while the disease progresses. The platelet count is low to greatly decreased. The leukocyte count varies but is usually moderately to extremely elevated, with 50 to 100 $\times$ 10^9/L possible, although the count may be normal or even decreased. Blast cells are present in the peripheral blood film; generally, a total of more than 60% blasts indicates an acute leukemic process. The bone marrow is hypercellular and consists predominantly of blast cells. Untreated acute leukemias can lead to death within 2 to 3 months. Death is often the result of hemorrhage, which increases in severity while the platelet count falls below 20 $\times$ 10^9/L, or the result of infection, which develops while the granulocyte count falls below 1.5 $\times$ 10^9/L. Treatment includes chemotherapy, transfusion therapy, and bone marrow transplantation.

Epidemiology

Leukemia can occur at any age, but certain forms appear to be age related. AML (Fig. 11.46) occurs at all ages but is a disease primarily of middle age. In contrast, ALL is generally a disease of children younger than 10 (seldom older than 20 years) and peaks between the ages of 3 and 7. ALL (Fig. 11.47) is the most prevalent form of malignancy in children. CML (Fig. 11.48) usually occurs between ages 20 and 50. CLL (Fig. 11.49) is generally a disease of later adult years, typically older than 50. Treatment is usually only for complications of the disease.

Etiology

The exact cause of leukemia is unknown. Evidence suggests hereditary factors and genetic predisposition. Environmental causes have also been cited, especially exposure to gamma radiation, producing genetic mutations or chromosome damage, such as the Philadelphia chromosome seen in CML. Various chemicals and drugs have also been implicated, and viruses have been related to leukemia in mice and other animals. The chronic myeloproliferative disorders are a group of myeloid neoplasms in which there is malignant clonal proliferation of predominantly myeloid cells in the marrow and blood. These may be cells of the granulocytic, erythrocytic, or megakaryocytic cell lines. Diseases

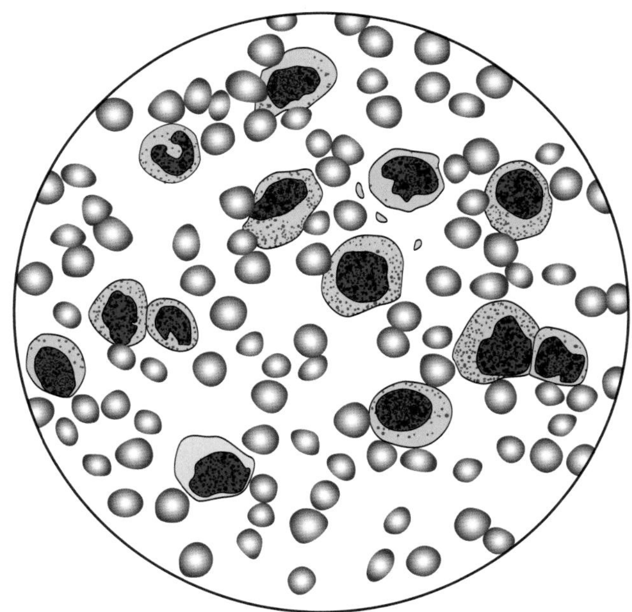

Fig. 11.46 Acute myeloid leukemia. Increased numbers of immature cells are seen in acute leukemias. The predominating cells in this peripheral blood smear are myeloblasts and promyelocytes. The number of platelets (thrombocytes) is severely decreased. (Simulates magnification 1000×) (From Turgeon M: *Clinical hematology,* ed 5, Philadelphia, 2011, Lippincott Williams & Wilkins, Fig. 19.2, p. 309.)

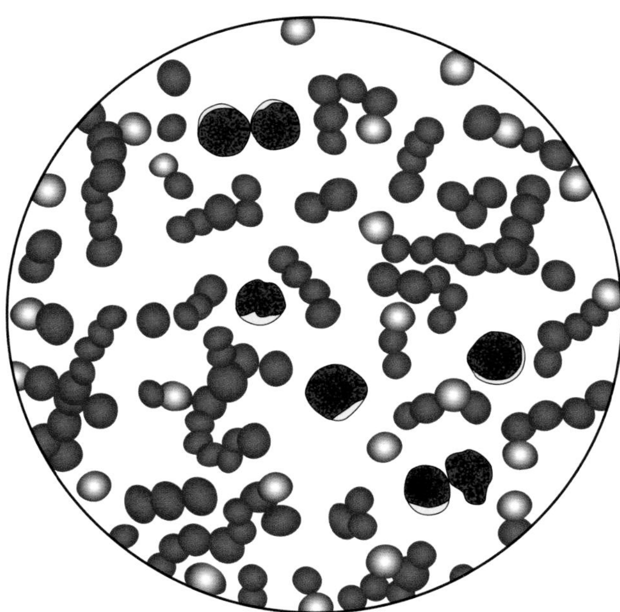

Fig. 11.47 Acute lymphoblastic leukemia. Increased numbers of immature cells are seen in acute leukemias. The predominating cell in this peripheral blood smear is the lymphoblast. Blood platelets (thrombocytes) are completely absent from this field of the smear. (Simulates magnification 1000×) (From Turgeon M: *Clinical hematology,* ed 5, Philadelphia, 2011, Lippincott Williams & Wilkins, Fig. 19.17, p. 318.)

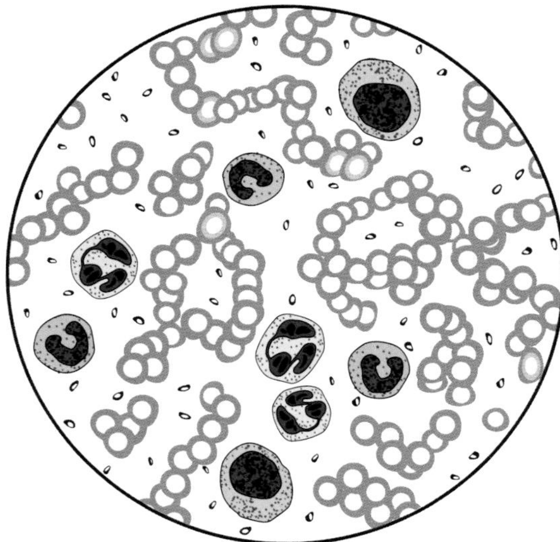

Fig. 11.48 Chronic myelogenous leukemia. Most of the cells in this field are mature granulocytes (band forms and segmented neutrophils). An increased number of platelets (thrombocytes) is also seen in this field of the smear. (Simulates magnification 1000×) (From Turgeon M: *Clinical hematology,* ed 5, Philadelphia, 2011, Lippincott Williams & Wilkins, Fig. 21.4, p. 366.)

include CML (neutrophilic), polycythemia vera (erythrocytic), and essential thrombocythemia (megakaryocytic).

Signs and Symptoms

Chronic leukemias (myeloproliferative or lymphoproliferative disorders) begin slowly and insidiously, and may exist for a long

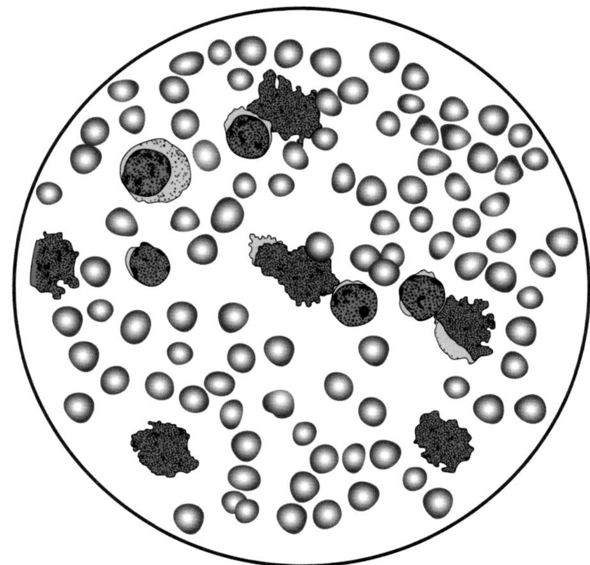

Fig. 11.49 Chronic lymphocytic leukemia. Mature cells predominate in the chronic leukemias. In this blood smear, a typical increase in the number of smudge cells is seen. (Simulates magnification 1000×) (From Turgeon M: *Clinical hematology,* ed 5, Philadelphia, 2011, Lippincott Williams & Wilkins.)

time without symptoms. Symptoms develop slowly and include fatigue, night sweats, weight loss, and fever.

Anemia usually develops late in the disease, but hemolytic anemia may develop while the disease progresses. The platelet count is usually normal and may even increase in CML; in the later stages, however, both thrombocytopenia and anemia usually occur. The WBC count is usually greatly increased, often higher than 100×10^9/L, but it can be normal or even decreased. Morphologically, fewer than 10% myeloblasts will be seen in the peripheral blood in CML, and the blood tends to look similar to bone marrow because it contains all granulocyte developmental stages plus basophilia, an important finding. In CLL, very few to no lymphoblasts are seen in the peripheral blood. The blood characteristically shows a monotonous picture of lymphocytes that are all similar in size and morphology. In addition, many damaged or smudge cells may be present because the lymphocytes tend to be fragile.

Laboratory Testing

Traditionally, morphologic criteria have been used to classify leukemias. The use of cytochemical and histochemical staining techniques and immunologic markers now makes it possible to identify abnormal hematopoietic precursors with more assurance. A testing battery of special studies using staining and immunologic methods is employed as part of the complete workup for a patient with leukemia. In the past, special stains were used; these included myeloperoxidase, Sudan black stain, leukocyte alkaline phosphatase activity, TdT enzyme activity, nonspecific and specific esterase activity, and the periodic acid–Schiff reaction. These tests are used to classify the acute leukemias in the French-American-British system. Today, flow cytometry is used to identify the presence of specific cluster designation cell surface membrane markers that are diagnostic.

Prognosis

The average length of survival for patients with an acute leukemia, if untreated, is measured in months. Drug therapy and bone marrow transplantation may extend a patient's life span. The average length of survival for patients with CML averages 3 to 4 years. However, since the introduction of imatinib (Gleevec, Novartis Pharmaceuticals, Basel, Switzerland), many patients in the chronic phase of CML have achieved at least one remission, which has extended life expectancy.

CML tends to proceed to an acute or accelerated stage called a *blast crisis,* and patients eventually die of hemorrhage or infection, as in acute leukemia. CLL has an average survival of about 10 years, although prolonged survival for up to 35 years is possible, and about 30% of patients die of causes unrelated to the disease. Infection is the most common cause of death related to CLL.

Other Malignant Changes

Malignant hematologic conditions other than leukemia include plasma cell dyscrasias (multiple myeloma, primary macroglobulinemia, Fc fragment or heavy-chain disease), Hodgkin disease (or malignant lymphoma, Hodgkin type), non-Hodgkin malignant lymphomas, and some unusual tumors closely resembling hematologic malignancies.

CASE STUDIES

CASE STUDY 11.1

A 25-year-old woman has a 2-month history of difficulty in breathing and extreme fatigue. She has been on a "fad" diet for the past 6 months.

Physical examination revealed no enlargement of the spleen or liver. Laboratory data are:

Hb: 6.0 g/dL
Hct: 18%
WBC count: 3.3×10^9/L
WBC differential:
- Neutrophils: 10%
- Lymphocytes: 80%
- Monocytes: 10%
- Eosinophils, basophils: 0%

RBC count: 2.00×10^{12}/L
- RDW: 12
- Platelet count: 13.0×10^9/L
- Reticulocyte count: 0.6%

Multiple Choice Questions

Answers are in Appendix A.

1. This patient's MCV is ___ fL.
   a. 90
   b. 85
   c. 80
   d. 75
2. This patient's MCH is ___ pg.
   a. 30
   b. 28
   c. 26
   d. 24
3. This patient's difficulty in breathing and extreme tiredness are most directly caused by:
   a. Low hemoglobin
   b. Low platelet count
   c. Low reticulocyte count
   d. Low white cell count

Critical Thinking Group Discussion Questions

1. Describe the factors that will assist you in classifying this anemia morphologically.
2. What is the most probable type of anemia seen in this patient, and what laboratory value supports this type of anemia?

Note: Answers to narrative questions posted on EVOLVE instructor site.

CASE STUDY 11.2

An 80-year-old man is seen for an annual physical examination. He complains of shortness of breath on exertion and is often tired. His stool is black. Laboratory data are:

Hb: 8.2 g/dL
Hct: 30%
WBC count: 4.2×10^9/L
WBC differential:
- Neutrophils: 60%
- Lymphocytes: 31%
- Monocytes: 7%
- Eosinophils: 2%
- Basophils: 0%

RBC count: 4.0×10^{12}/L
RDW: 20%
Platelet count: 400×10^9/L
Reticulocyte count: 1.2%
Stool occult blood: Positive

Multiple-Choice Questions

Answers are in Appendix A.

1. This patient's MCV is:
   a. 95 fL
   b. 85 fL
   c. 75 fL
   d. 65 fL

Continued

CASE STUDY 11.2—cont'd

2. This patient's MCV is:
   a. Within normal limits
   b. Below the reference range
   c. Above the reference range
   d. Unable to determine the reference range
3. How would you classify this anemia morphologically?
   a. Hypochromic-microcytic
   b. Hypochromic-macrocytic
   c. Normochromic-normocytic
   d. Normochromic-microcytic

Critical Thinking Group Discussion Questions

1. What is the most probable type of anemia seen in this patient?
2. What is the cause of the anemia seen in this patient?

Note: Answers to narrative questions posted on EVOLVE instructor site.

CASE STUDY 11.3

A 65-year-old woman is seen in clinic. She complains of extreme fatigue, difficulty in breathing, and an extremely sore tongue. Laboratory data are:

Hb: 8.7 g/dL
Hct: 25.5%
WBC count: 4.0×10^9/L
WBC differential:
  Neutrophils: 65%
  Lymphocytes: 31%
  Monocytes: 4%
RBC count: 1.97×10^{12}/L
  RDW: 19%
  Platelet count: 134×10^9/L
  Reticulocyte count: 0.3%

Multiple-Choice Questions

Answers are in Appendix A.

1. What is this patient's MCV?
   a. 132
   b. 129
   c. 108
   d. 100
2. How would you classify this anemia morphologically?
   a. Microcytic
   b. Macrocytic
   c. Normochromic
   d. Unable to tell
3. The most probable type of anemia seen in this patient is:
   a. Aplastic anemia from bone marrow depletion
   b. Megaloblastic anemia from folate or vitamin B_{12} deficiency
   c. Hemolytic anemia
   d. Iron deficiency anemia

Critical Thinking Group Discussion Questions

1. Given the hematologic results provided, what types of alterations in erythrocyte size or color would you not expect to find on a Wright-stained blood film from this patient?
2. What is the interpretation of this patient's total leukocyte count?

Note: Answers to narrative questions posted on EVOLVE instructor site.

CASE STUDY 11.4

A 20-year-old female university student is seen in the student health clinic. She has a general feeling of sickness, an extremely sore throat, and swollen lymph nodes in her neck. Blood is drawn for a CBC, and her throat is swabbed for a rapid strep test and culture. Laboratory data are:

Hemoglobin: 13.5 g/dL
RBCs: 3.9×10^{12}/L
RBC indices: All within normal limits
WBC count: 14.5×10^9/L
WBC differential:
  Neutrophils: 7%
  Lymphocytes: 89%
  Monocytes: 3%
  Eosinophils: 1%
  Basophils: 0%
Platelet estimate: Normal, with normal morphology
Rapid throat culture: Negative; culture pending

Multiple-Choice Questions

Answers are in Appendix A.

1. Based on the laboratory results provided, which of the following applies?
   a. Absolute lymphocytosis
   b. Absolute neutropenia
   c. Absolute granulocytosis
   d. None of the above
2. Which of the following leukocyte changes would you expect to find on a Wright-stained blood film from this patient?
   a. Toxic granulation of neutrophils
   b. Hypersegmentation of neutrophils
   c. Variant lymphocytes
   d. Hypochromic red blood cells
3. This patient's quantitative platelet count is estimated at:
   a. 50 to 100×10^{12}/L.
   b. 100 to 150×10^{12}/L.
   c. 150 to 350×10^{12}/L.
   d. More than 450×10^{12}/L.

Critical Thinking Group Discussion Questions

1. What is the estimated hematocrit percentage for this patient?
2. What is the disease most likely exhibited by this patient?

Note: Answers to narrative questions posted on EVOLVE instructor site.

CASE STUDY 11.5

A 65-year-old man has chills, high spiking fevers, cough, and signs of consolidation in the left lower lobe of his lung. Blood is drawn for a CBC, sputum is collected for Gram stain and culture, and a chest x-ray film is obtained. Laboratory data are:

Hemoglobin: 14.5 g/dL
Hematocrit: 42%
RBC indices: All within normal limits
WBC count: 24.0×10^9/L
WBC differential:
  Segmented neutrophils: 33%
  Band neutrophils: 61%
  Lymphocytes: 6%
Platelet estimate: Normal with normal morphology
Sputum Gram stain: Many Gram-positive cocci in pairs; culture pending

Multiple-Choice Questions

Answers are in Appendix A.

1. As determined by the laboratory results provided and your calculations, which of the following apply?
   a. Absolute lymphocytosis
   b. Absolute neutrophilia
   c. Neutropenia
   d. Reactive lymphocytosis
2. Which of the following leukocyte changes could you expect to find on a Wright-stained blood film from this patient?
   a. Hypersegmentation of neutrophils
   b. Variant lymphocytes
   c. Toxic granulation of neutrophils
   d. Hypochromia
3. This patient's red cell morphology on a peripheral blood smear will appear to be:
   a. microcytic-hypochromic
   b. macrocytic- hypochromic
   c. normocytic-normochromic
   d. normocytic-hypochromic

Critical Thinking Group Discussion Questions

1. The patient appears to be suffering from a _____ infection. This type of infection is supported by _____ laboratory results.
2. The disease most likely exhibited by this patient is ________. This diagnosis is supported by ________ laboratory results.

Note: Answers to narrative questions are posted on the EVOLVE instructor site.

REFERENCES

1. McPherson RA, Pincus MR, editors: *Henry's clinical diagnosis and management by laboratory methods*, 22 ed., Philadelphia, 2011, Elsevier/Saunders.
2. Profiles, neutrophil counts, ratio better identify meningococcal infection than total WBC, *MLO Med Lab Obs* 45(12):18, 2013.
3. Clinical and Laboratory Standards Institute: Laboratory documents: development and control; approved guideline, ed 5, Wayne, Pa, 2006, GP2-A5.
4. Clinical and Laboratory Standards Institute: Method for reticulocyte counting (automated blood counters, flow cytometry, and supravital dyes): approved guideline, ed 2, Wayne, Pa, 2004, H44-A2.
5. Vennapusa B, et al: Erythrocyte sedimentation rate (ESR) measured by the Streck ESR-auto plus is higher than with the sediplast Westergren method, *Am J Clinical Pathology* 135:386–390, 2011.

BIBLIOGRAPHY

Baron MH, Isern J, Fraser ST: The embryonic origins of erythropoiesis in mammals, *Blood* 119(21):4828–4837, 2012.

Brants A: Detection of hemoglobinopathies and thalassemias using automated separation systems, *MLO Med Lab Obs* 46(1):24–26, 2014.

Clinical and Laboratory Standards Institute: Procedure for determining packed cell volume by the microhematocrit method: approved standard, ed 3, Wayne, Pa, 2000, H07.

Clinical and Laboratory Standards Institute: Procedures and devices for the collection of diagnostic capillary blood specimens: approved standard, ed 6, Wayne, Pa, 2008, GP42.

Clinical and Laboratory Standards Institute: Reference procedures for the quantitative determination of hemoglobin in blood: approved standard, ed 3, Wayne, Pa, 2000, H15.

Epelman S, Lavine KJ, Randolph GJ: Origin and Functions of Tissue Macrophages, *Immunology* 41(1):21–35, 2014.

Levine RA: Dry hematology: its development, function, and role in point of care testing, *MLO Med Lab Obs* 45(2):14–16, 2013.

Patel N: Automation in hematology, *MLO Med Lab Obs* 46(1):6–11, 2014.

QBC star centrifugal hematology system, QBC Diagnostics 2005. www.qbcdiagnostics.com. Accessed May 8, 2006.

Teshima DY: EDTA in transit: degenerative changes in blood cell morphology, *MLO Med Lab Obs* 49(7):12–14, 2017.

Titus K: Acute leukemia workups, from top to bottom, *CAP Today* 31(5):1, 2017.

Turgeon M: *Clinical hematology,* ed 6, Philadelphia, 2017, Lippincott Williams & Wilkins.

Westergren A: The techniques of the red cell sedimentation reaction, *Am Rev Tuberc Pulmonary Dis* 14:94, 1926.

REVIEW QUESTIONS (ANSWERS IN APPENDIX A)

Hematopoiesis: Overall Blood Cell Maturation and Function

1. The blood cells responsible for carrying oxygen are:
   a. Erythrocytes
   b. Leukocytes
   c. Thrombocytes
   d. Either a or b

Erythrocytes

2. When seen on a Wright-stained peripheral blood film, a young red cell that has just extruded its nucleus is referred to as a:
   a. Normoblast (metarubricyte)
   b. Orthochromatic cell

c. Polychromatophilic cell
d. Reticulocyte

3. The approximate life span in peripheral blood of a red blood cell is:
   a. Months to years
   b. 120 days
   c. 1 to 3 days
   d. About 10 hours
   e. Less than 8 hours
4. Which of the following is essential to the oxygen-carrying capacity of a molecule of hemoglobin?
   a. Globin
   b. Heme
   c. Iron
   d. None of the above
5. A hemoglobin variant resulting in sickle cell anemia in the homozygous state is:
   a. Hemoglobin A
   b. Hemoglobin C
   c. Hemoglobin F
   d. Hemoglobin S
6. The principal form of hemoglobin found in the blood of normal adults is:
   a. Hemoglobin A
   b. Hemoglobin C
   c. Hemoglobin F
   d. Hemoglobin S
7. The principal form of hemoglobin during intrauterine life and at birth is:
   a. Hemoglobin A
   b. Hemoglobin C
   c. Hemoglobin F
   d. Hemoglobin S
8. An irreversible combination of hemoglobin with a sulfa group, incapable of transporting oxygen or reverting to functional hemoglobin, is:
   a. Carboxyhemoglobin
   b. Hemiglobincyanide (cyanmethemoglobin)
   c. Methemoglobin
   d. Sulfhemoglobin
9. Hemoglobin bound to carbon monoxide with an affinity 100 times that of oxygen is:
   a. Carboxyhemoglobin
   b. Hemiglobincyanide (cyanmethemoglobin)
   c. Methemoglobin
   d. Oxyhemoglobin
10. Hemoglobin containing iron in a ferric, rather than a ferrous, state is:
    a. Methemoglobin
    b. Oxyhemoglobin
    c. Reduced hemoglobin
    d. Sulfhemoglobin
11. The form of hemoglobin that normally transports carbon dioxide from the tissues to the lungs is:
    a. Carboxyhemoglobin
    b. Methemoglobin
    c. Oxyhemoglobin
    d. Reduced hemoglobin
12. The form of hemoglobin that normally transports oxygen from the lungs to the tissues is:
    a. Carboxyhemoglobin
    b. Methemoglobin
    c. Oxyhemoglobin
    d. Reduced hemoglobin

Leukocytes

13. The approximate life span in peripheral blood of a neutrophil (PMN) is:
    a. 120 days
    b. 1 to 3 days
    c. About 10 hours
    d. Less than 8 hours

Lymphocyte Maturation and Function

14. A white blood cell (WBC) count and WBC differential are performed. WBC count: 7.0×10^9/L; of 100 WBCs classified: 70% neutrophils, 20% lymphocytes, 7% monocytes, 2% eosinophils, and 1% basophil. The absolute lymphocyte count is:
    a. 1.40×10^9/L
    b. 2.10×10^9/L
    c. 3.55×10^9/L
    d. 3.99×10^9/L

Thrombocytes

15. Thrombocytes are also known as:
    a. Megakaryocytes
    b. Platelets
    c. Meta-megakaryocytes
    d. Poikilocytes

Clinical Hematology Procedures

16. The anticoagulant of choice for a complete blood count (CBC) is:
    a. EDTA
    b. Heparin
    c. Sodium citrate
    d. Oxalate
17. The use of daily hemoglobin control solution with automated equipment will detect which of the following?
    a. Accuracy of the measuring device used
    b. Deterioration of the hemoglobin reagent
    c. Technical skill of the technologist
    d. Both a and b
18. What is the unit of measurement for hematocrit (conventional)?
    a. Cells $\times 10^9$ per liter
    b. Cells $\times 10^{12}$ per liter
    c. Grams per deciliter
    d. Liters per liter
19. What is the unit of measurement for hemoglobin?
    a. Cells $\times 10^9$ per liter
    b. Cells $\times 10^{12}$ per liter
    c. Grams per deciliter
    d. Liters per liter

20. What is the unit of measurement for packed cell volume (SI units)?
    a. Cells × 10^9 per liter
    b. Cells × 10^{12} per liter
    c. Grams per deciliter
    d. Percent
21. What is the unit of measurement for platelet count?
    a. Cells × 10^9 per liter
    b. Cells × 10^{12} per liter
    c. Grams per deciliter
    d. Liters per liter
22. What is the unit of measurement for red cell count?
    a. Cells × 10^9 per liter
    b. Cells × 10^{12} per liter
    c. Grams per deciliter
    d. Liters per liter
23. What is the unit of measurement for white cell count?
    a. Cells × 10^9 per liter
    b. Cells × 10^{12} per liter
    c. Grams per deciliter
    d. Liters per liter
24. Assuming normochromic and normocytic red cells, a blood sample with a hemoglobin of 15 g/dL would be expected to show a hematocrit of:
    a. 25%
    b. 35%
    c. 45%
    d. 55%

Additional Hematology Procedures

25. Which of the following hematologic tests may not be part of the usual complete blood count?
    a. Hematocrit
    b. Hemoglobin
    c. Platelet estimate
    d. Reticulocyte count
26. Which of the following is a nonspecific screening test for inflammation?
    a. Erythrocyte morphology
    b. Erythrocyte sedimentation rate
    c. Leukocyte morphology and differential
    d. Platelet count
27. Which of the following tests is used to evaluate the response to vitamin B_{12} therapy in the treatment of pernicious iron deficiency anemia?
    a. Erythrocyte sedimentation rate
    b. Leukocyte morphology and differential
    c. Platelet count
    d. Reticulocyte count

Red Blood Cell Indices

28. The MCV (SI) units of measurement are:
    a. Femtoliters (fL)
    b. Picograms (pg)
    c. Grams per deciliter (g/dL)
    d. Percent (%)
29. The MCH (SI) units of measurement are:
    a. Femtoliters (fL)
    b. Picograms (pg)
    c. Grams per deciliter (g/dL)
    d. Percent (%)
30. The MCHC (SI) units of measurement are:
    a. Femtoliters (fL)
    b. Picograms (pg)
    c. Grams per deciliter (g/dL)
    d. Percent (%)

    Questions 31–34: Identify the common abbreviation for the following definitions of red blood cell (RBC) indices.
31. Hemoglobin concentration or color of the average RBC:
    a. MCH
    b. MCHC
    c. MCV
    d. RDW
32. Measure of the degree of RBC size variability:
    a. MCH
    b. MCHC
    c. MCV
    d. RDW
33. Volume or size of the average RBC:
    a. MCH
    b. MCHC
    c. MCV
    d. RDW
34. Average concentration of hemoglobin in a given RBC volume:
    a. MCH
    b. MCHC
    c. MCV
    d. RDW

Microscopic Examination of the Peripheral Blood Film

35. Which of the following stains is classified as a Romanowsky stain?
    a. Brilliant cresyl blue
    b. New methylene blue
    c. Wright-Giemsa
    d. Prussian blue

    Questions 36–41: For blood films stained with polychrome Romanowsky-type stain, identify the dye component for the following cell components.
36. Azurophilic granules are:
    a. Acidophilic (eosin)
    b. Basophilic (methylene blue)
    c. Acidophilic (eosin) and basophilic (methylene blue)
    d. Methylene azure (polychrome methylene blue)
37. Cytoplasmic RNA is:
    a. Acidophilic (eosin)
    b. Basophilic (methylene blue)
    c. Acidophilic (eosin) and basophilic (methylene blue)
    d. Methylene azure (polychrome methylene blue)
38. Eosinophilic granules are:
    a. Acidophilic (eosin)
    b. Basophilic (methylene blue)

c. Acidophilic (eosin) and basophilic (methylene blue)
d. Methylene azure (polychrome methylene blue)

39. Hemoglobin is:
a. Acidophilic (eosin)
b. Basophilic (methylene blue)
c. Acidophilic (eosin) and basophilic (methylene blue)
d. Methylene azure (polychrome methylene blue)

40. Neutrophilic granules are:
a. Acidophilic (eosin)
b. Basophilic (methylene blue)
c. Acidophilic (eosin) and basophilic (methylene blue)
d. Methylene azure (polychrome methylene blue)

41. Nuclear DNA is:
a. Acidophilic (eosin)
b. Basophilic (methylene blue)
c. Acidophilic (eosin) and basophilic (methylene blue)
d. Methylene azure (polychrome methylene blue)

42. What is the most probable cause of faded or washed-out appearance of all cells?
a. Improper washing or old stain
b. Overfixing, overstaining, underwashing; too-alkaline stain or buffer, or too-thick blood film
c. Overwashing, understaining, underfixing
d. Understaining, overwashing; too-acid stain, buffer, or water

43. What is the most probable cause of the gross appearance of slide being excessively blue, with blue-red erythrocytes and dark, granular leukocytes?
a. Improper washing or old stain
b. Overfixing, overstaining, underwashing; too-alkaline stain or buffer, or too-thick blood film
c. Overwashing, understaining, underfixing
d. Understaining, overwashing; too-acid stain, buffer, or water

44. What is the most probable cause of the gross appearance of the slide being excessively red with bright-red erythrocytes, pale-blue white cell, and brilliant-red eosinophilic granules?
a. Improper washing or old stain
b. Overfixing, overstaining, underwashing; too-alkaline stain or buffer, or too-thick blood film
c. Overwashing, understaining, underfixing
d. Understaining, overwashing; too-acid stain, buffer, or water

45. What is the most probable cause of large amounts of precipitated stain?
a. Improper washing or old stain
b. Overfixing, overstaining, underwashing; too-alkaline stain or buffer, or too-thick blood film
c. Overwashing, understaining, underfixing
d. Understaining, overwashing; too-acid stain, buffer, or water

Questions 46–51: Identify the morphologic appearance of RBCs related to the following causes or descriptions of anemia.

46. Acute blood loss (trauma):
a. Hypochromic-microcytic
b. Macrocytic
c. Normochromic-normocytic
d. Microcytic

47. Anemia associated with increased plasma volume (pregnancy and overhydration):
a. Hypochromic-microcytic
b. Macrocytic
c. Normochromic-normocytic
d. Microcytic

48. Anemia associated with aplastic anemia from bone marrow suppression:
a. Hypochromic-microcytic
b. Macrocytic
c. Normochromic-normocytic
d. Microcytic

49. Anemia associated with iron deficiency caused by diet or blood loss:
a. Hypochromic-microcytic
b. Macrocytic
c. Normochromic-normocytic
d. Microcytic

50. Anemia associated with thalassemia and other hemoglobinopathies:
a. Hypochromic-microcytic
b. Macrocytic
c. Normochromic-normocytic
d. Microcytic

51. Anemia associated with vitamin B_{12} or folate deficiency:
a. Hypochromic-microcytic
b. Macrocytic
c. Normochromic-normocytic
d. Microcytic

52. What is the term for erythrocytes that show normal color or staining reaction?
a. Normochromic
b. Normocytic
c. Orthochromatic
d. Polychromatophilic

53. What is an increased variation in size of erythrocytes on the blood film?
a. Anisocytosis
b. Microcytosis
c. Macrocytosis
d. Poikilocytosis

54. What is an increased variation in the shape of erythrocytes on the blood film?
a. Anisocytosis
b. Microcytosis
c. Orthochromia
d. Poikilocytosis

55. The presence of anisocytosis and poikilocytosis is reflected in which of the following red cell indices?
a. MCV
b. MCH
c. MCHC
d. RDW

56. The presence of polychromasia on a Wright-stained peripheral blood film is associated with which of the following untreated anemias?
a. Aplastic anemia
b. Hemolytic anemia

c. Iron deficiency anemia
d. Megaloblastic anemia

57. Which of the following leukemias is most frequently associated with the presence of the Philadelphia chromosome?
   a. Acute lymphocytic
   b. Acute myelogenous
   c. Chronic lymphocytic
   d. Chronic myelogenous
58. Which of the following types of leukemia is most associated with children ages 2 to 10 years?
   a. Acute lymphoblastic
   b. Acute myelogenous
   c. Chronic lymphocytic
   d. Chronic myelogenous
59. The presence of Auer rods in the peripheral blood is associated with which of the following cells?
   a. Lymphoblast
   b. Myeloblast
   c. Reactive lymphocyte
   d. Shift cell
60. A patient being treated for metastatic carcinoma was found to have a white cell count of 5×10^9/L with 5 metarubricytes (nucleated red cells) per 100 WBCs. What is the corrected white cell count for this patient?
   a. 2.1×10^9/L
   b. 2.4×10^9/L
   c. 4.8×10^9/L
   d. 5.2×10^9/L

Turgeon: Linné & Ringsrud's Clinical Laboratory Science, 8th Edition

STUDENT PROCEDURE WORKSHEET 11.1

Packed Cell Volume of Whole Blood (Hematocrit): Centrifugation Method

Student Learning Outcomes

See Chapter 11 of *Linné & Ringsrud's Clinical Laboratory Science: Concepts, Procedures, and Clinical Applications,* 8th edition, for a complete discussion of this procedure. After reading Chapter 11, and at the completion of the laboratory exercise and review questions, the student will be able to:

- Perform a spun microhematocrit procedure.
- Explain the principle of the procedure.
- Discuss procedural sources of error.
- State the reference range of hematocrit values for men, women, and children.
- Complete the end-of-procedure review questions with a grade of 80% or higher.

Principle

The packed cell volume (PCV), hematocrit, is a measurement of the ratio of the volume occupied by the red blood cells (RBCs) to the volume of whole blood after centrifugation in a sample of capillary or venous blood expressed as a percentage. Clinically, the hematocrit is used to screen for anemia or other red cell volume alterations. In conjunction with an erythrocyte count, the hematocrit is used to calculate the mean corpuscular volume (MCV). The hematocrit is also used in conjunction with the hemoglobin concentration to calculate the mean corpuscular hemoglobin concentration (MCHC).

Specimen

Anticoagulated venous blood or capillary blood collected directly into heparinized capillary tubes can be used. Specimens should be centrifuged within 6 hours of collecting. Hemolyzed specimens cannot be used for testing.

Equipment and Supplies

1. Capillary tubes, either plain or heparin-coated
2. Clay-type tube sealant
3. Microhematocrit centrifuge
4. Microhematocrit reading device

Calibration

The calibration of the centrifuge should be checked regularly for timer accuracy, speed, and maximal packing of cells.

Quality Control

Commercially available whole blood can be used to check the accuracy of normal and abnormal levels.

Reporting Results

The microhematocrit can be expressed as a percentage or a decimal fraction, such as 45% or 0.45 L/L.

Reference Range

Adult Males	41.5%-50.4%
Adult Females	36.0%-45.0%
Pediatric (3-6 mo)	29-41%

Procedure Notes

Sources of Error

Erroneous results can be caused by inclusion of the buffy coat in reading the packed column, hemolysis of the specimen, and inadequate mixing. If the centrifugation time is too short or the speed is too low, an increase in trapped plasma (1%-3%) will occur in normal blood. Increased amounts of trapped plasma can produce errors in patients with an erythrocyte abnormality, such as sickle cell anemia. Do not allow the tubes to remain in the centrifuge for more than 10 minutes after the end of centrifugation because the interface between the plasma and the cells will become slanted, and an inaccurate reading will result.

Clinical Applications

The microhematocrit is used for detecting anemia, polycythemia, hemodilution, or hemoconcentration.

References

Clinical and Laboratory Standards Institute: Procedure for determining packed cell volume by the microhematocrit method: approved standard, ed 3, Wayne, Pa, 2000, H7-A3.
Turgeon M: Clinical hematology, ed 5, Philadelphia, 2012, Lippincott Williams & Wilkins.

Instructions for the Procedure

Read the list of required equipment, supplies, and reagents and the procedural steps. Follow the procedural steps in exact order.

SEQUENCE	PROCEDURAL STEP	INSTRUCTOR-OBSERVED ACCEPTABLE PERFORMANCE (CHECK IF ACCEPTABLE)
1	Assemble equipment and supplies.	
2	Wash your hands and put on gloves and eye protection as directed.	
3	Well-mixed anticoagulant blood should be drawn into two microhematocrit tubes by capillary action. Free-flowing capillary specimens should be collected directly into heparinized capillary tubes. NOTE: The tubes should be filled to about three fourths of their length. Wipe off the outside of the tubes with a suitable wipe.	
4	Seal one end of each tube with a small amount of claylike material by placing the dry end of the tube into the sealant, holding the index finger over the opposite end to prevent blood from leaking out of the tube onto the sealant.	
5	Place the filled and sealed capillary tubes into the centrifuge (see Fig. 11.50). The sealed ends should point toward the outside of the centrifuge. The duplicate samples should be placed opposite the other to balance the centrifuge. Record the position number of each specimen.	

(Continued)

Turgeon: Linné & Ringsrud's Clinical Laboratory Science, 8th Edition

STUDENT PROCEDURE WORKSHEET 11.1

SEQUENCE	PROCEDURAL STEP	INSTRUCTOR-OBSERVED ACCEPTABLE PERFORMANCE (CHECK IF ACCEPTABLE)
6	Securely fasten the flat lid on top of the capillary tubes. Close the centrifuge top and secure the latch. Set the timer for 5 minutes. The fixed speed of centrifugation should be 10,000 to 15,000 rpm.	
7	After the centrifuge has stopped, open the top and remove the cover plate. Within 10 minutes, read the microhematocrit on a reader. Measure the microhematocrit by adjusting the top of the clay sealant to the 0 mark and reading the top of the red cell column. Do not include the buffy coat in reading the packed erythrocyte column. A capillary tube reader with an ocular that has cross-markings produces the most accurate reading.	
8	Discard used lancets in a sharps container and discard gauze and other contaminated supplies into a biohazard container.	
9	Clean equipment and return to proper storage.	
10	Clean work area with disinfectant solution.	
11	Remove gloves and discard into biohazard container. Wash hands using proper procedure.	

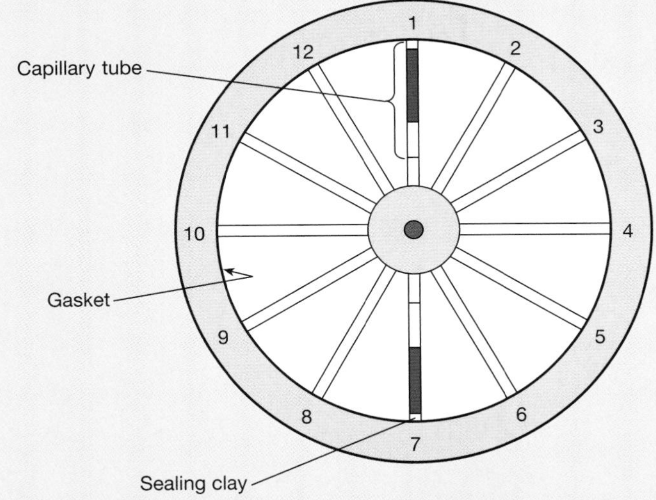

Fig. 11.50 Placement of the capillary tubes in microhematocrit centrifuge. Centrifuge must be balanced by placing tubes directly across from each other, as shown for places 1 and 7.

Results of Unknown Specimens

SPECIMEN IDENTIFICATION	RESULTS

Review Questions

Questions 1-5: Match the following situations regarding spun microhematocrit determinations with results (a, b, or c).

1. ___ Capillary blood is drawn into a heparinized anticoagulated microhematocrit tube.
2. ___ Inadequate sealing of the microhematocrit tube.
3. ___ Inclusion of the buffy coat in the measured packed cell volume.
4. ___ Use of a hemolyzed blood sample.
5. ___ Anticoagulated venous blood is drawn into an anticoagulated microhematocrit tube.

a. Falsely high
b. Falsely low
c. Unaffected

Procedural Evaluation

Student's Name ______________________________ Grade__________

Instructor's Signature ___________________________ Date__________

Comments:

Turgeon: Linné & Ringsrud's Clinical Laboratory Science, 8th Edition

STUDENT PROCEDURE WORKSHEET 11.2

Making a Blood Film: Push-Wedge Slide Method

Student Learning Outcomes

- Prepare an acceptable push-wedge blood film.
- Name and explain corrective actions for unsatisfactory blood films.
- Complete the end-of-procedure review questions with a grade of 80% or higher.

Principle

A properly prepared blood film is necessary for an accurate evaluation of a blood specimen.

Specimen

Equipment and Supplies

1. Clean glass slides (plain or with one frosted end)
2. No. 2 lead pencil

Procedure Notes

1. The push-wedge method is recommended by the Clinical Laboratory Standards Institute (CLSI) as the reference method for differential leukocyte counting.
2. Normally, two smears are prepared. If free-flowing capillary blood is used, more than two smears may be desired.

Visual Examination of a Good Smear

An ideal smear:

1. Progresses from being thick at the point of origin to thin with a uniform edge at the termination point.
2. Does not touch the outer borders of the slide or run off the sides or ends of the slide.
3. Appears smooth without waves of gaps.
4. Does not have any streaks, ridges, or troughs, which indicate an increased number of leukocytes carried to that area.
5. Is prepared with a proper amount of blood and spread to occupy approximately two thirds of the length of the glass slide.

Causes of a Poor Blood Smear

1. Prolonged storage of anticoagulated whole blood specimens can cause cellular distortion.
2. Delayed preparation of a blood smear causes larger cells, such as neutrophils and monocytes, to be disproportionately located at the feathered edge when examined microscopically.
3. Dirty slides can cause uneven preparation of a blood film.
4. Improper angle of the pusher slide can cause too thick a smear if increased too much or too long a smear if decreased too much.
5. Preparing the smear too slowly which produces irregularities and the distribution of cells on a slide.
6. High humidity will prolong the drying time of blood smears and produce distortion of erythrocytes.

Instructions for the Procedure

Read the list of required equipment, supplies, and reagents and the procedural steps. Follow the procedural steps in exact order.

SEQUENCE	PROCEDURAL STEP	INSTRUCTOR-OBSERVED ACCEPTABLE PERFORMANCE (CHECK IF ACCEPTABLE)
1		
2		
3		
4		
5		

(Continued)

Turgeon: Linné & Ringsrud's Clinical Laboratory Science, 8th Edition

Reference

Turgeon ML: *Clinical hematology*, ed 5, Philadelphia 2012, Lippincott Williams & Wilkins.

STUDENT PROCEDURE WORKSHEET 11.2

SEQUENCE	PROCEDURAL STEP	INSTRUCTOR-OBSERVED ACCEPTABLE PERFORMANCE (CHECK IF ACCEPTABLE)
	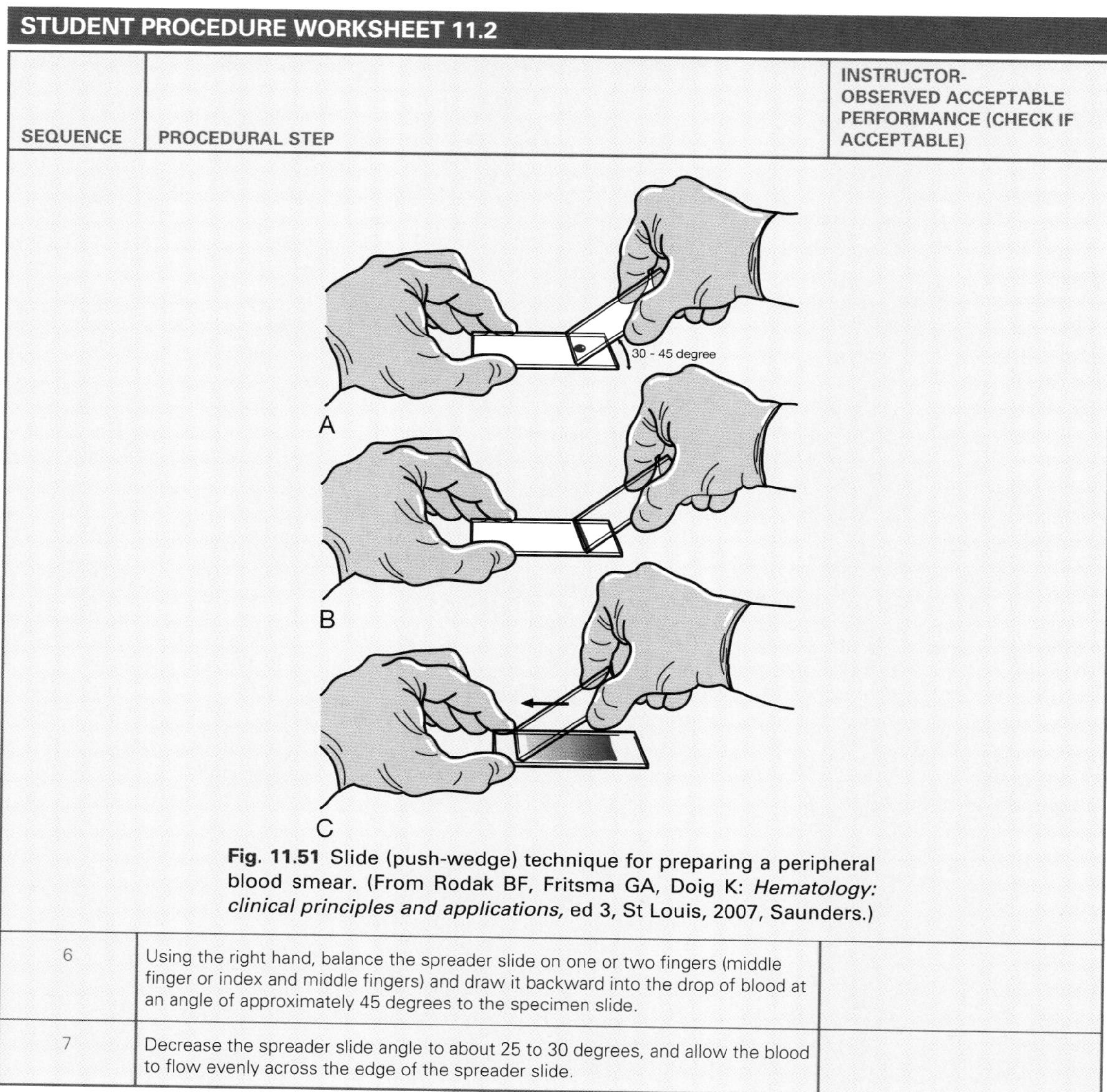 **Fig. 11.51** Slide (push-wedge) technique for preparing a peripheral blood smear. (From Rodak BF, Fritsma GA, Doig K: *Hematology: clinical principles and applications,* ed 3, St Louis, 2007, Saunders.)	
6	Using the right hand, balance the spreader slide on one or two fingers (middle finger or index and middle fingers) and draw it backward into the drop of blood at an angle of approximately 45 degrees to the specimen slide.	
7	Decrease the spreader slide angle to about 25 to 30 degrees, and allow the blood to flow evenly across the edge of the spreader slide.	

(Continued)

Turgeon: Linné & Ringsrud's Clinical Laboratory Science, 8th Edition

Reference

Turgeon ML: *Clinical hematology*, ed 5, Philadelphia 2012, Lippincott Williams & Wilkins.

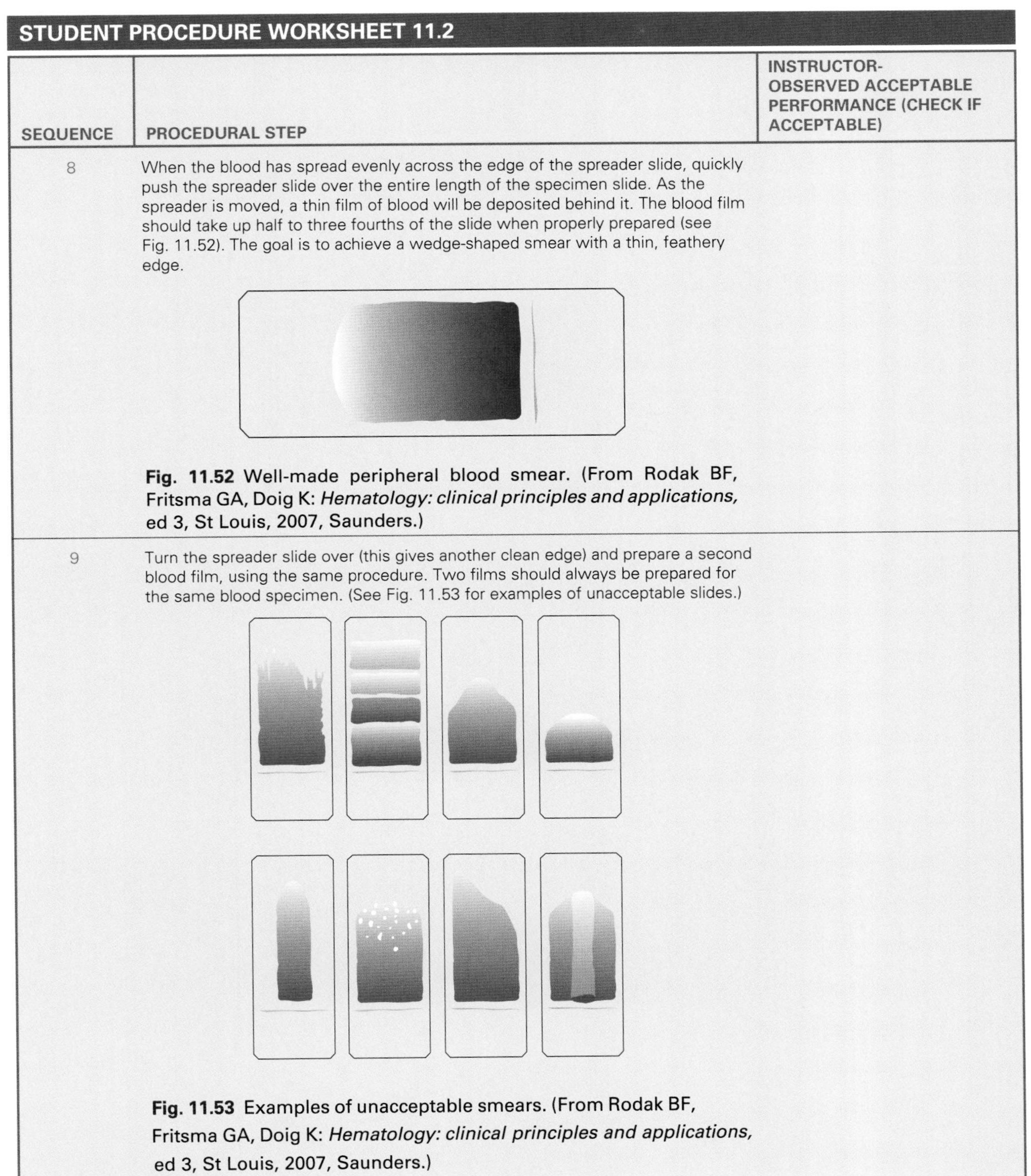

STUDENT PROCEDURE WORKSHEET 11.2

SEQUENCE	PROCEDURAL STEP	INSTRUCTOR-OBSERVED ACCEPTABLE PERFORMANCE (CHECK IF ACCEPTABLE)
8	When the blood has spread evenly across the edge of the spreader slide, quickly push the spreader slide over the entire length of the specimen slide. As the spreader is moved, a thin film of blood will be deposited behind it. The blood film should take up half to three fourths of the slide when properly prepared (see Fig. 11.52). The goal is to achieve a wedge-shaped smear with a thin, feathery edge. **Fig. 11.52** Well-made peripheral blood smear. (From Rodak BF, Fritsma GA, Doig K: *Hematology: clinical principles and applications,* ed 3, St Louis, 2007, Saunders.)	
9	Turn the spreader slide over (this gives another clean edge) and prepare a second blood film, using the same procedure. Two films should always be prepared for the same blood specimen. (See Fig. 11.53 for examples of unacceptable slides.) **Fig. 11.53** Examples of unacceptable smears. (From Rodak BF, Fritsma GA, Doig K: *Hematology: clinical principles and applications,* ed 3, St Louis, 2007, Saunders.)	

(Continued)

Turgeon: Linné & Ringsrud's Clinical Laboratory Science, 8th Edition

Reference

Turgeon ML: *Clinical hematology*, ed 5, Philadelphia 2012, Lippincott Williams & Wilkins.

STUDENT PROCEDURE WORKSHEET 11.2

SEQUENCE	PROCEDURAL STEP	INSTRUCTOR-OBSERVED ACCEPTABLE PERFORMANCE (CHECK IF ACCEPTABLE)
10	Dry the blood film immediately. If it is not dried quickly, the blood cells will shrink and appear distorted.	
11	Label the film by writing the name of the patient and the date in the dried blood at the thick end of the film, using a lead pencil.	
12	Discard used lancets in a sharps container and discard gauze and other contaminated supplies into a biohazard container.	
13	Clean equipment and return to proper storage.	
14	Clean work area with disinfectant solution.	
15	Remove gloves and discard into biohazard container.	
16	Wash hands using proper procedure.	

(Continued)

STUDENT PROCEDURE WORKSHEET 11.2

Results of Blood Smear Preparation

SPECIMEN IDENTIFICATION	ACCEPTABLE RESULTS (YES/NO)

Review Questions

1. ___ Blood film covers half to three quarters the length of slide
2. ___ Defined border at end of blood film (no feather edge)
3. ___ Chipped slide
4. ___ Dirty slides or excess fat in lipemic specimen or very high white cell count
5. ___ Large drop of blood, large angle, and slow stroke
6. ___ Small drop of blood, small angle, and fast stroke

a. Good blood film
b. Neutrophils accumulate in feather edge
c. Unusually thick blood film
d. Unusually thin blood film
e. Vacuoles or bubbles in blood film

Procedural Evaluation

Turgeon: Linné & Ringsrud's Clinical Laboratory Science, 8th Edition

STUDENT PROCEDURE WORKSHEET 11.3

Staining Blood Films with Wright-Giemsa

Student Learning Outcomes

See Chapter 11 of *Linné & Ringsrud's Clinical Laboratory Science: Concepts, Procedures, and Clinical Applications*, 8th edition, for a complete discussion of this procedure. After reading Chapter 11, and at the completion of this laboratory exercise and answering the review questions, a student should be able to:

- Properly stain a blood smear.
- Explain precautions and sources of error when staining a blood film.
- Complete the end-of-procedure review questions with a grade of 80% or higher.

Principle

A properly stained blood film is essential to a quality evaluation of the peripheral blood smear. Blood and other types of specimens can be stained using Romanowsky-based stains, such as Wright-Giemsa stain. Bone marrow specimens may be stained with Romanowsky-based stain.

Specimen

A glass slide with a properly prepared peripheral blood smear.

Equipment, Supplies, and Reagents

1. Prepared Wright-Giemsa stain or prepare by diluting preweighed vials in methyl alcohol according to the manufacturer's directions
2. A staining rack of Coplin staining jars are needed
3. Filter paper, funnel, and suitable dispensing bottle
4. Buffer (pH 6.4)

Procedure Notes

Sources of Error

1. Failure to filter stain daily or before use can produce sediment on blood films. Heavy amounts make it impossible to see the blood film; small amounts of sediment can be mistaken for platelets when the blood smear is examined microscopically.
2. Inaccurate buffer pH can produce too bright or too dark staining reactions. If pH is too acidic, the blood cells are too red; if the pH is too alkaline, the blood smear will be too blue when examined microscopically.
3. Improper timing or buffering can produce faded or altered colors of the blood cells. Too short a staining time produces a blood smear that is too red; too long of a staining time will produce a stain that is too dark.
4. Deteriorated stain or an incorrect ratio of stain and buffer can produce washed-out cellular colors.

Clinical Applications

A properly stained blood smear is examined microscopically to evaluate the structure and appearance of erythrocytes, an estimated quantity and appearance of platelets, and the comparative percentage of leukocytes in a specimen.

Reference

Turgeon ML: *Clinical hematology*, ed 5, Philadelphia, 2011, Lippincott Williams & Wilkins.

Instructions for the Procedure

Read the list of required equipment, supplies, and reagents and the procedural steps. Follow the procedural steps in exact order.

SEQUENCE	PROCEDURAL STEP	INSTRUCTOR-OBSERVED ACCEPTABLE PERFORMANCE (CHECK IF ACCEPTABLE)
1	Assemble equipment and supplies. Wash your hands and put on gloves and eye protection as directed.	
2	Optional: In some laboratories, blood smears are fixed separately in alcohol before the staining procedures to enhance the retention of granules in blood cells. The usual fixative is methyl alcohol. Slides can be placed in anhydrous and acetone-free methanol for 1 minute or longer.	
3	Place the dried blood film on a level staining rack, with the film side up and the feather edge away from you. Allow the dried film to set at least 5 minutes before staining is begun.	
4	Fix the film by flooding the slide with the filtered stain. The amount of stain is important. There must be enough to avoid excessive evaporation, which would result in precipitation of stain on the slide. NOTE: Wright or other Romanowsky-based stains are dissolved in methyl alcohol; therefore fixation normally takes place when the stain is applied to the blood smear.	
5	Allow the stain to remain on the slide for 3 to 5 minutes. This is the fixation period. Determine the exact timing for each batch of stain used.	

(Continued)

Turgeon: Linné & Ringsrud's Clinical Laboratory Science, 8th Edition

STUDENT PROCEDURE WORKSHEET 11.3

SEQUENCE	PROCEDURAL STEP	INSTRUCTOR-OBSERVED ACCEPTABLE PERFORMANCE (CHECK IF ACCEPTABLE)
6	Without removing the Wright-Giemsa stain, add phosphate buffer, using about 1 to 1.5 times as much buffer as stain on the slide so that a layer piles up but none spills off. Add the buffer dropwise; then blow on the surface to mix the stain and buffer. A metallic greenish sheen should form on the surface when the slide is buffered adequately.	
7	Allow the stain and buffer mixture to remain on the slide for 10 to 15 minutes. During this time, the staining takes place as a result of the combination of dye and buffer at the correct pH.	
8	Wash the slide with a steady stream of deionized water. Precipitation of the metallic scum on the film must be avoided. This is done by first flooding the slide with water, then washing and tipping the slide simultaneously. If this is not done and the dye is poured off the slide before it is washed, the insoluble metallic scum will settle on the blood film.	
9	Wipe the dye from the back of the slide when it is still wet by rubbing with a piece of moist gauze.	
10	Place the slide in a vertical position to air-dry, with the feather edge (thin edge) up. Never blot a blood film dry. The heaviest part of the film is at the bottom to allow precipitated stain to flow away from the edge, which will be used for examination of the blood film.	
11	Do not use the slide for microscopic examination until it is dry.	
12	Discard used lancets in a sharps container and discard gauze and other contaminated supplies into a biohazard container.	
13	Clean equipment and return to proper storage.	
14	Clean work area with disinfectant solution.	
15	Remove gloves and discard into biohazard container.	
16	Wash hands using proper procedure.	

Results of Blood Smear Staining

SPECIMEN IDENTIFICATION	ACCEPTABLE RESULTS (YES/NO)

(Continued)

Turgeon: Linné & Ringsrud's Clinical Laboratory Science, 8th Edition

STUDENT PROCEDURE WORKSHEET 11.3

Staining Blood Films with Wright-Giemsa

Review Questions

1. Why would the erythrocytes on a stained peripheral blood film appear to be too red?

2. If the cells on a stained peripheral blood film appear to be very dark, what is the cause?

3. What can variations in cellular appearance can a buffer with a pH of 6.4 that is more acidic or more alkaline produce on a stained blood film?

Procedural Evaluation

Student's Name ______________________________ Grade___________

Instructor's Signature ___________________________ Date___________

Comments:

Turgeon: Linné & Ringsrud's Clinical Laboratory Science, 8th Edition

STUDENT PROCEDURE WORKSHEET 11.4

Leukocyte Differential Count

Student Learning Outcomes

See Chapter 11 of *Linné & Ringsrud's Clinical Laboratory Science: Concepts, Procedures, and Clinical Applications*, 8th edition, for a complete discussion of this procedure. After reading Chapter 11, and at the completion of this laboratory exercise and answering the review questions, a student should be able to:

- Correctly stain a peripheral blood smear.
- Name the type and percentage of normal leukocytes found in peripheral blood of adults and children.
- Complete the end-of-procedure review questions with a grade of 80% or higher.

Principle

A stained blood smear is examined to determine the percentage of each type of normal leukocyte present and assess the erythrocyte and platelet morphology. Increases of normal leukocytes or the presence of immature erythrocytes in peripheral blood are diagnostically important. Various anemias can exhibit abnormalities in the appearance of erythrocytes. Platelet quantities and size irregularities are suggestive of various thrombocyte disorders.

Specimen

Peripheral blood, bone marrow, or body fluid sediments, such as cerebrospinal fluid. Unstained smears can be stored indefinitely.

Reagents, Supplies, and Equipment

1. Manual cell counter designed for differential leukocyte counts
2. Microscope, immersion oil, and lens paper

Quality Control

A set of reference slides and other proficiency testing methods should be used for quality assurance to document the expertise of the hematologist in microscopy. Questionable or abnormal smears should be referred to a supervisor for verification.

Reporting Results

Reference values may vary. Pediatric values are different from adult reference values.

Average	Neutrophils (Bands, Segs)	Lymphocytes	Monocytes	Basophils	Eosinophils
Adults	59%	34%	4%	0.3%	2.7%
Pediatric (1 year)	31%	61%			
Pediatric (10 years)	54%	38%			

Note: Pediatric values an approximate Neutrophil:Lymphocyte Ratio. Other types of WBCs would contribute to a total of 100%. (From Rodak BF, Fritsma GA, Doig K: *Hematology: clinical principles and applications*, ed 3, St Louis, 2007, Saunders.)

Procedure Notes

A well-prepared and well-stained specimen smear is essential to the accuracy of the differential cell count. The knowledge and ability of the morphologist are critical to high quality results. All the leukocytes should appear evenly distributed in the usable fields of the film. Erythrocytes should be barely touching each other in an acceptable field for observation of erythrocytes and leukocytes.

Reference

Turgeon ML: *Clinical hematology*, ed 5, Philadelphia, 2011, Lippincott Williams & Wilkins.

Instructions for the Procedure

Read the list of required equipment, supplies, and reagents and the procedural steps. Follow the procedural steps in exact order.

SEQUENCE	PROCEDURAL STEP	INSTRUCTOR-OBSERVED ACCEPTABLE PERFORMANCE (CHECK IF ACCEPTABLE)
1	Assemble equipment and supplies.	
2	Wash your hands and put on gloves and eye protection as directed.	
3	Use a correctly prepared and stained smear.	
4	Focus the microscope on the 10 × (low-power) objective. Scan the smear to check for cell distribution, clumping, and abnormal cells. Add a drop of immersion oil, and switch to the 100 × (oil-immersion) objective.	
5	Determine a suitable area to begin the count. Extend the examination from the area where approximately half the erythrocytes are barely overlapping to an area where the erythrocytes touch each other. If an area is too thick, cellular details such as nuclear chromatin patterns are difficult to examine. In areas that are too thin, distortion of cells makes it risky to identify a cell type.	

(Continued)

Turgeon: Linné & Ringsrud's Clinical Laboratory Science, 8th Edition

STUDENT PROCEDURE WORKSHEET 11.4

SEQUENCE	PROCEDURAL STEP	INSTRUCTOR-OBSERVED ACCEPTABLE PERFORMANCE (CHECK IF ACCEPTABLE)
6	Count the leukocytes using a tracking pattern (Fig. 11.54). Each cell identified should be immediately recorded as a neutrophil (band) or polymorphonuclear neutrophil (PMN), lymphocyte, monocyte, eosinophil, or basophil. (See Tables 11.3 and 11.4 and text discussion for a brief leukocyte morphology reference.) **Fig. 11.54** Pattern for performing a white blood cell differential.	
7	Abnormalities of leukocytes, erythrocytes, and platelets should be noted. Nucleated erythrocytes are not included in the total count but are noted per 100 white blood cells (WBCs). A total of at least 100 leukocytes should be counted.	
8	Express the results as a percentage of total leukocytes counted.	
9	Discard any used gauze and other contaminated supplies into a biohazard container.	
10	Clean equipment and return to proper storage.	
11	Clean work area with disinfectant solution.	
12	Remove gloves and discard into biohazard container.	
13	Wash hands using proper procedure.	

Unknown Specimens

SPECIMEN IDENTIFICATION	RESULTS

(Continued)

Turgeon: Linné & Ringsrud's Clinical Laboratory Science, 8th Edition

STUDENT PROCEDURE WORKSHEET 11.4

Leukocyte Differential Count

Review Questions

1. Describe the normal morphology of segmented neutrophils, band neutrophils, lymphocytes, monocytes, eosinophils, and basophils.

CELL TYPE	NUCLEAR APPEARANCE	CYTOPLASMIC APPEARANCE
Segmented neutrophil		
Band neutrophil		
Lymphocyte		
Monocyte		
Eosinophil		
Basophil		

Procedural Evaluation

Student's Name ______________________ Grade__________

Instructor's Signature ______________________ Date__________

Comments:

12

Hemostasis and Blood Coagulation

http://evolve.elsevier.com/Turgeon/clinicallab

CHAPTER CONTENTS

LEARNING OUTCOMES

Hemostatic mechanism
- Correlate the three components of the hemostatic system.
- Differentiate between the primary and secondary forms of hemostasis.

Quantitative platelet disorders
- Explain the role of platelets in hemostasis and associated disorders.

Qualitative platelet disorders
- Name and briefly explain the nature of qualitative platelet disorders.

Coagulation
- List and describe the role of various coagulation factors.

Pathways for coagulation cascade
- Break down the activity of the extrinsic pathway of coagulation.
- Break down the activity of the intrinsic pathway of coagulation.
- Differentiate the three major steps of the mechanism of coagulation.

Fibrinolysis
- Describe the process of fibrinolysis.

Protective mechanisms against thrombosis
- List the biological activities responsible for protecting the body against thrombosis.

Tests for hemostasis and coagulation
- Differentiate the characteristics and applications of the common laboratory tests used for coagulation and hemostasis.
- Describe the use of coagulation point-of-care tests.

Case studies
- Analyze the patient history, clinical signs and symptoms, and laboratory data for the stated case studies, answer the related critical thinking questions, and conclude the most likely diagnosis.

Review Questions
- Demonstrate comprehension of the chapter content by completing the end-of-chapter review questions with a grade of 80% or higher.

Note:
- indicates MLT and MLS core content
- indicates MLT (optional) and MLS advanced content

KEY TERMS

activated partial thromboplastin time (APTT)
coagulation
disseminated intravascular coagulation (DIC)
extrinsic system of coagulation
fibrinolysis
hemophilia
hemostasis
international normalized ratio (INR)
intrinsic system of coagulation
platelets
primary hemostasis
prothrombin
prothrombin time
secondary hemostasis
thrombin
thrombus

Hemostasis is the cessation of blood flow from an injured blood vessel. The process of hemostasis balances numerous interdependent coagulation factors that prevent bleeding and involves a complex interaction among blood vessels, platelets, plasma coagulation factors, and inappropriate clotting.

The result of activation of the hemostatic system is the formation of the *hemostatic plug* or thrombus (clot) at the site of injury to the blood vessel. Hemostasis also prevents pathologic or harmful clotting by controlling limitations on formation of the hemostatic plug.

Primary hemostasis begins with endothelial damage and results in the formation of a platelet plug. The most immediate response of the body to bleeding is vasoconstriction; the damaged blood vessel constricts, decreasing the blood flow through the injured area. Platelet adhesion is essential to the formation of a platelet plug. Platelets must be available in adequate numbers and must be functioning normally for this to occur.

Secondary hemostasis results in the formation of a blood clot because coagulation factors present in the blood interact, forming a fibrin network and a thrombus to stop the bleeding completely. Slow lysis of the thrombus (fibrinolysis) begins, and final repair to the site of the injury takes place.

HEMOSTATIC MECHANISM

The hemostatic mechanism is the entire process by which bleeding from an injured blood vessel is controlled and finally stopped (Fig. 12.1). It is a series of physical and biochemical changes normally initiated by an injury to the blood vessel and tissues and culminating in the transformation of fluid blood into a thrombus that effectively seals the injured vessel. The entire hemostatic mechanism can be divided into the following three components:
- Extravascular effects
- Vascular effects
- Intravascular effects

An unbalanced system or mechanism produces bleeding or thrombosis. These conditions can result from a defect in any of the phases of repair, as follows:
1. Vascular system itself may be prone to injury.
2. Platelets may be inadequate in number or function to form the temporary platelet plug.
3. Fibrin clotting mechanism may be inadequate.
4. Fibroblastic repair may be inadequate.

Excessive abnormal bleeding is usually the result of a combination of defects.

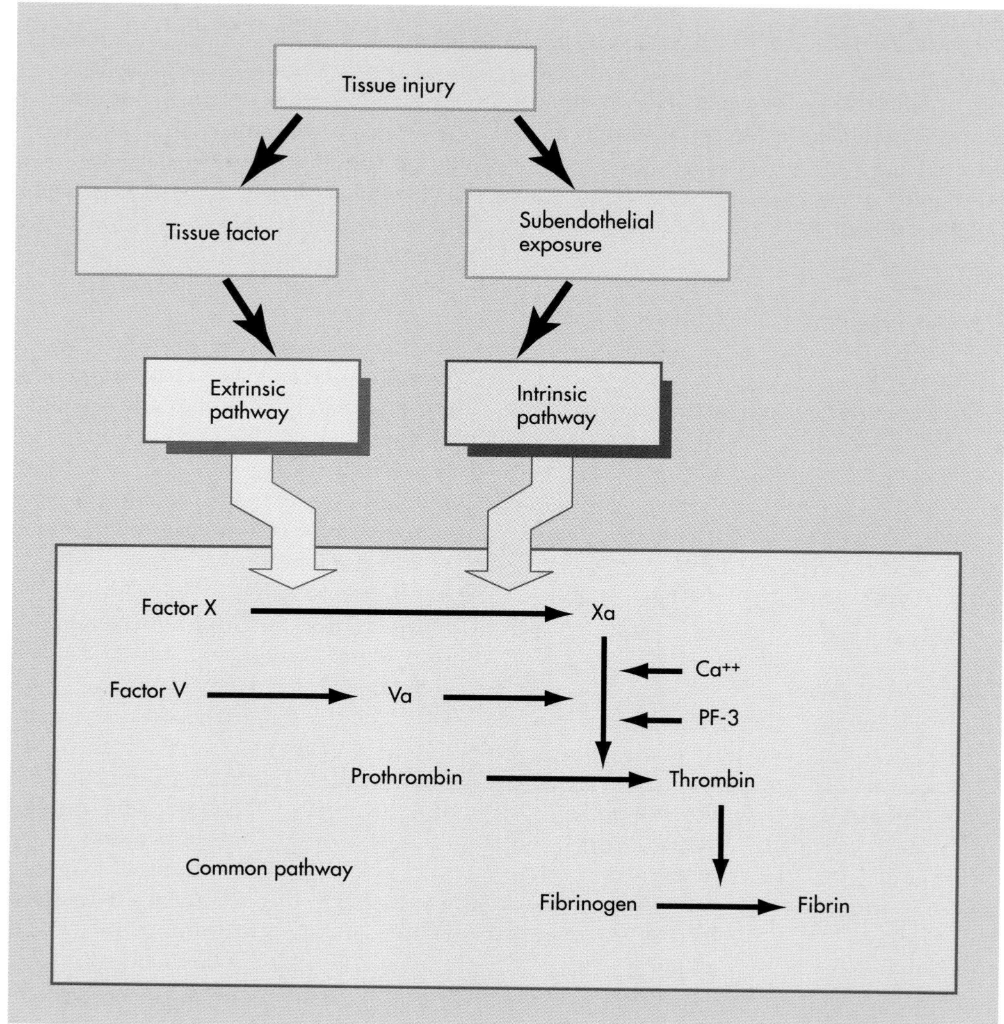

Fig. 12.1 Overview of coagulation. Relationships among the three pathways—common, extrinsic, and intrinsic—emphasizing the major events of the common pathway. *PF-3,* Platelet factor 3. (Redrawn from Powers LW: *Diagnostic hematology,* St Louis, 1989, Mosby.)

Extravascular Effects

The tissue surrounding the blood vessels constitutes the extravascular component. Extravascular effects consist of (1) the physical effects of the surrounding tissues (such as muscle, skin, and elastic tissue), which tend to close and seal the tear in the injured vessel, and (2) the biochemical effects of certain tissue factors that are released from the injured tissue and react with plasma and platelet factors. These latter coagulation factors are found in the extrinsic system of coagulation.

Vascular Effects

The blood vessels themselves constitute the vascular component. The inner monolayer of cells of the blood vessel, the vascular endothelium, is important to hemostasis. This layer of cells provides an inert surface protecting the circulating procoagulants from inappropriate activation until coming in contact with subendothelial collagen. Trauma or injury can disrupt the endothelium and expose the underlying basement membrane of the vessel that contains collagenous material. When circulating platelets make contact with this collagenous material, biochemical and structural changes occur and result in the formation of platelet aggregates and fibrin clots. Platelet aggregates (platelet plug) can plug gaps in the endothelial lining and prevent more stimulation by the collagen layer.

Vascular effects also involve the blood vessels themselves, which constrict almost instantaneously when injured (vasoconstriction). This phenomenon tends to last a relatively short time, but it may be enhanced and prolonged by local release of a vasoconstricting substance, serotonin. Serotonin is released from the platelets as they adhere to the margins of the injury in the wall of the blood vessel. It promotes local, direct, biochemically stimulated narrowing of the torn blood vessel and of locally intact blood vessels in the same vicinity as the injury.

Intravascular Effects

The intravascular component of the hemostatic mechanism includes the platelets and plasma coagulation proteins that circulate in the blood vessels. The intravascular coagulation factors participate in an extremely complicated sequence of physiochemical reactions that transform the liquid blood into a firm fibrin clot. This process requires the initiation of a platelet plug, which is followed by reinforcement with fibrin derived from the activation of the **intrinsic system of coagulation**. All the coagulation factors necessary for the intrinsic system are contained within the blood. Many natural inhibitors and accelerators are brought into action during this time.

Functions of Platelets

Platelets have three important functions, as follows:

1. To react to injury of vessels by forming an aggregate plug of platelets that can physically slow down or stop blood loss
2. To help activate and participate in plasma coagulation to serve more effectively as a barrier to extensive blood loss
3. To maintain the endothelial lining of the blood vessels

To provide normal primary hemostasis, there must be an adequate number of normally functioning platelets. In the past, the bleeding time (BT) test was used as a general screening test for platelet function, but that has largely been replaced by more specific platelet function tests.

Formation of Platelet Plug

When endothelial cells are damaged or displaced or become degenerate, the platelets in the bloodstream are exposed to the underlying collagen. The contact with collagen results in activation or changes in platelet function, which in turn result in platelet adherence to the damaged area of the blood vessel. Fibronectin is secreted by endothelial cells and platelets and assists in bonding platelets to the collagen substrate. An additional protein factor, von Willebrand factor (VIII:vWF), acts as the glue necessary for optimal platelet-collagen binding to occur. Adherence to the collagen initiates platelet activation. On activation, platelets take on a different shape, becoming more spherical with long, irregular arms. This greatly increases the surface area of the platelet and facilitates interaction with other platelets and proteins in the coagulation cascade process. Platelets also aggregate with one another because of changes that occur on their outer coats, a phenomenon known as *platelet aggregation*. The mass of platelets grows and forms the primary hemostatic plug in vivo. This plug must be stabilized by the fibrin strands produced during plasma protein coagulation for more lasting, rather than temporary, effects.

Platelets in Coagulation

The role of platelets in the coagulation process is varied. Platelets secrete substances that serve to promote vasoconstriction, platelet aggregation, and vessel repair. During platelet activation, alterations result in the formation of receptors capable of binding several plasma proteins, most importantly fibrinogen.

Platelet factor 3 (PF3) is a phospholipoprotein (phospholipid) that resides on or within the plasma membrane of the platelets. PF3 is required in the activation of certain coagulation factors. One important function of this activation process is facilitating the formation of **thrombin**.

The endothelium of blood vessels is repaired and maintained with help from products that are secreted by the platelets, such as platelet-derived growth factor.

QUANTITATIVE PLATELET DISORDERS

The reference range of circulating platelets ranges from $150 \times 10^9/L$ to $450 \times 10^9/L$. When the quantity of platelets decreases to levels below this range, a condition of thrombocytopenia exists. If the quantity of platelets increases, thrombocytosis is the result. Disorders of platelets can be classified as quantitative (thrombocytopenia or thrombocytosis) or as qualitative functional disorder (see automated platelet functional analysis).

QUALITATIVE PLATELET DISORDERS

Malfunctioning of platelets is a qualitative disorder. This type of disorder is suggested by a prolonged BT or other clinical expression of bleeding, even though the patient's platelet count and coagulation assay results are normal. Most frequently, these disorders are acquired, but they can be inherited. Types of platelet dysfunction can include the following:

- Drug-induced dysfunction, most commonly due to aspirin ingestion
- Uremia due to renal dysfunction
- Liver disease, e.g., cirrhosis or hepatic dysfunction
- Acquired or inherited von Willebrand disease
- Paraneoplastic platelet dysfunction associated with plasma cell dyscrasias, e.g., multiple myeloma

Thrombocytopenia

A correlation exists between severe thrombocytopenia and spontaneous clinical bleeding. If platelets are absent or severely decreased below $100 \times 10^9/L$, clinical symptoms usually include the presence of petechiae or purpura. Petechiae appear as small, purplish hemorrhagic spots on the skin or mucous membranes; purpura is characterized by extensive areas of red or dark-purple discoloration.

Thrombocytopenia can result from a wide variety of conditions, such as after the use of extracorporeal circulation in cardiac bypass surgery or in alcoholic liver disease. Heparin-induced thrombocytopenia (HIT) and associated thrombotic events, relatively common side effects of heparin therapy, can cause substantial morbidity and mortality. Thrombocytopenia in itself rarely poses a threat to affected patients, but disorders associated with it—which include deep venous thrombosis, **disseminated intravascular coagulation (DIC)**, pulmonary embolism, cerebral thrombosis, myocardial infarction, and ischemic injury to the legs or arms—can produce severe morbidity and mortality.

Serum from patients with HIT contains immunoglobulin G that, in the presence of small amounts of heparin, activates normal platelets and causes them to aggregate and release the contents of their granules, including serotonin.

Most thrombocytopenic conditions can be classified into the following major categories:

1. Disorders of production
2. Disorders of destruction and disorders of utilization
3. Disorders of platelet distribution and dilution

Thrombocytosis

Thrombocytosis is generally defined as a substantial increase in circulating platelets over the reference range upper limit of 450×10^9/L.

COAGULATION

When a blood vessel is injured, coagulation is the mechanism that allows plasma proteins, coagulation factors, tissue factors, and calcium to work together on the surface of the platelets to form a fibrin clot. Most clinical conditions requiring coagulation studies involve the intrinsic system of coagulation. This section discusses the coagulation factors and their nomenclature.

The blood coagulation mechanism involves many coagulation factors; knowing which factor is not performing its proper function is critical. The proper formation of a blood clot after a scratch or cut depends on healthy functioning of all the coagulation factors. In an individual with a weakness or deficiency in one or several coagulation factors, severe trauma from serious injury or surgical treatment can result in collapse of the clotting mechanism. This will result in a most drastic manifestation, severe hemorrhage. Some persons have a clotting mechanism that is adequate for everyday living, but during such common surgical procedures as dental extraction or tonsillectomy, they experience severe bleeding.

It is generally agreed that all the elements necessary for clot formation are normally present in the circulating blood, and that the fluidity of blood depends on a balance between the coagulant and anticoagulant.

The mechanism of coagulation takes place in the following major steps, with the formation of a fibrin thrombus being the major goal:

1. Formation of thromboplastin
2. Formation of thrombin
3. Formation of fibrin
4. Fibrinolysis

Coagulation Factors

The coagulation factors are fundamentally protein, with the exception of calcium and the phospholipid of the platelets.

The coagulation factors are divided into three categories: substrate, cofactors, and enzymes. Fibrinogen (factor I) is considered the substrate because the formation of a fibrin clot from fibrinogen is seen as the major goal of the coagulation process. *Cofactors* are proteins that accelerate the reactions of the enzymes involved in the process. Cofactors include coagulation factors III (tissue factor), V (labile factor), and VIII (antihemophilic factor) and high-molecular-weight kininogen (HMWK, Fitzgerald factor). Most of the remaining coagulation factors are enzyme precursors, or zymogens, which become active enzymes after proteolytic or structural change. Except for coagulation factor XIII (fibrin-stabilizing factor, fibrinase), which is a transamidase, the enzyme factors functioning in coagulation are serine proteases, which require vitamin K for proper formation. This becomes important when discussing anticoagulation with warfarin. Except possibly for coagulation factor VIII, coagulation proteins usually are produced in the liver. Other factors are produced in endothelial cells and the megakaryocytes.

The process of coagulation is a series of biochemical reactions in which inactive zymogens are converted to active enzyme forms, which then activate other zymogens. The coagulation process is a true coagulation cascade of factor activities, all interrelated to other factors. It is a carefully controlled process that responds to injury while continuing the maintenance of blood circulation.

Nomenclature

To standardize the complex nomenclature used by researchers involved in coagulation studies, the Scientific and Standardization Committee of the International Society on Thrombosis and Haemostasis (ISTH) has established an ongoing updating process.[1] Twelve coagulation factors are described and designated by Roman numerals; other coagulation factors are known by name only (Table 12.1).

TABLE 12.1 Coagulation Factors

Factor[a]	Name	Synonym(s)
I	Fibrinogen	
II	Prothrombin	
III	Tissue thromboplastin	Tissue factor
IV	Ionized calcium	
V	Labile factor	Proaccelerin, accelerator globulin
VI	An obsolete term for activated factor V (Va)	Accelerin
VII	Proconvertin	Stable factor
VIII:C	Antihemophilic factor	Antihemophilic globulin, antihemophilic factor A, subunit VIII:C
VIII:vWF	von Willebrand factor	Subunit VIII:vWF
IX	Plasma thromboplastin component	Antihemophilic factor B, Christmas factor
X	Stuart-Prower factor	Stuart factor
XI	Plasma thromboplastin antecedent	Antihemophilic factor C
XII	Hageman factor	Glass factor, contact factor
XIII	Fibrin-stabilizing factor	Fibrinase
Other Essential Coagulation Reactants		
	Prokallikrein (the proenzyme to tissue kallikrein)	Prekallikrein, Fletcher factor
	High-molecular-weight kininogen	HMW kininogen, Fitzgerald factor
	Fibronectin	
	Phospholipid	Phospholipoprotein
	Phospholipoprotein of platelets	
	Active form of kallikrein	
	Kininogen	
	Antithrombin III	
	Protein C	
	Protein S	

[a]When factors have been activated, they have the designation "a" after the Roman numeral.

Roman numerals have been assigned to the various coagulation factors in the order of their discovery and do not indicate anything about the sequence of the reactions. No coagulation factor has been assigned Roman numeral VI. The numerals are used to denote the coagulation factors as they exist in the plasma, except for coagulation factor III, tissue thromboplastin, which is not normally present in plasma but is found in tissue. Factor III is not a single substance but a variety of substances, which is why the ISTH committee made "tissue thromboplastin" the standard designation and relegated factor III to an historical reference.

The lowercase "a" denotes activated forms and cofactors for the coagulation factors. All coagulation factors except tissue thromboplastin (factor III) circulate in an inactive, or precursor, form. In addition to the coagulation factors denoted by Roman numerals, other essential coagulation reactants participate in the coagulation process.

Fibrinogen (Factor I)

Fibrinogen is the soluble precursor of a clot-forming protein, fibrin, and is involved in the common pathway of both extrinsic and intrinsic clotting. Fibrinogen is a globulin with a molecular weight of 340,000 daltons (D). It is present in the plasma of normal persons at a concentration of 200 to 400 mg/dL. A minimum of 50 to 100 mg/dL is required for normal coagulation.

Fibrinogen is synthesized by the liver but does not require vitamin K for its production. In severe liver disease, a moderate lowering of the plasma fibrinogen level may occur, although rarely to the degree that results in hemorrhage.

By the action of thrombin, two peptides are split from the fibrinogen molecule, leaving a fibrin monomer. Fibrin monomers aggregate to form the final polymerized fibrin clot.

Fibrinogen is relatively unaffected by heat and storage (is stable) but may be irreversibly precipitated at 56°C. It has a half-life of 120 hours.

Prothrombin (Factor II)

Thrombin is generated from a precursor, **prothrombin**, and is involved in the common pathway of both extrinsic and intrinsic clotting. Prothrombin is synthesized by the liver through the action of vitamin K. It is a protein (globulin) with a molecular weight of about 70,000 D and is normally present in the plasma in a concentration of approximately 8 to 15 mg/dL. Prothrombin is utilized in the clotting mechanism to such a degree that little remains in the serum. In normal plasma, there is an excess of prothrombin relative to the amount of thrombin needed to clot fibrinogen. A wide margin of safety has been provided for this important substance. About 20% to 40% of the normal concentration must be present to ensure hemostasis. Prothrombin is heat stable and has a half-life of 70 to 110 hours.

Tissue Thromboplastin (Factor III)

Thromboplastin, or *tissue factor,* is the name given to any substance capable of converting prothrombin to thrombin. In coagulation, two separate mechanisms utilize thromboplastin: as intrinsic or blood thromboplastin and as extrinsic or tissue thromboplastin. All injured tissues yield a complex mixture of as-yet unclassified substances that possess potential thromboplastic activity. During clotting of whole blood, platelets appear to be the source of thromboplastin.

Tissue thromboplastin is a high-molecular-weight lipoprotein that is found in almost all body tissues. The molecular weight depends on the type of tissue from which the particular thromboplastin is derived, and ranges from 45,000 to more than 1 million D. Tissue thromboplastin is found in brain, lung, vascular endothelium, liver, placenta, and kidneys.

Ionized Calcium (Factor IV)

Calcium in the ionized state is essential for coagulation. The term *ionized calcium* is now used for calcium when it participates in this process; this was formerly called "factor IV." Ionized calcium is necessary to activate thromboplastin and to convert prothrombin to thrombin; the exact mechanism by which calcium acts is not completely understood. Only a small amount of ionized calcium is required for blood coagulation. Ionized calcium is essential for clotting, which makes possible the use of anticoagulants that bind calcium; by binding of calcium, fibrin formation cannot take place, and clotting does not occur.

Calcium appears to function mainly as a bridge between the phospholipid surface of platelets and several clotting factors. Binding sites on several factors allow bridging with the calcium-phospholipid complex.

Factor V (Proaccelerin or Labile Factor)

Factor V is essential for the prompt conversion of prothrombin to thrombin in the clotting of whole blood and is involved in the common pathway of both extrinsic and intrinsic clotting pathways. It is synthesized in the liver; acquired deficiencies have been observed in liver disease. When factor V levels decrease to 5% to 25% of normal, bleeding occurs. Factor V is a globulin of about 330,000 D. It is labile, its activity being destroyed in the clotting process. The activity of factor V in plasma deteriorates even when the plasma is frozen; it is the most unstable of the coagulation factors and is also known as *labile coagulation factor.* Its activity decreases within a few hours when human blood or plasma is stored at or above room temperature. It has a half-life of about 25 hours in the plasma.

Factor VII (Proconvertin, Stable Factor, Serum Prothrombin Conversion Accelerator)

Factor VII is neither destroyed nor consumed in the clotting process and is known as *stable factor.* It is present in both plasma and serum and is essential only for the extrinsic clotting pathway. It is a beta (β-) globulin of 60,000 D. It is synthesized in the liver and requires vitamin K for its production. For normal coagulation, minimum levels are 5% to 10% of the normal amount. An acquired deficiency of factor VII results from any disorder that decreases its synthesis in the liver. It has a very short biological half-life, 4 to 6 hours, which results in a rapid disappearance from the blood when factor VII production is halted. This may occur during drug therapy with warfarin or in a congenitally deficient patient. Factor VII remains at a high level in stored blood as well as in serum. Factor VII activates tissue thromboplastin and accelerates the production of thrombin from prothrombin. Its presence can be monitored by the prothrombin test.

Factor VIII (Antihemophilic Factor, VIII:C, VIII:vWF, Factor VIII Clotting Activity)

Factor VIII is actually a combination of two functional subunits circulating as a complex: coagulation factors VIII:C and VIII:vWF. The entire circulating molecule can be designated *VIII/vWF.*

Factor VIII:C. Factor VIII:C represents the ability of the factor VIII molecule to correct coagulation abnormalities associated with classic hemophilia A. A hereditary deficiency of VIII:C corresponds with classic hemophilia A; deficiencies can be acquired as well. The subunit designated coagulation factor VIII:C acts in the intrinsic clotting pathway as a cofactor to factor IXa in the conversion of X to Xa. This unit is measured by the factor VIII assay and the activated partial thromboplastin time (APTT) test.

Factor VIII:VWF. The other factor VIII subunit, called *factor VIII:vWF,* facilitates platelet adherence to subendothelial surfaces. Factor VIII:vWF is necessary for normal platelet adhesion. It is the portion of the molecule responsible for binding platelets to endothelium and supports normal platelet adhesion and function. This subunit is not involved in the coagulation pathway. It is present in plasma, platelets, megakaryocytes, and endothelial cells.

The larger part of the factor VIII complex is made up of the VIII:vWF subunit. It is strongly antigenic, and a portion of the molecule participates in platelet aggregation induced by the antibiotic ristocetin. Laboratory tests using immunoassay measure antigenic activity, whereas the basis of another test is the portion of the molecule that makes possible platelet aggregation in the presence of ristocetin.

The production site of factor VIII is not certain; possible sites are endothelial cells and megakaryocytes for the VIII:vWF subunit. Factor VIII is a β-globulin of more than 1 million D. It is lost rapidly from the bloodstream; the VIII:C subunit has a half-life of 6 to 10 hours. This rapid clearance occurs in normal persons as well as in those with a congenital deficiency of the factor (classic hemophilia A).

Hemophilia A. *Hemophilia* refers to a sex-linked recessive coagulation disorder. The terms *antihemophilic factor* and *antihemophilic globulin* have been used to designate the procoagulant present in normal plasma but deficient in the plasma of patients with hemophilia. It has been demonstrated that the coagulation defect can be corrected by the use of normal plasma-mixing study. Mixing normal plasma with plasma from a patient with hemophilia A will correct the deficiency of AHF that exists in this patient's plasma. Further, mixing normal plasma with patient plasma is a convenient way to differentiate factor deficiency from an acquired deficiency caused by antibody deactivation or specific pathologic factor inhibitors.

The term *hemophilia A,* the classic form of the disorder, is adopted to designate the hereditary disease caused by a deficiency in the factor VIII:C subunit. Patients with severe hemophilia A have a history of bleeding into joints and intramuscular hemorrhage. These patients usually have normal levels of the VIII:vWF subunit and a normal BT.

Von Willebrand disease (vWD) is hereditary and is found in several different subtypes; the clinical manifestations will vary with the severity of the disease. Symptoms can include abnormal bleeding in childhood, easy bruising, bleeding gums, gastrointestinal bleeding, and abnormal bleeding after dental procedures. Patients with vWD have a deficiency of von Willebrand factor (VIII:vWF subunit of coagulation factor VIII); this factor is required for normal platelet adhesion to endothelium in the hemostatic process.

Factor IX (Plasma Thromboplastin Component)

Factor IX is a stable protein factor, either an α- or β-globulin, of 55,000 to 62,000 D. It has a half-life of about 20 hours, is not consumed during clotting, and is not destroyed by aging. It is present in both serum and plasma, and there is probably no significant loss of the factor in blood or plasma stored at 4°C for 2 weeks. Factor IX is an essential component of the intrinsic thromboplastin-generating system. It is synthesized in the liver and requires vitamin K for its production.

Hemophilia B. The disease resulting from a deficiency of factor IX is known as *hemophilia B.* It is inherited as a sex-linked recessive disorder, and its clinical symptoms are similar to those of hemophilia A. Hemophilia B can be classified as *mild, moderate,* or *severe,* paralleling the level of coagulation factor IX present.

Factor X (Stuart-Prower Factor)

The relatively stable factor X is not consumed during the clotting process and therefore is found in both serum and plasma. It is an α-globulin of 59,000 D that requires vitamin K for its synthesis in the liver. Factor X is essential to the intrinsic pathway, working with other substances to generate thromboplastin that converts prothrombin to thrombin. It helps to form the final common pathway through which products of the intrinsic and extrinsic thromboplastin-generating systems act. Factor X is stable for several weeks to 2 months when stored at 4°C. It has a half-life of 24 to 65 hours.

Factor XI (Plasma Thromboplastin Antecedent)

Factor XI is a β-globulin of 160,000 to 200,000 D. Its synthesis takes place in the liver, and vitamin K is not required for its production. It circulates as a complex with another protein, HMWK. Only part of factor XI is consumed during the clotting process, so it is present in the serum as well as in the plasma. It is essential for the intrinsic thromboplastin-generating mechanism.

Factor XII (Hageman Factor)

Factor XII is a stable gamma (γ-) globulin of 80,000 D. It is not consumed during the clotting process and is found in both serum and plasma. It is synthesized in the liver and does not depend on vitamin K for its synthesis. Factor XII is converted to an active form when it comes in contact with glass and therefore also is known as the *contact factor* or *glass factor.* The natural counterpart of glass is not known, but platelets or damaged endothelium may be involved in this primary activation process. Factor XII is involved in the initial phase of the intrinsic coagulation pathway. Deficiency of this factor does not place a patient at risk for abnormal bleeding.

Factor XIII (Fibrin-Stabilizing Factor, Fibrinase)

Factor XIII is an α-globulin of high molecular weight. Its site of production is not fully known but is believed to be in the liver for the plasma factor. Platelet factor XIII is synthesized by megakaryocytes. Evidence indicates that factor XIII is an enzyme (fibrinase) that catalyzes the polymerization of fibrin; polymerizing the fine fibrin clots produces a stable fibrin clot. This factor is inhibited by ethylenediaminetetraacetic acid (EDTA).

Factor XIII is used up in the polymerization of fibrin. It acts to stabilize the fibrin clot and further acts to assist in linking the endothelial cell protein fibronectin to collagen and fibrin residues; this is extremely important in tissue growth and repair. Deficiencies cannot be detected by routine testing methods.

Prokallikrein (Prekallikrein, Fletcher Factor)

Prokallikrein (PK) is a precursor for a serine protease, kallikrein, which also activates plasminogen. PK is involved in the intrinsic coagulation pathway. Kallikrein is a chemotactic coagulation factor used to recruit phagocytes, and it can stimulate the complement cascade. PK is found in the plasma in association with HMWK. It is produced in the liver but is not dependent on vitamin K for its synthesis. PK is the precursor for the plasma zymogen, which converts to active kallikrein.

High-Molecular-Weight Kininogen (Fitzgerald Factor)

HMWK can be acted on to yield kinin. It serves as a cofactor for reactions involving coagulation factor XII and activation of coagulation factor VII. HMWK is involved in the intrinsic coagulation pathway. It is the precursor molecule of bradykinin, an important inflammatory mediator involving vascular permeability and dilation, pain production at sites of inflammation, and synthesis of prostaglandin. HMWK is produced in the liver and is not dependent on vitamin K for its synthesis.

Properties of Coagulation factors

Coagulation factors can be divided into three groups based on their properties: fibrinogen, prothrombin, and contact.

Fibrinogen group. The fibrinogen group (thrombin sensitive) consists of coagulation factors I, V, VIII, and XIII. Thrombin acts on all these factors. Thrombin enhances factors V and VIII by converting them to active cofactors. It also activates factor XIII and converts fibrinogen (factor I) to fibrin. All these factors are consumed in the coagulation process. Coagulation factors V and VIII are relatively labile and are not present in stored plasma. In addition being present in plasma, fibrinogen factors are also found within platelets.

Prothrombin group. The prothrombin group (vitamin K dependent) consists of coagulation factors II, VII, IX, and X. Vitamin K is essential for synthesis of all these factors. Warfarin-type drugs such as Coumadin, which inhibit vitamin K, cause a decrease in these factors. Factors VII, IX, and X are not consumed in the coagulation process and are present in serum as well in plasma. These factors are stable and are well preserved in stored plasma.

Contact group. The contact group consists of coagulation factors XI and XII, PK (Fletcher factor), and HMWK (Fitzgerald factor). These factors are not consumed in the coagulation process, are not dependent on vitamin K for their synthesis, and are relatively stable.

Mechanism of Coagulation

The complex mechanism of coagulation takes place in three major stages.

Stage 1: Generation of Thromboplastic Activity

The thromboplastic activity necessary to convert prothrombin to thrombin is produced in stage 1 through the interaction of platelets with coagulation factors XII, XI, IX, and VIII (intrinsic pathway) or through the release of tissue thromboplastin from the injured tissues (extrinsic pathway). Plasma coagulation factor VII is activated by the tissue thromboplastic substances released by the injured tissue and initiates the extrinsic pathway. Various tests will detect stage 1 deficiencies, but the test of choice for screening and identifying them is the APTT test.

Stage 2: Generation of Thrombin

The plasma or tissue thromboplastin, plus factor VII produced in stage 1, in the presence of factors V and X converts prothrombin to the active enzyme thrombin. Laboratory tests are available to detect deficiencies in stage 2. The one-stage prothrombin time (PT) test detects deficiencies best in stages 2 and 3. Abnormal formation of a clot results from a deficiency of any of the coagulation factors or from the presence of an inhibitor or anticoagulant. The anticoagulants EDTA, oxalate, and citrate remove calcium to prevent clotting in vitro. Heparin and warfarin (Coumadin) prevent the conversion of prothrombin to thrombin, also preventing the clotting mechanism from functioning in vivo.

Stage 3: Conversion of Fibrinogen to Fibrin

Thrombin converts fibrinogen to fibrin, and a fibrin clot is formed that is stabilized by the presence of factor XIII. The thrombin time (TT) test measures the concentration and activity of fibrinogen in stage 3.

The presence of calcium ions is necessary in all three stages of the clotting mechanism.

PATHWAYS FOR COAGULATION CASCADE

The final product in the clotting process is the production of a stable fibrin clot (see Fig. 12.1). A series of events must take place involving many reactions and feedback mechanisms before the clot is formed. By means of the intrinsic or extrinsic pathway, or both, leading to a common pathway, the various precursors, factors, and other reactants respond normally in an orderly, controlled process—the coagulation cascade.

Intrinsic versus Extrinsic Coagulation Pathway

All factors required for the intrinsic pathway are contained within the blood. The extrinsic pathway is activated by tissue thromboplastin (factor III), which is released from the damaged cells and tissues outside the circulating blood.

Intrinsic Pathway (Activation of Factor X)

In the intrinsic pathway, the circulating blood contains all the necessary components that lead to the activation of factor X (Fig. 12.2). It is thought that tissue injury, after exposure to foreign substances such as collagen, activates the intrinsic pathway. Injury to endothelial cells can begin this process. In this pathway a complex involving factors VIII and IX, in association with calcium and phospholipid on the platelets, ultimately activates factor X. To accomplish this, factor IX is first activated by the action of factor XIa (in the presence of calcium ions), which has previously been activated by factor XII. Factors XI and XII are known as *contact factors* because their activation is initiated by contact with subendothelial basement membrane that is exposed at the time of a tissue or blood vessel injury.

Although the complex reactions that occur in the intrinsic pathway take place relatively slowly, they account for the majority of the coagulation activities in the body. A laboratory test that monitors the intrinsic pathway leading to fibrin clot formation is the APTT. The APTT measures factors XII, XI, X, IX, VIII, V, II, and fibrinogen.

Extrinsic Pathway (Activation of Factor X)

The term *extrinsic* is used to indicate the pathway taken when tissue thromboplastin, a substance not found in the blood, enters the vascular system and, in the presence of calcium and factor VII, activates factor X (Fig. 12.3). Factor VII is activated to its VIIa form in the presence of ionized calcium (factor IV) and tissue thromboplastin (factor III). Factor VIIa activates coagulation factor IX to IXa, which in turn activates factor X to Xa. Thromboplastin is released from the injured wall of the blood vessel. Only activated factor VII is needed in the extrinsic pathway, bypassing factors XII, XI, IX, and VIII (used in the intrinsic pathway to activate factor X to its activated form, Xa). In addition to quickly providing small amounts of thrombin, which leads to fibrin formation, the thrombin generated in the extrinsic pathway can enhance the activity of factors V and VIII in the intrinsic pathway. To monitor the extrinsic pathway leading to fibrin clot formation in the laboratory, the PT test is performed. The PT measures factors VII, X, V, II, and I.

Common Pathway (Formation of Fibrin Clot From Factor X)

By means of the extrinsic or the intrinsic pathway, or both, the common pathway, the activation of factor X to Xa, occurs. The

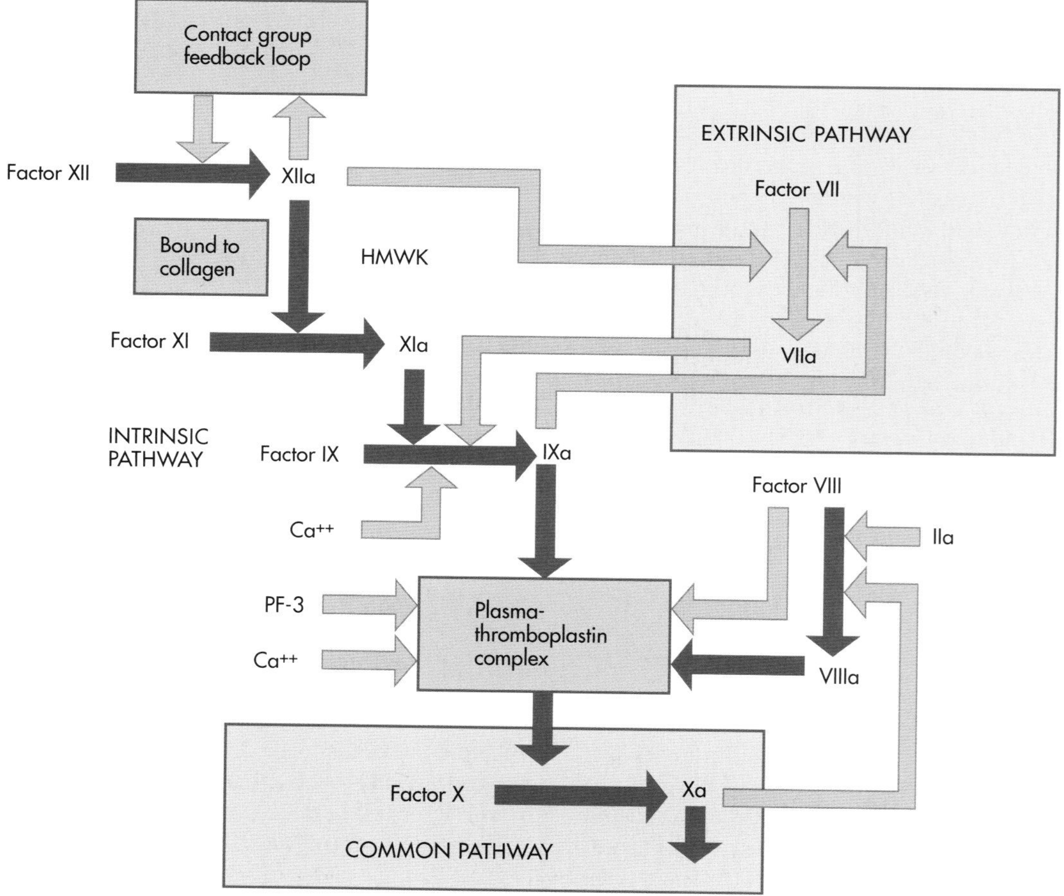

Fig. 12.2 Major reactions of the intrinsic pathway. Generation of factor IXa and the plasma-thromboplastin complex (a, activated). *HMWK,* High-molecular-weight kininogen; *Ca^{++},* ionized calcium; *PF-3,* platelet factor 3. (Redrawn from Powers LW: *Diagnostic hematology,* St Louis, 1989, Mosby.)

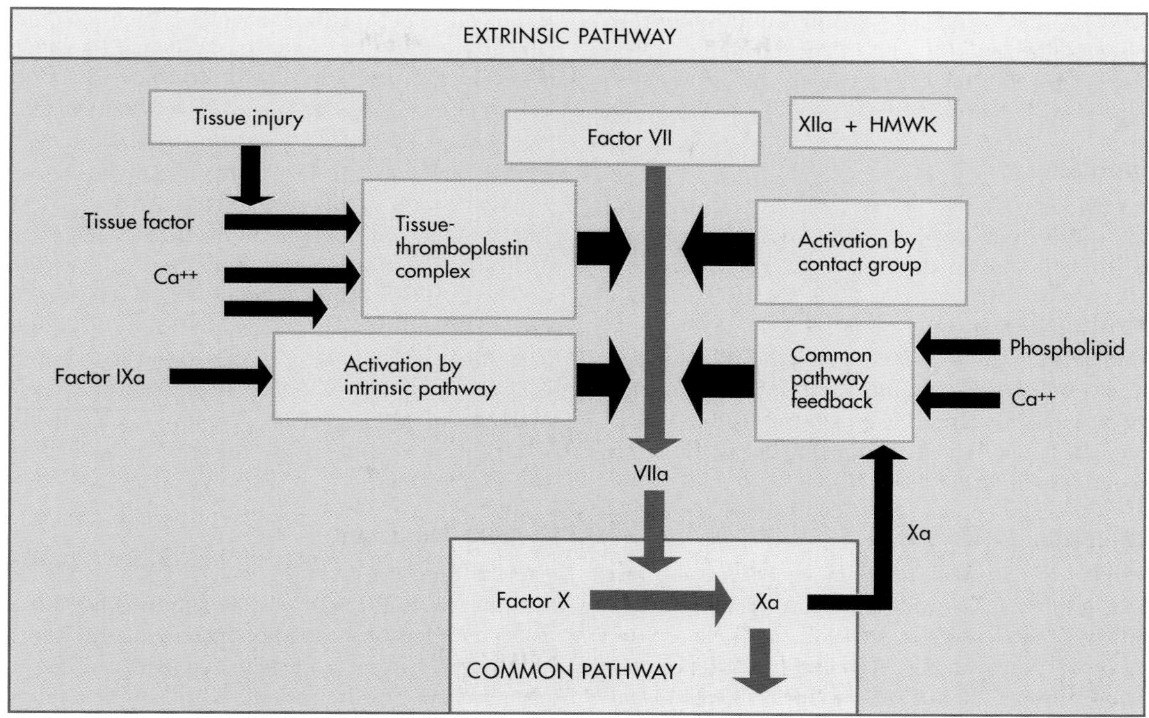

Fig. 12.3 Major reactions of the extrinsic pathway. Generation of factor VIIa after activation of tissue factors. (Redrawn from Powers LW: *Diagnostic hematology,* St Louis, 1989, Mosby.)

activation of factor X is the point where the two pathways converge to form the common pathway. Once Xa is formed, another cofactor, V, in the presence of calcium and PF3, converts prothrombin (factor II) to the active enzyme, thrombin. The activation of thrombin is slow, but once generated, it further amplifies the coagulation process. Thrombin acts to convert fibrinogen to fibrin. Activation of factor XIII during this process results in the formation of a stronger, more durable clot.

Fibrin Clot and Clot Retraction

The result of converting fibrinogen to fibrin is a visible fibrin clot. The fibrin clot is formed loosely over the site of injury, reinforcing the platelet plug and closing off the wound. After a time, the clot begins to retract and becomes smaller—clot retraction. This retraction is attributed to the action of the platelets and other cells that have been trapped in the clot. The fibers of fibrin are pulled closer together by cytoplasmic processes initiated by the platelets. Clot retraction also can be observed in a test tube (in vitro). The liquid remaining after the clot has retracted is serum. Normal clot retraction in vitro should be complete by 4 hours at 37°C.

FIBRINOLYSIS

Besides having a system for clot formation, the body also has a means by which the fibrin clot may be removed and the flow of blood reestablished. The mechanism for clot removal is not completely understood.

As soon as the clotting process has begun, fibrinolysis is initiated to break down the fibrin clot that is formed. Normally, the fibrinolytic system functions to keep the vascular system free of fibrin clots or deposited fibrin. Evidence indicates that the fibrinolytic system and the coagulation system are in equilibrium in normal persons. As a general rule, fibrinolysis is increased whenever coagulation is increased.

The active enzyme that is responsible for digesting fibrin or fibrinogen is plasmin. Plasmin is not normally found in the circulating blood but is present in an inactive form, plasminogen. Plasminogen is converted to plasmin by certain proteolytic enzymes. These plasminogen activators are found in small amounts in most body tissues, in very low amounts in most body fluids, and in urine. The decomposition products of fibrin and fibrinogen, called fibrin degradation products or fibrin split products, are formed during fibrinolysis and are removed from the blood by the mononuclear phagocytic system. As breakdown products of fibrin, D-dimers result only when fibrin that has been stabilized by factor XIII cross-linking has been digested.

PROTECTIVE MECHANISMS AGAINST THROMBOSIS

To maintain a balance, the body has a number of proteins that inhibit coagulation and help prevent unwanted thrombus formation. In the blood circulation, the predisposition to thrombosis depends on the balance between procoagulant and anticoagulant factors. Several important biological activities normally protect the body against thrombosis, as follows:

1. Normal flow of blood
2. Removal of activated clotting factors and particulate material

3. Natural in vivo anticoagulant systems: antithrombin III (AT-III), heparin cofactor II (HC-II), and protein C and its cofactor, protein S
4. Cellular regulators

Normal Blood Flow

Normal flow of blood prevents the accumulation of procoagulant material, which reduces the possibility of local fibrin formation.

Removal of Materials

Activated clotting factors are removed by hepatocytes. This process and naturally occurring inhibitors limit intravascular clotting and fibrinolysis by inactivation of such factors as XIa, IXa, Xa, and IIa. Removal of particulate material is also important in preventing the initiation of coagulation.

Natural Anticoagulant Systems

The in vivo existence of natural anticoagulant systems is essential to prevent thrombosis. These natural anticoagulants include AT-III, HC-II, and proteins C and S.

Deficiencies of AT-III, protein C, or protein S, or deficiencies of their inhibitors (antibodies), will contribute to a hypercoagulable state. Enzyme-linked immunosorbent assay (ELISA) tests will reveal deficiencies of these proteins.

Antithrombin III

AT-III is considered the major inhibitor of thrombin. It inhibits thrombin formation by forming a stable, one-to-one complex with thrombin. AT-III is the principal physiologic inhibitor of thrombin and factor Xa. AT can be determined by measuring the inhibitory effect on either thrombin or factor Xa as the target enzyme.

AT-III is also known to inhibit factors IXa, XIa, and XIIa.

The AT-III laboratory assay relies on the principle that in the presence of heparin, thrombin is neutralized at a rate that is proportional to AT-III concentration. After defibrination, plasma is assayed in a two-stage procedure that uses standardized amounts of heparin, fibrinogen, and thrombin. The resulting clotting time is interpreted using a calibration curve.

Heparin Cofactor

AT-III heparin cofactor and HC-II are two heparin-dependent thrombin inhibitors present in human plasma. Heparin is produced endogenously by mast cells, and heparin-like molecules are found in the endothelium.

Protein C and Protein S

Protein C is synthesized in the liver and circulates as an inactive zymogen. Protein C is converted to an active form, activated protein C (APC), by thrombin in the presence of thrombomodulin, which is found on the endothelial cells. APC in the presence of the cofactor protein S cleaves factor Va and factor VIIIa into their inactive Vi and VIIIi forms (*i* indicating *inactive*). Its interaction with protein C and protein S shows that thrombin acts not only as a procoagulant, but also as an anticoagulant. The coagulometric protein C assay is based on an APTT reaction in which the APC inactivates the accelerators factor Va and factor VIIIa, prolonging the clotting time with increasing protein C levels. The chromogenic protein C assay allows a direct determination of the enzymatic activity.

APC resistance, also known as *factor V Leiden,* is a genetic variation of the factor V protein that alters the binding site for APC and prevents APC from inactivating factor Va. The heterozygous form of this genetic variation occurs in up to 20% of people tested and can account for 20% to 50% of cases of inherited thrombophilia.

The ProC Global is an APTT-based screening assay for the protein C system that determines the ratio of a dilute APTT in the presence of protein C activation versus no protein C activation. ProC AcR is a similar, more specific assay for the determination of APC resistance/factor V Leiden that uses a dilute Russell viper venom time in the presence and absence of a protein C activator.

Cellular Regulators

Cellular regulators include enzymes, which are cellular proteases that block the activation or action of plasmin. In addition, cells that regulate coagulation include not only hepatic cells but also monocytes, macrophages, and platelets. The production of protein S cofactor by endothelial cells is believed to play a significant regulatory role in the initiation, propagation, and suppression of hemostasis and thrombosis.

Therapeutic Anticoagulant Therapy

Anticoagulants are included in a family of drugs called *antithrombotics.* These include oral antiplatelet drugs (such as aspirin and clopidogrel), intravenous antiplatelet membrane glycoprotein receptor drugs (such as abciximab, eptifibatide, and tirofiban), and the thrombolytics.

Anticoagulant therapy is either therapeutic or prophylactic. This therapy can be used for patients with coronary artery disease complicated by cardiac insufficiency with anticoagulation or for the prevention of ischemic stroke in patients with chronic atrial fibrillation or artificial heart valves.

Deep venous thrombosis (DVT) is a common disorder in which a blood clot forms inside a blood vessel and obstructs blood flow, resulting in blockage of the vessel. Although the incidence of DVT is 1 or 2 patients/1000 patients each year, the incidence of thrombotic events increases with age and rises to about 1 patient/100 patients older than 75 years. DVTs are associated with oral contraceptives, various forms of immobilization, pregnancy, trauma, surgery, malignant neoplasms, older age, and genetic risk factors, most frequently Factor V (Leiden) and Factor II G20210A mutations.

In addition, anticoagulation is used for the prevention of venous thromboembolism (VTE) in the form of deep venous thromboses (clots in major leg veins) or pulmonary emboli (clots in the vasculature of the lungs), or is used subsequent to orthopedic surgery, neurosurgery, or a complicated pregnancy.[2–4]

Antithrombolytic drugs include the following:

- Anti-Xa anticoagulants (such as heparin and its analogs)
- Warfarin, a vitamin K antagonist
- Direct thrombin inhibitors (DTI) such as new oral anticoagulants

Heparin

Heparin therapy can consist of unfractionated heparin (UFH) or low-molecular-weight heparin (LMWH) derived from UFH. LMWH has a predictable dose-response relationship that makes it safer and easier to administer than UFH. LMWH is used as initial therapy to induce a quick anticoagulation response in conditions such as deep vein thrombosis. LMWH does not need to be used regularly, except in some patients with a coagulopathy or with a condition such as pregnancy or renal or hepatic disease.

Direct-Acting and Novel Anticoagulants

Direct-acting novel, oral anticoagulants (DOACs or NOACs) are intended to replace warfarin treatment. Two broad classes of DOACs include: oral direct thrombin inhibitors e.g. dabigatran and oral direct factor Xa inhibitors, e.g. rivaroxaban and apixaban. DTIs, dabigatran, bind and inhibit thrombin without involving another coagulation protein. Unlike heparins, DTIs are small molecules that inhibit thrombin directly, with no need for a cofactor. DTI action results in specific binding of free and fibrin-bound thrombin, thereby preventing fibrin formation; in thrombin-mediated activation of factors V, VIII, XI, and XIII; and in thrombin-induced platelet aggregation.[5]

Rivaroxaban – the first oral, direct Factor Xa inhibitor is a small-molecule that binds directly and reversibly to Factor Xa. Rivaroxaban competitively inhibits Factor Xa and is more than 10,000-fold more selective for Factor Xa than other related serine proteases, and it does not require cofactors (such as antithrombin) to exert its anticoagulant effect. Unlike indirect Factor Xa inhibitors, rivaroxaban inhibits both free and clot-bound Factor Xa, as well as prothrombinase activity, thereby prolonging clotting times. Apixaban is an orally active inhibitor of coagulation factor Xa with anticoagulant activity. Apixaban also directly inhibits factor Xa, thereby interfering with the conversion of prothrombin to thrombin and preventing formation of cross-linked fibrin clots.

These oral anticoagulants can be be reliably measure with the activated partial thromboplastic time (APTT) or the prothrombin time (PT). In fact, the benefit of these drugs is promoted to be the lack of laboratory testing to monitor. A direct thrombin inhibitor can be measured by diluting a patient blood plasma specimen !:4 with normal plasma followed by the performance of a standard thrombin time. The factor Xa inhibitors can be measured quantitatively by liquid chromatography.

TESTS FOR HEMOSTASIS AND COAGULATION

Screening Tests for Disorders of the Hemostatic System

Diagnosis of disorders of the hemostatic system should begin with a physical examination and clinical history of the patient and family members. It also is important to include a complete drug history, which often will provide information about the type of disorder that may be affecting the patient. Hemostatic disorders can be secondary to several primary diseases, such as liver disorders, renal failure, and certain carcinomas. Screening tests for hemostasis and coagulation include tests for the condition of the blood vessels (vascular coagulation factors), for platelets, and for the coagulation and fibrinolytic systems—divided according to the main lines of defense against hemorrhage (see Hemostatic Mechanism). A comprehensive and carefully obtained clinical history is considered the most valuable screening test.

Formerly, tests for the vascular factors included the capillary fragility test (also known as the *cuff test, tourniquet test,* or *capillary resistance test*) and BT tests. Current tests for platelets include the platelet count, platelet aggregation assays, and platelet adhesiveness studies. There are various tests for the coagulation factors involved in coagulation (Table 12.2).

Tests for Platelet Function

Platelet dysfunction may be acquired, inherited, or induced by platelet-inhibiting agents. It is clinically important to assess platelet function as a potential cause of a bleeding diathesis, especially in critically ill patients who may develop life-threatening hemorrhages. The most common causes of platelet dysfunction are related to uremia, liver disease, vWD, and exposure to agents such as acetylsalicylic acid (ASA, aspirin). Current methods to assess platelet function include platelet aggregation studies and whole-blood in vitro test systems such as the closure time (CT).

Platelet Closure Times

CT is a test system to assess platelet-related primary hemostasis with greater accuracy and reliability than BT. The CT assay is an important aid in the assessment of platelet dysfunction and bleeding risk caused by uremia, vWD, congenital platelet disorders, and exposure to agents such as aspirin. CTs are indicated when a disorder of platelet function is suspected by a personal or family history of easy bruising, nosebleeds (epistaxis), menorrhagia, or postoperative bleeding, especially after dental extraction or tonsillectomy. CT is not recommended as a screen for potential bleeding risk. CTs may be prolonged when the platelet count is less than $100{,}000/mm^3$, even if platelet function is normal. In addition, CT will be prolonged when hematocrit levels are less than 35%, because of the contributory effect of red blood cells on platelet behavior. These restrictions should be considered before performing CT testing.

Suspected vWD, inherited platelet disorders, and evaluation of acquired disorders of platelet function (hepatic disease, renal disease, drug effects) are appropriate clinical reasons for CT screening. It also may be useful to monitor the response of therapeutics, such as desmopressin (DDAVP) infusions, renal dialysis, and platelet/antiplatelet drug therapy. Abnormal CTs, indicating possible defective platelet function, should be further investigated with standard platelet aggregation tests.

CTs are performed on a PFA-100, an instrument and test cartridge system in which the process of platelet adhesion and aggregation after vascular injury is simulated in vitro. This system allows for rapid evaluation of platelet function on samples of anticoagulated whole blood. Membranes consisting of collagen/epinephrine and collagen/adenosine-5′-diphosphate and the high shear rates generated under standardized flow conditions result in platelet attachment, activation, and aggregation,

TABLE 12.2 Example Laboratory Tests for Hemostasis and Coagulation

Screening Test*	Factor Assessment	Reference Value	Diagnostic and Therapeutic Purpose
Activated partial thromboplastin time (APTT)	Measures plasma factors: inhibition or deficiencies in intrinsic (stage 1) and common pathways: • intrinsic pathway factors XI, IX, and VIII • common pathway coagulation factors X, V, II, and fibrinogen (factor I) • factor XII and other "contact factors" (prekallikrein and high-molecular-weight kininogen)	25–40 seconds	Prolongation of the APTT can occur as a result of an acquired or congenital deficiency of one or more coagulation factors, or the presence of an inhibitor of coagulation such as heparin, a lupus anticoagulant, a nonspecific inhibitor such as a monoclonal immunoglobulin, or a specific coagulation factor inhibitor. Shortening of the APTT usually reflects either elevation of factor VIII activity in vivo, which is most commonly associated with acute or chronic illness or inflammation, or spurious results associated with either difficult venipuncture and specimen collection or suboptimal specimen processing. Monitors heparin therapy.
Note: The APTT does not measure factors in the extrinsic coagulant pathway, including factor VII and tissue factor, nor the activity of factor XIII (fibrin-stabilizing factor)			
Prothrombin time (PT)	• identifies stage 2 deficiency of factor VII • identifies stage 3 deficiencies (factors X, V, II, I)	10–13 seconds (depending on method)	Prolonged results can be diagnostic of liver disease or acute disseminated intravascular coagulation. Monitors warfarin therapy based on INR calculated from the prothrombin assay result. Therapeutic INR is 2–3.
Thrombin time (TT)	Plasma factors: measures concentration and activity of fibrinogen in stage III	13–15 seconds	This assay has been replaced in most circumstances. A functional fibrinogen assay (with or without a fibrinogen antigen assay) for evaluating fibrinogen. Increased value when functional fibrinogen levels are <100 mg/dL.
Fibrinogen	Plasma factors: deficiencies of fibrinogen, alteration in conversion of fibrinogen to fibrin	200–400 mg/dL	Deficiency may be noted in liver disease or acute disseminated intravascular coagulation.
Specific Factor Assays	**Plasma Factors**		
Factor VIII:C	Deficiency: hemophilia A		Classic hemophilia
Factor VIII:vWF	Deficiency: von Willebrand disease		Von Willebrand disease
Factor IX	Deficiency: hemophilia B		Christmas disease
	Anti–factor Xa		Monitoring of low-molecular-weight heparin, if necessary

*Procedures are posted on EVOLVE.
APTT, Activated partial thromboplastin time; *INR,* international normalized ratio.

building a stable platelet plug at the aperture. The time required to obtain full occlusion of the aperture is reported as the CT in seconds.[6]

Platelet Aggregation Studies

The response of platelets during the hemostatic process includes a change in shape, an increase in surface adhesiveness, and the tendency to aggregate with other platelets to form a plug. Measurement of platelet aggregation is an essential part of the investigation of any patient with suspected platelet dysfunction. An aggregating agent is added to a suspension of platelets in platelet-rich plasma (PRP), and the response is measured turbidometrically as a change in the transmission of light. The various commercially available instruments devised to conduct this test are called *aggregometers* or *platelet function analyzers.* The platelet function CT automates the measurement of aggregation in the presence of various aggregating reagents.

When an aggregating reagent (such as thrombin, adenosine diphosphate [ADP], epinephrine, serotonin, arachidonic acid, ristocetin, snake venoms, or collagen) is added to PRP while being stirred in a cuvette at a constant temperature, platelets start to aggregate, and the transmission of light increases. The PRP appears turbid at the beginning of the test. With the addition of the aggregating reagent, larger platelet aggregates begin to form, and thus the PRP begins to clear, while a corresponding increase in light is transmitted. The increased change in optical density or transmission of light is recorded as a function of time on a moving strip recording. The platelet response curve consists of distinct phases that vary with the concentration and type of aggregating reagent used. The response curve can indicate whether an observed clinical picture is caused by a platelet dysfunction or vWD.

Automated Platelet Function Analysis

Light transmission aggregometry (LTA) is the gold standard for platelet function testing for diagnostic and therapeutic analyses. LTA is the only platelet function test endorsed by platelet experts.

Impedance platelet counting uses two separate anticoagulated samples, one of which contains ADP and collagen. The platelet count is measured in an impedance hematology analyzer, and the percent aggregation is calculated.[7]

Platelet aggregation under flow conditions can measure quantitative, qualitative, and vWF defects. Citrated whole blood is aspirated under constant vacuum through apertures coated with platelet agonists. These agonists include epinephrine/collagen and collagen/ADP. The platelets undergo adherence, activation, and aggregation, ultimately plugging the aperture. The time required for closure is measured and the results evaluated to identify inherited dysfunction such as Glanzmann thrombasthenia and Bernard-Soulier syndrome. vWD can be detected and DDAVP monitored in patients who are responsive to desmopressin therapy (stimulates release of vWF). This test system is insensitive to defects or deficiencies in the classic coagulation factors or fibrinogen. In a similar process, nonanticoagulated whole blood is passed through small holes in a blood conduit. In one hole, a collagen fiber is present to activate the platelets, and CT is measured. This system simulates in vivo clotting and platelet function under physiologic conditions.[8]

Tests for Plasma Coagulation Factors

Clotting Assays

Clotting tests are still the most often performed assays in the hemostasis laboratory. Common screening tests of the plasma coagulation system are the Activated Partial Thromboplastin Time (APTT), Prothrombin Time (PT), and Thrombin Time (TT) (see Table 12.2). Once it has been determined by the screening tests that the patient has a coagulation disorder, the exact coagulation factor deficiency or abnormality can be identified.

In the monitoring of anticoagulant therapy, measurement of prothrombin is most often done when the patient is receiving warfarin. The newest way of monitoring heparin therapy is to monitor factor Xa.

Chromogenic Methods

The introduction of synthetic chromogenic substrates was a milestone for the investigation of individual coagulation inhibitors. The chromogenic assay allows a direct determination of the activity of the substrate.

The determination of inhibiting activity of anticoagulants on factor Xa is one of the most traditional chromogenic substrate methods. In this assay, activation of factor X in the sample is induced with one factor X–activating enzyme. The activated factor is directly detected with a chromogenic substrate. Preliminary studies suggest that the anti–factor Xa chromogenic assays are potential candidates for measuring rivaroxaban blood concentration, if required.

The manual methods for coagulation tests have been replaced by automated and semiautomated equipment. Automated methodology is based on manual methods. Several instruments are available that can do coagulation tests for PT and APTT. Two nonautomated techniques for performing plasma-clotting tests are discussed in this section: assay for prothrombin and APTT.

Specimens for Coagulation Tests

The ultimate goal of coagulation testing is to reflect the patient's actual state of hemostatic function in vivo. Clinical and Laboratory Standards Institute (CLSI) guidelines cover the essentials for the proper collection, transport, and processing of blood specimens for coagulation testing.[9]

For various reasons, coagulation assays are highly vulnerable to preanalytical variations in sample collection, processing, and storage.[10] Any factor that causes the test to misrepresent the actual state of coagulation function in the patient can lead to adverse outcomes for the patient.

Blood must be drawn carefully to avoid the following:

1. Contamination of the specimen with tissue thromboplastin
2. Contact with the surface of an inappropriate specimen container
3. Use of an inappropriate anticoagulant
4. Improper temperature conditions
5. Any technique that would produce hemolysis of the specimen

Anticoagulants in specimen collection. Screening coagulation assays are performed on plasma that has been processed from blood anticoagulated with a 3.2% sodium citrate solution. The citrate reversibly binds calcium ions and prevents the various steps in the coagulation process, beginning with the activation of factors IX and VII. Binding the calcium does not inhibit the contact phase of coagulation, so it is critical that no activation of this process be made while the blood is being collected or processed. An example of contact-phase effects is premature activation of factors XI and XII if blood comes in contact with glass. For this reason, only nonreactive materials can be used for collection tubes or testing steps when performing coagulation tests.

The ratio of blood to anticoagulant is critical for clotting tests, necessitating the use of only evacuated-tube systems with the proper vacuum; expiration dates must be observed, and outdated tubes must not be used. By a long-established convention for coagulation tests, nine volumes of carefully drawn blood are mixed with one volume of citrate anticoagulant (1:10 ratio). The standard ratio of anticoagulant to sample is 1:10 for persons with hematocrit between 20% and 60%. Ratios must be changed for persons who are extremely polycythemic. For specimens from patients with extremely high hematocrit, when there is a reduced plasma volume, the use of a reduced anticoagulant volume is needed. CLSI recommends that "the final concentration in the blood should be adjusted in patients who have hematocrits above 0.55 L/L (55%)."[9] Clots are unacceptable in a specimen because clots change the activity of clotting factors.

Collection and storage technique. When multiple tubes of blood are collected, the tube for coagulation testing should be collected first or only after tubes with no additives are collected. This is to prevent carryover from tubes with other anticoagulants.

A clean, rapid venipuncture is necessary to prevent tissue thromboplastin from contaminating the blood sample. Tissue thromboplastin (in the tissue juices) can be found in blood samples when the vessel has been cut or traumatized, and even a slight amount can alter coagulation test results for both normal and abnormal samples. Hemolyzed red blood cells act similar to tissue thromboplastin in activating plasma coagulation factors. Hemolysis of the sample must be avoided. Temperature also affects hemostasis; for example, factors V and VIII are very labile if left at room temperature for any length of time, and factors VII and XI are activated prematurely by cold temperatures. For PT testing, the specimen tube may be stored at room temperature for up to 24 hours; for an APTT, the specimen tube can be stored at room temperature for up to 4 hours.

A clean entry into the vein must be made. The blood should flow quickly and smoothly into the container. If obtaining a blood specimen is difficult, a discard tube should be partially filled before the anticoagulant specimen tube is obtained. It is not necessary to draw a discard tube before the coagulation tube, as was once the standard. If a butterfly collection system is used, a discard tube must be drawn initially to prevent air in the tubing from entering the evacuated tube. Entry of air into the evacuated tube causes a reduction in the amount of blood drawn into the tube because of reduced vacuum in the tube.

Specimen processing. Once the sample is drawn, some changes can begin quickly in vitro. Transportation to the laboratory for testing should be done as quickly and carefully as possible. CLSI allows PT specimens to remain uncentrifuged for up to 24 hours (as long as the tube stays capped). Specimens to be tested for APTT should be centrifuged and the plasma tested or separated from the cells within 60 minutes of being drawn, if the patient is receiving heparin. Otherwise, CLSI states that the APTT specimens do not need to be centrifuged for up to 4 hours. The tubes should be kept stoppered during centrifuging and until the plasma is removed for testing. The platelet-poor ($<10 \times 10^9$/L) plasma-anticoagulant mixture should be separated from the cellular elements unless testing is done immediately; when immediate testing is done, the plasma may remain on the packed cells.

It is important to check the sample for microclot formation. If present, specimens are unacceptable for testing because clotting has been initiated. Specimens that have visible hemolysis are also unacceptable for testing because of possible coagulation factor activation and interference in endpoints for many of the analytical testing instruments being used. Most instruments using an optical detector may also have problems with endpoint determinations using samples that are extremely icteric or lipemic. The plasma to be tested should be kept refrigerated in a tightly covered clean tube until it is tested.

Performance of Coagulation Assays

General guidelines apply to most coagulation tests. A manufacturer's specific instructions for each instrument must be followed explicitly. For coagulation assays, an ongoing program of quality control (QC) should be in place and carefully followed to comply with Clinical Laboratory Improvement Amendments of 1988 (CLIA '88) regulations. Records must be maintained for documentation purposes.

Quality Control

Normal and abnormal controls should be run when testing is begun each day and at the beginning of each new work shift or with each test run of assays. Control specimens are reconstituted daily from a lyophilized aliquot, or frozen controls are used. Controls must be used within their established viability periods, usually 8 to 16 hours. Once a control is thawed or reconstituted, it should not be refrozen or reused. Control samples should be handled and tested under conditions similar or identical to those for the patient samples being tested. Patient values are not reported unless the control values are within the established reference range. Laboratories must develop their own reference ranges representing a normal population for the particular facility. Reference ranges should be reestablished when a new lot of reagents is implemented, with major changes in collection techniques, or when new instruments are introduced into the laboratory.

Prothrombin Assay

The PT clotting assay is a screening assay for the function of the extrinsic (and final common) pathway. It is used to obtain an overview of factors VII, X, V, thrombin, and fibrinogen (Student Procedure Worksheet 12.1). The original assay for PT was devised on the assumption that when an optimal amount of calcium and an excess of thromboplastin are added to decalcified plasma, the rate of coagulation depends on the concentration of prothrombin in the plasma.

The assay measures the functional activity of the extrinsic (and common) coagulation pathway. PT tests generation of thrombin (stage 2) and conversion of fibrinogen to fibrin (stage 3) of the clotting mechanism. The PT screens for deficiencies of factors I, II, V, VII, and X. A normal PT assay shows that the factors of stages 2 and 3 of the coagulation mechanism are probably not disturbed.

In clotting tests, the time between the addition of a thromboplastin reagent and the formation of the fibrin clot or fibrin monomers is measured. The increasing viscosity and turbidity of the sample allow the detection of clot formation using mechanical or optical endpoint detection respectively. The normal reference interval for the PT is generally 10 to 13 seconds but varies with the type of thromboplastin used in the procedure and the method (electromechanical or optical). Therapeutic range is considered to be longer than 25 seconds.

The measurement of PT is the method of choice for monitoring anticoagulant therapy with vitamin K antagonists (warfarin-type oral anticoagulant drugs), especially for preventing postoperative thrombosis and pulmonary embolism, and to screen for coagulation factor deficiencies in hemorrhagic diseases (see Table 12.3). If the degree of anticoagulation is insufficient, rethrombosis or embolism can occur, but an excess of anticoagulation can produce a fatal hemorrhage.

The reagents necessary for the prothrombin assay are primarily calcium chloride and thromboplastin. Thromboplastin reagents with an assigned international sensitivity index (ISI) are used. Each prothrombin control must be prepared before use according to the manufacturer's directions. Control values and limits will vary with the brand of control used. The laboratory will establish its own range for the control specimens. Proper use of the control can detect (1) deterioration of the thromboplastin and (2) use of an improper incubation temperature.

Automated prothrombin assays. Automated or semiautomated assays are employed for conducting coagulation testing. The endpoint of the reaction is the formation of a fibrin clot. The older Fibrometer (BBL Microbiology Systems, BD), which is still used in many student laboratories and as a backup instrument in many laboratories, is a semiautomated electromechanical (amperometric) instrument for fibrin clot detection. It consists of a Fibrometer coagulation timer, a thermal

TABLE 12.3 Comparison of Selected Coagulation Test Results and Applications

Assay	Possible Deficient Factors, if abnormal	Possible Clinical Disorders
Activated Partial Thromboplastin Time (APTT)	V, VIII, IX, X, XI or XII, II and I	Deficiency, dysfunction or inhibition of factors V, VIII, IX, X, XI or XII, II and I. Disseminated Intravascular Coagulation (DIC) Increased fibrin degradation products (FDPs or FSPs) High doses of heparin Lupus anticoagulant Vitamin K deficiency or antagonist The PT is a more sensitive.
Prothdrombin Time (PT)	V, VII, X, II, I	Deficiency, dysfunction or inhibition of factors V, VII, X, II, I Disseminated Intravascular Coagulation (DIC) Increased fibrin degradation products (FDPs or FSPs) Hepatic failure High doses of heparin Lupus anticoagulant (High Levels) Vitamin K deficiency or antagonist

Reference: Turgeon, ML. Clinical Hematology, ed.6, LWW, pp. 692-698, 2018.

preparation block or incubator, and an automatic pipetting system. The Fibrometer consists of a timer, several warming wells, and a clot detector (probe arm with electrodes).

Optical automated or semiautomated coagulation systems are available. Clot formation is timed automatically and is detected by a photocell that reads the optical density change when the clot is formed. The unit contains a heating block that brings the reagents and plasma samples to 37°C during the testing process. These analyzers automatically pipette the necessary reagents and samples or require manual pipetting before analysis. All routine coagulation assays may be performed with these instruments, including PT, APTT, specific coagulation factor assays, TT, and fibrinogen tests. Reagents are stored at room or refrigerator temperature. Refrigeration helps to maintain reagent integrity.

Limitations

Underfilling of specimen tubes can also result in a prolonged PT. In addition, the clinical condition of polycythemia can produce a prolonged PT because of a distortion of the blood to anticoagulant ratio of 9:1.

PT results can be shortened because of prolonged plasma storage due to activation of Factor VII.

Reporting prothrombin results: international normalized ratio. Numerous patient-specific factors influence warfarin sensitivity. These factors include age, body mass, hepatic function, nutritional status, and genetic variation in the cytochrome P-450 complex and vitamin K epoxide reductase complex 1.

The international normalized ratio (INR) is the current method of reporting results for patients receiving warfarin anticoagulant therapy. Warfarin has a narrow therapeutic window that requires frequent INR monitoring to minimize hemorrhagic and thromboembolic complications. Therapeutic range is considered to be longer than 25 seconds. Most adult patients receiving warfarin are required to maintain therapeutic INR values between 2 and 3 (2.5–3.5).

The World Health Organization (WHO) originally helped devise use of the INR for patients receiving long-term anticoagulant therapy to ensure that tests done in different laboratories would yield comparable results. Manufacturers of thromboplastin reagents provide the ISI for each lot of reagents. The ISI is obtained by comparing the manufacturer's thromboplastin reagent with the WHO international reference thromboplastin with an assigned ISI value of 1.0.

The INR is the ratio between the sample PT over the mean normal PT (MNPT) raised to the power of a calculated ISI of the standardized thromboplastin reagent: INR = (patient PT/MNPT) ISI. The INR reference range is 0.9 to 1.13 in those age 1 year or older, and increasing INR values correspond to increased anticoagulation. The INR is elevated with deficiencies in coagulation factors in the extrinsic pathway. These deficiencies most often result from the use of oral anticoagulant therapy, which depletes the vitamin K–dependent coagulation factors (II, VII, IX, X), or from liver disease.

Activated Partial Thromboplastin Time

The APTT, as with the PT assay, is automated using the same instrumentation. However, in the APTT assay an activator, calcium chloride, is mixed with a phospholipid component of thromboplastin (a platelet substitute) before its addition to the plasma being tested. Only a partial component of thromboplastin is used, thus giving the test its name. The APTT test is the most useful routine screening procedure for factor deficiencies of the intrinsic and common pathways. The APTT adds the kaolin, an activator of factor XII, which allows more complete activation, shortens the clotting times, and improves reproducibility over the formerly used "partial thromboplastin time" test.

The APTT measures deficiencies mainly of factors VIII, IX, XI, and XII but can detect deficiencies of all factors except VII and XIII. The tests are based on the observation that when whole thromboplastin is used, as for prothrombin assays, the times obtained for hemophilic plasma are about the same as those for normal plasma. With a partial thromboplastin solution or platelet substitute, the times obtained for hemophilic plasma are much longer than those for normal plasma.

The principal use of the APTT test is in the management of patients receiving standard heparin or UFH therapy. The sensitivity of the thromboplastin reagent must be evaluated before this test is used as a heparin control. Most thromboplastin reagents are insensitive to LMWHs. Anti-Xa assays should be used to monitor LMWH. LMWH generally does not require monitoring, except in extremes of patient weight, pregnancy, renal disease, and children.

A phospholipid substitute for platelets acts as a partial thromboplastin. It is more sensitive to the absence of coagulation factors involved in intrinsic thromboplastin formation than are the more complete tissue thromboplastins used in prothrombin assays.

Activation in the procedure is obtained by separate addition of a kaolin suspension. Kaolin ensures maximal activation of the coagulation factors. Addition of kaolin speeds up the slow contact phase of the coagulation cascade. Activators used can vary with the manufacturer of the reagents being used. By activation of the contact coagulation factors, more consistent and reproducible results are achieved.

The APTT test result will be prolonged in contact and intrinsic coagulation factor deficiencies (see Table 12.3). The presence of an inhibitor, such as the lupus anticoagulant, in the patient's plasma may also be the cause of a prolonged APTT. The APTT is used to monitor heparin concentration during intravenous administration. The APTT is not sensitive to minor abnormalities in some common-pathway coagulation factors but is useful to screen mild to moderate deficiencies of factors VIII and IX and the contact coagulation factors. Deficiencies of these coagulation factors represent the most common and potentially serious disorders. If an abnormal APTT is determined, differential studies should be done for specific coagulation factor deficiencies.

The principle of the APTT test holds that during anticoagulation, the calcium present in the blood is bound to the anticoagulant. After centrifugation, the plasma contains all the intrinsic coagulation factors except calcium (removed during anticoagulation) and platelets (removed during centrifugation). Under carefully controlled conditions and with properly prepared reagents, calcium, a phospholipid platelet substitute (the partial thromboplastin), and an activator (kaolin) are added to the plasma to be tested. The time required for the plasma to clot is the APTT. The normal times proposed by the reagent manufacturer should be followed.

Normal control results must always fall within the acceptable control range; if not, a problem exists with the reagents, the equipment, or the technique being used. When the control is out of range, the entire test must be repeated. Most laboratories also include controls in the "high" and "low" ranges at least once a day. The ranges for controls are established by the laboratory before each new lot is placed into service.

Precautions and technical factors. Use of kaolin provides maximal activation of the coagulation factors and therefore more consistent and reproducible results. Kaolin in suspension settles out very quickly; when kaolin is used, it is necessary to mix the solutions vigorously before any pipetting is done. Many automated instruments provide continual mixing. Citrated blood should be centrifuged within 1 hour of collection. Plasma allowed to sit longer than the recommended time can lead to abnormal results.

Reporting results. APTT tests are reported in seconds to the nearest tenth of a second, along with the control specimen reference values established for the laboratory. Results must be clearly marked for "patient" or "control." Generally, a normal APTT is less than 35 seconds, with a range from 25 to 40 seconds. Control plasmas must be run every 8 hours, and their values must fall within the laboratory's reference range. Deviations in control results can be caused by deterioration over time, temperature changes, different reagent lots, the technique being used, or instrument malfunction, if automation or semiautomation is being employed.

Limitations

Several interferences reduce APTT sensitivity or heparin resistance. Inflammation accompanied by hyperfibrinogenemia, or VIII:vWF, reduces the APTT response to heparin. AT may become depleted with prolonged therapy or in patients with inherited or acquired underlying AT deficiency. APTT remains within the reference interval or is only slightly prolonged despite increased doses of heparin. APTT can shorten 1 hour after collection because of in vitro platelet factor 4 release. This will interfere with APTT and chromogenic anti-Xa heparin assay.

LMWH is not monitored routinely but must be assayed if the patient has fluid imbalance or unstable coagulation, renal disease, liver disease, diabetes, or chronic inflammation.

Mixing Studies

When a patient has an abnormally increased PT or APTT, laboratories should perform a mixing study. An equal volume of the patient's citrated plasma is mixed with normal pooled plasma, and the PT or APTT is repeated on a 1:1 mix. If an assay is now corrected and within the reference range for the assay, the initial result was caused by a deficiency or dysfunction of one or more clotting factors. If the mixing study continues to yield abnormal results, an inhibitor is such as heparin, direct-acting oral anticoagulants, or autoantibodies against coagulation factors or phosopholipid-binding proteins, present in the patient's plasma. If a 1:1 mix result decreases significantly but remains above the reference internal, it is considered to lack correction.

D-Dimer Assay

The D-dimer assay is actually two different tests, with each having a specific application and each being completely misleading when used for the wrong application. D-Dimer is the cross-linked breakdown product of fibrin. A normal D-dimer levels essentially rules out DIC (excellent negative predictive value). Using an immunoturbidimetry method, the reference value is 0.0-0.4 μg FEU/mL. There are two analytical avenues of testing for D-dimer: ELISA and particle agglutination. Particle agglutination is used for detecting D-dimers associated with DIC and does not require a high degree of sensitivity because they are being generated systemically. The particle agglutination tests generally detect D-dimers at about 500 ng/mL. ELISA testing for D-dimer is a more sensitive order of magnitude, detecting less than 10 ng/mL. This level of sensitivity is necessary to rule out VTE. Using a particle agglutination test to rule out VTE will result in many false-negative results, and using ELISA D-dimer testing for diagnosing DIC will result in false-positive results.

The D-dimer test has attracted attention lately because age-adjusted (patients over 50 years) D-dimer cutoff are part of an

American College of Physicians (ACP) clinical guideline for ruling out acute pulmonary embolism. The ACP guideline states that age-adjusted D-dimer thresholds, defined as the patient's age times 10 ng/mL rather than a generic cutoff of 500 ng/mL in patients older than 50 years. The ACP guideline didn't stipulate the type of unit for the age adjusted D-dimer cutoff, which could be fibrinogen equivalent units (FEU) or D-dimer units (D-DU). Two FEUs are equal to one D-DU.[11]

Anti-Xa Assay

Anti-Xa is the preferred choice for monitoring unfractionated heparin (UFH) therapy and sometimes to monitor low molecular weight heparin (LMWH) therapy. The anti-Xa assay is a direct concentration measurement method compared with indirect methods such as APTT. Occasionally, the anti-Xa assay is ordered to monitor and adjust UFH levels. This chromogenic method usually contains exogenous factor Xa and AT, both in excess, as well as a chromogenic substrate for factor Xa. Heparin in a patient's specimen complexes with AT, and this complex inhibits factor Xa. Any residual factor Xa cleaves the chromogenic substrate and releases a yellow chromophore.

Report anti-Xa as units per milliliter of anti-Xa activity; therapeutic range of anti-Xa is 0.3 to 0.7 U/mL for UFH. Anti-Xa determination may be helpful in urgent surgery, compromised kidney function, or dehydration.

Thrombin Time

TT is an older clotting screening test for fibrinogen polymerization and is performed by adding a low concentration of thrombin to plasma. This produces the formation of fibrin. The assay measures the ability of fibrinogen to form fibrin strands in vitro. The assay is independent of endogenous thrombin and any of the other clotting factors. It is particularly sensitive to heparin. A modification of the TT assay is the quantitative fibrinogen assay. This assay requires the addition of exogenous thrombin with diluted plasma. The results are reported in milligrams per deciliter (mg/dL) and are determined from a standard curve generated from a calibrator plasma.

Activated Clotting Time

The activated clotting time (ACT) assay uses whole blood mixed with a clot activator. Clotting usually takes 70 to 180 seconds when measured mechanically or electrochemically. This method can be performed at the point of care when high-dose heparin anticoagulation during cardiopulmonary bypass surgery or cardiac catheterization is performed.

Fibrinogen

Several fibrinogen assays exist, including an immunological mass assay based on enzyme-linked immunoabsorbent (ELISA), radial immunodiffusion and electrophoresis methods. Immunological assay measure protein (antigen) concentration not functional activity. A gravimetric assay also exists. The Clauss assay is the most commonly performed fibrinogen assay and it is a modified thrombin time (TT).

Fibrinogen assays are conducted for the diagnosis of clinical conditions such as hypo- or dysfibrinogenemia, disseminated intravascular coagulation (DIC), and primary fibrinolysis.

Other Tests for Coagulation

Other tests for specific coagulation factors include the following:

- Prothrombin consumption test
- Thromboplastin generation test
- Plasma recalcification time (plasma clotting time)
- Russell viper venom time
- Reptilase time
- vWF and other coagulation factor assays
- Assays for the hypercoagulable state, AT-III, protein C and APC, protein S, and circulating lupus anticoagulant

Point-of-Care Tests for Coagulation Assays

Because turnaround time is of great importance in certain clinical situations, point-of-care testing (POCT) is used for some coagulation assays. During surgical procedures for patients receiving heparin anticoagulant therapy, POCT tests for ACT can be performed. Studies have shown that frequent home monitoring of oral anticoagulant therapy time reduces the number of major bleeds or thrombotic events. A POCT INR testing has several disadvantages due to the interference from severe anemia (hematocrit below above 25%) or polycythemia (hematocrit above about 55%); coadministration of other anticoagulants with warfarin, e.g., low molecular weight heparin (LMWH); fibrinogen level; and antiphospholipid inhibitors. Even without known interfering conditions, significant discrepancies between clinical INR and point-of-care values are common, especially when clinical INR >3.0).

Coagulation Analyzers

Some POCT analyzers use only capillary blood, and others use capillary blood, whole blood, plasma, or all three. Coagulation analyzers can be used in surgical suites, intensive care units, dialysis units, or other patient care units (Table 12.4). Fresh whole blood is added to a sample well on a test cartridge, which is inserted into the instrument after a prompt signal appears. The blood sample is drawn by capillary action into the test channel, where it mixes with the reagents. An electro-optical system detects the point at which blood flow ceases and the clot forms; this is the endpoint of the assay. The result appears in a display window. Results with whole blood are higher than for the typical laboratory analyzers, which use plasma. Results are converted to equivalent plasma values, and INRs are given for prothrombin assays. Coagulation POCT results should be included in the patient's chart in the same manner as for traditional coagulation test results.

The Siemens Healthineers Xprecia Stride Coagulation analyzer is an example of a handheld device that delivers PT/INR testing for POCT monitoring and management of oral anticoagulation therapy with warfarin. This device uses fresh capillary whole blood, results in INR. It uses the same Dade reagents that are used by Siemens central laboratory analyzers. Handheld shown to be equivalent to a reference laboratory hemostasis systems.

Quality Control

QC programs must be used with any POCT coagulation analyzer. CLIA '88 regulations mandate that two levels of control,

TABLE 12.4 Examples of Blood Coagulation Analyzers

Sysmex	Detection methods: clotting, chromogenic, and immunologic	Multiple reagents	Systemic, CA-500 (www.medicalsiemens.com)
Prothrombin time with INR	Reflectance photometry	Single-use cartridge	CoaguChek S (www.rochediagnostics.com)
Prothrombin time with INR, activated partial thromboplastin time, activated clotting time	Optical motion detection	Single-use tube containing an activator and a magnet	Hemochron Response 401/801[a] CoaguChek Pro (www.rochediagnostics.com)
Prothrombin time (PT)/INRatio Monitor	Platelet aggregation thromboelastography	Electrochemical test strip	HemoSense (www.hemosense.com)

INR, International normalized ratio.
[a]Three types of activator tubes are available. Equipment is able to perform thrombin time, heparin-neutralized thrombin time, high-dose thrombin time, fibrinogen, and protamine dose assay.
Data from College of American Pathologists: Chemistry analyzers for low-volume laboratories, *CAP Today* 27(8):35–47, 2013.

normal and abnormal, be assayed during each 8-hour shift for automated coagulation systems, traditional methods, and POCT. The manufacturers of these coagulation POCT analyzers are working to improve their electronic QC, but currently conventional liquid coagulation controls remain the type acceptable for CLIA '88. Use of liquid controls is expensive for POCT coagulation assays because the control specimen is viable for only a specific time, usually 8 to 16 hours. Also, often only a few patients are tested by POCT during this time, in contrast to traditional in-laboratory coagulation testing, in which many tests are performed during an 8-hour shift. Each time a control specimen or patient specimen is tested, a test cartridge is used, increasing the cost.

Problems and Drawbacks

Reagents for coagulation POCTs are considerably more expensive than reagents for conventional coagulation assays. Another potential drawback of coagulation POCTs is that data can be lost or potentially never transferred to the patient's permanent record; this uncertainty must be weighed against the advantages of almost instantaneous data and the analyzers' ease of use. Validation of coagulation point-of-care analyzers can be daunting. Calibration to dissimilar laboratory-based methods requires comparison of laboratory wet reagents to POCT dry reagents with different reaction kinetics. The coefficient of variation of the INRs generated on a POCT instrument may range from 9% to 13%, whereas plasma-based assays typically do not exceed 5%. For this reason, clinicians require that the POCT be done on one instrument consistently, and that if the INR must be generated on an alternate system, its respective interval must be consulted.

Training of Users

It is important that any person who is to use the coagulation POCT analyzers be adequately trained in their use and that the training be documented. Ideally, users should be trained under the auspices of the laboratory, and the QC measures should be monitored by laboratory staff. Some manufacturers of coagulation POCT analyzers provide users, including physicians, patients (in their homes), and other health care workers, with a system of quality management. This includes in-depth training in the use of the analyzer and technical support, if needed, in the future. Training must include information about the importance of good specimen collection techniques and the use of QC measures.

CASE STUDIES

CASE STUDY 12.1

A 23-year-old man has a long history of abnormal bleeding into his joints. The following laboratory results are reported:
Prothrombin assay: Normal
APTT: Greatly prolonged
Factor VIII assay: Greatly decreased
Factor IX assay: Normal
Platelet count: Normal

Multiple Choice Questions

Answers are in Appendix A.

1. If the APTT is prolonged but the partial thromboplastin time is normal, a deficiency of what factor can be suspected?
   a. IX
   b. VIII
   c. II
   d. I
2. Based on the patient's history and laboratory results, which of the following disorders is most likely for this patient?
   a. Classic hemophilia A
   b. Classic hemophilia B
   c. Von Willebrand disease
   d. Severe liver disease

Critical Thinking Group Discussion Questions

1. What is the biological cause of a greatly decreased factor VIII level?
2. What technical errors could produce a decreased factor VIII?

Note: Narrative answers are published on the EVOLVE instructor site.

CASE STUDY 12.2

A 45-year-old woman has severe liver disease with jaundice, purpura (bleeding into the tissues), and a platelet count of 120 × 10^9/L.

Multiple Choice Questions

Answers are in Appendix A.

1. Which of the following coagulation profiles is most likely for this patient?
   a. APTT normal, PT increased
   b. APTT increased, PT increased
   c. APTT normal, PT normal
   d. APTT normal, PT decreased
2. A patient with severe liver disease can exhibit:
   a. Abnormal platelet function
   b. Abnormal synthesis of factor VIII
   c. Abnormal synthesis of factor II
   d. Increased levels of fibrin split products

Critical Thinking Group Discussion Questions

1. What abnormality does purpura reflect?
2. Severe liver disease can influence the synthesis of which coagulation factors?

Note: Narrative answers are published on the EVOLVE instructor site.

CASE STUDY 12.3

A 25-year-old man was admitted to the hospital for surgical repair of an abdominal hernia. He was in good physical condition, but his family history included minor bleeding problems among some of his relatives. The following laboratory results are reported:

PT: Normal
APTT: Prolonged
Factor VIII assay: Normal
Factor VIII:C: Normal
Factor VIII:vWF: Normal
Factor IX assay: Decreased
Platelet count: Normal
Platelet aggregation test: Normal

Multiple Choice Questions

Answers are in Appendix A.

1. A family with a history of minor bleeding problems suggests a:
   a. Genetic condition in males of the family
   b. Genetic condition in females of the family
   c. Non–gender-related genetic condition in the family
   d. Prevalence of liver disease in the family
2. The family history of bleeding is related to:
   a. Inadequate platelet count
   b. Inadequate platelet function
   c. Blood vessel weakness
   d. Coagulation factor deficiency

Critical Thinking Group Discussion Questions

1. Describe the genetic inheritance of various familial bleeding disorders.
2. Based on the history and laboratory results, what bleeding disorder might this patient have?

Note: Narrative answers are published on the EVOLVE instructor site.

REFERENCES

1. Blombäck M, Abildgaard U, van den Besselaar AM, et al: Nomenclature of quantities and units in thrombosis and haemostasis (recommendation 1993), *Thromb Haemost* 71(3):375–394, 1994.
2. Fritsma GA: Monitoring the anti-Xa anticoagulants, from heparin to Eliquis, *Clin Lab Sci* 26(1):49–53, 2012.
3. Fritsma GA: Anticoagulant therapy overview, *Clin Lab Sci* 26(1):39–42, 2012.
4. Tran HAM, Ginsberg JS: Anticoagulant therapy for major arterial and venous thromboembolism. In Colman RW, Marder VJ, Clowes AW, et al, editors: *Hemostasis and thrombosis: basic principles and clinical practice*, ed 5, Philadelphia, 2006, Lippincott Williams & Wilkins.
5. Fritsma GA: Monitoring the direct thrombin inhibitors, *Clin Lab Sci* 26(1):54–57, 2012.
6. Hassett AC, Bontempo FA: Closure time platelet function screening, transfusion medicine update, Institute for Transfusion Medicine, www.itxm.org, 2005.
7. Lennon MJ, Gibbs NM, Weightman WM, et al: A comparison of Plateletworks and platelet aggregometry for the assessment of aspirin-related platelet dysfunction in cardiac surgical patients, *J Cardiothorac Vasc Anesth* 18:136, 2004.
8. Mammen EF, Comp PC, Gosselin R, et al: PFA-100 system: a new method for assessment of platelet dysfunction, *Semin Thromb Hemost* 24:195, 1998.
9. Clinical and Laboratory Standards Institute: *Collection, transport, and processing of blood specimens for coagulation testing and performance of coagulation assays: approved guideline*, ed 4, 2003. Wayne, PA, H21-A4.
10. Lawrence JB: CE update, *Lab Med* 34(1):49–57, 2003.
11. Lusky K: In hemostasis, two hot-button testing issues: CAP TODAY, 31(12):1–38, 2017.

BIBLIOGRAPHY

Accumetrics: Verify now aspirin, San Diego, 2005.

Adcock DM, Tiefenbacher S, Pruthi RK: The value of the chromogenic activity assay in diagnosis and therapeutic monitoring of hemophilia, *Med Lab Observer* 49(2):8–14, 2017.

Allen T: Thromboelastometry: its methodology, application and benefits, *MLO Med Lab Obs* 46(2):26–29, 2014.

American Proficiency Institute: Overview of Coagulation Testing, Am Soc of Clin Path, Clinical Laboratory, www.ascp.org, accessed May 2017.

Bostic G, Thompson R, Atanasoski S: et. al.: Quality Improvement in the Coagulation Laboratory: Reducing the Number of Insufficient Blood Draw Specimens for Coagulation Testing, Lab, *Medicine* 46 (4):347–355, 2015.

Botero JP: Diagnostic considerations with inherited platelet disorder testing, *Med Lab Obs* 50(2):8–12, 2018.

Cheng X, et al.: Prevalence, profile, predictors, and natural history of aspirin resistance measured by the Ultegra rapid platelet function assay-ASA in patients with coronary heart disease: clinical studies/outcomes, presentation number C-25, International Federation of Clinical Chemistry (IFCC)/American Association for Clinical Chemistry (AACC) meeting, Fla, 2005, Orlando.

Clinical and Laboratory Standards Institute: *Assays of von Willebrand factor antigen and ristocetin cofactor activity:* approved guideline, 2002, Wayne, Pa, H51-A.

Clinical and Laboratory Standards Institute: Point-of care monitoring of anticoagulation therapy: approved guideline, 2004, Wayne, Pa, H49-A.

Clinical and Laboratory Standards Institute: Procedures for validation of INR and local calibration of PT/INR systems: approved guideline, 2004, Wayne, Pa, H54-A.

Clinical and Laboratory Standards Institute: Performance of the bleeding time test: approved guideline, ed 2, 2005, Wayne, Pa, H45-A2.

Codina S: Post-transfusion purpura, *ASCLS Today* 27(2):4–5, 2013.

Favaloro EJ, McVicker W, Lay M, et al: Harmonizing the International Normalized Ratio (INR), *Am J Clin Pathol* 145(2):191–202, 2016.

Ford A: Hemophilia diagnosis: how to test, what to know, CAP TODAY, 31(3):5–6, 2017.

Harris NS, Winter WE: The international normalized ratio, *Clin Lab News* 36(11), 2010.

Harris NS, Bazydlo LA, Winter WE: *Coagulation tests, Clin Lab News 38(1),* 2012.

Johnson SA: Point of Care or Clinical Lab INR for Anticoagulation Monitoring: Which to Believe, *Cl Lab News* 43(4), 2017.

Katz B, Marques MB: Point-of-care testing in oral anticoagulation: what is the point, *MLO Med Lab Obs* 36(3):30–35, 2004.

Lenk E, Spannagl M: Platelet function testing–guided antiplatelet therapy, *J Int Fed Clin Chem* 24(3–4):1–7, 2013.

Mani H, Wagner C, Lindhoff-Last E: Influence of new anticoagulants on coagulation tests, www.siemens.com/diagnostics, 2011.

McMorran BJ, Wieczorski L, Drysdale KE, et al: Platelets reveal a new weapon in the fight against malaria, *Science* 338:1348–1351, 2012.

McGlasson DL: Monitoring Coumadin: the original oral anticoagulant, *Clin Lab Sci* 26(1):43–47, 2013.

Riley P: Measuring, monitoring heparin, *Advance Med Lab Professionals* 25(2):10–12, 2013.

Tomic BV, Gvozdenov MZ, Pruner IB, et al: Are Prothrombic Mutations a Time-to-Event Risk Factor? *Laboratory Medicine* 48(4):326–331, 2017.

Turgeon ML: Clinical hematology: theory and procedures, *ed 6,* Philadelphia, 2018, Lippincott Williams & Wilkins.

Winter WE, Flax SD, Harris NS: Coagulation Testing in the Core Laboratory, *Laboratory Medicine* 48(4):295–312, 2017.

REVIEW QUESTIONS (ANSWERS IN APPENDIX A)

Hemostatic Mechanism

1. *Hemostasis* is defined as a process to:
   - **a.** Localize an injury
   - **b.** Restore normal anatomy
   - **c.** Stop bleeding from an injured blood vessel
   - **d.** Facilitate the removal of a clot
2. Which of the following peripheral blood cells is involved in hemostasis?
   - **a.** Thrombocytes
   - **b.** Lymphocytes
   - **c.** Erythrocytes
   - **d.** Granulocytes
3. Primary hemostasis results in:
   - **a.** Formation of a thrombus
   - **b.** Retraction of the clot
   - **c.** Formulation of a platelet plug
   - **d.** Presence of vitamin K

Quantitative Platelet Disorders

4. For the control of bleeding, all the following characteristics are true *except:*
   - **a.** PF3 is important in activation of some coagulation factors.
   - **b.** Platelet adhesion is essential.
   - **c.** VIII:vWF acts as a glue for platelet-collagen binding to occur.
   - **d.** It is not necessary for platelets to aggregate with one another.

Qualitative Platelet Disorders

5. A disorder associated with platelet dysfunction despite a normal platelet count is:
   - **a.** Von Willebrand disease
   - **b.** Hemophilia
   - **c.** Dermatitis
   - **d.** Autoimmune disorders

Coagulation

6. All the following factors will be inhibited by warfarin-type drugs *except:*
   - **a.** II
   - **b.** VII
   - **c.** VIII
   - **d.** X
7. Hemophilia A is a disorder associated with a deficiency of:
   - **a.** Factor VIII
   - **b.** Factor IX
   - **c.** Circulating platelets
   - **d.** Vitamin K–dependent coagulation factors
8. Which factor is part of the common coagulation pathway?
   - **a.** VIII
   - **b.** X
   - **c.** XI
   - **d.** XII

9. Which factor is used only in the extrinsic coagulation pathway?
   a. III
   b. V
   c. XII
   d. VIII
10. Which factor is used only in the intrinsic coagulation pathway?
   a. XII
   b. V
   c. VII
   d. I
11. Fibrinogen is synthesized in the:
   a. Liver
   b. Endothelium
   c. Platelets
   d. Plasma

Pathways for Coagulation Cascade

12. The extrinsic pathway of coagulation is triggered by the entry of _____ into the circulation.
   a. Membrane lipoproteins (phospholipoproteins)
   b. Tissue thromboplastin
   c. Ca^{2+}
   d. Factor VII
13. The intrinsic pathway of coagulation begins with the activation of _____ in the early stage.
   a. Factor II
   b. Factor I
   c. Factor XII
   d. Factor V
14. The final common pathway of the intrinsic-extrinsic pathway is
   a. Factor X activation
   b. Factor II activation
   c. Factor I activation
   d. Factor XIII activation

Fibrinolysis

15. Fibrinogen is converted to fibrin monomers by
   a. Prothrombin
   b. Thrombin
   c. Calcium ions
   d. Factor XIIIa

Protective Mechanisms Against Thrombosis

16. Clot removal is accomplished by which of the following systems?
   a. Fibrinolysis
   b. Hemostasis
   c. Anticoagulation
   d. Thrombosis
17. Protective mechanisms against thrombosis include all the following *except:*
   a. Normal blood flow
   b. Natural in vivo anticoagulants (such as AT-III)
   c. Cellular regulators that block the activation or action of plasmin
   d. Antibodies produced by lymphocytes to block thrombin

Tests for Hemostasis and Coagulation

18. Which of the following is the anticoagulant of choice for routine coagulation assays?
   a. Heparin
   b. Sodium oxalate
   c. Sodium citrate
   d. Lithium oxalate
19. The prothrombin assay requires that the patient's citrated plasma be combined with which of the following?
   a. Thromboplastin
   b. Calcium chloride and thromboplastin
   c. Calcium chloride
   d. Kaolin
20. What does the silicate (kaolin) do in the test system for APTT?
   a. It binds calcium so that clotting does not occur.
   b. It activates tissue thromboplastin.
   c. It facilitates platelet adherence to endothelial surfaces.
   d. It allows more complete activation of coagulation factor XII, thus shortening the clotting times.
21. Which factor is measured by the prothrombin assay?
   a. II
   b. VI
   c. VIII
   d. IX
22. Which factor is measured by the prothrombin assay?
   a. III
   b. IV
   c. VIII
   d. X
23. Which of the following is the most accurate POCT coagulation assay used to monitor heparin?
   a. Prothrombin time
   b. Activated partial thromboplastin time
   c. Bleeding time
   d. Platelet count

Turgeon: Linné & Ringsrud's Clinical Laboratory Science, 8th Edition

STUDENT PROCEDURE WORKSHEET 12.1

Prothrombin Time[1]

Student Learning Outcomes

See Chapter 12 of *Linné & Ringsrud's Clinical Laboratory Science: Concepts, Procedures, and Clinical Applications*, 8th edition, for a complete discussion of this procedure. After reading Chapter 12, and at the completion of this laboratory exercise and answering the review questions, a student should be able to:

- Describe the procedure and sources of error in prothrombin time (PT) testing.
- Complete the end-of-procedure review questions with a grade of 80% or higher.

Principle

The procedure that was used before semiautomated methods became available involves adding plasma to an excess of extrinsic thromboplastin-calcium substrate. Thromboplastin is derived from tissues that supply phospholipoprotein (such as animal brain). The length of time required to form a fibrin clot is measured in seconds.

Specimen

Prothrombin assays should be done within 24 hours of blood collection, if the specimen remains capped. After that time, plasma must be frozen. Freezing should occur at – 20 °C for up to 2 weeks and – 70 °C for up to 6 months. The blood for this test must be free of clots; if any clots are present, a new specimen must be drawn. The ratio of anticoagulant to blood specimen should be 1:10.

Equipment, Supplies, and Reagents

1. Thromboplastin (reconstitute according to manufacturer's directions)
   Note: When the thromboplastin-calcium reagent is used, it is important to mix the suspension very well.
2. 12 × 75–mm test tubes
3. Pipettes 0.1 mL (100 μL)
4. 37 °C heat block or water bath
5. Stopwatch
6. Nichrome loop or magnifying glass

Quality Control

Normal and abnormal citrated test plasma should be tested with each patient assay or test batch.

Reporting Results

The reference range for PT values is 10 to 15 seconds. Record and report, if necessary, both the patient result and the normal control result in seconds. Currently, the PT result is used to calculate the INR value. Many automated instruments calculate the INR internally.

Clinical Applications

The PT procedure is used to monitor oral anticoagulant therapy (such as warfarin).

Procedure Notes

The PT assay depends on the activity of factors VII, V, X, II, and I. A deficiency of any of these factors may produce a 3- to 4-second prolongation in the test.

Reference

Turgeon, ML: *Clinical hematology*, ed 6, Philadelphia, 2018 Precautions and Technical Factors, Lippincott Williams & Wilkins.

Instructions for the Procedure

The PT procedure is typically performed using automated equipment. In addition to laboratory instrumentation, many models of handheld point-of-care instruments are often used. In some cases, however, a manual procedure similar to the one described here might be the only alternative.

Read the list of required equipment, supplies, and reagents and the procedural steps. Follow the procedural steps in exact order.

SEQUENCE	PROCEDURAL STEP	INSTRUCTOR-OBSERVED ACCEPTABLE PERFORMANCE (CHECK IF ACCEPTABLE)
1	Prewarm plasma separated from erythrocytes at 37 °C for a minimum of 2 minutes and a maximum of 10 minutes.	
2	Prewarm thromboplastin at 37 °C for a minimum of 2 minutes and a maximum of 60 minutes.	
3	Add 0.1 mL of plasma to 0.2 mL of thromboplastin. NOTE: Pipette quickly, and start stopwatch simultaneously.	
4	Using a nichrome loop technique, the loop is swept through the mixture at two sweeps/second until the first thread of fibrin appears. The tube may also be tilted using a magnifier to observe fibrin clot formation.	
5	Repeat the procedure in duplicate for all patient specimens and controls. The duplicate results should be within 1 second of one another.	

(Continued)

[1]Semiautomated activated partial thromboplastin time (APTT) and prothrombin time (PT) procedures using the Fibrometer are posted on EVOLVE.

Turgeon: Linné & Ringsrud's Clinical Laboratory Science, 8th Edition

STUDENT PROCEDURE WORKSHEET 12.1

Prothrombin Time

Review Questions

1. Which of the following is a source of error that can affect the PT assay?
   a. Improper specimen storage
   b. Improperly reconstituting and storing test reagents
   c. Improper temperature of test reaction
   d. All the above

2. The PT assay requires:
   a. Proper specimen storage
   b. The use of sodium citrate to anticoagulate the whole-blood specimen
   c. Proper reaction temperature
   d. All the above

Procedural Evaluation

Student's Name ______________________________ Grade___________

Instructor's Signature __________________________ Date___________

Comments:

13

Renal Physiology and Urinalysis

http://evolve.elsevier.com/Turgeon/clinicallab

CHAPTER CONTENTS

LEARNING OUTCOMES

Overview of Urinalysis
- Compare the characteristics of historical and modern urinalysis.
- Discuss the components of a quality assessment system for urinalysis.

Renal Anatomy and Physiology
- Describe the basic anatomic components of the urinary system and the function of each.

Composition of Urine
- Contrast the clinical usefulness of urinalysis, and classify tests pertaining to diseases or conditions affecting the kidney or urinary tract and metabolic disease.

Collection and Preservation of Urine Specimens
- Differentiate various urine specimen requirements for a routine urinalysis, including preservation and storage requirements.
- Categorize various types of urine collection, including midstream clean-catch, quantitative, and timed specimens, and compare the differences.

Physical Properties of Urine
- Correlate normal and abnormal physical properties that might be encountered in urine specimens, with physical findings and chemical and microscopic findings.
- Define the term *specific gravity.*
- Correlate the relationship between urine volume and specific gravity.

Chemical Tests in Routine Urinalysis
- Discuss the chemical composition of normal urine.
- For each of the analytes discussed in this chapter, evaluate the following: clinical importance, principle of the test, specificity and sensitivity, interferences, and additional considerations.

- Integrate the pathophysiology and significance of proteinuria due to glomerular damage, tubular damage, prerenal disorders, lower urinary tract disorders, asymptomatic proteinuria, and consistent microalbuminuria.
- Integrate the pathophysiology of hematuria, hemoglobinuria, and myoglobinuria, and explain how to differentiate among the respective analytes when a positive reagent strip test for blood is seen.
- Integrate the pathophysiology and clinical importance of tests for nitrite and leukocyte esterase and how they relate to each other.
- Integrate the pathophysiology and clinical importance of bilirubin and urobilinogen, and identify the laboratory findings in various types of jaundice.

Microscopic Analysis of Urine Sediment

- Describe conditions when urine should be examined microscopically.
- Correlate various urine sediment constituents that might be encountered, including pathophysiology and clinical importance.

Constituents of Urine Sediment

- Describe the formation and significance of casts and how they are classified and reported.
- List the normal crystals encountered in acid and alkaline urine, describe the most frequently encountered forms of each, and identify any associated disorders.
- Name the most common chemical compositions of renal calculi.
- List the abnormal crystals of metabolic and iatrogenic origin, describe the most frequently encountered forms of each, and identify any associated disorders.
- Correlate the relationships among sediment, chemical, and physical findings in the urine.
- Recognize discrepant results when reviewing urinalysis findings (physical, chemical, and sediment), before results are reported.

Automation in Urinalysis

- Compare the characteristics of various semiautomated, automated, and microscopic urinary sediment analyzers.

Case Studies

- Analyze the patient history, clinical signs and symptoms, and laboratory data for the stated case studies, answer the related critical thinking questions, and conclude the most likely diagnosis.

Review Questions

- Demonstrate comprehension of the chapter content by completing the end-of-chapter review questions with a grade of 80% or higher.

Note:

- • indicates MLT and MLS core content
- ❖ indicates MLT (optional) and MLS advanced content

KEY TERMS

antidiuretic hormone (ADH)
casts
epithelial cells
glomerular filtrate
glomerulus
nephron
osmolality
renal threshold
specific gravity
urobilin
urobilinogen
urochrome

OVERVIEW OF URINALYSIS

History of Urinalysis

Hippocrates, Aristotle, and the ancient Egyptians inferred diagnoses from urine evaluation, but it was not until the Middle Ages that "uroscopy" reached diagnostic dominance. A major reason for its rise to prominence was the publication of Johannes de Ketham's *Fasciculus Medicinae* in 1491. This was the first illustrated medical book printed. It depicts a urine wheel: a large circle surrounded by thin-necked, urine-filled flasks. This wheel shows how the color and consistency of urine could be matched to a diagnosis. Disease was thought to result from the imbalance of *humors,* reflected by one of the urine colors. In the corners of the urine wheel, four small circles contain descriptions of the four temperaments (humors):[1]

1. Sanguineous (blood)
2. Choleric (yellow bile)
3. Phlegmatic (phlegm)
4. Melancholic (black bile)

Modern Urinalysis

Urine yields a great amount of valuable information quickly and economically. In general, a urine screening test is one of the most common laboratory tests (Box 13.1).

The physical, chemical, and microscopic analysis of urine is known as *urinalysis.* Many of the routine tests are relatively simple to perform using chemically impregnated strips. When manually performed, a test strip is immersed into a urine specimen, and a color reaction is observed by visual comparison with a color chart at an appropriate time. Many companies have developed automated urine analyzers that integrate and perform all three of these urinalysis components. Semiautomated or fully automated systems are used in laboratories with a high volume of tests.

Quality Assessment and Quality Control

The urinalysis laboratory, as with all departments of the clinical laboratory, requires a quality assessment program to ensure that results of testing are meaningful. For many years, preanalytical improvements have centered on blood specimens. Urine

BOX 13.1 Purposes for Urinalysis

- To aid in the diagnosis of disease
- To monitor wellness (screening for asymptomatic, congenital, or hereditary disease)
- To monitor therapy (effectiveness or complications)

collection and processing often have lagged behind and represent areas with opportunity for improvement.[2]

The preanalytical stage of urine testing consists of the following six phases:

1. Test ordering
2. Sample collection
3. Specimen transport to the laboratory
4. Specimen receipt in the laboratory
5. Preparation of samples for testing
6. Transportation of samples to the section of the laboratory where testing occurs

Each of these phases contains between two and five steps, so the average preanalytical urine testing workflow consists of at least 22 steps. Common areas of preanalytical variability in urine testing include patient-related factors, specimen collection, specimen identification and labeling, specimen transfer and transport, and specimen processing.[2] The effect on the outcomes of urine testing is described in more detail later.

The specifics of a given quality assurance program must meet the requirements of the Clinical Laboratory Improvement Amendments of 1988 (see Chapter 3). Quality assessment elements include record keeping, the procedure manual, materials and equipment, proficiency testing, and continuing education and training.

The use of multiple-reagent strips generally ensures rapid and reliable screening of all specimens, providing a greater range of abnormal constituents than was possible before these strips came into routine use. Tests must be performed in a technically correct manner, and the reagent strips and tablets must be stored properly so that they react as they were designed to react; this is ensured by the use of control specimens.

Control solutions must be used each day by each shift of workers. Several commercial quality control products are suitable for laboratory use. Most are obtained in *lyophilized* form (freeze-dried human urine) and require reconstitution before use. Positive and negative controls are available, and both should be used in the routine testing program. The products are assayed for expected results with common reagent strips and methods. The assayed values available for a product will be a factor in determining which product a laboratory uses.

Urinalysis control solutions may be used both as a check on the urinalysis reagents and procedures and as a means of evaluating the ability of the laboratory personnel to perform and interpret the tests correctly. New bottles of reagent strips and tablets should be tested when first opened. All previously opened bottles of reagent strips and tablets should be tested at the beginning of each shift. Controls should be included whenever new reagents are used. Control solutions should be employed that check for both false-negative and false-positive results, the relative sensitivity at different concentrations, and the stability of the reagents.

Results should be recorded or documented in such a way as to ensure that the laboratory remains in control and that problems are corrected when detected. The notation system used will vary from laboratory to laboratory; control results may be tabulated on daily and weekly graphs similar to those used for clinical chemistry analyses. Control specimens should be tested as follows:

1. Test all opened bottles of reagent strips or tablets each morning.
2. Test each new bottle on opening.
3. Record data on the record sheet daily.

All bottles should be covered tightly when not in use. The manufacturer's directions for storage should be carefully followed. If any discoloration appears on the reagent strips or tablets, discard the bottle immediately. Record the date when a bottle is first opened. Note the expiration date, and do not use any product after that date.

Although now infrequently used, refractometers should be checked when used for accuracy, and the data should be recorded in an acceptable manner. The method of checking refractometers is described later (see Specific Gravity).

Probably the earliest but still the most useful tool in the quality control of urinalysis is a final inspection of all the results of the urinalysis before these are reported on the patient's laboratory record. Correlation of expected findings is discussed in this chapter whenever applicable. To inspect the testing output correctly for correlated results, laboratory staff must know the limitations of the tests and the reasons for their use. Physical properties, chemical test results, and constituents seen in the urine sediment should be correlated, and if discrepancies are seen, they should be corrected or explained before results are reported.

RENAL ANATOMY AND PHYSIOLOGY

Renal Anatomy

In general, urine can be considered a fluid composed of the waste materials of the blood. It is formed in the kidney and excreted from the body by way of the urinary system.

Anatomy of the Kidney

The urinary system[3] consists of two kidneys located in the retroperitoneal space on either side of the vertebral column (between T11–12 and L3), two ureters, the bladder, and the urethra (Fig. 13.1). Blood enters the kidney through the renal artery. This artery branches into smaller and smaller units, finally becoming the afferent arterioles entering the glomerular tuft. Blood leaves the glomerulus through the efferent arterioles. These arterioles run close to the corresponding renal tubules of the **nephron** so that reabsorption and secretion between the blood and **glomerular filtrate** can occur. The kidney is a highly vascular organ. Normally, one-fourth of the cardiac output is contained within the kidneys at a given time.

Gross examination of the kidneys reveals two bean-shaped, reddish-brown organs. Each kidney weighs about 150 g. Much of the medial border is occupied by an indentation, the hilum, through which the renal vessels, nerves, lymphatics, and the renal pelvis enter or leave the renal sinus, the space enclosed by the renal parenchyma. The bisected kidney through the hilum shows that the parenchyma consists of an outer cortex, which forms a continuous subcapsular band of tissue, and an inner medulla, which is discontinuous, interrupted by projections of the cortex toward the renal sinus, the renal columns (columns of Bertin). The medulla consists of several triangular structures, the

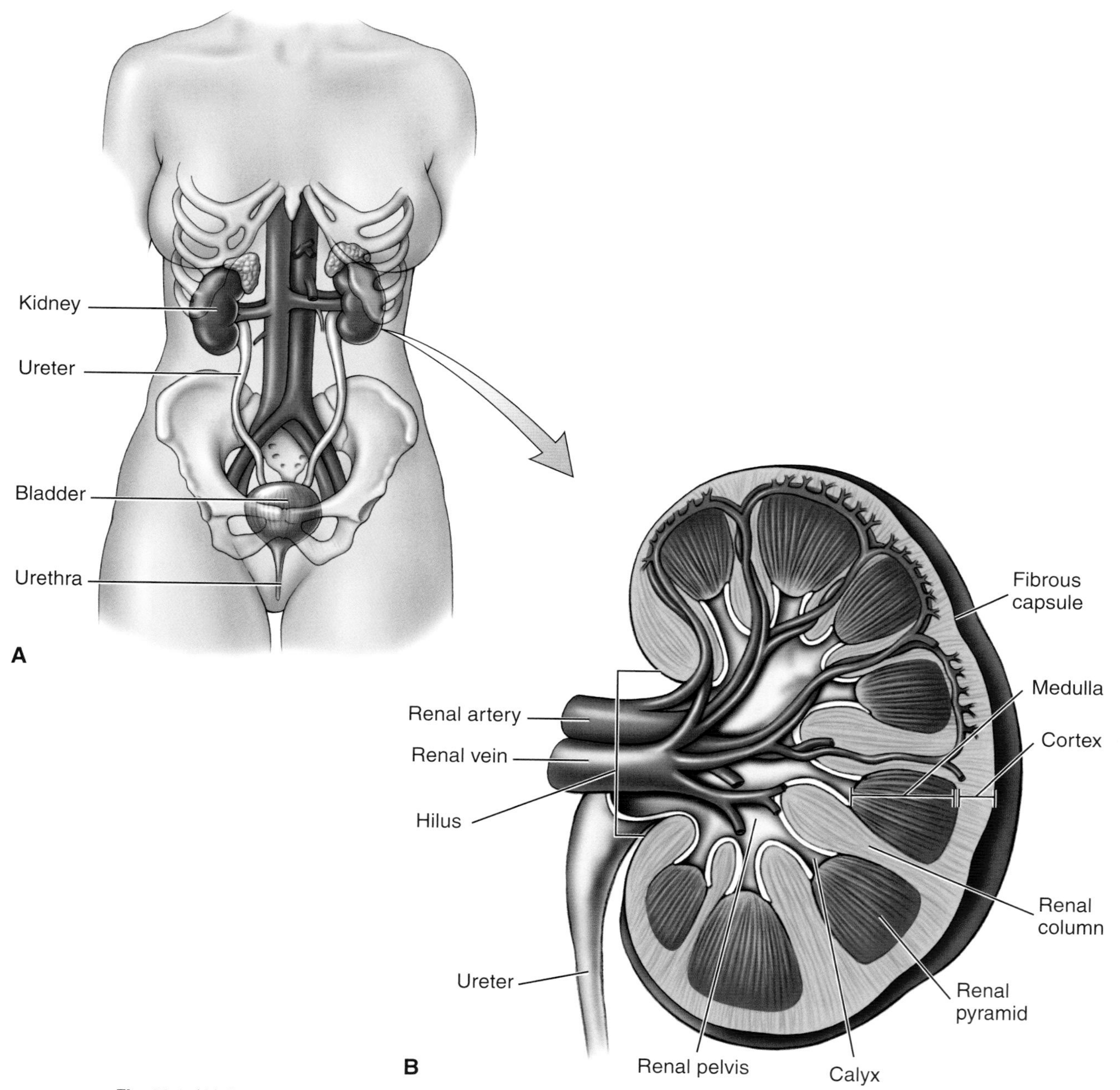

Fig. 13.1 (A) Organs of urinary system; (B) internal structure of kidney. (From Herlihy B: *The human body in health and illness,* ed 5, St Louis, 2014, Elsevier, p 462.)

pyramids, with their bases toward the cortex and their tips, called *papillae,* projecting into minor calyces.

Renal Physiology

The functional unit of the kidney is the nephron, where urine is formed (Fig. 13.2). The formed urine flows from the kidney into the ureter and is passed to the bladder for temporary storage. It is eliminated from the body through the urethra.

The kidney may be described as having the following main functions:

1. Removal of waste products, primarily nitrogenous wastes from protein metabolism, and acids
2. Retention of nutrients such as electrolytes, protein, water, and glucose
3. Acid–base balance
4. Water and electrolyte balance
5. Hormone synthesis, such as erythropoietin, renin, and vitamin D

These functions are carried out by means of filtration, reabsorption, and secretion.

Glomerulus

Each nephron consists of a tuft of anastomosing capillaries called the glomerulus. Blood enters the glomerulus from the

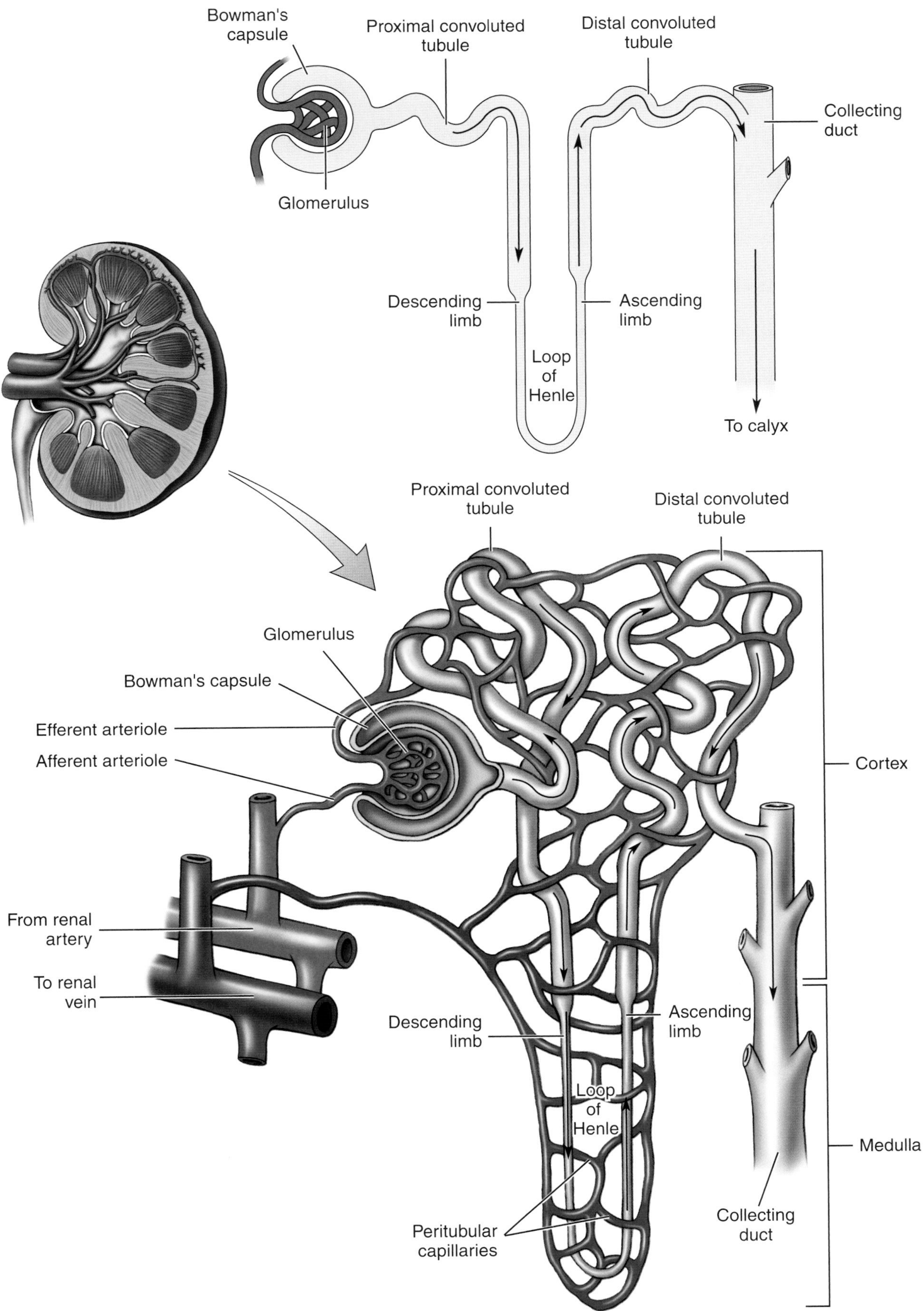

Fig. 13.2 Nephron Unit Tubular and Vascular Structures. (From Herlihy B: *The human body in health and illness,* ed 5, St Louis, 2014, Elsevier, p 464.)

renal circulation through the afferent arteriole and leaves through the efferent arteriole. Urine formation begins with the glomerulus, the structure that delivers the blood to the nephron; it is the "working portion" of the kidney.

Glomerular (Bowman's) Capsule

As blood circulates through the glomerulus, it is filtered into Bowman's capsule. The glomerular capillaries are covered by the inner layer of Bowman's capsule, forming a semipermeable membrane that allows passage of all substances with molecular weights less than about 70,000 daltons. The fluid that passes through this membrane is basically blood plasma without proteins and fats. It is an ultrafiltrate of blood and is called the *glomerular filtrate.* Because it has most of the solutes of plasma, the glomerular filtrate is iso-osmolar with plasma. That is, it has about the same osmolality as plasma, 232 to 300 mOsm/L, with a specific gravity of about 1.008. The formation of the glomerular filtrate is the first step in urine formation. About 180 L of glomerular filtrate are produced daily, but only 1 or 2 L of urine are eliminated from the body. Therefore most of the glomerular filtrate is reabsorbed back into the blood.

Proximal Convoluted Tubule

Reabsorption from the renal tubules back into the blood begins at the proximal convoluted tubule, where about 80% of the fluid and electrolytes filtered by the glomerulus is reabsorbed.

Reabsorption may be active reabsorption, with an expenditure of energy required for the analyte to be reabsorbed, usually against a concentration gradient, from a region of lower concentration to a region of higher concentration. Alternately, the reabsorption may be passive reabsorption, in which case an analyte moves passively down a concentration gradient, from a region of higher to a region of lower concentration. In addition, an analyte can move passively along with another analyte that may be actively reabsorbed.

Most of the water in the glomerular filtrate is passively reabsorbed, along with sodium ions, which are actively reabsorbed by the sodium pump mechanism. Chloride, bicarbonate, and potassium ions, together with 40% to 50% of the urea present in the filtrate, are passively reabsorbed with water at the proximal tubules. Other analytes that are actively reabsorbed in the proximal convoluted tubules include glucose, protein as albumin (a small amount of albumin is filtered into Bowman's capsule and subsequently reabsorbed), amino acids, uric acid, calcium, potassium, magnesium, and phosphate.

The proximal tubule has a limit to the amount of an analyte that will be completely reabsorbed from the glomerular filtrate. This is referred to as the renal threshold. This differs with each analyte. When the plasma concentration of an analyte is greater than its renal plasma threshold, it will remain in the glomerular filtrate and be excreted in the urine. For example, the renal plasma threshold for glucose is about 180 mg/dL. When a patient with diabetes mellitus has a blood glucose concentration greater than 180 g/dL, excess glucose will be eliminated in the urine.

The proximal convoluted tubules are also a site of active secretion of body wastes. The secretion includes hydrogen ions, phosphate, organic acids, and certain drugs such as penicillin. Hydrogen ions are secreted in exchange for sodium ions, which are reabsorbed with bicarbonate into the plasma. This exchange depends on the presence of the enzyme carbonic anhydrase, which is present in proximal and distal renal tubular cells and red blood cells (RBCs).

Solutes and water are reabsorbed in equal proportions at the proximal tubules, so the tubular fluid is still iso-osmolar with plasma when it leaves the proximal tubules.

Loop of Henle

The descending and ascending loops of Henle function to reduce the volume of the urine while reabsorbing or recovering sodium and chloride. The descending portion of the loop is the concentrating portion. The interstitial fluid outside the tubules in the medulla of the kidney becomes hypertonic as a result of increased concentrations of sodium, chloride, and urea in the tubules. This occurs because the descending portion is freely permeable to water but not to solutes. As the loop passes farther into the medulla, water moves from the loop into the interstitium. This further concentrates the urine in the tubule. The water released into the interstitium is then reabsorbed back into the blood vessels that accompany the tubules. In other words, as the fluid (to be urine) moves down the descending loop, water moves out and into the bloodstream in a countercurrent mechanism.

The ascending loop of Henle serves as the diluting segment because of the ability to actively secrete sodium and chloride but prevent water loss. Therefore the fluid within the tubule loses sodium and chloride and eventually is either hypertonic or isotonic compared with plasma when it reaches the distal convoluted tubule.

Distal Convoluted Tubule

There are two main functions of the nephron at the distal tubule. The final reabsorption of sodium occurs at this point (maintaining water and electrolyte balance), and excess acid is removed from the body (acid–base balance).

Sodium is actively reabsorbed with some bicarbonate at this point. The primary mechanism for sodium reabsorption is by the sodium–potassium pump under the control of the hormone aldosterone. Aldosterone is released from the adrenal medulla in response to angiotensin II, which is a product of the renin response to either hypotension or low plasma sodium. Aldosterone stimulates the active absorption of sodium ion in exchange for potassium that is excreted by tubular cells (the sodium–potassium pump). Overall, there is an increase in plasma sodium and water, with a decrease in body potassium levels.

When it is necessary to retain more sodium ions, ammonia is formed from glutamine and combines with hydrogen ions to form ammonium ions. This allows for a greater exchange of hydrogen ions for sodium ions. The pH of the final urine is affected by the distal tubules, especially by an excretion of hydrogen and ammonium ions in exchange for sodium. In general, the blood pH is maintained within very narrow limits at about 7.4, whereas urine generally has a pH of 5 or 6. Water is also reabsorbed under the influence of antidiuretic hormone (ADH).

Collecting Tubules

The collecting tubules are the site for the final concentration of urine. The fluid that will eventually be urine is still isotonic when it leaves the distal tubule and enters the collecting ducts. Although the collecting ducts are permeable to water, reabsorption is under the control of ADH, or vasopressin, a hormone produced by the pituitary gland. ADH is produced in response to increased plasma osmolality and has the effect of preventing excess excretion of water (antidiuresis). A lack of ADH results in the production of more dilute urine (diuresis).

Ureters, Bladder, and Urethra

The fluid that leaves the collecting ducts and enters the ureters is now urine. There are two ureters, narrow tubes that carry urine from the kidneys to the bladder. Muscles in the ureter walls continually tighten and relax, forcing urine downward, away from the kidneys. If urine backs up or is allowed to stand still, a kidney infection can develop. About every 10 to 15 seconds, small amounts of urine are emptied into the bladder from the ureters.

The bladder is a triangle-shaped, hollow organ located in the lower abdomen. It is held in place by ligaments that are attached to other organs and the pelvic bones. The bladder's walls relax and expand to store urine and contract and flatten to empty urine through the urethra. Two circular sphincter muscles keep urine from leaking by closing tightly like a rubber band around the opening of the bladder. Innervation of the bladder alerts a person when it is time to urinate, or empty the bladder.

The urethra is a hollow tube that allows urine to pass outside the body. The brain signals the bladder muscles to tighten, which squeezes urine out of the bladder. At the same time, the brain signals the sphincter muscles to relax to let urine exit the bladder through the urethra. When all the signals occur in the correct order, normal urination occurs.

Histology

All the structures that make up the urinary system, from the glomerular capsule to the terminal portion of the urethra, are lined with epithelial cells. Each portion of the urinary system is characterized by a specific type of epithelial cell. These cells generally are classified as either *renal* (meaning from the kidney or nephron itself), *transitional,* or *squamous* epithelial cells (see Microscopic Analysis of Urine Sediment). A few of these cells are constantly sloughed off into the urine, but increased numbers or cytologic changes of any of these cells may have clinical significance and may be important in determining the cause of renal dysfunction.

COMPOSITION OF URINE

The composition of urine varies greatly, depending on such factors as diet, nutritional status, metabolic rate, general state of the body, and state of the kidney or its ability to function normally.

Urine is a complex aqueous mixture consisting of 96% water and 4% dissolved substances, most derived from the food eaten or waste products of metabolism. The dissolved substances consist primarily of salt (sodium and some potassium chloride) and urea, the principal end product of protein metabolism.

In addition to urea, the principal organic substances found in urine are uric acid and creatinine. Urea, uric acid, and creatinine are nitrogenous waste products of protein metabolism that must be eliminated from the body because increased levels are toxic. Urea makes up about half the dissolved substances in urine; it is the end product of amino acid and protein breakdown. The amount of creatinine excretion is related to the muscle mass of the body, not diet. Each individual excretes a constant amount of creatinine daily; therefore urine creatinine measurements are used to assess the completeness of timed urine collections. Blood (plasma) creatinine levels are used to indicate renal function because creatinine is normally filtered through the glomerulus, and none is reabsorbed back into the blood. An increase in the plasma creatinine indicates impaired glomerular filtration and thus impaired renal function. The glomerular filtration rate is calculated from the urine and plasma creatinine levels, together with 24-hour urine volume and patient's height and weight.

In addition to sodium and chloride, the main inorganic substances present in urine include potassium, calcium, magnesium, and ammonia, plus phosphates and sulfates.

Normal Urine

Normal urine contains a few cells from the blood and lining of the urinary tract but little or no protein and no casts (although a few *hyaline casts* may be present). The reference values shown in Table 13.1 are typical of what may be "normally" encountered when the urine is examined for physical and chemical properties. Any of the substances tested for in routine urinalysis may be present in various disease states (Box 13.2).

Normal but concentrated urine typically crystallizes certain chemicals out of solution at room or refrigerator temperature. A routine urinalysis usually shows crystals of uric acid or its salts, the urates, at an acid pH, whereas phosphates typically crystallize out of solution in concentrated urine of an alkaline pH. Such crystallization appears grossly as cloudiness or turbidity of the urine, and the crystals are identified morphologically by microscopic examination. Although they are the primary

TABLE 13.1 Urine Reference Values (Physical and Chemical)

Property	Reference Value
Color	Yellow
Transparency	Clear
pH	5–7
Specific gravity	1.003–1.035 (adult random urine)
Protein, albumin	Negative Trace (in a concentrated specimen)
Blood (hemoglobin)	Negative
Nitrite	Negative
Leukocyte esterase	Negative
Glucose	Negative
Ketones	Negative
Bilirubin (conjugated)	Negative
Urobilinogen	<1 mg/dL

BOX 13.2 Clinical Usefulness of Routine Urinalysis

Indicators of State of Kidney or Urinary Tract
Appearance (color, transparency, odor, foam)
Specific gravity
Chemical tests (protein, blood, nitrite)
Leukocyte esterase
Urinary sediment (cells, casts, certain crystals)

Indicators of Metabolic and Other Conditions or Disease
pH (crystal identification; occasionally for acid–base status)
Appearance (pigments, concentration/dilution)
Glucose and ketones (diabetes mellitus)
Bilirubin (jaundice, liver disease)
Urobilinogen (hemolytic anemias, some liver diseases)

Indicators of Other Systemic (Nonrenal) Conditions or Disease
Hemoglobin (intravascular hemolysis)
Myoglobin (rhabdomyolysis)
Light-chain proteins (multiple myeloma, other γ-globulinopathies)
Porphobilinogen (some porphyrias)

TABLE 13.2 Changes in Urine Left at Room Temperature

Constituent	Observed Change	Mechanism of Change
pH	Increased (alkaline)	Breakdown of urea to ammonia
Cells	Decreased number	Lysis
Casts	Decreased number	Lysis—dissolution
Glucose	Decreased	Glycolysis (by bacterial action)
Ketones	Decreased	Conversion of diacetic acid to acetone and evaporation of acetone from specimen
Bilirubin	Decreased (color change from yellow to green)	Oxidation to biliverdin
Urobilinogen	Decreased (color change from colorless to orange-red)	Oxidation to urobilin

Modified from Ringsrud KM, Linné JJ: *Urinalysis and body fluids: a color text and atlas,* St Louis, 1995, Mosby.

constituents of urine, urea and sodium chloride do not crystallize out of urine specimens.

Identification of a Fluid as Urine

It is sometimes necessary to determine whether a specimen is urine or a body fluid such as amniotic fluid. This is done by measuring urea, creatinine, sodium, and chloride levels, which are all significantly higher in urine than in other body fluids.

COLLECTION AND PRESERVATION OF URINE SPECIMENS

Important considerations in the proper collection and handling of urine for routine examination include the container used, the collection procedure, and the conditions of storage and preservation from the time of collection until the specimen is tested. For routine urinalysis, the urine specimen must be collected in a suitable, clean, dry container. In most cases, the first specimen freely voided in the morning is preferred, although a specimen collected 2 to 3 hours after eating is preferable for testing of glucose. The specimen must be examined when fresh, ideally within 30 minutes, or suitably preserved, such as by refrigeration for up to 6 to 8 hours. Changes in urine left at room temperature more than 2 hours are detailed in Table 13.2.

Types of Urine Specimens

Clinical information obtained from a urine specimen is influenced by the collection method, timing, and handling. Various types of collection and transport containers for urine specimens are available. A specimen must be carefully collected, preserved, and processed before analysis in order for the reported results to be reliable. If urine testing cannot be performed within 2 hours of collection, the specimen should be stored at 4°C as soon as possible after collection. Specimens can be stored under refrigeration for 6 to 8 hours, with no gross alterations in constituents.

Random Specimen

A random urine specimen is the most common type for analysis.[4] Random specimens, or specimens collected at any time, can give an inaccurate view of a patient's health because the specimen is too diluted and analyte values are artificially lowered. Although there are no specific guidelines on how the collection should be conducted, avoiding the introduction of contaminants into the specimen is recommended. This requires explicit instructions to patients about not touching the inside of the cup or cup lid with any part of the body.

First Morning Specimen

The first urine voided in the morning is the specimen of choice for urinalysis and microscopic examination. This urine is generally more concentrated because of the length of time the urine is allowed to remain in the bladder overnight. The specimen contains relatively high levels of cellular elements and analytes such as glucose and protein. Any urine that is voided from the bladder during the 8-hour (typically overnight) collection period should be pooled and refrigerated so that a true 8-hour sample is obtained. To test for the presence of urine sugar, the best specimen to use is one voided 2 to 3 hours after a meal. This is the one exception to the recommended use of the first morning specimen.

Midstream Clean-Catch Specimen

Midstream clean-catch urine is the preferred type of specimen for culture and sensitivity (C&S) testing because of the reduced incidence of cellular and microbial contamination. Patients are required first to cleanse the urethral area and then to void the first portion of the urine stream into the toilet. These first steps significantly reduce the incidence of contamination of the urine specimen. A midstream sample of urine is then collected into a clean container. This method of collection can be conducted at any time of day or night.

24-Hour or Timed Specimen

The most common tests requiring the 24-hour urine specimen include those measuring creatinine, urine urea nitrogen, glucose, sodium, potassium, and substances such as catecholamines and 17-hydroxysteroids that are affected by diurnal variations. The bladder is emptied before beginning the timed collection. Then for the duration of the designated 24-hour period, all urine is collected and pooled into a collection container, with the final collection at the end of the period. Usually the specimen is refrigerated. Accurate timing is critical to determining the concentration of various analytes and calculated ratios.

Catheter Collection Specimen

Catheter collection is an assisted procedure conducted when a patient is confined to bed or cannot urinate independently. A health care provider can use an existing catheter or can insert a Foley catheter into the bladder through the urethra to collect the urine specimen.

Suprapubic Aspiration Specimen

The suprapubic aspiration method is used when a bedridden patient cannot be catheterized or a sterile specimen is required. The urine specimen is collected by needle aspiration through the abdominal wall into the bladder.

Pediatric Specimen

For infants and small children, a special urine collection bag is adhered to the skin surrounding the urethral area. Once the collection is completed, the urine is poured into a collection cup or transferred directly into an evacuated tube with a transfer straw. Urine collected from a diaper is not recommended for laboratory testing, because contamination from the diaper material may affect test results. If a 24-hour pediatric specimen is required, a special tube can be attached to the bag, which in turn is connected to a collection bottle.

Containers for Urine Collection

It is essential that the containers used to collect the urine specimen be clean, dry, and free of particles or interfering substances.[4] Containers should not be reused. Several types of containers are suitable for this purpose. Disposable inert plastic containers with leak-resistant lids, plastic bags, or jars are most often used.

Any bedpans that are used to collect voided urine must be scrupulously clean and free of cleaning agents or bleach. Labels must remain fixed to the urine specimen container at all times and must be on the container, not on the lid.

Urine Collection Cups

Urine collection container cups come in a variety of shapes and sizes, with either snap-on or screw-on lids. Clinical and Laboratory Standards Institute (CLSI) guidelines for urine (GP16-A2) recommend the use of a primary collection container that holds at least 50 mL, has a wide base, and has an opening of at least 4 cm.[4] The wide base prevents spillage, and a 4-cm opening is an adequate target for urine collection.

Leak-resistant cups should be used to protect health care personnel from exposure to the specimen and protect the specimen from exposure to contaminants. Some urine transport cup closures have special access ports that allow closed-system transfer of urine directly from the collection device to the tube.

Urinalysis Tubes

Evacuated tubes, similar to those used in blood collection, are filled through a straw device from cups with integrated transfer devices built into their lid, or from direct sampling devices, and are used to access catheter sampling ports. Becton Dickinson (BD) manufactures a plastic urine preservative tube. This tube contains chlorhexidine, ethylparaben, and sodium propionate and maintains sample integrity for up to 72 hours without refrigeration.

For testing purposes, conical-bottom test tubes provide the best sediment collection for microscopic analysis. Some tubes are specially designed to be used with a pipettor that allows for standardized sampling. Fill volumes of urinalysis tubes usually range from 8 to 15 mL.

24-Hour Collection Containers

Urine collection containers for 24-hour specimens should hold up to 3 L and may be colored to protect light-sensitive analytes such as porphyrins and urobilinogen from degradation.

If a preservative is required,[4] the least hazardous type should be selected and added to the collection container before the urine collection begins. Common 24-hour preservatives are hydrochloric acid, boric acid, acetic acid, and toluene. Warning labels should be placed on the container. A corresponding material safety data sheet should be given to the patient, and the health care provider should explain any potential hazards.

Urine Culture Containers

The CLSI guidelines recommend sterile collection containers for microbiology specimens. These containers should have secure closures to prevent specimen loss and to protect the specimen from contamination.

Urine Transport Tubes

Transport tubes should be compatible with automated systems and instruments used by the laboratory. Collection containers and transport tubes should be compatible with the pneumatic tube system if one is used for urine specimen transport in the facility. A leakproof device in this situation is critical.

Urine Volume for Routine Urinalysis

The minimum volume for routine urinalysis is usually 12 mL, but 50 mL is preferable. The minimum amount necessary for the usual processing procedure is 12 mL; the urine is placed in a disposable centrifuge tube, centrifuged, and concentrated 12:1 so that 1 mL of sediment is retained for the microscopic analysis of the sediment. This volume also allows for a convenient, standardized volume of urine for assessment of physical properties, such as color and transparency, which are often observed in the centrifuge tube.

Smaller volumes may be accepted for chemical analysis from oliguric patients or from infants. If only 3 mL of urine is collected, a 12:1 concentration of sediment may still be made. In some situations, a drop of unconcentrated urine placed on the desired portion of a reagent strip or observed microscopically may be the only option available.

Collection of Urine Specimens

Routine Specimens. A specimen for urinalysis should be collected in a clean, dry container, and the specimen should be fresh. For routine screening, a freshly voided, random, preferably midstream (freely flowing) urine specimen is usually suitable. For most routine urinalysis, including protein content and urinary sediment constituents, the concentrated first morning specimen is the most satisfactory one to use.

Occasionally, a catheterized specimen may be needed. This type of specimen is obtained by a physician or designee and is obtained by introducing a catheter into the bladder, through the urethra, for the withdrawal of urine. Catheterization may be required under special circumstances or for obtaining a sterile urine specimen for bacteriologic examination. The risk of introducing infection is always present when an invasive procedure such as catheterization is performed. Under most conditions, a free-flowing (midstream) voided specimen is satisfactory for bacteriologic cultures.

When both a bacteriologic culture and a routine urinalysis are needed on the same specimen, the culture should always be done first, then the routine tests, to avoid contamination of the specimen before culturing on bacteriologic media.

Collection of Timed Urine Specimens. The patient is carefully instructed about details of the urine collection process if the collection will be done on an outpatient basis. The bladder is emptied at the starting time, such as 8 a.m., and this time is noted on the collection container. The first urine voided at the beginning of the collection is always discarded. All subsequent voidings are collected and put into the container, up to and including the urine voided at 8 a.m. the following day. This last urine specimen will complete the 24-hour collection.

For timed collections of other than 24 hours, the sample-collection principle applies. These timed collection specimens are preserved by refrigeration between collections, with the appropriate chemical preservative added to the container before the beginning of the collection process. The total volume of the timed collection sample is measured and recorded, and the sample well mixed, before a measured aliquot is withdrawn for analysis.

Collection of Urine for Culture. A clean-catch, midstream urine specimen is desirable for culture. It is important that the glans penis in the male and the urethral orifice in the female be thoroughly cleaned with a mild antiseptic solution by means of sterile gauze or cotton balls. The patient should be instructed to urinate forcibly and allow the initial stream of urine to pass into the toilet or bedpan. Throughout the urination process for the female, the labia should be separated so that no contamination results. The midstream specimen should be collected in a sterile container, and no portion of the perineum (female) should come in contact with the collection container. After the specimen has been collected, the remaining urine is discarded.

Preservation of Urine Specimens

If a fresh specimen of urine is left at room temperature for a period, the urine rapidly undergoes changes. Decomposition of urine begins within 30 minutes after collection. Specimens left at room temperature will soon begin to decompose, primarily because of the action of urea-splitting bacteria, which produces ammonia. On combining with hydrogen ions, ammonia forms ammonium ions, causing an increase in urine pH, which will contribute to the decomposition of casts and certain cells, if present in the urine. The various laboratory tests planned for a urine specimen should be performed promptly after collection. No longer than 1 or 2 hours should elapse before the tests are done, unless the urine is preserved in some way.

The best method of preservation is immediate refrigeration during and after collection. The specimen may be kept 6 to 8 hours under refrigeration with no chemical preservative added, with no gross alterations. Specimens can be frozen (at 24–16°C) after collection. Several chemical preservatives are available as additives for routine urine specimens.[5] Preservatives have different roles but usually are added to reduce bacterial action or chemical decomposition or to solubilize constituents that might otherwise precipitate from the solution. Specimens for some types of analysis should not have preservatives added because of the possibility of interference with analytical methods. Generally, the length of preservation capacity ranges from 24 to 72 hours.

In addition to refrigeration or freezing, common chemical preservatives are hydrochloric acid, boric acid, and acetic acid. Boric acid allows urine to be kept at room temperature while still providing results comparable to those of refrigerated urine. Other preservatives include the following:[6]

- Toluene, a solution lighter than urine or water, prevents the growth of bacteria by excluding contact of urine with air. A thin layer of toluene is added, just enough to cover the surface of the urine. The toluene should be skimmed off or the urine pipetted from beneath it when the urine is examined. Toluene (toluol) is the best all-around preservative because it does not interfere with the various tests done in the routine urinalysis.
- Formaldehyde (formalin), a liquid preservative, acts by fixing the formed elements in the urinary sediment, including bacteria. It may interfere with the reduction tests for urine sugar, however, and may form a precipitate with urea that interferes with the microscopic examination of the sediment. Preservative tablets that produce formaldehyde are commercially available. The tablets are more convenient to use than the liquid formalin and do not interfere with the usual chemical and microscopic examination.
- Thymol, a crystalline substance, works to prevent the growth of bacteria. Thymol may interfere with tests for urine protein and bilirubin.
- The BD Vacutainer Plus Plastic UA Preservative Tube contains a proprietary additive (chlorhexidine, ethylparaben,

sodium propionate) that maintains sample integrity of up to 72 hours without refrigeration. When a specimen is directly transferred from a collection cup into a preservative tube, it provides a stable environment for the specimen until testing can be conducted and reduces the risk of bacterial overgrowth or specimen decomposition.

- Specialized additives include nitric acid for mercury analysis, sodium bicarbonate and ethylenediaminetetraacetic acid for porphyrins, and sodium bicarbonate for urobilinogen analysis.[4]
- The most common preservative of urine for C&S testing is boric acid, which comes in tablet, powder, or lyophilized form. Clinical evidence suggests that nonbuffered boric acid may be harmful to certain organisms and that buffered boric acid preservatives can reduce the harmful effects of the preservative on the organisms.[4] C&S preservatives are designed to maintain the specimen in a state equivalent to refrigeration by deterring the proliferation of organisms that could result in a false-positive culture or bacterial overgrowth.
- Preserved urine specimens can be stored at room temperature until time of testing. Product claims regarding the duration of preservative potency should be obtained from the particular manufacturer.

Specimen Preservation Guidelines[4]

1. CLSI guidelines for microbiological urine testing recommend refrigeration of specimens at 2°C to 8°C or the use of chemical preservatives if the specimen cannot be processed within 2 hours of collection.
2. Chemical preservatives should be nonmercuric and environmentally friendly. The American Hospital Association and the US Environmental Protection Agency issued a Memorandum of Understanding for the "virtual elimination of mercury containing waste from the health care industry waste stream" (see http://www.epa.gov/mercury).
3. To ensure accurate test results, the proper specimen-to-additive ratio must be maintained when using a chemical preservative. Maintaining the correct ratio is especially important when transferring samples into a preservative tube. The indicated fill lines on the tube are used to ensure proper fill.
4. An evacuated tube system is designed to achieve proper fill volume to ensure the proper specimen-to-additive ratio and proper preservative function. Evacuated systems also reduce the potential exposure of the health care worker to the specimen.

Labeling and Processing of Urine Specimens

As with any type of laboratory specimen, certain criteria must be met for proper collection and transportation of urine specimens.

Labels

Include the patient name and identification information on labels. Make sure that the information on the container label and the requisition match. If the collection container is used for transport, the label should be placed on the container, not on the lid, because the lid can be mistakenly placed on a different container. Ensure that the labels used on the containers are adherent under refrigerated conditions.

Collection Date and Time

Include the date and time of the urine collection on the specimen label. This will confirm that the collection was done correctly. For timed specimens, verify start and stop times of collection. Document the time at which the specimen was received in the laboratory for verification of proper handling and transport after collection.

Collection Method

The method of collection should be checked when the specimen is received in the laboratory to ensure the type of specimen submitted meets the needs of the test ordered.

Proper Preservation

Check whether there is a chemical preservative present or whether the specimen has not been refrigerated for longer than 2 hours after collection. Verify that the method of preservation used is appropriate for the selected test.

Light Protection

Verify that specimens submitted for testing of light-sensitive analytes are collected in containers that protect the specimen from light.

PHYSICAL PROPERTIES OF URINE

The first part of a routine urinalysis usually involves an assessment of physical properties, including volume, color, transparency, and odor (Table 13.3). Another physical property, specific gravity, is discussed later in this section. Simple observations are extremely useful both for the eventual diagnosis of the patient and for the laboratory personnel who perform the complete urinalysis. Such tests often give clues leading to findings in subsequent portions of the urinalysis. For example, if a urine specimen is cloudy and red, the presence of RBCs will probably be revealed by microscopic analysis of the urine sediment. If RBCs are not found, all parts of the urinalysis must be carefully rechecked for accuracy. Chemical tests for blood (hemoglobin) might be falsely negative when ascorbic acid is present in urine; however, the presence of blood might be indicated by an abnormal red color and confirmed by the presence of RBCs in the urine sediment. If hemoglobin is present without RBCs, the only indication of ascorbic acid interference might be the abnormal color of the urine.

Certain tests are performed when abnormal physical properties are observed. For example, a chemical test for the pigment bilirubin is necessary when it is suspected on the basis of the abnormal color of the urine. In several situations the laboratory evaluates the complete urinalysis for reliability before reporting results to the physician, or abnormal constituents are found in subsequent tests because abnormal physical properties were noted.

Volume

Normal Volume

Although it is a physical property, the volume of the urine is not measured as part of a routine urinalysis. In certain conditions, the volume of urine excreted in 24 hours is a valuable aid to clinical diagnosis. In normal adults with normal fluid intake, the

TABLE 13.3 Physical Properties of Urine

Physical Property	Description	Possible Cause
Normal color	Yellow	Urochrome, uroerythrin, urobilin
Abnormal color	Pale	Dilute urine
	Amber (dark yellow or orange-red)	Concentrated urine or bilirubin
	Brown (yellow-brown or green-brown)	Bilirubin or biliverdin
	Orange (orange-red or orange-brown)	Urobilin (excreted colorless as urobilinogen)
	Bright orange	Azo-containing dyes or compounds
	Red	Blood or heme-derived pigment, urates or uric acid, drugs, foodstuffs
	Clear red	Hemoglobin
	Cloudy red	Red blood cells
	Dark red-brown	Myoglobin
	Dark red or red-purple	Porphyrins
	Black (dark brown and black)	Melanin, homogentisic acid, phenol poisoning
	Green, blue, or orange	Drugs, medications, foodstuffs
Normal transparency	Clear	Normal or dilute urine
Abnormal transparency	Hazy, cloudy, turbid	Mucus, phosphates, urates, crystals, bacteria, pus, fat, casts
Normal odor	Aromatic	Normal
Abnormal odor	Ammoniacal, putrid or foul	Breakdown of urea by bacteria (old urine)
		Urinary tract infection
	Sweet or "fruity"	Ketone bodies
	Sweaty feet, maple syrup, cabbage or hops, mousy, rotting fish, rancid	Specific amino acid disorder for each

average 24-hour urine volume is 1200 to 1500 mL, although the normal range is 600 to 1600 mL. The total volume of urine excreted in 24 hours must be measured when quantitative tests are performed because it enters into the calculation of test results.

Under normal conditions, a direct relationship exists between urine volume and water intake. That is, if water intake is increased, the kidney will protect the body from excessive retention of water by eliminating a larger volume of urine than normal. Conversely, if water intake is decreased, the kidney will protect the body against dehydration by eliminating a smaller amount of urine.

Abnormal Volume

Patient conditions that can result in abnormal urine volumes include the following:

- *Polyuria:* Consistent elimination of an abnormally large volume of urine, more than 2000 mL/24 hours
- *Diuresis:* Any increase in urine volume, even if the increase is only temporary
- *Oliguria:* Excretion of an abnormally small amount of urine, less than 500 mL/24 hours
- *Anuria:* Complete absence of urine formation
- *Nocturia:* Excretion of more than 400 mL urine at night

Color

The color of normal urine seems to result from the presence of three pigments: urochrome, uroerythrin, and urobilin. **Urochrome** is a yellow pigment and is present in larger concentrations than the other two pigments of uroerythrin, a red pigment, and **urobilin**, an orange-yellow pigment. The color of normal urine varies considerably, even in one person in a single day. Numerous words have been used to describe the range of normal color. In general, normal urine is some shade of yellow. The terms *yellow, straw,* and *amber* may be used. *Straw* is generally used to describe a lighter-colored urine with normal yellow pigment. *Amber* refers to a darker color, with red or orange pigments in addition to yellow. Abnormalities in color may have various possible causes (see Table 13.3).

Pale urine suggests that the urine is dilute; urine that is more highly colored has a greater concentration of normal waste products because its volume is diminished.

Transparency

When voided, urine is normally clear; most urine will become cloudy when allowed to stand. Cloudiness of a specimen when voided is usually of clinical significance and should not be disregarded. Numerous words describe the degree of transparency of a urine specimen. According to CLSI, standardized terms such as *clear, hazy, cloudy,* and *turbid* should be used to reduce ambiguity and subjectivity. Schweitzer and colleagues[7] advocate the use of a limited number of descriptors, as follows:

- *Clear:* No visible particulate matter is present.
- *Hazy:* Some visible particulate matter is present; newsprint is not distorted or obscured when viewed through the urine.
- *Cloudy:* Newsprint can be seen through the urine, but letters are distorted or blurry.
- *Turbid:* Newsprint cannot be seen through the urine.

Table 13.4 summarizes common constituents that cause cloudiness in urine, either normal or possibly significant or pathologic.

Odor

Normal urine has a characteristic, faintly aromatic odor because of the presence of certain volatile acids (see Table 13.3). If urine is allowed to stand, it acquires the strong odor of ammonia. This

TABLE 13.4 Common Constituents Causing Cloudiness in Urine

Generally Normal	Possibly Pathologic
Amorphous phosphates and urates	Amorphous urates
Normal crystals	Abnormal crystals
	Red blood cells
	White blood cells
	Casts
	Fat (lipids)
Epithelial cells (squamous, transitional)	Epithelial cells (renal, transitional, malignant)
Bacteria (old urine)	Bacteria (fresh urine)
	Other microorganisms (yeast, fungi, parasites)
Mucus	
Sperm, prostatic fluid	Chyluria (lymph, rare)
Powders, antiseptics	Fecal matter (from fistula)

is caused by the breakdown of urea by bacteria to form ammonia.

Specific Gravity

Urine is a mixture of substances dissolved and suspended in water. In normal urine, these dissolved substances are primarily urea and sodium chloride. Specific gravity is a measure of the amount of dissolved substances in a solution compared with distilled water with a specific gravity of 1.000. The specific gravity of urine is used as a measure of the ability of the kidney to regulate the composition and osmotic pressure of the extracellular fluid by concentrating or diluting the urine.

Specific gravity is defined as the weight of a solution compared with the weight of an equal volume of water. More specifically, it is the ratio of the density (weight per unit volume) of a solution to the density (weight per unit volume) of an equal volume of water at a constant temperature. Because it is a ratio, specific gravity has no units. It is always reported to the third decimal place.

Clinical Aspects

Clinically, the specific gravity of urine may be used to obtain information about two general functions: the state of the kidney and the patient's state of hydration.

If the kidney is performing adequately, it is capable of producing urine with a specific gravity ranging from about 1.003 to 1.035. If the renal epithelium is not functioning adequately, it will gradually lose the ability to concentrate and dilute the urine. The ability to concentrate urine is one of the first functions lost when the kidney is impaired. Deficiency or failure to respond to ADH will also result in failure to concentrate urine. The specific gravity of the protein-free glomerular filtrate is about 1.008. Without any active work on the part of the kidney, this will increase to 1.010 as a result of simple diffusion as the filtrate passes through the kidney tubules. Thus, if the kidney has completely lost its ability to concentrate and dilute the urine, the specific gravity will remain at 1.010. If it is known that the kidney is functioning adequately, the state of hydration may be reflected by the specific gravity. For example, if the urine is consistently very concentrated, dehydration is implied.

Although normal specific gravity may range from 1.003 to 1.035, the specific gravity of a 24-hour collection is usually between 1.016 and 1.022 with normal diet and fluid intake. Because the specific gravity reflects the amount of dissolved substances present in solution, it varies inversely with the volume of urine (this is because a fairly constant amount of waste is produced each day). If the urinary volume increases because of increased water intake, and the amount of waste produced remains constant, the specific gravity of the urine decreases. In other words, if the urinary volume is high, the specific gravity is low, and vice versa, assuming the kidney is functioning normally. With an individual on a restricted fluid diet for 12 hours, the normal kidney is capable of concentrating urine to a specific gravity of about 1.022 or more. A person without fluids for 24 hours should produce urine with a specific gravity of 1.026 or more. If the individual is placed on a very high-fluid diet, the normal kidney is capable of diluting the urine to a specific gravity of about 1.003. The concentrated first urine specimen passed in the morning should have a specific gravity greater than 1.020 if the kidney is functioning normally.

Two frequently observed cases in which specific gravity does not vary inversely with urinary volume are diabetes mellitus and certain types of renal disease. With diabetes mellitus, an abnormally large urinary volume associated with an abnormally high specific gravity is observed. This is caused by the presence of large amounts of dissolved glucose, which raises the specific gravity of the urine. In certain types of renal disease, such as glomerulonephritis, pyelonephritis, and various anomalies, there is a combination of low specific gravity and low urinary volume. This results from the inability of the renal tubular epithelium either to excrete normal amounts of water or to concentrate the waste products. The specific gravity in these cases may eventually be fixed at about 1.010.

The loss of concentrating ability is seen in diabetes insipidus, an impairment of ADH. This rare condition results in extremely large volumes of urine with very low specific gravity, ranging from 1.001 to 1.003.

Abnormally high specific gravity values, usually greater than 1.035 and up to 1.050 or more, may also be encountered after certain diagnostic x-ray procedures in which a radiographic dye is injected intravenously to obtain a pyelogram of the kidney. Such high specific gravity readings will be accompanied by delayed false-positive reactions for protein with the sulfosalicylic acid (SSA) procedure, and the dye may crystallize out of the urine as an abnormal, colorless crystal resembling plates of cholesterol.

Measures of Urine Solute Concentration (Specific Gravity and Osmolality)

Although specific gravity is a convenient measure of the urine solute concentration, it is not the only one available. Other measures are osmolality, refractive index, and ionic concentration. All the methods of measuring solute concentration are influenced by the number of molecules present in solution, in addition to the size and ionic charge.

Osmolality by Osmometer. Measuring osmolality by osmometer is another method of determining solute concentration. Osmolality is a measure of the number of solute particles per unit amount of solvent; thus it depends only on the number of particles in solution. It is determined with an osmometer by measuring the freezing point of a solution because the freezing point is depressed in proportion to the amount of dissolved substances present. In normal persons with a normal diet and fluid intake, the urine will contain about 500 to 850 mOsm/kg of water. Osmolality is preferred to specific gravity as a measurement of urine concentration. Urine and plasma osmolality as a ratio is used to evaluate renal tubular concentration, which depends on the patient's state of hydration.

Specific Gravity as Refractive Index by Refractometer. A previously popular method for measurement of solute concentration, reported in the urinalysis laboratory as specific gravity, is refractive index. The refractive index of a solution is the ratio of the velocity of light in air to the velocity of light in solution. This ratio varies directly with the number of dissolved particles in solution. Although not identical to specific gravity, refractive index corresponds with specific gravity. Measurement is made with a refractometer that is calibrated to give results in terms of specific gravity (Fig. 13.3). The specific gravity scale by refractometer is valid only for urine.

Few normal urine specimens have values greater than 1.035. Higher values suggest the presence of unusual solutes in the specimen, such as increased amounts of glucose or protein, or radiopaque compounds. Beyond a value of 1.035, the refractive index correlates poorly with the specific gravity.

Quality Control. The refractometer should be checked daily or at time of use with deionized or distilled water and with a solution of known specific gravity. The distilled water should read 1.000 $\pm$ 0.001. The instrument contains a zero set screw to adjust the reading to water. Follow the manufacturer's directions.

Use of Reagent Strips for Specific Gravity

Reagent strips have extensively replaced the refractometer. These strips actually measure ionic concentration, which relates to specific gravity. Values are reported as specific gravity. However, substances that are dissolved in the urine must ionize to be measured by this method. The waste products that constitute normal urine constituents and that indicate the concentration and dilution ability of the kidney do ionize. Certain substances that may be present in urine, such as glucose or certain radiopaque dyes, do not ionize; therefore specific gravity results obtained with a refractometer will be significantly higher than with the reagent strip if the urine contains significant quantities of a nonionizable, dissolved substance.

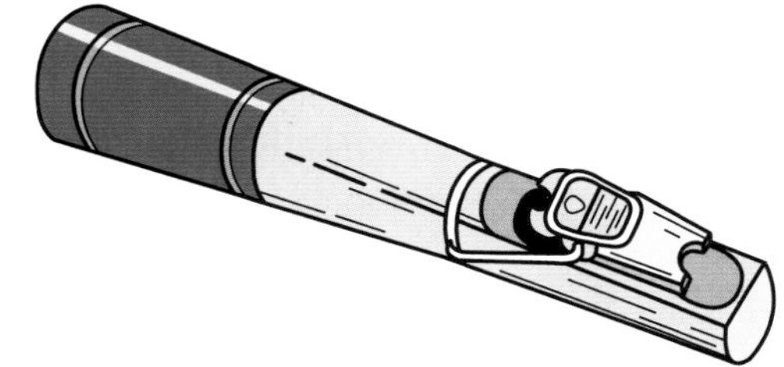

Fig. 13.3 Refractometer.

Principle. The reagent strips for specific gravity actually measure ionic concentration. Reagent strip tests for specific gravity are based on a pK_a change of certain pretreated polyelectrolytes in relation to the ionic concentration of urine. The polyelectrolytes in the reagent strip contain acid groups that dissociate in proportion to the number of ions in solution. This produces hydrogen ions, which reduce the pH (hydrogen ion concentration). The pH change is indicated by the color change of an acid-base indicator. The system is buffered so that any change in color is related to pK_a change, and not pH of the urine itself. Therefore reagent strips measure only ionizable substances. (The pK_a is the negative logarithm of the ionization constant of an acid.)

Readings are made at 0.005 intervals from 1.000 to 1.030 by comparison with a color chart. Therefore precision is significantly less than by refractometer, which is read at 0.001 intervals. Reagent strip tests generally correlate to within 0.005 of the refractometer. Urine with a specific gravity greater than 1.025 is not reliably measured with ionic concentration methodology and should be tested with the refractometer. The procedure for measuring urine specific gravity with reagent strips is the same as that used for all reagent strips (Student Procedure Worksheet 13.1).

Corrections and Limitations. Dissolved substances must ionize to be detected by the reagent strips for specific gravity. Substances that do not ionize, such as glucose and radiopaque dyes, will not affect the reagent strips, giving different values from those obtained with a refractometer. Although this may give a better picture of the concentrating ability of the kidney, to interpret specific gravity results properly, it is important that the clinician understand which methodology is used by the laboratory and whether the results are "corrected" or not.

Highly buffered alkaline urine may cause low readings, and 0.005 may be added to readings from urine with a pH of 6.5 or greater. Automated instruments apply this correction. Unlike readings with the refractometer, elevated specific gravity readings may be obtained in the presence of only moderate (100–750 mg/dL) amounts of protein. Urine specimens containing urea at concentrations greater than 1 g/dL will cause low readings relative to more traditional methods.

CHEMICAL TESTS IN ROUTINE URINALYSIS

Reagent Strip Tests

Chemical tests in routine urinalysis are generally done by using multiple-reagent strips (Student Procedure Worksheet 13.1, Fig. 13.26). Specialized tests for ascorbic acid, microalbumin, and creatinine as available as single chemical tests. Many chemical tests have become routine as they have been added to the readily available multiple-reagent strips. Different combinations are available for use in different clinical situations. For example, in an obstetric clinic, tests for glucose, protein, blood, and leukocyte esterase are especially desirable. In certain cases, positive findings in the chemical screen may require confirmation with other chemical tests or may indicate the likelihood of certain findings in the microscopic examination of the urine sediment.

Most of the chemical tests done as part of the routine urinalysis use dry reagent strips. Reagent strips are available both as single tests for a specific chemical substance and as combinations of single tests, referred to as *multiple-reagent strips.*

Reagent strips are plastic strips that contain one or more chemically impregnated test sites on an absorbent pad. When the chemicals on the test site come into contact with urine or a control solution, a chemical reaction occurs. The reaction is indicated by a color change, which is compared with a special color chart that is provided with the reagent strip, usually printed on the bottle. Results can be read visually or in special instruments that automatically read specific reagent strips.

The intensity of the color formed is generally proportional to the amount of substance present in the specimen or control when observed at a specific time. Some areas are used as screening tests; others are used to estimate (semiquantitate) the amount of substance present and are reported in a plus system or in numeric values such as mg/dL or g/dL. The method of reporting results will vary from laboratory to laboratory.

Advantages to dry reagent strip tests over the more traditional chemical tests on which they are based include the following:

1. Convenience: rapid results with a minimum of time and personnel
2. Cost-effectiveness
3. Stability
4. Relative ease in learning to use
5. Disposability
6. Smaller sample volumes required
7. Space savings: storage, use, and cleanup

Because of the apparent ease of use, reagent strip tests are candidates for abuse. Reliable, reproducible results depend on correct technique. Manufacturers' directions must be followed exactly. Any person using reagent strips should understand the principle and specificity of each chemical test area, should be aware of precautions or limitations and interferences that occur, and should know the sensitivity and significance of positive or negative results.

In certain cases, additional confirmatory tests may be used when positive results are obtained with the reagent strip tests. These are usually in the form of tablet tests.

Manufacturer's Directions

It is imperative that the specific directions of the manufacturer be followed for all reagent strip tests. Tests are continually changed and reformulated in this highly competitive market. Each container of reagent strips is supplied with a product insert. This contains the most up-to-date information for the successful performance of the test in question. Inserts include directions for use, warnings, procedure limitations, specimen-handling information, storage, and expected values. Information on interfering substances that may produce false-negative or false-positive reactions is also included. For each new lot number of reagent strips, the laboratorian should study the product insert, compare it to the previous insert, noting any changes, and file it with the laboratory procedure manual.

In this discussion, tests are arranged in order of clinical utility or physiologic significance, not in the order in which they are placed on a reagent strip. Chemical tests indicating disease of the kidney or urinary tract—pH, specific gravity, protein, blood, nitrite, and leukocyte esterase—are described first. Chemical tests indicating metabolic and other diseases are then described: glucose, ketones, bilirubin, and urobilinogen. Many reagent strips include a test for specific gravity, as described previously. Each parameter is described in terms of clinical importance, principle of the test, specificity (what is being tested), sensitivity (minimum detectable level), and interferences (false-positive and false-negative reactions).

Sampling or Wetting

The specimen to be tested must be fresh or adequately preserved, well mixed (not centrifuged), and at room temperature. The first step in using the reagent strip is adequately sampling the specimen or wetting the reagent strip. Although this sounds easy, it is a common source of error. The strip must be adequately moistened so that all test areas of the strip are brought into contact with the sample. Care must be taken not to leave the strip in contact with the sample too long, or chemicals will be leached out of the strip and unavailable for the chemical reaction to occur. Therefore the strip is inserted into the specimen only briefly, for 1 second or less. Another problem is runover between chemicals on adjacent pads. This is avoided by drawing the edge of the strip along the edge of the urine container as it is removed, touching the edge of the strip to absorbent paper, and holding the strip horizontally while waiting for and reading results.

Storage and General Precautions

Reagent strips must be kept in tightly capped containers. They will deteriorate rapidly when exposed to moisture, direct sunlight, heat, or volatile substances.[7] Each container contains a desiccant, or drying agent, within the product to protect it from moisture; the desiccant should not be removed. Store containers at recommended temperatures, generally at room temperature, under 30°C, but not refrigerated or frozen. Keep strips in their original containers. Do not mix strips from different containers. Remove only the number of strips needed at a time, and close the container tightly. Do not touch the test areas. Keep the test areas away from detergents, bleach, or other contaminating substances.

Stability

Each container of reagent strips is marked with a lot number and an expiration date. Do not use strips after the expiration date. Write the date opened on each container. Once the container is opened, use strips within 6 months. Watch test areas for possible deterioration by comparing the color of the dry reagent with the color of a negative test block on the color chart. If deterioration is suspected, test the strip with a known control solution. Discard the entire bottle of strips if any reagent pads are discolored or when quality control is consistently out of range.

Timing

Read the results at the time stated by the manufacturer for each chemical test. This is absolutely necessary if results are to be semiquantitated. Different results will be seen for the same specimen at different times. An advantage of using an automated or semiautomated instrument to read reagent strips is that it controls the exact time at which all the chemical reactions are read.

Reading Results

Whenever results depend on a color comparison, individual interpretation is a possible source of error. Adequate light is essential in visual interpretation. Hold the strip next to the most closely matched color block for each chemical test (see Fig. 13.26). Be sure to follow the manufacturer's instructions to orient the reagent strip correctly to the color chart when reading results. The use of automated or semiautomated instruments will eliminate individual differences in color interpretation and improve the reproducibility of results. Report results in a consistent manner as established for your institution.

Although multiple-reagent strips were developed to be read visually, several instruments have been developed to measure electronically the intensity of the color reactions produced on the reagent strips. These reflectance photometers measure the intensity of light produced by the chemical reaction between the analyte in question and the chemicals impregnated on each test portion of the reagent strip. The intensity of light produced is proportional to the amount of analyte in the specimen being tested. Actual instruments vary in the way the strips are inserted into the instrument, the degree of automation, and the manner in which patient specimens are identified and results are displayed or printed. The advantages of semiautomated and automated systems include more reproducible readings and printed results that decrease the incidence of transcription (clerical) errors. Results can also be interfaced with the laboratory computer system to further minimize clerical errors and save time in reporting results.

Controls

Several commercial control products are readily available either lyophilized or as a liquid. Manufacturers' directions for reconstitution and use should be followed. Generally, a negative control and a positive control should be used to test every parameter of the reagent strip in use. Reagent strips should be tested at least once each day or shift that the test is performed and whenever a new bottle of reagent strips is opened. Acceptable results are generally within one color block of the assigned target, as stated by the manufacturer. The only acceptable result for a negative control solution is negative. CLSI emphasizes that quality control should adhere to all local, state, and federal regulation as well as the manufacturer's instructions.

pH

One function of the kidney is to regulate the acidity of the extracellular fluid. Some information about this function, as well as other information, may be obtained by testing the urinary pH.

The pH is the unit that describes the acidity or alkalinity of a solution. In ordinary terms, *acidity* refers to the "sourness" of a solution, whereas *alkalinity* refers to its "bitterness." Lemon juice is an example of a sour, or acidic, solution; baking soda (sodium bicarbonate) is a bitter, or alkaline, substance in solution. In chemical terms, acidity refers to the hydronium ion (H_3O^+) concentration of a solution, and alkalinity refers to its hydroxyl ion (OH^-) concentration. These concentrations are usually expressed in terms of pH.

All solutions can be placed somewhere on a scale of pH values from 0 to 14. Some solutions, however, are neither acidic nor basic. These solutions are neutral and are placed at 7 on the pH scale. Water is an example of a neutral solution; its pH is 7. Water is neutral because the concentration of hydronium ions is equal to the concentration of hydroxyl ions.

A solution with more hydronium ions than hydroxyl ions is an acidic solution. On the pH scale, an acidic solution has a value ranging from 0 to 7. The farther it is from 7, the greater the acidity. For example, solutions of pH 2 and pH 5 are both acidic, but a solution of pH 2 is more acidic than a solution of pH 5. In simpler terms, a solution of pH 2 is more "sour" than a solution with a higher pH value. For example, lemon juice has a pH of about 2.3, whereas orange juice has a pH of about 3.5.

An alkaline solution has a pH value greater than 7. It can be any value from 7 to 14; the farther it is from 7, the greater the alkalinity, or the more "bitter" the solution.

Clinical Importance

Regulation of the pH of the extracellular fluid is an extremely important function of the kidney. Normally, the pH of blood is about 7.4 and varies no more than 0.05 pH unit. If the blood pH is 6.8 to 7.3, marked acidosis will be seen clinically; if it is 7.5 to 7.8, marked alkalosis will be observed. A pH of less than 6.8 or greater than 7.8 will result in death. The carbon dioxide produced in normal metabolism results in a tremendous amount of acid, which must be eliminated from the blood and extracellular fluid, or death will result. This acid is normally eliminated from the body by the lungs and the kidneys.

Because the kidney is generally working to eliminate excess acid, the pH of urine is normally between 5 and 7, with a mean of 6. The kidney is capable of producing urine ranging in pH from 4.6 to 8. The urine is normally acidified through an exchange of hydrogen ions for sodium ions in the distal convoluted tubules. In renal tubular acidosis, this exchange and the ability to form ammonia are impaired, resulting in a relatively alkaline urine. Certain metabolic acid–base disturbances may also be reflected in measurements of urinary pH as the kidney attempts to compensate for changes in blood pH. Such acid–base disturbances are classified as *metabolic* or *respiratory* acidosis and alkalosis, and measurements of titratable acidity, ammonium ion, and bicarbonate concentration are used in these distinctions.

Although the kidney is essential in controlling the pH of blood and extracellular fluid, measurements of urinary pH are not necessarily used to obtain information about this role. The routine urinalysis includes a measurement of urinary pH for the following reasons:

1. Freshly voided urine usually has a pH of 5 or 6. However, on standing at room temperature, urea is converted to ammonia

by bacterial action. The production of ammonia raises the hydroxyl ion concentration, resulting in an alkaline urine specimen. Therefore unless it is known that a urine specimen is fresh, an alkaline pH probably indicates an old urine specimen.

2. Alkalinity of freshly voided urine, especially if persistent throughout the day, may indicate a urinary tract infection (UTI). Other urinalysis findings in infection include positive reagent strip tests for nitrite and leukocyte esterase and large numbers of bacteria and possibly white blood cells (WBCs; neutrophils) in the urine sediment.
3. The urinary pH helps in the identification of crystals of certain chemical compounds that are often seen in the urine sediment. Certain crystals are associated with acid urine, pH less than 7, and others with alkaline urine, pH 7 and greater. Knowledge of the urine pH is important in the identification of crystals and may be the major reason for testing the pH of a urine specimen.
4. If the urine specimen is dilute and alkaline, various formed elements, such as casts and RBCs, will rapidly dissolve.
5. Persistently acidic urine may be seen in a variety of metabolic disorders, especially diabetic acidosis resulting from an accumulation of ketone bodies in the blood.
6. Persistently alkaline urine may be seen in some infections, in metabolic disorders, and with the administration of certain drugs.
7. It is sometimes necessary to control the urinary pH in the management of kidney infections, in patients with renal calculi (stones), and during the administration of certain drugs. This is done by regulating the diet; meat diets generally result in acidic urine and vegetable diets in alkaline urine.

Reagent Strip Tests for pH

Principle. Reagent strip tests use a methyl red and bromthymol blue double-indicator system that measures urine pH in a range from 5 to 9. They are available as multiple-reagent strips in combination with other tests for urine constituents. The methyl red is used to indicate a pH change from 4.4 to 6.2, with a color change from red to yellow. Bromthymol blue indicates a pH change from 6 to 7.6, as seen by a color change from yellow to blue.

Interferences. No interferences are known. The pH value is not affected by the buffer concentration of the urine.

Additional Comments. The specimen must be tested when fresh because bacterial growth may result in a significant shift to an alkaline pH, giving falsely alkaline values. Be careful not to wet the reagent strip excessively so that the acid buffer from the protein area runs into the pH area, causing an orange discoloration.

Protein

Clinical Importance

In the detection and diagnosis of renal disease, probably the most significant finding involves urinary protein. The presence of protein, when correlated with certain chemical tests, especially tests for blood, nitrite, and leukocyte esterase, and findings in the microscopic analysis of the urine sediment, is part of the eventual diagnosis.

The occurrence of protein in the urine is termed *proteinuria*. Proteinuria is an abnormal condition, probably the most important pathologic condition found in a routine urinalysis. In general, proteinuria may result from the following:

1. Glomerular damage
2. Tubular damage
3. Prerenal disorders or overflow from excessive production of low-molecular-weight proteins such as hemoglobin, myoglobin, or immunoglobulins
4. Lower urinary tract disorders
5. Asymptomatic disorders

Proteinuria may be classified as to the amount (quantity) or degree of protein excreted per day (24 hours), as follows:

Amount of Proteinuria	Grams of Protein Excreted Daily
Mild (minimal)	<1 g/day
Moderate	1–3 or 4 g/day
Large (heavy)	>3 or 4 g/day

Note that the amount of protein per 100 mL in a random urine specimen is related to 24-hour urine volume. Thus heavy proteinuria, with 3 g of protein eliminated daily and a 24-hour urine volume of 1500 mL, would correspond to 200 mg protein/dL in a random urine specimen. If the 24-hour urine volume were 500 mL, there might be 600 mg protein/dL.

Normally, the glomerular filtrate, the initial stage in the formation of urine, is an ultrafiltrate of blood plasma without cells, larger protein molecules, or certain fatty substances. Normal urine contains less than 10 mg/dL of protein as albumin. This is not detectable by normal tests for urinary protein. The normal glomerular membrane allows the passage of proteins with molecular weights of 50,000 to 60,000 D or less. Albumin has a molecular weight of about 67,000 D. This is a fairly small molecule, and some albumin is normally filtered through the glomerulus. However, this is normally reabsorbed in the convoluted tubules. Therefore proteinuria (measurable amounts of protein in urine) may be the result of increased permeability of the glomerulus or decreased reabsorption by the renal tubules.

Tamm–Horsfall protein is a high-molecular-weight glycoprotein (mucoprotein) that is normally secreted by renal tubular epithelial cells. It is a product of the kidney and is not present in the blood plasma. This is the protein that forms the basic matrix of most urinary casts. Casts are an important pathologic urinary finding and are associated with proteinuria. The occurrence of casts with proteinuria distinguishes an upper urinary tract (kidney) disorder from a disorder of the lower urinary tract (bladder).

The implications of protein in the urine in association with renal disease are extremely serious, and prompt diagnosis and treatment are vitally important. In addition, the loss of protein from the blood plasma will result in severe water balance problems because the osmotic pressure of the blood is largely dependent on the concentration of plasma proteins. This is readily seen in the edema often associated with kidney disorders.

Although proteinuria is indicative of renal disease, additional tests are needed for the final diagnosis. These include observations of the urine sediment (especially for the presence and types of casts), a determination of the amount of protein excreted daily by quantitative tests, the type of protein by electrophoresis, and the patient's clinical history.

Glomerular Damage

Proteinuria (generally albuminuria) is a consistent finding in glomerular disease. If the glomerular membrane is damaged, larger protein molecules find their way into the glomerular filtrate and are detected in the urine. This increased glomerular permeability usually begins with the passage of the smaller albumin molecules, and the larger globulin molecules remain in the blood plasma.

A variety of causes, including toxins, infections, vascular disorders, and immunologic reactions, may result in glomerular damage and increased filtration with proteinuria. Poststreptococcal acute glomerulonephritis is an example of glomerular proteinuria. This is an immunologic sequela of a bacterial infection, usually a throat infection caused by group A β-hemolytic streptococcus. Urinalysis findings include proteinuria, hematuria (RBCs), and casts (RBC, blood, or granular).

Early in cases of glomerular damage, only the small protein molecules (albumin) are filtered through the glomerulus. As the glomerular damage progresses, virtually all proteins present in the plasma find their way into the urine. Albumin is responsible for the osmotic pressure. Decreased amounts result in generalized swelling or edema throughout the body. In the nephrotic syndrome, heavy (massive) proteinuria (3 or 4 g/day) is seen. So much protein is lost from the body through the urine that the ability of the liver to synthesize sufficient albumin to maintain the normal blood albumin is lost, and hypoalbuminemia results. In addition to massive proteinuria, the nephrotic syndrome is associated with the presence of free fat, tubular epithelial cells containing fat (oval fat bodies [OFBs]), and fatty casts in the urine sediment.

Tubular Damage

A very small amount of protein (albumin) does find its way into the glomerular filtrate. In normal situations, all this protein is reabsorbed back into the blood through the renal convoluted tubules. Although the concentration of protein that normally filters into the glomerular filtrate is extremely small, and only 1 in 180 parts of the glomerular filtrate is eliminated from the body as urine (the rest is reabsorbed), failure to reabsorb any protein from this large volume of glomerular filtrate will result in fairly large amounts of protein in the urine. In other words, another cause of proteinuria is decreased reabsorption of protein by the renal tubular cells. The amount of proteinuria in tubular damage is generally mild to moderate. Examples of tubular proteinuria include pyelonephritis, acute tubular necrosis, polycystic kidney disease, heavy metal and vitamin D intoxication, phenacetin damage, hypokalemia, Wilson disease, galactosemia, Fanconi syndrome, and posttransplantation syndrome.

Acute pyelonephritis is an infection of the pelvis and parenchyma of the kidney. It is usually the result of infection ascending from the lower urinary tract into the kidney. In addition to moderate proteinuria, urinalysis findings may include nitrite, leukocyte esterase, WBCs (neutrophils), and casts (WBC, cellular, granular, or bacterial). The presence of casts in the urine locates the infection in the kidney.

Drug-induced acute interstitial nephritis (an allergic response) is also associated with moderate proteinuria. The presence of eosinophils is especially characteristic, together with neutrophils, RBCs, and cellular or granular casts.

Only mild proteinuria may be seen with acute renal failure or acute tubular necrosis. However, the sediment may contain renal tubular epithelial cells and casts (epithelial, granular, or waxy).

Prerenal Disorders

Prerenal or overflow disorders may result in proteinuria from disorders in body sites other than the kidney. Overflow from excessive production of low-molecular-weight proteins such as hemoglobin, myoglobin, or immunoglobulins may result in such proteinuria. The presence of light-chain immunoglobulins (Bence Jones protein) associated with multiple myeloma is an example.

Prerenal proteinuria may also be the result of a change in hydrostatic pressure in the kidney glomerulus. Increased blood pressure may force more proteins than normal through the glomerulus, resulting in the mild proteinuria seen with hypertension, congestive heart failure, and dehydration.

Lower Urinary Tract Disorders

Infections of the lower urinary tract may result in a mild proteinuria. The proteinuria may result from infection of the ureters or bladder with exudation through the mucosa (lining). Other urinalysis findings include positive chemical tests for nitrite (depending on the infecting organism) and leukocyte esterase, and the presence of WBCs and bacteria in the sediment. Casts are not present in lower UTIs; casts originate in the kidney.

Asymptomatic Proteinuria

In certain situations, small amounts of urinary protein may occur transiently in normal persons. In particular, urinary protein may be found in young adults after excessive exercise; after exposure to cold; or in orthostatic proteinuria, which occurs in those engaged in normal activity and disappears when they lie down.

In general, the proteinuria associated with renal disease is consistent, whereas that found in normal persons is transient. The long-term significance of asymptomatic proteinuria is unclear. To determine the cause of the proteinuria, it is often necessary to determine quantitatively the amount of protein in a 24-hour urine collection. Tests for orthostatic proteinuria are made on urine collections obtained both when the patient is at rest (first morning, collected immediately after rising) and after the patient has been walking and standing, but not sitting, for about 2 hours.

Consistent Microalbuminuria

Although screening tests for proteinuria should not be so sensitive that they detect the very small amount of protein that may be normally present in urine, it is sometimes desirable to detect the consistent passage of very small amounts of protein (microproteinuria). This is especially true of patients with diabetes mellitus. In these patients, it is thought that the early development of renal complications can be predicted by the early detection of consistent microalbuminuria. This early detection is desirable because better control of blood glucose levels may delay the progression of renal disease. The methodology for the detection of microalbuminuria includes nephelometry, radial immunodiffusion, and radioimmunoassay. With Chemstrip Micral Urine Test Strips (Roche Diagnostics) for microalbumin, albumin present in the patient's urine binds specifically with a soluble antibody-gold conjugate present on a zone of the test strip. This test strip is useful in monitoring the progression of nephropathy in diabetic patients once it has been diagnosed, but it is not suitable as a diagnostic test.

Reagent Strip Tests for Protein

Principle. Reagent strip tests for urinary protein involve the use of pH indicators, substances that have characteristic colors at specific pH values. At a fixed pH, certain pH indicators will show one color in the presence of protein and another color in its absence. This phenomenon is referred to as the "protein error of indicators." The pH of the urine is held constant by means of a buffer, so any change of color of the indicator will indicate the presence of protein.

Specificity. The reagent strip tests for urinary protein are more sensitive to albumin than to other proteins such as globulin, hemoglobin, Bence Jones protein, and mucoprotein. If these proteins are present in the urine without albumin, false-negative results may be obtained. In other words, a negative reagent strip does not rule out the presence of protein. Therefore depending on the patient population, it may be necessary for a given laboratory to test all urine specimens with both a reagent strip and a precipitation method for urinary protein so as not to miss certain abnormal proteins, such as those seen in new, undiagnosed cases of multiple myeloma.

Sensitivity (Minimum Detectable Level): Manufacturer's Values for Urinary Protein.

Multistix/Albustix	15–30 mg/dL albumin
Micro-Bumintest	4–8 mg/dL albumin
Chemstrip	6 mg/dL albumin (in 90% tested)

Interferences. If the urine is strongly pigmented, there may be interference with the color reaction. Bilirubin or drugs that give a vivid orange color, such as phenazopyridine (Pyridium) and other azo-containing compounds, may result in this interference.

False-Positive Results.

- If the urine is exposed to the reagent strip for too long, the buffer may be washed out of the strip, resulting in the formation of a blue color whether protein is present or not.
- If a urine specimen is exceptionally alkaline or highly buffered, the reagent strip tests may give a positive result in the absence of protein.
- Contamination of the urine container with residues of disinfectants containing quaternary ammonium compounds or chlorhexidine may show a positive result because of increased alkalinity.
- Chemstrip products may give false-positive results during therapy with phenazopyridine and when infusions of polyvinylpyrrolidone (blood substitutes) are administered.

False-Negative Results. When proteins other than albumin are present, the reagent strip will give a negative result in the presence of protein.

Additional Comments. The reagent strip tests for protein are not affected by turbidity, radiographic contrast media, most drugs and their metabolites, or urine preservatives, which occasionally affect other protein tests.

The color must be matched closely with the color chart when results are being read. The protein portion of the reagent strip is difficult to interpret, especially at the trace level. When results are in doubt, the slightly more sensitive SSA protein test or a test for microalbuminuria such as Micro-Bumintest (Bayer) might be helpful.

Blood (Hemoglobin and Myoglobin)

Clinical Significance

Together with tests for protein and the microscopic analysis of the urine sediment, tests for blood in the urine are used as indicators of the state of the kidney and urinary tract. Chemical tests for blood in urine react with RBCs, hemoglobin, and myoglobin (muscle hemoglobin). Although the chemical tests are more sensitive to the presence of hemoglobin and myoglobin than to intact RBCs, most positive reactions are actually caused by the presence of RBCs (erythrocytes). Blood may represent bleeding at any point from the glomerulus to the urethra, and the actual location is important to the diagnosis and treatment of the patient. Although the chemical detection of blood in urine is a serious finding, the presence of a few RBCs in urine is normal, and hematuria may be associated with benign conditions.

It is clinically significant to differentiate between RBCs and hemoglobin in the urine. Because tests for hemoglobin are positive in the presence of both free hemoglobin and erythrocytes, it would seem that this differentiation is made mainly by the finding of RBCs in the microscopic analysis of the urine sediment. The presence of hemoglobin and the absence of RBCs in the urine does not necessarily mean that the hemoglobin was originally free urinary hemoglobin. RBCs rapidly lyse in urine, especially when the specific gravity is low (<1.010). Therefore urine should be fresh when examined for the presence of RBCs.

Hematuria

Hematuria is the presence of RBCs in the urine. It results from many conditions, including lesions of the kidney and bleeding at any other point in the urinary tract. It may be an early sign of kidney or bladder tumor (benign or malignant) or may result from stone formation in the kidney or bladder. Hematuria may be a sign of glomerular damage or interstitial nephritis (infection of the kidney) or may be seen with a lower UTI such as cystitis (bladder infection). Generalized bleeding disorders or anticoagulant therapy may also result in hematuria.

Hematuria is a sensitive early indicator of renal disease and should not be missed. Although blood will not be present in every voided specimen in every patient with renal disease, occult blood (blood that is not grossly visible but is found by laboratory tests) may be present in almost every renal disorder. There may be little correlation between the amount of blood and the severity of the disorder, but its presence may be the only indication of renal disease. Hematuria is associated with glomerular damage and is typically seen in glomerulonephritis. Other laboratory findings besides hematuria indicate the presence of renal disease. Protein is usually present along with blood, and the presence of casts (especially RBC casts) and dysmorphic RBCs in the urine sediment is particularly useful.

Hemoglobinuria

Hemoglobinuria, or the presence of free hemoglobin in the urine, results from a variety of conditions and disease states. It may be the result of hemolysis in the bloodstream (intravascular hemolysis), in the kidney or lower urinary tract, or in the urine sample itself. The detection of intravascular hemolysis is important because the passage of free hemoglobin through the glomerulus and subsequent uptake by renal proximal convoluted epithelial cells are damaging to the nephron. Hemoglobin is carried in the bloodstream bound to a protein, haptoglobin. This hemoglobin–haptoglobin complex is a large molecule that is not filtered through the glomerulus. However, there is a limited amount of haptoglobin in the blood, and once it is saturated, the excess hemoglobin is filtered through the glomerulus into the renal tubules. Some of the excreted hemoglobin is absorbed into the renal tubular cells, converted to ferritin and hemosiderin, and subsequently excreted several days after an acute hemolytic episode. These hemosiderin- containing cells and granules may be observed in the urine sediment, especially when stained with Prussian blue.

Hematologic disease states resulting in hemoglobinuria include hemolytic anemias, hemolytic transfusion reactions, paroxysmal nocturnal hemoglobinuria, paroxysmal cold hemoglobinuria, and favism. Severe infectious diseases such as yellow fever, *Bartonella* infection, and malaria also result in hemoglobinuria, as do poisonings with strong acids or mushrooms, severe burns, and renal infarction. Finally, significant amounts of free hemoglobin occur whenever excessive numbers of RBCs are present as a result of various renal disorders, infectious or neoplastic diseases, or trauma in any part of the urinary tract.

Myoglobinuria

Myoglobinuria is the presence of myoglobin in the urine; it is a rare finding. Chemical tests for occult blood are equally sensitive to the presence of hemoglobin and myoglobin. Myoglobin is released after rhabdomyolysis, acute destruction of muscle fibers. Myoglobinuria may result from traumatic muscle injury such as occurs in motor vehicle crashes, excessive unaccustomed exercise, and beating or other crush injury. It is also seen in certain infections, after exposure to toxic substances and drugs, and in rare hereditary disorders.

The detection of myoglobinuria is important because myoglobin is rapidly cleared from the blood and excreted into the urine as a red-brown pigment. Large amounts of myoglobin are damaging to the kidney and may result in anuria. It seems that myoglobin is more damaging than hemoglobin to the kidney.

Differentiation of Hematuria, Hemoglobinuria, and Myoglobinuria

The differentiation of these conditions may be difficult. It is done with a combination of gross observations of urine and serum (or plasma) and certain chemical tests (Table 13.5). The occurrence of blood in urine will result in coloration ranging from normal to smoky, pink, amber, red to red-brown, brown, or frankly bloody. In general, with hemoglobin and myoglobin, the urine specimen is brown or red-brown. Although the presence of RBCs would result in cloudiness, and hemoglobin or myoglobin by itself would leave a clear specimen, other constituents often accompany all three entities, leading to cloudiness of the specimen. A gross observation of the serum or plasma accompanying these specimens is useful. If the urine contains only RBCs, the serum would have a normal color. If intravascular hemolysis has occurred, the serum would appear to be hemolyzed (red). If rhabdomyolysis occurs, the myoglobin released into the blood is rapidly cleared into the urine, and the serum appears normal in color.

In all three cases, the reagent strip test for blood is positive. If present, RBCs should be detectable in the microscopic examination of the urine sediment. With both hemoglobin and myoglobin, RBCs would be absent, or very few would be present. In the case of rhabdomyolysis resulting in myoglobinemia and myoglobinuria, greatly elevated serum creatine kinase (CK) is typical because of the destruction of muscle. CK levels are not affected as greatly by hemolysis. Unfortunately, myoglobin-induced renal failure may not be seen clinically until a week or more after the clinical event, and by then myoglobin is no longer present in the urine.

TABLE 13.5 Differentiation of Red Blood Cells, Hemoglobin, and Myoglobin in Urine

Finding	Red Cells	Hemoglobin	Myoglobin
Reagent strip for blood	Positive	Positive	Positive
Urine sediment for red cells	Present	Absent (few)	Absent (few)
Urine appearance	Cloudy red	Clear red	Clear red-brown
Plasma appearance	Normal	Pink to red (hemolysis)	Normal
Total serum creatine kinase (CK)	Normal	Slight elevation (10 times normal upper limit)	Marked elevation (40 times normal upper limit)
Total serum lactate dehydrogenase (LDH)	Normal	Elevated	Elevated
LDH_1 and LDH_2	Normal	Elevated	Normal
LDH_4 and LDH_5	Normal	Normal	Elevated

Modified from Ringsrud KM, Linné JJ: *Urinalysis and body fluids: a color text and atlas,* St Louis, 1995, Mosby.

Reagents Strip Tests for Blood

Principle and Specificity. Reagent strip tests for blood (hemoglobin, myoglobin) in urine make use of the peroxidase activity of the heme portion of the hemoglobin molecule. The reagent strips are impregnated with an organic peroxide, together with the reduced form of a chromogen. A positive reaction is seen when the peroxidase activity of the heme portion of the hemoglobin or myoglobin molecule catalyzes the release of oxygen from peroxide on the reagent strip. The released oxygen reacts with the reduced form of a chromogen, forming an oxidized chromogen, which is indicated by a color change. This reaction is summarized as follows:

Peroxide	Heme	Water
+	$\longrightarrow$	+
Reduced chromogen	(Peroxide activity)	Oxidized chromogen

The reagent strips are equally sensitive to hemoglobin and myoglobin. Intact RBCs are hemolyzed when they come into contact with the reagent strip, and the released hemoglobin reacts as described. It is essential that well-mixed urine be tested for the presence of blood. This is especially important when only a few intact RBCs are present in the urine specimen. If intact RBCs are allowed to settle and the supernatant urine is tested, false-negative results will be obtained.

Sensitivity (Minimum Detectable Level): Manufacturer's Values for RBCs/Hemoglobin.

Multistix/Hemastix	0.015–0.062 mg/dL hemoglobin (equivalent to 5–20 intact RBCs/µL)
Chemstrip	5 RBCs/µL, or hemoglobin corresponding to 10 RBCs/µL in 90% of urine specimens tested

Interferences.

False-Positive Results.

- Strong oxidizing cleaning agents, such as hypochlorite bleach, because of oxidation of the chromogen in the absence of peroxidase
- Microbial peroxidase activity associated with UTI
- The presence of blood as a contaminant from menstruation (no clinical significance)

False-Negative or Delayed Results.

- Ascorbic acid in urine specimens containing more than 25 mg/dL—this is seen after ingestion of large doses of vitamin C or when ascorbic acid is included as a reducing agent in certain parenteral antibiotics, such as tetracycline. Both Multistix and Chemstrip reagent strips claim no interference at reasonable or normally encountered levels. Chemstrip products include a blood-iodate scavenger to reduce false-negative results. Multistix products containing diisopropylbenzene dihydroperoxide as the organic peroxide are less subject to interference with ascorbic acid.
- Testing the supernatant urine from centrifugation or settling when only a few intact RBCs are present—urine must be well mixed when tested.
- Elevated specific gravity (high salt concentration) or elevated protein may reduce the lysis or RBCs necessary for a reaction to occur.
- When formalin is used as a urinary preservative
- Treatment with captopril (antihypertensive)
- Extremely high nitrite levels (>10 mg/dL), seen (rarely) in severe UTIs

Additional Comments. The presence of ascorbic acid in urine is a potential problem in the reagent strip tests for blood, as in any reagent strip test that depends on the release of oxygen and subsequent oxidation of a chromogen. When present in sufficient quantity, the ascorbic acid (a strong reducing agent) reacts with the released hydrogen peroxide (rather than the chromogen), causing inhibited (negative) results or a delayed color reaction.

When the reagent strip test for blood is negative but RBCs are observed in the urine sediment, the presence of ascorbic acid should be suspected. This may be confirmed by testing the urine with a reagent strip for ascorbic acid or by the patient's clinical history.

Confirmatory Tests.

- Microscopic examination of the urine sediment
- Reagent strip test for ascorbic acid if the test for blood is negative and RBCs are seen in the urine sediment or if blood is suspected on the basis of the appearance of the urine specimen

Nitrite

Clinical Importance

Tests for the presence of nitrite in the urine have been included in the routine urinalysis as a rapid method of detecting UTI. Screening tests for nitrite are most useful when combined with tests for leukocyte esterase, another indicator of UTI. The presence of urinary nitrite indicates the existence of a UTI. It is especially useful in detecting asymptomatic infections. When certain bacteria are present in the urinary tract, they will convert nitrate, a normal constituent of urine, to nitrite, an abnormal constituent. Nitrate converters are generally Gram-negative bacteria, such as the common *Enterobacteriaceae.* Gram-positive organisms such as enterococci and yeast do not generally convert nitrate to nitrite. However, there must also be sufficient nitrate (primarily derived from vegetables in the diet) in the urine for conversion to nitrite to take place.

Urine must be retained (incubated) in the bladder for a sufficient period (generally 4 hours) for this reaction to take place. Thus a first morning urine collection is the specimen of choice in testing for nitrite. A specimen collected at least 4 hours after previous voiding is also acceptable. Unfortunately, a common complaint with UTI is frequent urination, making the collection of an adequate specimen difficult.

The early detection of UTI is important for the prevention of kidney damage. It is believed that most UTIs begin in the lower urinary tract as a result of fecal contamination. Most infections are caused by organisms normally present in the feces, such as *Escherichia coli.* The infection is introduced into the normally sterile urinary tract through the urethra and ascends to the bladder, ureters, and finally the kidney. The early detection and subsequent treatment of UTI are important in preventing infection of the kidney and subsequent renal failure. From this discussion, it should be apparent that because of anatomic differences, UTI is much more common in women than men.

Traditionally, UTIs are diagnosed through quantitative urine culture, in which the organism that causes the infection is cultured and identified (see Chapter 15). Nitrite tests are screening tests that aid quantitative urine cultures. The existence of UTIs is also suggested by other findings in the routine urinalysis. Microscopic findings include the presence of WBCs and bacteria in lower UTIs; this plus the presence of casts, especially WBC or pus casts, indicates upper UTI (pyelonephritis). Chemical test results suggestive of UTI include the presence of leukocyte esterase and protein and a more alkaline urinary pH.

Reagent Strip Tests for Nitrite

Principle. Reagent strip tests for nitrite are based on the Griess test. This involves a diazo reaction. Nitrite will react with an aromatic amine (*p*-arsanilic or sulfanilic acid) in an acid medium to produce a diazonium salt. The diazonium salt is then coupled with another aromatic ring (quinoline) to give an azo dye, which is seen as a pink or red color.

Specificity. The Griess test is specific for nitrite.

Results. Results are reported as positive or negative. Any overall pink coloration is a positive reaction. Pink spots or pink edges are a negative reaction. The intensity of color formation does not necessarily indicate the degree of bacterial infection. Any pink coloration suggests a significant infection.

Sensitivity (Minimum Detectable Level)

Multistix	0.06–0.1 mg/dL nitrite ion
Chemstrip	As low as 0.05 mg/dL nitrite

Interferences

False-Positive Results

- Medications such as phenazopyridine or other azo-containing compounds or dyes that color urine red or that turn red in an acidic medium
- In vitro conversion of nitrate to nitrite as a result of bacterial contamination of the specimen; prevented by testing fresh urine specimens

False-Negative or Delayed Results

- Insufficient time in the bladder for the conversion of nitrate to nitrite, even with significant bacterial infection
- Insufficient dietary nitrate present for bacteria to reduce nitrate to nitrite, such as with starvation, fasting, or intravenous feeding
- Presence of bacteria that further reduce nitrite to nitrogen
- Sensitivity may be reduced in concentrated urine with low pH (<6). This is not typically seen with bacterial infection.
- Ascorbic acid in a concentration of 25 mg/dL or greater in specimens with small amounts of nitrite, resulting from the reduction of the diazonium salt by ascorbic acid

Additional Comments. The nitrite test is primarily useful if positive. If the nitrite test area shows a negative reaction, UTI cannot be ruled out. Organisms must contain the reductase enzyme necessary to reduce nitrate to nitrite. This is true of most of the Gram-negative enteric pathogens that cause UTIs. The Gram-positive enterococci and yeast, however, do not contain this enzyme. The urine must be retained in the bladder for 4 hours or more for adequate conversion of nitrate to detectable nitrite. Obtaining such specimens may be difficult because urgency and frequent urination are common in patients with UTIs. Thus lack of sufficient incubation time is a major obstacle to positive reagent strip results with significant infection.

Confirmatory Tests. Microscopic examination of the urine sediment, Gram stain, and quantitative urine culture can be used to confirm the nitrite test.

Leukocyte Esterase

Clinical Importance

Chemical tests for leukocyte esterase have been included on the urine reagent strip tests as another means of detecting UTI. Increased leukocyte esterase may be seen in conditions in which bacteria are not seen in the urine sediment or cultured. These include inflammatory conditions that may occur without bacterial infection, bacterial infection after treatment with antibiotics, and infections by organisms such as trichomonads and chlamydia, which are not seen on standard culture media.

These tests are based on the measurement of leukocyte esterase, which is present in azurophilic or primary granules of granulocytic leukocytes. These granulocytes include polymorphonuclear neutrophil (PMN) leukocytes, monocytes (histiocytes), eosinophils, and basophils. In practice, positive reactions occur with increased neutrophils. Conditions associated with sufficient quantities of other granulocytes to give positive reactions are extremely rare, if they ever occur. Lymphocytes and the various epithelial cells that make up the kidney and urinary tract do not contain leukocyte esterase and are not measured in this test.

The detection of leukocyte esterase as an indicator of infection is useful because neutrophils are generally increased in response to bacterial infection. When bacteria infect the urinary tract at any point from the urethra to the kidney, the number of WBCs, particularly neutrophils, is typically increased. Neutrophils are also seen in the urine sediment. However, a frequent problem is the rapid lysis of neutrophils in urine, a result of their phagocytic activity. Once lysed, they are not detectable in the microscopic analysis of the sediment. However, the test for leukocyte esterase depends on its release from the azurophilic or primary granules of granulocytes. Thus the leukocyte esterase test is positive whether lysed or intact cells are present in the urine.

Urine normally contains a few (up to five) WBCs per high-power field (hpf) in the microscopic analysis of the urine sediment. This normal occurrence of WBCs is not sufficient to cause a positive reaction with the leukocyte esterase test. The reaction requires 5 to 15 leukocytes/hpf to give a positive reaction. Therefore the absence of leukocyte esterase does not rule out a UTI. However, the presence of leukocyte esterase is helpful, especially with an elevated (alkaline) urine pH and the chemical detection of nitrite in the urine, together with the presence of bacteria and WBCs in the urine sediment. The finding of nitrite-positive and leukocyte esterase–positive urine using chemical screening tests is helpful in detecting UTIs, especially in combination with the presence of bacteria and leukocytes in the urine sediment. Identification of the organism requires a urine culture for bacteria.

Negative or low results for leukocyte esterase may be seen in the urine of immunosuppressed patients who have a significant bacterial infection, because of the inability to produce adequate granulocytes.

Reagent Strip Tests for Leukocyte Esterase

Principle. Reagent strip tests for leukocyte esterase use a diazo reaction, similar to the reagent strip tests for nitrite. The test area contains an ester that is hydrolyzed by leukocyte esterase to form its alcohol (which contains an aromatic ring) and acid. The aromatic ring is then coupled with a diazonium salt present in the test area, to form an azo dye, which is seen as the formation of a purple color. Chemstrips use an indoxyl ester, and Multistix use a pyrrole amino acid ester.

Specificity. The reaction is specific for esterase that is present in granulocytic leukocytes, primarily neutrophils in urine.

Sensitivity (Minimum Detectable Level): Manufacturer's Values for Leukocyte Esterase

Multistix	5–15 cells/hpf in clinical urine
Chemstrip	10–25 cells/μL

Interferences. The presence of substances that color urine, such as azo-containing compounds, nitrofurantoin, riboflavin, and bilirubin, may make color interpretation difficult.

False-Positive Results. Strong oxidizing agents such as chlorine bleach and urinary preservatives such as formalin (formaldehyde) may cause false-positive results; preservatives should not be used.

False-Negative or Reduced Results.

- Drugs (antibiotics) such as cephalexin, cephalothin, tetracycline, and gentamicin
- Elevated glucose (>3 g/dL)
- High specific gravity
- Oxalic acid (metabolite of ascorbic acid)
- High levels of albumin (>500 mg/dL)

Additional Comments. The presence of repeated trace and positive values are clinically significant and indicate the need for further testing to determine the cause of the presence of neutrophils (granulocytes) in the urine (pyuria). Tests may include microscopic analysis of the urine sediment, Gram stain, and quantitative urine culture. The test is not affected by the presence of blood, bacteria, or epithelial cells. Results of leukocyte esterase testing are especially useful when combined with reagent strip tests for nitrite.

Glucose (Sugar)

Clinical Importance

Chemical screening tests for glucose (dextrose) are generally included in every routine urinalysis. Unlike the parameters previously discussed, these tests are used to diagnose and monitor a metabolic condition, rather than a renal or urinary tract condition. The occurrence of glucose in the urine indicates that the metabolic disorder diabetes mellitus should be suspected, although several other conditions result in glucosuria.

Any condition in which glucose is found in the urine is termed *glycosuria* (or *glucosuria*). Tests for glucosuria were among the earliest laboratory tests. The "taste test" was used by the Babylonians and the Egyptians to detect diabetes by tasting for the presence of sugar (sweet) in what would normally be a salty solution, and Hindu physicians noticed that "honey urine" attracted ants.

The occurrence of measurable glucose in the urine is not normal. The blood glucose concentration normally varies between 60 and 110 mg/dL, depending on the method of analysis. After a meal, it may increase to 120 to 160 mg/dL. Normally, all the glucose in the blood is filtered by the glomerulus and reabsorbed into the blood. However, if the blood glucose concentration becomes too high, usually greater than 180 to 200 mg/dL, the excess glucose will not be reabsorbed into the blood and will be eliminated from the body in the urine. Other factors that might result in glucosuria are reduced glomerular blood flow, reduced tubular reabsorption, and reduced urine flow.

The lowest blood glucose concentration that will result in glycosuria is termed the *renal threshold,* which varies somewhat from person to person. The most common condition in which the renal threshold for glucose is exceeded is diabetes mellitus. In simplified terms, diabetes mellitus is a deficiency in the production of or an inhibition in the action of the hormone insulin. Insulin has the effect of lowering the blood glucose concentration. As a result of the deficiency of insulin, the blood glucose concentration exceeds the renal threshold, and glucose is spilled over into the urine.

Diabetic patients have used tests for urine glucose to self-monitor the adequacy of insulin control. Although these urine tests have been replaced by home blood glucose testing for unstable diabetic patients, urine glucose testing is less expensive, is noninvasive, and remains useful for patients who do not have to make frequent insulin dose adjustments. Tests for diabetes mellitus include tests for blood glucose as well as for urinary glucose. Additional tests, such as those for glycated hemoglobin (Hb A_{1c}), may also be used to monitor diabetes mellitus.

Although diabetes mellitus is suspected in patients with glycosuria, the occurrence of glycosuria is not diagnostic; glycosuria has many other causes. For example, glycosuria may be observed after large amounts of sugar or foods containing sugar are eaten, during acute emotional strain when the liver liberates glucose for energy, and after exercise. Glycosuria may also be associated with pregnancy, certain types of meningitis, hypothyroidism, certain tumors of the adrenal medulla, and some brain injuries.

In addition, certain abnormal conditions are characterized by the presence in the urine of sugars other than glucose. These are generally reducing sugars, which require detection by methods other than those employed in the reagent strip tests that are specific for glucose. Galactosuria is the presence of the sugar galactose in the urine. It results from a metabolic error whereby the enzyme galactose-1-phosphate uridyltransferase is lacking, so galactose is not metabolized, resulting in increased galactose in the blood (galactosemia) and urine. This condition results in permanent physical and mental deterioration, which may be controlled by early detection and dietary restriction of galactose. Therefore urine from young pediatric patients should be screened with a nonspecific copper reduction test for reducing substances that will detect galactose and other reducing sugars in addition to glucose. State-required newborn metabolic screening tests for inherited disease often include a test for galactosemia.

Other reducing sugars, such as lactose, may be seen in the urine late in pregnancy or early lactation. Lactose intolerance in infancy and failure to gain weight may occur because of intestinal lactase deficiency, and lactosuria may be seen.

Reagent Strip Tests for Glucose Oxidase

Principle and Specificity. The reagent strip tests for urinary sugar are specific for glucose because they are based on the use of the enzyme, glucose oxidase. An *enzyme* may be described as a "biological catalyst," a substance that must be present before a chemical reaction will occur. As with most enzymes, glucose oxidase is absolutely specific. It will react only in the presence of glucose, and it will not react with any other substance.

Reagent strip tests for urine glucose are double-sequential enzyme reactions. Glucose oxidase will oxidize glucose to gluconic acid and at the same time reduce atmospheric oxygen to hydrogen peroxide. In the presence of the enzyme peroxidase, the hydrogen peroxide formed will oxidize the reduced form of a dye to the oxidized form, which is indicated by the color change of an oxidation-reduction indicator. This reaction is diagrammed as follows:

Step 1:

$$\text{Glucose (in urine)} + O_2 \text{ (from air)} \xrightarrow{\text{Glucose oxidase}} \text{Gluconic acid} + H_2O_2$$

Step 2:

$$H_2O_2 + \text{Reduced form of dye} \xrightarrow{\text{Peroxidase}} \text{Oxidized form of dye} + H_2O$$

The glucose oxidase, the peroxidase, and the reduced form of the oxidation-reduction indicator are all impregnated onto a dry reagent strip. Reagent strips differ in the chromogen used as the oxidation-reduction indicator. They all contain glucose oxidase and peroxidase.

Laboratory personnel must remember that nonglucose-reducing substances (NGRSs) will not be detected by tests that are specific for glucose. Therefore specimens from infants and young pediatric patients and specimens in which NGRSs are suspected should be subjected to nonspecific (usually copper reduction) tests for reducing substances in addition to the specific tests for glucose.

Sensitivity (Minimum Detectable Level): Manufacturer's Values for Glucose

Multistix/Diastix	75–125 mg/dL glucose (as low as 40 mg/dL in dilute urine containing less than 5 mg/dL ascorbic acid)
Chemstrip	40 mg/dL in 90% of urine specimens tested

Interferences. Because reagent strip tests are all specific for glucose, most interferences lead to reduced or false-negative results.

False-Positive Results

- Contamination by bleach or other strong oxidizing agents may oxidize the reduced form of the dye present on the reagent strip, causing a color change in the absence of glucose. This shows the importance of using contamination-free urine containers and work surfaces.
- Trace values may be seen in very dilute urine specimens because of increased sensitivity at low specific gravity.
- Reagent strips exposed to air by improper storage have been shown to give false-positive results.[4]

False-Negative or Delayed Results

- Large urinary concentrations of ascorbic acid from therapeutic doses of vitamin C or from drugs such as tetracyclines, in which ascorbic acid is used as a reducing agent. Ascorbic acid blocks or delays the reaction by acting as a reducing agent reacting with the released hydrogen peroxide (rather than the chromogen in the reagent strip). Multistix products are inhibited by ascorbic acid concentrations of 50 mg/dL (500 mg/L) or greater in specimens containing small amounts (75–125 mg/dL) of glucose. Chemstrip is unaffected by ascorbic acid concentration less than 100 mg/dL (1000 mg/L). With questionable ascorbic acid interference, repeat tests on urine voided at least 10 hours after the last administration of vitamin C, or test for ascorbic acid.
- Ketone bodies at moderate levels (>40 mg/dL) in specimens containing small amounts (75–12 mg/dL) of glucose. This combination of high ketone and low glucose is unlikely in a diabetic patient.
- Sodium fluoride is an enzyme inhibitor; do not use as a preservative.
- Refrigerated specimens, because of decreased enzyme activity—urine must be at room temperature when tested.

When the presence of a reducing sugar other than glucose such as galactose is suspected in the urine, a nonspecific test (Clinitest) should be performed. The Clinitest method is a traditional procedure for the detection of reducing carbohydrates. The method detects the presence of any reducing substance to reduce copper II (cupric) ions to copper I (cuprous) ions in the presence of heat and alkali. A positive reaction is semiquantitated as a change in color ranging from blue to green, yellow, and orange, depending on the amount of sugar in the urine. This reagent tablet test will detect as low as 250 mg/dL of sugar.

Ketone Bodies

Clinical Importance

Ketone bodies are a group of three related substances: acetone, acetoacetic (or diacetic) acid, and β-hydroxybutyric acid. Their structural similarity is illustrated in Fig. 13.4. The ketone bodies are normal products of fat metabolism and are not normally detectable in the blood or urine.

In fat catabolism (phase of metabolism in which fats are broken down for energy), acetoacetic acid is produced first. It is converted either reversibly to β-hydroxybutyric acid or irreversibly to acetone. All three types of ketone bodies are utilized as a source of energy and are eventually converted to carbon dioxide

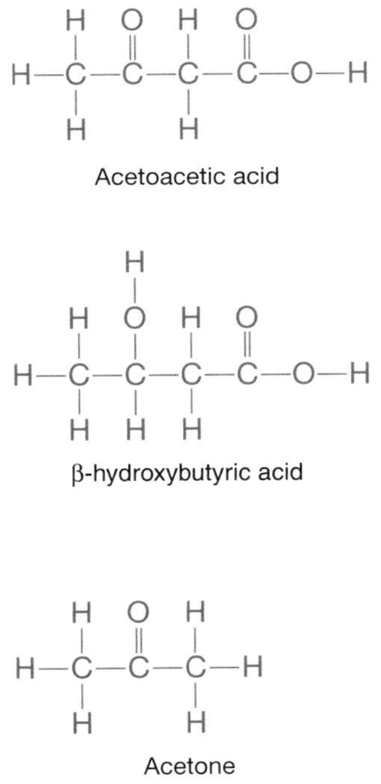

Acetoacetic acid

β-hydroxybutyric acid

Acetone

Fig. 13.4 Ketone bodies.

and water. When the body uses normal amounts of fat, the tissues are able to use the entire ketone production as an energy source. If more fat than normal is metabolized, however, the body is unable to use all the ketone bodies. The clinical result is an increased concentration of ketones in the blood (ketonemia) and urine (ketonuria). Ketosis is the combination of increased ketones in both the blood and the urine.

Whenever fat (rather than carbohydrate) is used as the major source of energy, ketosis and ketonuria may result. The two outstanding causes of ketone accumulation are diabetes mellitus and starvation. In diabetes mellitus the body is unable to use carbohydrate as an energy source and attempts to compensate by resorting to fat catabolism, which results in accumulation of the ketones. In starvation the body is depleted of stored carbohydrate and must resort to fat as an energy source. Similarly, ketosis is seen in patients with dehydration and conditions associated with fever, vomiting, and diarrhea. The same situation may occur in patients with severe liver damage. Most carbohydrate is stored as liver glycogen. In liver damage, there is no stored glycogen; thus the body must again resort to fat for energy. Also, a ketogenic diet will result in ketone accumulation. A ketogenic diet is high in fat and low in carbohydrates—specifically, a diet containing more than 1.5 g of fat per 1 g of carbohydrate. Low-carbohydrate diets used for weight reduction may be ketogenic diets.

Because the presence of ketone bodies in urine is an early indication of a lack of adequate insulin control, diabetic patients often use reagent strips that combine tests for glucose and ketones for home monitoring of their disease. The physiologic effect of ketone accumulation in the blood and urine (ketosis) is serious. Acetoacetic acid and β-hydroxybutyric acid contribute excess hydrogen ions to the blood, resulting in acidosis. Acidosis is an extremely serious condition and results in death if allowed to continue. Therefore the body attempts to compensate for excess acid in the blood by eliminating acid through the urine. The kidney is capable of producing urine with a pH as low as 4.5. Thus the occurrence of ketones in the urine is associated with a low urinary pH. Before insulin was used in the treatment of diabetes mellitus, acidosis was the cause of death in two-thirds of all patients. In the treatment of diabetes mellitus, it is important to control the amount of insulin so that ketosis and acidosis do not occur. A typical urine specimen from a patient with uncontrolled diabetes is pale and greenish, contains a large amount of sugar, has a high specific gravity by refractometer, has a low pH, and contains ketone bodies.

When ketones accumulate in the blood and urine, they do not occur in equal concentrations. Of the ketones, 78% are present as β-hydroxybutyric acid, 20% as acetoacetic acid, and only 2% as acetone. However, the reagent strip tests for ketones are most sensitive to the presence of acetoacetic acid. No simple laboratory tests exist for β-hydroxybutyric acid.

Reagent Strip Tests for Ketone Bodies

Principle. The reagent strip tests for ketone bodies are based on the Legal (Rothera) test, a color reaction with sodium nitroprusside (nitroferricyanide). Acetoacetic acid will react with sodium nitroprusside in an alkaline medium to form a purple color. If glycine is added, the test is slightly sensitive to acetone. Multistix and Ketostix have been formulated to react only with acetoacetic acid. They do not react with acetone. The Chemstrip products include glycine and detect both acetoacetic acid and larger amounts of acetone. None of the reagent strips detect β-hydroxybutyric acid.

Acetest Tablet Test. The Acetest (Bayer Diagnostics) is a tablet test for acetone and acetoacetic acid, based on a color reaction with sodium nitroprusside. The principle is virtually identical to that of the reagent strip tests. In addition to urine, Acetest tablets can be used to test whole blood, plasma, or serum. This test may be useful in testing urine containing interfering colors.

Interferences. The presence of various pigments, drugs, or substances causing abnormal, highly colored urine specimens presents problems in the reading of ketone results. False-positive reactions may result from the formation of a color that may be interpreted as positive, or true-positive reactions may be masked in these urine specimens.

False-Positive Results

- Specimens containing phthaleins (bromsulphalein, phenolsulfonphthalein), very large amounts of phenylketones, or the preservative 8-hydroxyquinoline
- Highly concentrated urine specimens (high specific gravity) or specimens containing large amounts of levodopa metabolites may give weak positive reactions.
- 2-Mercaptoethanesulfonic acid (mesna) or other compounds containing sulfhydryl groups—a positive reaction is seen initially, but the color fades to normal by the time specified for reading the color reaction. This interference is especially problematic when automatic reagent strip readers are employed because these instruments are programmed to

read the various chemical reactions more quickly than with visual readings. If such interference is suspected, reagent strips should be checked visually and the visual result reported. If the color persists and interference is still suspected, a drop of glacial acetic acid may be added to the test area on the reagent strip or the Acetest tablet. If the color is caused by a sulfhydryl group, it will fade, whereas color caused by diacetic acid will remain.

False-Negative or Reduced Results. Conversion of acetoacetic acid to acetone, with subsequent evaporation from the specimen, in improperly stored specimens may cause false-negative results. Urine specimens must be tested when freshly voided or immediately refrigerated.

Additional Comments. When a patient is monitored with repeated determinations of acetone and acetoacetic acid in plasma or urine, the concentrations of these compounds may start at very high levels and fall but may still give results that correspond to "large" on the color chart. Repeated reports of "large" do not reflect the changes as they occur. In some cases it is desirable to dilute subsequent specimens to monitor and observe a decrease in ketone excretion. The urine specimen is diluted 1:2, 1:4, and so on, until a "large" value is no longer seen. The report in such cases should state at what dilution a "large" value is no longer obtained such as large, 1:4 dilution moderate.

Bilirubin and Urobilinogen

As mentioned earlier, the routine urinalysis provides information on the function and disorders of the kidney and urinary tract, as well as other metabolic or systemic disorders. Tests for urine bilirubin and urobilinogen are used as indicators of liver function.

Normal Liver Function

The liver is a large and complex organ necessary for numerous body functions; it is responsible for metabolic, storage, excretory, and detoxifying processes. More specifically, the liver is a major factor in the metabolism of carbohydrates, lipids, and proteins, in terms of both intermediary metabolism and the synthesis of many essential compounds. Many enzymes and coenzymes needed for carbohydrate, lipid, and protein metabolism are present only in liver cells. Glycogen is formed, stored, and converted back to glucose in the liver. Energy derived from food is made available to the cells of the body through glycolysis of the high-energy bonds in adenosine triphosphate, which are formed by oxidative phosphorylation in the liver cells.

The liver is the site of detoxification of various substances. These toxic substances may be formed in normal body metabolism and converted or detoxified by the liver; an example is the formation of urea from the ammonia produced in protein metabolism. Toxic substances introduced into the blood from the intestine, such as dyes, heavy metals, or drugs, are excreted by the liver. The liver is essential in the formation and secretion of bile, bile pigments, and bile salts, which are necessary for digestion. These substances are derived from bilirubin, a major by-product of the destruction of RBCs. In addition, the liver is the site of formation and synthesis of many of the factors involved in the clotting of blood.

These important functions of the liver may be altered when the liver is diseased or damaged. Numerous laboratory tests are available to determine both the existence of liver disease and the extent, location, and type of damage so that appropriate treatment can be initiated. No one test will give a complete clinical view of liver function; instead, a carefully selected group of tests may be necessary, depending on the process in question. These include tests for the presence and concentration of bilirubin in the blood and the urine.

Normal Formation and Excretion of Bilirubin and Urobilinogen

Bilirubin is a normal product resulting from the breakdown of RBCs. Individual RBCs do not exist indefinitely in the body; they are degraded after approximately 120 days. As part of erythrocyte degradation, the heme portion of the hemoglobin molecule is converted to the bile pigment bilirubin by the mononuclear phagocytic system (MPS), primarily by MPS cells in the liver, spleen, and bone marrow. A total of approximately 6 g of hemoglobin is released each day as RBCs are eliminated from the body. The cells of the MPS initially phagocytose the RBCs, then convert the released hemoglobin through a complex series of reactions in which the heme portion of the molecule is finally converted to bilirubin.

Bilirubin is a vivid yellow pigment. An increase in the concentration of bilirubin in the blood indicates the presence of jaundice. Although it is useful in the bile, bilirubin is a waste product that must eventually be eliminated from the body. When formed by the MPS cells, bilirubin is not soluble in water. Therefore it is transported from the MPS cells through the blood to the liver cells linked to albumin as a bilirubin–albumin complex. This insoluble form of bilirubin is referred to as *free bilirubin* or *unconjugated bilirubin.*

Bilirubin is normally excreted from the body by the liver by way of the intestine. It is excreted by the liver rather than the kidney because the bilirubin–albumin complex cannot pass through the glomerular capsule of the kidney. When free bilirubin reaches the liver, it is made water soluble by conjugation with glucuronic acid and other hydrophilic substances to form bilirubin glucuronide.

The water-soluble bilirubin glucuronide, referred to as *conjugated bilirubin,* can be eliminated from the body by way of the kidney or the intestine. Normally, conjugated bilirubin is excreted by the liver into the bile and transported to the common bile duct and then to the gallbladder, where it is concentrated and emptied into the small intestine.

In the intestine, bilirubin is converted to **urobilinogen** by the action of certain bacteria that make up the intestinal flora. Urobilinogen is actually a group of colorless chromogens, all of which are referred to as *urobilinogen.* Part of the urobilinogen formed in the intestine is absorbed into the portal blood circulation and returned to the liver, where it is reexcreted into the bile and returned to the intestine. A very small amount of urobilinogen escapes this liver clearance and is therefore excreted from the body by way of the urine. This represents only about 1% of the urobilinogen produced in 1 day.

Part of the urobilinogen in the intestine is converted to stercobilinogen (colorless), which is oxidized to the colored stercobilin; this latter substance gives feces its normal color. The net effect is that, in normal circumstances, 99% of the urobilinogen formed from bilirubin is eliminated by way of the feces.

Urobilin (formerly known as *urochrome*) is a breakdown product of heme. Urobilin is produced when urobilinogen is oxidized by intestinal bacteria. Once urobilinogen is exposed to the environment on urination, it is oxidized to urobilin, which makes the urine appear dark in cases of common bile duct obstruction. Urobilin is a sensitive marker for biliary obstruction, as well as early acute hepatitis.

Urine normally contains only a very small amount of urobilinogen and no bilirubin. Unconjugated (albumin-bound) bilirubin cannot be excreted by the kidney and is absent in urine. However, conjugated bilirubin can pass through the renal glomerulus, and if it is present in an abnormal concentration in the blood, it will be excreted by the kidney.

Clinical Importance

Tests for urinary bilirubin and urobilinogen should be performed when indicated by the abnormal color of the urine or when liver disease or a hemolytic condition is suspected from the patient's history. Because these tests are part of most multiple-reagent strips, they are included in the routine urinalysis. The presence of bilirubin in the urine is an early sign of liver cell disease (hepatocellular disease) and of obstruction to the bile flow from the liver. It is especially useful in the early detection and monitoring of hepatitis, a highly infectious disease of particular importance to laboratory workers. The presence of urobilinogen in the urine is increased in any condition that causes an increase in the production of bilirubin glucuronide and any disease that prevents the liver from performing its normal function of returning urobilinogen to the intestine through the bile. Information about urinary bilirubin and urobilinogen, in addition to serum bilirubin levels, is useful in determining the cause of jaundice. (See also Chapter 10.)

Bilirubin

Clinical Significance. Tests for urinary bilirubin (along with urobilinogen) are important in the detection of liver disease and the determination of the cause of jaundice. Normally, there is no detectable bilirubin in the urine, even with the most sensitive methods. However, finding even very small amounts of bilirubin in urine is important because it may be present in the earliest phases of liver disease.

Jaundice is a condition that occurs when the serum bilirubin concentration becomes greater than normal and there is an abnormal accumulation of bilirubin in the body tissues. Bilirubin is a vivid yellow pigment, so its accumulation in the tissues results in yellow pigmentation of the skin, the sclera or white of the eyes, and the mucous membranes. The causes of jaundice are numerous and must be discovered as soon as possible so that treatment may be started. There are several classifications of jaundice; one describes three types: hemolytic (prehepatic), hepatic (hepatocellular), and obstructive (posthepatic). Table 13.6 summarizes laboratory findings in various types of jaundice.

Hemolytic (Prehepatic) Jaundice. Hemolytic jaundice, also known as *prehepatic jaundice,* occurs in conditions in which there is increased destruction of RBCs, such as hemolytic anemias and hemolytic disease of the newborn. The liver is basically normal, so there is an increased formation of conjugated bilirubin and subsequently of urobilinogen. Increased formation of urobilinogen from bilirubin results in increased levels of urobilinogen in the blood. The liver is overwhelmed by the increased production of bilirubin and urobilinogen and unable to excrete the urobilinogen back into the intestine. Therefore more urobilinogen is eliminated in the urine. However, all the bilirubin that is conjugated by the liver goes into the intestine, where it is converted to urobilinogen, and no bilirubin is found in the urine.

Hepatic (Hepatocellular) Jaundice. Hepatic jaundice, also called *hepatocellular jaundice,* results from conditions that involve the liver cells directly and prevent normal excretion of bilirubin. This type is probably the most varied and difficult jaundice to understand. Findings differ, depending on the disease or condition and the stage of disease, and include the following:

1. Failure to conjugate bilirubin, with increased concentration of free (albumin-bound) bilirubin in the blood
2. Failure to transport conjugated bilirubin into the bile canaliculi, with increased conjugated bilirubin backing up (regurgitating) into the blood and urine

TABLE 13.6 Laboratory Findings in Various Types of Jaundice

Type of Jaundice	Clinical Example	Blood Bilirubin (unconjugated)	Urine Bilirubin (conjugated)	Urine Urobilinogen	Color of Feces
Normal		0–1.3 mg/dL	Negative	<1 mg/dL	Normal, brown
Hemolytic (prehepatic)	Hemolytic anemia	Increased	Negative	Increased	Increased (dark brown)
	Hemolytic disease of the newborn				
Hepatic (hepatocellular)	Neonatal physiologic Hepatitis (viral, toxic) Cirrhosis	Increased (varies)	Increased (varies)	Increased or absent	Normal or pale
Obstructive (posthepatic)	Gallstones Tumor	Normal	Increased	None (decreased)	Pale, chalky white ("acholic")

Modified from Ringsrud KM, Linné JJ: *Urinalysis and body fluids: a color text and atlas,* St Louis, 1995, Mosby.

3. Failure of the liver to reexcrete the recirculated urobilinogen, with increased concentration of urobilinogen in the blood and the urine

Neonatal physiologic jaundice results when there is an enzyme deficiency in the immature liver and thus failure to conjugate bilirubin, resulting in increased unconjugated (free) bilirubin in the blood with no bilirubin in the urine.

Disturbances of the transport mechanisms by which conjugated bilirubin is passed into the bile canaliculi are characteristic of hepatocellular jaundice. In conditions such as viral hepatitis, toxic hepatitis (caused by heavy metal or drug poisoning), and cirrhosis, there is a diffuse overall hepatic cell involvement. In these cases, the bilirubin conjugated by the liver is not excreted into the bile; instead, conjugated bilirubin backs up into the blood and then can be eliminated by the kidney. Of the conjugated bilirubin that reaches the gut, urobilinogen is formed, part of which is absorbed into the portal circulation and returned to the liver for excretion. However, the diseased liver cells may be unable to remove the urobilinogen from the blood, resulting in excretion of urobilinogen into the urine. As the disease progresses to later stages, the liver is unable to form and pass conjugated bilirubin into the bile, so conjugated bilirubin regurgitates (backs up) into the blood and is eliminated from the body by way of the urine. Such patients would have little or no urobilinogen in the urine.

Obstructive (Posthepatic) Jaundice. Posthepatic jaundice, also known as *obstructive jaundice,* occurs when the common bile duct is obstructed by stones, tumors, spasms, or stricture. As a result, the conjugated bilirubin is regurgitated back into the liver sinusoids and the blood. If the blockage is sufficiently extensive, liver cell function may be impaired, and both free and conjugated bilirubin may be found in the blood. The conjugated bilirubin will be excreted by the kidney and therefore will be found in the urine. Conjugated bilirubin is unable to reach the intestine, so no urobilinogen is formed, and it is absent in the blood and urine. Because urobilinogen is not formed, urobilin is absent, and the stools have a characteristic chalky white to light-brown color, also referred to as *acholic.*

Reagent Strip Tests for Bilirubin

Principle. The reagent strip tests for bilirubin are based on a diazo reaction. Bilirubin is coupled with a diazonium salt in an acid medium to form azobilirubin. A positive reaction is seen as the formation of a colored compound. Tests differ in the diazonium salt used and thus the color produced.

Specificity. Tests are specific for bilirubin. However, the presence of other highly colored pigments in the urine causes problems in interpreting results. This is especially true when metabolites of drugs such as phenazopyridine are present. These metabolites give the gross urine specimen a characteristic vivid red-orange color that may be mistaken for bilirubin and may mask or give atypical color reactions on the reagent strip.

Sensitivity (Minimum Detectable Level): Manufacturer's Values for Bilirubin

Multistix	0.4–0.8 mg/dL
Chemstrip	0.5 mg/dL in 90% of urine specimens tested

Interferences. The reagent strip tests for bilirubin are difficult to read, and the color formed after reaction with urine must be carefully compared with the color chart supplied by the manufacturer. Proficiency in reading these results comes with experience and is essential for reliable results.

Atypical colors, which are unlike any of the color blocks, may indicate that other bile pigments derived from bilirubin are present in the urine and may be masking the bilirubin reaction. Testing the urine with a more sensitive test, such as the Ictotest tablet, may be indicated. Large amounts of urobilinogen may affect the color reaction but not enough to give a positive result.

False-Positive or Atypical Results

- Substances that color the urine red or that turn red in an acid medium, such as phenothiazine, chlorpromazine, and metabolites of phenazopyridine (Pyridium) or ethoxazene (Serenium)
- Metabolites of etodolac (Lodine)
- A yellow-orange to red color with indican (indoxyl sulfate)—indoles are formed from bacterial overgrowth in the gut or in surgically constructed urinary bladders made from intestine.

False-Negative or Decreased Results

- Oxidation of bilirubin to biliverdin, especially when exposed to ultraviolet light
- In vitro hydrolyzation of bilirubin diglucuronide to free bilirubin—tests are most sensitive to the conjugated form of bilirubin.
- Ascorbic acid in concentration of 25 mg/dL or more
- Elevated nitrite concentration, as seen in UTI, may decrease sensitivity.

Additional Comments. The presence of highly pigmented compounds may be mistaken for bilirubin in the gross urine specimen and may mask the reaction of small amounts of bilirubin. The Ictotest can be done when interpretation of the bilirubin pad on the chemical analysis strip is difficult or questionable to read.

Urine specimens must be tested when fresh, or bilirubin will oxidize to biliverdin. The test is specific for bilirubin; it will not react with biliverdin.

Urobilinogen and Porphobilinogen

Clinical Importance

Urobilinogen. Urobilinogens are normal by-products of erythrocyte degradation; they are formed from bilirubin by bacterial action in the intestine and are excreted in the feces as stercobilin. Increased destruction of RBCs may be accompanied by large amounts of urobilinogen in the urine. Urobilinogen is seen in the various hemolytic anemias, in pernicious anemia, and in the hemolytic phase of malaria. In the absence of increased erythrocyte destruction, the tests may be considered liver function tests. One of the first effects of liver damage is impairment of the mechanism for removing urobilinogen from the blood circulation and reexcreting it through the intestine. This results in removal of urobilinogen by the kidney and its presence in the urine. Tests for urinary urobilinogen are thus useful for the early detection of liver damage. Urobilinogen is found in the urine in conditions such as infectious hepatitis, toxic hepatitis, portal cirrhosis, congestive heart failure, and infectious mononucleosis.

Normally, 1% of all the urobilinogen produced is excreted in the urine, and 99% is excreted in the feces. Under certain conditions, however, urobilinogen is completely absent from the urine and the feces. When the normal intestinal bacterial flora is destroyed, as by antibiotic therapy, urobilinogen cannot be produced. Urobilinogen is also absent if the liver does not conjugate bilirubin, or if there is biliary tract obstruction, such as from gallstones, resulting in failure of conjugated bilirubin to reach the intestinal tract.

Porphobilinogen. Another substance that is related to urobilinogen is porphobilinogen. Porphobilinogen is a normal, colorless precursor of the porphyrins. The porphyrins are a group of compounds used in the synthesis of hemoglobin. The heme portion of hemoglobin is a type of porphyrin, namely, ferroprotoporphyrin-9. In normal persons, porphyrins are eliminated from the body in the urine and feces, mainly as coproporphyrin I, with a small amount of coproporphyrin III. However, certain errors of porphyrin metabolism lead to increased excretion of other porphyrins in the urine. These conditions are collectively called *porphyrias,* and in some porphyrias, porphobilinogen is present in the urine. *Porphobilinogenuria* is seen in acute attacks of acute intermittent porphyria, variegate porphyria, and hereditary coproporphyria. An acute attack may be precipitated by drugs affecting the liver, such as barbiturates, sulfa drugs, heavy metals, hydantoins, or hormones; by infection; and by diet. The discovery of porphobilinogen in urine is a critical value that can eliminate or reduce adverse effects from drugs or anesthetics.

Tests for urobilinogen that use the Ehrlich aldehyde reaction will detect urobilinogen and porphobilinogen, in addition to other Ehrlich-reactive compounds.

Reagent Strip Tests for Urobilinogen

Principle. The reagent strip tests for urobilinogen (unlike other reagent strip tests) differ in basic principle and specificity.

Multistix tests for urobilinogen are based on a modified Ehrlich aldehyde reaction. In this reaction, urobilinogen (also porphobilinogen and other Ehrlich-reactive compounds) reacts with *p*-dimethylaminobenzaldehyde in concentrated hydrochloric acid to form a colored (cherry-red) aldehyde. This is also the basis of the Watson–Schwartz test. An inverse Ehrlich aldehyde reaction is the basis of the Hoesch test, which is used for the detection of porphobilinogen in urine.

Chemstrip reagent strips employ a diazo reaction in which a diazonium salt reacts with urobilinogen in an acid medium to form a red azo dye.

Specificity. The Multistix reagent strips react with substances known to react with Ehrlich reagent. These substances include porphobilinogen and various intermediate Ehrlich-reactive substances, such as sulfonamides, *p*-aminosalicylic acid (PAS), procaine, and 5-hydroxyindoleacetic acid (HIAA). Therefore urine specimens that give a positive reaction with these reagent strips should be confirmed by using another method such as Chemstrip (specific for urobilinogen); Hoesch test for porphobilinogen; or Watson–Schwartz test for urobilinogen, porphobilinogen, and intermediate Ehrlich-reactive compounds.

The Chemstrip reagent strips react with urobilinogen and stercobilinogen. Differentiation between these two substances is not diagnostically important because stercobilinogen is found in feces, not urine. Porphobilinogen and other Ehrlich-reactive substances are not detected with some reagent strips. This is helpful because many interfering Ehrlich-reactive substances are often encountered in routine urinalysis. The existence of unsuspected or undiagnosed porphyria would be missed completely with this test.

Sensitivity (Minimum Detectable Level): Manufacturer's Values for Urobilinogen

Multistix	As low as 0.2 mg/dL
Chemstrip	Approximately 0.4 mg/dL

The absence of urobilinogen cannot be determined. Results of 1 mg/dL or less should be reported as normal, rather than negative. Normally, up to 1 mg/dL urobilinogen is present in urine.

Interferences. The presence of intermediate Ehrlich-reacting substances other than urobilinogen is a problem in any test based on the Ehrlich aldehyde reaction, such as Multistix. All strips are affected by highly colored pigments or their metabolites in the urine specimen. Strips based on the diazo reaction (Chemstrip) show interferences similar to reagent strip tests for bilirubin.

False-Positive Results.

- Intermediate Ehrlich-reacting substances, such as sulfonamides, PAS metabolites, procaine, and HIAA, will react in tests based on the Ehrlich aldehyde reaction (Multistix).
- Methyldopa (Aldomet) will give a strong color reaction with Ehrlich reagent.
- Highly colored pigments and their metabolites, including ethoxazene (Serenium), drugs containing azo dyes (such as phenazopyridine), nitrofurantoin, riboflavin, and *p*-aminobenzoic acid, may cause atypical or positive reactions with all reagent strips.
- Reactivity with Multistix increases with temperature and may give a false-positive reaction if the urine is tested at body temperature, because of a "warm aldehyde reaction." Test urine at room temperature (22–26°C).

False-Negative or Decreased Results

- Oxidation of urobilinogen (colorless) to urobilin, an orange-red pigment—the urine specimen should be tested as soon as possible after collection.
- Formalin as a preservative with all reagent strips
- Greater than 5 mg/dL nitrite with Chemstrip
- Although porphobilinogen may be detected with tests based on the Ehrlich aldehyde reaction, Multistix is not a reliable test for the detection of porphobilinogen.
- Tests based on a diazo reaction (Chemstrip) will not detect porphobilinogen in the urine.

Additional Comments. The absence of urobilinogen is not detectable with any reagent strip.

It is extremely important that fresh urine specimens be tested because urobilinogen is very unstable when exposed to room temperature or daylight. Urobilinogen, a colorless compound, is rapidly oxidized to urobilin, an orange-red pigment, which is not detected with either reagent strip test. This oxidation takes place so readily that most urine specimens that contain urobilinogen will show an abnormal color caused by partial oxidation to urobilin. The presence of urobilinogen and that of urobilin have the same clinical significance.

It is also extremely important that urine specimens be fresh and properly stored for testing for porphobilinogen. Porphobilinogen is a colorless compound that polymerizes (oxidizes) to a colored compound, porphobilin. Porphobilin gives a characteristic dark red or red-purple color, referred to as *port-wine red.* Fresh urine containing porphobilinogen is not usually colored, but some patients may have dark-red urine, or it may darken on standing as porphobilinogen polymerizes. To extend reactivity, the pH may be adjusted to 7 with sodium bicarbonate.

Summary

Table 13.7 summarizes the information in this section on chemical tests in routine urinalysis and provides additional testing data.

MICROSCOPIC ANALYSIS OF URINE SEDIMENT

Urine sediment refers to all solid materials suspended in the urine specimen. Microscopic examination of urine sediment is especially helpful in assessing the presence of kidney and urinary tract disease. The presence of certain findings in the microscopic examination will help explain abnormal physical and chemical tests.

The need for cost containment in health care has prompted some laboratories to omit the microscopic analysis of the urine sediment as part of every routine urinalysis. Various protocols now call for the microscopic analysis only when abnormal findings are seen in the physical and chemical analysis of the urine, or when determined by laboratory protocol (including the patient's condition or clinical history) or requested by the physician. CLSI emphasizes that each laboratory should decide whether to perform microscopic examinations based on its specific patient population.

Specimen Requirements

Type of Specimen

Although any freely voided collection is acceptable, the ideal specimen for microscopic analysis of the urine sediment is a fresh, voided, first morning specimen. A first morning specimen (an 8-hour concentration) is preferable because it is the most concentrated. This provides a greater chance of detecting abnormal constituents. In addition, the formed elements (cells and casts) are less likely to disintegrate in more concentrated urine.

Preservation

A fresh urine specimen is particularly important for reliable results. If the urine cannot be examined within 2 hours, it should be refrigerated as soon as possible after collection. Specimens

TABLE 13.7 Examples of Alternate Urinalysis Tests[a]

Substance	Test	Comments
Protein	Sulfosalicylic acid (SSA) test	Based on acid precipitation of protein with strong acid (SSA). Reagent strip test is most sensitive to albumin. SSA reacts with any protein; in addition to albumin: globulins, glucoproteins, and immunoglobulins.
Microalbuminuria	Micro-Bumintest (Bayer)	Tablet test for very small amounts of albumin; may be used to test for early presymptomatic diabetic nephropathy; principle as for reagent strip test but will detect as low as 4–8 mg albumin/dL.
Blood	Microscopic examination	If microscopic analysis shows more than two red blood cells per high-power field and reagent strip is negative, test for presence of ascorbic acid or otherwise account for discrepancy.
Hemoglobin, myoglobin	Centrifugation; then test supernatant with reagent strip test for blood	Separate hemoglobin from myoglobin by urine and plasma appearance, total serum creatine kinase (CK), total serum lactate dehydrogenase (LDH), and LDH isoenzymes.
Hemosiderin	Rous test	Based on positive Prussian blue reaction of hemosiderin with potassium ferrocyanide.
Glucose and other reducing substances	Clinitest (Bayer)	Tests for reducing substances in addition to glucose, based on reduction of copper II to copper I in presence of heat and alkali. Detects glucose, galactose, lactose, fructose, and pentose (L-xylulose) but not sucrose. False-positive results may be seen with large quantities of ascorbic acid, salicylates, and large quantities of some penicillins. Used routinely for pediatric specimens (<1 year old) to detect nonglucose reducing sugars.
Carbohydrates	Thin-layer chromatography	Common tests are for fructose, sucrose, dextrose, lactose, xylose, galactose, and arabinose because these are sugars most often found in urine.
Salicylates	Ferric chloride test	Rapid (spot) test for salicylate poisoning; also detects very large amounts of acetoacetic acid.
Bilirubin	Ictotest (Bayer)	Used when very small amounts of bilirubin are suspected because test more sensitive than reagent strip test; based on diazo reaction.
Urobilinogen, porphobilinogen	Watson–Schwartz test	This is Ehrlich aldehyde reaction. Will differentiate urobilinogen, porphobilinogen, and intermediate Ehrlich-reacting substances if Bayer reagent strip shows more than 1 Ehrlich unit.
Porphobilinogen	Hoesch test	Specific for porphobilinogen; based on inverse Ehrlich reaction.
Ascorbic acid	EM Quant (Merckoquant)	Use when interference is suspected from any of reagent strip tests that depend on presence of hydrogen peroxide; reagent strip tests for blood are especially susceptible.

[a]Some of the listed procedures are no longer performed in the United States but may be performed in developing countries.

left at room temperature for more than 2 hours are not acceptable. However, an "unacceptable" specimen should not be discarded until clinical personnel have been consulted and a mutually agreeable decision has been reached.

Although refrigeration prevents decomposition of urine sediment constituents, amorphous deposits of urates and phosphates tend to precipitate out of solution as the urine cools. These findings are important in that the deposits may obscure the presence of pathologic constituents.

If the specimen must be kept in the refrigerator for more than a few hours, a chemical preservative might be considered. Formalin may be used as a preservative to fix the various cellular elements and casts, but it interferes with many chemical tests. Other preservatives, such as toluene or thymol, may be used to prevent bacterial contamination. None of the preservatives is completely satisfactory; fresh collections are preferred. If preservatives that may interfere with various chemical tests are added, it is advisable to split the well-mixed specimen so that the sediment constituents are preserved, yet the chemical constituents are not affected.

Protection from Contamination

In addition to being a fresh first morning collection, the urine specimen should be clean and free of external contamination. This is sometimes a problem, especially with female patients, because vaginal contamination will result in the presence of epithelial cells, RBCs, and WBCs. In these patients, it may be necessary to use a clean-voided midstream specimen, which is also required for quantitative urine culture. It may also be necessary to pack the vagina or use a tampon in some cases to avoid vaginal and menstrual contamination.

Normal Sediment

Normally, urine contains minimal or no sediment, reflecting that normal urine is clear. However, a few constituents may be seen in any urine specimen. These generally consist of a few RBCs, WBCs, hyaline casts, epithelial cells, and crystals. Each laboratory must establish its own reference values for normal urine on the basis of methodology and patient population. The reference values in Table 13.8 are typical of what might be encountered in "normal" urine.

TABLE 13.8 Reference Values for Urine Sediment

Constituent	Reference Value
Red blood cells	0–2/hpf
White blood cells	0–5/hpf (female > male)
Casts	0–2 hyaline/lpf; identify with hpf
Squamous epithelial cells	Few/lpf
Transitional epithelial cells	Few/hpf
Renal tubular epithelial cells	Few/hpf
Bacteria	Negative
Yeast	Negative
Abnormal crystals	Negative
Sperm (males only)	Present

hpf, High-power field; *lpf,* low-power field.

Techniques for Examination of Urine Sediment

The urine sediment consists of a great variety of material. Some constituents are normal, whereas others are abnormal and represent serious conditions. It is important to learn to identify both the normal and the abnormal constituents. In general, normal constituents are more easily seen under the microscope and must be recognized so that they do not obscure the presence of the less obvious but more serious abnormal constituents. Recognition of abnormal constituents is extremely important in the diagnosis and treatment of various renal diseases. They often provide information about the state of the kidney and urinary tract. In addition, microscopic analysis of the sediment will help confirm and account for findings in the chemical examination of urine. For example, protein in the urine is often associated with the presence of casts and cellular elements in the sediment.

Traditionally, the urine sediment has been examined microscopically by placing a drop of urine on a microscope slide, applying a coverglass, and observing the preparation under the low-power (10 ×) and high-power (40 ×) objectives of a brightfield microscope.

Because the preparation is a wet mount, oil immersion cannot be used in this examination. The brightfield examination of unstained sediment is difficult, and various microscopic techniques, such as phase-contrast and polarizing microscopy, have been developed to aid in the identification of the various entities that might be present in the urine sediment. Other useful techniques in the examination of the urine sediment may include the use of stains and cytocentrifugation.

Microscopic Techniques

Brightfield Microscopy. Using the brightfield microscope is the traditional method of observation of the urine sediment and the most difficult. When the sediment is examined with brightfield illumination, correct light adjustment is essential. To give contrast between the unstained structures and the background liquid, the light must be sufficiently reduced by correct positioning of the condenser and the use of the iris diaphragm. As described in Chapter 5, the condenser should be left in a generally uppermost position (at most only 1–2 mm below the specimen) and the desired contrast achieved by opening or closing the iris diaphragm. The condenser should not be "racked down." The correct light adjustment requires care and experience. Correct light adjustment is essential, and various translucent elements that may occur in the urine sediment are easily overlooked with this technique. Of particular difficulty are hyaline casts, mucous threads, and various cells that have lost their hemoglobin content, such as RBCs.

If only a brightfield microscope is available, the use of a suitable stain is encouraged. Phase-contrast microscopy is helpful, and a combination of phase-contrast and brightfield microscopy is recommended. The hemoglobin pigment present in blood casts and RBC casts is more apparent with brightfield illumination, as are certain cellular details and the presence of highly refractile fat (free and in cells or casts). Most crystals are more easily visualized with brightfield microscopy or with both brightfield and polarizing microscopy.

Phase-Contrast Microscopy. Phase-contrast microscopy is useful in the examination of unstained urine sediment, particularly for delineating translucent elements such as hyaline casts and mucous threads, which have a refractive index similar to that of the urine in which they are suspended. Some laboratories use a phase-contrast microscope for the routine examination of the urine sediment. However, some elements are better visualized with brightfield, and the microscopist must be able to change from phase to brightfield with ease.

Plane-Polarizing Microscopy. Polarized light microscopy provides information on absorption color and differing refractive indices obtainable in brightfield microscopy, as well as optical properties of substances such as crystals. Crystal identification is of value in the examination of urine sediment and body fluids, including joint fluids.

Laboratory Procedure

Student Procedure Worksheet 13.2 uses a 12:1 concentration of the urine specimen and employs parts of the KOVA system. Well-mixed urine is measured and centrifuged in a special graduated centrifuge (KOVA) tube. The urine is decanted, and exactly 1 mL is retained for microscopic examination by using a special disposable pipette with a built-in plastic disk (KOVA Petter). Results are reported according to the system in Table 13.9. Directions are included for both standardized slides and traditional glass microscope slides with coverglasses, using both unstained and stained sediment. If a phase-contrast microscope is used, staining is generally unnecessary, but if only a brightfield microscope is used, staining is recommended.

Specimen Preparation (Concentration)

When the urine sediment is to be examined, a concentrated portion of the urine is used. The sediment is concentrated before examination to ensure detection of less abundant constituents. To concentrate the sediment, a well-mixed measured portion of urine is centrifuged. The clear supernatant is decanted, and the solid material, which settles to the bottom during centrifugation, is examined under the microscope. (The supernatant may be further tested for chemical constituents, such as urine protein.) The various parts of the sediment are identified and enumerated to give semiquantitative results. For these results to have meaning, a constant amount of urine must be centrifuged and a constant volume of supernatant removed.

TABLE 13.9 Reporting System for Urine Sediment

Sediment	Result
Average Number per Low-Power Field	
Casts (identify with high power)	Negative
Abnormal crystals	Negative
Squamous epithelial cells	
Mucus (if prominent)	
Average Number per High-Power Field	
Red blood cells	0–2
White blood cells	0–2
Normal crystals	Few
Epithelial cells (renal, oval fat bodies, transitional)	Few[a]
Miscellaneous (bacteria, yeast, *Trichomonas*, free fat)	Few
Sperm (males only)	Present

Magnification low-power (10 ×) objective × 10 × ocular = 100 × (*or* × 100). Magnification high-power (40 ×) objective × 10 × ocular = 400 × (*or* × 400).

[a]Some cells are present (*moderate,* easily seen; *many,* prominent).

Standardization

Various aids to standardization of the preparation and examination of the urine sediment are available. Complete systems or portions of systems may be used by a given a laboratory. Complete systems include specially designed, graduated centrifuge tubes with devices or pipettes that allow for the easy decanting of the supernatant urine and retention of an exact volume of undisturbed concentrated urine sediment. Systems differ in the final volume of urine sediment, although they generally begin by centrifuging 12 mL of well-mixed urine.

Traditionally, sediment was examined by placing a drop of concentrated sediment on a glass microscope slide and applying a coverglass. However, the size of the drop varied (it was generally not a measured drop), and results varied depending on the size of the coverglass used. Standardized systems employ specially designed slides of acrylic plastics with wells or applied coverglasses. They differ in the number of tests per slide, slide chamber volume (depth and surface area), availability of graded slides, and type of coverglass material (plastic or glass).

Commercial standardized systems to ensure comparison between laboratories and consistency within laboratories should be used. According to CLSI guidelines, the following factors must be standardized, regardless of whether a standardized system is used:

Urine volume: Standardized systems use 12 mL. Volumes of 10 and 15 mL are also used. The final concentration of sediment should be reported with results.

Time of centrifugation: Five minutes is recommended.

Speed of centrifugation: CLSI recommends a relative centrifugal force (RCF) of 400 *g*. Others recommend 450 *g* or 400 to 450 *g*. Normograms can be used to relate the revolutions per minute (rpm) to RCF by measuring the radius of the centrifuge head in centimeters from the center pin to the bottom of a horizontal cup, using the following formula:

$$\text{RCF}\,(g) = 11.8 \times 10^{-6} \times \text{Radius (cm)} \times \text{rpm}^2$$

Concentration factor of the sediment: This is based on the volume of urine centrifuged and the final volume of sediment remaining after the supernatant urine is removed. Standardized systems facilitate retention of a specific volume of urine sediment.

Volume of sediment examined: Standardized slides contain chambers that hold a specific volume of concentrated sediment. With a traditional slide and coverglass, the volume of concentrated sediment placed on the glass slide should be measured; 20 μL is typically used. The volume examined may be calculated based on the volume of sediment placed on the slide, size (area) of the coverglass, diameter of the microscope objective, and concentration of urine sediment used.

Reporting format: Every person in an institution who performs a microscopic examination of the urine sediment should use the same terminology, reporting format, and reference ranges.

CONSTITUENTS OF URINE SEDIMENT

In general, the constituents of the urine sediment are either biological or chemical. The biological part includes RBCs (erythrocytes), WBCs (leukocytes), epithelial cells, fat of biological origin, casts, bacteria, yeast, fungi, parasites, and spermatozoa. The chemical portion consists of crystals of chemicals and amorphous material. In general, it is less important than the biological portion. However, some abnormal crystals have pathologic significance. In addition, the constituents of the crystalline or chemical portion are sometimes so numerous that they tend to obscure the more important parts, which must be searched for with great care.

Cellular Constituents

Red Blood Cells (Erythrocytes)

Clinical Importance. A few RBCs are present in the urine of normal persons. The number varies, but generally five or fewer per high-power field (≤5/hpf) in the concentrated sediment is considered "normal."[2] As discussed earlier, the condition in which RBCs are found in the urine is termed *hematuria.* The degree of hematuria may vary from a frankly bloody specimen on gross examination to a specimen that shows no change in color. Hematuria may be the result of bleeding at any point along the urogenital tract and may be seen with almost any disease of the urinary tract, including renal disease or dysfunction, infection, tumor or lesions, stone formation, and generalized bleeding disorders, or it may result from anticoagulant usage. Hematuria is a sensitive early indicator of renal disease.

To determine the cause of hematuria, it is necessary to determine the site of bleeding. This involves various types of information, both laboratory and clinical. Part of this information will depend on other findings in the microscopic examination and other portions of the routine urinalysis. For example, bleeding through the glomerulus will often be accompanied by RBC casts, as seen in acute glomerulonephritis or disease of the glomerulus. This is an extremely serious situation, and RBC casts must be looked for carefully when erythrocytes are found. There may be little correlation between the amount of blood and the severity of the disorder, but the hematuria may be the only indication of renal disease. The occurrence of hematuria without accompanying protein and casts usually indicates that the bleeding is in the lower urogenital tract.

Microscopic Appearance. RBCs are not easy to find under the microscope. Their detection requires careful examination. The high-power objective is used, and the light must be reduced by proper adjustment of the condenser and iris diaphragm, or the RBCs will be missed. Their detection also requires continual refocusing with the fine adjustment of the microscope. The phase-contrast microscope is very useful in detecting RBCs. Even after hemolysis has occurred, the erythrocyte membrane is clearly visible with this technique.

In absolutely fresh urine, RBCs will be unaltered or intact and appear much as they do in diluted whole blood. They are seen as pale, yellowish-orange, intact biconcave disks that are especially apparent as they roll over. RBCs have a generally smooth appearance, as opposed to the granular appearance of WBCs, and are about 7 μm in diameter (Fig. 13.5A). However, RBCs rapidly undergo morphologic changes in urine specimens and are rarely observed as described. This is because urine is rarely an isotonic solution with RBCs (the solute concentration within the RBC is rarely the same as the solute concentration of urine). The urine may be more or less concentrated than the blood, and the changes described next will result.

When the urine is hypotonic or dilute, as evidenced by low specific gravity, the RBCs appear swollen and rounded because of diffusion of fluid into them. If the urine is hypertonic or concentrated (high specific gravity), the RBCs appear crenated and shrunken because they lose fluid to the urine (Fig. 13.5B). When crenated, the RBCs have little spicules, or projections, that cause them to be confused with WBCs. However, a crenated RBC is significantly smaller than a WBC and has a generally smooth, rather than granular, appearance. Also, when the urine is dilute and alkaline, the RBCs will often appear as shadow cells or ghost

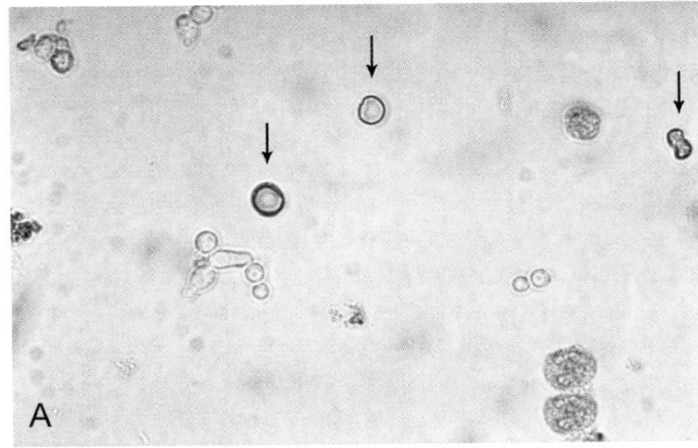

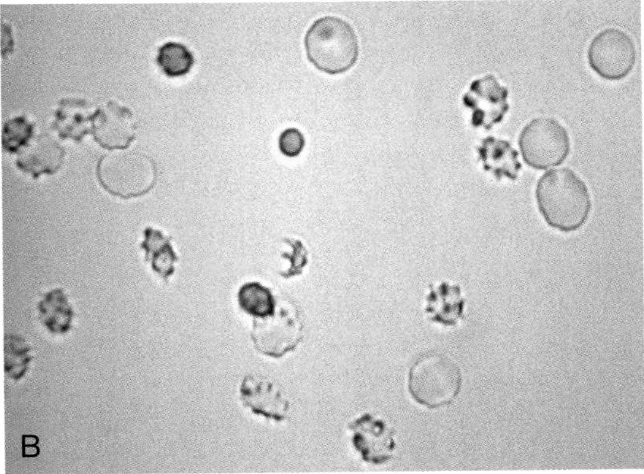

Fig. 13.5 Red blood cells (RBCs). (A) Three RBCs: two viewed from above appear as biconcave disks, and one viewed from the side appears hourglass-shaped *(arrows)*. Also present are budding yeast and several white blood cells. (Brightfield, Sedi-Stain, ×400.) (B) Crenated RBCs. RBCs in hypertonic urine (concentrated, high specific gravity). Many cells in this field of view have lost their typical biconcave shape and are crenated. (From Brunzel NA: *Fundamentals of urine and body fluid analysis,* ed 4, Philadelphia, 2018, Saunders.)

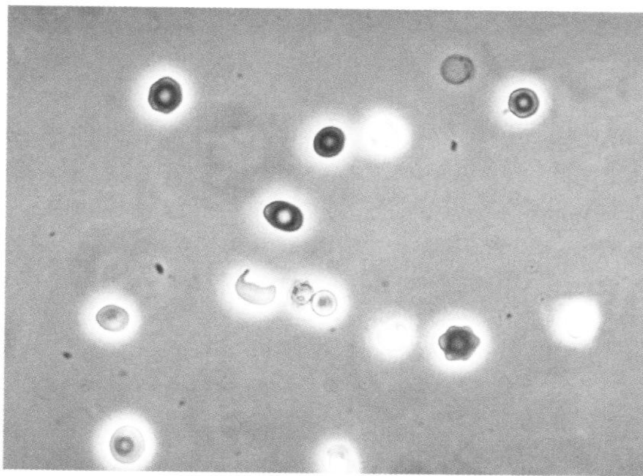

Fig. 13.6 Ghost red blood cell (RBC). Dysmorphic and crenated RBCs. A single ghost RBC is located at top of view. (Phase contrast, ×400.) (From Brunzel NA: *Fundamentals of urine and body fluid analysis,* ed 3, Philadelphia, 2012, Saunders.)

cells. In this situation the RBCs have burst and released their hemoglobin; all that remains is the faint, colorless cell membrane, a "ghost" or "shadow" of the original cell. This membrane is clearly visible with phase-contrast illumination. Ghost cells are often seen in old urine specimens. Eventually, even the ghosts will disappear as the cell completely disintegrates (Fig. 13.6).

Dysmorphic RBCs may also be seen. These distorted or misshapen RBCs may indicate the presence of glomerular disease. The distortion is best seen with phase-contrast illumination. It is also possible to see nucleated RBCs or sickle cells (in sickle cell disease) in urine, but this is extremely rare.

Structures Confused with Red Cells. RBCs not only are difficult to detect in a urine specimen but also are often confused with other structures found in urinary sediment. RBCs are often confused with WBCs (leukocytes), but the leukocyte is larger and has a generally granular appearance plus a nucleus. If morphologic differentiation is impossible, a drop of 2% acetic acid may be added to a new preparation or introduced under the coverglass. Acetic acid will lyse the RBCs and at the same time stain (or accentuate) the nuclei of leukocytes. With a Sternheimer–Malbin stain, RBCs in acidic urine may stain slightly purple or not at all. If the urine is alkaline, the alkaline hematin that is formed stains dark purple. The reagent strip tests for blood and leukocyte esterase are also helpful.

Yeast may also be confused with RBCs in urine, but yeast cells are generally smaller than RBCs, are spherical rather than flattened, and vary considerably in size within one specimen. In addition, because yeast reproduces by budding, the occurrence of buds or little outgrowths should identify yeast.

A very rare ovoid form of calcium oxalate may also be confused with RBCs, especially when viewed with brightfield illumination. However, calcium oxalate crystals are more refractile and, unlike RBCs, polarize light. Thus these crystals are easily differentiated with polarizing microscopy.

Bubbles or oil droplets are also confused with RBCs, especially by the inexperienced viewer. These vary considerably in size, are extremely refractive or reflective, and are obvious under the microscope.

Other Considerations. The presence of RBCs may be indicated by a tiny, red button of cells in the bottom of the centrifuge tube after centrifuging.

RBCs in the sediment should correlate with a positive reagent strip test for blood. Because chemical tests are more sensitive to hemoglobin than to intact RBCs, however, it is possible to have a negative reagent strip test when only a few intact cells are present and no hemolysis has occurred. This is rare. Reagent strip sensitivity is reduced in urine with high specific gravity; the RBC must lyse in order to react. In this situation, RBCs may be demonstrated by adding water to the sediment to lyse cells, then retesting with the reagent test for blood.

When large amounts of vitamin C are present, reagent strip results may be negative or delayed even though RBCs are seen in the sediment. In such cases the sediment result can be confirmed by the use of a reagent strip test for ascorbic acid. Another clue would be the gross appearance of the urine sediment or a red button of cells in the bottom of the centrifuge tube.

If the reagent strip test for blood is positive and RBCs are absent in the urine sediment, the presence of hemoglobin or myoglobin in the urine should be considered.

White Blood Cells (Leukocytes)

Clinical Importance. The presence of a few WBCs or leukocytes in the concentrated urine sediment is normal. Again, reference values vary, but more than a few (as many as 5/hpf) is considered abnormal. The term *white blood cell* or *leukocyte* in urine usually refers to the presence of a neutrophil (PMN); unless otherwise specified, it is assumed that this is what is meant. However, any WBC type present in blood can also be found in the urine sediment. The presence of lymphocytes and eosinophils is of particular diagnostic significance, as described later.

The presence of large numbers of WBCs in the sediment indicates inflammation at some point along the urogenital tract. The inflammation may result from a bacterial infection or other causes. The presence of WBCs is often associated with bacteria, but both bacteria and WBCs can be present alone, without the other. In bacterial infections, ingested bacteria may be seen within the cell. These cells are extremely labile and rapidly disappear from the specimen. If the leukocytes originate in the kidney, rather than lower in the urinary tract such as in the bladder, they may form cellular casts. Therefore the presence of casts (usually cellular or granular) along with WBCs and bacteria would help distinguish an upper (kidney) from a lower (bladder) UTI. Protein is usually present along with casts, and it may or may not be present in a lower UTI. The condition in which increased numbers of leukocytes are found in urine is termed *pyuria.* Pyuria may cause clouding of the urine, and when this is severe enough, the urine will have a characteristic milk-white appearance. Under the microscope, the WBCs may appear singly or in clumps. The presence of clumps is associated with acute infection.

Microscopic Appearance. Leukocytes must be searched for with the high-power objective, reduced light, and continual refocusing with fine adjustment. Typically, WBCs are about 10 to 14 μm in diameter, about twice the size of RBCs; however,

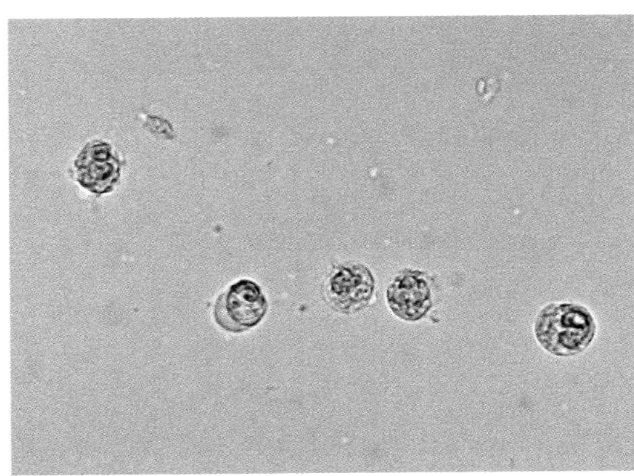

Fig. 13.7 Five white blood cells (WBCs). (From Brunzel NA: *Fundamentals of urine and body fluid analysis*, ed 4, Philadelphia, 2018, Saunders.)

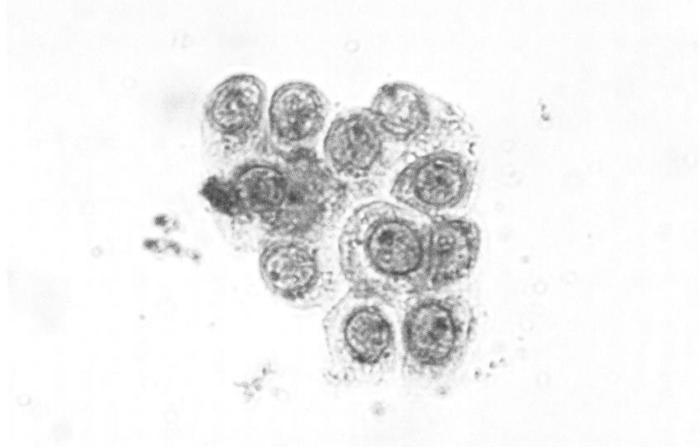

Fig. 13.9 Fragment of renal collecting duct epithelial cells. Stained with 0.5% toluidine blue. (Brightfield, ×400.) (From Brunzel NA: *Fundamentals of urine and body fluid analysis*, ed 4, Philadelphia, 2018, Saunders.)

this size difference may not be obvious, and WBCs often appear about the same size as RBCs. Leukocytes have thin cytoplasmic granulations and a nucleus. Even if the nucleus is not distinct, the center of the cell appears granular (Fig. 13.7). WBCs are fragile and will disintegrate in old alkaline urine specimens. Various stages of disintegration may be observed in a single urine specimen. Neutrophil leukocytes are especially vulnerable in dilute alkaline urine specimens, and about 50% can be lost within 2 to 3 hours if the urine is kept at room temperature. In addition, the lobed nucleus tends to consolidate, and the neutrophil appears as a mononuclear cell as the cell begins to degenerate. If the urine is dilute, the cell cytoplasm may expand out in petals, without granules, before the neutrophil disintegrates.

Phase-contrast microscopy is especially useful in the detection and identification of WBCs in the urine sediment (Fig. 13.8), as is the use of a stain such as the Sternheimer–Malbin stain. However, precipitation of the stain in the highly alkaline urines associated with WBCs and bacteria may pose a problem. When stained, neutrophilic leukocytes show a red-purple nucleus and violet or blue cytoplasm, although the same urine specimen may have a variety of staining reactions, and extremely fresh cells may fail to stain.

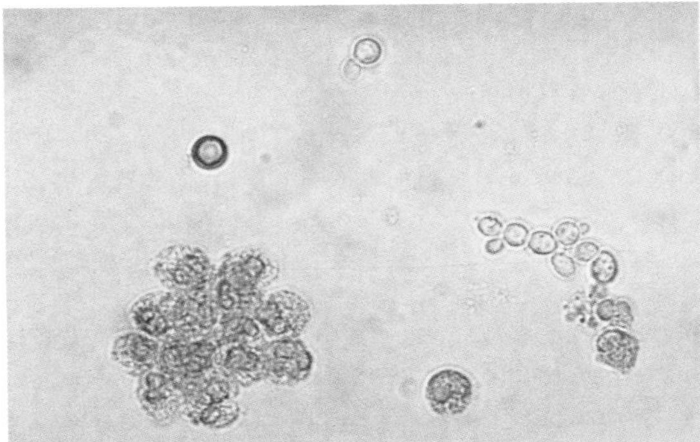

Fig. 13.8 Clump of white blood cells (WBCs). One red blood cell (RBC) and budding yeast are also present. (Brightfield, Sedi-Stain, ×400.) (From Brunzel NA: *Fundamentals of urine and body fluid analysis*, ed 4, Philadelphia, 2018, Saunders.)

Structures Confused with White Cells. Other structures may be mistaken for leukocytes. Most often this occurs with RBCs and epithelial cells. WBCs are generally larger than RBCs, appear granular, and have a nucleus. A 2% acetic acid solution may aid in the identification of WBCs. There are several different morphologic types of epithelial cells, but these generally are larger than WBCs and have smaller nuclei. Renal epithelial cells most resemble WBCs, although the nucleus is generally round, more distinct, and surrounded by more cytoplasm (Fig. 13.9).

Other Leukocytes in Sediment. Other WBC cell types may be seen in the urine sediment, as described next.

Glitter Cells. Glitter cells are larger, swollen neutrophilic leukocytes that appear in hypotonic urine with a specific gravity of about 1.010 or less. Their cytoplasmic granules are in constant random (Brownian) movement, giving a glittering appearance. These cells are especially striking under phase-contrast illumination. When stained, glitter cells have a light-blue or almost colorless cytoplasm, and the Brownian motion of the granules may or may not be observed. Once thought to indicate chronic pyelonephritis, glitter cells are also seen in dilute urine specimens from patients with lower UTIs.

Eosinophils. Eosinophils may be present in the urine sediment. They are morphologically similar to neutrophils and difficult to distinguish, especially with a wet preparation, under both brightfield and phase-contrast illumination. Eosinophils are typically larger than neutrophils and oval or elongated. The cytoplasmic granules may not be prominent, but the presence of two or three distinct lobes of the nucleus with fresh specimens is helpful. Cytocentrifugation is useful in confirming the presence of eosinophils. However, they do not stain as well with Wright stain as they do in blood smears. Use of special eosinophil stains, such as Hansel stain, is helpful. Increased eosinophils are associated with drug-induced interstitial nephritis, as seen with treatment with penicillins. Detection is important because the treatment is fast and effective (i.e., discontinuation of the drug).

Lymphocytes and Other Mononuclear Cells. A few small lymphocytes are normally present in urine, even though they are rarely recognized. They are difficult to distinguish from RBCs, especially with the normal wet preparation of the urine sediment, under both brightfield and phase-contrast illumination. These lymphocytes are only slightly larger than RBCs, with a single round nucleus and scant cytoplasm. The presence of many small lymphocytes is seen in the first few weeks after renal transplant rejection and is a useful early indicator of this rejection process. If their presence is suspected, identification of lymphocytes is most easily confirmed by cytocentrifugation and using Wright stain. Because they are not granulocytes, lymphocytes will not react with the reagent strips for leukocyte esterase.

Monocytes, histiocytes, and macrophages may also be present in the urine sediment. They are difficult to recognize on the standard wet preparation but are generally larger than, and resemble, aging neutrophils. Their cytoplasm is usually abundant, vacuolated, and granulated. These cells are granulocytes and are capable of reacting with the reagent strips for leukocyte esterase. However, the sensitivity of the strips may not be sufficient to detect these cells, which, even when present, are seen in relatively small numbers. Monocytes and histiocytes are associated with chronic inflammation and radiation therapy. Macrophages may be present with various inclusions within the cytoplasm. These include ingested fat, hemosiderin, RBCs, and crystals. As with lymphocytes, identification of other mononuclear cells is most easily confirmed by cytocentrifugation and Wright stain.

Epithelial Cells

Except for the single layer of renal epithelial cells lining the tubules of the nephron, the structures that make up the urinary system are lined by several layers of epithelial cells. The layer of epithelial cells closest to the lumen of organs such as the urethra and bladder (besides contaminating cells of the male and female genital tracts) is continually sloughed off (exfoliated) into the urine and replaced by cells originating from deeper layers. Therefore a few squamous epithelial cells are seen in most urine specimens. The single-layered renal epithelial cells are also sloughed into the urine. The identification of the various epithelial cell types may be difficult yet clinically significant. They include squamous, transitional (urothelial), and renal epithelial cells.

Squamous Epithelial Cells

Squamous epithelial cells line the urethra and bladder trigone in the female and the distal portion of the male urethra. They also line the vagina, and many of the squamous epithelial cells found in urine are the result of perineal or vaginal contamination in females or foreskin contamination in males. They are the most frequently encountered and the least significant type of epithelial cell in urine specimens. Squamous epithelial cells can be divided into intermediate and superficial squamous cells. They form the most superficial layer of cells that line the mucosa and are continually sloughed off and replaced by newer, deeper cells.

Squamous epithelial cells are very large, flat cells that consist of a thin layer of cytoplasm and a single distinct nucleus (Fig. 13.10). The nucleus is about the size of an RBC or lymphocyte, and the cell is about five to seven times the size of an RBC, about 30 to 50 μm. A thin flat cell, the squamous epithelial cell may be rectangular or round. Epithelial cells are large enough to be seen easily under low power and sometimes roll into cigar shapes, which are mistaken for casts. When stained, these cells show a purple nucleus and an abundant pink or violet cytoplasm. They are easily recognized until they begin to degenerate, when they may eventually appear as an amorphous mass.

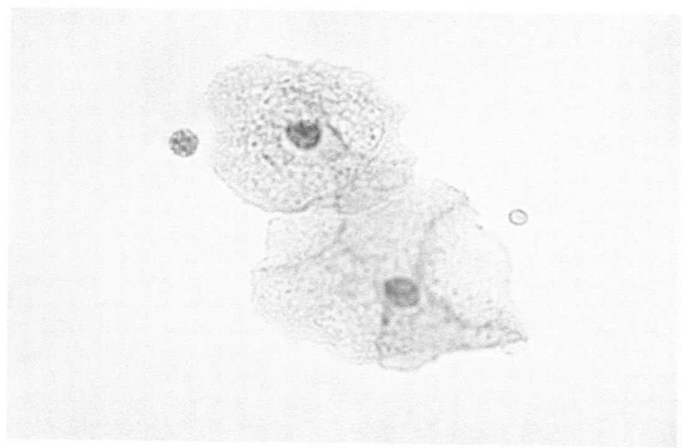

Fig. 13.10 Two squamous epithelial cells. Stained with Sternheimer-Malbin. (Brightfield, ×100.) (From Brunzel NA: *Fundamentals of urine and body fluid analysis,* ed 4, Philadelphia, 2018, Saunders.)

The presence of squamous epithelial cells is of little clinical significance unless they are present in large numbers. When the urine is contaminated by vaginal secretions or exudates, sheets of squamous epithelial cells accompanied by many rod-shaped bacteria or yeasts, or both, may be seen.

Clue Cells. Bacterial vaginosis (BV) is the most common cause of vaginal disease (vaginosis) in women of reproductive age. Detection of BV is important because it has been associated with an increased risk of sexually transmitted diseases (STDs), including human immunodeficiency virus (HIV) infection. Clue cells, a type of squamous epithelial cell of vaginal origin, may be observed in the examination of urine sediment. Clue cells are epithelial cells covered or encrusted with a bacterium, *Gardnerella vaginalis.* Most of the cell surface is covered with bacteria, and the bacteria should extend beyond the cytoplasmic margins for the cell to be called a clue cell. Free background bacteria in the sediment may be limited because of strong affinity of the epithelial cells for bacteria.

Transitional Epithelial (Urothelial) Cells

Transitional epithelial cells occur in multiple layers. They line the urinary tract, from the kidney pelvis in both females and males to the base of the bladder in the female and the proximal part of the urethra in the male. As the cell layers become deeper, the cells become thicker and rounded, increasingly resembling renal epithelial cells or WBCs. Their size varies with the depth and place of origin in the transitional epithelium. In general, however, transitional epithelial cells are about four to six times the size of an RBC (20–30 μm) and appear smaller and plumper than squamous epithelial cells. Urothelial cells are spherical or polyhedral in shape. Because they readily take on water, urothelial cells are often spherical from swelling, similar to a balloon of water. They are generally larger than renal tubular cells and have a round nucleus (sometimes two nuclei) similar in size and appearance to the nucleus seen in a squamous epithelial cell. The more superficial bladder epithelial cells are large, flat cells of a squamous nature. Transitional epithelial cells stain with a

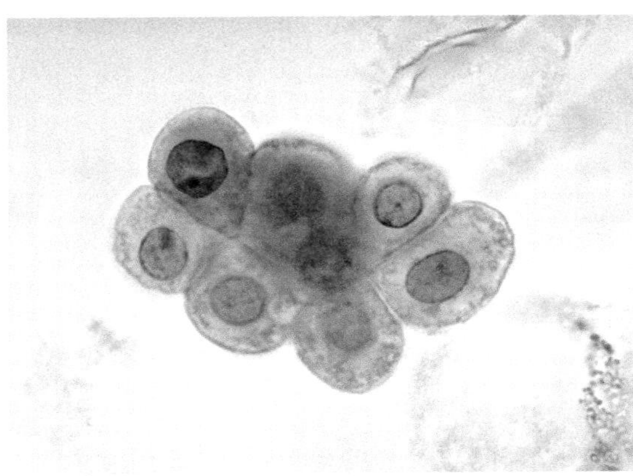

Fig. 13.11 Fragment of transitional epithelial cells. (From Brunzel NA: *Fundamentals of urine and body fluid analysis,* ed 4, Philadelphia, 2018, Saunders.)

dark-blue nucleus and varying amounts of pale-blue cytoplasm, which may have occasional inclusions. Some of these cells have tails and are indistinguishable from the caudate cells of the renal pelvis.

A few transitional epithelial cells are present in the urine of normal persons. Increased numbers are seen in the presence of infection. Clusters or sheets of these cells are seen after urethral or ureteral catheterization and with urinary tract lesions. Urothelial cells may show malignant changes, and such cells should be referred for cytologic examination. Radiation therapy may result in large cells with multiple nuclei and vacuoles (Fig. 13.11).

Renal Epithelial Cells

Renal epithelial cells are the single layer of cells that line the nephron from the proximal to the distal convoluted tubules, plus the cells lining the collecting ducts to the pelvis of the kidney. Their occurrence in urine is important because it implies a serious pathologic condition and destruction of renal tubules, as does the presence of epithelial casts. Identification of renal epithelial cells is difficult in wet preparations with either brightfield or phase contrast. Morphology varies, depending on the site of origin within the nephron. Intact renal epithelial cells are from three to five times the size of RBCs—that is, up to twice as large as a neutrophil. Cells from the proximal convoluted tubules are relatively large and elongated or oval, with a granular cytoplasm. The granularity makes the proximal tubular cells, in particular, appear as small or fragmented granular casts. The nucleus is extremely difficult to see in these renal epithelial cells in wet preparations. The use of cytocentrifugation and Wright staining will help visualize the nucleus and show these structures to be cells rather than casts, but the traditional cytologic examination with the Papanicolaou (Pap) stain is recommended.

Renal epithelial cells resemble both WBCs and smaller transitional epithelial cells. Morphologically, they closely resemble leukocytes, especially degenerating WBCs, but renal epithelial cells are typically larger and have a distinct single round nucleus. Renal cells of the collecting tubules tend to be polyhedral or cuboid; one side tends to be flat, unlike the rounded cell more typical of transitional epithelial cells. (Unlike transitional epithelial cells, renal cells do not absorb water and swell; therefore they tend to retain their polyhedral shape.) When these cells are stained, the nucleus stains a dark shade of blue-purple and the cytoplasm a lighter shade of blue-purple. Cytocentrifugation and a Pap stain are helpful.

As with all epithelial cells, renal epithelial cells will not react with the leukocyte esterase reagent strips; this may be helpful in distinguishing them from neutrophils. Renal epithelial cells are associated with the presence of protein in the urine and are often found in association with casts. The presence of epithelial or granular casts will help confirm their identification, and when renal cells are suspected, casts should be sought with great care. The phase-contrast microscope is particularly useful in such situations.

Renal Epithelial Fragments. These fragments or groups of three or more renal epithelial cells originate from the collecting ducts. Their presence is more serious than the presence of individual renal epithelial cells because they indicate renal tubular injury with disruption of the basement membrane.

Oval Fat Bodies. A special type of renal epithelial cell is filled with fat (lipid) droplets. OFBs are sometimes referred to as *renal tubular fat (RTF)* or *RTF bodies.* They indicate serious pathologic conditions and must not be overlooked when present in the urine sediment. The fat droplets are generally contained within degenerating or necrotic renal epithelial cells, although some OFBs may be macrophages that have filled with fat. The fat droplets contained within these cells are highly refractive, coarse droplets that vary greatly in size (Fig. 13.12). OFBs are more easily visualized with brightfield than phase-contrast microscopy. Although they are cells filled with fat, the cell nucleus is usually invisible.

Certain aids to the identification of OFBs are available. When stained with Sternheimer–Malbin, fat globules do not become colored but appear highly refractive in a blue-purple background. With fat stains such as Sudan III or oil red O, globules of triglyceride or neutral fat appear orange or red. Polarized light is useful for indicating the presence of cholesterol esters in the fat. Cholesterol esters show a typical Maltese cross pattern when viewed with polarizing filters. Triglycerides or neutral fat do not

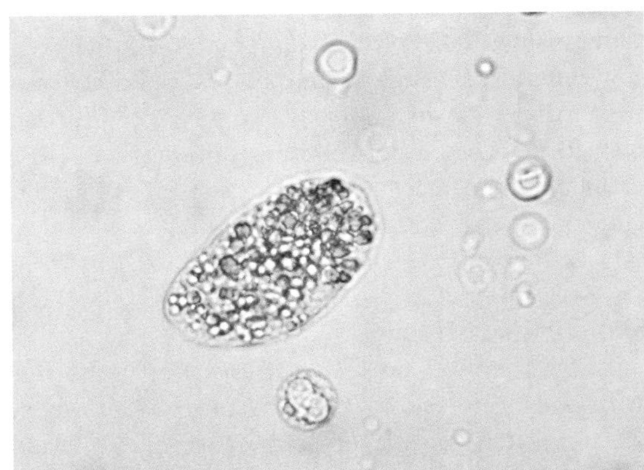

Fig. 13.12 Oval fat body. The cell has numerous highly refractile fat globules and other inclusions. (Brightfield, ×400.) (From Brunzel NA: *Fundamentals of urine and body fluid analysis,* ed 4, Philadelphia, 2018, Saunders.)

show this pattern with polarized light. The appearance of a Maltese cross pattern is also seen with starch, a common urine contaminant. Fat should be confirmed by careful microscopic examination or specific staining. OFBs are often seen along with fat droplets and fatty casts in the urine sediment, and the other two components should be searched for carefully when one is present.

The OFBs resulting from tubular epithelial degeneration of the nephron are associated with large amounts of protein in the urine, as in the nephrotic syndrome. The fatty material in the tubular cells may be the lipoprotein that passes through the damaged glomerulus in this syndrome. The lipoprotein may be ingested by the renal tubular cell, which metabolizes it into cholesterol. Clinically, the presence of neutral fat (triglyceride) and the presence of cholesterol are equal.

Fat Globules. Although not a cellular constituent, fat globules are discussed here because of their relationship to OFBs. Fat globules may be found in the urine sediment as highly refractive droplets of various sizes. When their source is biological (rather than contamination), a serious pathologic condition implying severe renal dysfunction exists. Such lipiduria is also associated with the nephrotic syndrome and its various causes, with diabetes mellitus, and with conditions that result in severe damage to renal tubular epithelial cells, such as ethylene glycol or mercury poisoning. Fat globules are found in association with OFBs and fatty casts. Fat stains orange or red with Sudan stains or oil red O. The identification may be aided by the use of polarized light; cholesterol will show a Maltese cross pattern. Fat in urine may also come from extraneous sources, such as unclean collection utensils or oiled catheters. This occurs less often with the use of disposable urine collection containers.

Hemosiderin. Occasionally, renal epithelial cells with granules of hemosiderin in the cytoplasm are seen in the urine sediment. This occurs several days after a hemolytic episode, when free hemoglobin has passed through the glomerulus into the nephron. The hemosiderin granules appear as yellow or colorless granules that are morphologically similar to amorphous urates. Unlike urates, they will stain blue with a Prussian blue for iron (Rous test). Besides their presence in desquamated renal epithelial cells, granules of hemosiderin may be seen as free granules in sediment, macrophages, and casts.

Viral Inclusion Bodies. Renal tubular epithelial cells may also be seen with viral inclusion bodies. This is especially characteristic of infection with cytomegalovirus (CMV). Viral inclusion bodies are difficult to recognize on wet preparations. Cytocentrifugation and Pap staining are helpful in recognizing this condition.

Casts

Formation and Significance

Casts are both the most difficult and the most important constituent of the urine sediment to discover. Their importance and their name derive from the manner in which they are produced. Casts are formed in the lumen of the tubules of the nephrons (working units of kidney) by solidification of material in the tubules. They are important because anything contained within the tubule is flushed out in the cast. Thus a cast represents a biopsy of an individual tubule and is a means of examining the contents of the nephron. It is believed that casts may be formed at any point along the nephron, either by precipitation of protein or by grouping together (conglutination) of material within the tubular lumen. In either case, the basic structure of the cast is a protein matrix. All casts have a matrix of Tamm–Horsfall mucoprotein (see earlier); in addition, plasma proteins may be present.

Before casts can form within the renal tubules, certain conditions must exist. Because the cast is made of protein, there must be a sufficient concentration of protein within the tubule. In addition, the pH must be low enough to favor precipitation, and there must be a sufficient concentration of solutes. For the same reasons, casts are not likely to be found in dilute alkaline urine because such conditions do not favor cast formation. This also means that the urine must be examined when fresh; as urine becomes alkaline with aging, the casts will disintegrate.

Because casts represent a biopsy of the kidney, they are extremely important clinically. Casts often contain RBCs, WBCs, epithelial cells, fat globules, and bacteria. These inclusions are not normally present within the renal tubule and represent an abnormal situation. The formation of casts implies at least a temporary blocking of the renal tubules. Although a few hyaline casts consisting only of precipitated Tamm–Horsfall mucoprotein may be seen in "normal" urine, increased numbers of casts indicate renal disease rather than lower urinary tract disease. The number of hyaline casts may increase in mild kidney irritation associated with dehydration or physical exercise. The presence of other types of casts represents a serious (pathologic) situation.

Identification and Morphology

Casts are extremely difficult to see and must be searched for carefully with reduced light and the low-power objective. Casts are found and enumerated under low power but must be identified as to type by means of the high-power objective. The refractive index of the cast is almost the same as that of glass, which means that the image is difficult to see under the microscope. For this reason, phase-contrast and interference-contrast microscopy are useful in the examination of the urine sediment. Phase-contrast microscopy gives sufficient contrast so that structures are not overlooked, and differential interference microscopy provides an appreciation of the shape and inclusions within these structures. Stains such as Sternheimer–Malbin are also particularly useful for the discovery of casts in the urine sediment. Casts that might otherwise be overlooked in brightfield examination, especially by the inexperienced observer, become obvious when so stained, although the presence of mucous strands in the sediment might be confusing, especially in searching for hyaline casts.

As might be imagined from the shape of the tubular lumen, casts are cylindrical bodies and have rounded ends. To be identified as a cast, a structure should have an even and definite outline, parallel sides, and two rounded ends. Although they vary somewhat in size, casts should have a uniform diameter (about seven or eight times the RBC diameter) and should be several times longer than wide.

Although casts should have parallel sides and two rounded ends, this is not always the case. Casts take on the shape of the tubule in which they are formed. They may be serpentine or convoluted and are often folded. One end may taper off to a tail or point. Such structures have been referred to as *cylindroids,* but they should be considered to be, and enumerated along with, hyaline casts. Cylindroids are often confused with strands of mucus, and care must be taken to avoid this mistake. In addition, casts may be fragmented or broken, and waxy casts typically show blunt rather than rounded ends. Judgment is necessary in the enumeration of such structures. The whole urine sediment picture must be considered so that important pathologic findings are reported. Conversely, the occurrence of only one questionable cast, with no other pathologic indicators, should not be reported.

Classification of Casts

Classification of casts is not always simple. In the laboratory, classification is done mainly on the basis of morphologic groupings, as follows:

- Hyaline
- Cellular
- Granular
- Waxy
- Fatty

Casts are long cylindrical structures that result from the solidification of material in the renal or tubular lumen of the kidney tubules. Casts are believed to arise either by precipitation of protein within the renal tubule or by conglutination (clumping) of material within the tubular lumen.

Either type of cast may contain inclusions. Casts formed by protein precipitation may trap any other substance that may be present, including leukocytes, fat, bacteria, RBCs, desquamated renal tubular epithelium, and crystals. Casts formed by either mechanism may appear coarsely or finely granular or waxy as cells disintegrate when the cast is retained in the tubule before being flushed out of the kidney. Structures will also disintegrate if the urine specimen stands.

Again, casts have a protein matrix, and the presence of casts in the urine is almost always accompanied by proteinuria. Tamm–Horsfall protein, the specific mucoprotein secreted by the renal tubular cells, has been identified immunologically and found to be present in all casts. Other immunoproteins have been identified in certain casts, although they are not found exclusively in any particular type of cast or disease state.

The following morphologic classification is based on appearance, physical properties, and existence of cellular components. The appearance of a cast when seen in the urine may not be the same as when it was originally formed in the renal tubule. If the cast is retained in the kidney (as in oliguric patients), its cells change in appearance. As the cells degenerate in the cast, their cytoplasm becomes granular. This is followed by loss of cell membranes, resulting in large or coarse granules. As these granules degenerate further, the cast shows smaller or fine granules. The final step in this degeneration is complete lack of structure, with the protein changed or coagulated into a thick, very refractive, opaque substance with a waxlike appearance, referred to as a *waxy cast.* These are the most serious casts pathologically because the formation of the waxy material implies a greatly lengthened transit time or a shutdown of the portion of the kidney where the structure evolved. Such casts are sometimes referred to as *renal failure casts.*

The width or diameter of a cast is important clinically. Most casts have a fairly constant diameter, as do the tubules in which they are formed, although casts from small children are narrower than those from adults. Narrow casts probably result from swelling of the tubular epithelium, as in an inflammatory process, with narrowing of the tubular lumen. They are not particularly important and tend to be of a hyaline type.

Broad casts are a much more serious finding. Their diameter is several times greater than normal, believed to result from their formation in dilated renal tubules or in collecting tubules. (Several nephrons empty into a common collecting tubule, which has a greater diameter than the renal tubule.) Severe chronic renal disease or obstruction (stasis) will often result in dilation and destruction of renal tubules. Cast formation in the collecting tubules must result from urinary stasis in the group of nephrons feeding a single collecting tubule. If not, the fluid pressure would be much too great for cast formation to occur. This cast formation represents serious stasis, and the presence of a significant number of broad casts in the urine sediment is considered a poor prognostic sign. Broad casts can be of almost any type, but because of the degree of stasis necessary for their formation, most tend to be waxy.

The types of casts encountered in the microscopic analysis of the urine sediment are described next in a morphologic classification (Box 13.3).

Hyaline Casts

Hyaline casts are colorless, homogeneous, nonrefractive, semitransparent structures (Fig. 13.13). They are the most

BOX 13.3 Morphologic Classification of Casts

- Hyaline cast
- Cellular cast
  - White blood cell (leukocyte, neutrophil, pus) cast
  - Red blood cell (blood, hemoglobin, hemoglobin pigment) cast
  - Epithelial cell cast
  - Bacterial cast
- Granular cast
- Waxy cast
- Fatty cast
  - Oval fat body cast
- Pigmented casts
  - Hemoglobin (blood) cast
  - Myoglobin cast
  - Bilirubin cast
  - Drug pigment cast
- Inclusion casts
  - (Granular cast)
  - (Fatty cast)
  - Hemosiderin cast
  - Crystal cast

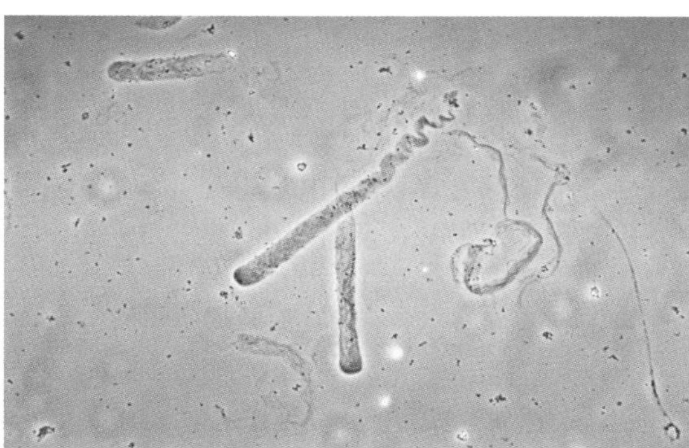

Fig. 13.13 Three hyaline casts. The cast with the tapered end is frequently called a *cylindroid.* (Phase contrast, ×100.) (From Brunzel NA: *Fundamentals of urine and body fluid analysis,* ed 4, Philadelphia, 2018, Saunders.)

difficult casts to discover under the microscope and the least important clinically. Hyaline casts require careful adjustment of light with the brightfield microscope; the light is adjusted to give contrast by lowering the condenser slightly and closing the iris diaphragm. Phase-contrast and interference microscopy are especially valuable tools in the search for hyaline casts. Stain is also useful; hyaline casts stain a uniform pale pink or pale blue. However, they may take up a minimum of stain and remain difficult to visualize. Hyaline casts also may be difficult to distinguish from mucous threads when they are present in the urine, both when stained and when observed by phase-contrast microscopy.

Hyaline casts result from solidification of Tamm–Horsfall protein, which is secreted by the renal tubular cells and may be seen without significant proteinuria. They will include any material that may be present in the tubular lumen at the time of formation, such as cells or cellular debris.

Although hyaline casts are generally of the classic shape for identification as a cast (i.e., parallel sides, uniform diameter, definite borders, and rounded ends), interesting modifications, representing molds of the tubular lumen where they are formed, may be observed. Some hyaline casts are broad, whereas others are thin and elongated; serpentine and folded forms are not unusual. As previously discussed, cylindroids are hyaline casts with one end that has not rounded off; they have the same significance and should be enumerated and reported as hyaline casts.

Hyaline casts are soluble in water and even more soluble in slightly alkaline solution. They are therefore more likely to be found in concentrated, acidic urine and may not form in advanced renal failure because of the inability to concentrate the urine or maintain the normal acid pH. In addition, hyaline casts dissolve if the urine stands and becomes alkaline. Hyaline casts may be further classified, according to their inclusions, as hyaline cellular (red, white, or epithelial), hyaline granular, and hyaline fatty casts.

Simple hyaline casts are the least important clinically, and a few, or less than two per low-power field (<2/lpf), may be seen in urine from normal persons. They may be seen in increased numbers after strenuous exercise; however, the sediment returns to normal in 24 to 48 hours. Simple hyaline casts may be seen in large numbers (20 or 30/lpf) in moderate or severe renal disease.

Cellular Casts

Cellular casts contain intact WBCs, RBCs, or epithelial cells. They are called *white cell* (or *pus*) casts, *RBC* (or *blood*) casts, and *epithelial* casts. Bacterial casts have also been described. A truly cellular cast appears to result from clumping, or conglutination, of cells rather than simply precipitation of protein and entrapment of cells, although they are still incorporated in a protein matrix. Alternatively, smaller numbers of the same cell types may be embedded in a hyaline cast.

Cellular casts indicate the presence of cells in the renal tubules. When this occurs, although causes vary with different degrees of severity, a serious situation exists.

It may be difficult if not impossible to distinguish the type of cell in a cast, especially when cells begin to deteriorate. In these situations the best indicator is probably the nature of other constituents in the urine sediment. Leukocytes and bacteria in the sediment would be associated with leukocyte (WBC) casts, whereas epithelial casts are more likely to be accompanied by cells appearing to be renal epithelium. Glitter cells are often seen when phagocytic neutrophils are present. When a morphologic distinction is impossible, the cast should be reported merely as a "cellular cast" rather than possibly misidentifying it. The clinician will use other findings in the urine specimen, both chemical and microscopic, to infer the cell type or source.

Cellular casts are more easily detected under the microscope than hyaline casts because the cells give them a definite structure compared with the homogeneous solidified protein of the hyaline cast. Cellular casts must still be sought with care, however, and proper illumination of the brightfield microscope is essential. Phase-contrast or interference microscopy and stains and cytocentrifugation are useful tools in the examination of the urine sediment for cellular casts.

White Blood Cell Casts. WBC casts are also referred to as *leukocyte casts* or *pus casts* when neutrophilic leukocytes are present. When leukocytes are present in a cast, it is obvious that the cells originated in the kidney. The leukocytes may enter the nephron from the blood by passing through the glomerulus into the glomerular capsule in glomerular diseases. More often, they probably enter the nephron from the blood by squeezing through the cells making up the renal tubules, often in response to a bacterial infection within the tubular interstitium. Such phagocytic neutrophils are typically seen in pyelonephritis, a renal infection of the interstitium. In such cases, leukocytes and bacteria are also present in the urine sediment. The presence of casts (particularly WBC casts), along with leukocytes and bacteria, is used to distinguish an upper from a lower UTI.

The WBC casts are seen fairly easily in the urine sediment with the brightfield microscope (Fig. 13.14). The cells are fairly prominent, and the characteristic multilobular nucleus can usually be seen. Small leukocytes stain purple to violet, whereas large cells may be pale blue, in a pink matrix. As the cells disintegrate within the cast, their cytoplasm becomes granular, cell borders merge, and nuclei become indistinct, resulting in a

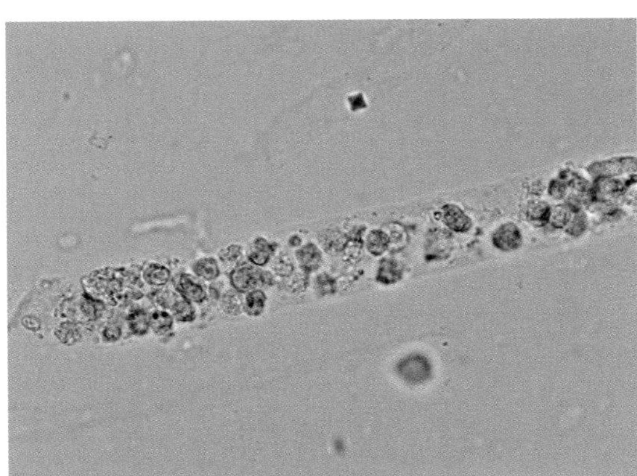

Fig. 13.14 White blood cell (WBC, leukocyte) cast. (Brightfield, ×400.) (From Brunzel NA: *Fundamentals of urine and body fluid analysis,* ed 3, Philadelphia, 2013, Saunders.)

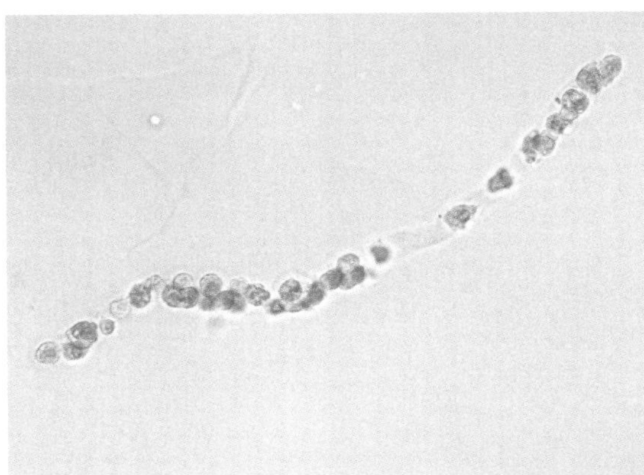

Fig. 13.15 Renal tubular epithelial cell cast. (Brightfield, ×400.) (From Brunzel NA: *Fundamentals of urine and body fluid analysis,* ed 4, Philadelphia, 2018, Saunders.)

granular cast when the cells are no longer distinguishable. The number of cells in a cast varies; some casts are packed with cells, and others show only a few cells in a hyaline matrix. WBC casts packed with cells still have a protein matrix and should have parallel sides and rounded ends. It is sometimes difficult to distinguish such a WBC cast from a clump of leukocytes (pseudoleukocyte cast), which may originate lower in the urinary tract. The presence of strands of mucus to which the WBCs adhere is another complication. However, it is still important not to report such pseudocasts as "casts," which implies renal involvement or disease.

Epithelial Cell Casts. As indicated earlier, to be called an *epithelial cell cast,* the epithelial cell must be renal tubular in origin. Epithelial casts represent a serious situation, although they are infrequently seen in the urine. They may be seen in cases of exposure to nephrotoxic substances, such as mercury or ethylene glycol (antifreeze), or in infections with viruses, such as CMV or hepatitis virus. Epithelial casts result from destruction or desquamation of the cells that line the renal tubules. These cells are responsible for the work done by the kidney. The damage may be irreversible, depending on the severity of the disease process. The time needed to replace renal epithelial cells, if the basement membrane is left intact, is unknown; however, cells do not show maximum concentrating ability for several months after severe loss of tubular epithelium.

The epithelial cast often appears to consist of two rows of renal epithelial cells, implying tubular desquamation (Fig. 13.15). However, the cells may also vary in size, shape, and distribution, showing a varying amount of protein matrix. A haphazard arrangement of cells in the cast in varying stages of degeneration implies cellular damage and desquamation from different portions of the renal tubule. The epithelial cast does not remain constant once formed, but rather undergoes a series of changes. These changes result from cellular disintegration as the cast remains within the kidney, because of decreased urine flow (stasis). Therefore a range of epithelial casts may be seen, from cellular to coarsely granular, finely granular, and finally waxy. The waxy type represents the most serious situation because prolonged blockage of renal flow is required for them to form. All these types of casts are often seen in the same specimen; such specimens are referred to as "telescoped" urine sediments. Epithelial casts may be difficult to distinguish from WBC casts, as previously discussed. When stained, the cells have a blue-purple nucleus and lighter blue-purple cytoplasm in a pink matrix. Phase-contrast and interference microscopy are also helpful in this examination, as is cytocentrifugation.

Red Blood Cell (Blood and Hemoglobin) Casts. The observation of RBC casts in the urine sediment is a significant diagnostic finding and indicates a serious renal condition. Their presence must not be missed. The RBCs enter the nephron by leakage through the glomerular capsule. It is possible that RBCs bleed into the renal tubules at a point beyond the glomerular capsule; however, this would be a much less common path because RBC casts are almost always associated with diseases that affect the glomerulus, such as acute glomerulonephritis and lupus nephritis. Once RBCs are present in the lumen of the nephron, they clump together to form RBC casts. RBC casts are probably the most fragile casts in the urine sediment, which may explain why they are rarely observed and why fragments are more often found. When physical conditions indicate that RBC casts may be present, it is imperative that the urine specimen be absolutely fresh and gently treated. The casts may be so fragile that they disintegrate under the microscope as the observer watches.

Blood (RBC) casts have a characteristic orange-yellow color caused by hemoglobin, which makes them unlike anything else seen in the urine sediment (Fig. 13.16). Stain may or may not be useful in the identification of blood casts; however, the casts may have intact RBCs, which stain colorless or lavender in a pink matrix. Both phase-contrast and interference microscopy are useful in detecting RBC casts. The characteristic color is best seen with brightfield observation of the unstained sediment.

The number of cells present in the blood cast is variable. Often, only a few intact cells are seen in a hyaline matrix; this may be referred to as a hyaline RBC cast. If many cells are clumped together to form the cast, the matrix is often not visible. These casts are more fragile and, unfortunately, more serious clinically.

RBC casts or casts derived from RBCs are often divided into RBC casts, blood casts, and hemoglobin casts. It is also possible to see mixed-cell casts, which are a combination of all types. The

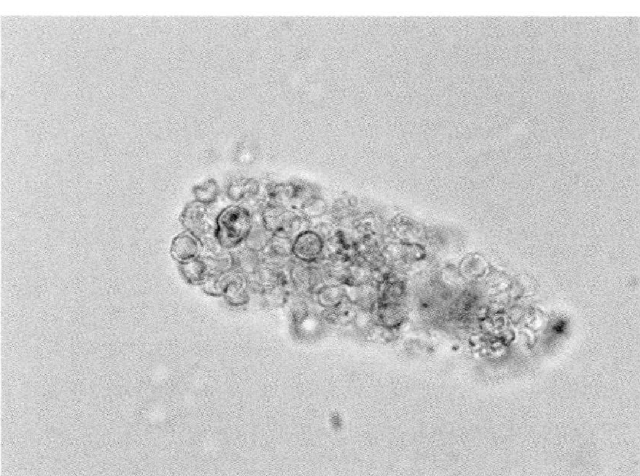

Fig. 13.16 Red blood cell (RBC, erythrocyte) cast, unstained. (From Brunzel NA: *Fundamentals of urine and body fluid analysis*, ed 4, Philadelphia, 2018, Saunders.)

RBC cast contains at least some recognizable RBCs. They may be present in a generally hyaline matrix or may appear as a solid mass of conglutinated RBCs with little or no matrix between the packed cells. When the RBCs degenerate, no longer showing a cell margin but remaining recognizable as probably being derived from blood, they are called a *blood cast.* (This is analogous to the cellular or coarsely granular cast derived from WBCs or epithelial cells.) The hemoglobin (pigment) cast shows a homogeneous matrix with no cell margins or recognizable RBCs. Both blood and hemoglobin casts have a characteristic orange-yellow color. The hemoglobin pigment cast is then analogous to the waxy cast, representative of urinary stasis, and a more chronic than acute condition.

The occurrence of RBCs within a cast, regardless of the number of cells, represents a serious situation. The finding of RBCs in the urine sediment, in conjunction with RBC casts of any type, indicates renal (usually glomerular) involvement.

Bacterial Casts. Casts made up of bacteria in a protein matrix have been described. Bacterial casts are an important finding and are diagnostic of acute pyelonephritis or intrinsic renal infections. They are probably mistaken for granular casts, which they resemble. The use of phase-contrast or interference-contrast microscopy and supravital stain is helpful. However, bacterial casts are most easily recognized if a dry or cytocentrifuged preparation is viewed with Gram stain. The bacteria in the cast may be packed closely together, sparsely distributed throughout, or concentrated in an area of a cast matrix. In addition to the bacteria, WBCs may be present within the cast.

Granular Casts

The granules seen in granular casts may result from the breakdown of cells within the cast or the renal tubule, or they may be aggregates of plasma proteins, including fibrinogen, immune complexes, and globulins in a Tamm–Horsfall matrix. Once all the cells have become granules, it is impossible to determine what type of cell was originally present in the renal tubule. Such a distinction is useful because RBC casts indicate glomerular injury, epithelial cell casts indicate renal tubular damage, and WBC casts indicate interstitial inflammation or infection. Often, casts are seen that are basically granular but show some cells in transition to granules. When cells are present, they should be identified if possible. Once again, phase-contrast and interference microscopy are helpful in this distinction, as is cytocentrifugation. The end product of this disintegration is the waxy cast.

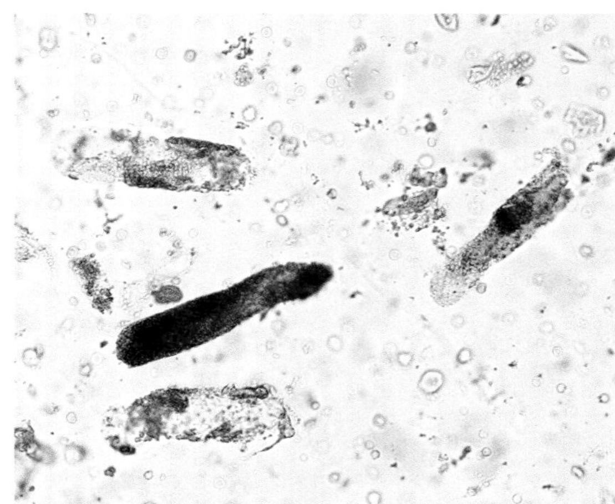

Fig. 13.17 Finely granular and coarsely granular casts. (From Brunzel NA: *Fundamentals of urine and body fluid analysis*, ed 4, Philadelphia, 2018, Saunders.)

The size of the granules within the granular cast varies; they become progressively smaller as the cells disintegrate. The number of granules also varies, and casts range from those that are completely filled with granules to those that are basically hyaline and contain only a few granules. Such granules may have been present in the renal tubule and trapped in a protein matrix as the cast was formed. Although granular casts are sometimes reported as coarsely or finely granular, the term *granular* is sufficient (Fig. 13.17). The distinction between coarsely and finely granular is subjective but relatively easily made. If the cast has a definite hyaline matrix with only a few granules, it is reported as *hyaline.* When large numbers of granules are present, it is described as *granular.* When many somewhat shortened granular casts are seen, the possibility that they are actually proximal renal tubular epithelial cells should be considered (see earlier discussion). They are more easily visualized with stained brightfield preparations, and cytocentrifugation and use of Wright and Pap stains are especially helpful.

Coarsely Granular Casts

Coarsely granular casts contain large granules that appear to be degenerated cells (Fig. 13.18). They tend to be darker, shorter, and more irregular in outline than finely granular casts. They show a darker color and large granules that make them easier to find than either hyaline or finely granular casts. Coarsely granular casts stain with dark-purple granules in a purple matrix.

Finely Granular Casts. Although finely granular casts look similar to hyaline casts, the presence of fine granules makes them more distinctive and easier to find. When viewed with phase-contrast or interference microscopy, hyaline casts generally show a fine granulation. They are usually grayish or pale yellow in the unstained sediment and stain with fine, dark-purple granules in a pale-pink or pale-purple matrix.

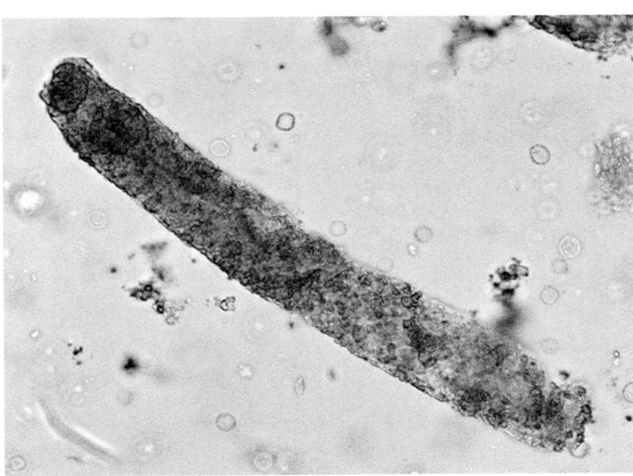

Fig. 13.18 Granular cast with coarse granules. (From Brunzel NA: *Fundamentals of urine and body fluid analysis,* ed 4, Philadelphia, 2018, Saunders.)

Waxy Casts

Waxy casts resemble hyaline casts, and they may be mistaken as such but are much more significant clinically. The waxy cast is homogeneous, as is the hyaline cast, but it is yellowish and more refractive, with sharper outlines. It appears hard, whereas the hyaline cast has a delicate appearance. Waxy casts tend to be wider than hyaline casts (they are described as "broad casts" or "broad waxy casts") and usually have irregular broken ends and fissures or cracks in their sides (Fig. 13.19). Fairly long forms are also seen. Phase-contrast and interference microscopy and staining are useful in the examination of waxy casts. They generally stain with greater intensity than hyaline casts, making them easier to visualize.

Waxy casts are thought to be the final step in the disintegration of cellular casts and are especially serious because they imply renal stasis. They are associated with severe, chronic renal disease and renal amyloidosis. Waxy casts are seen only rarely and in small numbers in acute renal diseases.

Fatty Casts

The importance and probable mechanism of formation of fatty casts are discussed with OFBs and fat globules (see previous sections). These three structures are often seen together in the same urine specimen, along with extremely large amounts of protein (>2000 mg/dL) and the pale, foamy appearance of the specimen associated with the nephrotic syndrome. They are also seen in diabetes mellitus with renal degeneration and in toxic renal poisoning, as from ethylene glycol or mercury.

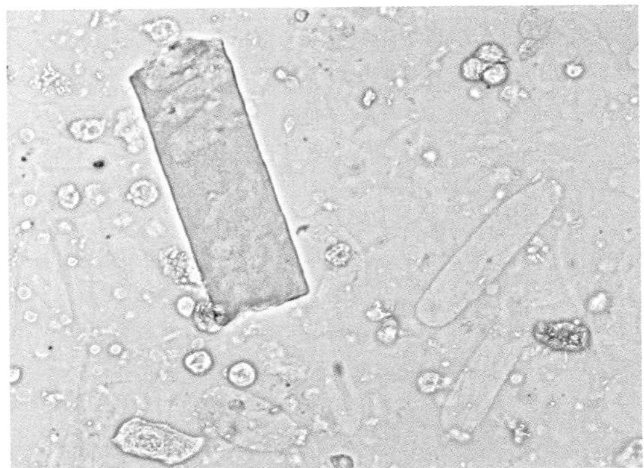

Fig. 13.19 Waxy cast. Single waxy cast and two hyaline casts. Note the difference in refractility between these two types of casts. (From Brunzel NA: *Fundamentals of urine and body fluid analysis,* ed 4, Philadelphia, 2018, Saunders.)

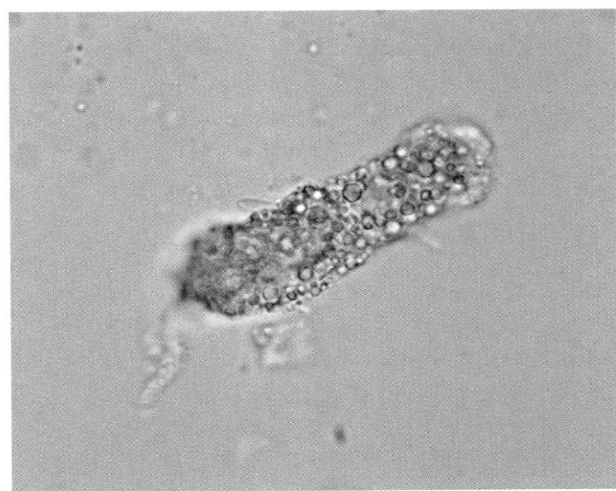

Fig. 13.20 Fatty cast. Note the globules and their characteristic refractility. (Brightfield, ×400.) (From Brunzel NA: *Fundamentals of urine and body fluid analysis,* ed 4, Philadelphia, 2018, Saunders.)

Fatty casts contain droplets of fat, which are highly refractile under the microscope (Fig. 13.20). Although phase-contrast and interference microscopy are useful, the characteristic refractile appearance of fat droplets might be better appreciated with the brightfield microscope. If the droplets are neutral fat or triglyceride, they will stain bright orange or red with Sudan III or oil red O stains. If cholesterol is present, the fat droplets will show a Maltese cross pattern with polarized light. With Sternheimer–Malbin the cast matrix will stain, but the refractile fat globules will not stain.

Fatty casts may be seen as a protein matrix almost completely filled with fat globules or as fat globules contained within a basically hyaline, cellular, or granular cast. In addition to free fat globules, intact OFBs may be seen within the cast matrix; these are sometimes referred to as *OFB casts.*

Other Casts

Various other structures found in the urine sediment may rarely be incorporated into the protein matrix of a cast. Pigmented casts may be seen, including hemoglobin (already described), myoglobin, bilirubin, and drugs such as phenazopyridine. Hemosiderin casts contain granules of hemosiderin. Crystal casts, which contain urates, calcium oxalate, or sulfonamides, have also been seen. However, these must not be mistaken for crystals adhering to strands of mucus; rather, the protein matrix must be visualized in a true crystal cast.

Structures Confused with Casts

Mucous Threads. The refractive index of mucous threads is similar to that of hyaline casts; however, mucous threads are long, ribbonlike strands with undefined edges and pointed or split ends. They also appear to have longitudinal striations.

Mucous threads are most apparent, and cause the most confusion, with phase-contrast or interference microscopy. They are often seen together with hyaline casts. Although difficult to distinguish, hyaline casts are generally more formed or structured than mucous threads.

Rolled Squamous Epithelial Cells. Squamous epithelial cells may be mistaken for casts when they have rolled into a cigar shape. However, they have pointed ends rather than rounded ones and are shorter than casts, and a single, round nucleus may be discovered with careful focusing.

Disposable Diaper Fibers. Diaper fibers are easily confused with waxy casts, appearing almost identically as highly refractile with blunt ends. They may be seen in urine specimens from infants or from geriatric patients or other adults who must use diapers. Unlike waxy casts, diaper fibers are rarely accompanied by other pathologic findings, especially proteinuria. The use of polarizing microscopy may be useful; waxy casts do not polarize light, whereas diaper fibers do (Fig. 13.21).

Other Structures. Bits of hair or threads of material fibers are also mistaken for casts by the beginner. However, these are extremely refractive structures that have nothing in common with the appearance of protein microscopically. Likewise, scratches on the glass slide or coverglass may be mistaken for casts at first. Again, they are much too definite and obvious to be important. Finally, hyphae of molds are sometimes mistaken for hyaline casts; this is similar to mistaking yeast for RBCs. Hyphae are much more refractive than hyaline casts and are jointed and branching, as may be observed on closer examination.

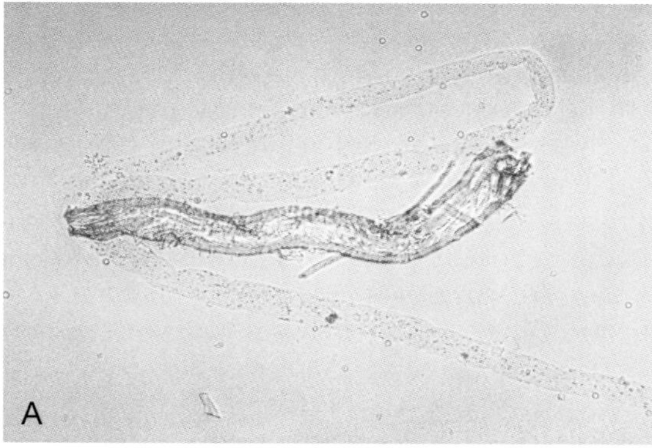

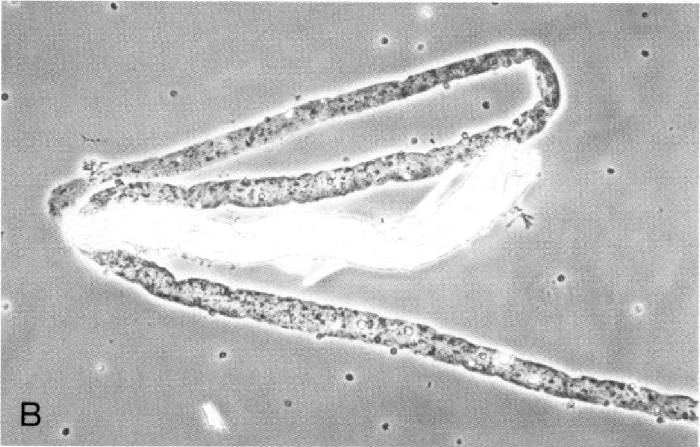

Fig. 13.21 **Hyaline cast and a fiber.** Note the difference in form and refractility. (A) Brightfield, ×100. (B) Phase contrast, ×100. (From Brunzel NA: *Fundamentals of urine and body fluid analysis,* ed 4, Philadelphia, 2018, Saunders.)

Crystals and Amorphous Material

Clinical Significance

As urine specimens stand, especially when refrigerated, many lose clarity and become cloudy because of the precipitation of amorphous material and crystals. The presence of crystals is generally important only when present in urine when voided (at body temperature).

If crystals are abundant, they will obscure such important structures as RBCs, WBCs, and casts. The more important structures must be sought with extreme care when crystals and amorphous materials are present. The use of a stain such as Sternheimer–Malbin may be especially useful in these situations.

The precipitation of certain crystals may accompany kidney stone formation (lithiasis). The chemical composition of stones depends on the chemical imbalance in the urine. The five most common types of stones are comprised of calcium—calcium oxalate and calcium phosphate, uric acid, struvite, and cystine. When crystals are seen in the urine of patients with lithiasis, the chemical composition of the calculi (stones) may be implied. This is one reason for the attention formerly given to urinary crystals. However, stone formation may exist without the presence of crystals in the urine, and crystals are often present without stone formation.

Amino acids such as cystine, leucine, and tyrosine may crystallize in urine and indicate serious metabolic or inherited disorders. Administration of sulfonamide drugs may cause the formation of sulfonamide crystals, especially in acidic urine. The formation of sulfonamide crystals within the kidney may result in blockage of renal output and severe renal damage. This problem was greater when sulfonamide drugs were first introduced. Current drugs are more soluble and thus less likely to precipitate. However, crystals are occasionally seen when high doses are given. More recently, crystals of the protease inhibitor indinavir sulfate have been associated with renal blockage and stone formation in individuals with HIV.

When the concentration of a salt in solution is greater than the salt's solubility threshold, crystals will precipitate out of solution. Therefore crystals are more likely to be seen in concentrated urine specimens with high specific gravity. This is often observed in the urine of persons with dehydration and fever.

Classification of Urine Crystals

The various crystals that are encountered in urine specimens are usually classified as *normal* or *abnormal.* These are further subclassified as normal *acid* crystals (crystals seen in normal urine of an acidic pH), normal *alkaline* crystals (crystals seen in normal urine of an alkaline pH), abnormal crystals of *metabolic* origin, and abnormal crystals of *iatrogenic* origin. *Iatrogenic* refers to crystals that result from medication or treatment, that is, inadvertently caused by the physician. The various crystals found in the urine sediment are categorized in Box 13.4. The crystals in each category are arranged in approximately the order of importance or frequency in which they are encountered.

Identification and Reporting of Urine Crystals

Identification of crystals is usually done on the basis of shape or morphology. This is aided by knowledge of the urine pH.

BOX 13.4 Crystals Found in Urine Sediment

Normal Acid Crystals
Amorphous urates
Uric acid
Acid urates
Monosodium or sodium urates
Calcium oxalate (also seen in neutral and alkaline urine)

Normal Alkaline Crystals
Amorphous phosphates
(Calcium oxalate)
Triple phosphates
Calcium carbonate

Abnormal Crystals of Metabolic Origin
Cystine
Tyrosine
Leucine
Cholesterol
Bilirubin
Hemosiderin

Abnormal Crystals of Iatrogenic Origin (Drugs)
Sulfonamides
Ampicillin
Radiographic contrast media
Acyclovir
Indinavir sulfate

Certain forms are seen in urine of an acid pH (generally $\leq$ 6.5), whereas others are associated with urine of an alkaline pH (generally $\geq$ 7.0). Although pH 7 is neutral, crystals present in urine of pH 7 are generally forms seen in a more alkaline pH.

The normal crystals are usually reported on the basis of morphology alone. They are observed with both low-power and high-power objectives, depending on size, and reported as few, moderate, or many per high-power field. Unlike the urine sediment constituents already described, crystals are characterized by *shape* rather than size. Although some crystals are typically large or small, crystals of chemicals such as uric acid may vary from extremely small crystals that can only be visualized with high power to extremely large forms that are easily seen with low power. The *color* of the crystals, both macroscopically (on the basis of urine appearance) and microscopically, is also helpful. In some cases, solubility with heat, acids, or alkalis is useful in the final identification.

The abnormal crystals generally require confirmation before they are reported to the clinician. They are observed under low and high power, depending on size, and reported on the basis of the average number per low-power field, as shown in Table 13.9. Confirmation may consist of a chemical test, such as a diazo reaction for sulfonamides or a cyanide nitroprusside reaction for cystine. When confirmatory chemical tests are unavailable, confirmation may consist of the patient's drug history or history of various imaging procedures, such as intravenous pyelography or computed tomography.

Most crystals are birefringent when viewed with polarized light. The strength of birefringence depends on both the chemical composition of the crystal in question and the thickness of the crystal. Thick crystals will show stronger birefringence than thin ones. As with synovial fluid crystals, phosphates or phosphate-containing crystals generally show weaker birefringence than urates or uric acid. The ability to polarize light is very helpful in the identification of crystalline structures versus structures of biological origin, such as cells, microorganisms, and casts, which do not polarize light.

Normal Crystals

Normal Acid Crystals (Fig. 13.22)

Amorphous Urates. Urates represent the amorphous material found in urine of an acid pH. Chemically, amorphous (without shape or form) urates are a sodium salt of uric acid (sodium, potassium, magnesium, or calcium). The urates show a characteristic yellowish red, shapeless granulation (Fig. 13.22*A*). When present in sufficient numbers, they form a fluffy pink or orange precipitate referred to as "brick dust." Amorphous urates tend to precipitate out of urine that is highly concentrated, as in dehydration and fever. When treated with ammonium hydroxide, urates will change to ammonium biurate, the ammonium salt of uric acid.

Although the appearance of the urine may be alarming to a patient, such specimens are of minimal concern clinically.

Uric Acid. Uric acid crystals have a variety of shapes and colors. Typically, they are yellow or reddish brown, similar to the chemically related amorphous urates (Fig. 13.22B). The typical shape is the whetstone. Other shapes include rhombic plates or prisms, somewhat oval forms with pointed ends ("lemon-shaped"), and barrel-shaped forms. Wedges, rosettes, irregular plates, and laminated forms are also seen. Uric acid crystals are usually recognized by color, but some, especially the rhombic plates, may appear colorless. Unusual crystals of an acid pH are generally forms of uric acid. A hexagonal form of uric acid may be mistaken for cystine crystals, which are abnormal and important to detect. Several of the sulfonamides may mimic uric acid.

Uric acid crystals are often seen in urine specimens, especially after the specimen has been standing. However, they are pathologic only when seen in fresh urine immediately after it is voided. As with amorphous urates, uric acid is soluble when heated to 60°C and when treated with 10% sodium hydroxide (NaOH).

Amorphous urates and uric acid, together with elevated serum uric acid, may be associated with gout or stone formation. The uric acid concentration in urine depends on dietary intake of purines and breakdown of nucleic acid. Therefore large amounts of urates or uric acid are often seen in the urine of patients with leukemia or lymphoma who are receiving chemotherapy.

Acid Urates. Acid urates are a rare form of uric acid seen in urine of acidic or neutral pH. Acid urates may be sodium, potassium, or ammonium urates and are observed as brown spheres or clusters that resemble the alkaline counterpoint of uric acid, ammonium biurate. They are often seen in urine together with amorphous urates. Acid urates have the same significance as amorphous urates or uric acid. Acid urates also resemble

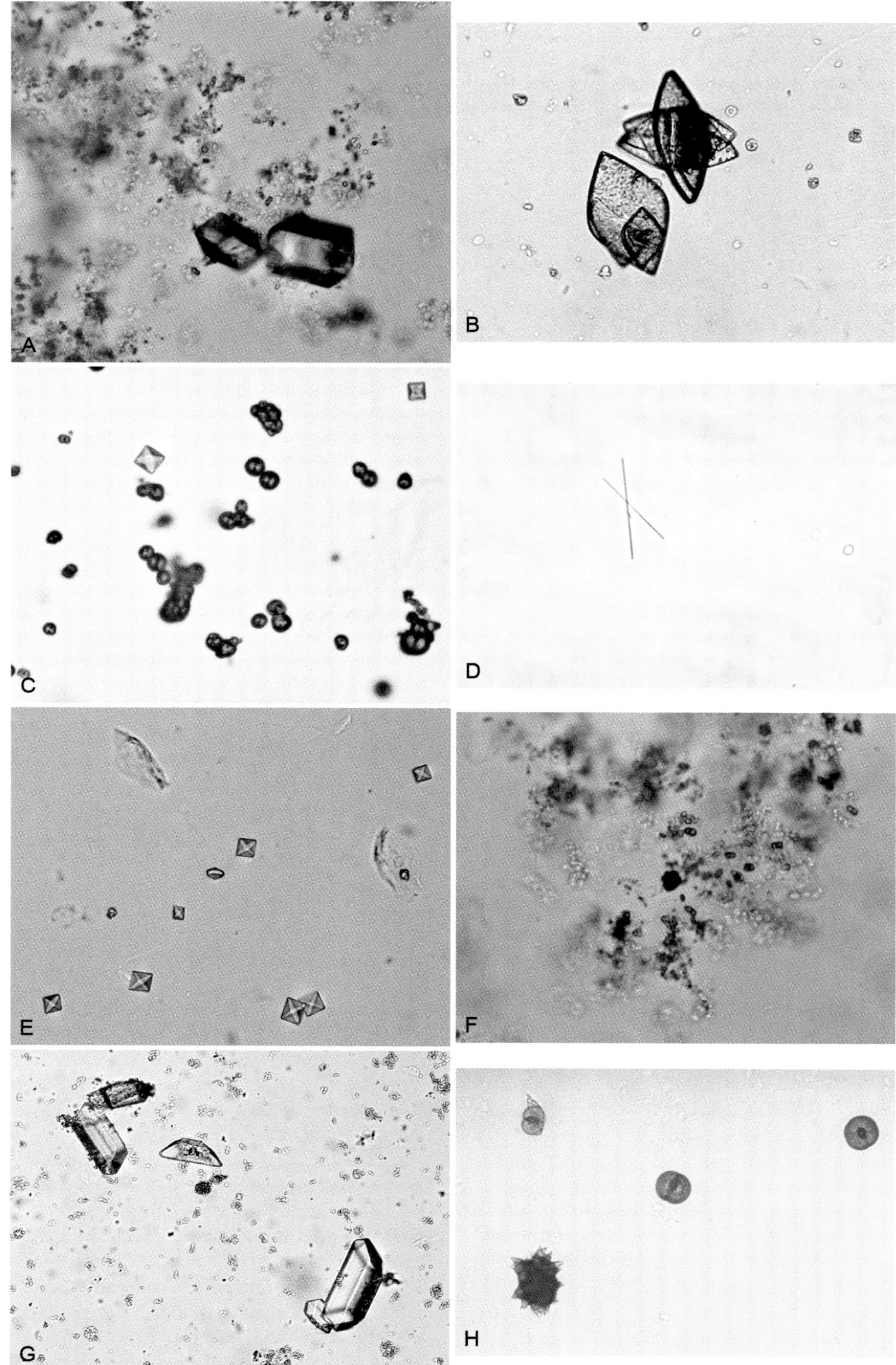

Fig. 13.22 Urinary crystals. (Brightfield magnification.) (A) Amorphous urates (×400); (B) uric acid crystals: common diamond shape; (C) acid urate crystals (×200); (D) monosodium urate (×200); (E) calcium oxalate crystals: octahedral (envelope) form of dehydrate crystals (×200); (F) amorphous phosphates (×400); (G) triple phosphate crystals: typical "coffin-lid" form (×100); (H) ammonium biurate crystals: spheres and "thorn-apple" form (×200);

continued

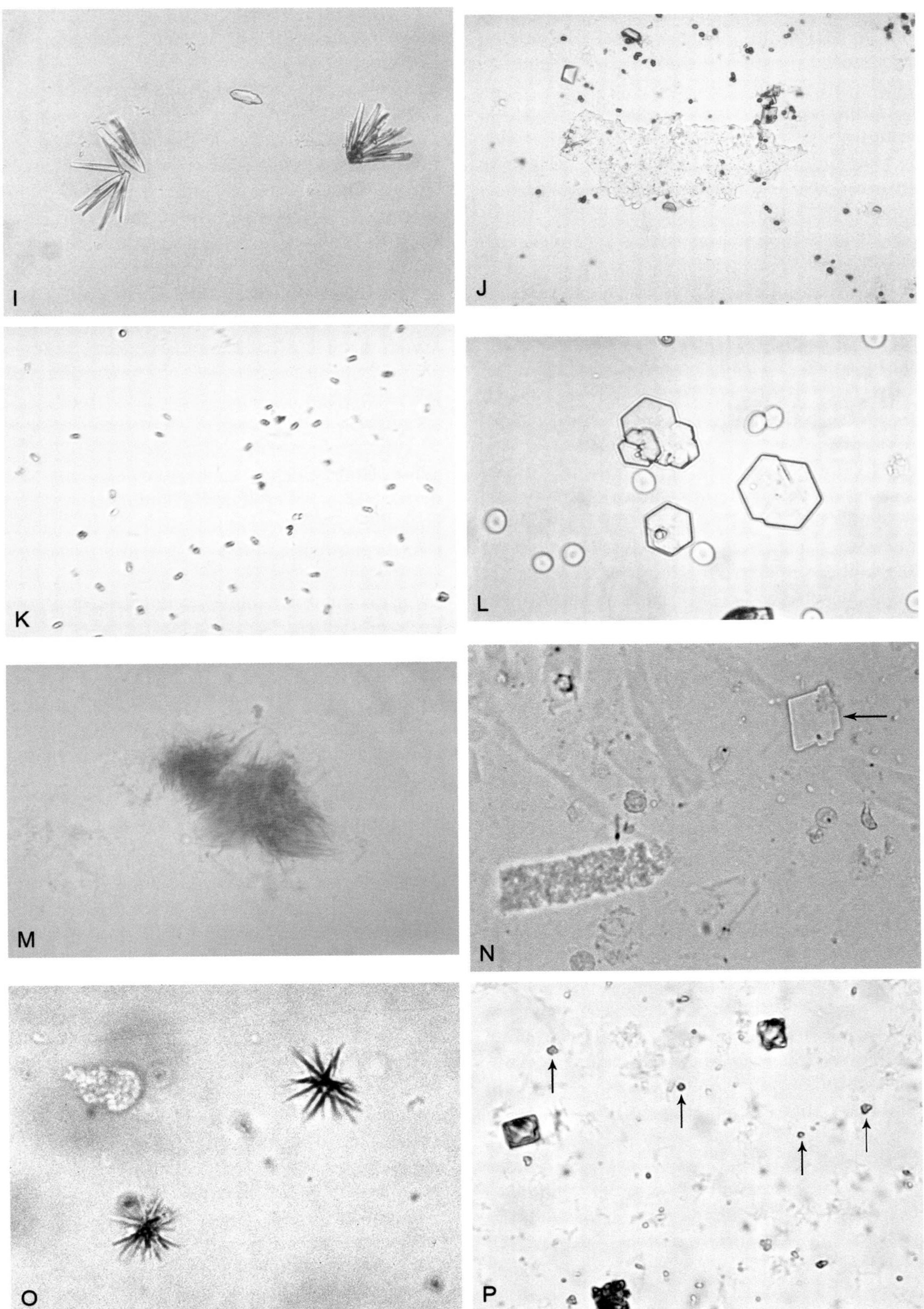

Fig. 13.22—cont'd (I) calcium phosphate crystals: prisms are arranged singly and in rosette forms (×100); (J) calcium phosphate sheet or plate (×100); (K) calcium carbonate crystals: numerous single crystals (dumbbell shape); (L) cystine crystals: thin, colorless, laminated hexagons (×400); (M) tyrosine crystals: fine, silky needles; (N) cholesterol crystal *(arrow)*; (O) bilirubin crystals; (P) hemosiderin granules in urine sediment appear yellow-brown; numerous granules and a clump are present in this field of view; arrows identify four granules. (From Brunzel NA: *Fundamentals of urine and body fluid analysis*, ed 4, Philadelphia, 2018, Saunders.)

sulfamethoxazole, an abnormal crystal of pathologic significance, and are important to recognize for this reason (Fig. 13.22C).

As with amorphous urates and uric acid, the acid urates are soluble at 60°C and in 10% NaOH and are changed to uric acid when treated with glacial acetic acid.

Monosodium or Sodium Urates. The sodium urates are another rare form of uric acid that might be seen in urine. Monosodium urate is the form of uric acid seen in the synovial fluid of patients with gout. If present in urine, it appears as tiny, slender, colorless needles (Fig. 13.22D).

Calcium Oxalate. Calcium oxalate crystals have a characteristic shape referred to as an "envelope." These octahedrons vary somewhat in size but are typically small, colorless, and glistening. Occasionally, they are seen as rectangular forms with pyramidal ends. Less frequently, calcium oxalate crystals may appear in a dumbbell or an ovoid shape similar to RBCs. Unlike RBCs, however, calcium oxalate will polarize light (Fig. 13.22E).

Although most common in acidic urine, calcium oxalate crystals may also be seen in neutral or alkaline urine specimens. They are of little clinical significance, although they may be present in association with stone formation. Calcium oxalate is the most common constituent found in kidney stones. A correlation exists between calcium stones and excess oxalate and uric acid in the urine. (Uric acid may be the nidus for stone formation.) Excess oxalate may result from ingestion of foodstuffs containing oxalic acid, such as spinach and rhubarb, and from ingestion of vitamin C, because oxalic acid is a breakdown product of ascorbic acid. Calcium oxalate crystals may also be seen in cases of ethylene glycol or methoxyflurane poisoning.

Normal Alkaline Crystals. These forms are the "normal" crystals seen in urine of an alkaline pH (generally ≥ 7.0). They are usually phosphate- or calcium-containing crystals. However, the alkaline counterpoint of uric acid, ammonium biurate, is also seen. Phosphates have little clinical significance, although they are associated with an alkaline pH and infection.

Amorphous Phosphates. The amorphous material found in alkaline urine is amorphous phosphate. Generally, the phosphates give a finer or more "lacy" precipitate than the amorphous urates and are colorless (Fig. 13.22F). Phosphates are the most common cause of turbidity in alkaline urine and are seen as a fine, white precipitate microscopically. They do not dissolve when heated but are soluble in acetic acid and dilute hydrochloric acid. Phosphates resemble, and are often seen with, bacteria; care must be taken not to overlook bacteria when phosphates are present.

Triple Phosphate. Triple (ammonium magnesium) phosphates (also referred to as *struvite*) are colorless crystals and typically show great variation in size, from tiny to relatively huge crystals. They have a characteristic "coffin-lid" shape that is impossible to miss (Fig. 13.22G). They may also be seen as large, long prisms that are difficult to distinguish from calcium phosphate. Both triple and calcium phosphates have similar clinical significance, and either may be reported as phosphates. Less often, triple phosphates occur in a fernlike form as they dissolve into solution. They are soluble in dilute acetic acid.

Ammonium Biurate. Ammonium biurate, a salt, is the alkaline counterpart of uric acid and amorphous urates in urine. The crystals are spherical with radial or concentric striations and long prismatic spicules, resembling thorn apples (Fig. 13.22H). They are yellow and may be mistaken for some forms of the sulfonamide drugs that may precipitate out of urine. Sulfa crystals, however, are usually seen in acidic urine. Ammonium biurates are often present in old alkaline urine specimens, especially those that contain unusual sediment constituents and have been retained for teaching purposes. They are much less frequently seen in fresh urine collections. They are soluble at 60°C with acetic acid and in strong alkali. Ammonium biurates will convert to uric acid with concentrated hydrochloric acid or acetic acid.

Calcium Phosphate. Calcium phosphates are colorless crystals occasionally seen in normal alkaline urine. Typically, they appear as slender prisms with a wedgelike end, occurring singly or arranged in rosettes (Fig. 13.22I). They may resemble, and appear with, triple phosphate crystals as long prisms of calcium monohydrogen phosphate, also known as *brushite.* Calcium phosphate may also appear as flat plates, which might be mistaken for large, degenerating squamous epithelial cells (Fig. 13.22J).

Calcium phosphate is insoluble when heated to 60°C, slightly soluble in dilute acetic acid, and soluble in dilute hydrochloric acid.

Calcium Carbonate. Calcium carbonate crystals are tiny, colorless granules that typically occur in pairs ("dumbbells") but also may occur singly (Fig. 13.22K). Because they are so small, calcium carbonate crystals represent part of the amorphous material seen in normal alkaline urine specimens. They are soluble in acetic acid with effervescence.

Abnormal Crystals

With only a few, very rare exceptions, the abnormal urinary crystals are seen in urine specimens of an acid pH, 6.5 or less. Normal crystals of urine may be reported on the basis of microscopic examination (morphology) and pH. However, the abnormal crystals require further confirmation. Whenever possible, this should be a chemical confirmation, although a history of medications or treatment procedures may be the only possible confirmation. Unlike the normal crystals, which are reported as few, moderate, or many, the abnormal crystals are reported as the number seen per average low-power field.

Abnormal crystals may be further classified as *metabolic* (physiologic) or *iatrogenic* (see Table 13.9). The abnormal crystals of metabolic origin are the result of certain disease states or inherited conditions. These include cystine, tyrosine, leucine, cholesterol, bilirubin, and hemosiderin. Iatrogenic crystals are the result of medication or treatment and thus are inadvertently caused by the physician. Examples of iatrogenic crystals include the various sulfonamides, ampicillin, radiographic contrast media, acyclovir, and indinavir sulfate.

Abnormal Crystals of Metabolic Origin.

Cystine. Cystine crystals are colorless, refractile, hexagonal plates that are often laminated (Fig. 13.22L). They may be seen in the urine of patients with the hereditary condition cystinuria.

This is an amino acid transport disorder affecting cystine, ornithine, lysine, and arginine. Of these amino acids, only cystine crystallizes out in the urine. This crystallization of cystine is serious because these patients tend to form cystine stones, which may lead to kidney damage. Patients with cystinuria must always be well hydrated to prevent such stone formation. The crystals may be mistaken for a form of uric acid that is also hexagonal.

Cystine crystals are most insoluble in urine of an acid pH. However, they remain insoluble up to pH 7.4. They are soluble in alkali (especially ammonia) and dilute hydrochloric acid. They are destroyed by the presence of bacteria because of the formation of ammonia. Cystine crystals are insoluble in boiling water, acetic acid, alcohol, and ether.

Tyrosine. Tyrosine crystals are rare but may be present as the result of inherited amino acid disorders (hereditary tyrosinosis, oasthouse urine disease) and, together with leucine, in patients with massive liver failure.

Tyrosine crystals are colorless, fine, silky needles arranged in sheaves or clumps and appear black as the microscope is focused (Fig. 13.22M). They occur in urine of an acid pH. Tyrosine is soluble in alkali and dilute mineral acid. Tyrosine crystals are relatively soluble when heated but are insoluble in alcohol and ether.

Leucine. Leucine crystals are yellow, oily-looking spheres with radial and concentric striations. They are of metabolic origin and extremely rare. Leucine and tyrosine crystals usually appear together and are associated with severe liver disease. Leucine is found in urine of an acid pH.

Cholesterol. Droplets of cholesterol that polarize as a Maltese cross are seen in the urine sediment as free fat, in OFBs, and in fatty casts. However, cholesterol crystals or plates are extremely rare in freshly voided urine sediment; they have rarely been seen after the specimen has been refrigerated. When seen, they have the same clinical significance as the more common globules or droplets.

As with most abnormal crystals, cholesterol crystals are associated with urine of an acidic or neutral pH. Cholesterol crystals are large, flat, hexagonal plates with one or more notched corners (Fig. 13.22N).

When apparent cholesterol crystals are seen in large numbers, the presence of another drug or its crystals should be suspected. Crystals of radiographic media such as meglumine diatrizoate are found in urine collected immediately after intravenous radiographic studies. They are morphologically similar to cholesterol but are associated with a very high specific gravity ($>$1.035 by refractometer) and a false-positive, delayed SSA test for protein. Radiographic media crystals should not be mistaken for cholesterol.

If present, crystals of cholesterol should be associated with other findings, such as free fat, OFBs, or fatty casts. They are more likely to be seen in urine specimens that have been retained and refrigerated.

Absolute chemical confirmation of cholesterol may be difficult. However, cholesterol crystals are very soluble in chloroform, ether, and hot alcohol.

Bilirubin. The presence of crystals of precipitated bilirubin is occasionally seen in the urine sediment of patients with bilirubinuria. This finding has about the same clinical significance as the chemical detection of bilirubin in urine, and these crystals should not be reported in the absence of bilirubin. Bilirubin crystals are seen as reddish-brown needles that cluster in clumps or as spheres (Fig. 13.22O).

Hemosiderin. The pathophysiology of hemosiderin is discussed in the section on renal epithelial cells. However, this abnormal crystal might be mistaken for amorphous urates, a common urine sediment finding.

Hemosiderin may be seen in acid or neutral urine a few days after a severe intravascular hemolytic episode. In unstained urine sediment, hemosiderin appears as coarse, yellow-brown granules. These may be seen as free granules or may be contained within renal epithelial cells, macrophages, or casts. Hemosiderin may be confirmed with the Rous test, a wet Prussian blue stain for iron (Fig. 13.22P). Cytocentrifuged preparations of the urine sediment may also be stained with Prussian blue, as in hematologic stains for iron content.

Abnormal Crystals of Iatrogenic Origin.

Sulfonamides. The presence of these iatrogenic crystals in the urine sediment is an important pathologic finding. Sulfonamides are likely to cause renal damage because the crystals precipitate in the nephron, causing bleeding (hematuria) and oliguria as a result of mechanical blockage of the renal tubules, which may lead to renal failure or shutdown. Precipitation or crystallization of the sulfonamides is prevented by adequate hydration of the patient and possibly alkalization of the urine with diet or medication. Current pharmacology uses more soluble forms of these drugs, and sulfonamide crystals are now an uncommon finding.

The sulfonamides are most likely to precipitate in urine with a low acid pH. The crystals are generally yellow to brown but may be colorless. Shape varies with the actual drug, and the various sulfonamides mimic various forms of uric acid, urates, and biurates. They have been described as colorless needles in sheaves or rosettes, arrowheads, or whetstones; as brownish shocks of wheat with central binding; as colorless to greenish-brown fan-shaped needles; and as dense brown or irregularly divided spheres.

Sulfamethoxazole. Sulfamethoxazole is the sulfonamide crystal found most often in the urine sediment. It is supplied as acetylsulfamethoxazole together with trimethoprim (Bactrim, Septra). Although this is a common drug, occasionally it has been seen to crystallize in urine after unusually high dosage. When present, sulfamethoxazole is seen as a dense brown or an irregularly divided sphere.

Acetylsulfadiazine. Acetylsulfadiazine is a dangerous form of sulfonamide because of its relative insolubility. It is now rarely used. It is seen as yellow-brown sheaves of wheat with eccentric binding.

Sulfadiazine. Sulfadiazine is another form of sulfonamide that is used only rarely. It appears as dense brown globules. These crystals are morphologically similar to ammonium biurates and acid urates.

Ampicillin. Ampicillin crystals appear as long, thin, colorless needles in acidic urine. They are seen only rarely, as the result of large doses of the drug, which may be necessary for treatment of bacterial meningitis.

Radiographic Contrast Media. Crystals of compounds used for diagnostic radiographic procedures, such as meglumine diatrizoate (Renografin, Hypaque), may be precipitated in the urine for a brief period after injection. Radiographic contrast crystals are primarily important because they might be misidentified as cholesterol crystals. Occasionally, their presence is of clinical importance, such as in dehydrated older adult patients, who may experience renal blockage from crystalline precipitation.

Crystals of meglumine diatrizoate may be seen in the urine sediment as flat, four-sided plates, often with a notched corner. They closely resemble cholesterol plates and should not be mistaken for them. They may also occur as long, thin prisms or rectangles.

The presence of radiographic contrast media should be suspected when many crystals resembling cholesterol plates are seen and the specific gravity by refractometer is extremely high (>1.035). Because contrast media do not ionize, however, the specific gravity by reagent strip is unaffected by their presence. When they are present, the urine may show a delayed false-positive SSA precipitation test for protein. This should not be mistaken for true protein precipitation. The presence of radiographic contrast crystals may be confirmed by a clinical history of recent imaging procedures.

Acyclovir. Acyclovir is another drug form that may be seen in the urine sediment in rare cases of patients treated with high doses. Unlike most abnormal crystals, which are seen in acidic urine, acyclovir crystals have been seen in urine of pH 7.5. They appear as colorless, slender needles that are strongly birefringent with polarized light. They may be confirmed by obtaining a drug history.

Indinavir Sulfate. With the use of protease inhibitors in the treatment of HIV infection, the presence of crystals of indinavir sulfate (Crixivan) has been observed. According to product literature, 4% of patients treated with indinavir sulfate have renal stone formation.[8] As with other drugs that might precipitate in the urine, it is important that patients be well hydrated to avoid crystallization of the drug. The presence of these crystals in the urine might be an early sign of stone formation, especially when the patient has clinical evidence of stones, such as pain and hematuria.

Crystals of indinavir sulfate are slender, colorless needles or slender rectangular plates that tend to be arranged in fan-shaped or starburst forms, bundles, or sheaves. They resemble some forms of sulfonamides. Unlike most abnormal crystals, indinavir sulfate is most insoluble at an alkaline pH. The crystals are strongly birefringent with polarized light. Confirmation may depend primarily on the patient's drug history of indinavir use. Confirmation is possible by mass spectrometry or high-performance liquid chromatography, but this is beyond the scope of the routine laboratory.

Other Cellular Constituents

Spermatozoa

Spermatozoa may be present in the urine of both men and women. Laboratory protocol should be established and followed as to when the presence of sperm is to be reported. In fertility studies and cases of possible sexual abuse, the presence of spermatozoa may be an important finding.

Spermatozoa are easily recognized by their oval body (head) and long, delicate tail. The head is about 4 to 6 μm long (smaller and narrower than RBC), and the tail is about 40 to 60 μm long. Spermatozoa may be motile in wet preparation (an aid to identification) or may be stationary. Phase-contrast microscopy is especially helpful in identification (Fig. 13.23).

Bacteria

Under normal conditions, the urinary tract is free of bacteria, but most urine specimens contain at least a few bacteria because of contamination when the urine is voided. Bacteria multiply rapidly when urine stands at room temperature. In specimens that are obtained in a manner suitable for urine culture and kept under sterile conditions, the presence of bacteria may indicate a UTI. In this case the bacteria are likely to be associated with the presence of WBCs, although this is not always true. Bacterial infection should be confirmed by quantitative urine culture.

Bacteria are recognizable morphologically in wet preparation under high power. They are extremely small, only a few micrometers long. They may be either rods or cocci and may occur singly, in pairs, in chains, or in tetrads. Rods are more easily recognized than cocci because of their larger size, although some rods are extremely short and difficult to distinguish from cocci. Bacteria are often motile, which helps in their identification. Occasionally, unusually long, rod-shaped forms with central swelling are seen. These protoplasts are the result of damage to the cell wall by antibiotics (especially penicillins) used in therapy.

Bacteria are most often seen in alkaline urine and may be confused with amorphous material at first, but this will not be a problem as the microscopist gains experience in

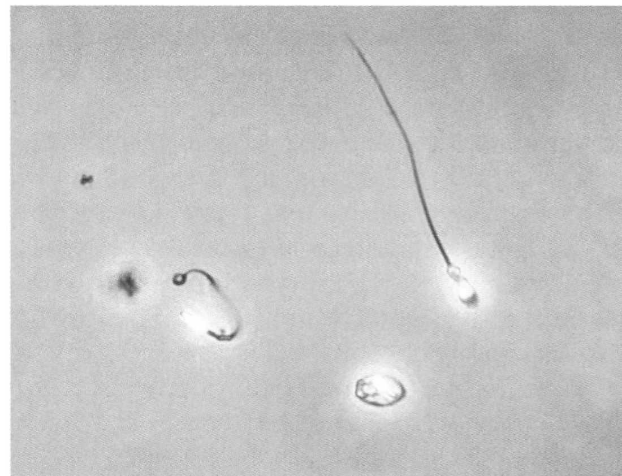

Fig. 13.23 Spermatozoa in urine sediment. One typical and two atypical forms. (Phase contrast, ×400.) (From Brunzel NA: *Fundamentals of urine and body fluid analysis,* ed 4, Philadelphia, 2018, Saunders.)

observation. Phase-contrast microscopy is very useful in the visualization of bacteria, which are difficult to see with brightfield illumination. Although not normally part of urinalysis, Gram-staining a drop of concentrated sediment is helpful in recognition of bacteria in difficult specimens. On Wright-stained cytocentrifuged preparations, all bacteria will stain deep blue-purple (basophilic).

In lower (bladder) UTIs, bacteria are generally but not always associated with the presence of WBCs (leukocytes, PMNs). Mild proteinuria and a positive reagent strip test for nitrites or leukocyte esterase may also be seen. With upper (kidney) UTIs, bacteria may be seen along with WBCs and casts (leukocyte, cellular, granular). The patient may have moderate proteinuria and a positive reagent strip test for nitrites or leukocyte esterase

Yeast

Yeast cells are occasionally seen in urine, especially from female and diabetic patients. They often are the result of contamination of the urine from a vaginal yeast infection. Yeast cells are associated with the presence of sugar in the urine. Sugar is the energy source for yeast cells, which grow and multiply rapidly when sugar is present. Therefore yeast cells are often discovered in the urine of diabetic patients, along with a high sugar content, low pH, and ketones. Yeast cells are also common contaminants from skin and air, and infections are seen in debilitated and immunosuppressed or immunocompromised patients.

Yeast cells are often mistaken for RBCs. They are generally smaller than erythrocytes and show considerable size variation, even within a specimen. Yeast cells have a typically ovoid shape, lack color, and have a smooth and refractive appearance. The most distinguishing characteristic is the presence of little buds, or projections, because of their manner of reproduction. Pseudomycelial forms of *Candida* species (type of yeast usually present) may also be seen. These are elongated cells that may be up to 50 μm long and resemble mycelia of true fungi. These pseudohyphae may be branched and have terminal buds (Fig. 13.24). They are clinically significant in the urine of debilitated patients with severe *Candida* infection, as seen in immunosuppressed patients. Other mycelial forms of yeast have been observed; these should not be mistaken for casts.

Parasites

Trichomonas Vaginalis. *Trichomonas vaginalis* is the parasite most frequently seen in urine specimens. This protozoan is primarily responsible for vaginal infections, but it can also infect the urethra, periurethral glands, bladder, and prostate. It generally resides in the vagina in women and prostate in men, where it feeds on the mucosal surface and ingests bacteria and leukocytes that may be present. The organism is motile, which is an aid to its identification. When an infection is suspected, direct swabs of the vagina or urethra are examined, although the organisms may be seen contaminating the urine sediment.

T. vaginalis is a unicellular flagellated organism, a protozoan. It has a characteristic pear-shaped appearance, with a single nucleus, four anterior flagella, and an undulating membrane, as well as a sharp, protruding posterior axostyle (Fig. 13.25). The most distinguishing feature of this trichomonad is its motility: a rapid, jerky, rotating, nondirectional motion that is easily recognized in wet preparations. The organisms are larger than typical leukocytes (up to 30 μm long) and may resemble transitional epithelial cells, especially when no longer motile. Phase-contrast microscopy is particularly useful in visualization, especially of the flagella. When stained, the cells lose their characteristic motility as they round up and die, appearing similar to degenerating transitional epithelial cell forms (see Chapter 15).

Other Parasites. Various other parasites may be seen in urine, mostly as the result of fecal or vaginal contamination. Some may be common to particular geographic areas and patient populations. All require special knowledge for identification, but parasites may be noticed initially during urinalysis and then referred to a microbiologist for identification.

Enterobius vermicularis, or pinworm, is a fairly common helminth infecting the intestinal tract that may occasionally be found in the urine in larval or egg (ova) form (see Chapter 15). Other

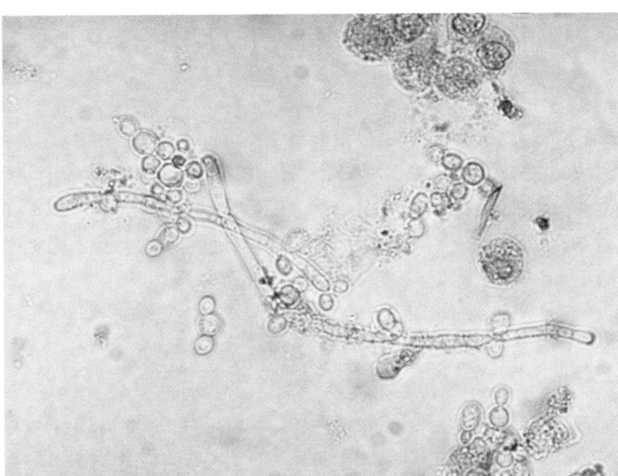

Fig. 13.24 Budding yeast and pseudohyphae. Leukocytes also present singly and as a clump. (Brightfield, Sedi-Stain, ×400.) (From Brunzel NA: *Fundamentals of urine and body fluid analysis*, ed 4, Philadelphia, 2018, Saunders.)

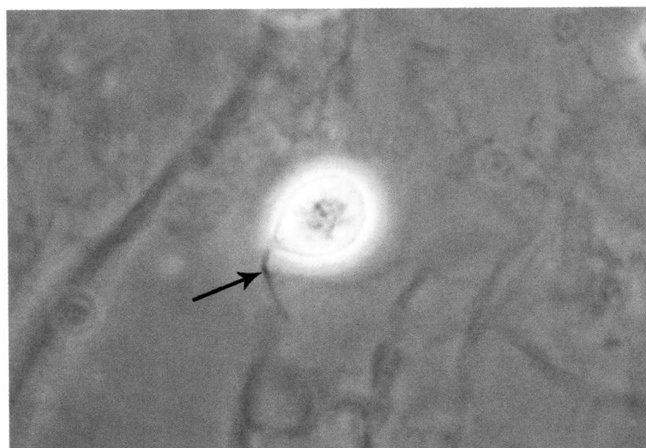

Fig. 13.25 *Trichomonas vaginalis* in urine sediment. Arrow points to the protruding posterior axostyle. (Phase contrast, ×400.) (From Brunzel NA: *Fundamentals of urine and body fluid analysis*, ed 4, Philadelphia, 2018, Saunders.)

parasites occasionally seen in urine include *Trichuris* (whipworm), *Schistosoma haematobium, Strongyloides,* and *Giardia,* as well as various amoebae. *S. haematobium* ova can be introduced directly into the urine from the bladder wall mucosa.

Various insects or "bugs" possibly seen in urine specimens include lice, fleas, bedbugs, mites, and ticks.

Tumor Cells

Tumor cells related to malignant conditions such as transitional cell carcinoma and other cell forms with altered cytologic features may be found in the urine sediment. These cell forms cannot be diagnosed from the usual sediment preparation but require special collection, cytocentrifugation, and stains and examination by qualified personnel in cytology. If tumor cells are suspected from the examination of the sediment, the specimen should be referred accordingly. The presence of RBCs in the chemical examination of the urine is an early diagnostic clue.

Contaminants and Artifacts

Many objects and structures in the urine sediment are contaminants or artifacts that distract the observer's attention from the important urinary constituents. These are the objects that beginning microscopists tend to see first when attempting a microscopic examination of the urine sediment. It seems to be a general rule that if an object is easy to see, it is unimportant.

Starch

Granules of starch are common contaminants in the urine sediment. They are the result of the use of barrier-protective gloves in all areas of the laboratory and medical care. *Starch* refers to cornstarch, a carbohydrate often used to line surgical or barrier-protective gloves. It is different from talc, or talcum, which is hydrated magnesium silicate, a chunky, irregular crystal.

Starch is a ubiquitous structure that is easily recognized, but it must not be confused with globules or droplets of cholesterol. Both starch and cholesterol globules are birefringent and polarize as a Maltese cross (white cross on a black background) when viewed with polarized light. Starch is most easily recognized with brightfield microscopy. It is seen as an irregular, generally round granule with a central dimple or slit. Even when viewed with polarized light, the Maltese cross formation produced by starch is more irregular than the very round, regular formation produced by droplets of cholesterol.

Fibers (Including Disposable Diaper Fibers)

Disposable diaper fibers are particularly troublesome in their resemblance to waxy casts. They may be seen in the urine of both infants and incontinent adults. They should be suspected when other findings associated with waxy casts, such as protein, are absent. As described earlier, diaper fibers will polarize light, but waxy casts will not.

Other contaminants may be introduced into the urine specimen on collection or by laboratory personnel during specimen processing or examination. These include cotton threads, wood fibers, synthetic fibers, and hair. These are all highly refractile structures that should not be mistaken for casts.

Air Bubbles

Air bubbles are highly refractile, structureless, and easily recognized. They may be introduced as the coverglass is applied to the urine sediment or as the sediment is introduced into the standardized slide.

Oil Droplets

Oil droplets may be the result of contamination from such lubricants as vaginal cream, catheter lubricant, and mineral oil. They may be confused with RBCs or fat globules of physiologic origin. Oil droplets are highly refractile and structureless.

Contaminating oil should be distinguished from fat of physiologic origin. True lipiduria is usually associated with other findings, such as proteinuria, fatty casts, and OFBs, as described previously.

Glass Fragments

Colorless, highly refractile, pleomorphic fragments of glass (probably from very small pieces of coverglass) might appear similar to crystals.

Stains

The various supravital stains used in the examination of the urine sediment may precipitate, especially when added to urine of an alkaline pH. This may be seen as an amorphous purple granulation or as brown-to-purple needle-shaped crystals in clusters. Sudan III fat stain may also precipitate as clusters of needle-shaped crystals that are bright red or red-orange. When such precipitation occurs, identification of pathologic structures that might be present is difficult.

Pollen Grains

Pollen grains may be seen as a urine contaminant, especially on a seasonal basis. They are fairly large and regularly shaped, with a thick cell wall. Pollen grains may resemble the eggs of some parasitic worms.

Fecal Contamination

The presence of fecal elements in urine is usually the result of contamination during collection. If there is a *fistula* (abnormal connection) between the colon and the urinary tract, fecal constituents may be seen in the urine. This is a serious pathologic condition that leads to recurrent UTI.

The presence of feces in the urine is usually observed as an overall yellow-brown color of the gross urine specimen. Microscopic findings include plant fibers, skeletal muscle fibers, and microorganisms. Rarely, columnar epithelial cells from the gut mucosa or squamous epithelial cells from the anal mucosa are seen.

When detection of a fistula is clinically indicated, patients may be fed activated charcoal, which is carefully searched for in the urine. The presence of charcoal in the urine demonstrates an abnormal connection between the gut and the urinary tract.

Specimen Changes on Standing

Changes may occur as the urine stands. RBCs become distorted because of the lack of an isotonic solution (see Table 13.2). Erythrocytes either swell or become crenated, which makes them difficult to recognize, and they finally disintegrate. WBCs rapidly disintegrate in hypotonic solutions. Casts disintegrate, especially as the urine becomes alkaline, because they must have sufficient acidity and solute concentration to exist. Other components that are found only in acidic urine will disappear as the urine becomes alkaline. The increase in alkalinity results from the growth of bacteria and production of ammonia. Finally, bacteria multiply rapidly, obscuring various components.

AUTOMATION IN URINALYSIS

Reagent strips were introduced to replace individual physical and manual chemical methods in the analysis of urine. Originally, reagent strip reactions were compared with a standardized color chart by a technologist. Today, semiautomated instruments and totally automated systems are available for routine testing in urinalysis and in some cases, microscopic examination (Table 13.10).

Semiautomated Systems

Semiautomated systems, the term that describes systems in which an analyzer is used to read the commercial reagent strip results of chemical examination using an instrument, use reflectance photometers for reading their respective reagent strips. Once the strip is placed in the analyzer, the microprocessor mechanically moves the strip into the reflectometer, turns on the light source needed, records the reflectance data, calculates the results, and removes the strip for disposal. If analysis is fully automated, for chemical analyses of glucose, ketones, proteins, and other constituents, the specimen is aspirated from the sample tube and added to a strip containing nine reactive reagent pads (for chemical and physicochemical tests) and one nonreactive pad (for color) per specimen. Use of this reflectance spectrophotometric instrument eliminates the need for "dipping" the reagent strip into the patient's urine

TABLE 13.10 Examples of Current Urine Analyzers

Name of Instrument	Manufacturer	Comments
Iris iChem 100	Beckman-Coulter, Inc.	Semiautomated. No microscopy analyzer.
Iris iChemVELOCITY	Beckman-Coulter, Inc.	Fully automated urinalysis chemistry solution measurements by light transmission (color), light scatter (turbidity/clarity), and refractive index (specific gravity). In addition to standard analysis, the iChemVELOCITY provides results for ascorbic acid levels in samples, a common urinalysis test interference factor.
Iris iRICELL 1500 2000, 3000	Beckman-Coulter, Inc.	Iris iRICELL 1500 is intended for low-volume laboratories (fewer than 70 urine tests per day). It integrates urine chemistry and microscopy in a fully automated instrument that tests urines and body fluids by a proprietary digital flow morphology technology using auto-particle recognition (APR) software for improved accuracy of results. Iris iRICELL 3000, designed for high-volume automation, uses the same technology as the Iris iRICELL 1500.
iQ200 series Iris iQ200SELECT Iris IQ200ELITE Iris iQ200SPRINT	Beckman-Coulter, Inc.	iQ200SELECT is available as either a stand-alone system or connected to an iChemVELOCITY urine chemistry system to form an automated iRICELL Workcell. It is designed for low-volume workloads. It automates up to 40 microscopic samples per hour. Using the Iris's proprietary digital flow morphology technology of APR software, urine particles are isolated, identified, and characterized on the screen. This autoclassification system virtually eliminates the need for manual microscopy. Iris iQ200ELITE is designed for medium- to high-volume workloads. The Iris iQ200SPRINT is one of the fastest high-capacity systems on the market.
Urine Albumin	HemoCue	Immunoturbidimetric reaction in microcuvettes read by photometer to detect low levels of urinary albumin. No microscopy analyzer.
URISED 3	Elektronika Kft	Urinary sediment optical system combining brightfield and phase-contrast microscopy.
URISYS 1100	Roche Diagnostics	Semiautomated instrument that uses reflectance photometer to detect glucose, bilirubin, ketones, occult blood, protein, nitrite, and leukocytes. No microscopy analyzer.
URISYS 2400 Cobas 6500 Urine Analyzer Series	Roche Diagnostics	Fully automated urine test strip analyzer with measurements by reflectance photometry and specific gravity (refractometer). Cobas 6500 provides fully automated urine test strip analysis with a throughput of up to 240 samples/hour. Uses reagent strip with ascorbic acid resistance.

Continued

TABLE 13.10 Examples of Current Urine Analyzers—cont'd

Name of Instrument	Manufacturer	Comments
		New technology of photometer for strip reading: an image sensor (camera chip) performs reflectance photometric measurements on each test pad of a test strip with four wavelengths. Twelve measured parameters: pH, leukocytes, nitrite, protein, glucose, ketones, urobilinogen, bilirubin, erythrocytes, gravity, color, and clarity. Uses digital imaging for microscopic examination. This new technology also allows the differentiation of intact and lysed erythrocytes up to 50 cells/μL and avoids the measuring failures caused by dust, low sample volume, or incorrect test strip positioning. The Cobas U 701 module provides fully automated urine microscopy analysis that captures, retains, and reports 15 images/sample. Eleven measured parameters: erythrocytes, leukocytes, squamous epithelial cells, nonsquamous epithelial cells, bacteria, hyaline casts, pathologic casts, crystals, yeasts, mucus, and sperm.
CLINITEK Status CLINITEK Advantus	Siemens Healthcare Diagnostics Inc.	Semiautomated. The CLINITEK Status+ Analyzer is a point-of-care urinalysis analyzer designed to read only Siemens Healthcare Diagnostics urine test strips and CLINITEST hCG cassettes. The CLINITEK Advantus Urinary Chemistry Analyzer provides an automated reading of the Multistix family of urinalysis tests. Semiquantitative tests include albumin, bilirubin, creatinine, glucose, ketone, leukocytes, nitrite, pH, protein, specific gravity, and urobilinogen. Other testing can include kidney disease testing by determination of the albumin-to-creatinine ratio, albumin-to-protein ratio, and pregnancy testing for human chorionic gonadotropin (hCG). The CLINITEK Status+ Urine Analyzer features new automatic checks (Auto-Checks). The analyzer automatically checks each test strip for humidity exposure, common sample interferences, and strip identification for Siemens test strips.
CLINITEK Atlas	Siemens Healthcare Diagnostics Inc.	Fully automated measurements by reflectance photometry (color), turbidimetry (clarity), and specific gravity (refractive index). No microscopy analyzer.
CLINITEK Novus Urine Analyzer		This analyzer combines dry-pad urine chemistry technology and a cassette test format to help ensure maximum productivity and standardized testing with other CLINITEK analyzers. This high-volume instrument measures specific gravity, blood, bilirubin, pH, leukocytes, color and clarity, protein, nitrite, glucose, urobilinogen, and ketones. An automated check for humidity exposure is included. No microscopy analyzer.
CLINITEK AUWi PRO System	Siemens Healthcare Diagnostics Inc.	This instrument combines dry-pad urine chemistry testing and sediment analysis for seamless integration of the CLINITEK Novus and the Sysmex UF-Automated Urine Chemistry Analyz1000i Urine Particle Analyzer. The UF-1000i offers the following measurement technologies: urine fluorescent flow cytometry, two stains with fluorescent dye, and a separate bacteria channel for improved discrimination. The UF-1000i identifies the formed elements—red blood cells, white blood cells, epithelial cells, hyaline casts, and bacteria—and flags pathologic casts, crystals, small round cells, sperm, yeast, and mucus.
Uri-Trak 120 Urine Analyzer	Stanbio	The Uri-Trak 120 Urine Analyzer uses Stanbio Uri-Chek 10SG urine test strips. The instrument is Clinical Laboratory Improvement Amendments of 1988 (CLIA 88) waived. It is capable of reading one strip at a time in the single-test option (60 strips/hour) or up to 120 tests per hour in continuous test mode.

specimen. It measures clarity, color, and specific gravity by refractive index. Samples are identified by bar code, and results may be interfaced to the laboratory computer for reporting.

Fully Automated Systems

Fully automated urine analyzers now play an important role in routine urinalysis in most large-volume laboratories. New analyzers and new associated modules on workstation platforms are dynamic and ever-changing. Systems for the chemical analysis of urine have similar formats, but approaches to the examination of urinary sediment vary among cuvette-based digital microscopy, digital flow microscopy, and flow cytometry.

A totally automated sample analysis with a fully automated urine chemistry analyzer begins with the urine specimen. Instruments of this type determine the physical characteristics of color, clarity, and specific gravity, but the methods used vary.

For example, color assessment can include an additional chemically impregnated pad on a reagent strip to determine color by reflectance photometry; other manufacturers use spectrophotometry at multiple wavelengths to determine color. Light scatter or light transmission is used to determine the clarity of the urine. Most fully automated urine analyzers use the refractive index for the determination of specific gravity. Once all of the testing is completed, the results are sent to data storage and are printed on a form or uploaded to the laboratory information system.

Automated Microscopy

Microscopic examination of urinary sediment can be automated through the use of digital imaging. Automated microscopy analyzers are newer innovations in urinalysis.

Manufacturers use various technologies for urinary microscopic analysis, such as digital flow microscopy or flow cell digital imaging followed by urine particle recognition using neural network software. Another type of urine microscopy analyzer technology is flow cytometry. This technology identifies and categorizes the particles in urine. A third type of urine microscopy analyzer is automated cuvette-based digital microscopy. This system takes digital images of entire microscopic fields of view of urine sediment on the bottom of a cuvette. Proprietary software then identifies and classifies the urinary sediment components.

CASE STUDIES

CASE STUDY 13.1

A 20-year-old female college student with a sore throat is seen in the student health service. A throat swab is cultured and reported positive for group A β-hemolytic streptococci. She is treated with an intramuscular injection of penicillin. Two weeks later, she wakes up in the morning and finds that she has decreased urine volume, and her urine is dark red. She also has a fever and swelling in her feet. She returns to the student health service, where urine is collected for urinalysis. The following urinalysis results were obtained:

Physical Appearance

Color: Red
Transparency: Cloudy

Chemical Screening

pH: 6.0
Specific gravity: 1.025
Protein (reagent strip): 100 mg/dL
Blood: Large
Nitrite: Negative
Leukocyte esterase: Negative
Glucose: Negative
Ketones: Trace
Bilirubin: Negative
Urobilinogen: Normal

Microscopic Examination (*hpf,* high-power field; *lpf,* low-power field):

RBCs: 10 to 25/hpf; dysmorphic forms present
WBCs: 0 to 2/hpf
Casts: 2 to 5 red blood cell casts/lpf
Crystals: Moderate amorphous urates

Multiple Choice Questions

Answers are in Appendix A.

1. Based on the patient's history and laboratory data, what is the most probable cause of her proteinuria?
   a. Glomerular damage
   b. Lower urinary tract disorder
   c. Prerenal disorders
   d. Tubular (or interstitial) damage
2. The presence of dysmorphic RBCs and RBC casts indicates which of the following?
   a. Bleeding from kidney stone formation
   b. Kidney disease located in the glomerulus
   c. Kidney infection
   d. Probable menstrual contamination
3. The trace reagent strip reaction for ketone and the presence of amorphous urates in the urine sediment of this patient are probably the result of which of the following?
   a. A false-positive ketone reaction caused by sensitivity of the test
   b. Dehydration caused by fever, with concentration of urine
   c. The presence of dysmorphic RBCs and RBC casts
   d. The presence of protein

Critical Thinking Group Discussion Questions

1. Based on the laboratory data, what is a likely diagnosis for this patient?
2. How does this patient's condition differ from the conditions of other patients who might have similar laboratory findings?

Note: Narrative answers are posted on the instructor EVOLVE website.

CASE STUDY 13.2

An 8-year-old girl complains of feeling like she needs to urinate all the time. Her urine burns when she does void, and it is cloudy. She is seen at her pediatrician's office, where urine is collected for routine urinalysis and culture. The following urinalysis results were obtained:

Physical Appearance
Color: Pale
Transparency: Cloudy

Chemical Screening
pH: 7.5
Specific gravity: 1.010
Protein (reagent strip): Trace
Blood: Negative
Nitrite: Positive
Leukocyte esterase: Positive
Glucose: Negative
Ketones: Negative
Bilirubin: Negative
Urobilinogen: Normal

Microscopic Examination
RBCs: 0 to 2/hpf
WBCs: 50 to 100/hpf; clumps of white cells seen
Casts: None seen
Crystals: Moderate amorphous phosphates
Bacteria: Many rods

Multiple Choice Questions
Answers are in Appendix A.

1. The positive reagent strip test for nitrite in this patient is probably caused by which of the following?
   a. Infection from Gram-negative bacteria
   b. Infection from Gram-positive bacteria
   c. Yeast infection
   d. Old urine specimen, unsuitable for examination
2. The positive reagent strip test for leukocyte esterase in this patient is caused by the presence of which of the following?
   a. Bacteria
   b. Protein
   c. Red blood cells
   d. White blood cells
3. This patient's alkaline pH is caused by the presence of which of the following?
   a. Bacteria
   b. Leukocyte esterase
   c. Nitrite
   d. Protein

Critical Thinking Group Discussion Questions

1. Based on the laboratory data, what is a likely diagnosis for this patient?
2. How does this patient's condition differ from the conditions of other patients who might have similar laboratory findings?

Note: Narrative answers are posted on the instructor EVOLVE website.

CASE STUDY 13.3

A 45-year-old man has been a paraplegic since being involved in a motorcycle accident 20 years ago. He has a history of recurrent urinary tract infections (UTIs) as a result of infection from an indwelling catheter. He now has severe back pain, with fever, chills, and vomiting. He has been exposed to "the flu" and seeks medical attention. A midstream urine specimen is collected for examination and culture. The following routine urinalysis results were obtained:

Physical Appearance
Color: Yellow
Transparency: Cloudy

Chemical Screening
pH: 6.5
Specific gravity: 1.010
Protein (reagent strip): 100 mg/dL
Blood: Moderate
Nitrite: Negative
Leukocyte esterase: Positive
Glucose: Negative
Ketones: Negative
Bilirubin: Negative
Urobilinogen: Normal

Microscopic Examination
RBCs: 2 to 5/hpf
WBCs: 10 to 25/hpf
Casts: 5 to 10 WBC casts/lpf
Bacteria: Moderate rods

Multiple Choice Questions
Answers are in Appendix A.

1. This patient's proteinuria is probably caused by which of the following?
   a. Glomerular damage
   b. Lower urinary tract disorder
   c. Prerenal disorder
   d. Tubular (or interstitial) damage
2. Concerning the positive leukocyte esterase and the negative nitrite in this patient, which of the following statements is correct?
   a. The leukocyte esterase test is probably a false-positive reaction.
   b. The negative nitrite reaction is probably caused by insensitivity of the test or lack of sufficient incubation of urine in the bladder.
   c. The positive leukocyte esterase reaction indicates that an upper UTI is present.
   d. The presence of a bacterial infection is ruled out because of the negative nitrite reaction.
3. Concerning the positive reagent strip test for blood and the relatively low level of RBCs seen in the urine sediment of this patient, which of the following statements is correct?
   a. The presence of hematuria is not consistent with the disease exhibited by this patient.
   b. The presence of protein is probably interfering with the chemical test for blood.
   c. The reagent strip test is extremely sensitive and consistent with the microscopic findings.
   d. The reagent strip test is probably falsely positive because of the presence of ascorbic acid.

Critical Thinking Group Discussion Questions

1. The presence of white blood cells, bacteria, and cellular casts in this urine specimen indicates what clinical condition?
2. How does this patient's condition differ from the conditions of other patients who might have similar laboratory findings?

Note: Narrative answers are posted on the instructor EVOLVE website.

CASE STUDY 13.4

A 12-year-old boy has a history of several infections in the past few months. He is now very lethargic and swollen, with generalized edema. He tells his mother that his urine is very foamy when he urinates and that he feels "awful." He is seen by his pediatrician, and urinalysis is performed, with the following results:

Physical Appearance

Color: Pale
Transparency: Cloudy
Foam: Abundant white foam

Chemical Screening

pH: 6.0
Specific gravity: 1.010
Protein (reagent strip): >2000 mg/dL
Blood: Trace
Nitrite: Negative
Leukocyte esterase: Negative
Glucose: Negative
Ketones: Negative
Bilirubin: Negative
Urobilinogen: Negative

Microscopic Examination

RBCs: 0 to 2/hpf
WBCs: 0 to 2/hpf
Casts: 5 to 10 fatty casts/lpf; 2 to 5 hyaline casts/lpf
Epithelial cells: Few renal epithelial cells; many oval fat bodies present
Other: Moderate free fat globules seen

Multiple Choice Questions

Answers are in Appendix A.

1. The abundant white foam in this urine specimen is caused by the presence of which of the following?
   a. Blood
   b. Casts
   c. Fat
   d. Protein
2. The edema seen in this patient is caused by the presence of which of the following?
   a. Blood
   b. Casts
   c. Oval fat bodies
   d. Protein
3. The presence of fatty casts, oval fat bodies, renal epithelial cells, and free fat in this case indicates which of the following?
   a. Lower UTI
   b. Allergic reaction
   c. Upper UTI
   d. Severe renal dysfunction, probably glomerular

Critical Thinking Group Discussion Questions

1. Based on the laboratory data, what is a likely diagnosis for this patient?
2. How does this patient's condition differ from the conditions of other patients who might have similar laboratory findings?

Note: Narrative answers are posted on the instructor EVOLVE website.

CASE STUDY 13.5

A 9-year-old boy has a history of a recent viral infection. He now feels faint and is feverish, and he is generally not well. He has to urinate frequently and is very thirsty. His breath smells fruity. He is seen in an urgent care clinic, where blood is drawn and urine collected for routine urinalysis. The following urinalysis results were obtained:

Physical Appearance

Color: Pale
Transparency: Clear

Chemical Screening

pH: 5.0
Specific gravity (refractometer): 1.029
Specific gravity (reagent strip): 1.005
Protein (reagent strip): Negative
Blood: Negative
Nitrite: Negative
Leukocyte esterase: Negative
Glucose: >2000 mg/dL
Ketones: Large
Bilirubin: Negative
Urobilinogen: Negative

Microscopic Examination

RBCs: 0 to 2/hpf
WBCs: 0 to 2/hpf

Multiple Choice Questions

Answers are in Appendix A.

1. The difference in the specific gravity values in this specimen is probably caused by which of the following?
   a. Ability of the refractometer to measure only nonionizing substances
   b. Difference in the principles of the methods
   c. Failure to use proper quality control
   d. Instrument error
2. This patient is at risk of losing consciousness as a result of which of the following?
   a. Diabetic coma
   b. Hypoglycemia
   c. Infection
   d. Kidney failure
3. Which of the following conditions is exhibited by this patient?
   a. Anorexia nervosa
   b. Diabetes insipidus
   c. Diabetes mellitus
   d. Galactosemia

Critical Thinking Group Discussion Questions

1. Why are ketone bodies present in such a large quantity?
2. How does this patient's condition differ from the conditions of other patients who might demonstrate the presence of ketone bodies?

Note: Narrative answers are posted on the instructor EVOLVE website.

REFERENCES

1. Angeletti LR, Gazzaniga V: Theophilus' Auctoritas: the role of De urinis in the medical curriculum of the 12th–13th centuries, *Am J Nephrol* 19:165–171, 1999.
2. Stankovic AK, DiLauri E: Quality improvements in the pre-analytical phase: focus on urine specimen workflow, *Clin Lab Med* 28(2):339–350, 2008.
3. Ringsrud KM, Linné JJ: *Urinalysis and body fluids: a color text and atlas,* St Louis, 1995, Mosby, 25–27. This section is reprinted with permission.
4. Clinical and Laboratory Standards Institute: *Routine urinalysis and collection, transportation, and preservation of urine specimens: approved guideline* (GP16-A2), ed 2, 2001, Wayne, Pa, Clinical and Laboratory Standards Institute.
5. Becton Dickinson: A comparative evaluation of spray coated urinalysis preservative tubes with current BD Vacutainer plus urinalysis preservative tubes for routine urinalysis testing on the Sysmex UF-50 and Siemens Clinitek Atlas systems. http://www.bd.com. Accessed December 2013.
6. Cohen HT, Spiegel DM: Air-exposed urine dipsticks give false-positive results for glucose and false-negative results for blood, *Am J Clin Pathol* 96:398, 1991.
7. Schweitzer SS, Schumann JL, Schumann GB: Quality assurance guideline of the urinalysis laboratory, *J Med Technol* 3(11):569, 1986.
8. Drug package insert: *indinavir sulfate,* West Point, Pa, 1996, Merck & Co.

BIBLIOGRAPHY

Altekin E, Kadiçesme O, Akan P: et. al.: New generation IQ-200 automated urine microscopy analyzer compared with KOVA cell chamber, *J Clin Lab Anal* 24(2):67–71, 2010.

Bayer Health Care Diagnostics Division: *Modern urine chemistry,* Tarrytown, NY, 2004, Bayer Health Care.

Brunzel NA: *Fundamentals of urine and body fluid analysis, ed 4,* St Louis, 2018, Elsevier, pp. 287–346.

Busby DE, Atkins RC: The detection and measurement of microalbuminuria: a challenge for clinical chemistry, *MLO Med Lab Obs* 37(2):8, 2005.

College of American Pathologists: Clinical microscopy [glossary entry]. In 1996 Proficiency Testing Program, Northfield, Ill, 1996, CAP, p 12.

Dumonceaux MD, Gamez M: Rediscovering urine chemistry—and und understanding its limitations, *MLO* 48(12):12–14, 2016.

Haber MH: *Urine casts: their microscopy and clinical significance,* ed 2, Chicago, 1976, American Society of Clinical Pathologists.

Haber MH: *Urinary sediment: a textbook atlas,* Chicago, 1981, American Society of Clinical Pathologists.

Haber MH: *A primer of microscopic urinalysis,* ed 2, Garden Grove, Calif, 1991, Hycor Biomedical.

Henry JB, Lauzon RL, Schumann GB: Basic examination of urine. In Henry JB, editor: *Clinical diagnosis and management by laboratory methods, ed 21*, Philadelphia, 2008, Saunders.

Kaplan LA, Pesce AJ: *Clinical chemistry: theory, analysis, and correlation, ed 5,* St Louis, 2010, Mosby.

Karcher DS, McPherson RA: Cerebrospinal, synovial, and serous body fluids and alternative specimens. In McPherson RA, Pincus MR, editors: *Henry's clinical diagnosis and management by laboratory methods, ed 22*, Philadelphia, 2011, Elsevier, pp 480–508.

Kulkarni S: Urine cultures, *CAP Today* 27(9):12–14, 2013.

Mahon CR, Smith LA: Standardization of the urine microscopic examination, *Clin Lab Sci* 3:328, 1990.

Midyett R: Urinalysis: Are we done spinning yet? *MLO* 48(12):15, 2016.

Nikon: Microscopy U: polarized light microscopy. http://www.microscopyu.com/articles/polarized/polarizedintro.html. Retrieved August 2005.

Schneider's Children's Hospital at North Shore Department of Urology: http://www.schneiderchildrenshospital.org/peds_html_fixed/peds/urology/urinaryant.htm, Retrieved August 2005.

Schumann GB, Schumann JL, Marcussen N: *Cytodiagnostic urinalysis of renal and lower urinary tract disorders,* New York, 1995, Igaku-Shoin Medical Publishers.

Wesarachkitti B, Khejonnit V, Pratumvinit B, et al: Performance evaluation and comparison of the fully automated urinalysis analyzers UX-2000 and Cobas 6500, *Lab Med* 47(2), 2016.

REVIEW QUESTIONS (ANSWERS IN APPENDIX A)

Overview of Urinalysis

1. The parts of a routine urinalysis include:
   a. Physical
   b. Chemical
   c. Microscopic
   d. All the above

Renal Anatomy and Physiology

2. The formation of urine begins in the:
   a. Nephron
   b. Glomerulus
   c. Ureter
   d. Bladder

3. What is the principal end product of protein metabolism in the urine?
   a. Uric acid
   b. Creatinine
   c. Glucose
   d. Urea

Composition of Urine

4. Which of the following is true about the first morning urine specimen?
   a. It contains high levels of analytes and cellular elements.
   b. It is preferred for culture and sensitivity testing.
   c. It is used for substances affected by diurnal variation.
   d. It is the most common type of specimen collected.

Collection and Preservation of Urine Specimens

5. After collection with no gross alterations, how long can urine be refrigerated?
   a. 2 to 4 hours
   b. 4 to 6 hours
   c. 6 to 8 hours
   d. 8 to 10 hours
6. Which of the following preservatives will allow urine to be kept at room temperature with results comparable to refrigeration?
   a. Hydrochloric acid
   b. Boric acid
   c. Toluene
   d. All of the above

Physical Properties of Urine

7. Anuria is:
   a. Any increase in urine volume, even temporary
   b. Complete absence of urine formation
   c. Consistent elimination of 2000 mL urine per 24 hours
   d. Excretion of 500 mL urine per 24 hours
8. Diuresis is:
   a. Any increase in urine volume, even temporary
   b. Complete absence of urine formation
   c. Consistent elimination of 2000 mL urine per 24 hours
   d. Excretion of 500 mL urine per 24 hours
9. Polyuria is:
   a. Any increase in urine volume, even temporary
   b. Complete absence of urine formation
   c. Consistent elimination of 2000 mL urine per 24 hours
   d. Excretion of 500 mL urine per 24 hours
10. A urine specimen with a strong ammonia odor is most often the result of:
    a. Breakdown of urea by bacteria
    b. The presence of higher quantities of acetone
    c. Ingestion of certain foodstuffs
    d. Urinary tract infection in an older specimen
11. If the kidney has completely lost the ability to concentrate or dilute urine, the specific gravity will remain at:
    a. 1.000
    b. 1.005
    c. 1.010
    d. 1.035

Chemical Tests in Routine Urinalysis

12. When urine decomposes, the pH:
    a. Becomes more alkaline
    b. Becomes more acidic
    c. Does not change
    d. Causes crystals associated with acidic urine to form
13. Urine pH is:
    a. An indicator of proteinuria
    b. Helpful in the identification of some types of crystals in the urine
    c. Unaffected by diet
    d. Unchanged for each individual
14. Detection of which of the following urine constituents is most helpful in the detection and diagnosis of renal disease?
    a. Blood
    b. Leukocyte esterase
    c. Nitrite
    d. Protein
15. Which of the following is correct regarding the presence of albumin in urine?
    a. It is associated with γ-globulinopathies such as multiple myeloma.
    b. It may be seen in urine as the result of intravascular hemolysis.
    c. Molecule is generally too large to be filtered through the glomerulus.
    d. It is the protein most often associated with glomerular damage.
16. Which of the following is correct regarding the presence of globulin in urine?
    a. It is associated with γ-globulinopathies such as multiple myeloma.
    b. It may be seen in urine as the result of intravascular hemolysis.
    c. Molecule is generally too large to be filtered through the glomerulus.
    d. It is the protein most often associated with glomerular damage.
17. Which of the following is correct regarding light-chain immunoglobulins (Bence Jones protein)?
    a. It is associated with γ-globulinopathies such as multiple myeloma.
    b. It may be seen in urine as the result of intravascular hemolysis.
    c. Molecule is generally too large to be filtered through the glomerulus.
    d. It is the protein most often associated with glomerular damage.
18. The reagent strip test for protein is more sensitive to which of the following than to other proteins?
    a. Albumin
    b. Hemoglobin
    c. Light-chain immunoglobulins
    d. Both a and b
19. Which of the following is *not* detected by the reagent strip test for blood?
    a. Hemoglobin
    b. Hemosiderin
    c. Myoglobin
    d. Red blood cells
20. Reagent strip tests that depend on the release of oxygen and subsequent oxidation of a chromogen, resulting in a color change, are subject to false-negative reactions because of the presence of:
    a. Ascorbic acid (<25 mg/dL)
    b. Azo-containing drugs or compounds
    c. Chlorine bleach
    d. Low specific gravity

21. Dipstick tests for nitrite tend to be:
    a. Positive when large numbers of Gram-positive bacteria are present
    b. Positive when large numbers of Gram-negative bacteria are present
    c. Negative in the presence of a urinary tract infection
    d. Falsely positive in the presence of a urinary tract infection
22. Reagent strip tests for urinary leukocyte esterase are most useful in the detection of:
    a. Immunosuppression
    b. Malignancy
    c. Renal transplant rejection
    d. Urinary tract infection
23. Reagent strip tests for urinary leukocyte esterase are most useful when results are evaluated together with the results for the reagent strip test for:
    a. Blood
    b. Nitrite
    c. Protein
    d. Specific gravity
24. A positive reagent strip test for glucose is most often associated with which of the following conditions?
    a. Anorexia nervosa
    b. Diabetes insipidus
    c. Diabetes mellitus
    d. Starvation
25. Which of the following is true about hematuria?
    a. Sensitive early indicator of renal disease
    b. Distorted or misshapen red cells that may indicate glomerular damage
    c. Presence associated with dilute or hypotonic urine
    d. Indicates a high level of protein

Microscopic Analysis of Urine Sediment

26. Normal urinary sediment can exhibit a:
    a. Few leukocytes
    b. Moderate number of squamous epithelia
    c. Rare hyaline case
    d. All the above

Constituents of Urine Sediment

27. Which of the following is true about a microscopic finding of dysmorphic red cells?
    a. Sensitive early indicator of renal disease
    b. Distorted or misshapen red cells that may indicate glomerular damage
    c. Presence associated with dilute or hypotonic urine
    d. Indicates a high level of protein
28. Which of the following is true about a microscopic finding of shadow or swollen red cells?
    a. Sensitive early indicator of renal disease
    b. Distorted or misshapen red cells that may indicate glomerular damage
    c. Presence associated with dilute or hypotonic urine
    d. Indicates a high level of protein
29. Which is suggested by the presence of neutrophils (PMNs) in a urine microscopic analysis?
    a. Indicates active kidney disease or tubular injury
    b. May be seen with infection and after urethral catheterization
    c. Type of leukocyte most often seen in urine; indicates inflammation somewhere in the urogenital tract
    d. Associated with the nephrotic syndrome
30. Which is suggested by the presence of oval fat bodies in a urine microscopic analysis?
    a. Indicates active kidney disease or tubular injury
    b. May be seen with infection and after urethral catheterization
    c. Type of leukocyte most often seen in urine; indicates inflammation somewhere in the urogenital tract
    d. Associated with the nephrotic syndrome
31. Which is suggested by the presence of renal epithelial cells in a urine microscopic analysis?
    a. Indicates destruction of renal tubules
    b. May be seen with infection and after urethral catheterization
    c. Type of leukocyte most often seen in urine; indicates inflammation somewhere in the urogenital tract
    d. Associated with the nephrotic syndrome
32. Which is suggested by the presence of transitional epithelial cells in a urine microscopic analysis?
    a. Indicates active kidney disease or tubular injury
    b. May be seen with infection and after urethral catheterization
    c. Type of leukocyte most often seen in urine; indicates inflammation somewhere in the urogenital tract
    d. Associated with the nephrotic syndrome
33. The presence of which of the following types of casts has the *least* clinical significance?
    a. Fatty
    b. Granular
    c. Hyaline
    d. Red or white cell
34. The presence of epithelial cell casts indicates:
    a. Acute glomerulonephritis
    b. Acute pyelonephritis
    c. Chronic renal disease or renal failure
    d. Nephrotoxic poisoning
35. The presence of fatty casts indicates:
    a. Acute glomerulonephritis
    b. Acute pyelonephritis
    c. Chronic renal disease or renal failure
    d. Diabetes type 1 with renal degeneration
36. The presence of hyaline indicates:
    a. Acute glomerulonephritis
    b. Acute pyelonephritis
    c. Diabetic nephropathy
    d. Strenuous exercise
37. The presence of red blood cell casts indicates:
    a. Acute glomerulonephritis
    b. Acute pyelonephritis

c. Chronic renal disease or renal failure
d. Nephrotoxic poisoning

38. The presence of waxy casts indicates:
a. Acute glomerulonephritis
b. Acute pyelonephritis
c. Chronic renal disease
d. Nephrotoxic poisoning

39. The presence of white blood cell casts indicates:
a. Acute glomerulonephritis
b. Pyelonephritis
c. Chronic renal disease or renal failure
d. Nephrotoxic poisoning

40. Which of the following is true about hemosiderin?
a. It is seen as free granules in cells or casts several days after an acute hemolytic episode.
b. Most of its abnormal crystals are seen in urine of an alkaline pH.
c. Most or its birefringent crystals are seen in urine.
d. It is made of calcium oxalate– or calcium-containing compounds.

41. Uric acid crystals in the urine sediment indicate that the patient probably has:
a. Gout
b. Rheumatoid arthritis
c. Urinary tract infection
d. Acute glomerulonephritis

Automation in Urinalysis

42. Urinary dipsticks are read in semiautomated equipment by:
a. Reflectance photometry
b. Digital imaging
c. Flow cell cytometry
d. Visual inspection

Turgeon: Linné & Ringsrud's Clinical Laboratory Science, 8th Edition

STUDENT PROCEDURE WORKSHEET 13.1

General Procedure for Urine Reagent Strips

Student Learning Outcomes

After reading Chapter 13 in *Linné & Ringsrud's Clinical Laboratory Science: Concepts, Procedures, and Clinical Applications*, 8th edition, and at the completion of the laboratory exercise and review questions, a student will be able to:

- Perform a routine chemical analysis of urine, and explain the diagnostic value of each of the chemically treated pads on the disposable urinalysis strip.
- Complete the end-of-procedure review questions with a grade of 80% or higher.

Principle

See specific reagent test strip content in chapter.

Equipment, Supplies, and Reagents

1. Disposable gloves, lab coat, and goggles
2. Disposable urinalysis strips in a sealed container
3. Watch with a second hand
4. Paper towels, pen

Specimen

Fresh urine specimen

Instructions for the Procedure

Read the list of required equipment, supplies, and reagents, and the procedural steps. Follow the procedural steps in exact order.

SEQUENCE	PROCEDURAL STEP	INSTRUCTOR-OBSERVED ACCEPTABLE PERFORMANCE (CHECK IF ACCEPTABLE)
1	Test fresh, well-mixed, uncentrifuged urine at room temperature.	
2	Completely immerse all chemical areas of the reagent strip briefly, not more than 1 second.	
3	Remove excess urine from the reagent strip. Draw the strip along the lip or rim of the urine container as it is removed, then touch the edge of the strip to absorbent paper or gauze.	
4	CAUTION: Avoid possible mixing of chemicals from adjacent reagent areas; hold the strip horizontally while waiting and reading results.	
5	Time and read each chemical reaction exactly as stated on the container.	
6	Use adequate light. Hold the strip close to the color block on the chart supplied by the manufacturer, and match carefully for each chemical test. Be sure the strip is properly oriented to the color chart.	
7	Read the results in consistent units as established for your laboratory.	

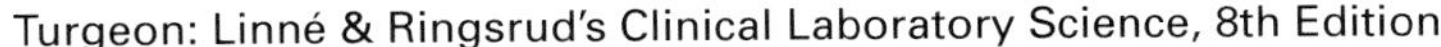
Turgeon: Linné & Ringsrud's Clinical Laboratory Science, 8th Edition

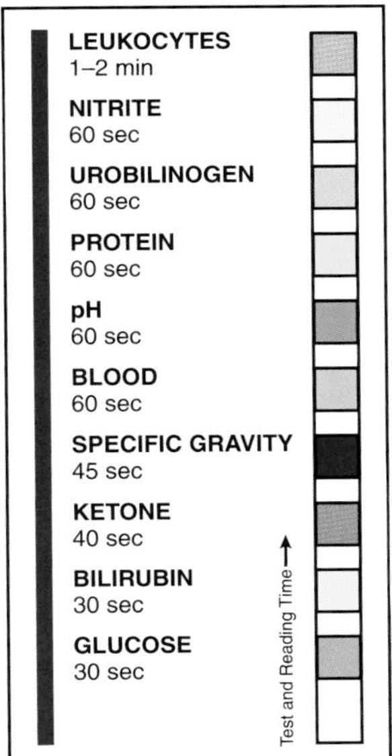

FIGURE 13-26 Reading reagent strips (orientation to bottle).

Results of Unknown Specimens

Specimen Identification	Results
______________________	______________________________
______________________	______________________________
______________________	______________________________

Instructor Initial, if acceptable______________

Procedural Evaluation

Student's Name ________________________ Grade _________

Instructor's Signature ____________________ Date _________

Comments:

Turgeon: Linné & Ringsrud's Clinical Laboratory Science, 8th Edition

STUDENT PROCEDURE WORKSHEET 13.1

General Procedure for Urine Reagent Strips

Review Questions

1. The term used to compare the density of urine to the density of distilled water is:
   a. Refractometry
   b. Specific gravity
   c. Hematuria
   d. Oligouria
2. The concentration of hydrogen ions in urine is expressed as:
   a. pH
   b. Specific gravity
   c. Nitrite
   d. Esterease
3. A positive nitrite test would indicate the presence of _______ in urine.
   a. Leukocytes
   b. Casts
   c. Bacteria
   d. Renal epithelium
4. An increase in _________ suggests renal disease.
   a. Protein
   b. Glucose
   c. pH
   d. Acetone

Turgeon: Linné & Ringsrud's Clinical Laboratory Science, 8th Edition

STUDENT PROCEDURE WORKSHEET 13-2

Microscopic Examination of Urine Sediment

Student Learning Outcomes

See Chapter 13 of *Linné & Ringsrud's Clinical Laboratory Science: Concepts, Procedures, and Clinical Applications*, 8th edition, for a complete discussion of this procedure. After reading Chapter 13, and at the completion of the laboratory exercise and review questions, a student will be able to:

- Microscopically examine and identify normal and abnormal structures in a sample of urine sediment.
- Complete the end-of-procedure review questions with a grade of 80% or higher.

Principle

Microscopic examination of urinary sediment for normal and abnormal structures.

Equipment and Supplies

1. Disposable gloves, lab coat, and goggles
2. Microscope slides
3. Paper towels, pen
4. Conical test tubes
5. Centrifuge
6. Stain (optional)

Specimen

Fresh urine specimen

Instructions for the Procedure

Read the list of required equipment and supplies and the procedural steps. Follow the procedural steps in exact order.

SEQUENCE	PROCEDURAL STEP	INSTRUCTOR-OBSERVED ACCEPTABLE PERFORMANCE (CHECK IF ACCEPTABLE)
General Procedure		
1	Pour about 5 mL of well-mixed urine into a labeled, graduated centrifuge (KOVA) tube.	
2	Centrifuge at a relative centrifugal force of 450 for 5 minutes. Let the centrifuge come to a stop without using the brake. Use of the brake will cause resuspension of the sediment and falsely low results.	
3	Quickly, decant the clear supernatant urine into a test tube; this will leave the sediment in the KOVA tube.	
4	Gently tap the centrifuge tube on the counter; this will resuspend the sediment. Carefully place a small drop on a standardized microscope slide. NOTE: If using a brightfield microscope, a supravital stain can be used. Add 1 or 2 drops of stain to the sediment and mix thoroughly. If the amount of original specimen is limited, or if the urine is very alkaline, split the concentrated sediment and stain only one portion.	
5	If traditional glass slides and coverglasses are used, place a drop of resuspended sediment on a glass microscope slide and cover with a 22 × 22–mm coverglass. The size of the drop and the size of the coverglass are important. The fluid should completely fill the area under the coverglass without overflowing the area or causing the coverglass to float. Take care that no bubbles appear when placing the coverglass over the sediment. If bubbles appear, a new preparation must be made on a clean slide. Bubbles are confusing and make enumeration impossible because they prevent random distribution of the substances to be counted.	
6	Place the preparation on the microscope stage, and focus. Adjust the light, using the low-power objective, by carefully positioning the condenser and iris diaphragm. The tendency is to have too much light, but the light must not be overly reduced. Be sure that the sediment itself is brought into focus, rather than the coverglass. It is easier to achieve focus with specimens that are stained. Finally, vary the fine adjustment continuously to maintain focus.	

(Continued)

Turgeon: Linné & Ringsrud's Clinical Laboratory Science, 8th Edition

STUDENT PROCEDURE WORKSHEET 13-2

SEQUENCE	PROCEDURAL STEP	INSTRUCTOR-OBSERVED ACCEPTABLE PERFORMANCE (CHECK IF ACCEPTABLE)
7	Be systematic in the examination. With standardized slides, scan the entire preparation. With traditional microscope slides and coverglasses, begin by looking around the four sides of the coverglass, then the center. First, look for the substances that are identified and graded under low power. Change to high power, refocus and readjust the light, and search for the substances that are identified and graded under high power. NOTE: All gradings are based on the average number of structures seen in a minimum of 10 microscope fields. Describe separately the structures searched for under low power and high power. Casts and cells are most important; look for these most carefully, observing the less important crystals and miscellaneous structures almost in retrospect.	
Low-Power Examination With the low-power (10 ×) objective, search for the following:		
1	*Casts.* With standardized slides, scan the entire area for the presence of casts. With traditional slides, look for casts around all four edges of the preparation, then in the center, because casts tend to roll to the edges of the coverglass. a. When a cast is discovered, change to high power to identify it. b. Grade and report casts on the basis of the average number seen per low-power field (see Table 13-9). c. If more than one type of cast is found in a single specimen, identify and grade each type separately.	
2	*Crystals and amorphous material.* Look for these structures in the same way as for casts. a. Normal crystals are reported as few, moderate, or many per high-power field, if present. However, crystals may be more apparent under low power. b. Abnormal crystals are graded as the average number seen per low-power field, when present (see Table 13-9). Abnormal crystals must be confirmed by chemical test or clinical history before they are reported. c. Crystals are generally identified by shape rather than size. Therefore a combination of low-power and high-power observation is necessary in the detection and identification.	
3	*Squamous epithelial cells.* When these are present, report as few, moderate, or many per low-power field.	
4	*Mucus (mucous threads).* These are reported as present when easily seen or prominent under low power. They are more apparent with phase-contrast microscopy.	
High-Power Examination With high-power (40 ×) objective, search for the following:		
1	*Red blood cells.* Grade and report based on the average number seen per high-power field (see Table 13-9). Report the presence of unusual forms, such as dysmorphic red cells, if encountered.	
2	*White blood cells.* Grade and report based on the average number seen per high-power field (see Table 13-9). These are usually neutrophils (PMNs). If unusual cell types, such as lymphocytes or eosinophils, are morphologically identifiable, report this finding.	

(Continued)

Turgeon: Linné & Ringsrud's Clinical Laboratory Science, 8th Edition

STUDENT PROCEDURE WORKSHEET 13-2

SEQUENCE	PROCEDURAL STEP	INSTRUCTOR-OBSERVED ACCEPTABLE PERFORMANCE (CHECK IF ACCEPTABLE)
3	*Normal crystals.* Identify and report as few, moderate, or many per high-power field for each type of crystal encountered.	
4	*Casts.* Identify with high power, but grade under low power.	
5	*Epithelial cells:* renal tubular, oval fat bodies (renal tubular cells with fat), and transitional. When these are present, estimate and report as few, moderate, or many per high-power field.	
6	*Miscellaneous.* This category includes various cell forms and other structures that may be encountered in the urine sediment, such as yeast, bacteria, trichomonads, and fat globules. When these are present, identify the cell or structure, and report as few, moderate, or many per high-power field. Report sperm as present in males only. It is considered a contaminant in routine urinalysis specimens from females and is not reported.	

REPRESENTATIVE GRADING SCALE FOR MICROSCOPIC STRUCTURES

STRUCTURE	QUANTITATION (REPRESENTATIVE NUMERIC RANGE)*
RBCs/hpf	0-5, 5-10, 10-25, 25-50, 50-100, > 100 (too numerous to count), with or without clumps
WBCs/hpf	0-5, 5-10, 10-25, 25-50, 50-100, > 100 (too numerous to count), with or without clumps
Epithelial cells/lpf	Specify type: 0-5 (rare), 5-20 = few, 25-100 = moderate, > 100 = many
Casts/lpf	Specify type (such as hyaline or granular): 0-5, 5-10, > 10
Crystals/hpf	Specify type: 0-5 (rare), 5-10 (moderate), > 20 (many)
Bacteria/lpf	Rare, few, many

hpf, high-power field; *lpf*, low-power field; *RBC*, red blood cell; *WBC*, white blood cell.
* Quantitate an average of 10 representative fields. Do not quantitate trichomonads, sperm, budding yeast, or mucus, but note their presence on the report.

Results of Unknown Specimens

Specimen Identification Results

______________________ ______________________________

______________________ ______________________________

______________________ ______________________________

Instructor Initial, if acceptable ______________

(Continued)

Turgeon: Linné & Ringsrud's Clinical Laboratory Science, 8th Edition

STUDENT PROCEDURE WORKSHEET 13-2

Microscopic Examination of Urine Sediment

Review Questions

Student's Name ______________________________ Date _____________

1. A microscopic examination of urine sediment should begin with:
   a. Low-power objective (10 ×) with bright illumination
   b. Low-power objective (10 ×) with low illumination
   c. High-power objective (40 ×) with bright illumination
   d. High-power objective (40 ×) with low illumination

2. The purpose of centrifuging and decanting a urine specimen before microscopic examination is:
   a. To dilute the urine
   b. To concentrate the urine
   c. To remove contamination from the urine
   d. To kill bacteria in the specimen

3. The most commonly found leukocyte in a urine sediment is a:
   a. Neutrophil
   b. Lymphocyte
   c. Monocyte
   d. Plasma cell

4. How many hyaline casts in a urine sediment would be considered normal?
   a. 0-1/lpf
   b. 5-10/lpf
   c. 10-20/lpf
   d. > 20/lpf

Procedural Evaluation

Student's Name ______________________________ Grade___________

Instructor's Signature ___________________________ Date___________

Comments:

14

Examination of Body Fluids and Miscellaneous Specimens

http://evolve.elsevier.com/Turgeon/clinicallab/

CHAPTER CONTENTS

LEARNING OUTCOMES

Overview of Body Fluids
- Name various types of body fluids and their synonyms.

Cerebrospinal Fluid
- Integrate the gross examination, cell counts, morphologic examination, and common chemical tests in the examination of cerebrospinal fluid.
- Differentiate a traumatic spinal tap from a hemorrhage tap on the basis of the gross appearance of the spinal fluid.

Serous Fluids: Pericardial, Pleural, and Peritoneal
- Identify the serous fluids, and describe the components of their routine examination.
- Define the term *effusion.*
- Differentiate a transudate from an exudate.

Synovial Fluid
- Define synovial fluid, and describe the components of a routine synovial fluid examination.

- Interpret the microscopic examination of synovial fluid for gout and pseudogout, using compensated polarizing microscopy for the identification of crystals.

Seminal Fluid

- Describe the components of a semen analysis, and state the normal reference range of cells in semen.

Amniotic Fluid

- Describe the function and properties of amniotic fluid.
- Discuss laboratory testing of amniotic fluid for fetal maturity.

Saliva

- Name three types of studies of saliva.

Automation in Body Fluid Analysis

- Name and compare the characteristics of various automated body fluid analyzers.

Case Studies

- Analyze the patient history, clinical signs and symptoms, and laboratory data for the stated case studies, answer the related critical thinking questions, and conclude the most likely diagnosis.

Review Questions

- Demonstrate comprehension of the chapter content by completing the end-of-chapter review questions with a grade of 80% or higher.

Note:

- indicates MLT and MLS core content

❖ indicates MLT (optional) and MLS advanced content

KEY TERMS

amniotic fluid
cerebrospinal fluid (CSF)
effusion
exudate
inflammatory
pericardial fluid
pleural fluid
semen
serous fluids
synovial fluid
transudate

OVERVIEW OF BODY FLUIDS

Circulating blood, urine, and body fluids in various body cavities are sterile under normal conditions. In various disorders and diseases, the quantity of these fluids can increase significantly (Table 14.1). Fluid specimens aspirated from different anatomic sites can be analyzed for the total number of red blood cells (RBCs) and white blood cells (WBCs), differentiation of white cell types, chemical composition, and microorganisms. Standard Precautions must be practiced when handling all types of body fluids.

The type of examination performed on the body fluid depends on the source of the specimen. The specimen must be fresh. Cell counts cannot be done on a clotted specimen; anticoagulants must be used to prevent coagulation of the specimen when a cell count is needed. Aliquots of many types of specimens, such as **cerebrospinal fluid (CSF)**, are sent to a particular division of the clinical laboratory: hematology, chemistry, microbiology, immunology, or cytology.

CEREBROSPINAL FLUID

CSF acts as a shock absorber for the brain and spinal cord. CSF circulates nutrients, lubricates the central nervous system (CNS), and may contribute to the nourishment of brain tissue. CSF is found inside all the ventricles, in the central canal of the spinal cord, and in the subarachnoid space around both the brain and the spinal cord (Fig. 14.1).

All CSF specimens must be immediately delivered to the laboratory for examination. The four or five collection tubes must be handled using Standard Precautions. Tubes are designated for routine testing in hematology, microbiology, clinical chemistry, and immunology/serology.

The CSF is normally clear, colorless, and sterile. The average, healthy adult has 90 to 150 mL of CSF, and the newborn infant, 10 to 60 mL. CSF has the following four main functions:

1. Serve as a mechanical buffer that prevents trauma
2. Regulate the volume of the intracranial contents
3. Provide nutrient medium for CNS
4. Act as an excretory channel for metabolic products of CNS

A physician performs a spinal tap, or lumbar puncture (LP), only if serious diagnostic concerns exist because LP involves potential harm to the patient. Indications for LP are as follows:

- Diagnosis of meningitis (bacterial, fungal, mycobacterial, amebic)
- Diagnosis of hemorrhage (subarachnoid, intracerebral, cerebral infarct)
- Diagnosis of neurologic disease such as multiple sclerosis, demyelinating disorders, and Guillain–Barré syndrome
- Diagnosis and evaluation of suspected malignancy such as leukemia, lymphoma, or metastatic carcinoma
- Introduction of drugs, radiographic contrast media, and anesthetics

The greatest risk of LP involves paralysis or death resulting from tonsillar herniation in patients with increased intracranial pressure. LP also carries a risk of infection.

Spinal fluid differs from serous and synovial fluids because of the selective permeability of the membranes and adjacent tissues containing CSF. This is referred to as the *blood–brain barrier (BBB).* As a result, CSF is not an ultrafiltrate of plasma. Rather, active transport occurs among the blood, CSF, and brain in both directions, giving differing concentrations of substances in each direction. For the CNS to become infected with bacteria, parasites, or a virus, the BBB must be penetrated.

TABLE 14.1 **Body Fluids**

Fluid	Infectious Diseases	Causative Organisms
Bronchoalveolar lavage (also bronchial washings)	Bronchitis	Viruses are a common cause.
	Bronchial washings	Bacteria, viruses, or parasites
Cerebrospinal fluid (CSF; also, spinal fluid, lumbar puncture fluid, ventricular fluid, meningeal fluid)	Neonatal meningitis	Bacteria; group B streptococci, *Escherichia coli, Listeria monocytogenes*
	Meningitis in children 4 mo–5 yr	Bacteria, *Haemophilus influenzae* type b (Hib)
	Meningitis in young adults	Bacteria, *Neisseria meningitides*
	Meningitis in young children and elderly patients	Bacteria, *Streptococcus pneumoniae*
	Encephalitis	Enteroviruses
Peritoneal fluid (also, dialysate fluid, paracentesis fluid, ascitic fluid)	Primary peritonitis in children	Bacteria; *S. pneumoniae* and group A streptococci, Enterobacteriaceae, other Gram-negative bacilli, staphylococci
	Primary peritonitis in adults	Bacteria; *E. coli* followed by *S. pneumoniae* and group A streptococci; tuberculosis is rare.
	Young women (sexually active)	Bacteria; *Neisseria gonorrheae* and *Chlamydia trachomatis*
	Immunocompromised patients or patients receiving prolonged antibacterial therapy	Yeast, *Candida* spp.
	Secondary peritonitis	Bacteria, anaerobes; Enterobacteriaceae, enterococci, or other streptococci. In pelvic inflammatory disease, gonococci, anaerobes, or chlamydiae are present. If bowel flora altered by antimicrobial agents, more resistant Gram-negative bacilli and *Staphylococcus aureus.* Also, *E. coli, Bacteroides fragilis* group, enterococci and other streptococci, *Bilophila* spp., other anaerobic Gram-negative bacilli, anaerobic Gram-positive cocci, clostridia
Pericardial fluid (also, fluid from heart, pericardiocentesis fluid)	Pericarditis	Usually, viruses; bacteria, fungi, and parasites are relatively uncommon causes.
Pleural fluid (also, chest fluid, thoracic fluid, thoracentesis fluid)	Pleural cavity infection	Bacteria are the most common cause.
Seminal fluid (also, semen)	None	Not usually cultured; not a source of sexually transmitted diseases
Synovial fluid (also, joint fluid)	Septic arthritis	Bacteria; *S. aureus* is most common cause.
	Adults (<30 years old)	Bacteria; *N. gonorrheae* is isolated most frequently.

Many drugs do not enter CSF from the blood. Electrolytes such as sodium, magnesium, and chloride are more concentrated in spinal fluid than in plasma or plasma ultrafiltrates, whereas bicarbonate, glucose, and urea are less concentrated in CSF. Protein enters CSF in very small amounts. Very few cells are found in normal spinal fluid.

Collection of Cerebrospinal Fluid

A certain degree of risk to the patient is inherent in the procedure for obtaining a specimen of spinal fluid. These specimens must be handled with the utmost care. In general practice, three or four sterile tubes containing about 5 mL each are collected during the spinal tap. These tubes are numbered in sequence of collection and immediately brought to the laboratory. In some cases, four tubes may not be collected, as with neonates or babies or a problematic tap.

The opening pressure is measured as the LP is done. It is important that any cell count or glucose determinations be done as soon as possible after collection to prevent deterioration of cells and potentially decreased glucose concentrations. As with other body fluids, CSF is potentially highly infectious, and it must always be collected and handled using Standard Precautions.

The tubes that are sequentially collected and labeled in order of collection are generally dispersed. The order for analysis (after gross examination of all tubes) may differ from one institution to another. Each laboratory has a protocol for the processing of spinal fluid. Students and new staff members need to familiarize themselves with the established protocol for that laboratory. An example of a typical sequence is as follows:

Tube 1: Chemical tests
Tube 2: Microbiology studies
Tube 3: Total cell counts and differential cell count
Tube 4: Immunology/serology studies and repeat RBC count

Routine and Special Examination of Cerebrospinal Fluid

Gross Appearance

All tubes collected by LP are evaluated as to gross appearance. Normal CSF is crystal clear and looks similar to distilled water. Color and clarity are noted by holding the sample beside a tube of water against a clean white paper or a printed page.

Turbidity and color. Slight haziness in the specimen or turbidity may indicate an increased WBC count. Turbidity in spinal fluid may result from the presence of large numbers of leukocytes

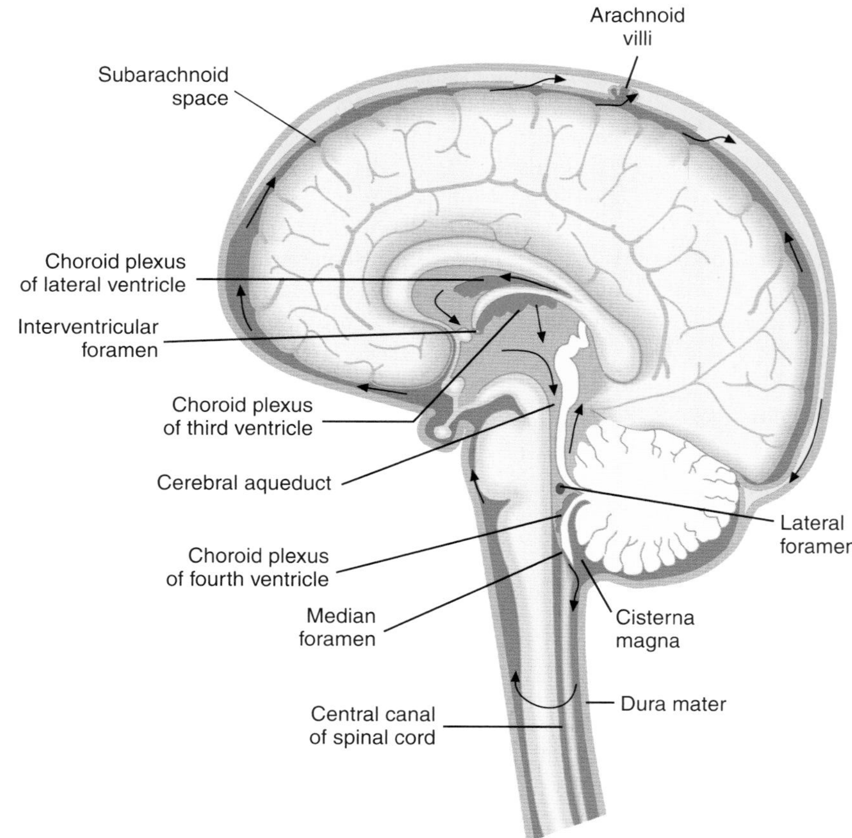

Fig. 14.1 Flow of cerebrospinal fluid (CSF) through the brain. CSF originates in the choroid plexus and then flows through the ventricles and subarachnoid space and into the bloodstream. (From Tille P: *Bailey & Scott diagnostic microbiology,* ed 14, St Louis, 2017, Elsevier/Saunders.)

TABLE 14.2 Traumatic Cerebrospinal Fluid Tap: Abnormal Color Associations

CSF color	Association	Comments
Bloody	Fresh subarachnoid hemorrhage	All collection tubes
Pale-pink to pale-orange xanthochromia	Recent subarachnoid hemorrhage	Oxyhemoglobin peaks in 24–36 hours and gradually disappears in 4–8 days.
Yellow xanthochromia	Old subarachnoid hemorrhage	Color by bilirubin, formed from hemoglobin from lysed red blood cells Appears about 12 hours after a bleeding episode, peaks in 2–4 days and gradually disappears in 2–4 weeks When CSF protein level > 150 mg/dL because of damage to blood–brain barrier, a yellow color similar to color of normal serum or plasma may be seen.

CSF, Cerebrospinal fluid.

(WBCs) or from bacteria, increased protein, or lipid. If radiographic contrast media have been injected, the CSF will appear oily, and when mixed, turbid. This artifactual turbidity is not reported.

Bloody fluid can result from a traumatic tap or subarachnoid hemorrhage. Any presence of color should be noted (Table 14.2). If blood in a CSF specimen results from a traumatic tap (inclusion of blood in specimen from LP itself), the successive collection tubes will show less bloody fluid, eventually becoming clear. Because hemolysis of erythrocytes (RBCs) will occur in vitro as well as in vivo, the examination of CSF for xanthochromia must be done within 1 hour of collection or false-positive results will be obtained.

Clots. In addition to the gross observations of turbidity and color, CSF should be examined for clotting. Clotting can result from increased protein. Gel formation on standing is caused by an increased fibrinogen content resulting from a "traumatic tap." Rarely, clotting may be associated with subarachnoid block or meningitis.

Red and White Blood Cell Counts

Cell counts on CSF are usually performed using automated equipment. Manual methods may be used under some circumstances; for example, inadequate specimen volume or cell numbers usually preclude the use of automated methods[1] (Student Procedure Worksheet 14.1).

The viscosity of some body fluids (especially joint fluids), variations in cell size (especially when tumor cells are present), and background debris, which is generally higher than cell counts, can create problems when using automated equipment. Fluids can be contaminated with pathogenic microorganisms, and special disinfecting procedures and disposable equipment are employed to prevent contamination. Semiautomatic micropipettes may be used to prepare dilutions, and disposable counting chambers may be used. Traditional hemocytometers must be thoroughly disinfected after use.

Normally, there are no RBCs in CSF. Again, RBCs may be present from the LP itself. The normal WBC count in CSF is 0 to 8 × 10^9 cells/L in adults and 0 to 30 × 10^9/L in neonates. Some laboratories use a reference range of 0 to 10 cells/µL. Increased WBC counts can be observed in infectious diseases such as meningitis and noninfectious conditions such as trauma and multiple sclerosis. Leukemic patients can have a normal WBC count but have immature blast cells present in their CSF.

Red Cell Counts in Subarachnoid Hemorrhage

Most cases of subarachnoid hemorrhage are diagnosed by computed tomography (CT) of the brain. If the CT result is negative, LP for CSF analysis is frequently performed. The diagnosis of subarachnoid hemorrhage includes the following:

- Elevated opening pressure
- Presence of RBCs
- Presence of xanthochromia

A CSF specimen from a traumatic tap can complicate the diagnosis of subarachnoid hemorrhage. A current trend is to perform an RBC count on both the first and last CSF tubes collected (tube 1 and tube 4). When an abnormal number of RBCs is demonstrated in tube 1 but tube 4 exhibits a decreased RBC count, this is strong evidence for a traumatic tap. If a specimen shows incomplete clearing, this probably represents a likely traumatic tap that may or may not be superimposed on a subarachnoid hemorrhage.[1]

Cytocentrifugation. Cytocentrifugation requires the use of a special cytocentrifuge such as the Cytospin (Shandon, Pittsburgh). It is a slow centrifugation method that provides better cell yield and morphologic preservation than ordinary centrifugation. Differentiation of cell types is best done by using 0.5 mL of specimen with a few drops of bovine serum albumin to preserve cellular morphology. The technique is relatively easy to learn and perform and gives an excellent yield with a small amount of sample. The sample is slowly centrifuged from 200 to 1000 rpm for 5 to 10 minutes. During centrifugation, the fluid portion of the specimen is absorbed into a filter paper, and the cellular portion is concentrated in a circle 6 mm in diameter on a microscope slide. The cytocentrifuged preparation is stained with Wright or a variety of stains for hematologic or cytologic studies.

Smears from centrifuged spinal fluid sediment. If a cytocentrifuge is not available, the CSF is centrifuged for 5 minutes at 3000 rpm. The supernatant is removed, and the sediment is used to prepare smears on glass slides. The smears are dried rapidly and Wright-stained. Recovery of cells is not as good as with other techniques, and the cells tend to be distorted or damaged.

Other concentration techniques. Special sedimentation methods and membrane filter techniques are also used. These are more time-consuming and expensive than cytocentrifugation and require more technical expertise. These methodologies are typically unavailable in small hospital laboratories.

Morphologic Examination

The protocol for performing a differential cell count on CSF varies among laboratories. Some laboratories do differential counts on all specimens; others use a minimum total cell count benchmark before performing a cell differential. Counts may be done on a smear made from the centrifuged CSF sediment, using recovery with a filtration or sedimentation method, or preferably on a cytocentrifuged preparation.

Differential cell count. Exactly 100 WBCs are counted and classified, and the percentage of each cell type is reported. Depending on the method of preparation, morphologic identification may be difficult. In some cases, cells can be identified only as "polynuclear" or "mononuclear." With other preparation techniques, identification is more specific. Any of the cells found in blood may be seen in CSF, including neutrophils, lymphocytes, monocytes, eosinophils, and basophils. A predominance of polynuclear cells usually indicates a bacterial infection (Fig. 14.2); the presence of many mononuclear cells (usually lymphocytes) indicates a viral infection.

Subarachnoid bleeding is associated with the microscopic observation of *erythrophagia,* the ingestion of RBCs by macrophages in the CSF.

In addition, cells that originate in the CNS may be seen. These include ependymal cells (Fig. 14.3), choroidal cells, and pia-arachnoid mesothelial cells. If any tumor cells or unusual cells are encountered, the CSF specimen should be referred for cytologic examination.

Routine Chemistry Tests

Several chemical determinations can be done on spinal fluid. The same chemical constituents are generally found in CSF and plasma, but because of the BBB and selective filtration, normal CSF values are different from plasma values. Abnormal CSF values may result from alterations in BBB permeability or from production or metabolism by neural cells in various pathologic

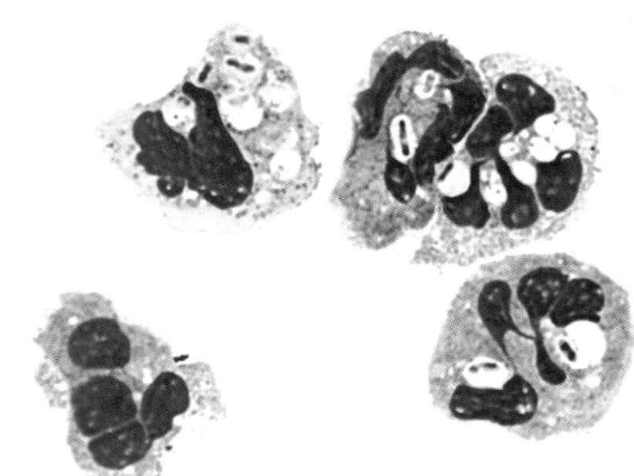

Fig. 14.2 Cerebrospinal fluid cells. (From Carr JH, Rodak BF: *Clinical hematology atlas,* ed 3, St Louis, 2009, Elsevier/Saunders.)

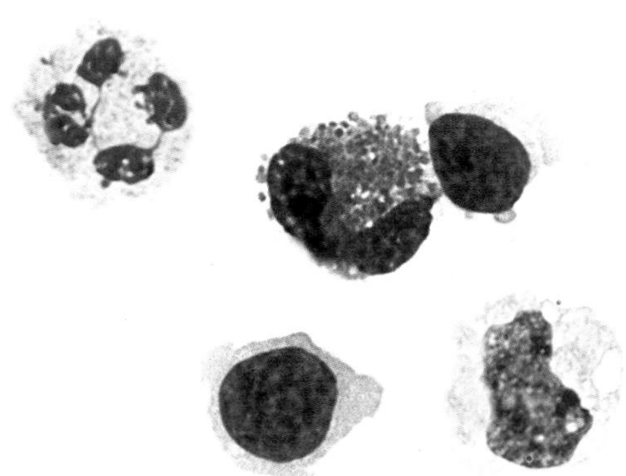

Fig. 14.3 Cerebrospinal fluid cells. (From Rodak BF, Fritsma GA, Doig K: *Hematology: clinical principles and applications,* ed 3, St Louis, 2007, Saunders.)

conditions. There are relatively few important CSF chemical findings. Some of the more routine analyses are described here.

Protein. Protein tests and protein electrophoresis are common analyses and of diagnostic significance for a variety of conditions and disease states. Protein fractions in CSF are generally the same as in plasma, but the ratios vary. The normal CSF protein varies with methodology and site of collection, with a reference range of approximately 20 to 40 mg/dL (12–60 mg/dL). Increased CSF protein levels are the most common pathologic finding and are seen with meningitis, hemorrhage, and multiple sclerosis. Low values are associated with leakage of fluid from the CNS because of damage to the BBB. Electrophoresis may be done when evaluation of CSF protein fractions is needed.

Glucose. The glucose level in spinal fluid should be measured immediately. The accepted reference value is 40 to 80 mg/dL. It is about two-thirds of the blood glucose value. For example, a patient with a 100 mg/dL blood glucose value would have a calculated CSF reference value of 67 mg/dL. Both levels should be measured simultaneously because the difference between these values is clinically significant. Bacteria and cells use glucose. The glucose level in CSF is especially reduced in bacterial meningitis but not in viral meningitis, primary brain tumor, or vascular accidents. Glucose is decreased in metastatic tumor and insulin shock and elevated in diabetic coma.

Lactate. Determination of lactate levels in CSF can be used in the diagnosis and management of meningitis, although its usefulness is controversial and method dependent. A lactate level greater than 25 mg/dL is seen in bacterial, fungal, and tubercular meningitis and is more consistent than a decrease in glucose level. The elevated serum lactate levels remain during initial treatment, but a fall indicates successful treatment. Increased lactate levels occur in oxygen deprivation and are seen in any condition involving decreased oxygen flow to the brain.

Biomarkers for Alzheimer Disease

Alzheimer disease represents a growing problem as the overall population ages. Identification of biomarkers for the disease has become increasingly important for risk prediction and diagnosis and to identify patients at high risk of disease development who may be eligible for inclusion in clinical trials of novel therapies.

CSF biomarkers amyloid beta (Aβ), hyperphosphorylated tau, and total tau have been the most extensively studied markers of Alzheimer disease.[2] Laboratory assays for these biomarkers have problems associated with absorption of Aβ to laboratory test tubes, a high degree of batch-to-batch variation, and the lack of certified reference material. Research into increased automation and implementation on routine diagnostic platforms to support cost-effective and reliable introduction of the tests on a wider scale is expected to expand the use of these and additional biomarkers.

Microbiological Examination

Gram stain and culture are done. CSF specimens are normally sterile. Gram stain is most useful in the diagnosis of acute bacterial meningitis because the organisms can actually be seen in the Gram-stained specimen. Tuberculosis (acid-fast stain) and *Cryptococcus* infections (India ink preparations) may also be detected with microscopic CSF examination. CSF cultures, both bacterial and viral, may be part of the routine protocol.

Serology Tests

The Venereal Disease Research Laboratories test is a well-known serologic test for syphilis that is done on spinal fluid (see Evolve for procedure). The frequently used rapid plasma reagin for syphilis testing is only applicable to serum. The fluorescent treponemal antibody absorption test is more sensitive but less specific in CSF.

SEROUS FLUIDS: PERICARDIAL, PLEURAL, AND PERITONEAL

The fluids of the pericardial, pleural, and peritoneal cavities are called serous fluids. They normally are formed continuously in the body cavities and are reabsorbed, leaving only very small volumes. The normal appearance of these fluids is pale and yellow colored. The fluid becomes more turbid as the total cell count rises, an indication of inflammation. Increases in the amounts of these body cavity fluids formed are seen in inflammation and when the serum protein level falls.

Serous fluids are aspirated by a physician if they are mechanically inhibiting the function of the associated organs, as well as for diagnostic purposes. The specimen is collected into various containers, depending on the laboratory testing to be done. An ethylenediaminetetraacetic acid (EDTA) tube is used for cell counts and smear evaluation; sterile tubes are used for cultures; and oxalate or fluoride tubes are used for protein, glucose, or other chemistry tests. If a large volume of fluid is aspirated, fluid is collected in a container with an appropriate additive to prevent clotting. If the fluid clots, it is useless for many analyses.

Serous fluids have a composition similar to that of serum and are the fluids contained within the closed cavities of the body. These cavities are lined by a contiguous membrane that forms a double layer of mesothelial cells called the *serous membrane.* The cavities are the pleural, pericardial, and peritoneal cavities.

A small amount of serous fluid fills the space between the two layers and serves to lubricate the surfaces of these membranes as they move against each other. The fluids are ultrafiltrates of plasma that are continuously formed and reabsorbed, leaving only a very small volume within the cavities. An increased volume of any of these fluids is referred to as an **effusion**.

Transudates and Exudates

Normal serous fluids are formed as an ultrafiltrate of plasma as it filters through the capillary endothelium and are called **transudates**. Normally, serum protein exerts colloidal osmotic pressure and helps impair movement of fluid into the serous cavity. If plasma protein levels decrease, the colloidal osmotic pressure falls, and effusion results, as movement of the transudate into the serous cavity increases. Serous fluid formation is also affected by capillary pressure and permeability.

An increase in serous fluid volume (effusion) occurs in many conditions. In determining the cause of an effusion, it is helpful to determine whether the effusion is a transudate or an **exudate**. In general, the effusion is a transudate (ultrafiltrate of plasma) because of a systemic disease. An example of a transudate is ascites, an effusion into the peritoneal cavity, which might be caused by liver cirrhosis or congestive heart failure. Transudates may be the result of a mechanical disorder affecting the movement of fluid across a membrane.

Exudates are usually effusions that result from an **inflammatory** response to conditions that directly affect the serous cavity. These inflammatory conditions include infections and malignancies.

Although it may be difficult to determine whether an effusion is a transudate or an exudate, the distinction is important from a practical standpoint. If the effusion is a transudate, further testing is generally unnecessary. If it is an exudate, however, further testing is required for diagnosis and treatment. If infection is suspected, Gram stain and culture are indicated; suspected malignancies might require cytologic tests and biopsy.

Serous effusions have been classified as transudates or exudates on the basis of the amount of protein. Generally, effusions with total protein content less than 3 g/dL are considered transudates, and those with total protein more than 3 g/dL are exudates. Unfortunately, there is considerable overlap in separating the effusions. A more reliable method of distinguishing transudates and exudates is the simultaneous measurement of the fluid and serum for protein and lactate dehydrogenase (LDH). The appearance of the fluid, cell counts, and spontaneous clotting are also useful in the differentiation. Table 14.3 summarizes these findings.

Description of Specific Serous Fluids

Pleural Fluid

Normally, about 1 to 10 mL of **pleural fluid** moistens the pleural surfaces. It surrounds the lungs and lines the walls of the thoracic cavity. If inflammation occurs, the plasma protein level falls, congestive heart failure is present, or lymphatic drainage decreases, there can be an abnormal accumulation of pleural fluid.

Pericardial Fluid

The pericardial space enclosing the heart normally contains about 25 to 50 mL of a clear, straw-colored ultrafiltrate of plasma called **pericardial fluid**. This fluid forms continually and is reabsorbed by the nearby lymph vessels (lymphatics), leaving a small but constant volume. When an abnormal accumulation of pericardial fluid occurs, it fills up the space around the heart and can mechanically inhibit its normal action (cardiac tamponade). In these patients, immediate aspiration of the excess fluid is indicated.

Peritoneal Fluid

Normally, less than 100 mL of clear, straw-colored peritoneal fluid is present in the peritoneal cavity (abdominal and pelvic cavities). An abnormal accumulation of peritoneal fluid is indicated by severe abdominal pain and may be caused by a ruptured abdominal organ, hemorrhage resulting from trauma, postoperative complications, or an unknown condition. The excess fluid is aspirated. Such an accumulation must always be considered in the light of other findings.

Collection of Serous Fluids

Serous fluids are collected under strictly antiseptic conditions. The aspiration may be for diagnostic purposes or for mechanical reasons to prevent an excess accumulation of fluid from inhibiting the actions of the lungs or heart. A pleural effusion may

TABLE 14.3 Differentiation of Serous Effusions: Transudate Versus Exudate[a]

Observation or Test	Transudate	Exudate
Appearance	Watery, clear, pale yellow Does not clot	Cloudy, turbid, purulent, or bloody May clot (fibrinogen)
White cell count	Low, < 1000 cells/μL, with more than 50% mononuclear cells (lymphocytes, monocytes)	500–1000 cells/μL or more, with increased polymorphonuclear neutrophil leukocytes (PMNs) Increased lymphocytes with tuberculosis or rheumatoid arthritis
Red cell count	Low, unless from traumatic tap	>100,000 cells/μL, especially with a malignancy
Total protein	<3 g/dL	>3 g/dL (or greater than half the serum level)
Lactate dehydrogenase	Low	Increased (>60% of the serum level because of cellular debris)
Glucose	Varies with serum level	Lower than serum level with some infections and high cell counts

[a]Note that some values are variable between the two effusions. Clinical considerations must always be used in combination with the laboratory findings.
Modified from Ringsrud KM, Linné JJ: *Urinalysis and body fluids: a color text and atlas,* St Louis, 1995, Mosby.

compress the lungs, a pericardial effusion may cause cardiac tamponade, and ascites (peritoneal effusion) may elevate the diaphragm, compressing the lungs. At least three anticoagulant tubes of fluid are generally collected and used, as follows:

1. EDTA tube for gross appearance, cell counts, morphology, and differential
2. Suitably anticoagulated tube such as heparin for chemical analysis
3. Sterile heparinized tube for Gram stain and culture

Additional tubes, or the entire collection with a suitable preservative, are collected for cytologic examination for tumor cells. Sequentially collected tubes are observed for a possible traumatic tap.

In some extreme cases, serous fluid may be collected into a sterile bag containing anticoagulant or a suitable preservative and transported to the laboratory for examination.

Routine Examination of Serous Fluids

The routine examination of serous fluids generally includes an observation of gross appearance; cell counts, morphology, and differential; and Gram stain and culture. Certain chemical analyses and cytologic examination for tumor cells and tumor markers are performed when indicated.

Gross Appearance

Normal serous fluid is pale and straw colored; this is the color seen in a transudate. Turbidity increases as the number of cells and the amount of debris increase. An abnormally colored fluid may appear milky (chylous or pseudochylous), cloudy, or bloody on gross observation. A cloudy serous fluid is often associated with an inflammatory reaction, either bacterial or viral. Blood-tinged fluid may result from a traumatic tap, and grossly bloody fluid may be seen when an organ, such as the spleen or liver, or a blood vessel has ruptured. Bloody fluids are also seen after myocardial infarction and in malignant disease states, tuberculosis, rheumatoid arthritis (RA), and systemic lupus erythematosus (SLE).

Clotting

To observe the ability of the serous fluid to clot, the specimen must be collected in a plain tube with no anticoagulant. The ability of the fluid to clot indicates a substantial inflammatory reaction.

Red and White Blood Cell Counts

Cell counts are done on well-mixed anticoagulated serous fluid in a hemocytometer. The fluid may be undiluted or diluted, as indicated by the cell count. The procedure is essentially the same as that described for CSF red and white cell counts. If significant protein is present, acetic acid cannot be used as a diluent for WBC counts because of the precipitation of protein. In this case saline may be used as a diluent, and the RBC and WBC counts are done simultaneously. The use of phase-contrast microscopy is helpful in performing these counts.

Leukocyte (WBC) counts greater than 500 cells/µL are usually clinically significant. If there is a predominance of neutrophils (polynuclear), bacterial inflammation is suspected. A predominance of lymphocytes suggests viral infection, tuberculosis, lymphoma, or malignancy. WBC counts greater than 1000/µL are associated with exudates.

Erythrocyte (RBC) counts greater than 10,000 cells/µL in pleural fluids may be seen in an effusion associated with malignancies, infarcts, and trauma.

Morphologic Examination and White Cell Differential

Morphologic examination and WBC differential for serous fluid are essentially the same as those described for CSF. Again, slides prepared by cytocentrifugation are preferred to smears prepared after normal centrifugation. Slides are generally Wright-stained, and a differential cell count is done. The WBCs generally resemble those seen in peripheral blood, with the addition of mesothelial lining cells. Generally, 300 cells are counted and differentiated as to the percentage of each cell type seen. If any malignant tumor cells are seen or appear to be present, the slide must be referred to a pathologist or qualified cytotechnologist.

Microbiological Examination

Microbiological examination of serous fluid includes Gram stain and culture on all body effusions of unknown cause (see Chapter 15).

Chemical Analysis

Protein. Total protein is measured in the fluid and the plasma. The level and ratio are helpful in distinguishing an exudate from a transudate. Protein electrophoresis is used in some cases.

Lactate dehydrogenase. LDH is also measured in the fluid and the plasma. The level and ratio, together with the total protein levels and ratios, are used to distinguish an exudate from a transudate. Increased LDH levels are caused by cellular debris from infection or malignancy.

Glucose. In bacterial infections, serous fluids have a lower concentration of glucose than blood. Glucose level is decreased because bacteria use glucose as a metabolic substrate. Glucose determinations on serous fluids should be accompanied by a simultaneous blood glucose collection.

Other tests. Determinations of amylase, lipase, other enzymes, ammonia, and lipids, among others, are also done in various conditions.

SYNOVIAL FLUID

Synovial fluid is the fluid contained in joints (Fig. 14.4). Arthrocentesis constitutes a liquid biopsy of the joint. Normal joints have very little synovial fluid. Aspiration of this fluid from the joints by arthrocentesis provides information about joint diseases. A variety of disorders, such as RA and gout, produce changes in the number and types of cells, the chemical composition, and crystals in the fluid. In addition, arthrocentesis may alleviate elevated intraarticular pressure.

Synovial membranes line the joints, bursae, and tendon sheaths. Normal synovial fluid is an ultrafiltrate of plasma with the addition of a high-molecular-weight mucopolysaccharide called *hyaluronate* or *hyaluronic acid.* The presence of

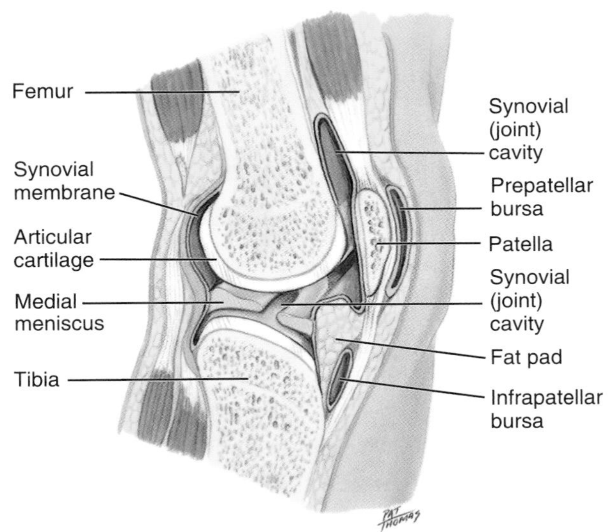

Fig. 14.4 Schematic representation of the knee. (From Applegate E: *The anatomy and physiology learning system,* ed 2, Philadelphia, 2000, Saunders.)

hyaluronate differentiates synovial fluid from other serous fluids and spinal fluid. Hyaluronic acid is responsible for the normal viscosity of synovial fluid, which serves to lubricate the joints so that they move freely. Hyaluronate is secreted by the synovial fluid cells (synoviocytes) that line the joint cavity. This normal viscosity is responsible for some difficulties in the examination of synovial fluid, especially in performing cell counts.

Normal Synovial Fluid

Normal synovial fluid is straw colored and viscous, resembling uncooked egg white (*syn,* "with"; *ovi,* "egg"). About 1 mL of synovial fluid is present in each large joint, such as the knee, ankle, hip, elbow, wrist, and shoulder.

In normal synovial fluid, WBC count is low, less than 200 cells/μL, and most WBCs are mononuclear, with less than 25% neutrophils. RBCs and crystals are normally absent, and the fluid is sterile. Because the fluid is an ultrafiltrate of plasma, normal synovial fluid has essentially the same chemical composition as plasma without the larger protein molecules. A small amount of protein is secreted by the synovial cells, resulting in less than 3 g/dL of total protein.

Aspiration and Analysis

Synovial fluid differs from other body cavity fluids because of the importance of finding crystals in the specimen and because it is normally very viscous.

The aspiration and analysis of synovial fluid may be done to determine the cause of joint disease, especially when accompanied by an abnormal accumulation of fluid in the joint (effusion). The joint disease might be crystal induced, degenerative, inflammatory, or infectious. Morphologic analysis for cells and crystals, together with Gram stain and culture, will help in the differentiation. Aspiration is also done for effusions of unknown etiology and for pain or decreased joint mobility. Effusion of synovial fluid is usually present clinically before aspiration, and therefore it is often possible to aspirate 10 to 20 mL of the fluid for laboratory examination. The volume, normally about 1 mL, may be extremely small, however, so the laboratory receives only a drop of fluid in the aspiration syringe.

In the management of joint disorders, the differential diagnosis is essential so that the correct treatment can be instituted. Analysis of synovial fluid can be invaluable, providing an immediate diagnosis in some disorders and valuable information on other joint diseases. If fluid volume or resources are limited, the most important aspects of analysis are microbiological study and examination for crystals with compensated polarized light microscopy.

Classification of Synovial Fluid in Joint Disease

The differential diagnosis of diseased synovial fluid usually classifies the fluid as noninflammatory, inflammatory, infectious, crystal induced, or hemorrhagic. Although the disease states in these groups overlap, this classification is helpful.

Noninflammatory Fluid

Noninflammatory synovial fluid is seen in degenerative joint disease, such as osteoarthritis and traumatic arthritis. The fluid is usually clear and viscous; WBC count is less than 2000 cells/μ L, with less than 25% neutrophils. The glucose and protein contents are approximately the same as in normal synovial fluid. Collagen fibrils or cartilage fragments may be seen, especially with phase-contrast microscopy.

Inflammatory Fluid

Inflammatory effusions are associated with immunologic disease, such as RA and lupus arthritis. The fluid is cloudy and yellow, has low viscosity, and has a moderately high WBC count, 2000 to 20,000 cells/μL, with more than 50% neutrophils. The glucose content is normal and protein content high. The fluid may form spontaneous fibrin clots.

Infectious Fluid

Infectious infusions suggest a bacterial infection. The fluid is generally cloudy and has low viscosity. The fluid may be yellow, green, or milky. WBC count is very high, 500 to 200,000 cells/μL, with more than 90% neutrophils. The glucose content is characteristically very low. The protein content is high, and fibrin clot formation is common. Most infections are bacterial. *Staphylococcus aureus* and *Neisseria gonorrheae* are most common, although streptococci, *Haemophilus, Mycobacterium tuberculosis,* fungi, or anaerobic bacteria are also seen. The most common type of organism found varies with patient age.

Crystal-Induced Fluid

Crystal-induced effusions are seen in gout and pseudogout. The fluid is yellow or turbid and has a fairly high but variable WBC count, 500 to 200,000/μL, with an increased percentage of neutrophils (up to 90%). Crystals of monosodium urate (MSU) are seen with gout and calcium pyrophosphate dihydrate (CPPD) crystals with pseudogout. Crystals are recognized by morphology and appearance when examined by polarized microscopy, with the addition of a full-wave compensator.

Hemorrhagic Fluid

Hemorrhagic effusions are characterized by the presence of RBCs from bleeding or hemorrhage in the joint. This may be the result of tumor or traumatic injury such as fracture. Coagulation deficiencies such as hemophilia and treatment with anticoagulants may also result in hemorrhagic effusions.

Collection of Synovial Fluid

Synovial fluid is collected by needle aspiration, which is called *arthrocentesis.* Only experienced persons should collect synovial fluid, under strict sterile conditions with a disposable needle and plastic syringe to avoid contamination with confusing birefringent material. The fluid should be collected both anticoagulated and nonanticoagulated. Ideally, the fluid should be divided into the following three parts:

1. Sterile tube for microbiological examination
2. Tube with liquid EDTA (preferred) or sodium heparin for microscopic examination
3. Plain tube (without anticoagulant) for clot formation, gross appearance, and chemical and immunologic procedures (this should be a plain tube without a serum separator)

Normal synovial fluid does not clot. To test for clot formation, the fluid must be collected in a plain tube without anticoagulant. However, infectious and crystal-induced fluids tend to form fibrin clots, making an anticoagulant necessary for adequate cell counts and an even distribution of cells and crystals for morphologic analysis. If an anticoagulant is used, sodium heparin or liquid EDTA is the additive of choice. There is some disagreement as to whether anticoagulated or plain tubes should be used for analysis of crystals; the decision may need to be individualized. Ideally, both tubes would be made available so that if artifactual anticoagulant crystals are suspected, the plain clot tube could be examined.

Although an anticoagulant will prevent the formation of fibrin clots, it will not affect viscosity. Therefore, if the fluid is highly viscous, it can be incubated for several hours with a 0.5% solution of hyaluronidase in phosphate buffer to break down the hyaluronate. This reduces the viscosity, making the fluid easier to pipette and count.

Routine Examination of Synovial Fluid

The routine examination of synovial fluid should include (Kurec, 2012) gross appearance (color, clarity, and viscosity), (Teunissen & Willemse, 2013) microbiological studies, (American College of Obstetricians and Gynecologists (ACOG), 2013) WBC and differential counts, (4) polarizing microscopy for crystals, and (5) other tests as necessary. The most important tests are the microbiological studies, especially Gram stain, and the crystal analysis. If the quantity of aspirated fluid is limited, these should be done first.

Gross Appearance

The first step in the analysis of synovial fluid is to observe the specimen for color and clarity. Noninflammatory fluid is usually clear. To test for clarity, read newspaper print through a test tube containing the specimen. As the cell and protein contents increase or crystals precipitate, the turbidity increases, and the print becomes more difficult to read. In a traumatic tap of the joint, blood will be seen in the collection tubes in an uneven distribution, which diminishes as the aspiration continues. It may also be seen as an uneven distribution with streaks of blood in the aspiration syringe. A truly bloody fluid is uniform in color and does not clot. Xanthochromia in the supernatant fluid indicates bleeding in the joint, but this is difficult to evaluate because the fluid is normally yellow. A dark-red or dark-brown supernatant is evidence of joint bleeding rather than a traumatic tap.

Viscosity

Viscosity is most easily evaluated at the arthrocentesis by allowing the synovial fluid to drop from the end of the needle. Normally, synovial fluid will form a string 4 to 6 cm long. If it breaks before it reaches 3 cm in length, the viscosity is lower than normal. Inflammatory fluids contain enzymes that break down hyaluronic acid. Anything that decreases the hyaluronic acid content of synovial fluid lowers its viscosity.

Viscosity has been evaluated in the laboratory by means of the mucin clot test. However, this test is of questionable value because the results rarely change the diagnosis and are essentially the same as with the string test for viscosity.

Red and White Blood Cell Counts

The appearance of a drop of synovial fluid under an ordinary light microscope can be helpful in estimating the cell counts initially and in demonstrating the presence of crystals. The presence of only a few WBCs per high-power (40 ×) field suggests a noninflammatory disorder. A large number of WBCs would indicate inflammatory or infected synovial fluid. The total WBC count and differential count are important in diagnosis (Student Procedure Worksheet 14.2).

WBC counts less than 200/μL, with less than 25% polymorphonuclear cells (neutrophils, PMNs) and no RBCs, are normally observed in synovial fluid. Monocytes, lymphocytes, and macrophages are seen. A low WBC count (200–2000/μL) with predominantly mononuclear cells suggests a noninflammatory joint fluid, whereas a high WBC count suggests inflammation, and an extremely high count with a high proportion of PMNs strongly suggests infection.

Morphologic Examination

As with CSF, cytocentrifuged preparations of synovial fluid are preferred for the morphologic examination and WBC differential. These preparations may also be used for crystal identification. The procedure is generally the same as that described for CSF. Slides should be prepared as soon as possible after collection to prevent distortion and degeneration of cells. Digestion with hyaluronidase may be necessary with highly viscous fluids. If neutrophils are increased, they are especially prone to disintegration, making them difficult to recognize.

If a cytocentrifuge is not available, smears are made, as for CSF, from normally centrifuged sediment. Smears should be thin because hyaluronic acid will distort the cells. Smears are sometimes prepared from the fluid at aspiration. The smears are air-dried and Wright-stained.

Lupus erythematosus (LE) cells may be found in stained slides from patients with SLE and occasionally in fluid from patients with RA. The in vivo formation of LE cells in synovial fluid probably results from trauma to the WBCs.

Eosinophilia may be seen in metastatic carcinoma to the synovium, acute rheumatic fever, and RA. It is also associated with parasitic infections and Lyme disease and has also occurred after arthrography and radiation therapy.

Microscopic Examination for Crystals

A drop of synovial fluid is placed on a slide and a coverglass applied, as for the examination of urine sediment (see Chapter 13). To avoid confusion from extraneous particles that might polarize, it is recommended that slides and coverglasses be cleaned with alcohol and carefully dried with gauze or lens paper just before examination. Also, the coverglass should be immediately sealed with clear fingernail polish to reduce drying from evaporation. If nail polish is used, the slide should be allowed to dry for 15 minutes before microscopic examination to prevent damage to the objective. An unsealed preparation can be examined during this waiting period if desired. Any crystals at the junction of the nail polish and synovial fluid should be ignored.

The unclotted synovial fluid is first examined with an ordinary brightfield or, preferably, phase-contrast microscope. Crystals are reported as being present or absent and, if present, as intracellular, extracellular, or both. The initial examination is followed by compensated polarized light microscopy. After examination of the wet preparation, a cytocentrifuged preparation may also be examined for the presence and identity of crystals.

Brightfield or phase-contrast microscopic examination. Needle-shaped, intracellular MSU crystals seen in a simple wet preparation of synovial fluid are characteristic of gouty arthritis. Pseudogout, a crystal-deposition disease distinct from gout, is demonstrated by the presence of rhomboid CPPD crystals (see later discussion).

Cholesterol crystals are a rare finding in synovial fluid from persons with RA and are not seen in normal synovial fluid. Lipid crystals showing a Maltese cross formation with polarized light have also been reported as causing acute arthritis. These should not be confused with starch (a common contaminant) or with a rare form of MSU seen as a spherulite or "beach ball."

Crystals of hydroxyapatite have been reported as causing apatite gout. They are too small to be seen with ordinary microscopy. Clumps of these crystals, however, may be seen as spherical microaggregates.

Crystals of calcium oxalate may occur in oxalate gout, in patients receiving chronic renal dialysis, or in the rare primary oxalosis.

Polyester fibers have been seen in the synovial fluid of patients who have had joint replacement, indicating deterioration of the artificial joint. These birefringent fibers are difficult to evaluate in the synovial fluid, especially on cytocentrifuged preparations that contain fibers derived from the filter paper.

Iatrogenic or extraneous crystals may be present in the synovial fluid. Starch might be introduced from gloves. These crystals show a Maltese cross pattern that might be confused with lipid droplets of cholesterol or spherulites of urates. Other substances lining gloves appear as tiny rectangles that might be mistaken for CPPD.

If the joint has been treated with corticosteroids, crystals may be seen that resemble both MSU and CPPD. The crystals are generally extracellular and show numbers significantly greater than is typical of MSU or CPPD, but identification without the clinical history is difficult. Other substances that might be present and confusing are collagen fibrils, fibrin strands, and fragments of cartilage.

Table 14.4 summarizes the crystals seen in synovial fluid, and Table 14.5 details artifacts and contaminants.

Polarized light microscopy. More definitive microscopic identification of crystals in synovial fluid can be made with the use of polarized light (see Chapter 5). Both wet and cytocentrifuged preparations may be examined for the presence and identity of crystals. A polarizing microscope with a first-order red compensator (quartz compensator) is used. To set up the microscope, a polarizing filter (called a *polarizer*) is placed between the light source (bulb) and the specimen. A second polarizing filter (called an *analyzer*) is placed above the specimen, between the objective and the eyepiece. One of the polarizing filters (usually the polarizer) is rotated until the two are at right angles to each other. This is seen as the extinction of light through the microscope; one sees a black field because all light waves are canceled when the filters are at right angles to each other (see Fig. 5.11).

Certain objects or crystals have the ability to rotate or polarize light so that they are visible when viewed through crossed polarizing filters. This property is called *birefringence,* and objects are termed *weakly birefringent* or *strongly birefringent* depending on how completely they polarize light. Strongly birefringent crystals appear bright (white) against a dark background; weakly birefringent crystals appear less bright.

Monosodium urate. In synovial fluid, MSU crystals appear as strongly birefringent, needle-shaped or rod-shaped crystals 1 to 30 μm in length (Fig. 14.5). MSU crystals may be intracellular or extracellular, and this distinction is recorded. The presence of intracellular crystals is characteristic of acute gout; extracellular crystals imply a more chronic condition. Crystals from a tophus may be quite large. MSU crystals are found in almost 100% of patients with acute gouty arthritis and in 75% of those with chronic gout.

Calcium pyrophosphate dihydrate. CPPD crystals are also found in synovial fluid. These crystals are weakly birefringent, rod-shaped, rectangular, or rhomboid and are occasionally needle-shaped. CPPD crystals may be very short and chunky, varying from 1 to 20 μm in length and up to about 4 μm in width. These crystals are characteristic of pseudogout, also referred to as *pyrophosphate gout* or *calcium pyrophosphate dihydrate crystal deposition disease.* Pseudogout is seen in patients with degenerative arthritis and in arthritides associated with hypothyroidism, hyperparathyroidism, hemochromatosis,

TABLE 14.4 Clinically Significant Crystals in Synovial Fluid

Crystal	Morphology	Strength of Birefringence	Crystal Color When Parallel to Slow Wave	Crystal Size (mm)	Comments
MSU	Long, slender needles	Strong	Yellow	1–30	Seen in gout
CPPD	Short, chunky rectangles or rhomboids	Weak	Blue	1–20	Seen in pseudogout (or more)
Hydroxyapatite	Shiny clumps	Difficult to detect	N/A	0.5–1	Need electron microscope to visualize
Cholesterol plates	Large, flat, notched plates	Variable	Variable	10–100	Extremely rare, chronic effusion
Fat droplets (cholesterol)	Round spheres	Strong	Blue-yellow Maltese cross	2–15	Maltese cross appearance similar to starch
Cartilage fragments	Irregular	Strong	Variable	10–50	No definite crystal morphology
Polyethylene "wear" fragments	Long threads	Strong	Variable	Variable	Appearance similar to Cytospin filter paper fibers
Calcium oxalate	Bipyramidal (octahedrons)	Strong/variable	N/A	2–10	Seen in oxalate gout, especially with renal dialysis
Hematin	Vivid yellow-brown; diamond shape	Weak	Might confuse with CPPD; use brightfield to avoid confusion	—	Seen 2–4 weeks after hemorrhage

CPPD, Calcium pyrophosphate dihydrate; *MSU,* monosodium urate; *N/A,* not applicable.

TABLE 14.5 Artifacts and Contaminants in Synovial Fluid

Crystal	Morphology	Strength of Birefringence	Crystal Color When Parallel to Slow Wave	Crystal Size (mm)	Comments
Corticosteroids	Variable Similar to MSU with blunt, jagged edges	Strong	Yellow	2–15 or more; variable	Common artifact from injection solution in alcohol Polarize like MSU Appear similar to MSU or CPPD
Starch	Variable Globule with irregular edges and central dimple	Strong	Blue-yellow Maltese cross	2–15	Common contaminant Maltese cross similar to cholesterol Use brightfield to identify
	Similar to tiny CPPD	—	Yellow	—	Similar to hydroxyapatite or CPPD
Filter paper fibers	—	Strong	Variable	10–50 or more	Similar to polyester fragments
Lipids from cells	—	Strong	Blue-yellow Maltese cross	≈ 1–2	Indicate degeneration of cells
Nail polish	—	—	—	—	Causes confusion; avoid edges of coverslip

CPPD, Calcium pyrophosphate dihydrate; *MSU,* Monosodium urate.

and other conditions. Symptoms of pseudogout resemble those of gout, RA, and osteoarthritis.

Compensated polarized light. MSU and CPPD crystals that have been identified by polarized light are further identified by adding a full-wave compensator. This is also referred to as a *first-order red plate* (filter) or a *full-wave retardation plate.* Morphology and intensity of birefringence, although helpful, are not sufficient in separating these crystals.

Birefringent crystals have different properties when viewed with polarized light with the addition of a compensator. When the compensator is in place, the background appears magenta rather than black. The compensator may be inserted above the analyzer or the polarizer. It is inserted in such a manner that the axis of slow vibration of the compensator (called the *slow wave*) is at an angle of 45 degrees to the crossed polarizers. In determining the type of crystal, the direction of the slow wave

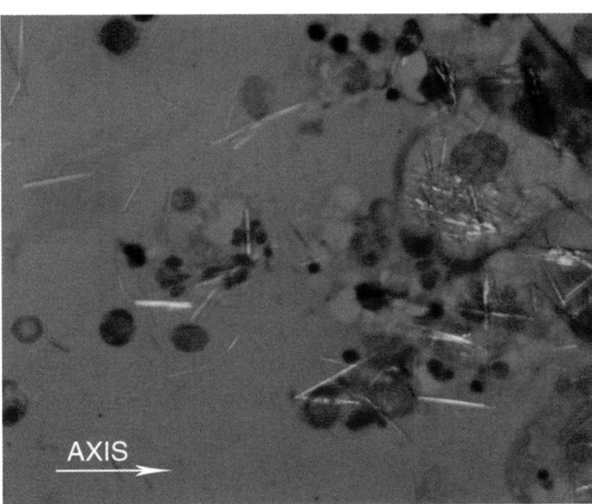

Fig. 14.5 Monosodium urate (MSU) crystals. In synovial fluid, fine, needlelike MSU crystals appear yellow, and calcium pyrophosphate crystals (rodlike) appear blue, when viewed using polarizing microscopy with longitudinal axis parallel to axis of the red compensator. (From Brunzel NA: *Fundamentals of urine and body fluid analysis,* ed 4, Philadelphia, 2018, Saunders.)

must be known. Crystals are identified by observation of the color of the long axis of the crystal in its relationship or orientation to the direction of the slow wave.

Crystals of MSU and CPPD have opposite characteristics when viewed with compensated polarized light. Crystals of MSU appear yellow when the long axis of the crystal lies parallel to the slow wave of the red compensator. These crystals appear blue when the long axis of the crystal lies perpendicular to the slow wave. This may be demonstrated by looking for crystals in the fluid that are so oriented, or by observing a crystal in a parallel orientation and then repositioning the slow wave at right angles to its original position. Alternatively, if the microscope has a rotating stage, the stage may be moved so that the crystal is rotated 90 degrees. In the case of MSU, the crystal will change from a yellow to a blue color. Crystals that appear yellow when parallel and blue when perpendicular to the slow wave exhibit negative birefringence. That is, the sign of birefringence is negative. The word *negative* should be avoided in reporting findings in synovial fluid so that it is not taken to mean the crystal in question is "absent." Crystals are reported as being "present" or "absent" and are identified as to crystal type.

In the case of CPPD, the crystal appears blue when the long axis of the crystal is parallel to the direction of the slow wave. The same crystal will appear yellow when it lies perpendicular to the slow wave, which can be demonstrated as previously described. The sign of birefringence in this case is positive (positive birefringence), which by definition is blue when the long axis is parallel to the slow wave. A determination of the type of birefringence with CPPD crystals may be troublesome because it may be very difficult to determine their long axis, which may be very short and almost square.

Microbiological Examination

Pathogenic organisms can be identified by the use of Gram stain and by culturing the synovial fluid. Cultures for suspected bacteria or mycobacterial or fungal infections are an essential part of the synovial fluid analysis. Gonococcal arthritis is a joint disease that may be difficult to diagnose unless special techniques and care are used.

Chemistry Tests

Glucose. The determination of glucose in the synovial fluid is valuable when infectious diseases are suspected. For example, a significantly lower glucose level in synovial fluid than in serum or plasma suggests infection of the joint. Samples of the patient's synovial fluid and blood must be obtained at the same time for a comparison of the two values to be valid.

Protein. Total synovial protein level is increased in several conditions. With inflammatory joint disease, such as RA, the total protein level approaches that of plasma. Normally, it is about a third of the plasma value. Values are also increased in gout and infectious arthritis.

Other tests. Other tests include LDH, uric acid, and lactate determinations.

Immunologic Tests

The synovial fluid normally contains a lower immunoglobulin concentration than plasma. This is not the case in RA, in which the level of immunoglobulin is about equal to that in plasma, which suggests the production of immunoglobulins in the affected joint.

Rheumatoid factor has been reported in the synovial fluid as well as in the serum of RA patients. The presence of rheumatoid factor in the synovial fluid but not in the serum can be helpful in the diagnosis of RA.

Other immunologic tests include antinuclear antibodies, which are associated with SLE, and the demonstration of decreased complement levels.

SEMINAL FLUID

The main function of seminal fluid is to transport sperm to female cervical mucus. After deposition in the female reproductive tract, sperm remain in seminal plasma for a short time while attempting to enter the mucus.

Semen Analysis

Seminal specimens are analyzed for male infertility. In addition to the traditional procedure that is described in this section, a new method has been developed.

Magnetic Resonance Spectroscopy Testing

This new magnetic resonance spectroscopy technique uses powerful magnets and works like radar by firing pulses of energy at the sperm specimen and then listening to the echoed signal given by the molecules in response. This technique has never been used to examine live sperm. The magnetic resonance spectroscopy technique detects differences in molecular composition as a novel biomarker between good and poor sperm specimens.

A major advantage of this approach is that unlike traditional staining or methods that break open the membranes of sperm cells to examine the contents, the low-energy pulses do not damage the sperm. Because of the viability of sperm after processing and examination, specimens can potentially be used for in vitro fertilization (IVF) treatment.

Traditional Seminal Analysis

A fresh specimen of semen is needed. The specimen may be collected in a clean, sterile, glass or plastic container. Ideally, seminal fluid should be analyzed within 30 minutes of collection. It is mandatory that the specimen be kept at 37°C and examined within 1 to 2 hours of collection. After 60 minutes of storage in a plastic container, sperm motility is significantly reduced. Most laboratories examine two specimens collected a few days apart. Collection, proper transport, and prompt examination are critical factors in the analysis of seminal fluid. Again, all persons must adhere to Standard Precautions when handling semen, blood, and other body fluids.

It is recommended that a 3- to 5-day period of sexual abstinence be observed before specimen collection; 2 days may be sufficient, but the period should not exceed 5 days. Condoms treated with spermicide or lubricants with spermicidal properties must be avoided during specimen collection. In addition, patients must be advised to keep the specimen warm if collected at home and to deliver it promptly to the laboratory.

Semen analysis is typically done for assessment of fertility or infertility, forensic purposes, determination of the effectiveness of vasectomy, and determination of the suitability of semen for artificial insemination procedures.

Semen (seminal fluid) consists of a combination of products of various male reproductive organs (Fig. 14.6). The total volume of semen is formed by secretions from various structures (Table 14.6). The reference range of a sperm count is 20 to 160 million/mL.

During ejaculation the products are mixed, producing the normal viscous semen specimen, or ejaculate. This ejaculated human semen is a viscous, yellow-gray fluid that forms a fairly firm, gel-like clot immediately after ejaculation. At room temperature, this clot liquefies spontaneously and completely within 5 to 60 minutes. If the liquefaction process requires more than 1 hour, the specimen is considered abnormal. Liquefaction must be complete before any laboratory analysis can be done.

Macroscopic Examination

Macroscopic examination of seminal fluid includes time for complete liquefaction, appearance, volume, viscosity (consistency), and pH.

Wet-Mount Analysis

Wet-mount analysis is used to determine the approximate sperm count and motility. A drop of the thoroughly mixed, liquefied semen specimen is placed on a clean glass slide under a coverslip. The volume of semen delivered onto the slide and the dimensions of the coverslip must be standardized. A standardized volume of 10 μL covered with a 22 × 22–mm coverglass will result in a fixed depth of about 20 μm and allow for an estimate of sperm number, morphology, motility, and velocity. The freshly made preparation is allowed to stabilize for 1 to 3 minutes before microscopic analysis. This is done by observing 10 to 20 microscope fields, using a 40× or 60× (high-power) objective.

Normally, mature sperm cells make up the majority of cells seen (Fig. 14.7). Other cells typically seen are epithelial cells from the male genital tract, immature germ cells, and WBCs. Percentages of the various types of cells are determined and reported. The approximate sperm count is reported as *few, several, many,* or *numerous.* Although subjective, this estimate should correlate with the actual chamber sperm count. The relative percentage of motile sperm is determined while the sperm count is estimated. Because mobility and velocity are temperature dependent, a microscope with a warm stage should be used. At least 200 motile and nonmotile sperm are counted in at least five different microscope fields, and the percentage of motile sperm is calculated as follows:

$$\%\,\text{Motility} = \frac{\text{Total sperm} - \text{Nonmotile sperm}}{\text{Total sperm}} \times 100$$

Normally, 50% or more sperm are motile.

Other Tests

Qualitative semen analysis is subjective and generally requires further testing, including tests or observations of agglutination, viability, counting-chamber sperm counts, and sperm antibody assays. In addition, sperm morphology can be evaluated by performing a differential count of morphologically normal and abnormal sperm types on a hematoxylin-eosin–stained smear.

The new Sperm-Chex and Sperm-Chex Post VC have stabilized sperm cells assayed for the Makler Counting Chamber. Two clinically significant levels of control simulate sperm cell concentrations. The stabilized control sperm cells have the same chamber-loading and optical characteristics as a patient sample. Sperm-Chex verifies the sperm analysis process and assesses the technologist's efficiency in sperm cell quantification and qualification. Sperm-Chex Post VC is a positive/negative postvasectomy sperm count control to validate the postvasectomy sperm count procedure.

AMNIOTIC FLUID

Amniotic fluid is the nourishing and protecting liquid contained by the amnion of a pregnant woman (Fig. 14.8). It consists of mostly water but also contains *proteins, carbohydrates, lipids/phospholipids, urea,* and *electrolytes,* all of which aid in the growth of the fetus. In the late stages of gestation, most of the amniotic fluid consists of fetal urine.

The volume of amniotic fluid increases until about 34 weeks' gestation, when the amount of amniotic fluid is about 800 mL. This amount decreases to about 600 mL at birth (about 40 weeks).

Amniotic fluid is continually being swallowed and "inhaled" and replaced by being "exhaled." It is essential that the amniotic fluid be breathed into the lungs by the fetus for the lungs to develop normally. The analysis of amniotic fluid, tapped from the mother's abdomen, is called *amniocentesis.*

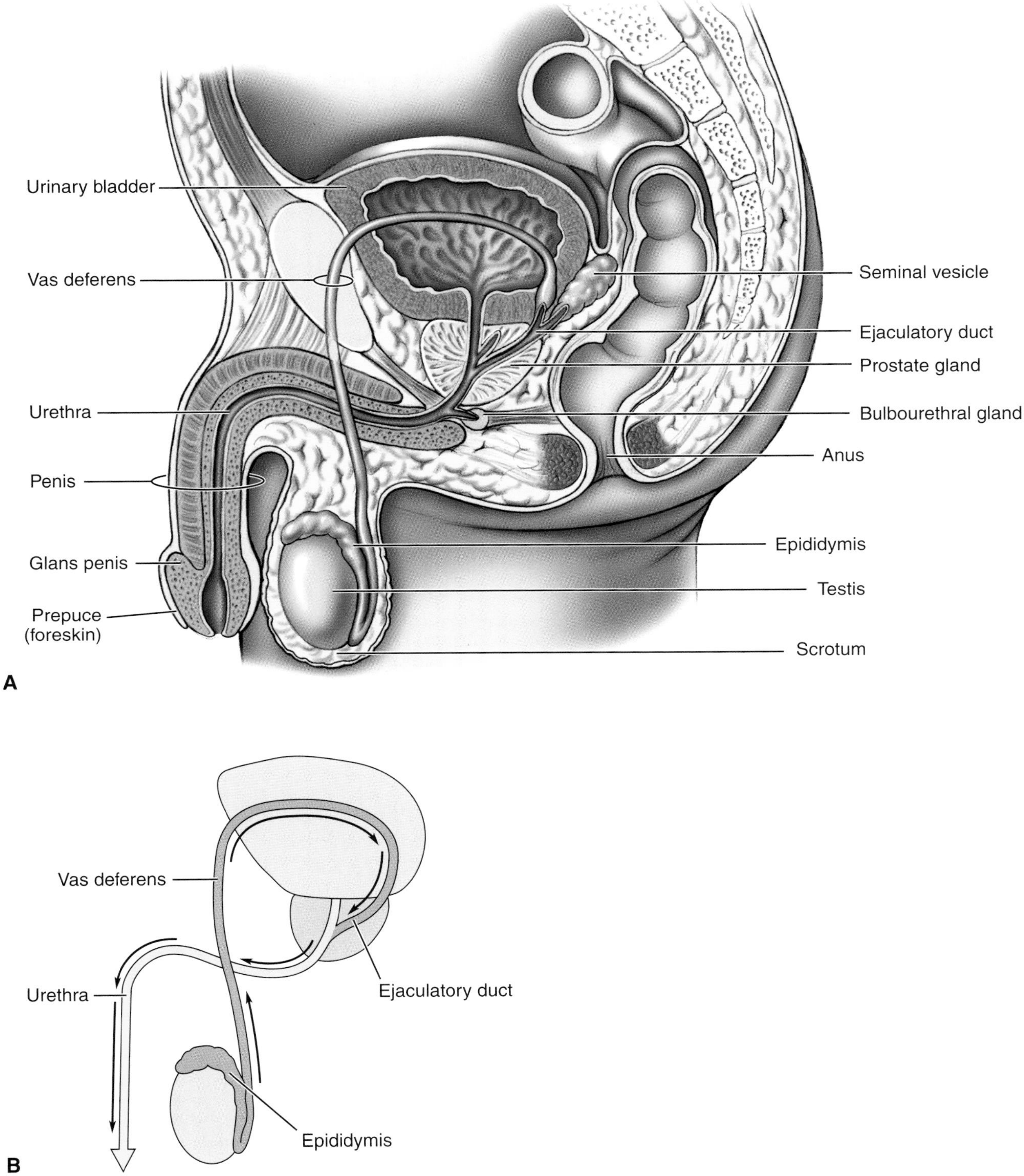

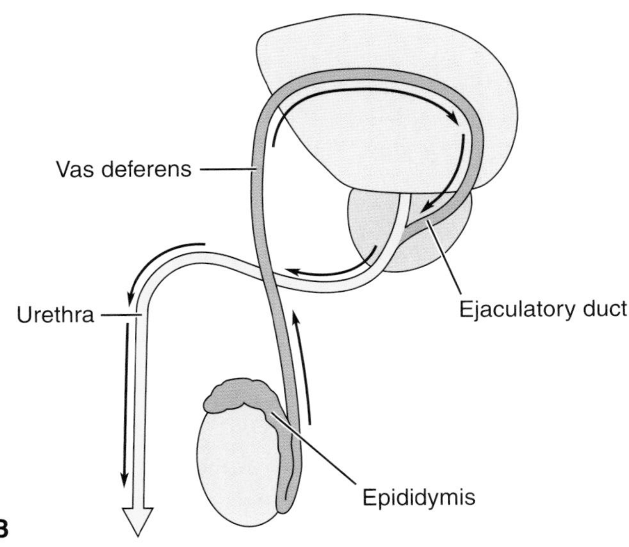

Fig. 14.6 Male reproductive system. (A) Male reproductive organs; (B) the pathway for semen (From Herlihy B: *The human body in health and illness,* ed 5, St Louis, 2014, Elsevier.)

Fetal Lung Maturity

Risk of respiratory distress syndrome (RDS) is inversely related to gestational age at birth. Newborn prematurity is associated with numerous complications, including neonatal RDS, a cause of infant morbidity and mortality. Since 2012, advances in neonatal care (e.g., surfactant replacement therapy and antenatal corticosteroid therapy) have significantly decreased infant mortality due to RDS. Amniocentesis for the determination of fetal lung maturity in well-dated pregnancies generally should not be used to guide the timing of delivery[3]. Fetal lung maturity

TABLE 14.6 Seminal Fluid: Structures and Secretions

Structure	Contribution to Total Volume of Semen (%)
Testes and epididymis	<5
Seminal vesicles	60
Prostate gland	30
Bulbourethral glands	<5
Sperm count	20–160 million/mL

From Patton KT, Thibodeau GA: *Anatomy & physiology*, ed 7, St Louis, 2010, Mosby.

can be hastened with antenatal corticosteroid injections at least 48 hours prior to a premature delivery and/or with intratracheal surfactant therapy in a preterm infant. The identification of those women who will deliver imminently is important to reduce morbidity and mortality in the neonate[4].

Amniotic fluid contains fetal cells that can be examined for genetic defects, and chemical analysis such as fibronectin and other assays can determine fetal lung maturity (FLM). Analysis of amniotic fluid does not necessarily reflect maturity in organ systems other than the lungs. FLM testing has limited value, according to the 2013 American College of Obstetrics and Gynecology (ACOG) guidelines,[3] which advise against delivery at < 39 weeks unless

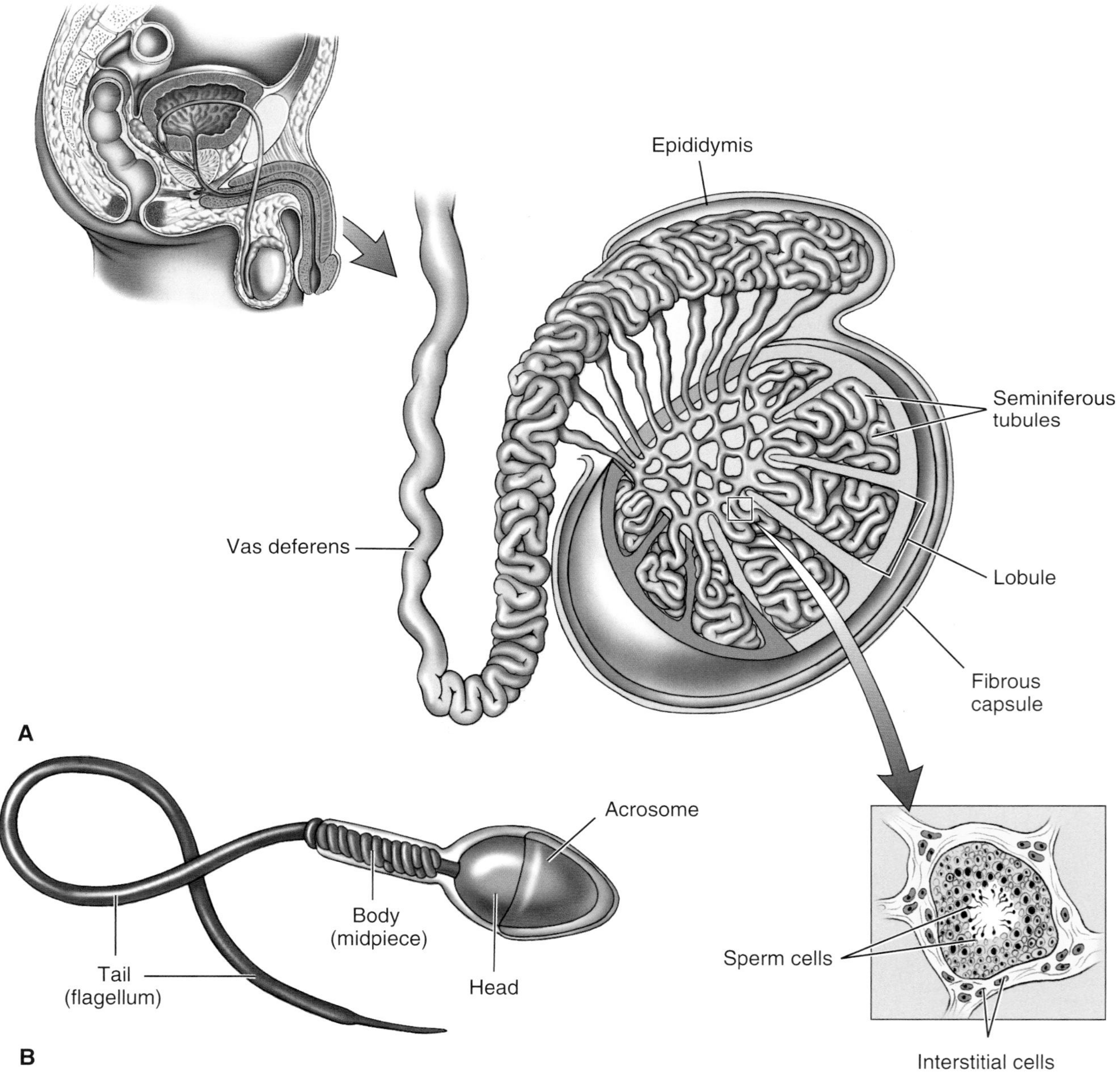

Fig. 14.7 Sperm formation. (A) Male gonad. The testis consists of lobules containing seminiferous tubules surrounded by interstitial cells. (B) Sperm. (From Herlihy B: *The human body in health and illness,* ed 5, St Louis, 2014, Elsevier.)

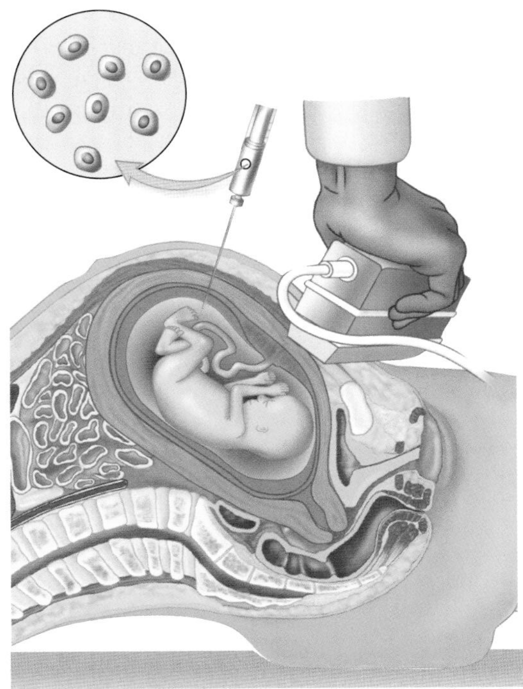

Fig. 14.8 Amniocentesis. (From Patton KT, Thibodeau GA: *Anatomy & physiology*, ed 7, St Louis, 2010, Mosby.)

medically mandated due to potential serious morbidity compared with those delivered at $\geq$ 39 weeks in spite of mature FLM tests.

Fetal Fibronectin

Fetal fibronectin (fFN) is the only test recommended by the American College of Obstetricians and Gynecologists for the prediction of preterm birth in women with and without symptoms of preterm labor[4]. However, many laboratories are discontinuing this assay because of the lack of diagnostic strength.[4] Fetal fibronectin (fFN) is a protein produced during pregnancy and functions as a biological glue, attaching the fetal sac to the uterine lining. An fFN test is performed if a woman is 26 to 34 weeks pregnant and is having symptoms of premature labor. The goal is to intervene to prevent the potentially serious health complications of a preterm baby.

A cervical or vaginal fluid sample is collected and analyzed for fFN. During the first trimester and for about half of the second trimester (up to 22 weeks' gestation), fFN is normally present in the cervicovaginal secretions of pregnant women. In most pregnancies, after 22 weeks, this protein is no longer detected until the end of the last trimester, 1 to 3 weeks before labor. The presence of fFN during weeks 24 to 34 of a high-risk pregnancy, along with symptoms of labor, suggests that the "glue" may be disintegrating ahead of schedule and alerts physicians to possible preterm delivery.

A laboratory assay positive result is expressed when the concentration of fFN is $\geq$ 0.05 μg/mL. A negative fFN result is highly predictive that preterm delivery will not occur within the next 7 to 14 days. A negative fFN can reduce unnecessary hospitalizations and drug therapies. High levels can have causes other than the risk of preterm delivery. The ACOG currently does not recommend routine fFN screening of pregnant women because its use has not been shown to be clinically effective in predicting preterm labor in low-risk, asymptomatic pregnancies.

Pulmonary Surfactants

RDS is caused by insufficient concentrations of pulmonary surfactants. This condition produces collapsed alveoli that are perfused but hypoventilated. The result is hypoxia, hypercapnia (a condition of abnormally elevated carbon dioxide [CO_2] levels in the blood), and respiratory acidosis.

Pulmonary surfactants are synthesized by type II pneumocytes and packaged into storage granules called **lamellar bodies** that function to decrease alveolar surface tension. These surfactants are as follows:

- Lecithin—detectable at week 28; surges at week 36
- Phosphatidylinositol—detectable at week 28; peaks at week 35
- Sphingomyelin—detectable at week 28
- Phosphatidylglycerol—detectable at week 36, with an increasing concentration until delivery

There continues to be a need for some laboratory testing in certain circumstances. The status of fetal lung maturity is reflected in the concentration of surfactant in the form of phospholipids and lamellar bodies present in amniotic fluid but it is a better indicator of maturity than immaturity.

SALIVA

Saliva, a clear, alkaline, and viscous fluid secreted by mucous glands of the mouth, can be used for various analyses. Microbial studies of viruses and bacteria and chemical testing of hormones, therapeutic drugs, and drugs of abuse can be performed on saliva. Saliva may be tested in the blood bank to detect secretors of certain antigens. The most common way of collecting a specimen is to have a patient chew on wax or absorbent dental cotton for several minutes and then collect the saliva.

AUTOMATION IN BODY FLUID ANALYSIS

Chemical analysis of body fluids (e.g., CSF) has been performed using chemistry automation for many years. Cerebrospinal fluid is the most challenging body fluid for such analysis because it requires the ability to count and differentiate WBCs down to a "normal" range, which is much lower than the diagnostic cutoff values used for other body fluids (e.g., serous fluids). The counting of cells in body fluids has traditionally been done by a manual counting method using a hemacytometer. This technique is subjective and is an extremely labor-intensive process. Precision at or around the cerebrospinal fluid WBC normal range is reduced even with the best flow cytometers, but manual microscopy is even less precise. Today, automated cell counting for body fluids is gradually replacing manual cell counting by hemacytometer. During the last decade, automated analyzers have become a popular method for first-line screening.

Automated Hematology Platforms

The addition of body fluid modes to some hematology analyzers adapts hematology automation technology and software to meet the particular requirements of body fluid analysis. However, the functional sensitivity for low cell counts currently limits the applicability of automated methods to certain types of body fluids. These analyzers offer the advantages of better precision, faster turnaround time, and reduced error.

Manual microscopy is still considered the gold standard despite its many limitations. Other types of specimens that laboratories may not want to analyze with hematology analyzers include purulent and flocculent specimens because there is concern that such specimens could clog flow cells or apertures. Additionally, crystals in synovial fluids may cause a falsely increased count and may need to be confirmed with a manual count.

Characteristics of Automated Hematology Platforms

The Abbott CELL-DYN Sapphire hematology analyzer for automated differentiation of cells in serous fluids was used to explore whether manual analysis of the raw data files could improve the differential count compared with reference microscopy. The standard Sapphire algorithm showed substantial deviations from the reference microscopic differentiation: polymorphonuclear cell counts were too high because they contained some monocytic cells. However, when an optimized manual gating strategy was used, a good correlation and negligible bias were found. It has been demonstrated that with a modified algorithm, the CELL-DYN Sapphire will provide reliable identification and enumeration of blood cells in peritoneal and pleural fluids.

The Siemens Advia 120 can analyze body fluids. Pretreating synovial fluid samples with hyaluronidase enzyme allows the specimens to be analyzed, with no significant differences found between manual and automated methods with respect to leukocyte counts and differentials. Results with pleural fluid samples indicated that leukocyte and differential counts obtained with the Advia 120 showed significant differences from results obtained with manual methods because of the high incidence of mesothelial, lymphoid, and other tumoral cells in that type of body fluid specimen. The use of hematology analyzers is questionable for these kinds of samples, especially from oncology patients with tumors.

Automated Urinalysis Platforms

In recent years, the addition of body fluid analysis to the capabilities of automated urinalysis analyzers has emerged. Technological advances have expanded the analytical capabilities to enable the processing of multiple types of specimens, including urine, CSF, peritoneal fluid, pleural fluid, synovial fluid, and lavages, on a single analyzer. Unlike hematology analyzers, which use particle counting and flow cell technology, automated urinalysis analyzers use digital imaging to perform counts. When digital imaging technology is used, there is reduced interference from background counts, and such analyzers have been judged to perform better than hematology analyzers with low cell counts. Performing automated body fluid counting on the same analyzer as that used for urinalysis can increase the testing volume, which can increase the cost-effectiveness for both low-volume laboratories and large laboratories.

Characteristics of Automated Urinalysis Platforms

The Beckman-Coulter Iris iQ200 Body Fluids Module provides laboratories with a standardized and fully automated method for the analysis of eight sample types (synovial fluid, CSF, pleural fluid, peritoneal fluid, peritoneal dialysate, peritoneal lavage, pericardial fluid, and serous fluid). This module provides true cell-count standardization and onscreen viewing of bacteria, crystals, and cellular abnormalities.

When CSF was evaluated with the new body fluids module for the Sysmex UF1000-i (UF1000i-BF) for analysis of WBCs and RBCs in CSF, it provided rapid and accurate WBC and RBC counts in clinically relevant values of CSF cells. The use of the UF1000i-BF may allow for replacement of routine optical counting, except for samples displaying abnormal WBC counts or abnormal scattergram distribution, for which differential cell counts may still be required. In addition, the Sysmex UF-1000i urinalysis analyzer can count total WBCs and RBCs in continuous ambulatory peritoneal dialysis (CAPD), ascites, and pleural fluids. The UF1000i-BF mode offers rapid and reliable total WBC and RBC counts for initial screening of pleural fluid. When using automated analyzers, however, the inspection of scattergrams is required to ensure the most accurate results are obtained.

CASE STUDIES

CASE STUDY 14.1

A 14-year-old high school student with fever, chills, and severe headache is seen in an urgent care clinic. He felt nauseated and vomited before reporting to the clinic. At the clinic, his temperature is 104°F; he has neck rigidity and complains of back pain. Some small petechial spots are noted on his chest and back and in the mouth. Blood is drawn for a complete blood count (CBC) and blood glucose, and a lumbar puncture is performed. Cerebrospinal fluid is collected sequentially in three sterile tubes and examined. The results are as follows:

Blood Results

White cell count: 25 × 10^9/L

Differential: 80% neutrophils, 10% lymphocytes, 10% monocytes

Glucose: 95 mg/dL

Cerebrospinal Fluid Results

CSF pressure: Increased

Gross appearance: All tubes equally cloudy, not bloody

Continued

CASE STUDY 14.1—cont'd

Glucose: 15 mg/dL
CSF white cell count: 12.0 × 10^9/µL; 90% neutrophils
Gram stain: Many Gram-negative cocci in pairs, some intracellular

Multiple Choice Questions
Answers are in Appendix A.

1. What type of infection is suggested by this patient's white cell count and differential on venous blood?
   a. Bacterial
   b. Viral
   c. Parasitic
   d. Cannot differentiate
2. What is the significance of the gross appearance of the spinal fluid in this patient?
   a. Indicates possible bleeding
   b. Indicates possible infection
   c. Is insignificant
   d. Either a or b
3. What is the significance of the CSF glucose in this patient?
   a. Possible viral infection
   b. Possible bacterial infection
   c. Possible hemorrhage
   d. All the above

Critical Thinking Group Discussion Questions

1. Based on the Gram stain, what is the likely diagnosis for this patient? Explain the reason for your answer.
2. How can this patient's diagnosis be differentiated from other similar clinical presentations?

Note: Narrative answers are published on the EVOLVE instructor site.

CASE STUDY 14.2

A 75-year-old woman has had a long history of joint pain in the large joints. She now has shoulder pain and a swollen and red knee joint. She has a slight fever and bilateral muscle weakness in the lower limbs. Blood is drawn for hematology, radiographs of her knee are taken, and arthrocentesis is performed on her knee.

Hematology Results
Hemoglobin: 11.9 g/dL
White cell count: 12.0 × 10^9/L

Radiographic Findings
Calcification in the cartilage and meniscus (chondrocalcinosis)

Synovial Fluid Findings
Appearance: Cloudy and watery
Microscopic examination: Many neutrophils; intracellular and extracellular crystals present, appearing as small, chunky rectangles that show weak birefringence and appear blue when parallel and yellow when perpendicular to the slow wave of vibration of compensated polarized light

Multiple Choice Questions
Answers in Appendix A.

1. The pattern of birefringence in this patient is consistent with:
   a. Calcium pyrophosphate dihydrate (CPPD)
   b. Cholesterol
   c. Hydroxyapatite (HA)
   d. Monosodium urate (MSU)
2. The disease exhibited by this patient is referred to as:
   a. Gout
   b. Osteoarthritis
   c. Pseudogout
   d. Rheumatoid arthritis
3. The defect in this disorder is a defect of:
   a. Urea metabolism
   b. Purine metabolism
   c. Pyrimidine metabolism
   d. Blood coagulation cascade

Critical Thinking Group Discussion Questions

1. Explain the pathophysiology (defect) that produces this patient's diagnosis.
2. Does this patient's diagnosis resemble any other metabolic defects?

Note: Narrative answers are published on the EVOLVE instructor site.

REFERENCES

1. Kurec A: Answering your questions, *MLO Med Lab Obs* 44(12):34, 2012.
2. Teunissen CE, Willemse EAJ: Cerebrospinal fluid biomarkers for Alzheimer's disease: emergence of the solution to an important unmet need, *J Int Fed Clin Chem* 24(3):1–7, 2013.
3. American College of Obstetricians and Gynecologists (ACOG): Medically indicated late-preterm and early-term deliveries, Committee Opinion 560, Am College of Obstetricians and Gynecologists, *Obstet Gynecol* 121(4):908–910, 2013.
4. Woodworth A: *Should We Still be Performing Fetal Fibronectin Testing in the Clinical Lab?* National Academy of Clinical Biochemistry (NACB), AACC Scientific Shorts, June, 2013.

BIBLIOGRAPHY

Aulesa C, Mainar I, Prieto M, et al: Use of the Advia 120 hematology analyzer in the differential cytologic analysis of biological fluids (cerebrospinal, peritoneal, pleural, pericardial, synovial, and others), *Lab Hematol* 9(4):214–224, 2003.

Brunzel NA: In *Body fluid: clinical importance and utility of cell counts,* Presented at American Association for Clinical Chemistry Annual Meeting, Orlando, Fla. 2005.

Brunzel NA: *Fundamentals of urine and body fluid analysis,* ed 4, St Louis, 2018, Elsevier.
Buoro S, Apassiti Esposito S, Alessio M, et al: Automated cerebrospinal fluid cell counts using the new body fluid mode of Sysmex UF-1000i, *J Clin Lab Anal* 30(5):381–391, 2016.
Butch AW: In *Performance of the Iris iQ200 for body fluid cell counting,* Presented at American Association for Clinical Chemistry Annual Meeting, Orlando, Fla. 2005.
College of American Pathologists: Hematology; clinical microscopy; body fluids [glossary entries]. In 1996 Proficiency Testing Program, Northfield, Ill, 1996, CAP.
de Graaf MT, de Jongste AH, Kraan J, et al: Flow cytometric characterization of cerebrospinal fluid cells, *Cytometry B Clin Cytom* 80(5):271–281, 2011.
Fleming C, Brouwer R, van Alphen A, et al: UF-1000i: validation of the body fluid mode for counting cells in body fluids, *Clin Chem Lab Med* 52(12):1781–1790, 2014.
Iris iQ200 Operators Manual. Rev A 07/2005. Chatsworth, Calif, Iris Diagnostics, Division of IRIS International, 2005.
Karcher DS, McPherson RA: Cerebrospinal, synovial, and serous body fluids and alternative specimens. In McPherson RA, Pincus MR, editors: *Henry's clinical diagnosis and management by laboratory methods*, 22 ed., Philadelphia, 2011, Elsevier/Saunders, pp 480–508.
Keuren JF, Hoffmann JJ, Leers MP: Analysis of serous body fluids using the CELL-DYN Sapphire hematology analyzer, *Clin Chem Lab Med* 51(6):1285–1290, 2013.
Kjeldsberg CR, Knight JA: *Body fluids: laboratory examination of amniotic, cerebrospinal, seminal, serous and synovial fluids,* ed 3, Chicago, 1993, American Society of Clinical Pathologists Press.
McCarty DJ, editor: *Arthritis and allied conditions: a textbook of rheumatology*, 12 ed., Baltimore, 1992, Lippincott Williams & Wilkins.
Ringsrud KM, Linné JJ: *Urinalysis and body fluids: a color text and atlas,* St Louis, 1995, Mosby.
Sandhaus LM: Body fluid cell counts by automated methods, *Clinics Lab Med* 53(11):1689–1706, 2015.
Schumacher RH Jr, Reginato AJ: *Atlas of synovial fluid analysis and crystal identification,* Philadelphia, 1991, Lea & Febiger.
Scott G: An automated approach to body fluid analysis, *MLO* 46 (6):20–22, 2014.
Technology Networks: New "sperm radar" test may uncover secrets about male infertility, https://www.technologynetworks.com. Retrieved June 2017.
Turgeon ML: *Clinical hematology,* ed 6, Philadelphia, 2018, Lippincott Williams & Wilkins.
Turgeon ML: *Immunology and serology in laboratory medicine,* ed 6, St Louis, 2018, Mosby.
Walker T, Nelson L, Dunphy B, Anderson D, Kickler T: Comparative evaluation of the Iris iQ200 Body Fluids Module with manual hemacytometer count, *Am J Clin Pathol* 131:333–338, 2009.
Yang D, Zhou Y, Chen B: Performance evaluation and result comparison of the automated hematology analyzers Abbott CD 3700, Sysmex XE 2100 and Coulter LH 750 for cell counts in serous fluids, *Clinica Chimica Acta* 419(18):113–118, 2013.

REVIEW QUESTIONS (ANSWERS IN APPENDIX A)

Overview of Body Fluids

1. Which of the following fluids is *not* an ultrafiltrate of plasma?
   a. Cerebrospinal fluid
   b. Peritoneal fluid
   c. Pleural fluid
   d. Synovial fluid

Cerebrospinal Fluid

2. Regarding gross appearance, normal spinal fluid is:
   a. Crystal clear
   b. Pale yellow
   c. Slightly cloudy
   d. Xanthochromatic
3. In cerebrospinal fluid (CSF) examination, which of the following characterizes bilirubin from past hemorrhage?
   a. Pale-pink or pale-orange xanthochromasia in supernatant
   b. Three sequentially collected tubes that are equally bloody
   c. Three sequentially collected tubes that are progressively less bloody, with the third being clear or almost clear
   d. Yellow xanthochromasia in supernatant fluid
4. Which of the following characterizes the normal CSF appearance?
   a. Cloudy fluid in all tubes
   b. Crystal-clear fluid in all tubes
   c. Pale-pink or pale-orange xanthochromasia in supernatant
   d. Three sequentially collected tubes that are equally bloody
5. In CSF examination, which of the following characterizes a fresh subarachnoid hemorrhage?
   a. Cloudy fluid in all tubes
   b. Crystal-clear fluid in all tubes
   c. Three sequentially collected tubes that are equally bloody
   d. Three sequentially collected tubes that are progressively less bloody, with the third being clear or almost clear
6. Which of the following characterizes a traumatic spinal tap?
   a. Cloudy fluid in all tubes
   b. Crystal-clear fluid in all tubes
   c. Three sequentially collected tubes that are equally bloody
   d. Three sequentially collected tubes that are progressively less bloody, with the third being clear or almost clear
7. A lower-than-normal CSF glucose level in relation to blood glucose is most characteristic of which of the following?
   a. Bacterial meningitis
   b. Brain tumor
   c. Diabetic coma
   d. Viral meningitis
8. Increased cerebrospinal fluid with increased CSF white cell count and a preponderance of neutrophils is most characteristic of which condition?
   a. Bacterial meningitis
   b. Tuberculosis
   c. Viral meningitis
   d. Yeast infection

Serous Fluids: Pericardial, Pleural, and Peritoneal

9. Exudate is:
   a. Normal serous fluid
   b. An effusion, usually the result of an inflammatory process
   c. An increase in serous fluid volume
   d. Found around the abdominal and pelvic organs
10. Serous fluids are:
    a. Normal body fluids
    b. An effusion, usually the result of an inflammatory process
    c. Found around the joints
    d. Normal fluids contained within the closed cavities of the body

Synovial Fluid

11. Synovial fluid is:
    a. Normal serous fluid
    b. An effusion, usually the result of an inflammatory process
    c. Found around the joints
    d. Normal fluid contained within the closed cavities of the body
12. Transudate is:
    a. Normal serous fluid
    b. An effusion, usually the result of an inflammatory process
    c. Found around the joints
    d. An increase in serous fluid volume
13. Degenerative joint disease is characterized by:
    a. Crystal-induced fluid
    b. Hemorrhagic fluid
    c. Infectious fluid
    d. Clear and viscous
14. Gout is characterized by:
    a. Crystal-induced fluid
    b. Hemorrhagic fluid
    c. Infectious fluid
    d. Inflammatory fluid
15. Hemophilia A is characterized by:
    a. Crystal-induced fluid
    b. Hemorrhagic fluid
    c. Infectious fluid
    d. Inflammatory fluid
16. Immunologic disease is characterized by:
    a. Crystal-induced fluid
    b. Hemorrhagic fluid
    c. Infectious fluid
    d. Inflammatory fluid
17. The viscosity of synovial fluid may be assessed by which of the following?
    a. Mucin clot test
    b. String test
    c. Specific gravity
    d. More than one of the above
18. The presence of monosodium urate (MSU) crystals in the synovial fluid is characteristic of:
    a. Gout
    b. Osteoarthritis
    c. Pseudogout
    d. Rheumatoid arthritis
19. The presence of calcium pyrophosphate dihydrate (CPPD) crystals in the synovial fluid is characteristic of:
    a. Gout
    b. Osteoarthritis
    c. Pseudogout
    d. Rheumatoid arthritis
20. The final identification of crystals in crystal-induced arthritis is best accomplished with:
    a. Brightfield microscopy
    b. Compensated polarized light microscopy
    c. Phase-contrast microscopy
    d. Polarized light microscopy

Seminal Fluid

21. For normal semen, all of the following statements are false *except:*
    a. Spermatozoa are the minority of cells seen.
    b. Qualitative semen analysis is subjective, and further testing is generally required.
    c. Qualitative semen analysis must take place before liquefaction of the specimen.
    d. For best results, semen specimens can be analyzed 8 hours after collection.

Amniotic Fluid

22. The chemical composition of amniotic fluid is mostly:
    a. Protein
    b. Carbohydrate
    c. Calcium
    d. Water

Saliva

23. Saliva can be used for all the following *except:*
    a. Microbial studies
    b. Tests for therapeutic drugs
    c. Tests for secretors of certain blood group antigens
    d. Detection of alcohol levels

Automation in Body Fluid Analysis

24. The most challenging body fluid for a hematology-automated platform because of the need to count and differentiate WBCs down to a 'normal range' is:
    a. Synovial fluid
    b. Seminal fluid
    c. Cerebrospinal fluid
    d. amniotic fluid
25. The technology used by automated urinalysis platforms is:
    a. Manual particle counting
    b. Semi-automated particle counting
    c. Flow cell technology
    d. Digital imaging

Turgeon: Linné & Ringsrud's Clinical Laboratory Science, 8th Edition

STUDENT PROCEDURE WORKSHEET 14-1

Counting Leukocytes in Cerebrospinal Fluid

Student Learning Outcomes

See Chapter 14 of *Linné & Ringsrud's Clinical Laboratory Science: Concepts, Procedures, and Clinical Applications*, 8th edition, for a complete discussion of this procedure.After reading Chapter 14, and at the completion of the laboratory exercise and review questions, the student will be able to:

- Describe how to perform a total cell count on a cerebrospinal fluid (CSF) specimen.
- Complete the end-of-procedure review questions with a grade of 80% or higher.

Principle

Microscopic counting of cells in CSF (erythrocytes and leukocytes) is useful in the diagnosis of cerebrospinal hemorrhage, inflammation, or infectious conditions.

Equipment, Supplies, and Reagents

1. 10% acetic acid
2. Neubauer counting chamber
3. Pasteur droppers and bulbs, safety glasses, lab coat, gloves

Specimen

Cell counts should be done as soon as possible after the specimen is obtained; cells lyse on prolonged standing, and the counts become invalid. If the cell count cannot be done immediately, the tubes should be refrigerated. At room temperature, 40% of white blood cells (WBCs) will lyse in 2 hours. With refrigeration, WBC lysis is not prevented but reduced to 15%. With refrigeration, red blood cells (RBCs) are relatively stable.[1]

Reference

MacDonnell K, Fan G: CSF cell count on clear fluid, *MLO Med Lab Obs* 42(5):50-51, 2010.

Instructions for the Procedure with Capillary Pipettes (Dilution 1:100)

The number of RBCs can be determined by placing a gently, well-mixed sample of undiluted CSF on the counting chamber and counting all cells within the nine-square ruled area on one side of the chamber. The WBC as described next is subtracted from the total cell count of the diluted specimen. This value represents the number of RBCs in the specimen and should be reported per microliter.

Read the list of required equipment, supplies, and reagents and the procedural steps. Follow the procedural steps in exact order.

SEQUENCE	PROCEDURAL STEP	INSTRUCTOR-OBSERVED ACCEPTABLE PERFORMANCE (CHECK IF ACCEPTABLE)
1	Don gloves and gown before testing.	
2	Mix the CSF by inversion. With a Pasteur pipette, transfer 9 drops of CSF to a small test tube. Add 1 drop of 10% acetic acid. Mix gently tapping the tube.	
3	Allow the mixture to stand for 5 minutes. Mix again.	
4	To a clean hemocytometer with coverslip, load each side of the chamber with a small amount of the diluted CSF. Allow the counting chamber to sit for a few minutes to allow cells to settle and RBCs to lyse completely.	
5	Place hemocytometer under low-power (10 ×) microscope objective. Erythrocytes should be absent or should appear as "ghost cells." The nucleus of segmented neutrophils will be bright, and the lymphocyte nucleus will be round.	
6	Count the WBCs of all 9 large squares of each 1 mm^2 surface. Average the count from both sides of the chamber.	

Calculation

Hemocytometer (Neubauer/Neubauer Improved)

Dilution 1:10

Total WBC count = average number of cells counted × 109

Example: If an average of 9 cells were counted, the total count is 9 × 109 = 10 WBCs/μL

Reference range: 0-5 cells/μL *or* 0-5 × 10^6/L

(Continued)

Turgeon: Linné & Ringsrud's Clinical Laboratory Science, 8th Edition

STUDENT PROCEDURE WORKSHEET 14-1

Results of Unknown Specimens

SPECIMEN IDENTIFICATION	RESULTS
Instructor Initial, if acceptable	

Review Questions

1. How are erythrocytes removed from the specimen for microscopic examination?

2. Why is laboratory examination of cerebrospinal fluid important in establishing a diagnosis?

Procedural Evaluation

Student's Name ______________________________ Grade__________

Instructor's Signature __________________________ Date__________

Comments:

Turgeon: Linné & Ringsrud's Clinical Laboratory Science, 8th Edition

STUDENT PROCEDURE WORKSHEET 14-2

Counting Leukocytes in Synovial Fluid

Student Learning Outcomes

See Chapter 14 of *Linné & Ringsrud's Clinical Laboratory Science: Concepts, Procedures, and Clinical Applications*, 8th edition, for a complete discussion of this procedure. After reading Chapter 14, and at the completion of the laboratory exercise and review questions, the student will be able to:

- Describe how and why the counting of leukocytes in synovial fluid is different from counting leukocytes in whole blood.
- Calculate the total leukocyte count in a synovial fluid.
- Complete the end-of-procedure review questions with a grade of 80% or higher.

Principle

Microscopic counting of white blood cells (WBCs) in lysis of the erythrocytes (RBCs). The Leuko-TIC Synovial Fluid (SF) contains no acetic acid because synovial fluids often contain substances that form precipitates with acetic acid such as hyaluronic acid. Precipitation produces clumped cells, but the method requires evenly dispersed cells.

Equipment, Supplies, and Reagents

1. Leuko-TIC SF units are ready for use with a dated shelf life at room temperature. Store vials in a dark place. Do not use if the reagent in the unit is not clear, blue, and free of particles. The manufacturer's package contains buffer, end-to-end volume capillaries, and chamber-filling capillaries.
2. Neubauer counting chamber
3. Optional capillary tube holder (Bioanalytic GmbH)
4. Gauze square (or Kimwipe)

Specimen

Fresh synovial fluid collected in K3EDTA blood collection tube is required. Mix gently and thoroughly before testing.

REFERENCE RANGE FOR SYNOVIAL FLUID	
Value 10^3/mL	**Condition**
0.3–1.0	Noninflamed
3.0–50.0	Inflamed
>50	Infectious

Reference

Leuko-TICS SF 1:100 Bioanalytic GmBH. www.bionalytic.de. Retrieved 2013.

Instructions for the Procedure with Capillary Pipettes (Dilution 1:100)

Read the package insert for preparation of 1:20 and 1:100 dilution preparation with an automatic pipette. Follow the procedural steps in exact order.

SEQUENCE	PROCEDURAL STEP	INSTRUCTOR-OBSERVED ACCEPTABLE PERFORMANCE (CHECK IF ACCEPTABLE)
1	Don gloves and gown before testing.	
2	Fill a 10 µL end-to-end volume capillary tube from end to end with well-mixed synovial fluid. CAUTION: Do not have bubbles in the tube with the specimen.	
3	Wipe the outside of the tube with gauze (or Kimwipe). CAUTION: Do not touch the fluid inside the capillary tube.	
4	Place the filled capillary tube into the opened vial. Close and shake until all the synovial fluid is washed out of the capillary tube.	
5	Wait for a minimum of 30 seconds for complete lysis of RBCs. Do not remove the capillary tube from the vial. NOTE: WBC count must be performed within 6 hours.	
6	Before the next step, shake the vial again. Use the filling capillary to fill the tube about ¼ to ½ its length. Stop the fluid from filling by placing a finger over the upper end of the tube.	
7	Hold the capillary tube at an angle of 45 degrees to carefully fill Neubauer counting chamber. Count the cells immediately. Count at 100 × magnification. With Leuko-TIC SF, WBCs appear as intact cells with a blue-stained nucleus.	

(Continued)

Turgeon: Linné & Ringsrud's Clinical Laboratory Science, 8th Edition

STUDENT PROCEDURE WORKSHEET 14-2

Calculation

Hemocytometer Neubauer/Neubauer Improved

Dilution 1:100

Count the WBCs of all 9 large squares of each 1 mm^2 surface. If the Neubauer Improved counting chamber is used, count cells up to the middle line.

Total count of the 9 large squares × 0.11111 = WBCs × 10^9/L SF units

Total count of the 9 large squares × 111.11 = WBCs/µSF units

For very high WBC concentrations in synovial fluid:

Total count of the 4 large squares each 1 mm^2 surface × 250 = WBCs/µSF units

Results of Unknown Specimens

SPECIMEN IDENTIFICATION	RESULTS
Instructor Initial, if acceptable	

Review Questions

1. What are the WBC count total values in an infection versus an inflammation?

2. Why does the counting fluid for synovial fluid lack acetic acid?

Procedural Evaluation

Student's Name ______________________________ Grade__________

Instructor's Signature __________________________ Date__________

Comments:

15

Introduction to Medical Microbiology

http://evolve.elsevier.com/Turgeon/clinicallab/

CHAPTER CONTENTS

LEARNING OUTCOMES

Introduction to Microorganisms
- Name the distinctive fields of study in microbiology.
- Compare a prokaryotic cell versus a eukaryotic cell.

Classification of Microorganisms: Taxonomy
- When given an example, identify the genus and species of a microorganism.

Microbiota (Normal Flora) and Pathogenic Microorganisms
- Differentiate microbiota (normal flora) associated with various body sites.
- Describe the benefit of probiotics.
- Define the terms *pathogen, nosocomial infection,* and *opportunistic pathogen.*
- Name various pathogenic bacteria, and state sites of infection.

Protection of Laboratory Personnel and Good Laboratory Practices
- Name at least two types of barrier precautions used in the laboratory.
- Define the terms *sterilization, disinfection,* and *antisepsis.*
- Describe the characteristics of a high-efficiency particulate air (HEPA) filter.

Specimens for Microbiological Examination
- Explain the importance of collection requirements for the various specimens used in microbiological studies.
- Compare the characteristics of various types of microbiology specimens.

Basic Equipment and Techniques Used in Microbiology
- Compare the knowledge gained as the result of microbial culture, characterization, and identification.

Identification of Bacteria
- Explain the principle of the Gram stain reaction for gram-positive and gram-negative bacteria.
- Prepare and examine a Gram-stained smear for common bacteria.
- Select and inoculate the appropriate media for frequently collected specimens: urine, throat swabs, genitourinary exudates, and blood.

Urine Cultures
- Explain the collection of an appropriate specimen for a urine culture, quantitatively plate it, and interpret results.

Throat Cultures
- Describe the collection process using a swab for a throat culture on sheep blood agar, plate it, and interpret results.

Genitourinary Cultures
- Explain the collection of genitourinary specimens for culture in the microbiology laboratory.

❖ Explain the major sexually transmitted diseases and the laboratory tests used in the microbiology laboratory.

Enteric Disease

❖ Compare various algorithmic approaches to the identification of causes of diarrhea.

Blood Cultures
- Explain the collection of blood for culture, and describe how to process and interpret the primary culture result.

Wound or Soft Tissue Cultures
- Define and differentiate the three major types of skin and tissue infections.
- Explain the primary difficulty associated with the collection, transport, and cultivation of infectious agents from skin and tissue infections.

Bacterial Disease
- Describe the purpose of antimicrobial susceptibility testing.

❖ Explain the factors that affect the proper selection of an antimicrobial agent.

Quality Control in the Microbiology Laboratory
- Name and describe the five categories of quality control testing in the microbiology laboratory.

Mycobacteria
- Describe the media and stains used to culture and stain tuberculosis organisms.
- Describe the appearance of tuberculosis organisms.

Tests for Fungi (Mycology)

❖ Explain the characteristics of fungi and the common methods used to detect fungi in the laboratory.

Tests for Parasites (Parasitology)
- Explain the specimen collection and identification process for common intestinal parasites.
- Describe the identification of the parasite that is considered to be a sexually transmitted disease.

Tests for Viruses (Virology)
- Describe the three major structural components that are included in the structure of a virus or virion.
- List the steps required for a virus to infect a host cell.

❖ Define the terms *viral tropism* and *cytopathic effect.*

❖ Describe cell culture, and explain the significance of using a shell vial over conventional cell culture.

Automation
- Define the abbreviation, MALDI-TOF.
- Explain the advantages of automated specimen processing.

Case Studies

❖ Analyze the patient history, clinical signs and symptoms, and laboratory data for the stated case studies, answer the related critical thinking questions, and conclude the most likely diagnosis.

Review Questions

❖ Demonstrate comprehension of the chapter content by completing the end-of-chapter review questions with a grade of 80% or higher.

Note:
- Indicates MLT and MLS core content;

❖ Indicates MLT (optional) and MLS advanced content.

KEY TERMS

acid-fast bacteria (AFB)
antisepsis
autoclave
cultures
disinfection
eukaryote
facultative anaerobes
Gram stain
hemolysis
matrix-assisted laser desorption/ionization time-of-flight mass spectrometer (MALDI-TOF)
microbiota
minimal bactericidal concentration (MBC)
nosocomial infection
opportunistic pathogen
pathogens
prokaryotes
sterilization

INTRODUCTION TO MICROORGANISMS

The field of medical or clinical microbiology involves the isolation and identification of infectious organisms and the development of effective ways to eliminate or control infectious organisms. The terms *microorganisms* and *microbes* indicate the need to use a microscope for observation of their structure.

Medical microbiology is generally divided into the study of bacteria, viruses, fungi, and parasites. The study of bacteria is

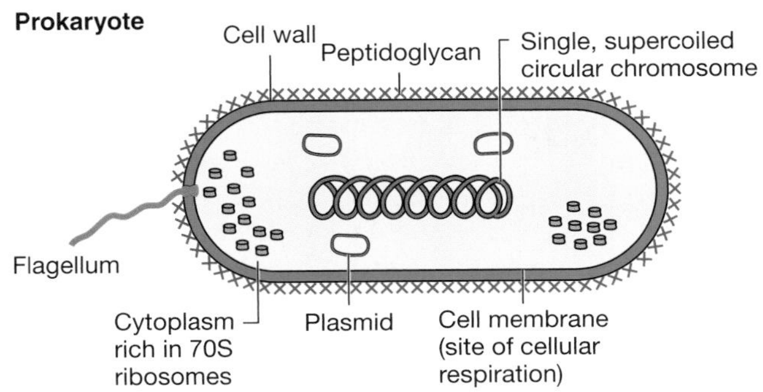

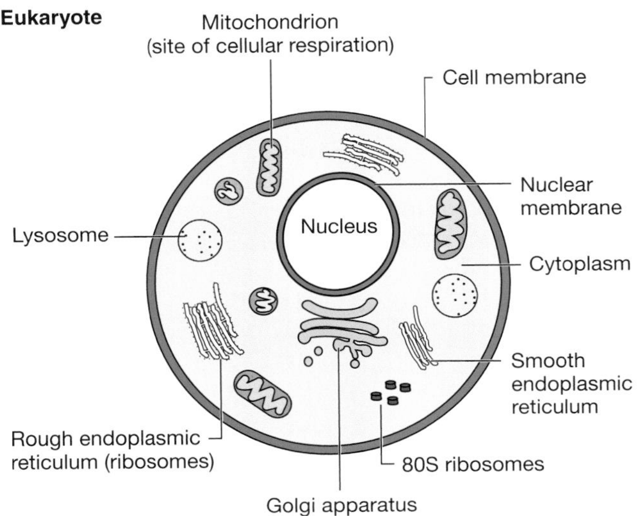

Fig. 15.1 Major features of prokaryotic and eukaryotic cells. (From Murray PR, Rosenthal KS, Pfaller MA: *Medical microbiology,* ed 5, Philadelphia, 2005, Mosby.)

bacteriology, the study of fungi is *mycology,* the study of parasites is *parasitology,* and the study of viruses is *virology.*

Prokaryotic and Eukaryotic Cell Differences

All living organisms can be classified according to their cellular makeup. Cells are defined as prokaryotic or eukaryotic (Fig. 15.1). Prokaryotes (Greek for "before nucleus") do not have a nucleus (membrane-bound organelle containing chromosomes) or any other membrane-bound organelles such as mitochondria. In addition, prokaryotes have smaller ribosomes, which are required for protein synthesis, compared with eukaryotic organisms. Prokaryotes' genetic material, DNA, typically consists of a single circular chromosome located in a nucleoid region within the cell. These organisms have a cell wall that contains peptidoglycan, a protein and carbohydrate structure, that aids in maintaining cell shape and prevents osmotic lysis. Bacteria are prokaryotic organisms.

Some bacteria are enclosed within a polysaccharide or protein capsule, often referred to as the *slime layer.* These capsules or slime layers provide the organisms with a means of adhering to biological and inorganic surfaces (catheters or needles), providing a means to enter the host and cause an infection. When multiple organisms are enclosed in a single slime layer or biofilm, a resulting polymicrobial infection may occur.

An important structure formed by some bacteria is the spore or endospore. Bacteria form spores during a process called *sporulation.* This process occurs when the environment is no longer suitable for growth or in a condition of nutrient depletion. Spores are resistant to heat, cold, drying conditions, and chemicals and therefore are able to survive under extremely unfavorable conditions. Spore-forming bacteria can revert to the vegetative or metabolically active state when the conditions become favorable for sustaining growth. This process is referred to as *germination.*

Some bacteria have external structures that are used for motility or attachment. Flagella are threadlike structures anchored within the cell membrane. The rotational motion (described as "runs" and "tumbles") of the flagella enables the bacterial cell to move. Flagella vary in their number and position on the bacterium. Pili are hairlike projections on the exterior of bacterial cells that promote adherence to surfaces. Adherence to tissue or artificial surfaces allows the organism to gain entry to begin the infectious process. Therefore pili are termed a *virulence factor* (factor that contributes to the disease process).

Eukaryotes (Greek for "true nucleus") are organisms composed of eukaryotic cells and include animals, plants, and fungi. Eukaryotic cells contain a membrane-bound nucleus, organelles such as mitochondria and lysosomes, a cytoskeleton, a cell membrane, and large ribosomes. The organism's DNA is enclosed within the nucleus, is typically arranged in multiple copies or chromosomes, and is packaged or organized by nuclear proteins, referred to as *histones.* The complexity of eukaryotic cells improves the efficiency of metabolic processes and allows the cells to grow larger, providing for tissue development and multicellular structures. In medical microbiology, the eukaryotes include the parasites and fungi.

CLASSIFICATION OF MICROORGANISMS: TAXONOMY

The scientific study of and the classification process is known as *taxonomy.* Taxonomy provides an orderly method for placing organisms into categories. Historically, the categories were based on morphologic and biochemical properties. More recently, advanced genetic testing has provided a more detailed and accurate method for classifying and grouping organisms. Taxonomy is also used as a standard method for developing a nomenclature of living things. Lastly, taxonomy provides a mechanism for the identification of living things and assigning them to a particular taxonomic group, such as bacteria, protozoa, or fungi. With the use of biological classification methods, it is possible for the laboratory microbiologist to identify microbes systematically through the use of morphologic, biochemical, and genetic characteristics.

All living things are classified using taxonomic grouping and hierarchic nomenclature. The scheme begins with the broadest relationship and progresses to members with the closest relationships and more detailed similarities. The classification scheme is divided into the following categories: kingdom, phylum, class, order, family, genus, and species (Fig. 15.2A). There are five kingdoms within the classification

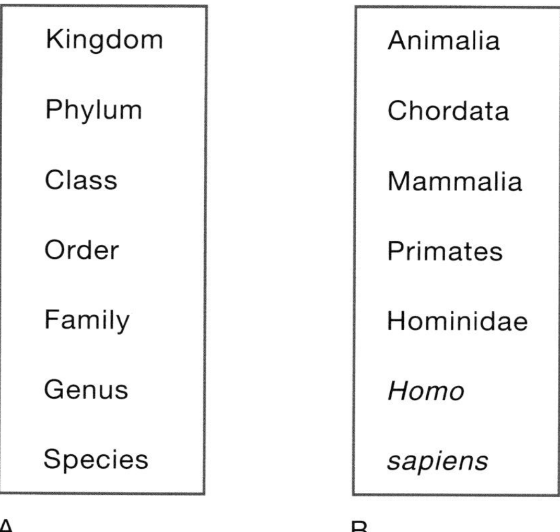

Fig. 15.2 Taxonomic hierarchy. (A) Categories of biological classification. (B) Biological classification of humans.

scheme: Animalia, Plantae, Protista, Fungi, and Monera (also referred to as *Prokaryotae*). Bacteria belong to the kingdom Monera, parasites to the kingdom Protista, and the yeasts and molds to the kingdom Fungi. All living things are systematically divided into related groupings within the classification scheme (Fig. 15.2B).

Medically important microorganisms include large groups of microorganisms, and the family division may be used to include all members. The family division precedes the genus designation; in other words, similar genera are grouped into families. An example is the family *Enterobacteriaceae,* which has more than 30 genera.

As part of the systematic classification, all organisms are designated with a minimum of a binomial (consisting of two names) nomenclature. Binomial nomenclature consists of the genus name and the species name. The genus is a broader classification. Members of the same genus share common features, but they differ from one another sufficiently to remain in a separate species classification; a genus can include several species, all of which differ somewhat from one another. Names are designated using Latin or Greek and are printed in italics. The genus name is always capitalized, and the species name is always lowercase. For example, the genus *Streptococcus* includes several species. It is common to see the genus name abbreviated within the literature, following the first use within the text. The genus may be abbreviated using the capital letter of the genus followed by the species designation, such as *S. pyogenes for Streptococcus pyogenes.* Another convention frequently used when discussing a genus without reference to a particular species is to abbreviate species to *sp.* (singular) and *spp.* (plural). An example is *Staphylococcus* spp. At other times, when there is a nonspecific or informal reference to all members of a group, no capital or italics is used; examples include staphylococci and β-hemolytic streptococci.

The species represents organisms with the closest physiologic and genetic relationship and is the basic unit of the biological world. Depending on the species, a microorganism may cause a different disease in humans and may be apparent in the naming of the organism.

Normal Flora (Microbiota)

Microorganisms are present under normal conditions in specific sites on or in the human body (Table 15.1). In areas of the body with expected **microbiota**, host microbiota and the immune system interact to maintain tissue homeostasis in healthy individuals. For example, microbiota benefit from this association because they derive essential food materials from the host. The host also benefits because the microorganisms synthesize and aid in the digestion of vitamins that are essential for human life. Among the gastrointestinal bacteria, some bacteria are known to provide health benefits to the host when

TABLE 15.1 Microbiota (Normal Flora) and Common Pathogens

Location	Normal flora/microbiota	Examples of common pathogens
Fluids		
Blood	Sterile	*Staphylococcus aureus* *Streptococcus pneumoniae* *Escherichia coli* *Clostridium* spp.
Cerebrospinal Fluid	Sterile	*Neisseria meningitidis*
Urine	Sterile	*Escherichia coli, Proteus* sp., *Pseudomonas* sp.
Sputum	Sterile	*Streptococcus pneumoniae* *Staphylococcus aureus*
Stomach	Sterile	*Helicobacter pylori*
Anatomic Body Locations		
Skin	*Staphylococcus* sp. coagulase negative	*Staphylococcus aureus*
Intestines	*E. coli, Pseudomonas* sp.	*Salmonella* sp., *Shigella* sp.
Throat	Alpha (α) *Streptococcus,* commensal *Neisseria* sp.	Group A β hemolytic *Streptococcus pyogenes*
Genitourinary	None	*Neisseria gonorrhoeae* *Chlamydia trachomatis* In vaginitis: *Gardnerella vaginalis, Trichomonas vaginalis,* or *Candida albicans*

acquired in adequate amounts and are called *probiotics.* Probiotics and other beneficial bacteria provide colonization resistance to pathogens. Beneficial microbes can also indirectly diminish pathogen colonization by stimulating the development of innate and adaptive immune systems, and as a function of the mucosal barrier. Disruption of the host microbiota, especially in the large intestine and colon, has been shown to be associated with many autoimmune diseases (see Chapter 16).

Some areas of the body or fluids should be sterile and lack microbiota. Sterile areas are the blood, cerebrospinal fluid (CSF), the lower respiratory tract, and the urinary bladder. The presence of microorganisms in these areas is harmful.

Pathogenic Microorganisms

Although microorganisms are generally beneficial and essential for life, some are harmful to the host. When microorganisms cause disease, they are referred to as **pathogens.** The ability to cause disease is called *pathogenicity.* It is important to be able to distinguish normal flora from pathogens in a specimen. Pathogenic microorganisms include bacteria, fungi, parasites, and viruses.

Health care–associated infections (HAIs) or **nosocomial infections** are infections that patients acquire during a course of treatment in a health care facility; the organism is neither present nor incubating in the patient before he or she is admitted to the hospital or health care facility. Often, the organisms associated with these infections are also more difficult to treat because of a high level of resistance to antibiotics.

If the patient develops symptoms of an infection within 48 hours after admission, the patient is considered to have acquired an HAI infection.[1] Infection control is essential to prevent HAIs. All types of health care facilities, such as nursing homes, assisted-living facilities, surgical centers, clinics, and hospitals, have active infection control programs. In contrast to HAIs, an individual who has not been hospitalized within the last 12 months or has not had any type of invasive medical procedure may acquire a community-associated infection (CAI). *Staphylococcus aureus* is a bacterium that has been identified as the causative agent of both HAI and CAI. The organism has developed resistance to many antimicrobial agents, making treatment difficult. Resistant isolates are called methicillin-resistant *S. aureus* (MRSA). The prevalence of hospital-acquired MRSA and community-acquired MRSA infections has steadily increased in association with clinical infections. CAIs are usually superficial in nature, including skin infections such as boils and abscesses.[2]

An **opportunistic pathogen** is an organism that does not usually cause an infectious disease in a person with an intact immune system but can cause disease when the host's immune system has been compromised by disease or another condition that has damaged or altered the immune status. The group of saprophytic fungi, organisms that derive nutrients from living or dying organic matter, includes both filamentous molds and microscopic yeast. Serious infections in immunocompromised patients are often associated with pathogenic or opportunistic fungi. Infectious microorganisms can be present in the hospital or treatment facility and become a major problem for immunocompromised patients.

Other pathogenic infections are caused by parasites that live in or on a host and cause damage to the host. Parasites are divided into protozoa such as *Giardia lamblia,* nematodes or roundworms such as *Enterobius vermicularis,* trematodes or flukes such as *Fasciolopsis buski,* and cestodes or tapeworms such as *Taenia solium.* A subgroup of parasites referred to as *ectoparasites* are invertebrate animals called *arthropods.* Arthropods such as mites, lice, and human crabs are capable of causing irritation and infection. Other arthropods rarely cause disease but serve as vectors for bacterial or parasitic infections. Malaria, *Plasmodium* spp., is an example of a parasitic disease transmitted by the *Anopheles* mosquito. A representative tickborne disease is Lyme disease, the etiologic agent being the spirochete *Borrelia burgdorferi,* a helical and motile bacterium. The spirochete is transmitted when the tick *Ixodes* spp. feeds on a blood meal from the host. Diagnosis of Lyme disease is based on the identification of antibodies specific to the infecting organism in the patient's serum or CSF (see Chapter 16).

Viral infections are common. Viruses cannot survive outside of a living host cell and must use a living cell to replicate and disseminate into nearby cells. Viruses are capable of infecting animals, plants, and bacteria.

PROTECTION OF LABORATORY PERSONNEL AND GOOD LABORATORY PRACTICES

The material or specimens examined in the microbiology laboratory often contain pathogenic organisms. All clinical laboratories have procedures that must be followed for the general safety and protection of the laboratory personnel. In addition to the typical hazards associated with handling blood and body fluids in a health care setting, microbiology laboratories pose additional concerns. Pathogenic agents are processed, cultivated, and analyzed in these laboratories, requiring extra precautionary measures, such as working under a biological safety hood. It is imperative to implement standardized safety measures when an infectious agent that is included in the Centers for Disease Control and Prevention (CDC) list of potential bioterrorism or select agents[3] (see Table 2-8 and Box 2-3) is suspected.

Classification of Biological Agents Based on Hazard to Personnel

The CDC, a branch of the US Department of Health and Human Services, classifies biological or etiologic agents based on the assessment of the relative risk that the organism or agent presents to the public health and national security.[4] The following discussion provides examples of the agents that may be encountered. Personnel must adhere to Standard Precautions (safe laboratory practice) when processing all patient specimens.

Biosafety Level 1

Biosafety Level 1 agents are well known, have relatively low risk of causing disease in healthy adults, and are of minimal hazard to laboratory personnel or the environment. Level 1 agents are used for laboratory instruction for introductory microbiology courses. Good standard working practices should be used in handling these agents, including using proper handwashing technique and proper personal protective equipment (PPE; standard gown and gloves), refraining from consumption of food and drink, and practicing proper disposal and decontamination within the laboratory. An example of a Biosafety Level 1 agent is *Bacillus subtilis*.

Biosafety Level 2

Biosafety Level 2 agents are those most often identified in patient specimens in the routine microbiology laboratory and pose a moderate threat to a healthy adult and the environment. They include all the common agents of infectious diseases. Laboratory personnel are trained to handle these pathogenic agents. In addition, the laboratory is equipped with additional safety equipment and procedures. These include (1) limited access to the laboratory, (2) precautions used to handle and dispose of contaminated sharps, and (4) the use of a biological safety cabinet when aerosolization of the agent is possible. Biosafety Level 2 agents include such organisms as *Salmonella* spp. and *Shigella* spp.

Biosafety Level 3

Agents in the Biosafety Level 3 category are not usually encountered in the routine microbiology laboratory. Agents in Biosafety Level 3 include certain arboviruses, arenaviruses, and cultures of *Mycobacterium tuberculosis* (specimen handling can be done at a Biosafety Level 2) and certain mold stages of systemic fungi. Laboratories where these agents are in use, including clinical, diagnostic, teaching, and research facilities, must have laboratory personnel with specific training in handling pathogenic and potentially lethal agents. All procedures manipulating infectious materials must be done in a biological safety cabinet with special engineering features for careful control of air movement. Personnel are required to wear protective clothing and other special barrier devices when working at Biosafety Level 3.

Biosafety Level 4

Biosafety Level 4 agents are not found in routine microbiology laboratories, pose a high risk of aerosol transmission, are frequently fatal, and have no treatment or vaccine. Access to laboratories working with Biosafety Level 4 material is highly controlled. All work is confined to a biological safety cabinet that has special engineering features for control of air movement. The Biosafety Level 4 laboratory has additional engineering features to prevent dissemination of these exotic agents into the environment. A Biosafety Level 4 agent includes the filoviruses, such as Ebola (hemorrhagic fever), and other arboviruses and arenaviruses not included in Biosafety Level 3. In the United States, the CDC is an example of a facility with a Biosafety Level 4 laboratory.

General Safety Practices in the Microbiology Laboratory

Access to the microbiology laboratory should be limited to individuals who understand the potential risk involved in exposure to infectious agents. Specific procedures considered high-risk work can be completed in a special laboratory with limited access.

The air-handling system of the microbiology laboratory is designed to move air from low-risk to high-risk areas. Ideally, air should not be recirculated after it has circulated in a high-risk area. If procedures generate aerosols considered infectious, a biological safety cabinet should be available for use. Airborne infectious particles are known as aerosols; several processes carried out in microbiological studies can create aerosols. Techniques such as mincing, vortexing, and preparation of direct smears have been known to produce aerosol droplets. These select procedures should be carried out in a biological safety cabinet. Several diseases may be contracted by inhalation of aerosols, including tularemia, tuberculosis, brucellosis, histoplasmosis, and legionnaires' disease.

It is essential that strict adherence to Standard Precautions be maintained. One important aspect of this is the conscientious use of barrier precautions or PPE, the most common being the use of gloves for handling patient specimens. Protective laboratory clothing, such as laboratory coats, should always be worn in the laboratory. These coats should be removed before leaving the laboratory.

Another important consideration is the transportation and handling of laboratory specimens. Specimen containers must always be transported to the laboratory in plastic, leakproof, sealed bags. The outside surface of the container should not be contaminated with specimen contents or other infectious materials.

Hands should be washed thoroughly before leaving the microbiology laboratory, according to the laboratory's established protocol; hands must also be washed in case of contamination. The microbiologist should not work with uncovered open cuts or broken skin; these should be covered with a bandage or some suitable material before putting on gloves. Each health care facility will have safety policies pertaining to the microbiology laboratory.

Waste Disposal and Disinfection Process

Any material that has become contaminated with an infectious agent must be decontaminated before disposal. All contaminated materials must be placed into clearly marked biohazard containers. These materials include media that have been inoculated, along with any remaining patient specimens. The biohazard bags or containers are then disposed of according to procedures established by the health care facility. Any sharp objects such as needles must be placed in puncture-resistant sharps containers for disposal before decontamination. The actual decontamination process may be completed by steam sterilization (autoclave), incineration, or burning.

The laboratory benchtops and equipment should be disinfected before and after use each day. Disinfectants such as phenol or a 10% bleach solution are typically used for cleaning. Diluted bleach is a very effective disinfectant. The longer the surface is allowed to remain wet with the cleaning agent, the more effective the disinfection will be. Disinfection is an ongoing process in the microbiology laboratory.

Incinerators and Flame Burners

Microbiology laboratories use incinerators to sterilize inoculating loops and needles. These units are electrical, as opposed to flame burners that operate on gas and may still be used in research or teaching laboratories. When inoculating loops or needles are sterilized, care must be taken to prevent splattering of material during the process.

Disinfection and Sterilization Techniques

It is essential to use sterile media for growing pure cultures of bacteria and to avoid contamination by microorganisms widely distributed in nature (organisms in the air, on the hands, and on laboratory equipment and supplies). In general, all equipment, labware, and media used in the microbiology laboratory must be sterile to ensure the preparation of pure cultures of microorganisms. Contaminated media must be placed in special biohazard bags before being discarded to prevent exposure to cleaning personnel and the environment.

Sterilization refers to the killing or destruction of all microorganisms, including bacterial spores. Sterilization may be achieved in various ways, generally involving physical means such as heat or filtration and chemical means such as oxidation.

Disinfection is the process of destroying pathogenic organisms, but not necessarily all microorganisms or bacterial spores (endospores). Physical (moist or dry heat) or chemicals (bleach, phenol, alcohols, aldehydes) may be used.

Antisepsis is the process used to decrease the number of microorganisms that are present on the skin. Typical antiseptic agents include iodine, alcohols, and chlorhexidine products. Alcohol is often used to disinfect the skin before drawing blood or venipuncture.

Use of Chemical Disinfectants

In microbiology laboratories, disinfection is required daily and when any spill occurs that may contain infectious microorganisms. Chemical disinfectants such as a 1:10 dilution of bleach or a 2% to 5% phenol solution are two types of disinfectants used to clean laboratory bench tops and other surfaces.

Use of Heat or Burning

Heat is a widely used and efficient physical means of sterilization. Heat may be employed in the form of dry heat or moist heat. Dry heat destroys bacteria by oxidation, whereas moist heat destroys organisms by denaturing proteins. The type of sterilization method that is used will depend on the nature of the material being treated.

Sterilization by Dry Heat. Dry-heat sterilization is carried out in a hot-air chamber similar to an oven. The temperature must be kept at 171°C for at least 1 hour. If the temperature is decreased, the time must be increased. Labware can be sterilized in this manner.

Sterilization by Moist Heat. One method of employing moist heat is by boiling water. Boiling in water is sufficient to kill vegetative forms of bacteria. Certain species of bacteria, including the genus *Bacillus,* have the ability to form spores under unfavorable conditions but return to the vegetative or active state when favorable conditions return. Spores are highly resistant forms of bacteria and thus pose a problem in sterilization.

The most effective means of sterilization with moist heat involves steam under pressure, using a special device called an autoclave. It is the method of choice for any material that is not damaged by moisture, high temperature, or high pressure. Most types of media used in microbiology are sterilized in the autoclave. Some equipment may also be sterilized in this manner. Contaminated materials or used media will also be sterilized using an autoclave and then discarded. An autoclave is a heavy metal chamber with a door or lid that can be fastened to withstand the internal steam pressure and has a pressure gauge, a safety valve, and a temperature gauge. The material is placed in a special autoclave bag or container and then expose to steaminat121°C for 15 minutes. This temperature is achieved by applying pressure. Generally, 15 lb/inch above atmospheric pressure is required to reach 121°C. These conditions will kill all forms of bacterial life, including spores. Temperature chart recorders must be used for documentation for autoclave maintenance and for quality assurance programs.

Use of Filtration

In the preparation of some microbiological media, the preceding methods of sterilization will result in deterioration of the media. In these cases, filtration through thin-membrane filters composed of plastic polymers or cellulose esters may be used as an alternate method of sterilization. Heat-sensitive solutions such as vaccines or antibiotic solutions can be sterilized by filtration.

High-efficiency particulate air (HEPA) filters are used to filter the air in biological safety cabinets. Isolation and operating rooms also use HEPA filters. These filters are capable of removing 99.97% of microorganisms larger than 0.3 µm.[5]

SPECIMENS FOR MICROBIOLOGICAL EXAMINATION

When a patient displays characteristic signs and symptoms associated with an infectious agent, identification of the causative agent is required to initiate effective treatment. It is important that the appropriate specimen is collected and provided for the laboratory. In addition to documenting the patient identification information, the date and time of collection, the individual who collected the specimen, and the ordering physician, documentation for all specimens sent to the microbiology laboratory should also include the source, such as wound, sputum, body fluid, and so on. If the information is available, it is also useful to indicate what antibiotics that the patient may have received.

The specimens are associated with the type of infection. For example, a patient with a possible kidney infection or urinary tract infection (UTI) will submit a urine specimen. If the patient has a sore throat, the throat will be swabbed, and this specimen will be submitted for testing. Gastroenteritis will require the examination of stool specimens. Examination of infected wounds will require swabs, aspirates, or appropriate material from the area of infection. Other sources from which material or swabs are submitted to the laboratory for culture and identification include blood and body fluids (pleural, peritoneal, cerebrospinal), genital area, ears, eyes, respiratory tract (upper and lower), and various tissues.

Specimen Collection Requirements for Culture

The microbiologist must be aware of the types of infective agents present in the specific specimen types. Likewise, for each source of infected material, the personnel collecting the specimen must have appropriate procedures to follow to ensure that the specimen will be optimal.

The treatment of a disease or infection often involves the use of antimicrobial agents that destroy various pathogens. Antibiotics are often administered before the causative agent is identified; standard identification procedures such as bacterial culture may take 24 hours or longer. If antibiotics are given before specimen collection, it may be impossible to recover the pathogenic bacteria, so the appropriate specimen should be obtained before antibiotics are administered.

It is important to remember that material should be collected for culture from the location where the suspected organism is most likely to be found. An example is a specimen from draining lesions containing *S. aureus*, a gram-positive coccus. This type of specimen should be collected with as little external contamination as possible from areas around the lesion. If the surrounding area is cultured along with the lesion, normal skin microbiota may grow in the culture. Another example is the collection of sputum to assist in the diagnosis of a lower respiratory tract infection. Sputum typically contains purulent material (white blood cells) and rare epithelial cells. Saliva from the oral cavity, which is not an acceptable specimen, can be differentiated from sputum by an increased number of epithelial cells and low numbers of white cells.

Pertinent information that accompanies the specimen such as source will help ensure that the correct medium for bacterial growth is inoculated for the identification of the pathogen.

Specimen Containers

Correct identification of a causative agent requires isolation and growth of a pure culture of the organism in the laboratory. The specimen must be collected in a sterile container and must not be contaminated during transfer to or isolation in the laboratory. It is also important, for the protection of laboratory personnel and others handling the specimen, that the specimen be placed in the appropriate container devoid of outside contamination. Proper transport procedures must be followed to minimize any risks to hospital personnel.

Various disposable containers have been manufactured for collecting microbiology specimens. A very useful supply used in microbiology is a swab that has a shaft and calcium alginate, Dacron, or rayon polyester tips. It is important to note that some organisms may fail to grow or tests may be inhibited by the type of swab used in the collection of the specimen. For example, when culturing the genital area for sexually transmitted organisms, wooden shafts should not be used to culture *Chlamydia trachomatis,* and cotton and calcium alginate can inhibit or be toxic to *Neisseria gonorrhoeae.* Genital swabs can be transported with charcoal, which acts as a detoxifying agent. These swab systems, tipped with the appropriate fiber and packaged in a capped sterile container, are available commercially and may be used for the collection of material from the throat, nose, eyes, or ears; from wounds and surgical sites; from urogenital orifices; and from the rectum. In addition, plastic swabs are recommended for collection of infectious agents from mucosal membranes for molecular assays as organisms are more easily removed from the plastic shafts. Calcium alginate swabs with aluminum wire shafts are not recommended for molecular testing.

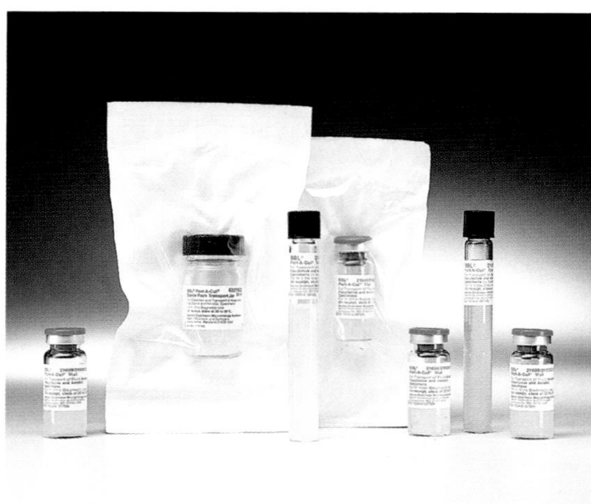

Fig. 15.3 Anaerobic transport system designed to support the viability of anaerobes present in liquid specimens. (Courtesy and copyright Becton, Dickinson and Company, Sparks, Md. Port-A-Cul is a trademark of Becton, Dickinson and Company.)

Several commercially available sterile, disposable culture units prolong the survival of microorganisms during transport. This is desirable when a significant delay occurs between collection, testing, and culturing. Swabs of infectious material can be prevented from drying out by immersion in a transport or holding medium until the culture is processed. Transport media are designed to sustain infectious agents without allowing appreciable growth and preventing death or loss of viability of the agent.

If the suspected organism is an anaerobe (killed by exposure to oxygen), conventional transport tubes should not be used. Some anaerobic transport systems are designed for liquid specimens and will support the viability of anaerobes (Fig. 15.3). The specimen is injected through the rubber stopper, avoiding the introduction of air. Atmospheric oxygen, which kills such organisms, must be kept out until the specimen has been processed in the laboratory. Swabs containing appropriate media and charcoal for maintaining pH are also available for collection of anaerobic organisms (see Requirements for Bacterial Cultivation).

Transport to the Laboratory

Once the specimen has been placed in the appropriate container, it should be delivered to the laboratory in a timely manner. Although many organisms remain viable for long periods after collection, some are fastidious, requiring special growth conditions, including rapid inoculation into a suitable nutrient medium. In fact, some organisms are so fragile that the appropriate collection device and nutrient media are supplied to the patient so that the specimen can be placed directly into the container.

Handling and Storing Specimens in the Laboratory

Immediate culture of freshly collected specimens is not always practical. Exceptions are those samples that must be immediately cultured (specimens that may contain gonococcal organisms) or certain meningitis-causing bacteria in CSF, such as meningococci *(Neisseria meningitidis),* that are susceptible to low temperatures. Most pathogenic organisms are not significantly affected by small changes in temperature but are susceptible to drying. Laboratory personnel are responsible for knowing which organisms require immediate inoculation and which can be safely stored until processed for culture or other tests.

Refrigeration will prevent overgrowth of other organisms (normal microbiota) present in the specimen. Refrigeration is particularly effective in controlling contamination by nonpathogenic organisms for urine, feces, sputum, and swabs from a variety of sources. It is not effective for anaerobic organisms, CSF, or genital cultures for *N. gonorrhoeae;* these specimens should be kept at room temperature until cultured. The microbiologist should be aware of all specimen collection and handling requirements needed for specific microorganisms or unique biological samples. Only when the specimens are properly collected and handled by the laboratory will the final results of the culture or test be valid. Serum samples for serology testing can be stored in the freezer for 1 week before testing.

Types of Microbiology Specimens Collected

Blood

Patients who are septic (organisms are multiplying in the bloodstream) or have a bacterium (organisms are present in the bloodstream) require a blood sample to be cultured in the microbiology laboratory. Special care must be taken to clean the venipuncture site or central intravenous port carefully to avoid possible contamination of the blood sample with normal microbiota from the skin or other contaminants. Cleansing of the skin or port with a 70% solution of alcohol removes dirt and lipids. A circular motion is used to mechanically remove dirt and contaminants. Some facilities require the use of a 1% to 10% povidone-iodine solution, followed by an alcohol rinse.[6] The specific protocol is determined by each facility.

Body Fluids

Collection of body fluids, such as abdominal, amniotic, ascitic, bile, joint, pericardial, or pleural fluids, should be obtained by needle aspiration after the skin is disinfected. Specimens should be placed in a sterile, screw-cap tube or anaerobic transport system.

Cerebrospinal Fluid

A physician collects CSF through a lumbar puncture. Rapid handling of CSF samples in the laboratory is extremely important. Meningitis is a life-threatening condition, and organisms recovered in meningitis are sensitive to temperature change. CSF is placed in sterile tubes. The tubes are immediately sent to the laboratory for testing, including culture and Gram stain. The optimal volume for a CSF specimen is 5 to 10 mL. CSF specimens greater than 1 mL should be centrifuged. The supernatant is removed and placed in a second sterile tube, leaving 0.5 mL to resuspend the sediment for Gram staining and culture.

Inner Ear

After cleaning the ear canal with mild soap, aspirate fluid with a needle if the eardrum is intact. If the eardrum is ruptured, use a swab to obtain a specimen. Place the aspirate or swab in a sterile, screw-cap tube or anaerobic transport media.

Respiratory

Good sputum samples depend on patient cooperation. The patient should not have ingested food for 1 to 2 hours before collection. Sputum is usually collected in the morning and should be sent to the laboratory and processed immediately. The patient should rinse the mouth with water before providing the specimen. Deep coughing will usually bring up a good sputum specimen. The sputum should be expelled into a wide-mouthed sterile container. Every attempt should be made to avoid contamination with saliva because this will reduce recovery because of contamination of or potential overgrowth in the culture by normal microbiota.

An acceptable or suitable sputum specimen that is free from contamination with saliva can be Gram-stained and checked microscopically for the presence of squamous epithelial cells. Finding an average of more than 10 squamous epithelial cells per low-power field indicates the specimen is not an acceptable specimen to culture.[7]

Additional lower respiratory specimens tested in the microbiology laboratory include bronchial washings, lavages, and brushings, which are collected by a physician in a procedure called *bronchoscopy.* These specimens are excellent for recovery of etiologic agents of pneumonia and should be processed promptly (smear and culture). Respiratory therapy technicians collect induced sputum specimens following a chemical breathing treatment that stimulates the patient to produce sputum. Bronchoscopy can be used when a patient cannot produce a sputum sample. Also, aspiration or suctioning can be used for specimen collection when the patient has a tracheostomy.

Upper respiratory specimens are often obtained using two swabs (dual collection swabs are commercially available) for throat culture and detection of group A β-hemolytic streptococci capable of causing pharyngitis (Fig. 15.4). The specimen is streaked onto sheep blood agar (SBA; a nutritionally rich media) or used in a rapid direct test utilizing extraction of the cell-wall polysaccharide antigen and its recognition by antibody. These rapid test results are available within minutes instead of hours (see Rapid Detection Methods). However, because of false-negative results using rapid methods, the second swab is inoculated to the SBA plate and incubated for 18 to 24 hours and reviewed for β-hemolytic colonies.

Scrapings

Corneal scrapings are collected using local anesthetic and inoculated directly to agar. Fungal scrapings of hair, nails, or skin need to be placed in a clean, screw-cap container for transport to the laboratory.

Stool

Stool specimens contain large numbers of bacteria (normal microbiota), requiring the microbiologist to differentiate nonpathogenic from pathogenic enteric organisms. Stool specimens should be cultured within 2 hours of collection. If this is not possible, transport media for stool samples can be used. Cary–Blair transport media preserves the viability of bacterial intestinal

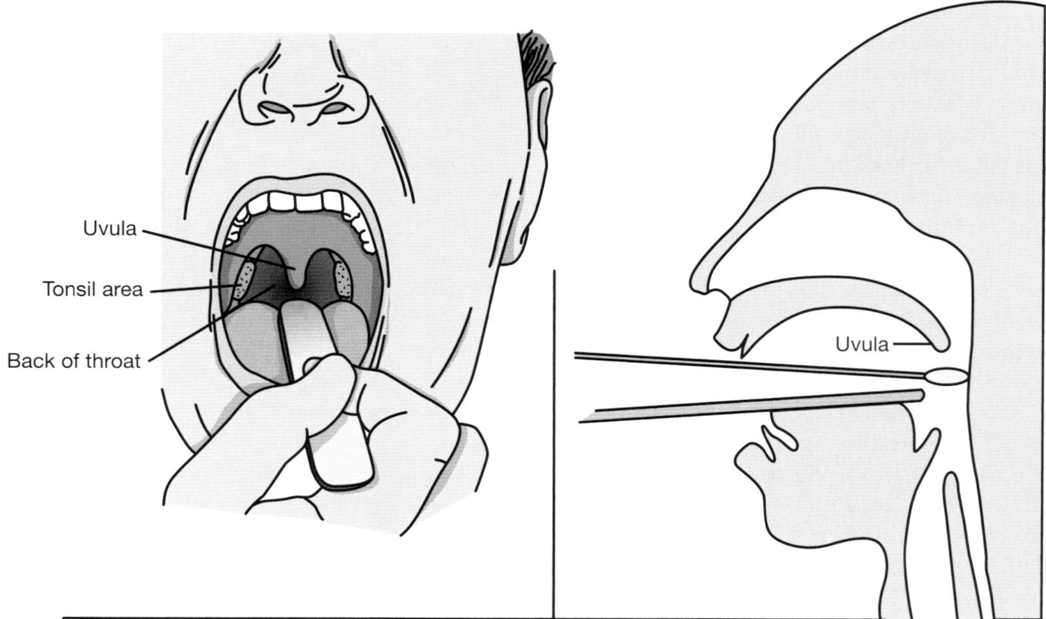

Fig. 15.4 Obtaining a throat culture.

pathogens. Swabs of the rectal area can be used for infants, but this is not the preferred method of collection for other age groups. Stool specimens are also collected for identification of parasites and viruses.

Swabs of Various Anatomical Sites

Swabs are used to collect cultures from various openings of the body, such as the outer ear, conjunctiva (eye), nose, throat, mouth, vagina, anus, and wounds. These swabs must be collected carefully and placed in the proper transport media before they are taken to the laboratory for processing. If swabs are not properly handled, the microorganisms are subject to drying and loss of viability, resulting in numbers insufficient for culture.

Urine

The collection of urine for microbiological studies requires patient compliance and a thorough understanding of the collection procedure. A clean-voided midstream sample, usually the first morning specimen, is suitable for culture, provided care has been taken to clean the urethral area before the collection.

Urine in the bladder is normally sterile. A sterile container must be used for urine collection for culture. When a patient is too ill or cannot void properly, a specimen is obtained by catheterization. After collection, specimens should be sent to the laboratory for immediate processing or refrigeration, or a preservative can be used to maintain bacterial counts.

A suprapubic specimen is the definitive method for collecting an uncontaminated urine specimen. A suprapubic aspiration is collected from a full bladder, primarily from infants and patients for whom the results of a voided specimen are difficult to interpret.

BASIC EQUIPMENT AND TECHNIQUES USED IN MICROBIOLOGY

Microbiologists use special equipment and techniques to grow and isolate pure cultures of microorganisms. Most work in the microbiology laboratory involves procedures to culture, characterize, and identify various microbes. The information gained through these procedures provides knowledge in three important areas:

1. Culture of organisms present in the patient specimens
2. Classification and identification of the isolated organisms
3. Interpretation of organism susceptibility patterns to determine the use of an appropriate antimicrobial agent

Such efforts require the use of specific techniques and equipment for specimen culture, serologic testing, molecular assays, and staining of slides for microscopic examination (see also Smear Preparation and Stains Used in Microbiology).

Inoculating Needle or Loop

The microbiologist uses an inoculating transfer needle or loop to spread the organism onto or place into artificial nutrient growth media. Needles and loops may be disposable or reusable. Disposable inoculating loops are calibrated to deliver accurate volumes of liquid specimens, are made of plastic, and can be discarded after use. Reusable loops or needles are typically made of platinum or an alloy such as Nichrome that can be sterilized by being heated to glowing without being damaged and that returns to room temperature fairly rapidly. An object that can be safely heated until it is red is sterilized almost instantaneously. The needle or loop is used to distribute specimens and transfer microorganisms from one medium to another or from a culture to a microscope slide. Because it can be sterilized quickly, the loop can be used repeatedly for this purpose. Before placing the needle or loop into the specimen or media, the needle or loop is sterilized in an incinerator, then used to perform the transfer, and then resterilized before it is set aside.

Incinerators

The incinerator burner is a common piece of equipment in the microbiology laboratory. Clinical laboratories use this sterilization method for inoculating loops and needles. Inserting the loop or needle into the central part of the burner, which is at a high temperature, results in sterilization. Research laboratories and educational institutions may still use open-flame sterilization, but open flames are prohibited in a diagnostic laboratory.

Solid and Liquid Media

Solid media can be prepared by adding agar to any nutrient liquid media. The liquid nutrients are mixed with the melted agar (heated to about 100°C) and poured into a Petri dish or agar plate. The plates are left to solidify. Once the medium has cooled and solidified, the Petri dish is inverted so that the lid is on the bottom, preventing the collection of condensation on the agar surface. The plates are also stored in an inverted position after inoculation; they are labeled on the bottom of the portion of the plate containing the medium (Fig. 15.5A). Slant cultures are solid media in a tube and can be used for storage, transportation, or biochemical testing. When preparing slants, the medium is dispensed into tubes and then autoclaved. The nutrient media and melted agar are allowed to solidify while set at an angle.

Liquid (broth) media are prepared by mixing nutrients to distilled water and placing the broth into test tubes (Fig. 15.5B). The broth tubes are then autoclaved or heated (100°C) for sterilization and cooled to room temperature before inoculation. Wound and anaerobic cultures are processed using solid and liquid media. When the microbiologist suspects that the pathogenic organism may be present in low numbers in the patient specimen, a broth media can be used to recover organisms of an insufficient number. Specific broths are used for this purpose and are generally referred to as *backup broth* or *enrichment media.* When bacteria grow in a broth medium, the appearance of the medium will change from clear to turbid. Blood cultures are another example of the use of liquid media. Blood is collected, placed into a broth medium (in bottles), and incubated; if positive, it can be Gram-stained and subcultured for identification.

Culturing Techniques

The dilution streak technique is a method used in microbiology to obtain isolated colonies and semiquantitation of bacterial colonies. A *colony* is a growth of bacteria that theoretically grew as a result of a single bacterium replicating into a large group of organisms visible on the agar plate. When plating a specimen on solid agar, the technique results in successively smaller quantities spread or streaked over four areas of the plate (quadrants) from the original material so that by the fourth quadrant, growth of isolated colonies is apparent. Some laboratories use a three-quadrant streak method to achieve isolation of colonies.

In general, a small amount of material (inoculum) is streaked onto the periphery of the plate, or the specimen can be dropped onto the periphery of the plate by a sterile pipette in the first or initial quadrant (Fig. 15.6). Streaking is achieved by drawing the sterilized inoculating loop back and forth across the surface of the medium, being careful to not return into or across previous streak lines. The first streak is continued across approximately one-quarter of the plate (first quadrant). The inoculating loop is sterilized and allowed to cool between all quadrants. The plate is then shifted about a one-quarter turn and streaked again, beginning at the periphery, overlapping the previously inoculated area a few times, and continuing across the second quadrant. The plate is turned once again and streaked a third time, beginning at the periphery, drawing the loop through the second streak a few times, and continuing across the third quadrant. The fourth quadrant is streaked beginning at the periphery, drawing the loop through the third streak a few times, and continuing across the fourth quadrant. The loop is sterilized and placed in a holder. In a specimen that has numerous bacteria present, isolated colonies will generally be visible in the fourth quadrant.

Incubators

Temperature is an important factor in recovering bacteria, and most human pathogens multiply best at 35°C to 37°C (body

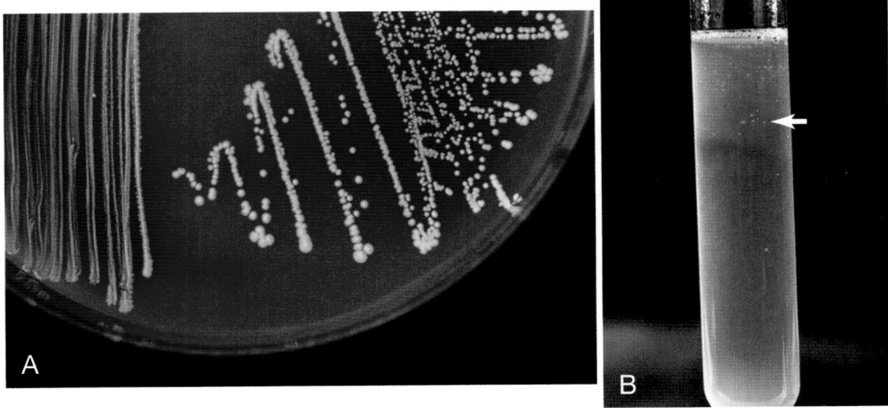

Fig. 15.5 (A) Example of bacterial growth on a solid blood agar plate. (B) Turbidity produced by bacteria growing in thioglycollate liquid broth. (From Mahon CR, Lehman DC, Manuselis G: *Textbook of diagnostic microbiology,* ed 5, Maryland Heights, Mo, 2015, Saunders.)

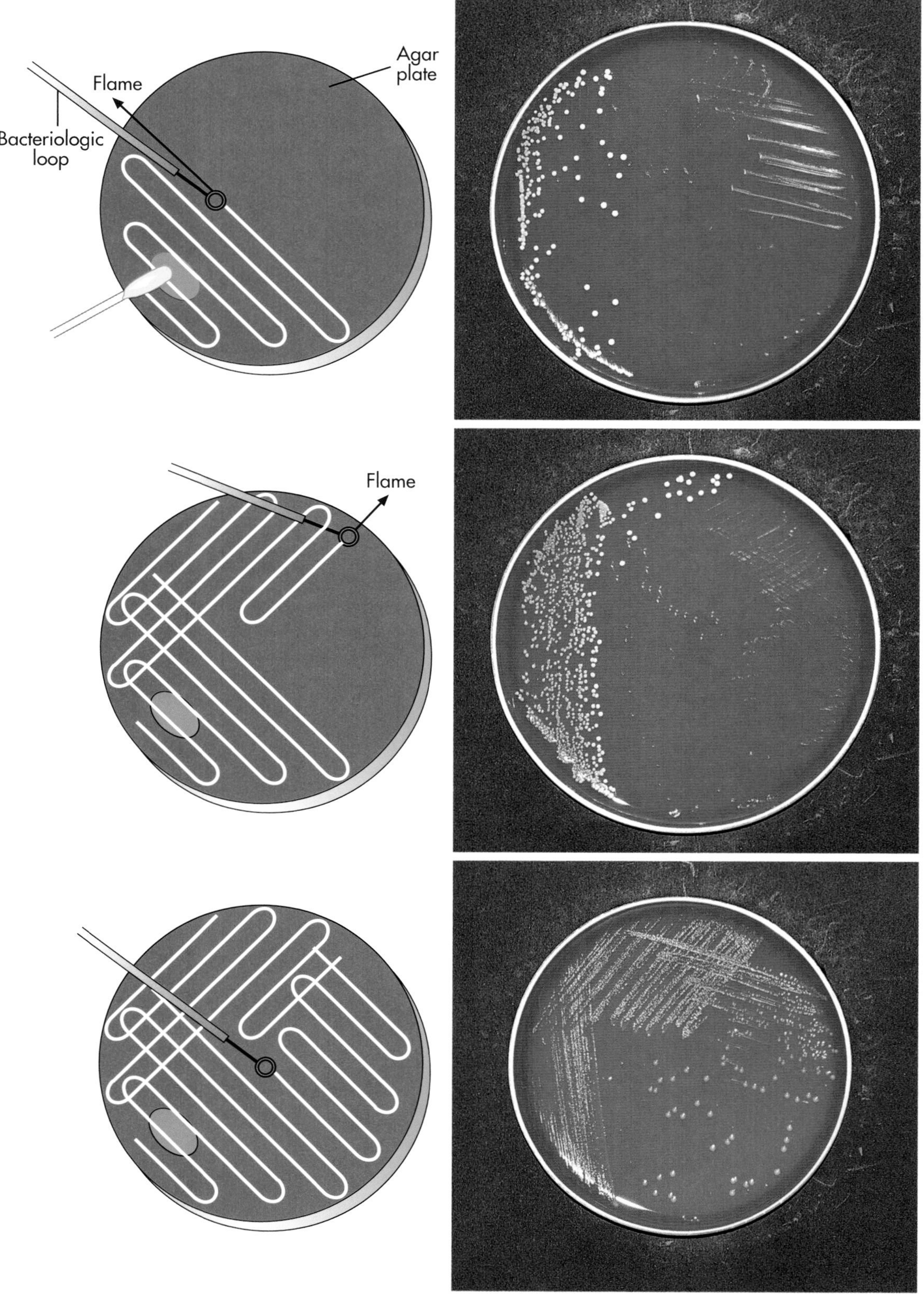

Fig. 15.6 Dilution streak technique. (From Tille PM: *Bailey and Scott's diagnostic microbiology*, ed 14, St Louis, 2017, Mosby.)

temperature). Incubators are chambers that have controlled environments. In the microbiology laboratory, routine incubators are set at 35°C ± 2°C, have 3% to 5% carbon dioxide (CO_2), and are humidified. Most bacteria demonstrate enhanced growth in the presence of CO_2; certain bacteria do not grow when CO_2 is absent. Some microbiology laboratories use a candle jar to create a CO_2 atmosphere (use only white, unscented candles). In most microbiology laboratories, two other incubators are set at 30°C, primarily for the cultivation of fungi, and 42°C for recovery of the intestinal pathogen *Campylobacter*.

IDENTIFICATION OF BACTERIA

Traditionally, organisms in microbiology have been classified based on the similarity of their morphologic or observable characteristics. This includes the macroscopic physical appearance (shape, color, and texture) of the organism's colonial morphology on artificial growth media and microscopic appearance, including cellular arrangement, shape, and biochemical staining characteristics (Gram stain). In addition to these phenotypic characteristics, organisms are also examined using methods that allow the observation of biochemical reactions or metabolic characteristics. Finally, within the last decade, genotypic characteristics, including the presence of specific genetic elements (deoxyribonucleic acid [DNA] or ribonucleic acid [RNA] sequences) within the organism's nucleic acids (genome), have been used to classify and identify infectious agents such as bacteria, viruses, parasites, and fungi.

Routine procedures such as specimen collection, media choice and inoculation, staining of slides, and microscopic examination of the slides are used to identify microorganisms. Monoclonal antibodies (single, specific antibody molecules) have been employed in many tests involving antigen–antibody reactions, which are described in this chapter and in Chapter 16. Direct molecular diagnostic techniques have added a new dimension to the microbiology laboratory. Genetic probes are also being applied; these known, labeled sequences of DNA or RNA are used to detect complementary sequences in target specimens. Currently in the microbiology laboratory, application of DNA probes includes the detection of bacterial, viral, fungal, mycobacterial, and parasitic pathogens.

To identify the etiologic agent of an infection correctly, the microbiologist must possess a general knowledge regarding the growth and nutritional requirements for microorganisms for optimal recovery and identification. The following sections discuss basic aspects of diagnostic microbiology, including routine specimen collection and identification processes for common bacteria, fungi, and parasites found in clinical specimens.

The principal role of laboratory personnel in microbiology is to isolate, identify, and provide interpretive information regarding the organisms that cause human disease. The identification of most bacteria involves microscopic observations (smear preparation and staining), bacterial cultivation, and biochemical tests. Table 15.2 contains microscopic and macroscopic (colony) morphology of gram-positive organisms routinely recovered in clinical microbiology. Table 15.3 lists the biochemical results for identification of gram-positive organisms. Fig. 15.7 depicts an algorithm for the identification of gram-positive cocci. Table 15.4 lists the biochemical results of select gram-negative organisms that are routinely recovered in clinical microbiology. Fig. 15.8 depicts an algorithm for the identification of gram-negative enteric bacilli.

Smear Preparation and Stains Used in Microbiology

Identification of a bacterium involves morphologic examination under the microscope. The cellular shape, arrangement, and

TABLE 15.2 Microscopic and Macroscopic (Colony) Morphology of Select Gram-Positive Cocci

Organism	Microscopic morphology	Macroscopic (colony) morphology
Staphylococcus aureus	Pairs and clusters	Medium to large; cream to yellow; translucent; smooth; slightly raised; predominantly β-hemolytic
Coagulase-negative staphylococci	Pairs and clusters	Small to medium; white; opaque; smooth; slightly raised or convex; γ-hemolytic
Group A β-hemolytic streptococci	Pairs and chains	Small; gray-white; transparent to translucent; matte or glossy; large zone of β-hemolysis
Group B β-hemolytic streptococci	Pairs and chains	Small; gray-white; translucent to opaque; glossy; flat; narrow zone of β-hemolysis
Group C β-hemolytic streptococci	Pairs and chains	Pinpoint to small; gray-white; transparent to translucent; glistening; large zone of β-hemolysis
Group F β-hemolytic streptococci	Pairs and chains	Pinpoint to small; gray-white; transparent to translucent; matte; small to large zone of β-hemolysis
Group G β-hemolytic streptococci	Pairs and chains	Pinpoint to small; gray-white; matte; large zone of β-hemolysis
Streptococcus pneumoniae	Lancet shaped pairs, short chains, possible halo around pairs (caused by capsule)	Small; gray; transparent to translucent; glistening; may be mucoid; umbilicated; α-hemolytic
Viridans streptococci	Pairs and chains	Pinpoint to small; gray; translucent; smooth to matte; domed; α-hemolytic
Enterococcus spp.	Pairs and chains	Small; cream to white; smooth; can exhibit α-, β-, or γ-hemolysis
Group D streptococci, not enterococci	Pairs and chains	Pinpoint to small; gray; smooth to matte; domed; α- or γ-hemolysis

TABLE 15.3 Testing for Identification of Select Gram-Positive Cocci

Organism	Hemolysis on BAP	Catalase	Coagulase	PYR	Bacitracin	Lancefield Typing	Optochin	Bile Solubility	Bile Esculin	Salt Tolerance (6.5% NaCl Broth)
S. aureus	β, δ	+	+[a]							
Coagulase-negative staphylococci	δ	+	−							
Group A β-hemolytic streptococci	β	−		+	+[b]	A				
Group B β-hemolytic streptococci	β	−		−	−[c]	B				
Group C β-hemolytic streptococci	β	−		−	−	C				
Group F β-hemolytic streptococci	β	−		−	−	F				
Group G β-hemolytic streptococci	β	−		−	−	G				
S. pneumoniae	α	−					+[d]	+		
Viridans streptococci	α	−		−			−[e]	−	−	−
Enterococcus spp.	α, β, δ	−[f]		+					+	+

[a]There are some animal isolates of the staphylococci that are tube coagulase-positive. *S. lugdunensis* and *S. schleiferi* may be positive with the slide coagulase test.
[b]Positive: any zone of inhibition around the disk (0.4 U).
[c]Negative: no zone of inhibition.
[d]Positive: zone of inhibition > 14 mm.
[e]Negative: no zone of inhibition.
[f]Some enterococci demonstrate pseudocatalase (weak release of bubbles).

staining characteristics of bacteria provide preliminary information as to the genus and species of the organism. Unstained bacteria placed on a glass slide and observed under the microscope will appear as transparent, colorless structures and may be homogeneous or granular. Staining provides a means for visualization and biochemical characterization based on cell-wall structure. Various staining procedures may be used, depending on the suspected infectious agent and specimen under examination (see Staining Techniques).

Smear Preparation

To visualize the presence of bacteria, the specimen is spread thinly on a glass microscope slide and allowed to air-dry. Heat fixing should not be used to dry the slides. Heating will result in distortion of the cell shapes and may result in a misinterpretation of the stain. The film should be thin enough that individual bacterial cells can be seen. If the material to be examined is a liquid, such as a broth culture, it may be transferred using a sterile swab, pipette, or inoculating loop and spread directly on the dry slide. If the sample is an isolated colony taken from an agar plate, a drop of sterile water may be used to suspend the bacteria and then spread over the slide.

Many specimens are sent to microbiology in a two-swab system: one for culture and the other for Gram stain. If the specimen is submitted to microbiology on a single swab, however, culture media must be inoculated first and then the swab rolled onto the surface of the dry, clean glass slide. Slides are not sterile and thus are prepared last after all other culture media are inoculated.

The material or specimen is spread thinly but evenly over the middle area of the slide. The material may be from a patient specimen, a suspension of bacteria in a liquid medium, or a colony from a solid medium. All slides prepared must be labeled with sufficient patient identification information. It is sometimes helpful to draw a circle, using a wax pencil, on the underside of the slide directly under the area where the specimen has been placed so the examination area may be found more easily under the microscope.

After the material has air-dried completely, it must be fixed to the slide. The fixing process prevents many of the bacterial cells from washing off the slide in subsequent staining operations. Fixation is achieved by heat or by placing the slide in 95% methanol for 1 minute.

Several staining procedures are used in the microbiology laboratory, but the Gram stain is used routinely and yields valuable information. Gram stains are also used for the examination of cultures to determine purity and for preliminary identification of bacterial microorganisms. Properly prepared and stained preparations of specimens may give clues as to which medium is needed for inoculation or help to identify additional biochemical tests useful in determining the organism present. Gram stain results on specimens such as CSF, sputum, and wound cultures can be of great value regarding preliminary information that allows the physician to begin treatment of the patient.

Types of Stains

To observe gross morphologic features, a simple stain such as methylene blue can be used. However, the most widely used

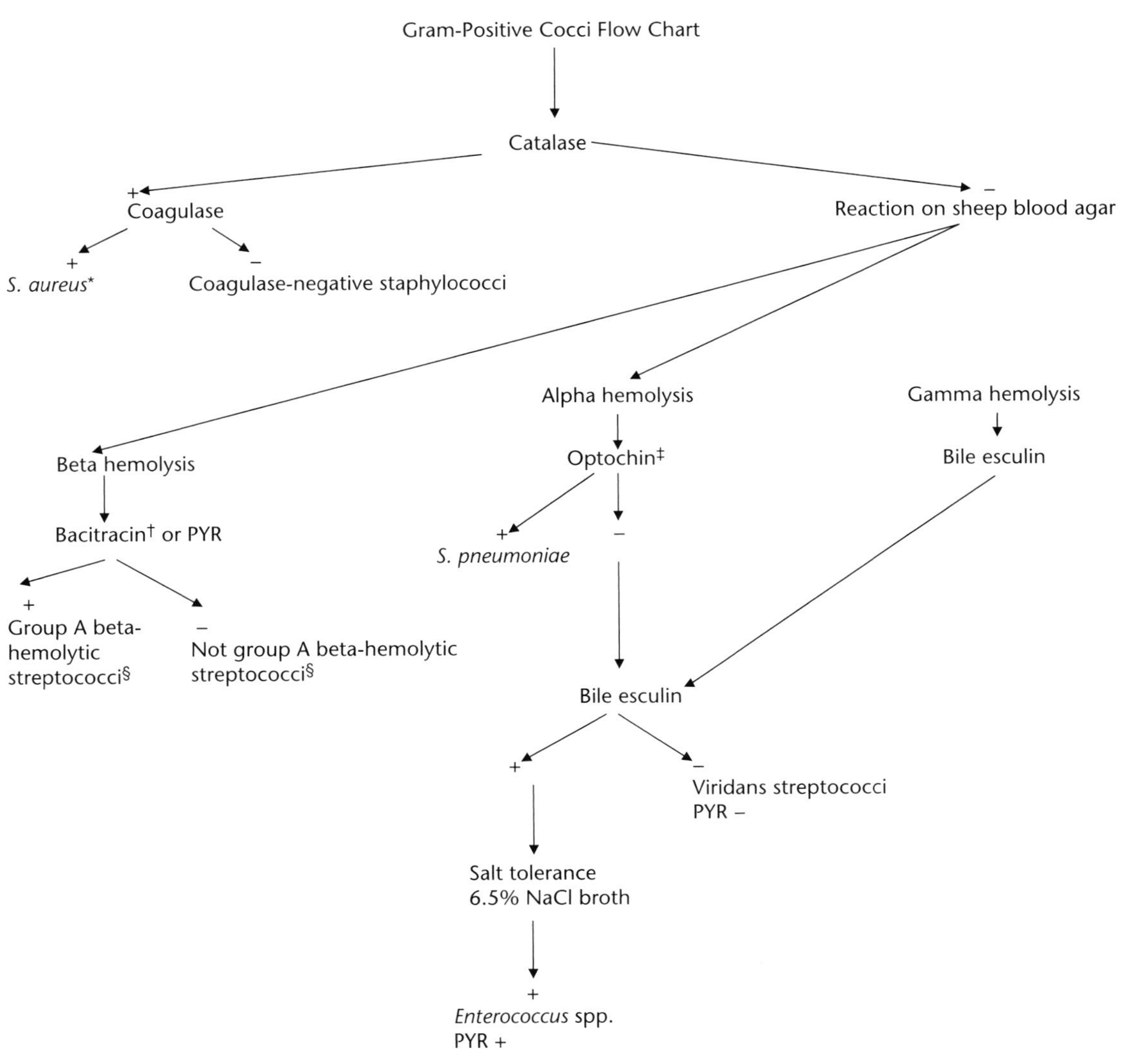

*There are some animal isolates of the staphylococci that are coagulase-positive. *S. lugdunensis* and *S. schleiferi* may be positive with the slide coagulase test.
†Positive: any zone of inhibition around the disc (0.04 U).
‡Positive: zone of inhibition >14 mm; zone of inhibition between 6 and 14 mm, perform bile solubility.
§Lancefield typing is performed to differentiate between beta-hemolytic streptococci.

Fig. 15.7 Algorithm for identification of select gram-positive cocci.

TABLE 15.4 Key Biochemical Reactions of Select Enteric Organisms

Organism	IND	CIT	H_2S	LDC	LDA	UREA	ODC	MOT	TSI	Gas
Escherichia coli	+	–	–	+	–	–	+	+	A/A	+
Shigella spp.	V	–	–	–	–	–	V	–	K/A	–
Edwardsiella tarda	+	–	+	+	–	–	+	+	K/A	+
Salmonella spp. (most)	–	+	+	+	–	–	+	+	K/A	V
Citrobacter spp.	V	+	V	–	–	V	V	+	V/A	+
Klebsiella pneumoniae	–	+	–	+	–	+	–	–	A/A	+
Enterobacter spp.	–	+	–	+	–	V	+	+	A/A	+
Serratia marcescens[a]	–	+	–	+	–	–	+	+	A/A	V
Proteus mirabilis	–	V	+	–	+	+	+	+	K/A	+
Proteus vulgaris	+	–	+	–	+	+	–	+	K/A	V
Morganella morganii	+	–	–	–	+	+	+	+	K/A	+
Providencia rettgeri	+	+	–	–	+	+	–	+	K/A	V
Providencia spp.	+	+	–	–	+	–[b]	–	+	K/A	V

CIT, Citrate utilization; *H_2S*, hydrogen sulfide; *IND*, indole; *LDA*, lysine deaminase; *LDC*, lysine decarboxylase; *MOT*, motility; *TSI*, triple-sugar iron agar; *UREA*, urease.
[a]If *Enterobacter* spp. and *Serratia marcescens* cannot be differentiated by the above tests, an additional gelatinase test can be performed; *S. marcescens* is positive, and *Enterobacter* is negative.
[b]*Providencia stuartii* is urease variable.

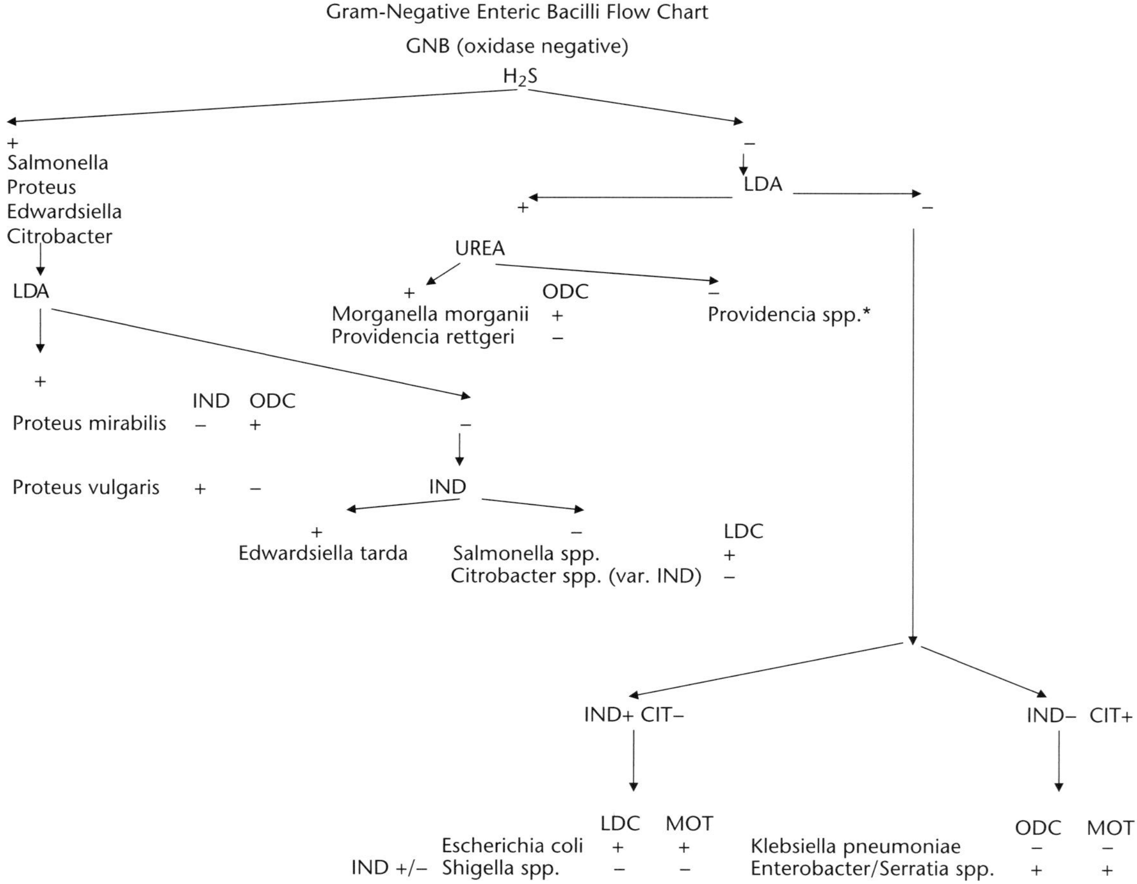

* *Providencia stuartii* is urea variable.

Fig. 15.8 Gram-negative bacilli algorithm for identification of select Enterobacteriaceae.

staining method in microbiology, the Gram stain, is a differential stain. The Gram stain separates bacteria into two groups based on their cell wall structure and staining characteristics as either gram positive (purple) or gram negative (pink). In addition to these two staining characteristics, observation of morphologic features, cell shape, and cellular arrangement is noted. Another differential stain is the acid-fast stain used to identify the organism responsible for tuberculosis. Organisms that require the acid-fast technique do not contain peptidoglycan, the compound responsible for the Gram-staining reaction. Other stains include capsule stains, flagella stains, stains for metachromatic granules, spore stains, and stains for fungi (see Staining Techniques).

Morphology of Bacteria

Each species of bacteria has a characteristic cell shape (Fig. 15.9). Spherical or round bacteria are *cocci* (singular *coccus*), rod-shaped bacteria are *bacilli* (singular *bacillus*), and spiral-shaped bacteria are *spirochetes* and *spirilla* (singular *spirochete* and *spirillum*). Within the group of cells classified as *bacilli,* there can be curved rods called *vibrios;* small round rods called *coccobacilli;* and long, thin, or fat bacilli. The particular cellular arrangement may be further classified according to whether the cells normally occur singly, in pairs, in chains, or in clusters. The prefix *diplo-* describes bacteria that occur in pairs, *strepto-* describes bacteria occurring in chains, and *staphylo-* refers to irregular clumps or clusters of bacterial cells. At times, certain bacteria will exhibit pleomorphism, or variation in form. In this case the bacteria will have a varied appearance on the same smear, such as long bacilli and coccobacilli in the same field of view in the microscope.

Although bacteria can be seen under brightfield microscope, they are extremely tiny cells. Bacteria are normally observed under oil immersion with a 100 × objective, giving a total magnification of 1000 times when the 10 × ocular is used. Bacteria are measured in micrometers (1 μm = 1/1000 millimeter) and vary in size. *Staphylococcus* ranges from 0.5 to1.5 μm in diameter; this is near the limit of resolution of the common light microscope, 0.2 μm. The bacilli show an even greater size variation. *Haemophilus influenzae* is a very small rod often referred to as a coccobacillus, about 0.2 μm wide by 0.5 μm long. *Bacillus anthracis* is a relatively large rod, 1 to 3 μm wide by 8 μm long. For comparison, a red blood cell (RBC) is approximately 7 μm in diameter. Morphology and staining characteristics of bacteria can provide the microbiologist with preliminary information related to the potential identification of the bacterium. For

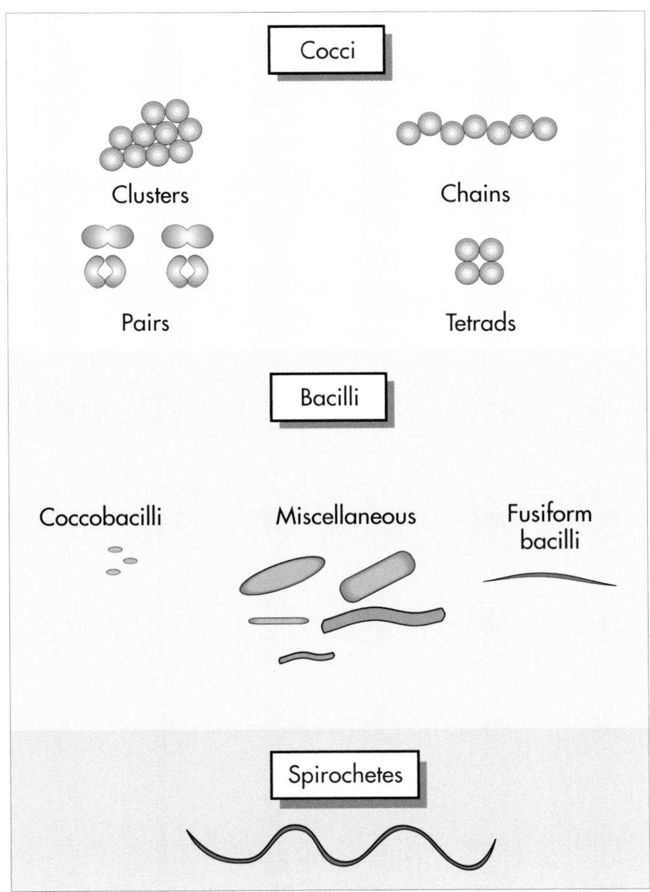

Fig. 15.9 Bacterial morphology. Diagram of microscopic shapes and arrangements of bacteria. (From Tille PM: *Bailey and Scott's diagnostic microbiology*, ed 14, St Louis, 2017, Mosby.)

the final identification, it is necessary to determine the cultural characteristics of the bacterium and to perform confirmatory biochemical or molecular testing.

Stains are chemical substances that contain dyes. Certain bacterial structures have affinities for particular dyes. Most microbiology laboratories purchase stains from commercial companies that are ready to use. Special stains are useful for identifying the morphology of bacteria and visualizing structures such as capsules, flagella, spores, and granules. Simple stains, such as methylene blue, or more complex differential stains are used to identify cellular details. The way bacteria retain differential stains, such as Gram stain, depends on the chemical composition of the cell wall. The cell walls of gram-positive organisms contain a large amount of heavily cross-linked peptidoglycans, whereas gram-negative organisms contain a small amount of peptidoglycan. Gram-negative organisms also possess a lipid layer on the periphery of the cell wall. Inside the cell wall of gram-negative and gram-positive organisms is a cell membrane, a lipid bilayer, that encloses the cytoplasm and controls the passage of nutrients and other molecules in and out of the cell.

Simple Stains. Simple staining procedures employing crystal violet, fuchsin, methylene blue, or safranin have limited use in the microbiology laboratory. These are termed *simple stains* because a single chemical stain is used, and all structures present are stained one color. When a simple stain is used, organisms should be observed for size, shape, cellular arrangement, and uniformity of staining.

Differential Stains. Differential stains are used to distinguish types of bacteria based on biochemical compositions. The most frequently used differential stain is the Gram stain.

Gram Stain. The Gram stain is used to differentiate bacteria that have similar morphologic features (Student Procedure Worksheet 15.1). The cell wall of the bacterium contributes to the Gram-staining reaction of the organism. The Gram stain method uses four different reagents: (1) the primary stain crystal violet; (2) Gram iodine, which serves as a mordant; (3) decolorization with an alcohol–acetone solution; and (4) a counterstain, safranin. A *mordant* is a substance that combines with a particular dye, forms an insoluble complex, and fixes or assists in the retention of the color in the substance.

The Gram stain method divides bacteria into two groups (Fig. 15.10). Bacteria that stain purple or blue as a result of retention of the crystal violet–iodine complex are termed *gram positive*. Bacteria that stain red or pink from the counterstain safranin are termed *gram negative*. The mechanism involved in retention of the crystal violet–iodine complex in gram-positive organisms but not in gram-negative organisms results from the difference in cell-wall structure between the two groups. Gram-positive cells have a thick peptidoglycan layer; gram-negative cells have a thinner peptidoglycan layer with an additional outer membrane similar to the inner cell membrane.

In the first step of the Gram stain procedure, all organisms stain violet by the primary stain, crystal violet. The Gram iodine is added and forms a crystal violet–iodine complex, which is fixed or retained in gram-positive but not in gram-negative organisms.

Decolorization with a mixture of acetone and 95% alcohol removes all color from gram-negative organisms but does not remove the color from the gram-positive bacteria, which remain purple or blue. When a slower decolorization is warranted, 95% alcohol can be used alone. Because the gram-negative organisms are colorless after this step, they are counterstained with safranin, staining the organisms pink so they can be visualized under the microscope.

Differentiation of bacteria is particularly helpful in determining the subsequent biochemical tests and culture media required for the growth and identification of the bacteria. It also provides a guide to treatment for patients because certain antibiotics are generally effective against gram-positive bacteria, whereas gram-negative bacteria are not as susceptible to their action, and vice versa.

Other Stains

1. Acridine orange. This is a fluorochrome dye that stains living or dead gram-positive and gram-negative bacteria. The dye binds to the nucleic acid of the cell and fluoresces as a bright orange when viewed with a fluorescent microscope.
2. Calcofluor white. This is a fluorochrome dye that binds to chitin in the cell wall of fungi. It fluoresces a bright apple-green or blue-white color when viewed under the microscope.

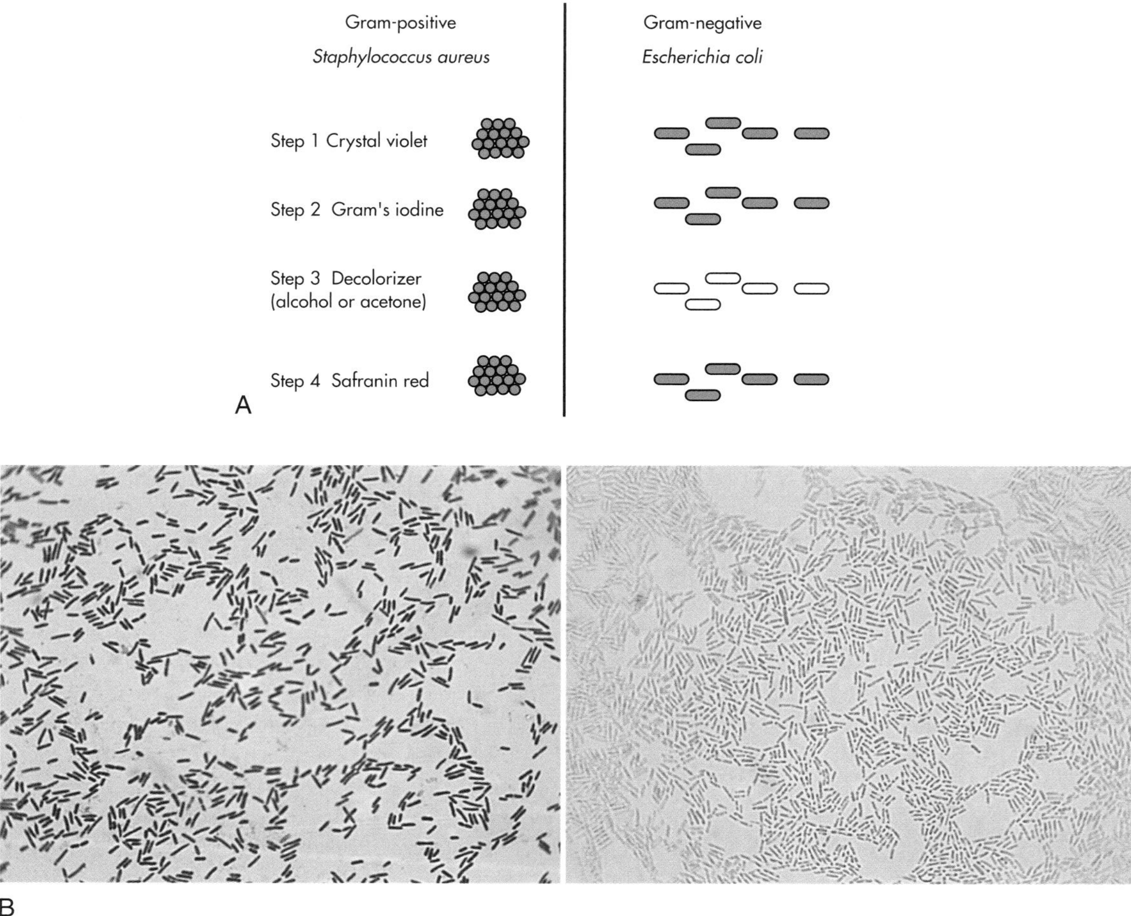

Fig. 15.10 Gram stain method. (A) In gram-positive bacteria such as *Staphylococcus aureus,* the crystal violet is retained in the thick peptidoglycan layer. These bacteria will appear purple/blue. In gram-negative bacteria such as *Escherichia coli,* the crystal violet–iodine complex is washed out during the decolorizing step, and then bacteria are counterstained with safranin. These bacteria will appear red/pink. (B) Gram stains of gram-positive *(left)* and gram-negative *(right)* bacteria observed under oil immersion. ([A] from Murray PR, Rosenthal KS, Pfaller MA: *Medical microbiology,* ed 5, St Louis, 2005, Mosby; [B] modified from Atlas RM: *Principles of microbiology,* St Louis, 1995, Mosby.)

3. Methylene blue. The traditional use for this stain is for detection of metachromatic granules in *Corynebacterium diphtheriae.*
4. Lactophenol cotton blue. This stain is used for detection of fungi grown in slide culture.
5. India Ink. This stain assists with viewing capsules around certain yeasts. The effect of the stain is to leave a clear capsule around the yeast against a dark background.
6. Endospore stain. The primary stain in the endospore stain is malachite green that is heated to steaming. This primary stain is removed after 5 minutes by washing the slide. A counterstain, safranin, is applied to the slide. The resulting view is of green endospores within a pink- or red-appearing bacterial cell.

Microscopy Techniques Used. Although brightfield microscopy is used for most routine microscopic examinations in the microbiology laboratory, the use of varying microscopy techniques is important in some microbiological assays.

Brightfield Microscopy. The brightfield microscope is used for most routine microscopy (see Chapter 5). With this type of illumination, the organism appears dark against a bright background. Gram stains are examined using an ordinary brightfield microscope and the oil-immersion objective (100 ×). Immersion oil decreases the amount of light refraction and improves the resolution of the image in all types of microscopy.

Fluorescent Microscopy. In fluorescence microscopy, the specimen is self-illuminating, and a light image is observed against a dark background. A special darkfield fluorescent microscope is used (see Chapter 5).

Immunofluorescent techniques are used in many laboratories for the identification of specific microorganisms. With this technique, it is possible to pretreat specific antibodies with fluorescent dye and then to react them with microorganisms. If the microorganism contains the complementary antigen for the specific antibody, the antibody–antigen will form a stable complex. The antibody–antigen complex is fluorescent and can be observed using the fluorescent microscope. This technique can be used to identify the bacterial pathogen *Legionella pneumophila* (legionnaires' disease) and various viral agents.

Bacterial Cultivation

The process of identification of microorganisms begins by inoculating various nutrient media designed to enhance the growth of the pathogenic organisms. The streak plate method previously described is used to separate organisms to obtain a pure culture isolate. Once a pure isolate is identified, the organisms can then be utilized in biochemical tests for identification purposes. In addition, pure culture is used to test for susceptibility and resistance to antimicrobial agents.

Primary Culture, Subculture, and Pure Culture

When culturing specimens, the primary culture plates are inoculated using the dilution streak technique to obtain isolated colonies. If the colonies on the primary plates appear as mixtures of more than one species of bacteria, a subculture (secondary streak plate) must be performed to separate the different types of bacteria. The growth of several colonies originating from a single colony, and thus a single cell, is known as a *pure culture* (Fig. 15.11). It is assumed that a colony arises when one parent bacterial cell multiplies many times, until a visible aggregate or colony forms.

Types of Culture Media

Many (but not all) microorganisms may be grown in the laboratory on artificial media. To grow or culture microorganisms, it is necessary to provide the proper nutrients and growth conditions. The growth of microorganisms on artificial material is referred to as *culture* of the microorganism, and the mixture of nutrients on which the microorganism is grown is the *culture medium.*

The isolation and identification of viable pathogenic organisms on culture media is the standard for diagnosis of many infectious agents. Serologic methods and molecular methods may be used when organisms are not cultivatable in the laboratory or require a more rapid identification. Choosing appropriate culture media is essential for the isolation, growth, and final identification of pathogenic organisms. The colonial characteristics of a particular bacterium, growth patterns, and biochemical reactions on the growth media are used to determine a presumptive identification.

The media used in microbiology are generally prepared from measured quantities of known substances that are formulated to give highly repeatable culture results. Media of this type are produced synthetically and consist of the specific amino acids, sugars, salts, vitamins, and minerals needed to ensure the proper growth of certain bacterial species. They are usually produced commercially and are used for diagnostic purposes. Commercially prepared media in disposable culture plates or tube have generally replaced on-site preparation. The Clinical and Laboratory Standards Institute (CLSI) publishes recommendations for manufacturers of commercial media[8] (see Quality Control of Media).

Agar is used in the preparation of solid media; it is a seaweed extract that is liquid when heated and solid when cooled. It does not affect bacterial growth and is an excellent base for nutrient media. Agar can be melted and poured into tubes or plates, where it will solidify when cooled. Plates and agar slants are prepared with agar as the base.

In addition to agar plates or Petri dishes to observe growth characteristics of the microorganisms, culture studies include the use of agar slants for maintenance of cultures, certain biochemical studies, or semisolid media for motility. Broths or liquid media are also used as culture media. Broths are meat extracts of protein materials, either peptone, an intermediate product of protein digestion, or digested protein. Broths are used for all wound and anaerobic cultures. They serve as a backup medium or enrichment broth if the suspect organism may be present in low numbers in the original specimen. The broth can be subcultured to agar plates for identification.

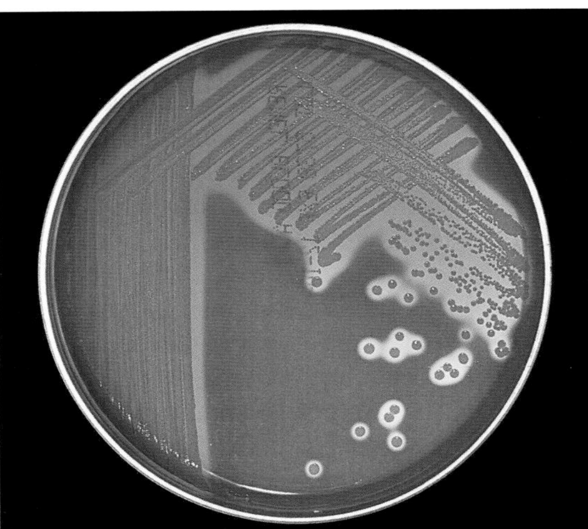

Fig. 15.11 Pure culture of *Staphylococcus aureus* on a sheep blood agar plate. Each colony began as an individual parent bacterial cell that multiplied many times to become visible. (From Tille PM: Bailey *and Scott's diagnostic microbiology,* ed 14, St Louis, 2017, Mosby.)

Colony Characteristics (Appearance) of Bacterial Cultures

When inoculated onto suitable semisolid or solid nutrient media with the proper temperature and moisture, bacteria rapidly multiply and form macroscopic colonies. For example, a single bacterium such as *Escherichia coli,* with a generation time of 20 minutes, would produce 1,073,741,824 (1×2^{30}) cells in 10 hours. Certain limiting factors, however, ultimately terminate growth. A culture that is a closed system will eventually stop growing as a result of exhaustion of essential nutrients, accumulation of toxic products, or development of an unfavorable pH.

The type of culture medium used (liquid or solid) can affect the appearance or growth of the colonies. In liquid media, bacterial growth does not have a characteristic appearance, and organisms cannot be separated from "mixed cultures." By contrast, on solid media the streak technique provides for the isolation of pure colonies, and the appearance of individual colonies is extremely useful in initially differentiating the bacterial species.

Bacteria multiply by binary fission. The bacterial cells divide and produce two daughter cells. Macroscopic bacterial colonies form in 24 to 48 hours. Different species of bacteria form colonies that differ in appearance; therefore colonial characteristics are useful in identifying the species of bacteria. Visible colonial characteristics that may be used for identification of the bacteria include the following:

1. Bacteria without slime capsules produce colonies that appear dry and rough.
2. Bacteria with slime capsules produce colonies that appear shiny and wet (mucoid).
3. Bacteria may possess a pigment that gives a characteristic color (white, red, yellow, orange) to the colony.
4. Bacteria may spread or swarm across the media, such as *Proteus vulgaris,* which indicates that they are motile.

Bacterial colonies should be observed for their characteristic morphology that includes relative size, shape or form, elevation, texture, and marginal appearance. This information, in addition to cellular morphology observed under the microscope, various staining reactions such as Gram stain, and results of biochemical tests performed, assists in the identification of a particular species of bacteria (see Tables 15.1 to 15.3 and Figs. 15.7 and 15.8).

Requirements for Bacterial Cultivation

Bacteria, as with all living things, have specific requirements to sustain life and reproduce. The culture requirements for bacteria include a source of nutrients, the proper temperature, an adequate supply of oxygen (or in some cases the absence of oxygen), and the correct pH.

Oxygen Requirements: Aerobes and Anaerobes. An important factor that must be considered in culturing microorganism is the presence or absence of oxygen. Pathogenic organisms are either obligate aerobes, using oxygen for their growth; obligate anaerobes, intolerant to oxygen; or microaerophiles, growing best in an atmosphere of reduced oxygen tension. Aerobes can be incubated in room air. Some fastidious organisms require an increased concentration of CO_2 and are referred to as *capnophilic.* Most clinically significant aerobes are really **facultative anaerobes**, which can grow under either aerobic or anaerobic conditions. Most of the common pathogenic bacteria grow well in the presence of oxygen.

Some pathogenic organisms are incapable of growth in oxygen and are classified as *obligate anaerobic organisms.* All specimens for anaerobic studies must be cultured as soon as possible after collection to avoid loss of viability. Special methods are required for the isolation and study of anaerobic bacteria. Anaerobes are able to derive energy from their food sources and are actually inhibited by atmospheric oxygen; to culture these anaerobes or anaerobic organisms, atmospheric oxygen must be excluded.

Specimens originating from sites where an anaerobic agent is suspected are cultured on both aerobic and anaerobic media. Enriched media as well as differential and selective media are inoculated (see Classification of Media). The enriched and selective media are needed because anaerobes are fastidious, and most anaerobic infections are polymicrobic or polymicrobial (mixed with aerobic and other anaerobic organisms). Inoculated plates are immediately placed in an anaerobic environment for incubation. Jars, chambers, or commercially produced pouches and bags can be used (Fig. 15.12). Anaerobic conditions can be attained by commercial hydrogen or CO_2 generator systems for use with jars and pouches. In anaerobic chambers, a gas mixture is used to keep an oxygen-free environment. Specimens and media are placed in the chamber by an airlock, therefore maintaining the anaerobic environment. Cultures are incubated for 48 hours at 35°C. Usually, these cultures are not exposed to oxygen until after 48 hours of incubation. If plates are in a chamber or an anaerobic bag, they can be observed after 24 hours without opening and exposure to oxygen.

Thioglycolate broth is used to grow anaerobic and aerobic organisms. It contains thioglycolate and 0.075% agar; both serve to create an anaerobic environment in the bottom of the tube (see Common Types of Media). Strict aerobes will grow at the top of the media, where oxygen is available. Prereduced media (oxygen has been removed) are commercially available for the isolation of anaerobic bacteria, and each facility has recommended enriched and selective media for primary plating of anaerobic specimens.

Nutrients. Different types of microorganisms require various types of nutrients for energy production and metabolism. Some grow on media containing simple mixtures of inorganic salts and are capable of synthesizing organic compounds. Others require complex mixtures of nutrients, including B vitamins and amino acids. In general, the culture medium must be able to supply carbon and energy sources, usually in the form of carbohydrates. Peptone is used in a variety of culture media because it contains nitrogen in a form (amino acids and simple nitrogen compounds) that can be used by most microorganisms. Certain bacteria require media to which serum, blood, or ascitic fluid has been added and is considered *nutritionally fastidious* (requiring additional growth factors or nutrients).

Temperature. All organisms have a minimum temperature below which development ceases, an optimum temperature at which growth is best or luxuriant, and a maximum temperature above which death occurs. Bacteria can grow at a wide range of temperatures. Pathogens generally have a narrow temperature range, with optimal growth at 35°C. Most cultures are incubated at 35°C. Because the heat of an incubator promotes drying, the incubator should always be equipped with containers of water or some other suitable source of humidity.

pH (Hydrogen Ion Concentration). Another factor affecting the growth or culture of microorganisms is the pH of the medium. A culture medium must contain the proper nutrients in the correct concentrations, but it must also have the correct degree of acidity or alkalinity. Most clinical pathogens prefer media that are near neutrality: pH range of 6.5 to 7.5.

The pH of media is controlled by the use of buffers, or substances that resist changes in pH. Buffers are especially useful for microorganisms that produce acid during metabolism. These microorganisms would kill themselves as a result of acid production if a suitable buffer were not present. Conversely, some bacteria produce alkaline products such as ammonia; these also must be buffered, or the culture becomes incapable of supporting growth.

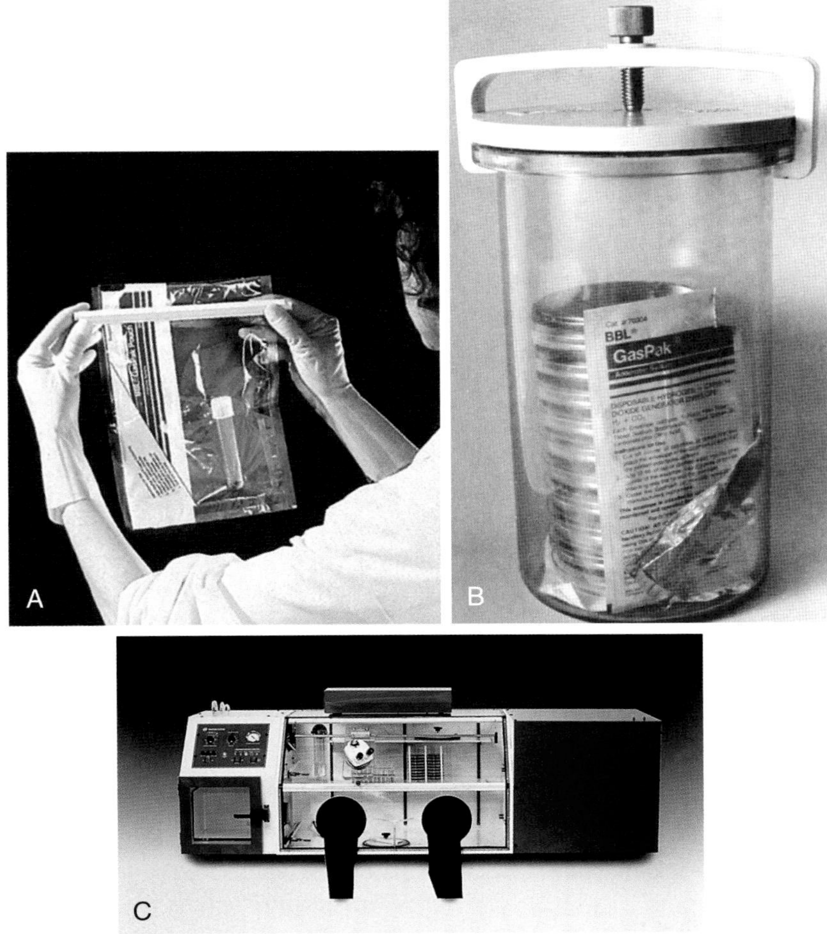

Fig. 15.12 Containers to create anaerobic atmospheres. (A) Anaerobic pouch. (B) Anaerobic jar. (C) Anaerobic chamber. ([A] courtesy and copyright Becton Dickinson and Company; [B] from Tille PM: *Bailey and Scott's diagnostic microbiology*, ed 14, St Louis, 2017, Mosby; [C] courtesy Anaerobe Systems, Morgan Hill, Calif.)

Sterile Conditions. To obtain a pure culture of a microorganism, the culture medium must be sterile. Not only is sterilization necessary for separation of the inoculated organism, but contamination by other microbes may influence or prevent the growth of the desired microorganism. Commercially prepared media are sterilized. If a laboratory makes media, sterilization is performed by use of the autoclave or heating to greater than 100°C for heat-sensitive nutrients.

Moisture. Water is necessary for metabolic reactions to take place in the bacterial cell and must be present in the medium for growth to occur. Dehydration of the media (loss of water) results in an increase in the relative concentration of the solutes within the media and reduces or inhibits bacterial growth. Incubator chambers are humidified to prevent drying of media.

Incubation Time and Temperature for Routine Cultures

Bacterial growth on artificial media or in culture typically requires 24 to 48 hours, although anaerobic cultures require longer incubation times, usually 3 to 5 days, to reach sufficient growth required for identification of the bacteria. Genital cultures are routinely kept 3 days before a final identification, or lack thereof, is reported to the physician. Although 2 days is generally required for identification, most bacteria can be visualized on media within 24 hours. Routine cultures are incubated at 35°C ± 2°C, with an atmosphere of 3% to 5% CO_2 and a source of humidity (see Incubators).

Storage of Media

Media are generally stored under refrigeration (4°C) to prevent deterioration and dehydration. Certain media require special storage; such information will be provided with the media. In general, a medium should be allowed to warm up to room temperature before it is inoculated, or microorganisms will not tolerate the temperature shock and will die.

Classification of Media

Different types of media are used in diagnostic microbiology to aid not only in supporting growth but also in identification. Therefore media are placed in categories according to their specific use: enrichment, supportive, selective, and differential.

Enrichment Media. Enrichment media permit one bacterial pathogen to grow in the presence of specific essential nutrients. An example of enrichment media is buffered charcoal–yeast

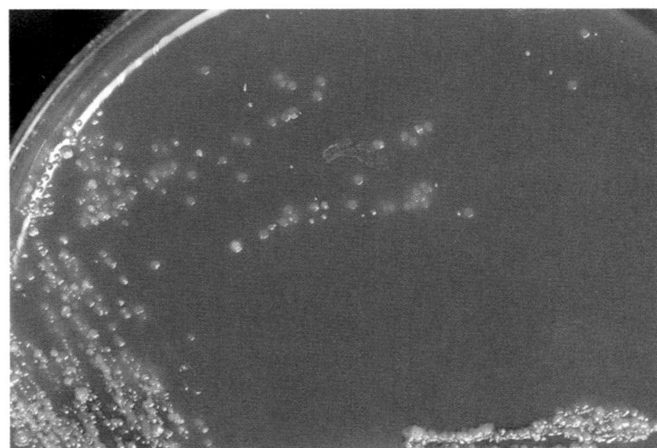

Fig. 15.13 Chocolate agar, an enrichment media. (From Mahon CR, Lehman DC, Manuselis G: *Textbook of diagnostic microbiology,* ed 5, Maryland Heights, Mo, 2015, Saunders, Fig 8-6, p. 173.)

extract agar that supports the growth of *L. pneumophila,* the causative agent of legionnaires' disease (Fig. 15.13).

Supportive Media. Supportive media contain nutrients permitting the growth of nonfastidious organisms. These media do not give one organism any growth advantage over another. The organism's metabolism affects the growth rate on the media.

Selective Media. Selective media are prepared by adding dyes, antibiotics, or other chemical compounds that inhibit certain bacteria while allowing others to grow. MacConkey agar (MAC) is a selective medium that contains crystal violet and bile salts to inhibit the growth of gram-positive bacteria (Fig. 15.14). In primary cultures, MAC is the most frequently used selective agar for recovery of gram-negative bacteria.

Differential Media. Differential media contain nutrients, energy sources, and color indicators that provide distinctive and easily recognizable characteristics as a result of the microorganism's metabolic and biochemical properties. MAC is a differential medium that contains lactose and neutral red for differentiation. Certain organisms ferment lactose to an acid product that changes the pH of the media. Colonies of an organism capable of fermenting lactose will appear a deep pink-purple color at an acid pH in the presence of the indicator, neutral red. Non–lactose-fermenting bacteria appear colorless or pale pink. Therefore microbiologists can differentiate between lactose-fermenting bacteria and non–lactose-fermenting bacteria based on colonial appearance on MAC. This is an important distinction because stool pathogens such as *Salmonella* and *Shigella* spp. are non–lactose-fermenting gram-negative organisms. As previously noted, MAC is a selective medium as well as a differential medium.

Various Types of Media

The eventual identification of a particular microorganism requires the examination of growth on various media (selective, enrichment, or differential). No single algorithm is universally employed in the identification of pathogens (see Biochemical and Enzymatic Tests). Descriptions and intended uses of various media can be found in either the Difco manual[9] or the REMEL technical manual.[10]

Chocolate Agar (Choc). Chocolate agar is an enrichment medium that promotes the growth of fastidious bacteria. Chocolate agar is prepared by adding blood to a nutrient base medium, then gently heating the preparation. The heat lyses the RBCs, causing the medium to turn brown, thus the name *chocolate.* This gives a richer medium than ordinary blood agar, releasing hemin (X factor) and nicotinamide adenine dinucleotide (NAD, or V factor) from the RBCs to enhance growth. The X and V growth factors are required for the growth of some fastidious organisms, such as *Haemophilus* spp. Chocolate agar is also used in the cultivation of the pathogenic *Neisseria* spp. These organisms are the causative agents of gonorrhea and meningitis. The organisms require a capnophilic atmosphere (3% to 7% CO_2) in addition to enrichment media for growth.

Colistin–Nalidixic Acid Agar with Blood. Colistin–nalidixic acid (CNA) agar is a selective and differential medium used to recover gram-positive bacteria. The antibiotics colistin and nalidixic acid inhibit most gram-negative organisms. The 5% sheep blood aids in the differentiation of hemolytic organisms (see Sheep Blood Agar).

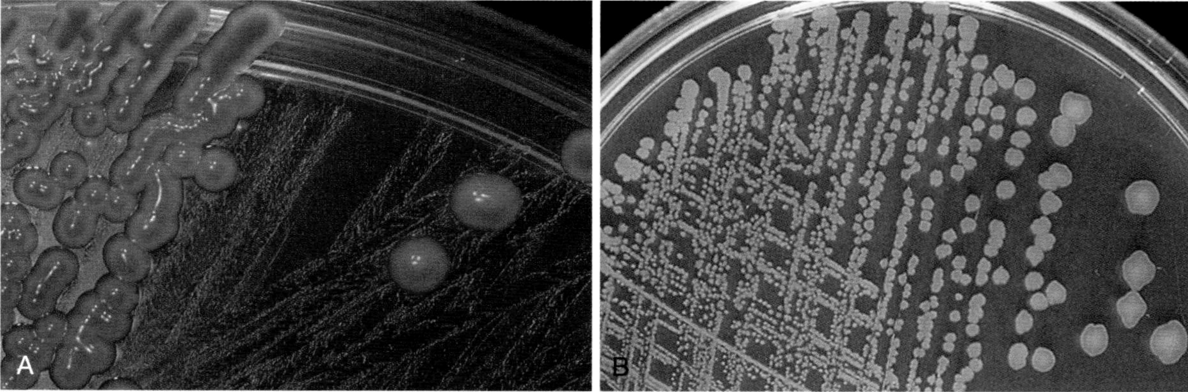

Fig. 15.14 MacConkey agar (MAC). MAC is a selective and differential medium used frequently for primary plating of specimens to isolate and differentiate gram-negative bacilli. (A) Gram-negative bacilli that ferment lactose will appear pink/red. (B) Gram-negative bacilli that do not ferment lactose will appear clear or slightly pink. (From Mahon CR, Lehman DC, Manuselis G: *Textbook of diagnostic microbiology,* ed 5, Maryland Heights, Mo, 2015, Saunders, Fig 8-2, 171.)

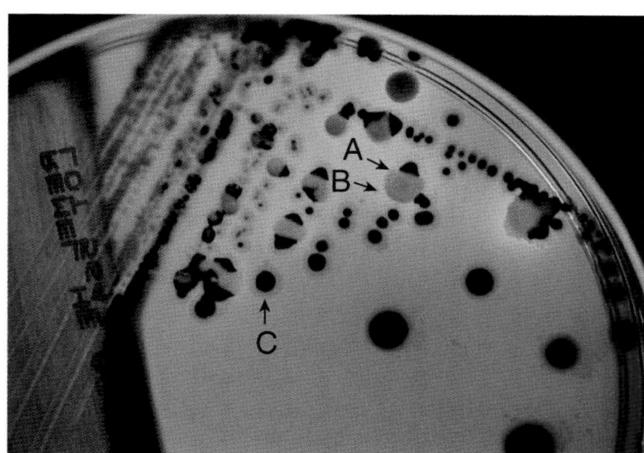

Fig. 15.15 Hektoen enteric (HE) agar. HE agar is a selective and differential medium for the isolation of enteric pathogens. (A) *Escherichia coli* is a lactose-fermenting gram-negative bacillus and appears yellow on HE. (B) *Shigella* spp. do not ferment lactose and will appear green or transparent. (C) *Salmonella* spp. are also non–lactose-fermenters but produce hydrogen sulfide (H_2S); therefore the colonies will appear green or transparent with black centers. (From Tille PM: *Bailey and Scott's diagnostic microbiology,* ed 14, St Louis, 2017, Mosby.)

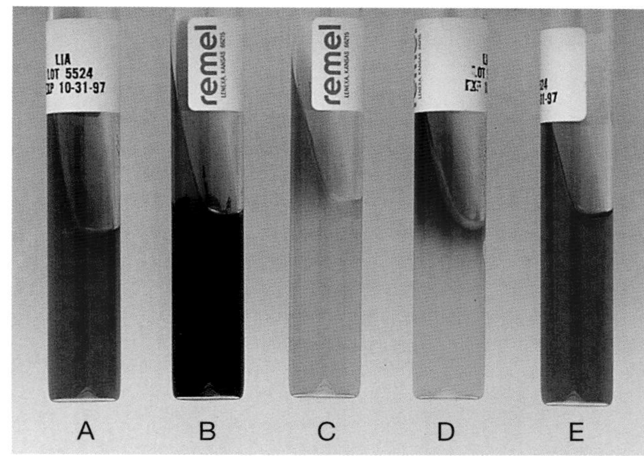

Fig. 15.16 Lysine iron agar (LIA). LIA tests for lysine deaminase (slant), lysine decarboxylase (butt), and H_2S production. (A) Alkaline slant/alkaline butt (K/K or purple/purple) is negative for lysine deaminase but positive for lysine decarboxylase. (B) Alkaline slant/alkaline butt, black precipitate (K/K H_2S +) is negative for lysine deaminase, positive for lysine decarboxylase, and positive for H_2S production. (C) Alkaline slant/acid butt (K/A or purple/yellow) is negative for both enzymes. (D) Red slant/acid butt (R/A) is positive for lysine deaminase and negative for lysine decarboxylase. (E) Uninoculated tube. (From Tille PM: *Bailey and Scott's diagnostic microbiology,* ed 14, St Louis, 2017, Mosby.)

Hektoen Enteric Agar. Hektoen enteric (HE) agar is a selective and differential media for the isolation of enteric pathogens such as *Salmonella* and *Shigella* spp. HE contains bile salts and two indicators, bromthymol blue and acid fuchsin, for the inhibition of gram-positive organisms. This medium inhibits the growth of most nonpathogenic enteric gram-negative bacilli and contains lactose for additional aid in differentiating pathogenic from nonpathogenic enteric bacteria (Fig. 15.15). Most nonpathogenic bacteria will ferment lactose, creating an acidic pH, and will appear yellow in the presence of the indicator bromthymol blue. *Salmonella* and *Shigella* spp. do not ferment lactose, and no color change will occur. Additional components, sodium thiosulfate and ferric ammonium citrate, are included in the medium for the detection of hydrogen sulfide (H_2S) production. Organisms that produce H_2S will form a black precipitate. Colonies of *Salmonella,* an H_2S producer, will appear green or transparent with black centers, and *Shigella,* a non–H_2S producer, will appear green or transparent.

Lysine Iron Agar. Lysine iron agar (LIA) contains lysine, peptones (nutrient source), glucose (small amount), ferric ammonium citrate (indicator), and sodium thiosulfate (sulfur source) (Fig. 15.16). This medium is used to determine whether an organism can decarboxylate lysine or deaminate lysine using the enzymes lysine decarboxylase or lysine deaminase, respectively. If the organism possesses lysine decarboxylase, the medium in the butt will appear purple (original color of medium). If the organism is lysine decarboxylase negative, the butt will appear yellow (see Biochemical or Enzymatic Tests).

An organism that is lysine deaminase positive will result in a burgundy-colored slant, and if negative, the slant will remain purple. An organism cannot be positive for both enzymes. Ferric ammonium citrate and sodium thiosulfate are present for detection of H_2S, as noted by a black color.

The LIA slants are inoculated by first stabbing the butt through the center, then streaking the slant surface. LIA aids in the differentiation of enteric pathogens from nonpathogenic organisms. Some nonpathogenic organisms that may be confused with *Salmonella* species are lysine-deaminase positive (burgundy slant), such as *Proteus.* Both *Salmonella* and *Shigella* are lysine-deaminase negative (purple slant), and *Salmonella* is lysine-decarboxylase positive (purple butt), further aiding in identification.

MacConkey Agar. MAC is both a selective and a differential medium for gram-negative bacilli and can be used in the primary plating of routine cultures.

Phenylethyl Alcohol Agar. Phenylethyl alcohol (PEA) agar is essentially SBA with added PEA. The medium inhibits the growth of gram-negative organisms, except *Pseudomonas aeruginosa,* and permits the growth of gram-positive cocci. PEA is also used to isolate anaerobic organisms, particularly when mixed with other flora. Therefore PEA is enriched and selective. Hemolysis cannot be observed on the PEA plate.

Selenite Broth. Selenite broth is an enrichment medium used for stool cultures (L-cystine for recovery of *Salmonella*). The selenite acts selectively to inhibit the growth of gram-positive organisms and coliform bacilli while favoring the growth of *Shigella* and *Salmonella,* two causative agents of gastroenteritis. The medium suppresses the growth of other organisms for 12 to 18 hours. After this time, coliform bacilli and enterococci grow rapidly, resulting in overgrowth. Therefore, after 18 hours of incubation, cultures grown in selenite broth must be subcultured to a suitable differential medium, such as HE or xylose–lysine–desoxycholate (XLD).

Sheep Blood Agar. SBA is an all-purpose medium that supports the growth of most bacteria. SBA is routinely used for primary plating and for subculturing. SBA is useful in distinguishing different types of organisms, such as streptococci, based on the ability of the organism to hemolyze the RBCs

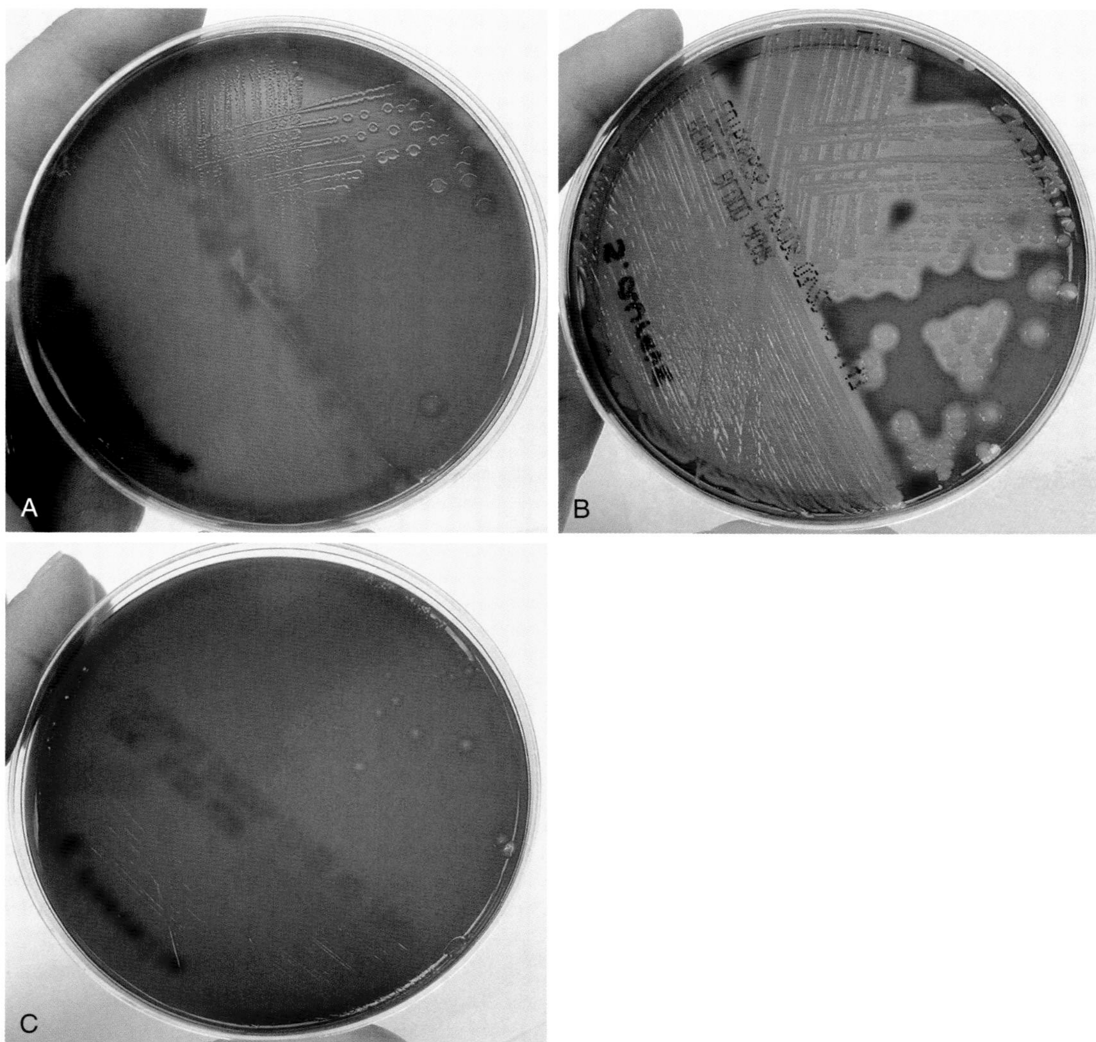

Fig. 15.17 Three characteristic types of hemolysis on sheep blood agar. (A) Alpha hemolysis of *Streptococcus pneumoniae.* (B) Beta hemolysis of *Staphylococcus aureus* (C) Gamma hemolysis of *Enterococcus faecalis.* (From Tille PM: Bailey *and Scott's diagnostic microbiology,* ed 14, St Louis, 2017.)

(erythrocytes) present in the medium. The medium is therefore not considered selective but is a differential medium. The three hemolytic patterns produced by various bacteria are alpha (α) hemolysis—green (or partial) hemolysis; beta (β) hemolysis—clear (or complete) hemolysis; and gamma (γ) hemolysis—no hemolysis (Fig. 15.17).

Thayer–Martin Agar (Modified Thayer–Martin Agar). Thayer–Martin agar is a selective and enriched medium used for the isolation of *N. gonorrhoeae* and *N. meningitidis.* It is a modification of chocolate agar, containing hemoglobin and a supplement (IsoVitaleX) that includes NAD and vitamins. Several antimicrobial agents are present in the medium to inhibit the growth of normal flora and fungi, such as *Candida albicans.*

Thioglycolate Broth (Thio Broth). Thioglycolate broth is a liquid medium that can be used to isolate a wide range of bacteria (see Fig. 15.5B). It is used as an enrichment broth for the cultivation of anaerobic organisms when additional supplements are added, such as vitamin K and hemin. It contains thioglycolate and agar to encourage anaerobic growth by decreasing oxygen (reduced state) tension in the bottom of the tube. The medium contains the indicator resazurin, which turns pink if the medium is oxidized. All cultures in which an anaerobic organism is suspected are inoculated into thioglycolate broth.

Triple-Sugar Iron Agar Slants. Triple-sugar iron (TSI) slants contain glucose, sucrose, and lactose (fermentable sugars), phenol red pH indicator, peptone (nutrient source), sodium thiosulfate (sulfur source), and ferric ammonium citrate (indicator) (Fig. 15.18). Proper inoculation of the media includes stabbing (use a straight inoculating needle) the butt through the center to the bottom, then streaking the slant.

The TSI medium aids the identification of gram-negative bacilli. It is used to test the ability of gram-negative bacilli to ferment glucose, sucrose, or lactose and produce H_2S. Fermentation of sugars is accompanied by acid production, which is indicated by a change in the color of the phenol red indicator from red to yellow (yellow in acid pH and red in alkaline

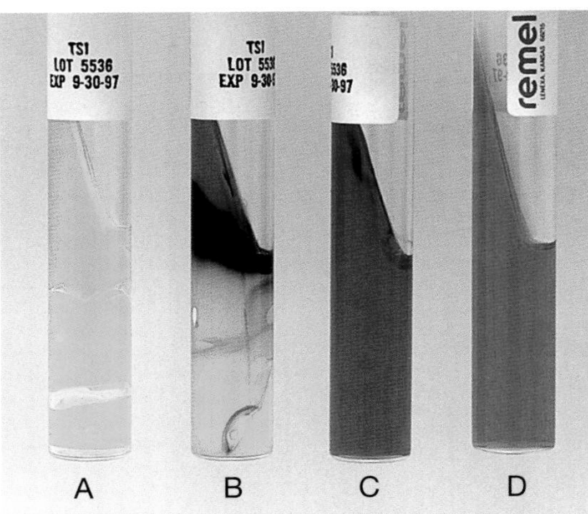

Fig. 15.18 Triple sugar iron (TSI) agar. TSI tests for fermentation of glucose (butt), lactose and/or sucrose (slant), H_2S production, and gas production. (A) Acid slant/acid butt with gas (A/A or yellow/yellow gas +) is fermentation of glucose, lactose and/or sucrose, and gas production. (B) Alkaline slant/acid butt with black precipitate (K/A or red/yellow H_2S +) is glucose fermentation and H_2S production. (C) Alkaline slant/alkaline butt (K/K or red/red) is no fermentation of the three sugars. (D) Uninoculated tube. (From Tille PM: *Bailey* and *Scott's diagnostic microbiology*, ed 14, St Louis, 2017, Mosby.)

pH). Ferric ammonium citrate and sodium thiosulfate are present for detection of H_2S, as noted by a black color. Bubbles or splitting of the agar indicates gas production (see Biochemical or Enzymatic Tests).

Other media similar to TSI include Kligler iron agar (KIA). This medium differs in that it tests the fermentation of glucose and lactose; sucrose is not included.

Urea Agar. Urea agar is used to test the ability of a microorganism to use urea. Breakdown of urea from the production of urease by the microorganism results in the conversion of urea into water, CO_2, and ammonia. The presence of ammonia raises the pH of the medium, as indicated by a color change of the phenol red indicator to a bright pink-red or magenta color. The organism is streaked onto the slant; the butt is not stabbed. Some organisms produce small amounts of ammonia, resulting in a pink color only in the slant; in others, both the butt and the slant will be pink.

Xylose–Lysine–Desoxycholate Agar. XLD agar is a selective and differential agar for the recovery of *Salmonella* and *Shigella* spp. The medium contains a phenol red indicator, desoxycholate, ferric ammonium sulfate, sodium thiosulfate, lysine, xylose, lactose, and sucrose. Desoxycholate inhibits gram-positive organisms and many nonenteric gram-negative bacilli. *Shigella* spp. do not ferment xylose, lactose, or sucrose and can be differentiated from other gram-negative enteric bacilli. Because *Shigella* spp. do not ferment these carbohydrates, the colonies appear transparent or red (color of medium). Nonpathogenic enteric organisms are capable of carbohydrate fermentation and appear yellow. *Salmonella* spp. produce the enzyme decarboxylase, which can break down the amino acid lysine. This reaction is called *decarboxylation* and can aid in differentiating *Salmonella* from other enteric organisms. The reaction yields colonies that are transparent or red. *Salmonella* spp. produce H_2S using sodium thiosulfate and react with the indicator ferric ammonium sulfate. This causes the transparent or red colonies to develop black centers.

Quality Control of Media

For commercially prepared media, the CLSI has developed recommendations for the use of abbreviated quality control (QC) testing.[8] If a manufacturer has followed the CLSI recommendations and can demonstrate that the performance of the media is consistent and adequate, the media do not require further QC testing in the clinical laboratory. Some commercially prepared media, however, require QC testing at the diagnostic laboratory, and the CLSI has identified these media. For this testing, QC organisms can be purchased that demonstrate the correct results; the relevant CLSI publication should be consulted for this information. All media prepared in the laboratory must be tested before being used for routine culture. The laboratory must maintain a stock of organisms for QC testing of the media for CLIA-mandated participation in quality assurance programs.

Biochemical or Enzymatic Tests

Many bacteria cannot be identified based on microscopic or culture characteristics alone. The biochemical properties and reactions of bacteria form the basis for an algorithm of identification procedures. Biochemical identification is an important function of the microbiology laboratory. Biochemical tests rely on bacterial physiology and the end products produced during metabolism of bacterial cells. Important biochemical reactions involve oxidation, fermentation, H_2S production, urea hydrolysis, and indole production.

In each biochemical procedure, the unknown bacterium causes a visible change in the medium, to which a specific test substance has been added. The change may be indicated by the formation of gas or by the formation of color. In some media, a pH indicator is used to demonstrate, for example, when an acid is produced during fermentation. Enzymatic breakdown of the amino acid tryptophan produces indole, which can be detected by the addition of an indicator and a resultant color change in the media. Biochemical tests may be completed individually or may be incorporated into culture media.

Colonies on primary cultures or colonies from subcultures can be used to perform biochemical tests. Some of these are rapid tests and take only minutes; others require hours of incubation. Together with macroscopic morphology (colonial characteristics) and microscopic morphology (cellular characteristics), biochemical testing provides additional information for the identification of microorganisms.

Modifications of the traditional biochemical tests have been made to facilitate inoculation of media, shorten the incubation time, automate procedures, and facilitate the identification of species based on reaction patterns.

In multitest systems, conventional biochemical tests are arranged in a series. A biocode is generated and a database accessed for identification of the organism (Fig. 15.19). Automated systems are used routinely and contain multiple-well systems in a card, cassette, or microtiter plate format.

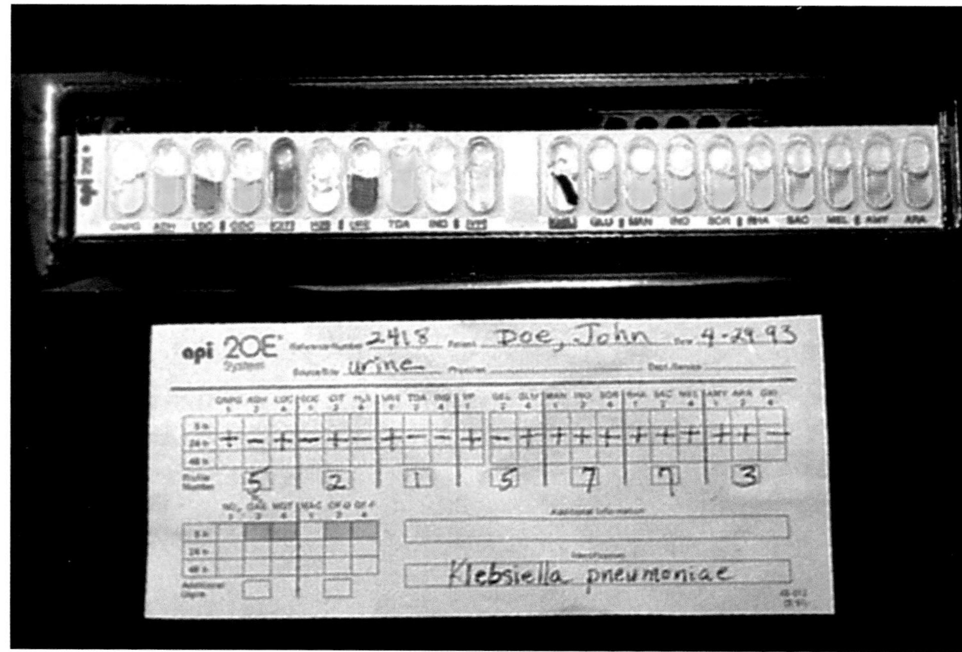

Fig. 15.19 Biochemical test panel used to identify bacteria (API; bioMérieux). Each cupule is a separate test that is scored positive or negative. These scores are added to generate a biocode that can be matched to a database of biocodes to give the identity of the organism tested.

The substrates are rehydrated and simultaneously inoculated with a suspension of the organism. In diagnostic microbiology laboratories, automated systems accommodate the identification of large volumes of isolates and simultaneously are capable of performing antimicrobial susceptibility testing. Automated systems can be interfaced with the laboratory computer information system for ease in reporting of results to the physician.

This section describes some of the more traditional biochemical tests that can aid in preliminary, presumptive, or final identification of organisms. These tests are reliable and inexpensive to perform.

Bile Esculin Agar

Bile esculin agar is used to aid in the identification of enterococci. The medium is supplemented with 40% bile, inhibiting the growth of most gram-positive organisms other than enterococci and some streptococci. The organisms such as enterococci capable of esculin hydrolysis will turn the indicator, ferric ammonium citrate, black.

Bile Solubility Test

Some organisms contain an active autocatalytic enzyme that will lyse the organism. With the addition of a bile salt, sodium desoxycholate, the lytic process is accelerated. When a drop of bile salt reagent is added to isolated colonies of *Streptococcus pneumoniae* on a blood agar, there will be visible autolysis of the colony within 30 minutes. *S. pneumoniae* gives a positive reaction, which is the disappearance of the suspected colony, leaving a flat area. Other streptococcal species will not be affected by the addition of the bile salt reagent.

Catalase Test

This reaction measures the presence of the enzyme catalase that converts hydrogen peroxide into oxygen and water. The catalase test is usually performed on a glass slide. A small amount of organism is placed on the slide, and a drop of 3% hydrogen peroxide is added to the sample. If bubbles of oxygen are immediately visible, the organism is positive for the production of catalase. The bubbles represent the release of oxygen in the enzymatic reaction. This test is often used to differentiate staphylococci from streptococci. All staphylococci are catalase positive and will produce oxygen gas. The genus *Streptococcus* does not produce catalase and consequently is catalase negative, producing no visible bubbling or lack of oxygen gas.

Citrate Utilization

Citrate agar is used to detect the use of sodium citrate as a sole source of carbon, and ammonium phosphate as a sole source of nitrogen. This test is useful in the identification of members of the Enterobacteriaceae. Most organisms capable of growth on this medium (slant) will turn the indicator, bromthymol blue, from green to blue. Some organisms can grow on this medium without turning the indicator blue (alkaline reaction). Therefore evidence of growth is considered a positive reaction (usually a longer incubation will result in an alkaline reaction).

Coagulase Test

S. aureus produces two forms of coagulase. The first, bound coagulase, or the clumping factor, can be detected by a rapid slide test. Clumping factor is bound to the cell wall and reacts with fibrinogen, causing visible clumping of bacterial cells in 10 seconds or less. A positive reaction is visible clumping,

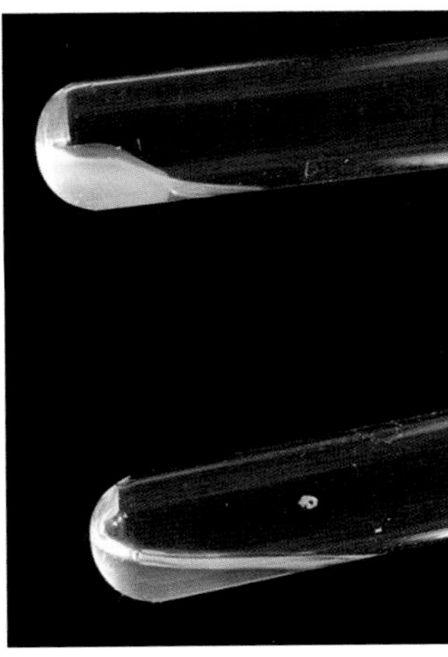

Fig. 15.20 Coagulase test. Tube coagulase test detects extracellular enzyme "free coagulase." *Top tube* is coagulase positive, showing a fibrin clot. *Bottom tube* is negative with no clot. (From Mahon CR, Lehman DC, Manuselis G: *Textbook of diagnostic microbiology*, ed 5, Maryland Heights, Mo, 2015, Saunders, Fig 14-6, p 322.)

and a negative test is a homogeneous suspension of the bacteria and the reagent. Commercial kits are available to test for clumping factor. If the test is weak or delayed, a tube test for unbound coagulase should be performed (Fig. 15.20A).

The second form of coagulase is the free, or unbound, coagulase. This test is carried out in a test tube and performed using rabbit plasma. The action of unbound coagulase causes a fibrin clot to form, and a positive test can be observed in 4 hours of incubation at 35°C. If the test appears negative, the time is extended to 24 hours. The test should initially be read at 4 hours because a positive test can revert to negative after 24 hours of incubation (Fig. 15.20B).

The coagulase test is used to differentiate *S. aureus* from other members of the genus *Staphylococcus*. *S. aureus* is a common cause of many serious infections, and rapid identification aids in the treatment of patients. Most other *Staphylococcus* species are coagulase negative, and because these staphylococci are usually members of the normal flora, they are together referred to as *coagulase-negative staphylococci*. If one of these members is isolated from a sterile source, the identification to species level can be performed if indicated. Coagulase-negative staphylococci are more frequently being identified in association with clinical infections in a variety of compromised patients.

Lysine Iron Agar

The LIA test, in conjunction with the TSI, is helpful in screening stool specimens for enteric pathogens. LIA tests for the presence of lysine deaminase and lysine decarboxylase (see Fig. 15.16). The formation of H_2S can also be determined, but TSI may be a more reliable medium. The medium is inoculated with an inoculating needle, by stabbing the butt of the medium through the center to the bottom of the tube and then streaking the slant (see Common Types of Media).

After incubation at 35°C for 18 to 24 hours in ambient air, reactions are noted. Reactions in the slant and butt are recorded as acid (A), alkaline (K), red (R), and the presence of H_2S

TABLE 15.5 Observations of Lysine Iron Agar (LIA)

Notation	Color Change	Metabolic Change
K/K	Purple slant, purple butt	Lysine decarboxylation
K/A	Purple slant, yellow butt	No enzymatic reactions, only glucose fermentation
R/A	Red slant, yellow butt	Lysine deamination
H_2S	Black in butt	H_2S production

A, Acid; *H_2S*, hydrogen sulfide; *K*, alkaline; *R*, red.

(blackening of the agar). An acid reaction is indicated by a yellow color and an alkaline reaction by a purple color. A *K/K reaction* (purple/purple) indicates a negative test for lysine deaminase (slant) and a positive test for lysine decarboxylase (butt). An *R/A reaction* (red/yellow) indicates a positive test for lysine deaminase (slant) and a negative test for lysine decarboxylase (butt). A *K/A reaction* (purple/yellow) indicates glucose fermentation and negative results for the two enzymes. H_2S is recorded as positive if a black precipitate is visible. Table 15.5 lists the various reactions and interpretations.

Oxidase Test

The oxidase tests determine the presence of cytochrome oxidase for the identification and differentiation of oxidase-negative Enterobacteriaceae from other gram-negative bacilli.

The presence of cytochrome oxidase is visualized by placing a small amount of the microorganism on a moistened piece of filter paper that contains 1% tetramethyl-*p*-phenylenediamine dihydrochloride, the substrate. An organism that produces oxidase will produce a color change of deep blue to purple within 10 seconds as a result of the conversion of the substrate to indophenol. A negative result is indicated by no color change.

PYR Test

PYR is a substrate, L-pyrrolidonyl-β-naphthylamide, that is broken down by the enzyme pyrrolidonyl arylamidase. It is a rapid test for the presumptive identification of *Enterococcus* spp. and group A β-hemolytic streptococci *(S. pyogenes)*. Commercially prepared filter paper impregnated with PYR is available. A small amount of the organism is applied to a prewetted piece of filter paper using a loop or wooden stick. The reaction is allowed to incubate for 2 minutes at room temperature. After incubation, a color-developing reagent, *N,N*-dimethylaminocinnamaldehyde, is added and observed for a color change within 1 minute. A positive test is indicated by the development of a bright-red color within 5 minutes. A negative test would be no color change or a yellow-orange color.

Rapid Urease Test

Organisms that produce the enzyme urease are able to hydrolyze urea-releasing ammonia as an end product. The production of ammonia results in an alkaline environment, thus causing the pH indicator phenol red to change from yellow to magenta. This test can be used to screen lactose-negative colonies identified on differential media, thereby assisting in the differentiation of the pathogenic urease negative *Salmonella* and *Shigella* spp. from the urease-positive nonpathogenic *Proteus* spp. Some diagnostic microbiology laboratories use this rapid test for detection of the yeast *Cryptococcus neoformans* (causative agent of pneumonia and meningitis) in sputum samples. It is a rapid method to screen sputum, and *C. neoformans* is positive, whereas other yeasts are usually negative.

Salt Tolerance Test

The salt tolerance test is used to determine whether an organism can grow in the presence of sodium chloride (NaCl). A heart infusion broth containing 6.5% NaCl is inoculated with an organism, and if the organism's growth is inhibited, the broth will remain clear. If an organism can grow in 6.5% NaCl, the broth will be cloudy or turbid. This test assists in the identification of enterococci capable of growth in 6.5% NaCl.

Indole Test

Organisms that produce the enzyme tryptophanase can break down the amino acid, tryptophan, to yield three possible end products, one of which is indole. The production of indole is detectable by Kovac's or Ehrlich's reagent that reacts with indole to produce a red-colored compound. Two forms of indole testing exist: tube indole and spot indole testing. The conventional tube method requires overnight incubation that identifies weak indole production compared to the rapid spot indole method.

In the rapid method, indole reagent containing the indicator (1% paradimethyl-aminocinnamaldehyde) is added to (and should saturate) the filter paper; a small amount of the isolated colony is placed on the filter paper. Indole-positive organisms will result in the rapid development of a blue color. This test can be used to differentiate swarming *Proteus* species and as a presumptive identification of *E. coli*. Positive organisms such as *E. coli* will produce a blue-green color on the filter paper, and negative organisms remain colorless.

Triple-Sugar Iron Agar and Kligler Iron Agar

TSI or KIA can provide initial presumptive identification of gram-negative bacilli, especially members of the Enterobacteriaceae family, the usual enteric intestinal pathogens screened. As previously described (see Common Types of Media), use of this medium can determine the primary characteristics of these organisms: ability to ferment the sugars glucose, lactose, and sucrose (KIA ferments only glucose and lactose); production of H_2S (visualized by black, iron-containing precipitate); and gas production (visualized by bubbles or splitting of medium). The medium is inoculated with a needle using a small amount of growth from a pure colony of the organism being tested, stabbing the butt of the medium through the center to the bottom of the tube, and then streaking the slant (see Fig. 15.18).

After incubation at 35°C for 18 to 24 hours in ambient air, reactions are noted and the organism presumptively identified based on fermentation reactions, H_2S production, and gas formation. Reactions in the slant and butt are recorded as acid (A) or alkaline (K), and the production of H_2S and gas (G) is noted.

TABLE 15.6 Observations of Triple-Sugar Iron Agar

Notation	Color Change	Metabolic Change
A/A	Yellow slant, yellow butt	Glucose fermented; lactose or sucrose or both fermented
K/A	Red slant, yellow butt	Glucose fermented; lactose and sucrose not fermented
K/K	Red slant, red butt	None of the three sugars fermented, or no reaction
H2S	Black in butt	H_2S production
G	Bubbles or splitting of agar in butt	Gas production

A, Acid; *G*, gas; *H_2S*, hydrogen sulfide; *K*, alkaline.

An acid reaction is indicated by a yellow color and an alkaline reaction by a red color. Table 15.6 lists various observations and interpretations.

Failure of the organism to ferment any of the three sugars results in a K/K reaction (or no reaction), indicated by a red slant and butt. A K/A reaction (red slant and yellow butt) results when only glucose is fermented. Organisms fermenting only glucose will initially give an A/A reaction or yellow slant and butt; the small amount of glucose present is used up as the incubation continues. The slant is under aerobic conditions and reverts to alkaline (or red) in 18 to 24 hours. In the butt, however, anaerobic conditions exist; there is no reversion to alkaline pH, and the acid (or yellow) reaction remains.

An A/A reaction (yellow slant and butt) results when glucose and lactose or sucrose are fermented. The medium contains 10 times more lactose and sucrose than glucose. Therefore organisms fermenting lactose or sucrose do not use up the sugars except after prolonged incubation. Fermentation of sucrose or lactose is indicated by acid (yellow) conditions in the slant. With prolonged incubation (48 to 72 hours), however, lactose and sucrose may also be used, and formerly acid reactions may revert to alkaline. Therefore the time of incubation is critical; the time recommended to obtain typical reactions is 18 to 24 hours.

URINE CULTURES

Urine cultures are used to diagnose bacterial infections of the urinary tract (bladder, ureter, kidney, and urethra). UTIs consist of two main types: (1) lower UTIs of the bladder or urethra, such as cystitis, an infection of the bladder; and (2) upper UTIs of the ureters and kidneys, such as pyelonephritis, an infection of the renal parenchyma (kidney). Routine urine cultures typically include the setup of one selective culture medium and one nonselective or supportive medium.

Collecting the Specimen

The urine specimen for culture must be collected in a clinically reliable manner; proper cleaning of the collection site, especially for female patients, is very important. Collecting a clean-catch, midstream urine sample uses the least invasive technique and consequently is most often performed. If a patient cannot urinate, a catheterized specimen can be obtained. Using straight catheters (in-and-out type) is more invasive than collecting clean-catch urine but eliminates contamination. If the catheterized specimen is from a patient with an indwelling Foley catheter, the urine from the tubing (not the bag) is sent to the laboratory (never the actual catheter). Urine is collected during cystoscopy as well and is sent to microbiology for culture.

The specimen must be collected into a sterile container and, if not cultured immediately, must be refrigerated to prevent bacterial growth. Urine is normally sterile within the bladder but is easily contaminated during the collection process.

Quantitative urine culture methods are required to differentiate infection from contamination. The presence of bacteria in clean-catch urine does not necessarily indicate a UTI unless the quantity of organism(s) is significant. Urine cultures are reported in colony-forming units per milliliter of urine (CFU/mL). An increased number of white blood cells (leukocytes) present (polymorphonuclear neutrophils [PMNs]) in the urine specimen, in conjunction with the results of the urine culture, is significantly more valuable for the diagnosis of infection. Table 15.7 provides interpretive guidelines for urine cultures and is used to assess the validity of the specimen.

Methods for Detection of Urinary Tract Infections

Rapid-Screening Test Strips

Rapid-screening test strips have been developed to test for UTIs. Nitrite tests have been incorporated into reagent strips used in many laboratories for routine urinalysis. Common organisms that cause UTIs, such as species of *Escherichia, Proteus, Klebsiella, Enterobacter,* and *Pseudomonas,* contain enzymes that reduce nitrate in the urine to nitrite. Organisms must possess the nitrate reductase enzyme necessary to carry out this process.

The rapid-screening test strips for UTIs are useful when the test for nitrite is combined with that for leukocyte esterase. Chemical test strips are available that combine nitrite and leukocyte esterase tests. Multiple-reagent test strips contain test pads for these constituents. Leukocyte esterase is an enzyme present in the granules of neutrophils. Neutrophils are generally increased in UTIs, so the presence of leukocyte esterase in the urine is an indicator of infection. The absence of leukocyte esterase, however, does not rule out UTI. The finding of nitrite-positive and leukocyte esterase–positive urine using chemical screening tests is helpful in detecting UTIs, especially in combination with the presence of bacteria and leukocytes in the urine sediment. Identification of the organism causing the infection requires a quantitative urine culture.

Quantitative Culture Methods

To determine a true UTI, quantitative methods are used to determine the number of CFUs/mL of urine specimen, and cultures are used to identify the organism(s) causing the infection.

Streak Plate Method. A streak plate method for quantitating the growth of microorganisms in the urine is typically used in clinical laboratories (Student Procedure Worksheet 15.2). A calibrated standardized inoculating loop containing 0.001 or 0.01 mL of urine is used to transfer the well-mixed specimen to streak the plates (Fig. 15.21). The larger volume (0.01 mL) delivers a greater amount of inoculums and can be used to gain more accurate quantitation, particularly in cystoscopy specimens where bacteria may be present in low numbers.

In common practice, a supportive medium such as SBA and a selective and differential medium (such as MAC or eosin methylene blue [EMB]) are streaked with the urine specimen. The drop of urine is spread as uniformly as possible on the plate (Fig. 15.22). After streaking and incubation, the number of colonies visible is multiplied by 1000 (for the 0.001-mL loop) or 100 (for the 0.01-mL loop) to calculate CFU/mL. Most bacteria will grow on SBA, which provides a total colony count. The selective medium indicates whether gram-negative bacilli are present. MAC also indicates whether the organisms are lactose positive or lactose negative. *E. coli,* one of the most common organisms identified in UTIs, accounts for a large percentage of UTIs in ambulatory and hospitalized patients. *E. coli, Klebsiella* spp., and *Enterobacter* spp. are lactose fermenters, whereas

TABLE 15.7 General Interpretive Guidelines for Urine Cultures

Result	Specific Specimen Type/Associated Clinical Condition, If Known	Workup
>104 CFU/mL of a single potential pathogen or for each of two potential pathogens	CCMS urine/pyelonephritis, acute cystitis, asymptomatic bacteriuria, or catheterized urines	Complete[a]
>103 CFU/mL of a single potential pathogen	CCMS urine/symptomatic males or catheterized urines or acute urethral syndrome	Complete
Three or more organism types with no predominating organism	CCMS urine or catheterized urines	None; because of possible contamination, ask for another specimen.
Either two or three organism types with predominant growth of one organism type and 104 CFU/mL of the other organism type (s)	CCMS urine	Complete workup for the predominating organism(s);[b] description of the other organism(s)
>102 CFU/mL of any number of organism types (setup with a 0.001- and 0.01-mL calibrated loop)	Suprapubic aspirates, any other surgically obtained urines (including ileal conduits, cystoscopy specimens)	Complete

CCMS, Clean-catch midstream; *CFU/mL,* colony-forming units per milliliter.
[a]A complete workup includes identification of the organism and appropriate susceptibility testing.
[b]Predominant growth = 10^4 to $> 10^5$ CFU/mL.
From Tille PM: *Bailey and Scott's diagnostic microbiology,* ed 13, St Louis, 2014, Mosby.

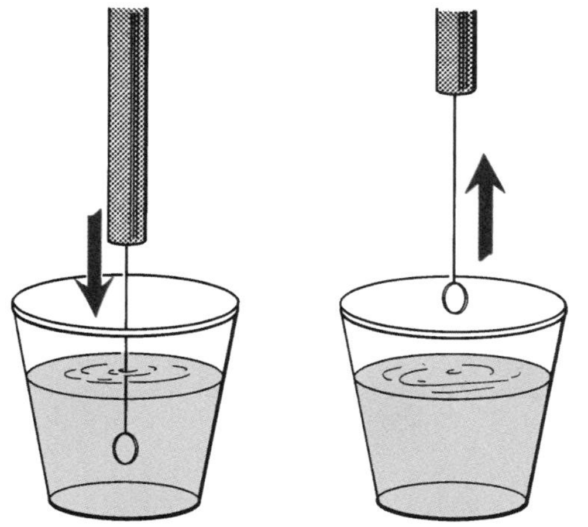

Fig. 15.21 Method for inserting a calibrated loop into urine to ensure that the proper amount of specimen will adhere to the loop. (From Tille PM: *Bailey and Scott's* diagnostic *microbiology,* ed 14, St Louis, 2017, Mosby.)

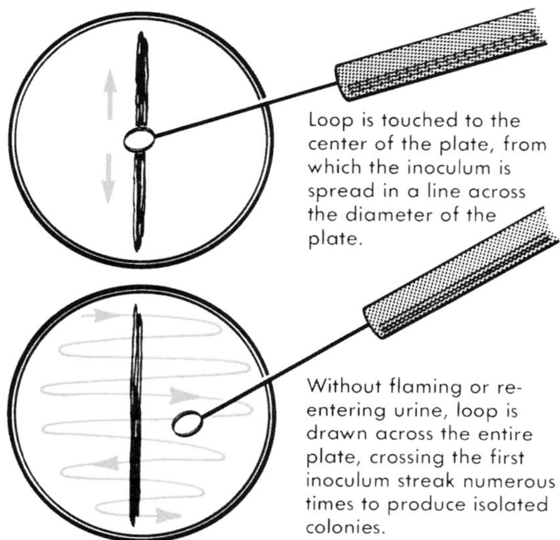

Fig. 15.22 Method for streaking a loopful of urine with a calibrated loop to produce isolated colonies and countable colony-forming units of organisms. (From Tille PM: Bailey *and Scott's diagnostic microbiology,* ed 14, St Louis, 2017, Mosby.)

Proteus spp. and *Pseudomonas aeruginosa* are lactose negative (do not ferment lactose). *Proteus* spp. may be recognized on SBA as spreading motile growth. Gram-positive organisms such as staphylococci and enterococci grow well on SBA but are inhibited and do not grow on MAC.

Interpreting Results of Quantitative Urine Cultures. Normal urine is sterile. Plates that contain no growth may be discarded and reported as no growth after 48 hours of incubation. In many UTIs, the laboratory findings show the presence of 100,000 (10^5) or more bacteria colonies per milliliter of urine specimen. After the incubation period, the number of colonies growing on the plates is counted and multiplied by 1000 (0.001-mL calibrated loop) to determine the number of microorganisms per milliliter of original urine specimen. A count of 100,000 CFU/mL urine or greater indicates a UTI in asymptomatic patients. A count of 1000 CFU/mL urine may be significant for a UTI in a symptomatic male patient. Therefore it is always important to combine the results of colony counts with the clinical information available. (See Table 15.7 for the interpretative guidelines for urine cultures.)

The growth characteristics of the colonies on the plates are also observed. As discussed previously, growth on MAC indicates a presumptive identification of gram-negative organisms. Any cultural observations should agree with the results of the Gram stain if one was performed. Further biochemical tests are used to identify the suspected organism.

Gram Stain of Urine Specimens

Gram stains are not done routinely on urine specimens, but if requested, the smear can be made directly from a well-mixed specimen. Using a sterile pipette, place 1 drop of urine on the slide and let air-dry. Fix the slide, perform the Gram stain, and observe using the 100 × oil-immersion objective. If at least one organism per field (after examining at least 20 fields) is seen, this correlates with a significant *bacteriuria* of greater than 100,000 CFU/mL urine.[11]

In patients with a severe UTI, progression to a bacteremia is possible. If this is suspected, a Gram stain result could aid in rapid diagnosis and direct treatment with the appropriate antimicrobial agent. In other patients, three or more morphologic types of bacteria may be detected, indicating a contaminated specimen from the perianal, vaginal, or urethral areas.

THROAT CULTURES

Throat cultures used primarily to differentiate the Lancefield group A β-hemolytic streptococcal *(S. pyogenes)* sore throat (pharyngitis) from a viral throat infection. Sore throats caused by group A streptococcus should be identified and treated. If an infection is untreated, sequelae may occur in some patients, leading to scarlet fever or acute rheumatic fever, followed by chronic rheumatic heart disease. Acute glomerulonephritis can also follow an untreated group A streptococcal throat infection but is often more common after a streptococcal skin infection.

Collecting the Specimen

As for all patient samples submitted to the clinical laboratory, proper collection of the sample is essential. Two sterile swabs are used to collect the specimen. The specimen is collected passing the swab over the rear pharyngeal wall and the tonsillar area within the patient's oral cavity (see Fig. 15.4 and Student Procedure Worksheet 15.3). Before culturing the specimen, one swab is used for rapid testing for group A β-hemolytic streptococci. If the rapid test is positive, a culture is not necessary. If the rapid test is negative, a confirmatory culture is completed with the second swab to ensure that the rapid test result was not a possible false-negative result. If only one swab is collected, an SBA plate is cultured first, and then the rapid test is performed. Transport to the laboratory should be within 2 hours in transport media, and specimens can be stored for 24 hours at room temperature.

Methods for Detection of Group A β-Hemolytic Streptococci

Rapid testing is routinely performed in most clinical laboratories. The rapid diagnosis of pharyngitis caused by group A β-hemolytic streptococci *(S. pyogenes)* can prevent complications such as scarlet fever. All negative rapid tests are confirmed by culture.

Rapid-Detection Methods: Nonculture Techniques

Numerous commercial products are available for the rapid detection of group A β-hemolytic streptococcal pathogens. The test results are available within 15 to 30 minutes, and antibiotic therapy can be started immediately. Systems for rapid streptococcal antigen detection include enzyme immunoassays, latex agglutination, and lateral flow assays.

Most rapid tests for group A β-hemolytic streptococci require extraction of any group A–specific antigen from the specimen on the throat swab. The group A–specific carbohydrate antigen is present in the cell wall of the streptococcal organisms. The swab is incubated with an enzyme or acid solution to extract the group A–specific carbohydrate antigen. Specific procedures will vary with the product, and the manufacturer's directions must always be followed carefully for optimal results. Controls should be used with all methods.

Most laboratory comparisons of conventional culture methods and rapid testing methods have shown excellent specificity. If results are positive using these methods, it is sufficient reason to begin antibiotic therapy because the rapid test is very specific for the group A β-hemolytic streptococcal antigen.

Many laboratories perform additional rapid antigen methods for detection of other pathogens, such as respiratory syncytial virus (bronchiolitis in infants) and influenza A and B (flu, respiratory illness) viruses. With increased surveillance for possible epidemic or pandemic (worldwide epidemic) influenza, the rapid detection of influenza A has become an important rapid test in the clinical microbiology laboratory.

Culture on Sheep Blood Agar

Culture on SBA will isolate bacterial pathogens from the pharyngeal area, if present. For recovery of other pathogens, such as *C. diphtheriae* or *N. gonorrhoeae,* special media must be used.

Interpreting Results of Throat Culture Plates. After suitable incubation has taken place, the colony morphology and the appearance of hemolysis on SBA are used in the identification of streptococci.

Appearance of Hemolysis. After incubation, hemolysis on SBA can be observed. Hemolysis is best determined by holding the culture plate directly in front of a light source. This phenomenon is useful in distinguishing different types of streptococci based on the hemolytic pattern or lysis of the RBCs (erythrocytes) present in the medium. As previously noted, hemolysis can be visualized in three distinct patterns, depending on the type of streptococci:

1. Alpha hemolysis is incomplete or partial hemolysis of the RBCs in the medium. Viridans streptococci (part of the normal flora of the throat) and *S. pneumoniae* (meningitis and pneumonia) exhibit this characteristic type of hemolysis, which is visualized macroscopically as a green discoloration of the medium surrounding the colony (see Fig. 15.17A).
2. Beta hemolysis is complete hemolysis of the RBCs in the medium. *S. pyogenes* (common throat pathogen) is β-hemolytic, and the hemolysis appears macroscopically as a clear zone surrounding the surface colonies or in stabs (produced during inoculation) in the blood agar; this represents complete hemolysis of RBCs in the media (see Fig. 15.17B).
3. Gamma hemolysis is no hemolysis of the RBCs in the medium. Macroscopically, there is no change in the color of the medium. Some *Enterococcus* spp. characteristically demonstrate no hemolysis (see Fig. 15.17C).

Throat cultures are used primarily to detect the presence of the Lancefield group A β-hemolytic streptococci. β-Hemolytic streptococci typically appear as small, gray-white, round colonies, with a large zone of β-hemolysis. Other pathogens may also be clinically significant. Normal throat cultures show a predominance of α-hemolytic streptococci (viridians streptococci) and commensal *Neisseria* spp. Other organisms can also constitute normal flora (Student Procedure Worksheet 15.4).

Identification of Group A β-Hemolytic Streptococci. The PYR test can be used to differentiate group A β-hemolytic streptococci from other β-streptococci (see Biochemical or Enzymatic Tests). Group A β-hemolytic streptococci are the only β-hemolytic streptococci with a positive reaction in this test. A pure culture must be used to avoid false-positive results caused by other organisms that may be in the normal flora. Other β-hemolytic streptococci, such as groups C and G, can cause pharyngitis (without the severe sequelae), but are PYR negative. Another organism that can be confused with group A β-hemolytic streptococci is *Arcanobacterium haemolyticum;* Gram stain results will rapidly differentiate the two because *A. haemolyticum* is a gram-positive bacillus.

Another test to identify group A β-hemolytic streptococci is by using bacitracin susceptibility. This traditional test has been performed for β-hemolytic streptococci by subculturing to SBA and adding the disk to the subculture or placing the disk in the primary throat culture plate in the first quadrant. The bacitracin disk (with 0.04 unit) is placed in the center of the inoculated area aseptically, and the plate is incubated at 35°C. Any zone of inhibition of growth around the disk is indicative of bacitracin susceptibility and a positive test for group A β-hemolytic streptococci.

Serology Tests. Many rapid products are available for testing cultures of β-hemolytic streptococci. These kits test for groups A, B, C, F, and G β-hemolytic streptococci by latex slide agglutination. Direct detection of the group A (or B, C, F, G) streptococcal antigens requires extracting the antigens. This method gives a definitive identification for the particular Lancefield group that agglutinates.

Bile Solubility or Optochin Susceptibility Tests. Throat cultures are primarily used to diagnose pharyngitis caused by group A β-hemolytic *S. pyogenes. S. pneumoniae* may be present in large numbers and is identified in sputum specimens, rather than throat cultures, as a common cause of pneumonia. If the culture is suspect, the bile solubility (see Biochemical and Enzymatic Tests) and optochin tests can be performed.

S. pneumoniae is an α-hemolytic streptococcus and can be differentiated from viridians streptococci (normal flora) by the addition of a desoxycholate (*S. pneumoniae* will be lysed by the bile salt; other α-streptococci will not). The optochin (ethylhydrocupreine hydrochloride) disk is applied to a pure subculture of the organism on SBA and incubated at 35°C with 3% to 5% CO_2 overnight. *S. pneumoniae* will be inhibited (zone of inhibition $\geq$ 14 mm) by the optochin impregnated in the disk.

If the bile salt detergent reagent is used, a drop of the reagent is added to isolated colonies on an SBA plate, and visible dissolution the *S. pneumoniae* colonies is noted within 30 minutes if they are present. The optochin disk, when used, is placed on a subculture of the suspected colonies on a blood agar plate, and the plate is incubated overnight. Zones of inhibition of 14 mm or larger are seen around the optochin disk as presumptive identification for *S. pneumoniae.*

Molecular Diagnostic Testing for Streptococci. Rapid nucleic acid testing is available and offers increased specificity over traditional identification schemes (see More Point-of-Care Rapid Testing Applications). Several assays that include polymerase chain reaction (PCR) or DNA probe hybridization assays are available for the detection of group B and group A streptococci. A fully integrated automated system has been developed for the detection of group B streptococcus DNA directly from a swab.

GENITOURINARY CULTURES

Microbiological examination of genitourinary tract specimens is used primarily to determine the cause of urethritis, vaginitis, and cervicitis. Organisms recovered from these sources are often sexually transmitted; *N. gonorrhoeae* and *C. trachomatis* are two examples. These infections can cause pelvic inflammatory disease, leading to infertility. Chlamydial infections have surpassed gonorrheal infections as the most prevalent sexually transmitted bacterial disease in the United States.

Other microorganisms that can cause vaginitis in females include *Gardnerella vaginalis* and *Trichomonas vaginalis*. A parasite and commonly recognized sexually transmitted organism, *T. vaginalis* can be identified in a wet mount of vaginal secretions (see Tests for Parasites). *G. vaginalis* can cause bacterial vaginosis (BV), a polymicrobial condition resulting from the disruption of the normal flora in the vagina (see later discussion). *G. vaginalis* is a short, gram-negative bacilli or coccobacilli. When the exfoliated vaginal epithelial cells are covered with tiny gram-variable bacilli and coccobacilli, they are known as "clue cells." Clue cells are coated with coccobacilli, and they alter the appearance of the squamous epithelial cell cytoplasm and may be described as refractile, stippled, or granular, with shaggy or bearded cell borders. Bacterial smears may also demonstrate mixed bacterial types because BV is a polymicrobic infection that may include anaerobic bacteria (small gram-negative bacilli), *Mobiluncus* spp. (curved gram-variable or gram-negative bacilli), and *G. vaginalis*. Smears, not culture, are diagnostic for BV.

Genitourinary fungal infections are also common and often the cause of vaginitis in women, especially those receiving antibiotic therapy that inhibits the growth of normal vaginal bacterial flora. A common fungal infection is caused by *Candida albicans* (see Tests for Fungi). Herpes simplex virus is another frequent cause of genitourinary infections.

Collecting the Specimen

It is essential that genitourinary tract specimens, usually from the vaginal cervix or inflamed perineal areas in women and the urethra in men, be appropriately collected so that the organisms may be detected. Specimens must be handled carefully to avoid any contamination with other viable infectious material.

Culture

For detecting chlamydial organisms from the endocervix, a swab is used to remove purulent discharge. A second swab is then collected by vigorously swabbing to recover epithelial cells. Generally, swabs for cell culture should have a plastic shaft, and the tip can be Dacron or rayon. Chlamydiae are obligate intracellular pathogens and do not grow in artificial media. Cell culture techniques are used to grow chlamydiae, with the McCoy line being the most popular. Once collected, the specimen should be placed in a transport medium, such as 0.2 M sucrose–phosphate or other suitable transport medium, and sent to the laboratory.

A separate sample must be collected for the detection of gonococcal organisms (see Gonorrheal Infections), in which case the specimen is preferably inoculated immediately onto the appropriate culture medium and a smear made for Gram stain. JEMBEC systems are used to culture *N. gonorrhoeae* directly (Fig. 15.23). The system includes a medium (modified Thayer–Martin) in a snap-top box and a CO_2-generating sodium bicarbonate pellet. The medium is inoculated with the swab in a W or Z pattern and placed in the bag provided, which should be sealed and sent to the laboratory. If not immediately plated, genitourinary specimens should be transported to the laboratory within 24 hours at room temperature. Commercially available systems for transport and storage of genitourinary tract specimens enhance the survival of the organisms, if present. Kits include collection swabs (preferably Dacron or rayon)

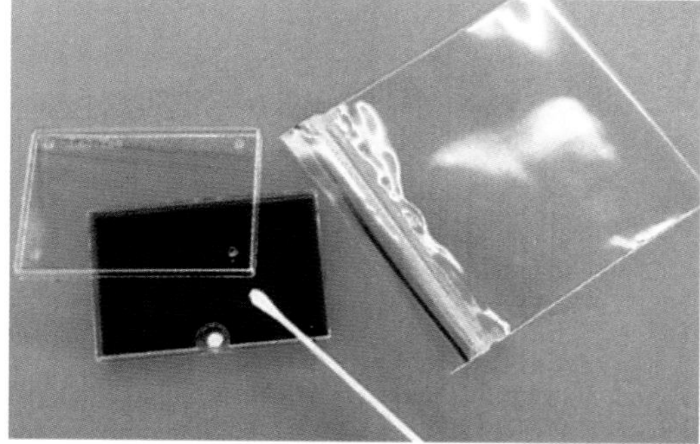

Fig. 15.23 JEMBEC plate for isolation of *Neisseria gonorrhoeae*. The system includes modified Thayer–Martin medium in a snap-top box and a carbon dioxide–generating sodium bicarbonate pellet. After inoculation, the medium is placed in a zip-locking plastic envelope. (From Tille PM: Bailey *and Scott's diagnostic microbiology,* ed 14, St Louis, 2017, Mosby.)

and transport tubes containing specially formulated media such as Stuart or Amies charcoal media.

Molecular Diagnostic Testing

Molecular assays that include hybridization and amplification methods have replaced serologic assays for the rapid diagnosis of infection with *C. trachomatis* and *N. gonorrhoeae*. PACE2 (Hologic Inc, Bedford, MA) is a hybridization method that allows detection of both pathogens from the same specimen. Viable organisms are not needed for this procedure, so transport is not an issue, which has facilitated specimen transport from distances. Disadvantages of this method are that no antimicrobial susceptibility testing is performed, and data for resistance surveillance are not available.

The PACE2 collection kits are available commercially and include two swabs, one to remove excess mucus and the second for collection. It is recommended the swab be rotated for 10 to 30 seconds in the endocervical canal to obtain sufficient sampling; the swab is then placed in a transport tube. Males should not urinate for 1 hour before collection. The swab should be inserted into the urethra 2 to 4 cm using a rotating motion, then placed in a transport tube. Transport is at 2°C to 25°C, as is storage, and testing should be done within 7 days. Additional molecular hybridization assays are available that detect bacterial ribosomal RNA using chemiluminescent DNA probes or RNA/DNA hybrids using antibody-mediated recognition.

Amplified assays are more sensitive than nonamplified assays. A nucleic acid–amplified method is APTIMA Combo2 (Hologic) for detection of *C. trachomatis* and *N. gonorrhoeae*. As with amplified assays, various commercial assays are currently available from various manufacturers and suitable for large-scale screening programs. For patients in whom treatment has failed, culturing *C. trachomatis* is recommended. Disadvantages of molecular methods include no antimicrobial susceptibility testing, and amplified methods cannot be used in legal cases. Urine can also be used as a source in the amplified method.

Endocervical swab collection follows the PACE2 protocol. If urine will be collected, the patient should not urinate for at least 1 hour before collection. A first-catch urine sample is collected (20 to 30 mL), and 2 mL of the specimen is transferred to a transport tube. Transport and storage are at 2°C to 30°C, and testing should be performed within 60 days of collection for swabs and 30 days for urine.

Methods for Detection of Common Genitourinary Tract Infections

The physician must alert the laboratory to the probable organisms causing the genitourinary infection so that the identification process can be initiated using the appropriate culture medium and assay protocol.

Gram Stain

Gram-stained smears from urethral discharge are examined for the presence of PMNs and gram-negative diplococci. Intracellular gram-negative diplococci (within PMNs) can be considered diagnostic evidence of gonococcal infection in men only. Vaginal flora contaminates smears in women, and the identification of diplococci should not be considered diagnostic because women harbor nonpathogenic strains; therefore intracellular organisms should not be reported, and a positive smear is considered presumptive evidence of gonorrhea.

Gonorrheal Infections

When *N. gonorrhoeae* is suspected, a special agar medium and CO_2 atmosphere for incubation are required for optimal recovery from the clinical specimen. Various supplemental media can also be inoculated. Modified Thayer–Martin agar is a selective medium for *N. gonorrhoeae* and contains various antimicrobials to inhibit the growth of other types of bacteria and fungi. Chocolate agar is also a supportive medium for *N. gonorrhoeae*, but it does not inhibit the growth of normal flora because it does not contain antibiotics.

After 24 to 48 hours of incubation on modified Thayer–Martin and chocolate agar, colonies of *N. gonorrhoeae* appear small, gray, translucent, and shiny. A Gram stain of *N. gonorrhoeae* would reveal characteristic gram-negative diplococci ("coffee bean"). In addition, presumptive identification of *N. gonorrhoeae* requires a positive oxidase test. Further testing may be required depending on the nature of the specimen.

Molecular diagnostic tests, nucleic acid methods, are widely used for diagnosing gonorrheal infections (see previous discussion).

Chlamydial Infections

Infection with *C. trachomatis* is a prevalent sexually transmitted disease in the United States. It is important that the specimen be collected properly from the appropriate site by using a technique that dislodges the necessary epithelial cells where the chlamydial organism resides. As with gonorrheal infections, nucleic acid methods are also widely used for chlamydial infections (see Molecular Diagnostic Testing).

If a culture is requested, the specimen must be transported to the laboratory immediately. *C. trachomatis* is a fastidious organism, requiring complex or extensive nutritional requirements. Nonculture methods other than nucleic acid testing include direct immunofluorescent antibody studies using monoclonal antisera and enzyme-linked immunosorbent assay.

Trichomonal and Yeast Infections

T. vaginalis can be observed on a direct wet mount of the vaginal fluid. This is the simplest and most rapid means of detection of this parasitic organism (see Tests for Parasites). Fungal elements can also be visualized at the same time. By addition of a 10% potassium hydroxide (KOH) reagent to the preparation, host cell protein is dissolved, allowing any fungal elements to be visualized (see Tests for Fungi). KOH also makes the discharge alkaline, causing it to emit a fishy, aminelike odor that is characteristically associated with BV.

Bacterial Vaginosis

BV is produced by a mixed infection with anaerobic and facultative organisms. These organisms live on or in a host but also survive independently. BV is characterized by a foul-smelling vaginal discharge, and Gram stain will show a mixed flora and decreased amount of *Lactobacillus* spp. (normal flora). The vaginal discharge can be examined microscopically for diagnosis of BV; in a wet preparation, sloughed epithelial cells, many of which are covered with tiny gram-variable bacilli and coccobacilli, may be visible (clue cells).

ENTERIC DISEASE

Infections of the intestinal tract can be caused by a variety of bacteria, viruses, or parasites. Infections are transmitted by contaminated food or water and typically produce diarrhea. The differential diagnosis of diarrheal disease can be difficult because of the many possible causes. The Infectious Diseases Society of America and ARUP Laboratories have algorithmic guidelines (Figs. 15.24 and 15.25) to assist in the workup of diarrheal illnesses.

Conventional Testing

Traditional testing methods for the detection of enteric pathogens use culture techniques. Routine stool cultures are commonly performed to detect the presence of *E. coli, Salmonella* species, *Shigella* species, and Campylobacter species. Conventional testing for gastrointestinal parasites includes microscopy and stool antigen tests. Antigen testing improves the detection of viral agents (norovirus, rotavirus), Shiga toxin–producing *E. coli,* and protozoan agents (*Giardia, Cryptosporidium, Entamoeba histolytica*). Antigen testing is not available for all pathogens.

Mass Spectrophotometry

Recently, mass spectrometry was introduced into the microbiology laboratory. In 2013, the matrix-assisted laser desorption ionization time-of-flight mass spectrometer (MALDI-TOF) was named as one of the "Top Ten Breakthrough Medical Technologies" of 2013. The benefits of MALDI-TOF include positive pathogen identification after only 18 to 24 hours even with a mixed-colonies culture. Anaerobic organisms provide an excellent example of the benefit of this technology. Because of the challenge of protecting the bacteria from oxygen exposure, rapid identification is important and can

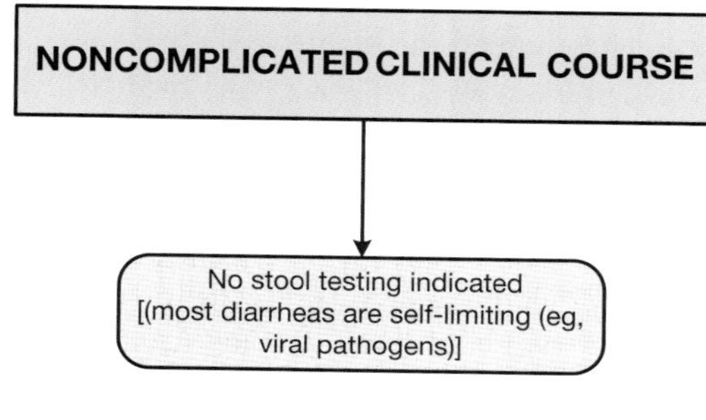

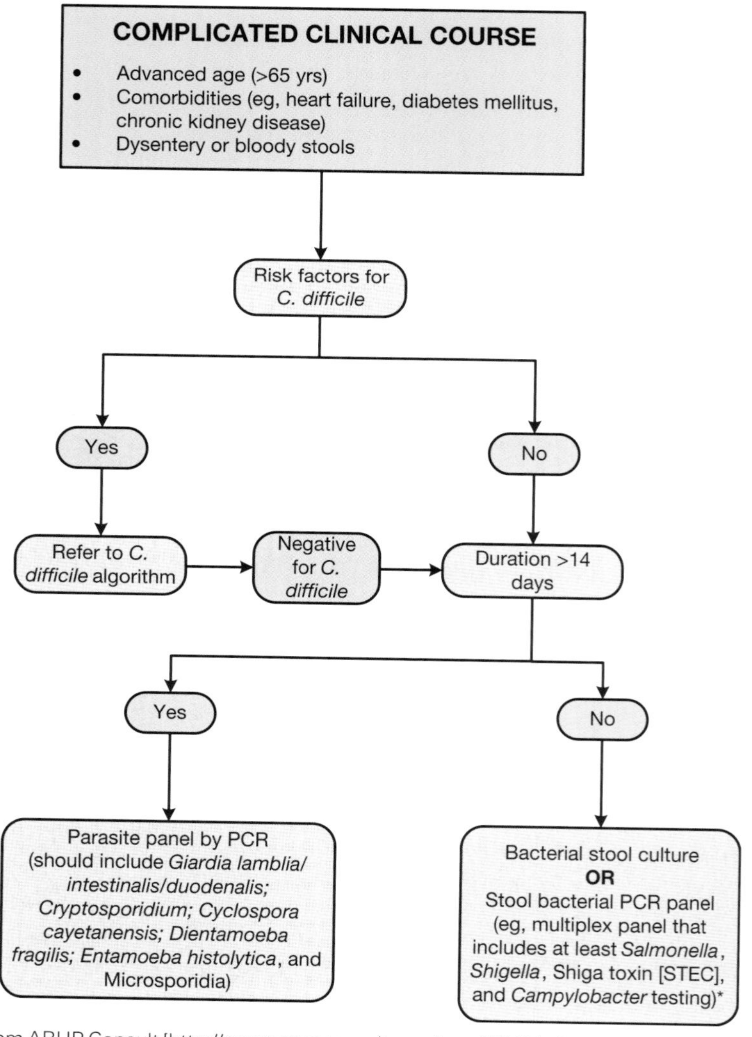

Fig. 15.24 Diarrhea in adults in primary care. (From ARUP Consult [http://www.arupconsult.com], an ARUP Laboratories test selection tool for healthcare professionals © 2006 ARUP Laboratories. All Rights Reserved. Revised 06/05/2015.)

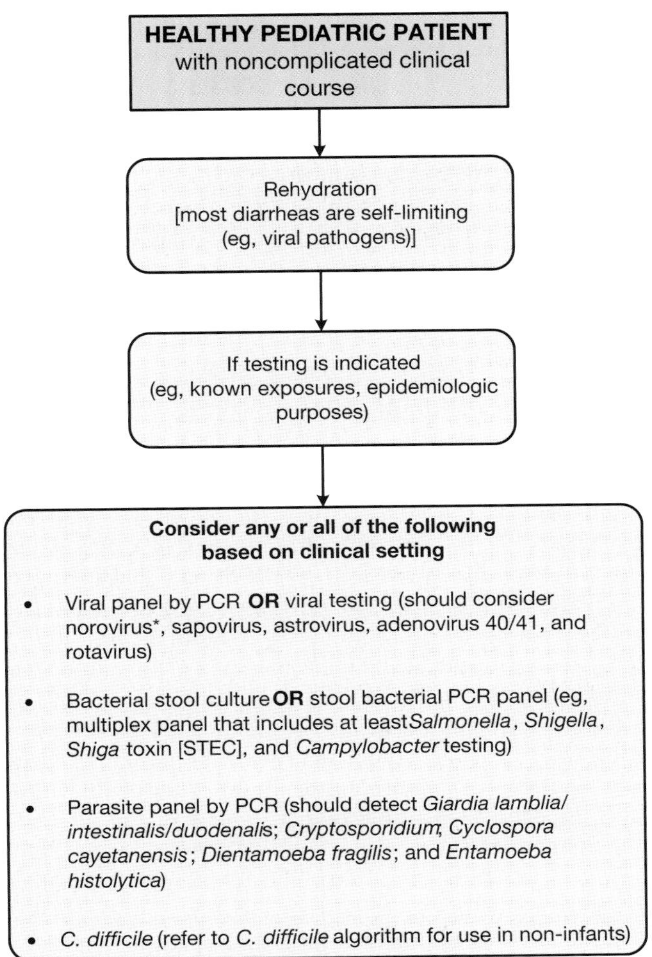

Fig. 15.25 Diarrhea in healthy pediatric patients. (From ARUP Consult [http://www.arupconsult.com], an ARUP Laboratories test selection tool for healthcare professionals © 2006 ARUP Laboratories. All Rights Reserved. Revised 8/9/2016.)

save the need for a second specimen or culture that prolongs patient treatment.

Molecular Diagnostics

Molecular testing is emerging as an important method of testing for increased detection of pathogenic bacteria, viruses, and mycobacterial infections. Molecular testing panels detect and identify multiple pathogenic gastrointestinal bacteria, viruses, and parasites simultaneously from a single patient specimen. A single panel can test for as many as 23 pathogens. Other testing panels are focused panels that use clinical algorithms for enteric bacteria versus parasites versus hospital-acquired *Clostridium difficile.*

BLOOD CULTURES

Blood is normally sterile. Infections involving bacteria in the bloodstream are serious.

Bacteremia can have serious consequences for the patient. Blood cultures can provide a clinical diagnosis of bacteremia. Bacteria can be detected in the blood in the absence of disease, especially after dental extractions or any incident involving a loss of integrity of the capillary endothelial cells; this is called a *transient bacteremia.* Septicemia or sepsis indicates a situation in which the bacteria are actively multiplying and metabolizing (producing toxins), causing harm to the host (patient). *Fungemia,* the presence of fungi in the blood, can be found in immunosuppressed hosts.

When a patient is septic, the bacteria can release *exotoxins* (toxins released to the surrounding environment) or *endotoxins* (part of the cell wall of gram-negative bacteria). Particularly in the case of endotoxins, a progressive syndrome, septic shock, can occur. Symptoms of septic shock are fever, chills, lowered blood pressure, respiratory distress, and disseminated intravascular coagulation (DIC). Endotoxins can activate complement and the clotting factors, leading to DIC. This is a serious complication of septic shock.

Organisms Commonly Isolated from Blood

Portals of entry for organisms that can cause bacteremia are the genitourinary tract (25%), respiratory tract (20%), abscesses (10%), surgical wound infections (5%), biliary tract (5%), miscellaneous sites (10%), and uncertain sites (25%).[12] Organisms commonly cultured from blood are gram-positive cocci such as *S. aureus,* coagulase-negative staphylococci, the viridans streptococci, *S. pneumoniae,* and *Enterococcus* spp. Common gram-negative organisms found in blood are *E. coli, Klebsiella pneumoniae, Pseudomonas aeruginosa, Enterobacter* spp., and *Proteus* spp. Two anaerobic groups also frequently recovered are *Bacteroides* and *Clostridium* spp.[12] Many of these organisms are likely to be found in the health care facility's environment and as normal flora; they may colonize the skin, oropharyngeal area, and gastrointestinal tract of hospitalized patients.

The incidence of bacteremia or septicemia has increased, most likely as a result of several factors: (1) the decreased immunocompetency status of several patient populations (patients live longer with proper therapy); (2) the increased use of invasive procedures such as intravenous catheters and vascular prostheses; (3) the prolonged survival of debilitated and seriously ill patients; (4) the increase in the aging population in general, and (4) the increased use of therapeutic drugs, such as broad-spectrum antibiotics, suppressing normal flora and facilitating the emergence of resistant strains of bacteria. These factors have made the interpretation of significant growth of microorganisms in the blood more difficult. Standard blood culture systems are usually sufficient to isolate most fungi.

Collecting the Specimen

Blood culture media has been developed as enrichment broths to enhance the growth of even a single organism. These media will also enhance the growth of contaminating organisms, making the collection process of paramount importance to reduce the introduction of contaminating organisms. The CLSI has published recommendations for the collection of blood for culture.[13] The timing of the collection is also critical. Transient bacteremia can occur incidentally after dental, colonoscopic, or cystoscopic procedures. In this case, bacteria may be present in the blood for a brief period after the procedure. Intermittent bacteremia can result from wound abscesses or other infections, and in this case, bacteria are present in the blood for a brief period, followed by a period with no bacteria present. For continuous bacteremia, in which the organisms are from an intravascular source and are present in the blood consistently, the timing is not as critical. Ideally, blood should be collected before any antimicrobial agents are administered because previous antimicrobial therapy may delay the growth of some organisms. A single culture is usually not sufficient to diagnose bacteremia.

Generally, two or three culture sets are drawn within 24 hours. The blood specimens can be drawn from separate sites or at timed intervals, depending on the patient's symptoms. Collecting more than three sets in a single day is discouraged; additional cultures do not add to the recovery of significant organisms. Typically, if subacute bacterial endocarditis is suspected, three sets are drawn within 24 hours, and if they do not grow, two or three additional sets are drawn in the next 24-hour period.[7]

The volume of blood being tested is a major factor in detecting bacteria in blood cultures; for adults, 10 to 20 mL of blood should be collected for each of the culture bottles. Smaller amounts are collected from children. Protocol for specific blood culture collection is established by each health care facility.

Cleansing the Collection Site

Because it is necessary to avoid any normal skin flora contaminating the collection, it is critical that extra precautions be taken to cleanse the venipuncture site when blood is collected for culture. Proper disinfection of the skin is essential. The skin is cleansed by using 70% alcohol and a povidone-iodine solution. Allow the iodine to dry for 1 minute. If the phlebotomist must palpate the vein after disinfection, the gloved finger must be disinfected in the same manner as the skin. An alternative disinfectant scrub is chlorhexidine gluconate, which can be used if a patient is allergic to the povidone-iodine solution. The cap or top of the blood culture bottle must also be disinfected prior to inoculation with alcohol. The blood is then transferred with the syringe into the blood culture bottles containing broth.

Culture Media for Blood

The medium into which the blood is drawn is of an enrichment media that encourages the growth and multiplication of all organisms present, even stray bacterial contaminants found as part of the normal skin flora.

The basic culture medium for blood is a liquid that contains both a nutrient broth and an anticoagulant. Most commercially available blood culture media contain trypticase soy broth, brain–heart infusion (BHI) agar, peptone supplement, or thioglycolate broth. In addition, an anticoagulant, 0.025% to 0.05% sodium polyanetholsulfonate (SPS), is used in blood culture bottles because it does not harm the bacteria.[12] A blood/medium ratio of 1:5 or 1:10 is adequate for most laboratories. Blood cultures are generally drawn in sets. Each set contains an aerobic and an anaerobic bottle.

In addition to the standard blood culture media, self-containing subculture systems are available that consist of a conventional blood culture bottle with an attached chamber containing a slide coated with agar. Special media for the isolation of *Mycobacterium* spp. and fungi are also available. To subculture, the bottle is inverted, allowing the broth contents to contact the agar without opening the bottle or inserting needles. An additional specialized blood culture system, the Isolator (Alere, Waltham, MA) is a stoppered vacutainer (vacuum venipuncture) tube that allows the specimen to be drawn directly into the tube. The tube contains a lysis agent and SPS as an anticoagulant. On vigorous vortexing, the pathogen is released from the cells, the tube is centrifuged, and the sediment is plated to regular culture media. This system improves the recovery of filamentous fungi.

Examination of Blood Cultures

Historically, blood culture bottles were visually examined daily, and blind subcultures to solid media were incubated to identify bacteria. Conventional blood culture techniques are labor intensive and time-consuming and are rarely used in a clinical laboratory. Automated systems are now widely used that are capable of rapid and accurate detection of organisms in blood specimens. These systems not only provide rapid identification of infectious organisms in the bloodstream but also can be used for the cultivation of sterile body fluids.

Automated systems continually monitor the growth within the broth by various methods. The Bactec (BD Diagnostic Systems, Sparks, MD) continuously monitors growth without visual inspection or subcultures and can automatically handle large numbers of blood culture bottles. Bottles are incubated in the incubator chamber, where constant rocking occurs to enhance growth. Some automated instruments now include small magnetic stir bars inside the bottles that provide for agitation and oxygenation. The Bactec chamber contains a detector that measures the CO_2 produced by bacterial metabolism. Gas-permeable sensors use fluorescence to detect the CO_2. The fluorescence is measured without entering the bottle. The system is alarmed to make personnel aware of positive samples. These systems improve the time to detection and show a reduced frequency of false-positive results. Other automated systems, such as the BacT/ALERT (bioMérieux, La Balme, France), measure CO_2-derived pH changes with a colorimetric sensor located in the bottom of each bottle. As CO_2 is generated and dissolves in water present in the matrix of the sensor, free hydrogen ions are generated, causing a color change in the sensor.

The blood culture bottles in the automated systems are subcultured and Gram-stained once they are flagged as positive. Organism identification proceeds using traditional algorithms applicable based on the growth characteristics of the organism on the subculture. The physician may also institute appropriate antibiotic therapy based on the Gram stain interpretation.

WOUND OR SOFT TISSUE CULTURES

The skin serves as an excellent barrier to microorganisms, protecting the internal organs and bloodstream from invasion. However, because of trauma, irritation, or natural openings such as pores, the skin remains at risk for infection. A wide array of organisms can cause infections of the skin. Therefore physicians will rely on the appearance of the rash, lesion, or wound to determine what type of procedure is needed for diagnosis, such as culture, biopsy, or surgical procedures.

Skin infections are typically divided into three general categories based on the level of invasion of the organism: (1) superficial infections of the epidermis and dermal layers, (2) infection of subcutaneous tissue, and (3) deep wound infections that may become systemic. Superficial infections of the skin or dermal layers are often a result of blockage of the hair follicle and can be characterized as folliculitis (minor infection of the follicle), furuncle (a boil or abscess that is painful), or a carbuncle that has spread deep into the subcutaneous tissue. Subcutaneous skin infections appear as abscesses (localized area filled with neutrophils and debris that may extend into subcutaneous tissue), ulcers (area that includes damage to tissue that spreads out from the infection), or boils (infection of the subcutaneous tissue around a hair follicle) and often contain mixed infections, including aerobic, facultative anaerobic, or strictly anaerobic organisms. Extensive soft tissue infections are serious and may cause systemic disease resulting in death. Such infections include necrotizing fasciitis (infection of the fascia overlying muscle tissue), gangrene (chronic necrotic tissue infection), and myositis (inflammation of the muscle). Finally, wound infections can be related to a postoperative procedure, bite wounds, or burns.

Organisms Commonly Isolated from Wounds or Soft Tissue Infections

One of the most common etiologic agents associated with superficial skin infections as well as subcutaneous or systemic infections is *S. aureus*. Occasionally, a member of the Enterobacteriaceae family may be isolated from a tissue infection. Common aerobic, facultative anaerobes or anaerobes that may be associated with tissue infections include *E. coli*, streptococci, *Peptostreptococcus* spp., clostridia, and a variety of gram-negative bacilli. *Pseudomonas aeruginosa* is often identified associated with infections from exposure in a hot tub, whirlpool, or swimming pool. Fungal organisms may also be associated with skin infections, including dermatophytes or organisms capable of dissemination, such as *C. neoformans, Blastomyces dermatitidis, Coccidioides immitis,* and *Histoplasma capsulatum.*

Collecting the Specimen

Proper collection of skin or wound infections may be difficult. The lesions are open and often contaminated with normal skin flora. It is essential to remove overlying skin and debris and collect material from the deepest area available. Appropriate collection may require debridement (surgical removal of necrotic tissue) or surgical extraction of a biopsy or purulent material from the infection. A Gram stain should be performed to initiate early treatment to prevent the spread of the organism to the patient bloodstream, resulting in a more serious bacteremia or septicemia. It is important to note that if anaerobes are suspected, an appropriate anaerobic swab and transport media should be used to sustain the viability of the organisms.

Culture Media for Wound and Tissue Infections

Typically, wound or tissue infections are inoculated onto a variety of media, including 5% SBA, MAC for the growth of gram-negative organisms, and chocolate agar for fastidious organisms. If an anaerobe is suspected, an additional anaerobic blood agar and special selective agars may be used to enhance the growth of anaerobes. Selective agars include one or all of the following: *Bacteroides* bile esculin agar, kanamycin-vancomycin laked (KVL) agar, and PEA. One additional chocolate plate is added to ensure that an organism isolated is a true anaerobe. This plate should be incubated in CO_2 to determine the aerotolerance of any organisms isolated on the anaerobic media. An enrichment broth, usually thioglycolate, is inoculated to enrich small amounts of organisms that may be present in tissue. Gram stain results, with colony morphology on aerobic and anaerobic media, provide a preliminary differentiation for most clinically relevant aerobes and anaerobes.

If a fungal infection is suspected, a skin scraping should be obtained and treated with 10% KOH and examined for the presence of fungal elements. Various fungal media are commercially available for the isolation and cultivation of the organisms and should include a medium with and without cycloheximide to inhibit fast-growing fungal isolates, as well as a medium with and without an antibacterial agent to suppress contaminating bacteria. Fungal cultures must be incubated at the optimal temperature for the suspect isolate, which is typically either 30°C or 37°C with sufficient humidity. Cultures may be retained for up to 21 days for some isolates before reporting the culture as negative. Limited serodiagnosis is available for a few select organisms, including *Cryptococcus, Blastomyces, Histoplasma,* and *Aspergillus.* Molecular methods are becoming more widespread in other areas of the laboratory, but none is accepted as a routine tool for the diagnosis of fungal infections.

BACTERIAL DISEASE

Diseases of a bacterial origin can be caused by gram-positive (Table 15.8) or gram-negative bacteria (Table 15.9). Another major grouping of bacterial diseases is associated with the oxygen requirements (anaerobic) of bacteria (Table 15.10).

Antimicrobial Susceptibility Tests

An important function of the medical microbiology laboratory is to test the isolated organisms for susceptibility to antimicrobial agents. The laboratory report showing susceptibility or resistance to a particular antibiotic largely determines whether the agent is used or withdrawn. In choosing an appropriate antimicrobial agent, the one with the most activity against the pathogen, the least toxicity to the host, the least effect on the normal flora, and the appropriate pharmacologic considerations, in addition to being the least expensive, should be selected to attain an effective outcome and treatment of the patient.

In doing tests for antimicrobial susceptibility, the laboratory must maintain a high level of accuracy in the testing procedures, results must have a high degree of reproducibility, and good correlation must exist between the results and the patient's clinical response.

TABLE 15.8 Summary of Gram-Positive Pathogenic Bacteria

Microorganism	Associated Sites of Infection or Disease
Aerobic, Gram-Positive Cocci	
Staphylococcus aureus	Skin and soft tissue wounds, skin (bullous impetigo), bacteremia, food poisoning, toxic shock syndrome
Staphylococcus saprophyticus	Urinary tract infections in young women
Staphylococcus lugdunensis	Heart (endocarditis), septicemia, meningitis, ski and soft tissue infections, urinary tract infections, septic shock
Staphylococcus warneri, Staphylococcus capitis, Staphylococcus simulans, Staphylococcus hominis, and *Staphylococcus schleiferi*	Septicemia, wound infections
Staphylococcus haemolyticus	Wounds, bacteremia, endocarditis, urinary tract infections
Methicillin-resistant *S. aureus* (MRSA)	Invasive abscesses, boils
Vancomycin-intermediate *S. aureus* (VISA)	In-dwelling catheters, peripheral vascular disease, persistent foot ulcers
Vancomycin-resistant *S. aureus* (VRSA)	
Micrococcus	In-dwelling catheters, knee aspiration, urinary tract infection in young women
Streptococcus pyogenes (Group A)	Throat (pharyngitis), skin and soft tissue infections
S. pyogenes (Group B)	In infants, fever, lethargy and difficulty breathing. In adults with chronic diseases, urinary tract infections, bloodstream (bacteremia), or lungs (pneumonia)
Streptococcus agalactiae	Neonatal bacteremia and meningitis
Streptococcus gallolyticus (formerly *Streptococcus bovis*)	Heart (endocarditis), urinary tract infections, (rarely) bloodstream (septicemia) and neonatal brain-covering meninges (meningitis)
Streptococcus pneumonia	Lungs (community-acquired pneumonia), brain-covering meninges (meningitis)
Enterococcus faecalis	Nosocomial urinary tract infections and bloodstream (bacteremia)
Enterococcus faecium	Nosocomial urinary tract infections and bloodstream (bacteremia)
Aerobic, Gram-Positive Bacilli	
Bacillus anthracis	Skin and soft tissue infections, pneumonia, bioterrorism agent
Bacillus cereus	Toxins can cause two types of illness: one type characterized by diarrhea and the other, called emetic toxin, by nausea and vomiting Eye infections
Bacillus spp.	Localized infections related to trauma (e.g., ocular infections), deep-seated soft tissue infections, and systemic infections (e.g., meningitis, endocarditis, osteomyelitis, and bacteremia)
Corynebacterium diphtheria	Diptheria[a]
Gardnerella vaginalis	Vaginitis
Lactobacillus	Blood (bacteremia)
Listeria monocytogenes	Meningitis, bacteremia
Nocardia sp.	Subcutaneous tissues, pneumonia
Aerobic, Gram-Negative Cocci	
Neisseria meningitidis	Meningitis
Neisseria gonorrhoeae	Gonorrhea
Moraxella catarrhalis	Upper respiratory tract

[a]Rare in the United States.

Susceptibility and Resistance

Antimicrobial susceptibility testing is performed on isolates from patients when clinically appropriate. A result of *susceptible* indicates that the patient most likely will respond to treatment with the antimicrobial agent. A result of *resistant* indicates that treatment with the agent will most likely fail. Each isolate is tested against a battery of antimicrobial agents when appropriate. An intermediate result can mean that a high dose (if possible with the agent) may be necessary for a successful treatment outcome.

Patterns of susceptibility and resistance are constantly changing. A number of drug-resistant organisms, including Enterobacteriaceae, *Campylobacter,* and *Candida,* show continually increasing levels of resistance. Some organisms are even resistant or becoming resistant to virtually all antibiotics, such as carbapenem-resistant Enterobacteriaceae (CRE) and multidrug-resistant *Acinetobacter.*

TABLE 15.9 Summary of Gram-Negative Pathogenic Bacteria

Microorganism	Associated Sites of Infection or Disease
Fastidious Gram Negative Coccobacillary	
Bordetella spp.	Respiratory system (whooping cough)
Brucella spp.	Ingestion of unpasteurized products, inhalation, wounds in skin/mucous membranes (brucellosis)
Francisella tularensis	Tick and deer fly bites, skin contact with infected animals, ingestion of contaminated water, inhalation of contaminated aerosols or agricultural dusts, laboratory exposure (tularemia)
Haemophilus influenza (serotypes B and non-B)	Respiratory system (flu)
H. influenza *Biovar aegyptius*	Respiratory system (flu)
Haemophilus spp.	Respiratory system (flu)
Legionella pneumophilia	Respiratory system (pneumonia)
Pasteurella multocida	Infected animal bite, scratch, or lick, but infection without epidemiologic evidence of animal contact may occur
Enterobacteriaceae	
Citrobacter spp.	A wide spectrum of infections in humans, such as infections in the urinary tract (most common), respiratory tract, wounds, bone, peritoneum, endocardium, meninges, bloodstream, and skin/soft tissues (including surgical site infection). Neonates, who may develop sepsis and meningitis (usually less than 2 months of age) and have a propensity for development of brain abscesses. *C. koseri* can cause an unusually severe form of neonatal meningitis, associated with necrotizing encephalitis and brain abscesses. Other high-risk groups are patients aged ≥ 65 years and immunocompromised patients.
Enterobacter aerogenes Enterobacter cloacae	Bacteremia, lower respiratory tract infections, skin and soft tissue infections, urinary tract infections (UTIs), endocarditis, intra-abdominal infections, septic arthritis, osteomyelitis, central nervous system (CNS) infections, and ophthalmic infections.
Escherichia coli	UTIs, diarrhea, bacteremia
E. coli (enterohemorrhagic *E. coli* due to Shiga toxin)	Subset of pathogenic *E. coli* that can cause diarrhea or hemorrhagic colitis in humans
E. coli (other diarrheagenic *E. coli*)	Watery or bloody diarrhea, abdominal cramps, with or without fever
Klebsiella pneumonia	UTIs, pneumonia, bacteremia
Klebsiella oxytoca	UTIs, pneumonia, bacteremia
Morganella morganii	Urinary tract, skin and soft tissue, hepatobiliary tract
Proteus mirabilis	UTIs
Proteus vulgaris	UTIs
Providencia species	Common cause of catheter-associated urinary tract infections, especially in the elderly with long-term indwelling urinary catheters, bacteremia
Salmonella species (*Salmonella enteric biovar typhi*)	Diarrhea, typhoid fever
Shigella species	Diarrhea
Serratia species	Nosocomial pneumonia
Yersinia enterocolitica	Enterocolitis, terminal ileitis, adenitis
Glucose Non-Fermenting Gram-Negative Rods	
Moraxella species	Acute otitis media (in children older than 3 months old), chronic and serious otitis media (fever, acute ear pain, irritability, and can escalate to sepsis and CNS infection), acute and chronic sinusitis (occasional fever, nasal or postnasal discharge, cough, sinus pain, and headache), upper and lower respiratory tract infections and sometimes systemic infections, meningitis, bacteremia, endocarditis, keratitis, arthritis
Pseudomonas aeruginosa	UTIs
Stenotrophomonas maltophilia	Occurs in a range of organs and tissues; commonly found in respiratory tract infections
Other Gram-Negative Bacilli	
Acinetobacter baumannii	Bacteremia, pneumonia/ventilator-associated pneumonia (VAP), meningitis, UTI, central venous catheter–related infection, and wound infection
Aeromonas species	Gastroenteritis, soft tissue and muscle infections, septicemia, skin diseases
Burkholderia cepacia	An important pathogen of pulmonary infections in people with cystic fibrosis (CF). Other pathogenic members include *Burkholderia mallei,* responsible for glanders disease (mostly in animals) and *Burkholderia pseudomallei,* the causative agent of melioidosis.

Continued

TABLE 15.9 Summary of Gram-Negative Pathogenic Bacteria—cont'd

Campylobacter jejuni	Gastrointestinal system, ranging from loose stools to dysentery)
Vibrio cholera	Gastrointestinal system, dysentery
HACEK[a] and Other Fastidious Gram-Negative Rods	
Aggregatibacter aphrophilus	Heart (infective endocarditis)
Aggregatibacter actinomycetemcomitans	Heart (infective endocarditis)
Cardiobacterium hominis	Heart (infective endocarditis)
Eikenella corrodens	Heart (infective endocarditis)

[a]*HACEK, Haemophilus* spp. (influenza, parainfluenzae, *Aggregatibacter* (*Hemophilus* spp.) *aphrophilus* (most commonly), *Aggregatibacter (Actinobacillus) actinomycetemcomitans, Cardiobacterium hominis, Eikenella corrodens,* and *Kingella* spp.

TABLE 15.10 Summary of Gram-Positive and Gram-Negative Anaerobic Pathogenic Bacteria

Anaerobic, Spore-Forming, or Non–Spore-Forming Gram-Positive Bacilli	
Bacteroides fragilis	Intraabdominal infections, abscesses
Clostridium perfringens	Soft tissue infections, food poisoning
Clostridium tetani	Tetanus
Clostridium difficile	Antibiotic-associated diarrhea
Actinomyces israelii[a]	Chronic localized or hematogenous anaerobic infection—actinomycosis
Propionibacterium acnes[a]	Acne, chronic blepharitis, endophthalmitis
Anaerobic Gram-Positive Cocci	
Peptostreptococcus sp.	Can occur in all body sites, including the central nervous system (CNS), head, neck, chest, abdomen, pelvis, skin, bone, joint, and soft tissues
Anaerobic Gram-Negative Rods and Cocci	
Bacteroides fragilis group	Polymicrobial infections such as intra-abdominal, obstetric-gynecologic, diabetic foot and skin, and skin structure infections; bacteremia
Bacteroides spp.	Abscess formation; polymicrobial infections involving the abdomen and pelvis, perirectal, skin and soft tissue, and solid organs; chronic sinusitis; chronic otitis media; dental infection; peritonsillar abscess; cervical adenitis; retropharyngeal space infection; aspiration pneumonia; lung abscess; pleural empyema; necrotizing pneumonia
Fusobacterium spp.	Infections may occur after surgical or accidental trauma, edema, anoxia, tissue destruction, and animal bites
Prevotella spp.	Chronic sinusitis, chronic otitis media, dental infection, peritonsillar abscess, cervical adenitis, retropharyngeal space infection, aspiration pneumonia, lung abscess, pleural empyema, necrotizing pneumonia
Veillonella spp.	Rarely implicated in cases of osteomyelitis and endocarditis

[a]Non–spore-forming bacilli.

Minimum Inhibitory Concentration and Minimum Bactericidal Concentration

The lowest concentration of an antimicrobial agent that will visibly inhibit the growth of the organism being tested is known as the *minimal inhibitory concentration (MIC).* This is detected by the lack of visual turbidity, matching that of a negative control included with the test. Many factors must be considered in choosing the specific antimicrobial agent; the MIC is one important consideration. MIC is determined by dilution antimicrobial susceptibility testing methods.

The ability of an antimicrobial agent to inhibit the multiplication of an organism is measured by the MIC. Because MIC is a measure of an organism's inhibitory status, when the antimicrobial agent is removed, the organism could begin to grow again. In this case the antimicrobial agent is called *bacteriostatic.* For certain infections, it may be necessary to determine the ability of the agent to kill the organism, or whether it is bactericidal. To determine this ability, a bactericidal activity test can be performed using a modification of the broth dilution susceptibility testing method; a **minimal bactericidal concentration (MBC)** is thus determined. The MBC results in a 99.9% reduction in the bacterial population.

Methods for Determination of Antimicrobial Susceptibility

Susceptibility and resistance are functions of the site of the infection, the microorganism itself, and the antimicrobial agent being considered. In other words, if the antimicrobial treatment is to be successful, the agent must be at the correct concentration at the infection site, and the organism must be susceptible to the agent. By using a standard method, the microbiology laboratory can produce consistent results to aid the physician in the therapeutic choice.

Two principal methods are employed to determine antimicrobial susceptibility: agar disk diffusion, or Kirby–Bauer method, employing antibiotic-impregnated disks; and dilution testing. Most microbiology laboratories use automated instrument methods and perform the disk diffusion when questions arise about automated-format results. The disk diffusion method is also used for some organisms that have fastidious requirements, with media modifications to accommodate their fastidious nature. An example is *S. pneumoniae,* which has become increasingly resistant. *S. pneumoniae* must be tested by disk diffusion with Mueller–Hinton (MH) or tryptic soy agar plus 5% v/v sheep blood and incubated with CO_2 for this organism to grow.

Each hospital laboratory, with the infectious disease department and pharmacy, must determine which of the many antimicrobial agents are appropriate for testing against the various organisms. The number of antimicrobials being tested against a single isolated organism usually is limited by the particular method being used. Disk diffusion plates (with 150 mm of agar) can usually accommodate 12 disks, whereas some of the commercially available panels can test more drugs on the same panel.

It is important to remember that any in vitro test (artificial environment in the laboratory) for antimicrobial susceptibility is an artificial measurement and provides an estimate of the effectiveness of an agent against a microorganism in vivo (conditions within the infected host). The only absolute test of antimicrobial susceptibility is the patient's clinical response to the dosage of the antibiotic.

The classic method for testing the susceptibility of microorganisms is the broth dilution method, yielding a quantitative result for the amount of antimicrobial agent needed to inhibit the growth of a specific microorganism, or the MIC. The CLSI has published the complete protocol for this method.[14] Laboratories have now adapted the broth-dilution methods to a microbroth method, which may be automated, because it saves time, is cost-effective, and promotes efficiency from replicate inoculation of the prepared systems being used.

The isolated organism being tested is first inoculated into a broth medium, whether a diffusion method or a macrodilution or microdilution method is used.

Preparation of Inoculum. The number of organisms in an inoculum can be determined in different ways. The standard method is to compare the turbidity of the test liquid medium with that of a standard that represents a known number of bacteria in suspension. Chemical solutions of standard turbidity have been prepared using barium sulfate. Tubes with varying concentrations of this chemical were developed by McFarland to approximate numbers of bacteria in solutions of equal turbidity, as determined by doing colony counts in a counting chamber[12] (see Disk Diffusion).

McFarland Standards. The standard used most frequently is the McFarland 0.5 standard, which contains 99.5 mL of 1% v/v sulfuric acid and 0.5 mL of 1.175% barium chloride to obtain a barium sulfate solution with a very specific optical density. This provides a turbidity comparable to that of a bacterial suspension containing approximately 1.5×10^8 CFU/mL.

Microdilution Method. The microdilution method uses plastic microdilution trays or panels and is used in many laboratories to give MIC results as part of the routine protocol for microbiology laboratory tests. This method permits a quantitative result to be reported (the MIC), indicating the amount of a drug needed to inhibit the microorganism being tested. Most laboratories purchase the microdilution panels commercially; the prepared wells each hold a small amount of the various concentrations of the antimicrobial agents being tested, with the necessary controls supplied for growth and sterility tests. These panels have been prepared under strict QC standards, which assure the laboratory of consistent performance when they are used according to the manufacturer's directions. Usually, various panels containing different drug combinations are available for testing groups of organisms.

Various automated systems are available that not only provide an identification biochemical reaction card but also include an antibiotic susceptibility reaction card or cassette. The Vitek System (bioMérieux) contains the antimicrobial agents in wells in a plastic card. The system includes a filler/sealer module, a reader incubator, a computer module, a data terminal, and a printer. The cards are incubated, and the wells are monitored for optical density. Results can be obtained in 6 to 8 hours for antimicrobial susceptibility testing. The Vitek System can be combined with identification testing, further simplifying the amount of work in a busy laboratory. Another automated system is the MicroScan Walkaway System (Siemens, Washington, DC). This system uses a broth microdilution format. The inoculation is manual; a multipronged device delivers diluted organism to each well of a microdilution tray. This tray is incubated, and susceptibility results are available in 3.5 to 5.5 hours. As with the Vitek System, MicroScan also offers identification testing in conjunction with susceptibility testing.

Disk Diffusion (Kirby–Bauer Method). Methods using disks impregnated with various antimicrobial agents and placed on an agar culture plate inoculated with the organism to be tested were used extensively before the advent of microdilution methodology.

For this test, the standardized inoculum is prepared as described and is swabbed over the surface of the agar plate. Paper disks containing a single concentration of the chosen antimicrobial agent are placed onto the inoculated surface, and the plate is incubated for 16 to 18 hours. The antimicrobial agent on the disk diffuses into the medium in a gradient extending from the disk in a circle, inhibiting the growth of the organism wherever the concentration of the agent is sufficient. Large zones of inhibition are an indication of more antimicrobial activity (Fig. 15.26). An area in which there is no zone indicates complete resistance to the drug. This test is also known as the *Kirby–Bauer method.*

With the disk diffusion method, several drugs can be tested against a single isolate at the same time. Bondi and colleagues[13]

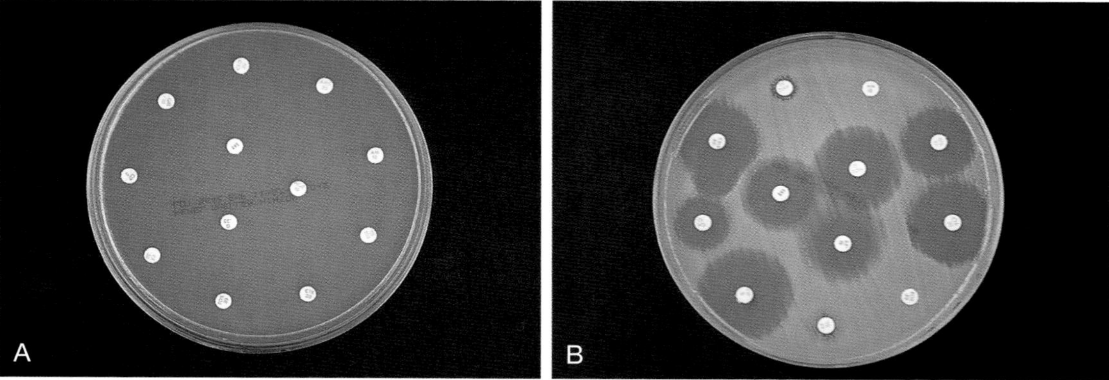

Fig. 15.26 Agar disk diffusion. (A) Mueller–Hinton agar has been inoculated with the test organism, and the antibiotic disks have been added to the media. No incubation has yet occurred. (B) After 16 to 18 hours of incubation, the zones of inhibition are apparent. The zones of inhibition are measured and compared to a table of values for each antibiotic. (From de la Maza LM, Pezzlo MT, Baron EJ: *Color atlas of diagnostic microbiology,* St Louis, 1997, Mosby.)

first described this method in 1947. In 1966, Bauer and associates[14] standardized the method and correlated it with MICs. They introduced standardized filter paper disks and enabled this method to yield qualitative results that correlated well with results obtained by MIC tests. The results can be correlated directly with MIC values, but clinical interpretation of this method depends on performing the test according to a standardized protocol.

Disks are commercially available for this method, and disk dispensers are used to distribute the appropriate disks on the inoculated plate. If there is a zone of inhibition around the disk containing the agent, the zone is measured with calipers and compared with the established breakpoints for susceptible, intermediate, or resistant. Much work has been done to standardize the disk procedure, and many laboratories use the Bauer modification.[14]

The disk diffusion test is more flexible than the commercially prepared microdilution panels, which are available in standard panels of antimicrobials. The disk diffusion method allows a laboratory to choose any number of appropriate antimicrobial agents; usually, 12 will fit on one plate. Because of this flexibility, it is also a cost-effective test.

The disk diffusion method is subject to CLSI requirements that cover disk concentrations, standardization of media, formula, pH, agar depth, inoculums density, temperature, zone sizes, interpretative tables, and reference strains of bacteria for controls.

Selection of Media for Plating. For antimicrobial susceptibility testing, MH agar plates are used. The plates should be stored in the refrigerator until used and should be checked periodically.

Handling and Storage of Antibiotic Disks. Disks for antimicrobial susceptibility testing are usually supplied in separate containers with a suitable desiccant to prevent deterioration. Most antimicrobial disks should be refrigerated until used, but some require freezing to maintain their potency. The manufacturer's instructions for storage and handling should be followed.

Preparation of Inoculum. A tube of trypticase soy broth (5 mL) is inoculated with a pure culture of the organism to be tested, using four or five isolated colonies of similar morphology, and is incubated at 35°C for 4 hours or until the culture is visibly cloudy. Most microbiologists use a second method in which colonies are picked from those grown overnight on nonselective media, suspended in broth or saline, and matched to the 0.5 McFarland standard.

The turbidity of the test organism is compared with that of a McFarland barium sulfate standard. The standard must be vigorously mixed before use. The turbidity of the broth culture may be adjusted by diluting with uninoculated broth. If the 4-hour broth tube does not have sufficient growth, it can be reincubated until adequate growth is observed.

The MH plates should be inoculated within 15 minutes of preparation of the inoculum.

Inoculation of Mueller–Hinton Agar Plate. A sterile swab is dipped into the standardized, well-mixed broth culture, and any excess fluid is removed from the swab by squeezing it on the side of the tube. The swab is streaked across the plate in three directions to ensure that the plate surface is covered with the inoculum. The disks should be applied within 15 minutes of inoculating the MH plate.

Application of Disks. The appropriate disks are applied to all the plates, using a disk dispenser if available. Each disk should be firmly pressed down onto the surface of the agar with flamed and cooled forceps to ensure complete contact with the agar. The disks should be distributed so that no two disks are closer than 24 mm from center to center. Once a disk has been placed, it should not be moved because diffusion of the antibiotic begins almost immediately. The plates are incubated at 35° C for 16 to 18 hours in ambient air.

Reading of Results. After incubation, the diameters of the zones of inhibition are measured with calipers or a zone reader and recorded to the nearest whole millimeter (see Fig. 15.26). Reading zone sizes can be visualized using reflective light and by placing the plates on a dark background. At times there may be a haze of growth produced by some bacteria, and transmitted light is better to read the zones of inhibition. Within the limitations of the test, the diameter of the inhibition zone is a measure of the relative susceptibility to a particular agent. The diameters are compared with a table of breakpoint values for each antimicrobial to see whether the organism is susceptible, intermediate, or resistant to that particular agent. These results are reported to the physician. The term *susceptible* implies that an infection caused by the strain tested may be expected to respond favorably to the particular antimicrobial agent. Resistant strains, on the other hand, are not inhibited by the usual therapeutic concentration of the antimicrobial agent.

QUALITY CONTROL IN THE MICROBIOLOGY LABORATORY

Control of Equipment

Equipment used in the microbiology laboratory can be easily controlled; for example, the temperatures of incubators, refrigerators, water baths, and freezers can be monitored daily. All monitoring data must be recorded as part of the laboratory's ongoing quality assurance program. Every laboratory handling biological material must have a biological safety cabinet for handling hazardous specimens and organisms.

Control of Media

Most media are purchased already prepared from commercial manufacturers. These media are generally of high quality and provide good batch-to-batch (lot-to-lot) consistency. Commercially prepared media must be stored and used in accordance with manufacturer's directions and must be used within the specified expiration dates. The QC measures used during the manufacture of commercial media should follow CLSI recommendations[8] (see Quality Control of Media). If the laboratory prepares the media, strict controls must be used in the preparation. The best way to control the quality of media is by performance testing: checking the media with cultures of known stock microorganisms. Control strains of bacteria are available commercially.

Control of Reagents and Antisera

Reagents should be tested daily (some tests not performed frequently can use controls during testing), using both positive and negative controls. New batches of reagents must also be tested in the same manner. Reagents should be dated when they are prepared, as with reagents in other areas of the laboratory. New reagents should be tested with known control cultures. Gram-staining reagents are examined during staining and reviewing of slides prepared with known suspensions of gram-negative and gram-positive organisms. In the same manner, acid-fast testing controls are prepared from acid-fast–positive and acid-fast–negative organisms.

Control of Antimicrobial Tests

Laboratories must periodically monitor their performance of methods used for antimicrobial testing, following CLSI recommendations.[12] Control organisms are specific strains of common organisms available for this purpose. These are maintained by subculturing daily to maintain organism viability. Typically, weekly QC is completed for disk diffusion and automated systems with known organisms that result in specific ranges of zones of inhibition or MICs, respectively.

Control of Specimens, Specimen Collection, and Specimen Rejection

If proper protocols and procedures are not in place regarding the collection of patient specimens and the procedures for handling these specimens in the laboratory, the identification of pathogens is not very useful, and quality assurance is not being practiced. Strict adherence to proper procedures for sample collection must be enforced and repeat collections made if the circumstances demand it.

If specimens are not collected appropriately (according to a standardized protocol), they should be rejected as unacceptable. If a new specimen cannot be collected, the person may request to process the original specimen. In this case, a statement should be included with the result regarding the inappropriate condition of the specimen. Specimens are rejected because of improper labeling or improper transport, transport medium, or transport temperature, as well as leaking containers. Sputum specimens are assessed for quality by Gram staining and viewing under low power for squamous epithelial cells. The presence of more than 10 cells per low-power field is evidence of contamination with saliva.[7]

MYCOBACTERIA

Mycobacteria is a family of *Actinobacteria,* a genus comprising more than 120 different species. They are acid-fast gram-positive bacilli that are obligate aerobic microorganisms. There are three main groups: *Mycobacterial tuberculosis* complex, *Mycobacterial leprae,* and nontuberculosis *Mycobacteria.* The mycobacterial diseases include tuberculosis, leprosy, *Mycobacteria* ulcer, and *Mycobacterium paratuberculosis.* Several species of *Mycobacteria* can cause disease in animals.

Laboratory Studies

Sputum species are the most common type of specimen for examination in the clinical laboratory.

Löwenstein–Jensen Medium

Löwenstein–Jensen (LJ) medium is used to cultivate and isolate *Mycobacterium* spp. It is an egg-based medium containing whole eggs, potato flour, and glycerol to support the growth of mycobacteria, typically within 18 to 24 days. The presence of malachite green in the medium inhibits the growth of other bacteria that may be present in the specimen. Specimens are inoculated onto LJ medium and incubated at 35°C with 5% to 10% CO_2 and high humidity, then observed weekly for 8 weeks. Alternate media used to cultivate *Mycobacterium* spp. include Middlebrook 7H10 and 7H11. Middlebrook media are agar based and result in growth in 10 to 12 days. Strains resistant to isoniazid (antimycobacterial agent) demonstrate improved growth on these media. Additional media formularies are available for use in semiautomated and fully automated systems for the growth of *Mycobacterium* spp.

Acid-Fast Stain

The acid-fast stain is used mainly to detect organisms that cause tuberculosis. Because of the possible aerosolization of these organisms, it is important to handle the specimens carefully, using a biological safety cabinet. These organisms would appear as partially staining, beaded gram-positive organisms in a routine Gram stain. Acid-fast staining organisms retain the primary dye, and decolorization is difficult, even with an acid–alcohol solution—thus the term **acid-fast bacteria (AFB)**. The acid-alcohol reagent decolorizes bacteria that do not have cell walls containing mycolic acid; AFB will be counterstained with a secondary color. The AFB (containing mycolic acid) will not decolorize and appear the color of the primary stain.

Acid-Fast Stain Using Kinyoun Carbolfuchsin Method

The Ziehl–Neelsen acid-fast method uses carbolfuchsin as the primary stain, heat to facilitate penetration of the stain, a mixture of 3% hydrochloric acid and 95% ethanol as the decolorizer, and methylene blue as the counterstain.

Kinyoun acid-fast modification uses a slightly different carbolfuchsin preparation, phenol to facilitate penetration of the stain, and either methylene blue or malachite green as a counterstain (see Evolve procedure). The Kinyoun method is referred to as the "cold" method because heat is not required because of the absence of phenol in the method. After the first step of the acid-fast staining procedure, all bacteria present on the slide appear red. Following decolorization with an acid–alcohol reagent, the AFB appear red, and all other bacteria are colorless. After counterstaining with methylene blue, the AFB appear red, and all other cells appear blue (if malachite green is used, all other cells appear green).

Another method of staining AFB is by using fluorochrome stains. Fluorochromes are dyes that absorb ultraviolet light and emit light of higher wavelengths. The acid-fast staining method using the fluorochromes auramine and rhodamine is a rapid screening method for detection of *Mycobacterium* spp., including *Mycobacterium tuberculosis,* the causative agent of tuberculosis.

Fluorescent microscopes have filters that excite fluorochromes and detect the emitted light (see Chapter 5). This method is more sensitive than the Ziehl–Neelsen and Kinyoun methods because the AFB will fluoresce and appear as bright yellow-orange against a dark background. The slides can also be rapidly screened under a lower magnification. The fluorochrome method uses auramine and rhodamine as the primary stains. The decolorizer is acid–alcohol reagent, and the counterstain is potassium permanganate (see Evolve procedure).

TESTS FOR FUNGI (MYCOLOGY)

The study of fungi (yeasts and molds) is called *mycology* and is carried out in the medical microbiology laboratory. If a laboratory processes mycology specimens and does not perform identification testing of fungi, the cultures can be referred to a reference laboratory.

Many immunosuppressed or otherwise compromised patients, such as those with human immunodeficiency virus (HIV), acquired immune deficiency syndrome (AIDS), or cancer, live longer lives with appropriate treatment. Transplantation (solid organ or bone marrow) requires immunosuppression, and great strides have been made in these areas to obtain successful patient outcomes. Opportunistic infections can occur in patients with diabetes mellitus or other chronic, debilitating diseases and in those with impaired immunologic function resulting from drug therapy with corticosteroids.

In recent years, more fungal infections have been identified in immunocompromised patients. When an organism is isolated in an immunocompromised patient, it must be considered a significant finding. Many fungi are considered opportunistic, causing disease under immune suppression. These infections can be difficult to treat because fungi are eukaryotic cells, having the same type of cell structure as mammalian cells and resulting in damage to the host while simultaneously destroying the infecting organism.

Genus-level and species-level identification of molds can be a very difficult procedure and is beyond the scope of this text. This section includes introductory information related to the collection of specimens, staining, media, general macroscopic and microscopic morphology, and common tests for yeast identification.

Characteristics of Fungi

Fungi differ significantly from bacteria and include both yeasts and molds. Fungi are eukaryotes, possessing a true nucleus with a nuclear membrane and mitochondria, whereas bacteria are prokaryotes, lacking these structures. In addition, fungal cell walls are not composed of peptidoglycan found in bacterial cell walls but contain alternate carbohydrates such as chitin. The fungi that are seen in the clinical laboratory, yeasts and molds, can be separated into the two groups based on the macroscopic appearance of the colonies formed.

Yeasts are single-celled organisms that reproduce by budding. Yeasts produce moist, opaque, creamy, or pasty colonies on Sabouraud media, whereas molds produce fluffy, cottony, woolly, or powdery colonies. All yeasts look similar microscopically and therefore need to be differentiated based on biochemical test results.

Molds have a basic structure that consists of tubelike filamentous projections called *hyphae.* Hyphae continue to grow, forming an intertwined mass collectively known as mycelia (singular *mycelium*). Vegetative hyphae make up the main body of the mold and are actively growing and feeding form of the mold. Aerial hyphae are extensions that rise above the main body and have reproductive structures (asexual spores) attached. These spores are not the same type of structure as bacterial endospores, which are not reproductive structures.

Some yeasts produce pseudohyphae, which are elongated buds that do not separate, similar to mycelia (Fig. 15.27). Pseudohyphae are constricted, unlike true hyphae, which have parallel walls and do not have constrictions. Types of mycelium can be recognized microscopically, which can assist in the early identification of molds. Molds have characteristic "fuzzy" or woolly appearance because of their mycelia.

Fungi as Source of Infection

Fungi normally live a nonpathogenic existence in nature, enriched by decaying nitrogenous material. Humans become

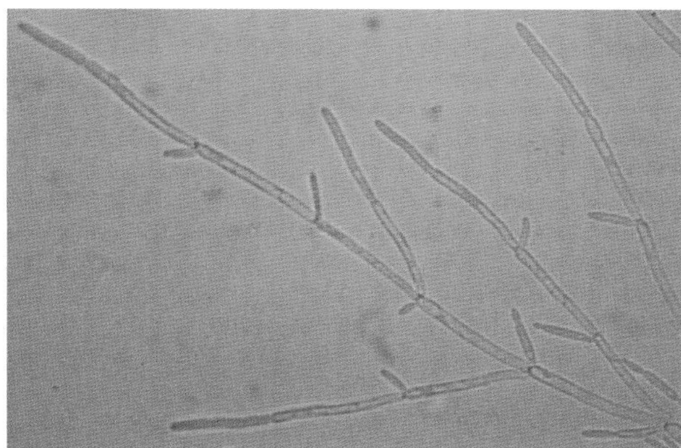

Fig. 15.27 Pseudohyphae consisting of elongated cells with constrictions at attachment sites. (From Mahon CR, Lehman DC, Manuselis G: *Textbook of diagnostic microbiology,* ed 5, Maryland Heights, Mo, 2015, Saunders, Fig 27-62, p 621.)

infected with fungi through accidental exposure by inhalation of spores or by their introduction into tissue through trauma. Any alteration in the immunologic status of the host can result in infection by fungi that are normally nonpathogenic; most yeast infections are opportunistic.

Candida species can be found on mucous membranes and skin without causing infection in healthy patients. The most frequently isolated yeast is *Candida albicans,* which can be part of the normal flora of the gastrointestinal tract in healthy individuals.

Candidiasis is a fungal infection caused by yeasts that belong to the genus *Candida.* There are over 20 species of *Candida* that can cause infection in humans, the most common of which is *C. albicans* (Table 15.11). Other types of fungi can also cause various infections in humans.

Other fungal infections (or mycoses) can be superficial, cutaneous, subcutaneous, or systemic (Table 15.12). A superficial mycosis is one confined to the outermost skin and hair layer, with symptoms of discoloration, scaling, or abnormal skin pigmentation. Cutaneous infections affect the keratinized layer of the skin, hair, or nails. Symptoms of these infections include itching, scaling, or ringlike patches (ringworm) of the skin; brittle or broken hairs; and thick, discolored nails. Subcutaneous infections affect the deeper layers of the skin, including muscle and connective tissue; these infections do not usually disseminate through the blood to other organs. Symptoms include ulcers that progress and do not heal and the presence of draining sinus tracts. *Systemic mycoses* affect the lungs and can disseminate to internal organs or the deep tissues of the body. The original site of these systemic infections is the lung, from which the organisms can disseminate through the bloodstream (hematogenous spread) to other sites in the body.

TABLE 15.11 Summary of Pathogenic Fungi—Yeasts

Microorganism	Sites of Infection or Disease
Candida albicans	Mouth and throat (thrush), vagina, or invasive in bloodstream
Candida auris	Bloodstream infections, wound infections, and ear infections. Several countries report severe illness in hospitalized patients. This yeast is often resistant to multiple antifungal drugs.
Cryptococcus neoformans	Oral, vaginal, pneumonia-like cryptococcal meningitis, coccidiomycosis
Cryptococcus gattii	Lungs and/or nervous system

TABLE 15.12 Summary of Pathogenic Fungi

Microorganism	Sites of Infection or Disease
Microsporum spp.	Lungs, inhalation of spores
Trichophyton spp.	Dermal infections (skin, hair, and nail diseases)
Epidermophyton floccosum	*E. floccosum* has keratinase that gives it the ability to break down keratin, a protein commonly found within the skin, nails, and hair. It is the only pathogenic species that is found worldwide, and its primary reservoir is humans. *E. floccosum* causes ringworm—tinea pedis, tinea cruris, tinea corporis, and onychomycosis (ringworm of the nail). It is spread by direct contact with the fungus where people share inanimate objects.
Zygomycetes	
Rhizopus spp.	Skin, paranasal sinuses, lungs, gastrointestinal system, subcutaneous, central nervous system, a systemic zygomycosis (mucormycosis)
Mucor spp.	Most *Mucor* species do not infect humans and warm-blooded animals because of their inability to grow in warm environments near 37°C. Thermotolerant species (e.g., *Mucor indicus*) sometimes cause opportunistic infections known as zygomycosis. Zygomycosis includes infections in mucous membranes, nasal passages and sinuses, eyes, lungs, skin, and brain, as well as renal and pulmonary infections and septic arthritis.
Lichtheimia spp.	Lungs, central nervous system, rhinocerebral, or cutaneous types of infection in animals and humans with impaired immunity
Opportunistic Molds/Septate Hyaline Molds	
Aspergillus (*Aspergillus fumigates, Aspergillus flavus, Aspergillus niger*)	Lungs (pulmonary), disseminated to visceral organs, brain, kidney, heart, bone, gastrointestinal tract, or eyes; also, paranasal sinuses and skin; immunocompromised patients due to AIDS, cancer, posttransplant chemotherapy, and antibiotics or immunosuppressant drugs
Penicillium	*Penicillium* species other than *Penicillium marneffei* are commonly considered as contaminants, but they are known to produce mycotoxins. For example, *Penicillium verrucosum* produces a mycotoxin, ochratoxin A, that is damaging to the kidney (nephrotoxic) and could be cancer causing (carcinogenic).
Fusarium spp.	*Mycotoxicosis* is the term used for poisoning associated with exposures to mycotoxins by ingestion, skin contact, or inhalation.
Other Fungi	
Pneumocystis jiroveci	Lungs (pneumonia) in immunocompromised patients

Infiltrates may be seen in the pulmonary system on x-ray films. Symptoms can be very general, such as fever and fatigue; other symptoms include a chronic cough and chest pain.

Collection of Specimens for Fungal Studies

Any tissue or body fluid can be cultured for fungi, and swabs are the least desirable specimen for culturing fungi. Other specimens collected for the identification of fungi include hair, skin, nails and nail scrapings, urine, blood or bone marrow, tissue, other ordinarily sterile body fluids, and CSF. Fungemia, or fungi in the bloodstream, is most often caused by *C. albicans*.

It is extremely important that specimens be appropriately collected from the proper site so that the fungi are recovered. It is also important that a specimen for fungal studies be transported to the laboratory as quickly as possible. Because many pathogenic fungi grow slowly, any delay in transporting or processing a specimen can compromise the quality of the specimen and the eventual prospects of isolating the causative organism.

Methods for Detection of Fungi

Because of the increase in the number of fungal infections, primarily in immunocompromised patients, there is an increased need for the detection of these infecting organisms for effective treatment and care of patients.

On receipt in the laboratory, specimens for fungal identification should be directly examined microscopically and cultured immediately to ensure the recovery of the suspected fungal organism from the specimen.

Direct Microscopic Examination of Fungi

Examination of the specimen microscopically is an important part of the microbiology laboratory's fungal identification process. It provides a rapid method, which in some cases leads to an immediate tentative diagnosis and result in the initiation of treatment. Direct microscopic examination in conjunction with several stains can be used for initial identification. Direct examination can also show specific morphologic characteristics and present a rationale for inoculation of required media. Initially, fungi are often visible in the routine Gram stain, but other direct stains or procedures can give more specific information regarding the identity of the infecting organism.

Gram Stain. A Gram stain typically is used for most clinical microbiological specimens. The Gram stain will detect most fungi, if present in the specimen (see Smear Preparation and Stains Used in Microbiology). Yeast will appear purple or blue/black and will often demonstrate budding cells or pseudohyphae when examined microscopically using the high-power (100 × magnification) oil-immersion objective (Fig. 15.28).

Potassium Hydroxide Preparation. KOH preparation is recommended for detecting fungal elements in the skin, hair, nails, and tissue. Addition of a 10% solution of KOH reagent clears the specimen, making the fungi easily visible. On a glass slide, a drop of the specimen is mixed with a drop of 10% KOH, a coverslip is applied, and the slide is scanned for fungal elements using the low-power objective. Any fungi present will be visible. The KOH reagent dissolves the keratin and cellular material in the specimen, releasing the fungal elements for visualization. If the specimen is extremely viscous, overnight incubation of the wet-mounted slide in a humidified chamber may be necessary. If the slide appears cloudy, warming may help to clear the slide in order to visualize the fungi.

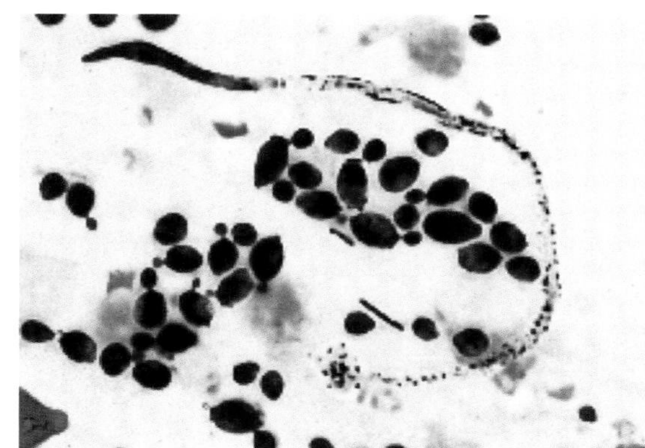

Fig. 15.28 Gram stain of yeast. Note: Yeast are not classified as gram positive because of absorption of Gentian Violet stain. (From Tille PM: Bailey *and Scott's diagnostic microbiology*, ed 14, St Louis, 2017, Mosby.)

Potassium Hydroxide with Calcofluor White. Calcofluor white, a fluorescent dye, can be mixed with KOH; a drop is mixed with the specimen on the glass slide, a coverslip applied, and a fluorescence microscope used for observation. Use of this preparation detects the presence of fungi (in 1 minute) by visualization of a bright apple-green or blue-white fluorescence, depending on the filters used in the microscope. The calcofluor white binds to cell walls of fungi. This method requires a fluorescence microscope, but fungi exhibit an intense, easily recognizable fluorescence with this type of microscopy.

India Ink. A drop of India ink may be added to a drop of CSF sediment from the centrifuged specimen and the specimen examined under high-power magnification. This is a negative staining method, whereby the budding yeast *C. neoformans* can be visualized surrounded by a large clear area against a black background and is presumptive evidence of infection with *C. neoformans* (Fig. 15.29). This clear area is caused by the capsule

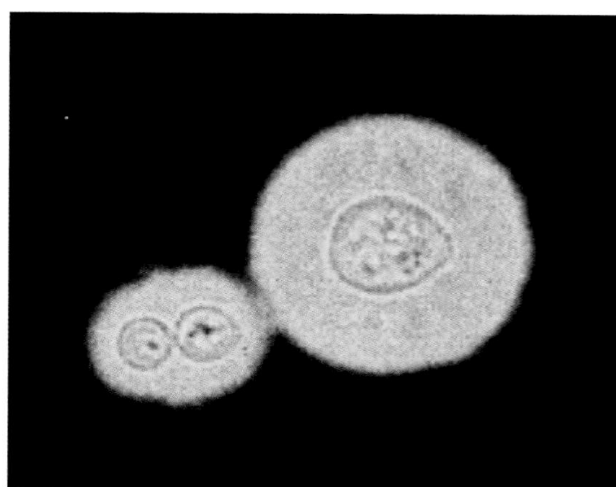

Fig. 15.29 India ink stain of *Cryptococcus neoformans*. (From Tille PM: Bailey *and Scott's diagnostic microbiology*, ed 14, St Louis, 2017, Mosby.)

that surrounds the yeast and is referred to as a *halo*. The India ink stain is a rapid test for *C. neoformans*, but the cryptococcal antigen test on CSF is more sensitive.

Acid-Fast Stain. The acid-fast stain used to detect mycobacteria but can also detect *Nocardia*. In mycology, the acid-fast stain is primarily used to differentiate *Nocardia* spp. from other actinomycetes. *Nocardia* spp. are gram-positive bacilli that appear as branching filamentous forms. They cause mycetomas (infection of subcutaneous tissues) and pulmonary infections. The subcutaneous infections resemble fungal infections of the same type.

Culture of Fungi

Specimens to be cultured for fungi should be inoculated on a general-purpose medium with and without cycloheximide (see next section). Mold cultures should be handled in a class II biological safety cabinet to prevent aerosol dissemination of fungal elements. Yeast cultures can be handled on a regular laboratory benchtop with no extra protection other than Standard Precautions. Laboratories will differ in the protocols used and the media required for fungal culture. Usually, a medium with and without cycloheximide can be used, with the addition of a blood-enriched medium.

Culture Media. Two general types of culture media are essential to ensure the primary recovery of all clinically significant fungi from clinical specimens: a nonselective media and a selective media.

The best-known medium is Sabouraud agar (SAB). This agar is sufficient for the recovery of dermatophytes from cutaneous specimens and yeasts from vaginal cultures. However, it is not recommended as a primary isolation medium because it is insufficiently rich to recover certain fastidious pathogenic species, particularly most of the dimorphic fungi.

Sabouraud's heart infusion (SABHI) agar can be used for primary recovery of saprophytic and dimorphic fungi, particularly fastidious strains. Agar with a combination of SAB and BHI agar, called SABHI, has proven to be useful for the isolation of clinically significant fungi.

Sabouraud's dextrose agar (2%) is most useful as a medium for the subculture of fungi recovered on enriched medium to enhance typical sporulation and provide the more characteristic colony morphology.

Most specimens for fungal identification are also contaminated with bacteria and other rapidly growing fungi, and it is important that antibacterial and antifungal agents be included in the culture medium. Some fungi are also sensitive to the presence of these antibiotics, and it is recommended that one SAB without antibiotics be inoculated simultaneously with a SAB containing antibiotics.

Addition of the antimicrobial agents cycloheximide to inhibit nonpathogenic or saprophytic fungi and chloramphenicol to inhibit bacterial growth is recommended. Mycosel/Mycobiotic agar is generally Sabouraud's dextrose agar with cycloheximide and chloramphenicol added. It is used for the primary recovery of dermatophytes.

Other types of media with specific objectives include the following:

- Brain–heart infusion (BHI) agar is a nonselective fungal culture medium that permits the growth of virtually all clinically relevant fungi. It is used for the primary recovery of saprophytic and dimorphic fungi.
- Czapek's agar is used for the subculture of *Aspergillus* species for their differential diagnosis.
- Dermatophyte test medium (DTM) is a specialized agar used in medical mycology. It is based on Sabouraud's dextrose agar with added cycloheximide to inhibit saprotrophic growth; antibiotic to inhibit bacterial growth; and phenol red, a pH indicator.
- Inhibitory mold agar (IMA) is used for primary recovery of dimorphic pathogenic fungi. Saprophytic fungi and dermatophytes will not be recovered.
- Niger seed agar is used for the identification of *C. neoformans.*
- Potato dextrose agar (PDA) is a relatively rich medium for growing a wide range of fungi.
- Potato flake agar is used for primary recovery of saprophytic and dimorphic fungi, particularly fastidious and slow-growing strains.

Examination of the Culture

Fungal cultures are incubated at 30°C for 4 to 6 weeks and examined weekly or twice weekly for growth before being reported as negative. Characteristic gross culture growth and microscopic features are observed to determine whether the isolate is a mold or yeast. Gross features, such as colony color, texture, and growth rate, are standard observations that lead to the identification of the fungus.

Agar plates are recommended because they provide improved aeration, but many laboratories use screw-capped agar tubes to minimize aerosolization of fungal spores, reducing the risk of exposure to laboratory personnel.

Microscopic Examination of Isolated Microorganism. Once the organism has been isolated, a direct mount is examined microscopically. Identification of yeasts requires that specific microscopic features be present, as well as the use of biochemical tests to confirm the species identification. Identification of molds also requires that specific microscopic morphologic features be present (see Characteristics of Fungi).

Yeasts are unicellular microorganisms that reproduce asexually by budding; the appearance of the colony is a collection of distinct, individual organisms that resemble the appearance of bacterial colonies on the agar surface. On culture media, *C. albicans* colonies appear heaped and dull. Some yeast may have pseudohyphae, which project from the edges of the colony as filamentous extensions. In contrast, molds are filamentous fungi with tubelike filamentous projections or hyphae. Hyphae continue to grow, forming an intertwined mass (mycelia). Different types of hyphae, reproductive structures, and colonial morphology can be examined to identify the various types of molds. Identification can be difficult, and laboratories that perform identification of molds have experienced staff to accomplish this task.

Germ-Tube Test. The germ-tube test is a simple, rapid test used to identify *C. albicans*. This test is based on the ability of

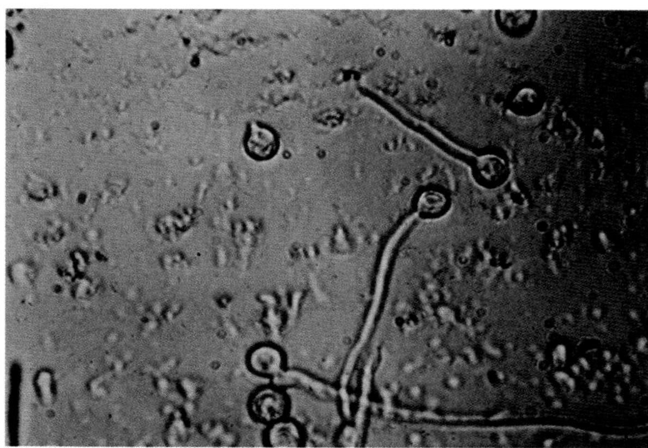

Fig. 15.30 Germ tube test. Germ tubes are true hyphae that are produced by *Candida albicans*. A positive germ tube has no constriction at its base (unstained, ×1000). (From Mahon CR, Lehman DC, Manuselis G: Textbook of diagnostic microbiology, ed 5, Maryland Heights, Mo, 2015, Saunders, Fig 27-59, p 620.)

C. albicans to produce germ tubes from their yeast cells when placed in 0.5 mL of sheep or rabbit serum and incubated at 35°C for no longer than 3 hours. It is important that the incubation time be limited to 3 hours because other species will begin to form structures resembling germ tubes with prolonged incubation. After incubation, a small amount of the serum is placed on a microscope slide, a coverslip is applied, and the specimen is examined under low-power magnification. A *germ tube* is a hyphalike extension of the yeast cell without having any constrictions at the point where the extension originates.[12] Germ tubes are the beginnings of true hyphae (Fig. 15.30).

Biochemical Screening Methods

Biochemical tests are necessary for yeast identification, but microscopic confirmation is also important. For rapid testing of yeasts, the germ tube (positive test: *C. albicans*) and urea agar (positive test: *C. neoformans*) are typically used (see Culture Media). Commercially available yeast identification systems are used in many laboratories, in conjunction with the morphology of yeast on cornmeal agar with Tween 80. These methods are usually rapid, and the results are available within 72 hours. These systems use a large database of information based on thousands of yeast biotypes and consider a number of variations and reaction patterns. One method uses a number of biochemical tests, monitoring reactions through various indicator systems after adding a reagent to certain substrates. This system is designed to provide identification within 4 hours. Some systems take longer for the final identification process. In general, these commercial identification systems are easy to use and interpret.

TESTS FOR PARASITES (PARASITOLOGY)

Human parasitic infections can be caused by a variety of parasites. These infections occur worldwide, although these problems arise more often in tropical areas. Parasites live in or on their hosts, at the expense of the host. Some parasites cannot survive without their designated host. Other parasites can exist in a free-living state as an intermediate state before transmission to a suitable host. Still others live commensally, a situation in which the parasite and the host exist together with no harm coming to the host; the relationship is beneficial to both. Many of the diseases diagnosed in parasitology (study of parasites) are serious infections and have a negative effect on the host.

Parasites as Source of Infection

As a result of increased travel to tropical areas, and because of the great influx of refugee populations, many organisms endemic elsewhere are being identified in patients in the United States. In addition, the increasing number of compromised patients poses a greater risk for certain parasitic infections (Table 15.13).

TABLE 15.13 Examples of Human-Disease–Causing Parasites

Category	Associated Disease
Blood and tissue protozoa *Plasmodium* spp. *Trypanosoma cruzi* *Trypanosoma brucei*	• Malaria • Chagas disease • African sleeping sickness
Intestinal and urogenital protozoa *Cryptosporidium* *Entamoeba histolytica* *Giardia* *Trichomonas vaginalis*	Diarrheal disease (cryptosporidiosis), dysentery, and invasive extraintestinal amebiasis (amebic liver abscess most common). *E. histolytica* is the only amebic species capable of invading tissues and causing disease. Intestinal infection with bouts of watery diarrhea (giardiasis—one of the most common causes of waterborne disease in the United States). Trichomoniasis—a sexually transmitted disease of the vagina.
Intestinal and tissue helminths Intestinal nematodes *Ascaris lumbricoides* *Enterobius vermicularis* (pinworm) *Ancylostoma duodenale, Necator americanus* (hookworm, round worm) *Schistosoma* (trematodes, flatworms) *Schistosoma haematobium, Schistosoma japonicum,* and *Schistosoma mansoni;* two other species, more localized geographically, are *Schistosoma mekongi* and *Schistosoma intercalatum.* *Taenia saginata* (beef tapeworm), *Taenia solium* (pork tapeworm), and *Taenia asiatica* (Asian tapeworm) *Trichinella spiralis* (nematode) *Trichuris trichiura* (nematode, whipworm)	• Most cases are asymptomatic, but infected persons may present with pulmonary or potentially severe gastrointestinal complaints. • Anal infection • Intestinal disorder with symptoms including diarrhea and anemia • Schistosomiasis—intestinal and urogenital. Inflammation in the intestine, rectum, or bladder causing tissue masses, granulomas, and stiffening of the tissue (fibrosis). *T. solium* tapeworm infections can lead to cysticercosis, the development of extraintestinal encysted larval forms of *T. solium* in various organs, including the brain (neurocysticercosis). Encapsulates in host muscle tissue with neurologic and cardiac involvement. Common intestinal helminthic infection

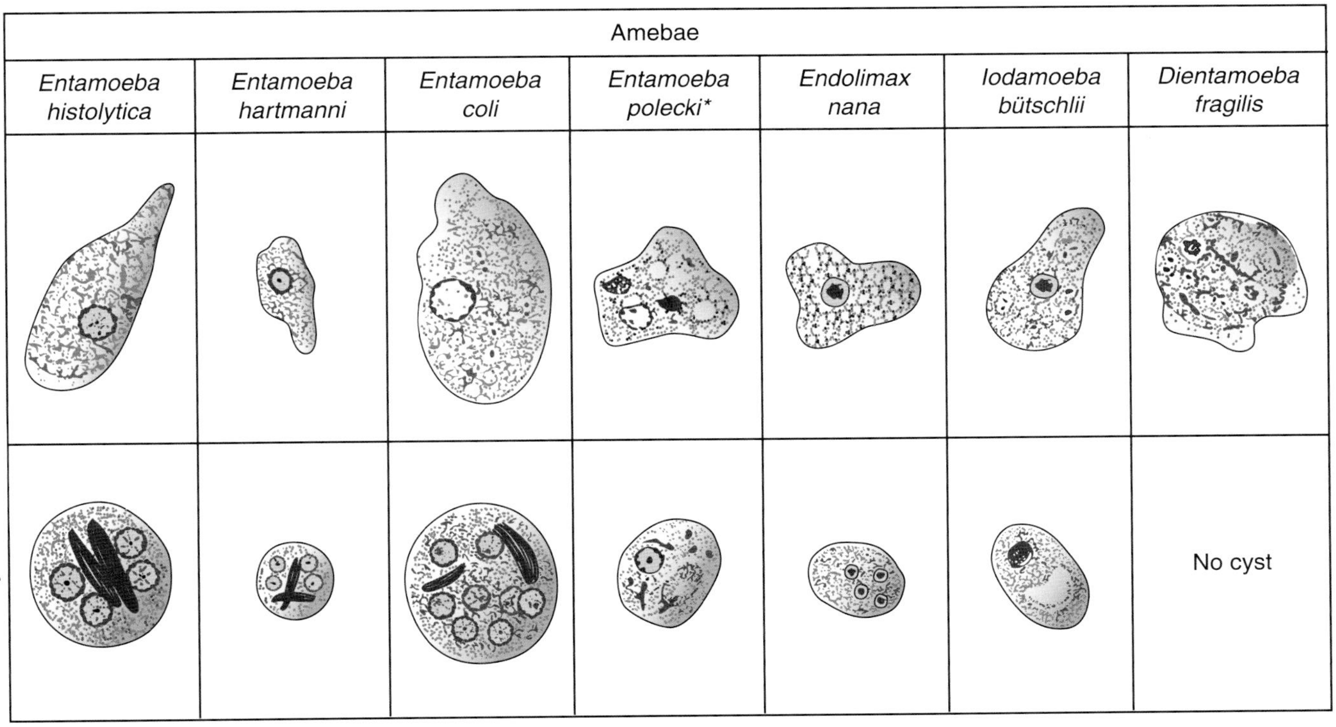

Amebae

Entamoeba histolytica | *Entamoeba hartmanni* | *Entamoeba coli* | *Entamoeba polecki** | *Endolimax nana* | *Iodamoeba bütschlii* | *Dientamoeba fragilis*

Trophozoite

Cyst

No cyst

*Rare, probably of animal origin

Fig. 15.31 Amebae found in human stool specimens. (*Dientamoeba fragilis* is a flagellate.) (From McPherson RA, Pincus MR: *Henry's clinical diagnosis and management by laboratory methods*, ed 22, Elsevier, 2011, Philadelphia, Fig 62-10, p 1210.)

Human parasites belong to separate subdivisions within the taxonomic kingdom Animalia. These include the subkingdom Protozoa (amebae, flagellates, ciliates, sporozoans, coccidia, microsporidia), the phylum Nematoda (roundworms), and the phylum Platyhelminthes (flatworms), which can be further separated into the trematodes (flukes) and cestodes (tapeworms). Parasites can also belong to the phylum Arthropoda, which includes insects, spiders, mites, and ticks.

Parasitic infections are diagnosed microscopically by the cysts (inactive stage) or trophozoites (actively feeding and reproducing forms) of amoebae (Fig. 15.31) and *Ciliate, Coccidia, Blastocystis hominis* species (Fig. 15.32) and the flagellates found in stool specimens of humans. Most protozoa have two developmental stages, the cyst, found in formed stool, and the trophozoite, found in loose or watery stools. Finding protozoan cysts usually indicates that the infection is in an inactive or carrier state, whereas finding trophozoites usually indicates an active infectious disease.

In addition, parasites can be directly identified by microscopically observing ova (parasite eggs), larvae (immature form), or adult parasites, usually the helminths (Fig. 15.33). Various immunologic tests are now available to detect parasitic infections. It is important that the infecting organism be identified specifically because treatment depends on the type of parasite and the site of infestation. Any identification process depends on correct specimen collection and adequate fixation. Specimens for parasitic identification include stool, urine, blood, sputum, and tissue biopsies.

The patient's symptoms and clinical history, including travel, are significant sources of information to be shared with the clinical laboratory. Good lines of communication between the laboratory and the physician will ensure that the appropriate specimen is collected and handled properly. The field of medical parasitology is vast, so medical parasitology textbooks should be consulted for in-depth studies. Excellent resource textbooks and other references contain the specific morphologic criteria needed to identify the more common parasites. The focus of this section is to introduce basic information on parasitology, such as collection, processing of ova and parasite (O&P) examinations, and common parasite identification.

Collection of Specimens for Parasite Identification

Specimens for parasite identification come primarily from the intestinal tract as fecal specimens, from the urogenital tract as a vaginal or urethral discharge or as a prostatic secretion, from sputum, from CSF, or from biopsy material from other body tissues. Blood can also be examined for parasites such as *Plasmodium,* a malarial parasite. Each specimen may harbor various life-cycle stages for individual parasites specific to the location in the host. Inadequate or improper specimen collection may result in misidentification of the infecting organism.

Stool Specimens

Identification of intestinal parasites, particularly protozoa, requires that specific collection protocol be followed to identify the organism properly. A single stool specimen may not be

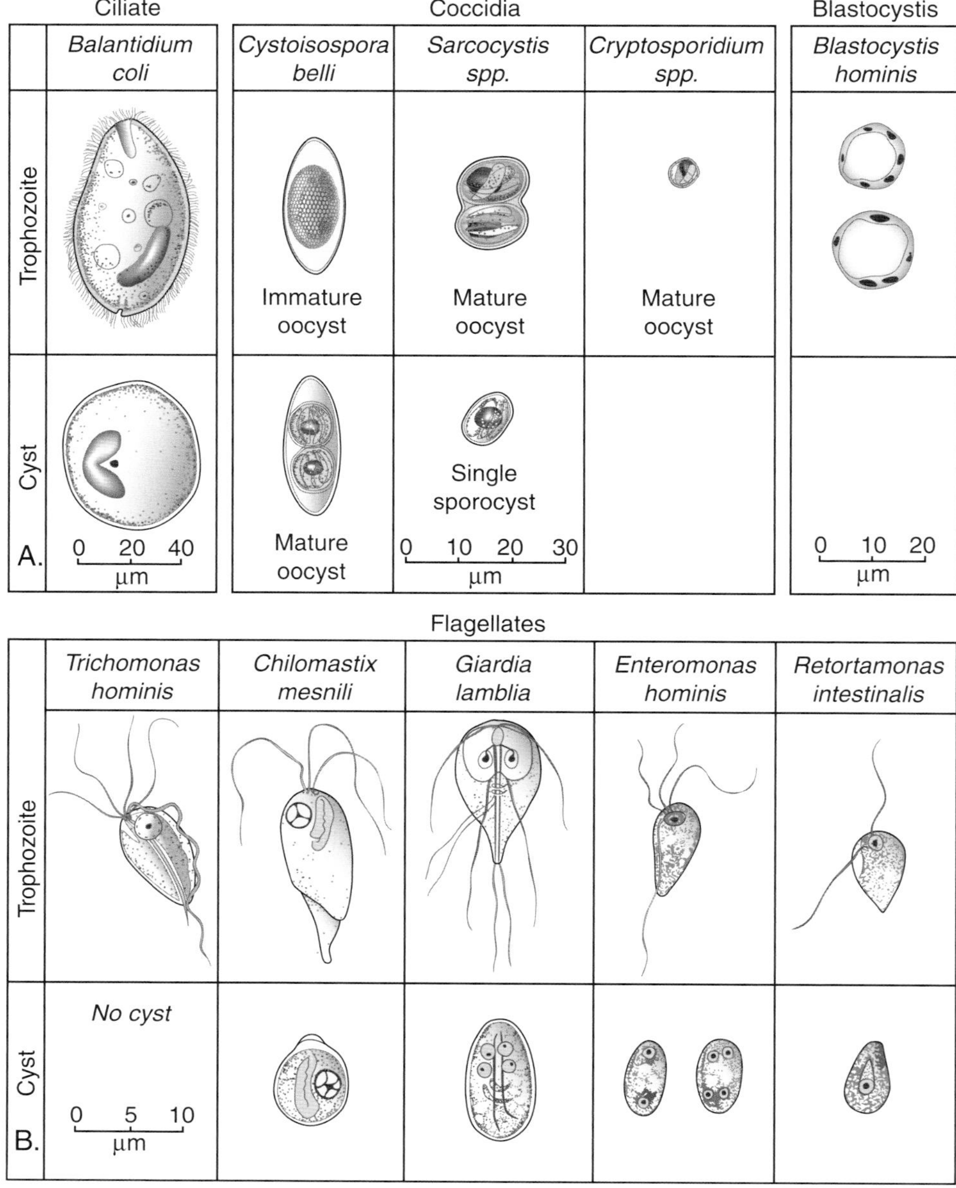

Fig. 15.32 (A) *Ciliate, Coccidia,* and *Blastocystis hominis* spp. found in stool specimens of humans. (B) Flagellates found in stool specimens of humans. (Adapted from Brooke MM, Melvin DS: *Morphology of diagnostic stages of intestinal parasites of man,* Publication No (CDC) 848116, Washington, DC, 1984, US Department of Health and Human Services. In McPherson RA, Pincus MR: *Henry's clinical diagnosis and management by laboratory methods,* ed 22, Elsevier, 2011, Philadelphia, Fig 62-13, p 1214.)

sufficient to isolate an intestinal parasite, for example, because many intestinal parasitic organisms shed eggs or cysts intermittently. The recommended protocol is to collect three stool samples 1 or 2 days apart, but all within a 10-day period, to provide optimal detection of intestinal parasites.

Collection of stool samples for parasites should always be done before radiologic studies involving barium sulfate; the use of barium will affect the sample for at least a week. Certain medications can also affect the detection of parasites in stool samples.

A clean, dry, waterproof container with a tight-fitting lid is an appropriate collection container for a stool sample for parasite identification. Contaminating the specimen with water or urine should be avoided. The sample should be sent to the laboratory as soon as possible; commercial transport systems are available that will preserve the stool sample when the specimen cannot be transported quickly. Any stool sample should be handled carefully because it is a potential source of infection.

Blood Specimens

Thick and thin smears are made to allow for better detection of parasites found in blood, such as *Plasmodium* spp. (malaria). The thick smear is used to screen a larger volume of blood; the thin smear does not distort the morphologic characteristics

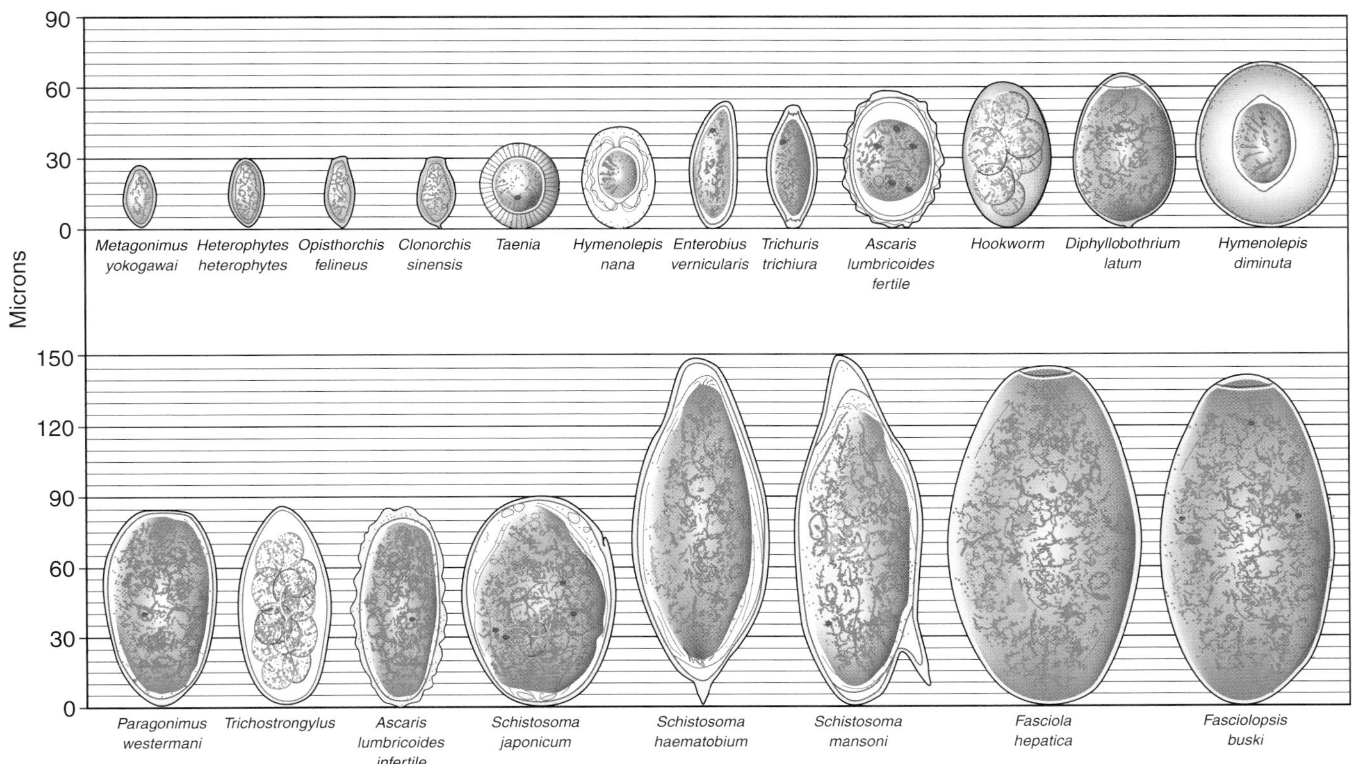

Fig. 15.33 Relative sizes of helminth eggs. (Courtesy Centers for Disease Control and Prevention, Parasitology Training Branch, Atlanta. In McPherson RA, Pincus MR: *Henry's clinical diagnosis and management by laboratory methods,* ed 22, Elsevier, 2011, Philadelphia, Fig 62-16, p 1219.)

of the organism used to identify the parasite. The Giemsa hematologic stain can be used to detect blood parasites (see Blood and Tissue Microorganisms).

Methods for Detection of Parasites

Methods for parasite detection vary with the specimen and its source. Because many parasitic infections are diagnosed through identification of eggs or larvae in a stool sample, methods of detection in stool are discussed more completely than detection using other specimens. Examination of a direct wet mount of a stool specimen is used to detect the presence of motile protozoan trophozoites and flagellates. A fecal concentration method, either sedimentation or flotation, can be used to enhance the detection of smaller numbers of parasites. Commercial products are available for the specimen collection and detection of some parasites. Permanent stained smears are made to confirm identification. Quality assurance of detection and identification results begins with the use of properly collected specimens (see Common Parasites Identified).

Wet Mount, Direct Smear

A fresh specimen is necessary for microscopic observation of motile trophozoites and larvae in a direct wet mount. A smear is prepared by mixing a small amount of the sample with a drop of physiologic saline on a glass slide with a coverslip. This is repeated using iodine, and both slides are examined for trophozoites, helminth ova (eggs), larvae, and protozoan cysts. Motility is also observed.

Common Parasites Identified

Trichomonas Vaginalis

T. vaginalis can inhabit the urogenital system of both males and females. It is considered a pathogenic parasite; *T. vaginalis* is the cause of vaginitis, urethritis, and prostatitis. *T. vaginalis* infection is usually considered a sexually transmitted disease. The motile trophozoite is found in freshly voided urine of both genders, in prostatic secretions, and in vaginal wet preparations (Fig. 15.34). Diagnosis is made by observation of the motile trophozoite, a pear-shaped elongated form, in fresh urine and urogenital specimens. The parasites move with a jerky and undulating motion; they are approximately the size of a neutrophil.

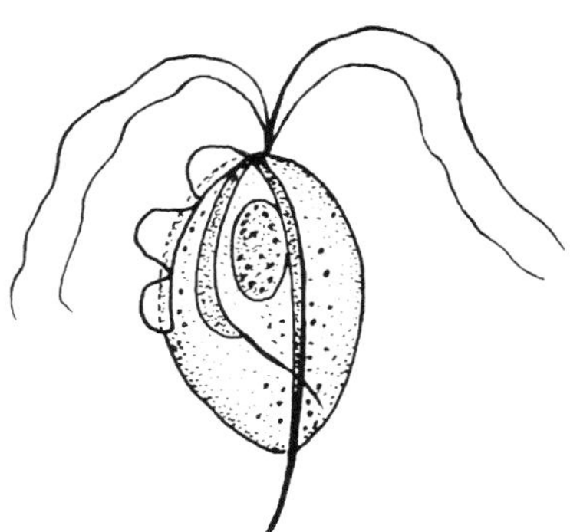

Fig. 15.34 *Trichomonas vaginalis* trophozoite. (From Tille PM: Bailey *and* Scott's *diagnostic microbiology,* ed 13, St Louis, 2014, Mosby.)

Motile trophozoites of *T. vaginalis* can be identified microscopically in fresh urine specimens and fresh genital secretions. Specimens that are not examined immediately may contain organisms; however, their morphology generally has changed, becoming "rounded up" and resembling a white blood cell or a transitional epithelial cell. For this reason, proper specimen collection and immediate transportation to the laboratory for analysis are important in the identification process.

A number of commercial products are available for rapid antigen detection of *T. vaginalis*. The OSOM *Trichomonas* Rapid Test (Sekisui Diagnostics, Framingham, MA) is a dipstick method that is both rapid and easy to perform (Fig. 15.35A). These antigen-detection methods are more sensitive than the wet preparation for *T. vaginalis* described earlier.

The most sensitive method for identification of *T. vaginalis* is culture, and commercial products are available for this purpose.[7] One product is a self-contained system, the InPouch TV System (BioMed Diagnostics, White City, OR), used for detection of the organism by both culture and direct microscopic examination (Fig. 15.35B). An open plastic viewing frame comes with the system, which allows for correct positioning and viewing of the pouch under the microscope.

Intestinal Ova and Parasites

Intestinal parasitic infections are diagnosed through identification of their eggs (ova) or larvae in a fecal sample. Stool specimens for examination must be preserved or fixed immediately. Most commercial collection kits for these tests contain the appropriate preservative and pH indicator. The preservative-fixative for specimens to be tested for ova and parasites is formalin or polyvinyl alcohol (PVA). These can be toxic and difficult to dispose of; newer commercial products are available that are considered safer environmental replacements for PVA. These commercial products are EcoFix (Meridian Diagnostics, Cincinnati, OH) and Proto-Fix (Alpha-TecSystems, Vancouver, WA). It is important to be aware of possible collection problems, such as with barium (radiologic studies), mineral oil, bismuth, some antidiarrheal preparations, antimalarials, and some antibiotics. Contamination with urine should also be avoided.

Macroscopic Examination. Macroscopic examination includes observation of the consistency of the specimen. A fecal specimen of normal consistency, in which the moisture content is decreased, will more likely yield cyst stages because the protozoan parasite has encysted to survive. In a soft or liquid sample, the trophozoite stages are more likely to be found. Occasionally, adult helminths can be seen on the surface of the feces. The presence of blood should be noted; dark feces may indicate bleeding in the upper gastrointestinal tract, whereas bright-red feces indicates bleeding in the gastrointestinal tract.

Microscopic Examination. Direct wet mounts of the specimen are observed to detect helminth eggs and motile trophozoite stages of the protozoa. It is not sufficient to identify the protozoa by using only the direct wet-mount preparation. Permanent-stained smears should also be examined to confirm the identification of the parasitic organism.

The microscopic identification of intestinal protozoa and helminth ova is based on recognition of specific morphologic characteristics. A brightfield microscope with a good light source and equipped with a calibrated ocular micrometer to measure the size of the ova and parasites is essential for proper identification.

To observe the sample microscopically, a small amount of the sample is mixed with a drop of physiologic saline on a glass slide, and a coverslip is applied over the mixture. Correct light adjustment, as for unstained urine sediment, is needed to see the motile trophozoite stages of the protozoa, which will appear pale and transparent.

After examination of the wet preparation, a drop of weak iodine solution can be placed at the edge of the coverslip. This stained preparation will assist in the identification of protozoan cysts that stain with iodine. The cysts appear with a yellow-gold

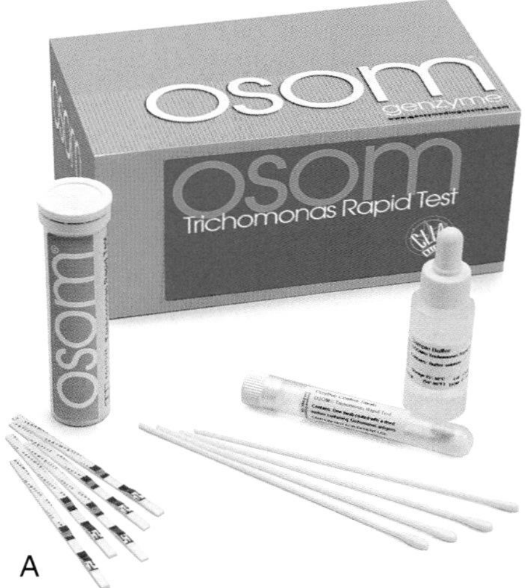

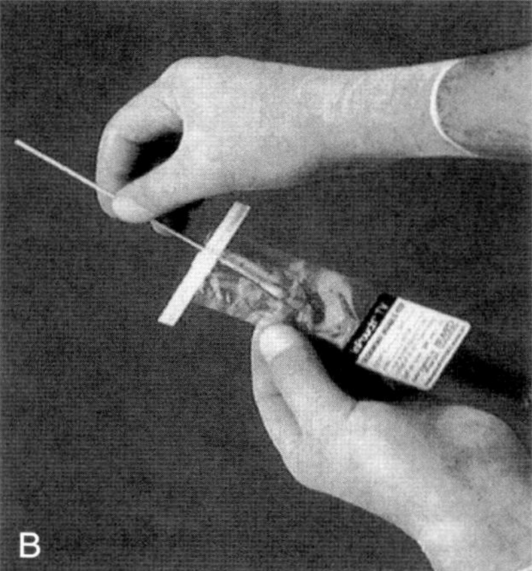

Fig. 15.35 *Trichomonas vaginalis.* (A) Rapid test for the identification of *T. vaginalis.* (B) Self-contained system for culturing *T. vaginalis.* (From Tille PM: *Bailey and* Scott's *diagnostic microbiology,* ed 13, St Louis, 2014, Mosby.)

cytoplasm, brown glycogen material, and paler refractile nuclei. Other stains are used to reveal nuclear detail in the trophozoite stages of the protozoa. A permanent-stained smear is used to confirm the identification of intestinal protozoa.

Concentration Procedures. Concentration of fecal material should be included in a complete O&P examination. Concentration procedures allow the visualization of small numbers of parasitic organisms that may be missed in a direct mount. Various concentration procedures are used, most often sedimentation or flotation techniques.

Sedimentation procedures use gravity or centrifugation and enhance the recovery of protozoa, eggs, and larvae.

Flotation procedures separate protozoan cysts and certain helminth eggs. A reagent with a high specific gravity is used, such as zinc sulfate. The parasitic elements will be located in the surface layer of the mixture, and the debris will be in the bottom layer. Some helminth or protozoan eggs do not concentrate well with the flotation method.

Permanent Stained Smears. Confirming the identification of intestinal protozoa requires the preparation of a permanent-stained smear. Permanent smears also provide a permanent record of the examination. To prepare slides for staining, fixation and preservation are first required. Commercial preparations are available, and stool can be added directly; then the permanent slide can be made from this preparation. Permanent stains used include iron hematoxylin and trichrome. Trichrome stains are most often used.

Molecular Diagnostic Testing. Nucleic acid–based amplification methods have been developed for the identification of the pathogenic protozoan *Entamoeba histolytica.* However, these tests are not widely used. Caution should be exercised when interpreting the results because stool specimens may contain inhibitors that interfere with the amplification method.

Direct Antigen Detection. Many commercial kits are available to detect antigens for both *Giardia lamblia* and *Cryptosporidium* in the same product kit. *G. lamblia* is one of the most common parasites causing infection in the United States, and *Cryptosporidium* is an important parasite in waterborne outbreaks. An O&P examination can be lengthy, and the use of these commercial products can save time in identification. The sensitivity of these kits is comparable to microscopy, and many clinical laboratories have adopted their use.

Enterobius vermicularis (Pinworm)

E. vermicularis, the pinworm, is a common parasite in children worldwide. It is a roundworm whose adult female migrates during the night, depositing her eggs in the perianal region. A fecal sample is not the optimal specimen because the eggs may not be observed in feces. Most laboratories use the clear cellophane tape method to collect and prepare the specimen for examination.

Cellophane Tape Collection Method. The cellophane tape method is often used to collect the pinworm specimen. A piece of clear cellophane tape (not frosted tape), with the sticky side toward the patient, is pressed against the skin across the anal opening to collect any eggs, using even, thorough pressure. The sticky side of the tape is then placed down against the surface of a clean glass slide with a glass coverslip. The slide should be labeled with the patient's name and additional identifying data. Commercial collection kits are available with sticky paddles, simplifying the collection process. These specimens must be collected when the patient awakens in the morning, before bathing, defecating, or urinating. Negative findings must be confirmed with repeat testing on subsequent days. The slide is scanned for the characteristically shaped eggs of the organism, using low-power and high-power magnification. *E. vermicularis* eggs are ellipsoid (football shaped), with one slightly flattened side (Fig. 15.36).

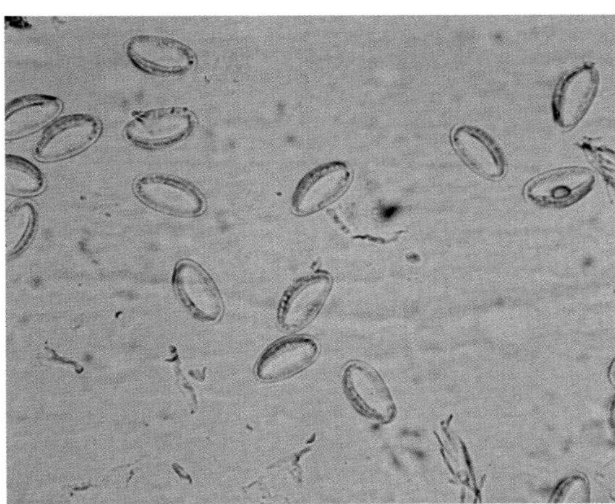

Fig. 15.36 Cellophane tape preparation of *Enterobius vermicularis* (pinworm) eggs. (From Tille PM: *Bailey and Scott's diagnostic* microbiology, ed 14, St Louis, 2017, Mosby.)

Blood and Tissue Microorganisms

Malaria is one of the most common infectious diseases worldwide, and its rapid laboratory diagnosis is important. Diagnosis depends on clinical symptoms (headache, fever, chills, sweats, nausea) and identification of the *Plasmodium* malarial parasites in the RBCs. The malarial parasite enters the human through the bite from an infected *Anopheles* mosquito.

Tickborne infectious agents can cause disease; these infections include babesiosis, Lyme disease, and ehrlichiosis. Babesiosis is a disease that clinically resembles malaria. *Babesia* organisms are tickborne sporozoan parasites. Diagnosis of babesiosis is made through identification of *Babesia* parasites in the RBCs. In Lyme disease the etiologic agent is the bacterium *Borrelia burgdorferi.* Transmission occurs by inoculation through the bite of a tick of the genus *Ixodes.* Diagnosis of Lyme disease depends on finding antibodies in the serum or CSF. Ehrlichiosis is another infectious process that is tickborne. The organism *Ehrlichia chaffeensis* is a gram-negative, obligate intracellular parasite that multiplies in monocytic white cells (human monocytic ehrlichiosis). Diagnosis is made by direct visualization of clusters (morulae) of the organisms in white cells using Giemsa stain, by indirect immunofluorescence for detection of antibodies, and with PCR techniques. Human granulocytic ehrlichiosis, now called *human granulocytic anaplasmosis,* is caused by *Anaplasma phagocytophilum.*

Malarial Parasites. The malarial parasites enter the bloodstream and invade RBCs. Thin and thick smears are prepared, stained with Wright or Giemsa, and examined for the blood parasites. The thick smears are more difficult to interpret but increase the sensitivity. The thin smears are used to better identify the species of the malarial parasite. Correct therapy depends on identification of the specific species of malarial organism present in the blood.

TESTS FOR VIRUSES (VIROLOGY)

The study of submicroscopic, obligate intracellular infectious agents is called *virology*. These infectious particles are among the smallest infectious agents and are capable of infecting plants, animals, and bacteria. The viral particles are so small that they are not visible under a standard microscope. Viruses have very specific and limited host range; viruses have a tropism for infection of a specific host cell type that depends on cellular and viral receptor interaction.

Viral agents are ubiquitous and can be found in every environment. Vaccination or immunization has proven successful in the prevention of a variety of viral agents. However, viruses are capable of undergoing genetic changes, resulting in a new or "novel" viral agent. These genetic changes may result from major changes that alter the viral antigens (antigenic shift) or minor changes that occur over time (antigenic drift). In 1918, a deadly outbreak of influenza virus, the Spanish flu, was a result of a novel influenza virus of avian origin. The virus adapted to human infection and then was able to be transmitted from human to human and covered a large geographical region, extending worldwide and resulting in a pandemic. Although immunization is successful for many viruses, others, such as HIV, influenza, and hepatitis, continue to pose many challenges in the control, prevention, and treatment of human infections.

Characteristics of Viruses

Viruses differ from all the organisms already discussed in this chapter. Viruses cannot replicate outside of another living host cell. The virus relies on host cell machinery to reproduce the viral particles for propagation, transmission, and infection. Virus particles are referred to as *virions* and consist of three major parts:

1. An inner nucleic acid core that may consist of either DNA or RNA
2. A capsid or protein coat that protects and contains the nucleic acid
3. Possibly an outer lipid layer, or envelope, that surrounds the nucleocapsid (capsid containing nucleic acid)

Unlike bacterial taxonomy, viral taxonomy incorporates a variety of categories, including information related to transmission, host tropism, pathology, host size, shape and structure, physical properties, and disease pathology. Because of the complexity of viral structure, many texts limit the viral classification to viral morphology, method of replication, genome organization, and whether or not the virus has an envelope.

Viruses as a Source of Infection

Viruses are obligate intracellular pathogens requiring a host cell for propagation and completion of the viral infectious cycle. The virus must first attach (adsorption) to the host cell using specific host–viral receptor interactions. Once attached, the virus penetrates the host cell in a variety of ways, depending on the viral structure. Some viruses simply inject their nucleic acid into the host cell, whereas others use the cellular machinery to induce endocytosis in the entire viral particle. Still others, such as the enveloped virus, fuse the viral envelope with the host cell membrane, resulting in the release of the viral capsid into the cell. Once the viral capsid is inside the cell, the viral capsid is either removed (uncoating) by simple dissociation or by degradation by viral or host enzymes. The viral nucleic acid is now available for replication, transcription, and translation of viral proteins using the host enzymes. This process is referred to as the *macromolecular synthesis* of the virus. Finally, the viral particles are assembled into viral particles and then released by breaking through the cell membrane, resulting in lysis (lytic virus) of the host cell or budding through the cell membrane, picking up a viral envelope without cell death.

Once a virus infects a host, the resultant infection is classified as an acute viral infection with apparent signs and symptoms; as a latent infection that has no signs and symptoms although the virus is still present in the host; or as a chronic, persistent state in which low levels of viral particles present and the host may or may not display signs and symptoms of infection. In addition, a virus may cause a pathogenic stimulation of the host's immune system, resulting in a condition of autoimmune pathogenesis. This typically occurs long after the resolution of an acute viral infection. Occasionally, a virus may promote transformation or uncontrollable growth of host cells, resulting in a tumor or cancer. These viruses are referred to as *oncogenic viruses*.

Collection of Specimens for Viral Identification

Specimen collection for the identification of a suspected viral agent can be confusing. Often, the suspected viral agent causes clinical symptoms similar to other organisms such as bacteria. In addition, although many viruses enter through the respiratory tract, they may infect tissues and cause symptoms significantly different from the primary site of entry.

Specimens for the identification of viral agents should be collected as soon as possible following the onset of patient signs and symptoms. In addition, variations in devices and containers are available that may enhance the recovery and detection of the viral agent. All respiratory specimens are typically acceptable for the identification and recovery of most viruses. However, they are also often contaminated with normal oral bacterial microbiota. In general, nasopharyngeal aspirates improve recovery of respiratory viruses over nasopharyngeal or throat swabs. Bronchial washings or lavages are excellent specimens for detecting viruses that infect the lower respiratory tract. Stool specimens are preferred for the isolation of rotavirus and enteric adenovirus over rectal swabs. Some human viruses can also be detected in the patient's urine in low numbers. As a result, three specimens and a minimum volume of up to 10 mL from a clean-catch first morning urine should be used. Because the urine pH or bacterial contamination may interfere with viral recovery, centrifugation or filtering of the specimen and neutralization are recommended. Sterile body fluids that may contain viruses, including blood, bone marrow, CSF, and pericardial or peritoneal fluids, are collected by the physician and sent to the laboratory. Tissue specimens are also collected by the physician during surgical procedures and may be useful for detecting viruses that infect the lungs, brain, or gastrointestinal tract. Cervical specimens may be collected using a swab or a brush and should be placed in transport media to maintain the integrity of the virus. Finally, some viruses are detectable from open skin lesions, such as herpes simplex virus or varicella zoster virus, by collecting vesicle fluid and cells scraped from the lesion. However, once the lesion is encrusted, viral recovery becomes problematic.

Methods for Detection of Viruses

Cell Culture

Viruses are obligate intracellular pathogens; therefore detection in living cells using cell culture for multiplication and replication of viruses is often used for rapidly growing viruses. It is important to use the appropriate host cells and the correct nutrient media to maintain the cells.

Following inoculation of the appropriate cell culture, cells are incubated for 1 to 4 weeks depending on the suspected viral agent. Periodically, the cells are inspected using an inverted light microscope to visualize the cytopathic effect (characteristic viral inclusion or change in cellular structure) resulting from the virus infecting the cells. To decrease the time from specimen collection to identification, a modified rapid shell vial technique is often used in place of conventional cell culture. A shell vial contains a round coverslip at the bottom of a small tube. The appropriate cells and nutrient medium are added. During the 1- to 2-day incubation required for identification of the virus, a monolayer of cells forms on top of the coverslip. The coverslip is then stained using virus-specific immunofluorescent conjugates for identification (see Fig. 15.34).

Immunodiagnosis (Antigen or Antibody Detection)

Various high-quality immunotechniques are available for the detection of viruses. These include fluorescent antibody, latex agglutination, and enzyme immunoassay.

Molecular Diagnostic Testing

Molecular assays, including hybridization and amplification methods, have replaced serologic assays for the rapid diagnosis of a variety of infectious diseases. Nucleic acid probes for the detection of viral agents are often useful when the amount of the virus is sufficient, when the viral culture is too slow or not possible, and when immunoassays lack sufficient sensitivity or specificity.

There are 28 molecular flu assays cleared for marketing by the US Food and Drug Administration (FDA), including two assays with test times of 15 to 20 minutes that have been granted waived status under the terms of the Clinical Laboratory Improvement Amendments of 1988 (CLIA '88). These tests are being used by health care providers in a wide range of settings to test for influenza, but there is a potential trade-off between accuracy and speed (Table 15.14).

TABLE 15.14 Laboratory Testing Trade-Offs

Test	Testing Time	Comments
Culture of specimen	4–5 days (traditional testing)	Time to results is 48–72 hours for newer "shell viral" platforms
Direct fluorescent antibody (DFA) testing	1–2 hours	Complex to administer; requires additional reagents and equipment
Rapid influenza testing (first generation)	Within 30 minutes	Generally high specificity Often poor to moderate sensitivity
Polymerase chain reaction (PCR) and related amplified molecular tests	Requires repeated, time-consuming thermocycling	Improved sensitivity Requires complex instrumentation

Adapted from Moore N: Rapid point-of-care assays for influenza testing, *MLO Med Lab Obs* 48(11):18–20, 2016.

One of the most popular molecular diagnostic testing systems is the BioFire FilmArray (bioMérieux), a user-friendly multiplex PCR method that provides results in approximately 60 minutes. The FilmArray now has four FDA-cleared panels: the Respiratory Panel, the Blood Culture Identification Panel, the Gastrointestinal Panel, and the Meningitis/Encephalitis Panel.

FilmArray Torch is a fully integrated, random-access system compatible with all existing FilmArray panels. FilmArray 2.0 has LIS-interfacing capabilities to enable simplified test ordering and send-outs, quicker turnaround times, and increased accuracy by minimizing manual data entry. FilmArray EZ Configuration is a CLIA-waived system for near-patient molecular testing. The EZ configuration is designed for use with Respiratory Panel (RP) EZ.

Another testing system that is FDA 510(k) cleared and CLIA waived for the detection of influenza is the cobas Influenza A/B (Roche Diagnostics, Risch-Rotkreuz, Switzerland) nucleic acid test for use on the cobas Liat System. This system is an automated multiplex real-time PCR (RT-PCR) assay for the rapid in vitro qualitative detection and discrimination of influenza A virus and influenza B virus RNA in nasopharyngeal swab specimens from patients with signs and symptoms of respiratory infection in conjunction with clinical and epidemiological risk factors. The test is intended for use as an aid in the differential diagnosis of influenza A and influenza B in humans and is not intended to detect influenza C.

The cobas Influenza A/B & RSV nucleic acid test for use on the cobas Liat System is an automated multiplex RT-PCR assay for the rapid in vitro qualitative detection and discrimination of influenza A virus, influenza B virus, and respiratory syncytial virus (RSV). RNA in nasopharyngeal swab specimens is evaluated from patients with signs and symptoms of respiratory infection in conjunction with clinical and epidemiological risk factors. The test is intended for use as an aid in the differential diagnosis of influenza A, influenza B, and RSV in humans and is not intended to detect influenza C.

More Point-of-Care Rapid Testing Applications

The test systems available today are technically mature and offer good to very good performance. For HIV, malaria, group A

TABLE 15.15 Advantages and Disadvantages of Rapid Microbiological Tests

Advantages	Disadvantages
• Facilitates immediate initiation of specific antibiotic therapy • Reduction in unnecessary antibiotic consumption • Reduction in selection pressure • Immediate recognition of infection chains • Reduction in preanalytical interference • Extension of diagnostic instrumentation; independent of culture • Better compliance with patients who are difficult to reach	• Poorer performance of older POCT systems (before the introduction of immunochromatographic techniques) • Lack of data on pathogen sensitivity • Increased risk of operator becoming infected • Requires adequate operator qualifications • Double or multiple infections more likely to be overlooked than in culture • Necessity of performing measures for quality control

POCT, Point-of-care testing.

streptococci, and legionellae, point-of-care testing (POCT), when indicated, is on a par with conventional procedures. The information yielded by rapid tests for pneumococci and for influenza tends to be supplementary in nature. The rapid test for group B streptococci is unsuitable for routine use because its sensitivity is still too low compared with bacterial culture. POCT can be successful only if the tests are performed correctly by trained personnel, quality management procedures are followed, and the severity of illness and the epidemiological circumstances are taken into account when interpreting the results.

POCT continues to increase for bacteria, parasites, and viruses. The available POCT has addressed diagnosis related to infectious diseases—mostly as test strips or easy-to-operate cassette systems. Immunochromatography test strips to detect infectious pathogens are technically fully developed and exhibit a series of specific advantages, but they also have disadvantages (Table 15.15).

Rapid Testing for Streptococcal Infections. For beta-hemolyzing streptococci, rapid tests are available for directly detecting the antigens of group A streptococci (GAS; *S. pyogenes*) and of group B streptococci (GBS; *Streptococcus agalactiae*). The tests are based on the extraction of the C-antigen from the cell wall, followed by detection with an immunological reaction. If GAS are directly detected during the examination of a tonsillitis patient, it is then possible to decide whether antimicrobial therapy is necessary.

The GBS are a major cause of neonatal infections in industrial countries. Although there has been considerable progress in their diagnosis and treatment, GBS infections lead to high morbidity and mortality. The most efficient strategy to reduce the frequency and severity of neonatal infection is currently thought to be culture detection of group B streptococci from rectovaginal screening swabs in weeks 35 to 37 of pregnancy and intrapartal chemoprophylaxis with ampicillin. If testing by culture is not available, routine use of the GBS rapid test is currently not recommended by obstetrical societies.

The cobas Liat Strep A, a strep A nucleic acid test, is a qualitative in vitro diagnostic test for the detection of *S. pyogenes* (group A β-hemolytic *Streptococcus;* strep A) in throat swab specimens from patients with signs and symptoms of pharyngitis. The cobas Liat Strep A assay utilizes nucleic acid purification and PCR technology to detect *S. pyogenes* by targeting a segment of the *S. pyogenes* genome.

Rapid Testing for Pneumococci and Legionellae. Rapid tests are available for the diagnosis of respiratory infections. These include detection of the antigens of influenza, pneumococci, and legionellae. The greatest benefits of these systems are the improvement in diagnostic yield (pneumococci, legionellae) and in the time saved in diagnosis. The sensitivity of the pneumococcal antigen test (Binax NOW, Abbott, Abbott Park, IL) is dependent on the severity of the pneumonia. The sensitivity of this test is 94%. Legionellae are important pathogens of both community-acquired and nosocomial pneumonia. Legionella can only be detected by culture in a few patients and usually requires 3 to 7 days for identification. The development of rapid testing for influenza virus (see Molecular Diagnostic Testing) was greatly accelerated by the recognition that early therapy (within 48 hours) with neuraminidase inhibitors is more likely to be successful. Currently available tests have moderate to high levels of sensitivity and specificity depending on the selected "gold standard."

Rapid Testing for Human Immunodeficiency Virus. Bedside rapid tests to detect HIV antibodies are now an equivalent alternative to the conventional antibody screening tests. Rapid testing is valuable in limited-resource countries (e.g., Africa), in patients who are difficult to reach (e.g., drug addicts or homeless persons), for the critical period in which a decision has to be made about prophylaxis after exposure, and after a birth where the HIV status of the mother is unknown. It is essential that positive rapid test results be confirmed by an alternate rapid test or by a conventional test (e.g., Western blot).

Rapid Testing for* Plasmodium falciparum *(Falciparum Malaria). An infection with *Plasmodium falciparum* (falciparum malaria) can be detected with highly reliable rapid tests for two specific antigens: histidine-rich protein 2 (HRP2) and parasite-specific lactate dehydrogenase (pLDH). These are an alternative to conventional diagnosis by light microscopy (thick drops and blood smear). False positives are possible, for example, because of rheumatoid factor. False negatives are also possible, usually if the parasitemia is very low (< 100/μL). It is also a problem that the rapid test sometimes fails in spite of high parasite density.

AUTOMATION

Implementation of automation in clinical microbiology has lagged behind other laboratory disciplines. Robotics and computer processing revolutionized chemistry and hematology instruments decades ago. But clinical microbiologists continue to process specimens manually and identify bacteria using methods from the 19th century.

Specimen Processing

Automation in clinical microbiology is challenging because of the variety of specimens and the diversity of identification methods. Microbiology specimen types include blood, sterile body fluids, tissues, urine, catheter tips, other prosthetic devices, and lower respiratory tract specimens, among others. A challenge in processing microbiology specimens is that specimens are collected and transported with the use of a wide variety of containers. Specimen handling and processing have been the last aspects of microbial testing to undergo change. Currently available specimen processors are the Autoplak (NTE-SENER, Cerdanyola del Vallès, Spain), the InoqulA (BD Kiestra, Becton Dickinson [BD], Rutherford, NJ), the Innova (BD), the PreLUD (I2A, Montpellier, France), the Previ-Isola (bioMérieux), and the WASP (Copan, Murrieta, CA). Each of these instruments is capable of automating the processing of a variety of liquid-based specimens, but only two main manufacturers, BD Kiestra and Copan, currently provide extended automated systems including specimen processors, conveyors, incubators, and digital imaging.

Mass Spectrophotometry (MALDI-TOF)

In recent years, matrix-assisted laser desorption ionization-time of flight mass spectrometry (MALDI-TOF MS) has emerged as a potential tool for microbial identification and diagnosis. Mass spectrometry is an analytical technique in which chemical compounds are ionized into charged molecules, and the ratio of their mass to charge (m/z) is measured. This new technology can be used for early identification and diagnosis of diseases caused by bacteria, viruses, or fungi. Specimens such as blood, urine, cerebrospinal fluid or stool can be used as the source of microorganisms. In addition to microbial identification, MALDI-TOF can be used for microbial strain typing, epidemiological studies, detection of biological warfare agents, detection of water- and food-borne pathogens, and the detection of antibiotic resistance. This process is rapid, sensitive, and economical in terms of both labor and costs. In several studies[15] MALDI-TOF was found to be equal or even surpassed the conventional diagnostic methods in speed and accuracy in detecting blood stream infections; minimal processing time and identified bacteria from urine samples in the presence of even more than two uropathogens; and rapid identification of enteric pathogens. MALDI-TOF has become a valuable tool for the microbiology laboratory and could potentially replace molecular identification techniques.

Total Microbiology Laboratory Automation

Total laboratory automation (TLA) systems are available to handle specimens, streak plates, incubate, and digitally image cultures. Some current microbiology TLA systems in use or in development (listed in alphabetical order by manufacturer) are as follows: BD Kiestra (BD), TLA full microbiology laboratory automation (FMLA; bioMérieux), and WASPLab (Copan). Certain common elements exist or are envisioned for all systems. These include conveyor/track systems to move plates to and from incubators, digital cameras to capture plate images at specified intervals, automated incubators with digital reading stations, and proprietary software to facilitate these processes. These systems use various versions of computer-driven robotic plate management to automate specimen processing and workup.

A criticism of total automation systems is that the systems are built around classic techniques—growing colonies on agar plates with at least a 24-hour incubation period—instead of new revolutionary techniques (e.g., growing microbes on film or using imaging to detect growth of cells rather than colonies). Software innovations have demonstrated that WASPLab software can read chromogenic plates to detect MRSA with 100% success and detect positive results that technologists missed. In addition, WASPLab has been modified to count colonies from urine specimens and potentially distinguish different colony types on blood plates.

CASE STUDIES

CASE STUDY 15.1

A mother brings her 10-year-old daughter to the clinic; the child is complaining of a sore throat and has a low-grade fever (99.6°F). The mother states that the child has had a runny nose and a cough for the last few days. On examination, the physician notes that the child's pharynx appears red and that her tonsils are slightly swollen; no exudate is noted. Blood is drawn for a complete blood count (CBC), and a rapid strep test is sent to the microbiology laboratory. Laboratory data follow:

Hemoglobin: Normal
White blood count: Slightly elevated
Rapid strep test: Negative
Confirmation culture: Negative for group A β-hemolytic streptococci

Multiple Choice Questions

Answers are in Appendix A.

1. What is the most likely diagnosis for this patient's condition?
   a. Viral infection, the cause of most cases of pharyngitis
   b. Streptococcal pharyngitis, to be treated with antibiotics for 10 days
   c. Acid-fast organisms that would not be detected
   d. No infection
2. What would be the follow-up testing for this patient?
   a. No follow-up microbiology tests are needed.
   b. Have her return in 24 hours and repeat the CBC.
   c. Repeat the throat culture.
   d. Treat with antibiotics and then repeat the rapid strep test.

Critical Thinking Group Discussion Questions

1. What are the clinically relevant signs and symptoms in the case history?
2. What are the clinically relevant laboratory findings to support this diagnosis?

Note: Narrative answers posted on EVOLVE instructor site.

CASE STUDY 15.2

An 80-year-old man presents to the emergency department (ED) complaining of right-sided chest pain when he breathes and a productive cough. A sputum sample collected from the patient revealed rust-colored sputum. He also states that his symptoms began abruptly with chills the day before this visit to the ED; he had previously been healthy. Examination by the physician identifies coarse breathing sounds in the right anterior chest. A chest radiograph shows a right-upper-lobe infiltrate. The patient currently has a fever of 102°F. Blood is drawn for a CBC. The sputum sample is Gram-stained and cultured. Laboratory data follow:

Complete Blood Count

Hemoglobin: 14.5 g/dL (normal)
White blood count: Elevated
Differential: 90% neutrophils (normal range 25% to 60%)

Sputum

Gram stain: Gram-positive lancet-shaped diplococci (cocci in pairs)
Culture report: Streptococcus pneumoniae

The diagnosis is pneumonia caused by *S. pneumoniae.*

Multiple Choice Questions

Answers are in Appendix A.

1. The observation of which cells on the Gram-stained smear will assure the laboratory that a sputum specimen has been collected and tested?
   a. Greater than 10 squamous epithelial cells per low-power field (10 ×)
   b. Fewer than 10 squamous epithelial cells per low-power field (10 ×)
   c. Greater than 10 columnar epithelial cells per low-power field (10 ×)
   d. Greater than 10 gram-positive diplococci per low-power field (10 ×)
2. What characteristics of this patient would coincide with pneumonia caused by this organism?
   a. The patient is otherwise healthy.
   b. The patient is most likely a smoker.
   c. The patient is an older adult.
   d. The patient is likely not providing all the details.

Critical Thinking Group Discussion Questions

1. What clinically relevant signs and symptoms support the diagnosis?
2. What laboratory findings support the diagnosis?

Note: Narrative answers posted on EVOLVE instructor site.

CASE STUDY 15.3

A 20-year-old woman presents to her family practice physician for a routine pelvic examination. It has been several years since her last visit to this clinic, when she was diagnosed and treated for a nongonococcal sexually transmitted disease (STD). She is sexually active with her fiancé and has had sexual encounters with others in the past. She is currently considering the potential for becoming pregnant. There are no apparent physical abnormalities, but the physician decides to culture the cervical discharge for gonorrhea and to perform a DNA test (Genprobe) for chlamydia and gonorrhea. A serum sample is also collected for HIV testing. All laboratory tests are normal, with the exception of the test for chlamydia, which is positive.

NOTE: Symptoms of chlamydial infections include dysuria and vaginal/urethral discharge, symptoms similar to those of gonorrhea. Many infected patients exhibit no symptoms of a chlamydial infection.

Multiple Choice Questions

Answers are in Appendix A.

1. Which of the following is the test of choice for the laboratory diagnosis of chlamydial infections?
   a. Nucleic acid amplification
   b. Immunofluorescent antibody test
   c. Enzyme immunoassay (EIA)
   d. Culture
2. If the patient is experiencing no symptoms, what would be the concern for the physician to order the laboratory tests in this case?
   a. To prevent unwanted transmission of the organism to the fiancé.
   b. The organism present could lead to future infertility.
   c. The patient could develop more serious infection prior to symptoms.
   d. All of the above statements are valid concerns in this case.

Critical Thinking Group Discussion Questions

1. What are some of the significant clinical findings that would lead to the diagnosis of an STD?
2. What are some of the significant laboratory findings that would lead to the diagnosis of an STD?

Note: Narrative answers posted on EVOLVE instructor site.

CASE STUDY 15.4

A disoriented 58-year-old man with a history of poorly controlled diabetes mellitus and chronic obstructive pulmonary disease presents to the ED. The patient has been smoking cigarettes for many years. He has been taking steroid medications for his pulmonary disease. Physical examination shows that he is slightly febrile, lethargic, and in respiratory failure. A diagnosis of meningitis is being considered. A lumbar puncture is done, and cerebrospinal fluid (CSF) is collected for a smear and culture.

Laboratory Data

A CSF specimen is collected and sent to the laboratory. A cytocentrifuged preparation of the CSF is stained, using calcofluor white for yeast by staining the yeast cell walls. The smear shows encapsulated, thick-walled budding yeasts. A cryptococcal antigen test is completed and is positive. The culture of CSF identifies *Cryptococcus neoformans.*

Multiple Choice Questions

Answers are in Appendix A.

1. Fungi are widespread in the environment but rarely cause central nervous system (CNS) infection. *C. neoformans* is the most common cause of fungal meningitis. It is especially common among immunocompromised patients. This type of infection is known as which of the following?
   a. Nosocomial infection
   b. Opportunistic infection
   c. Community-associated infection
   d. Health care–associated infection
2. What additional laboratory test could have been completed for a presumptive identification of *C. neoformans*?
   a. Gram stain
   b. Acid-fast stain
   c. India ink prep
   d. Trichrome stain

Critical Thinking Group Discussion Questions

1. What clinically relevant observations support the diagnosis of meningitis associated with the infectious organism?
2. What laboratory testing supports the diagnosis of meningitis associated with the infectious organism?

Note: Narrative answers posted on EVOLVE instructor site.

CASE STUDY 15.5

An 18-year-old female college student complains of fever, chills, headache, and vomiting. She presents to the college health service ED, where she is examined. She appears lethargic, and her temperature is 102°F. Blood is drawn for a CBC and culture, urine is collected for analysis, and a serum chemistry profile is ordered. A lumbar puncture is performed, and cloudy cerebrospinal fluid (CSF) is collected. Laboratory data follow:

Complete Blood Count

WBC count: 20.0 × 10^9 (normal range 5 to 10 × 10^9)
Differential: Marked neutrophilia with shift to immature forms (shift to the left)

CSF Results

WBC count: 1200 cells/mL with 95% neutrophils (reference value: 0 to 5 lymphocytes)
Glucose: 25 mg/dL (decreased, compared with blood glucose value)
Protein: 150 mg/dL (increased)

Other data

Gram stain: Many neutrophils, gram-negative diplococci in pairs
Urinalysis: Increased protein, few RBCs, few granular casts
Serum chemistries: Within reference values

NOTE: *Haemophilus influenzae* (gram-negative coccobacillus) type B was the most common cause of meningitis in children 1 to 6 years of age before the current vaccine became available. *Streptococcus pneumoniae* (gram-positive diplococci) is a causative agent of meningitis in adults. *Neisseria meningitidis* (gram-negative diplococci) is most frequently identified as the causative organism for meningococcal infections in adolescents and young adults and has occurred in epidemics in the United States.

Multiple Choice Questions

Answers are in Appendix A.

1. From the patient's history and laboratory results, all of the following findings in the blood and CSF substantiate a bacterial rather than a viral meningeal infection *except* which one?
   a. Decreased CSF glucose
   b. Increased WBCs in CSF, with neutrophils predominating
   c. Gram stain showing gram-negative diplococci
   d. Increased protein, few RBCs, few granular casts in urine
2. What laboratory media would be required to isolate a pure culture of the suspected infectious agent?
   a. Sheep blood agar, MacConkey agar, and eosin methylene blue
   b. Sheep blood agar, Thayer–Martin agar, and MacConkey agar
   c. Sheep blood agar, MacConkey agar, and chocolate agar
   d. Sheep blood agar, SXT agar, and chocolate agar

Critical Thinking Group Discussion Questions

1. What characteristics of the patient presented in the case history would provide clues as to the potential infectious agent?
2. Explain why the physician ordered the chemistry panel in conjunction with the other tests.

Note: Narrative answers posted on EVOLVE instructor site.

CASE STUDY 15.6

A 52-year-old woman presents with a localized swelling and purulent abscess in her right hand and enlarged lymph nodes in her axial region (under the armpit). She sustained a small puncture wound while replanting rose bushes 1 week earlier. She has repeatedly cleaned and dressed the wound with antibiotic treatment, with no success. The physician collects an aspirate from the abscess. Gram stain reveals gram-positive cocci in clusters. Laboratory data follow:
Catalase: Positive
Coagulase: Latex positive

Multiple Choice Questions

Answers are in Appendix A.

1. From the patient's history and laboratory results, which organism is the most likely cause of the infection?
   a. *Micrococcus luteus*
   b. *Staphylococcus aureus*
   c. *Staphylococcus epidermidis*
   d. *Sporothrix schenckii*
2. What other clinical condition could arise from this injury if treatment were not initiated?
   a. No concerns; infections are self-limiting.
   b. Patient may develop a bacteremia, resulting in a more serious infection.
   c. Patient may develop necrotizing fasciitis, resulting in loss of a limb.
   d. Patient will become colonized and will have recurrent infections.

Critical Thinking Group Discussion Questions

1. What culture media would be appropriate for culture and identification of the suspected isolate? Why?
2. What antibiotics would be used to treat this infection? Could there be any treatment problems with this isolate?

Note: Narrative answers posted on EVOLVE instructor site.

REFERENCES

1. Centers for Disease Control and Prevention: *Division of Healthcare Quality Promotion, National Center for Preparedness, Detection, and Control of Infectious Diseases: Healthcare-associated infections (HAIs),* http://www.cdc.gov/HAI/burden.html.
2. Centers for Disease Control and Prevention: *Division of Healthcare Quality Promotion, National Center for Preparedness, Detection, and Control of Infectious Diseases: Community-associated MRSA,* http://www.cdc.gov/HAI/organisms/organisms.html#s.
3. Centers for Disease Control and Prevention: National Select Agent Registry. http://www.selectagents.gov. Accessed April 1, 2014.
4. Versalovic J: *Manual of clinical microbiology, ed 10,* Washington, DC, 2011, ASM Press.
5. Department of Energy: *Specification for HEPA filters used by DOE contractors, DOE-STD 3020-97,* Washington, DC, 1997, US Department of Energy.
6. Clinical and Laboratory Standards Institute: *Quality control for commercially prepared microbiological culture media: approved standard, ed 3, CLSI Document M22-A3,* Wayne, Pa, 2004, Clinical and Laboratory Standards Institute.

7. Pezzlo MT: Laboratory diagnosis of urinary tract infections: current concepts and controversies, *Infect Dis Clin Pract* 2(469), 1993.
8. Tille PM: *Bailey and Scott's diagnostic microbiology, ed 13,* St Louis, 2014, Mosby.
9. Clinical and Laboratory Standards Institute: *Principles and procedures for blood cultures: approved guideline, CLSI Document M47-A,* Wayne, Pa, 2007, Clinical and Laboratory Standards Institute.
10. Emergency Nurses Association: Clinical practice guideline: prevention of blood culture contamination, December 2012, Accessed April 1, 2014.
11. Clinical and Laboratory Standards Institute: *Analysis and presentation of cumulative antimicrobial susceptibility test data: approved standard,* CLSI Document M39:A3, Wayne, Pa, 2013, Clinical and Laboratory Standards Institute.
12. Clinical and Laboratory Standards Institute: *Performance standards for antimicrobial disk susceptibility tests: approved standard, CLSI Document M02-A10,* Wayne, Pa, 2013, Clinical and Laboratory Standards Institute.
13. Bondi A, Spaulding EH, Smith ED, et al: A routine method for the rapid determination of susceptibility to penicillin and other antibiotics, *Am J Med Sci* 214:221, 1947.
14. Bauer AW, Kirby WWM, Sherris JC, et al: Antibiotic susceptibility testing by a standardized single disc method, *Am J Clin Pathol* 45:493, 1966.
15. Singha N, Kuman M, Kanaujia PK, Virdi JS: MALDI-TOF mass spectrometry: an emerging technology for microbial identification and diagnosis, *Front Microbiol* 6:791, 2015.

BIBLIOGRAPHY

American Proficiency Institute: Future testing for enteric pathogens, APIM153887151, http://www.ascp.org. Accessed May 2017.

Bourbeau PP, Ledeboer NA: Automation in clinical microbiology, *J Clin Microbiol* 51(6):1658–1665, 2013.

Clinical and Laboratory Standards Institute: *Performance standards for antimicrobial disk susceptibility testing, CLSI Document M02-A10,* Wayne, Pa, 2013, Clinical and Laboratory Standards Institute.

Ford A: No perfect approach to detecting *C. dif* infection, *CAP TODAY* 31(5), 2017.

Gen-Probe: *Package insert, APTIMA Combo 2 assay,* San Diego, 2009, Gen-Probe.

Gen-Probe: *Package insert, PACE 2 assay,* San Diego, 2008, Gen-Probe.

Kirkwood J: Automation and the future of microbiology laboratories, *J Clin Microbiol* 54(4):620–624, 2016.

Larone DH: *Medically important fungi, ed 4,* Washington, DC, 2002, ASM Press.

Murray PR, Rosenthal KS, Pfaller MA: *Medical microbiology,* ed 5, St Louis, 2005, Elsevier Mosby.

Paxton A: In flu season management, POC molecular to the fore, *CAP TODAY* 31(5), 2017.

Tille PM: *Bailey and Scott's diagnostic microbiology, ed 13,* St Louis, 2014, Mosby.

Valdez M: How MALDI-TOF MS has changed the microbiology, *Med Lab Observer (MLO)* 49(6), 2017.

Versalovic J, Caroll KC, Funke G, et al: *Manual of clinical microbiology, ed 10,* Washington, DC, 2011, ASM Press.

REVIEW QUESTIONS (ANSWERS IN APPENDIX A)

Introduction to Microorganisms

1. Host microbiota:
   - **a.** Interact with the immune system
   - **b.** Challenge the immune system
   - **c.** Disrupt the usually present microorganisms
   - **d.** Compete for available vitamins
2. The term *probiotic* refers to:
   - **a.** Bacteria that provide health benefits
   - **b.** Viruses that provide health benefits
   - **c.** Antagonistic bacteria
   - **d.** Antagonistic parasites
3. Areas of the body or body fluids that should lack microbiota are:
   - **a.** Large intestine and urinary bladder
   - **b.** Throat and small intestine
   - **c.** Cerebrospinal fluid and blood
   - **d.** Skin and blood
4. The term *pathogen* refers to:
   - **a.** Disease-causing microorganisms
   - **b.** Cancer-causing agents
   - **c.** Health care–associated infections
   - **d.** Community-associated infections
5. An opportunistic microorganism can cause infections:
   - **a.** In healthy individuals
   - **b.** In a person with an intact immune system
   - **c.** If the immune system is damaged
   - **d.** Only caused by parasites
6. The Gram stain is based on the chemical composition of:
   - **a.** The nucleus of a microorganism
   - **b.** A viral shell
   - **c.** A bacterial cell wall
   - **d.** a Parasitic cell wall

Classification of Microorganisms: Taxonomy

7. In the microorganism *Streptococcus pyogenes,* the term *Streptococcus* designates the:
   - **a.** Kingdom
   - **b.** Family
   - **c.** Genus
   - **d.** Species

Protection of Laboratory Personnel and Good Laboratory Practices

8. Biosafety Level 2 agents:
   - **a.** Have a low risk of causing disease in healthy adults
   - **b.** Are most often identified in patient specimens in the routine microbiology laboratory and pose a moderate threat to a healthy adult

c. Require laboratory personnel to have specific training in handling pathogenic and potentially lethal agents
d. Pose a high risk of aerosol transmission, are frequently fatal, and have no treatment or vaccine

9. Microbiology laboratory-acquired infections from an aerosol:
a. Occur in persons who are new to the job
b. Can occur from an accidental needle puncture wound
c. Can cause disease with an organism of low infectivity
d. Are associated with improper venting of air in the laboratory setting

10. Prevention of aerosolization can best be accomplished by:
a. Disinfecting the work areas with a bleach solution
b. Using puncture-proof sharps discard containers
c. Using a biological safety cabinet when working with specimens
d. Discarding all specimen-contaminated materials in a biohazard bag

11. Sterilization refers to:
a. Process of killing or destroying all microorganisms, including bacterial spores
b. Process of destroying pathogenic organisms, but not necessarily all microorganisms or bacterial spores (endospores)
c. Process used to decrease the number of microorganisms that are present on the skin
d. Process of cleaning laboratory work surfaces daily

Specimens for Microbiological Examination

12. If specimen processing for culture or other testing is delayed, which method provides a safe method for temporary storage of most pathogenic organisms or specimens until they can be cultured or tested?
a. Refrigeration at 4°C to 6°C
b. Refrigeration at 0°C to 4°C
c. Incubation at 37°C
d. Incubation at 56°C

Basic Equipment and Techniques Used in Microbiology

13. A colony is:
a. A growth of bacteria that results from a single bacterium
b. A diversified group of bacteria
c. Gram-positive bacteria
d. Viruses growing in liquid culture

Identification of Bacteria

14. Media that contain dyes, antibiotics, or other chemical compounds that inhibit certain bacteria while allowing others to grow are called:
a. Enrichment media
b. Differential media
c. Supportive media
d. Selective media

15. Media that contain factors such as carbohydrates that give colonies of particular organisms distinctive characteristics are called:
a. Enrichment media
b. Differential media
c. Supportive media
d. Selective media

16. Media that are used to permit the normal rate of growth of most nonfastidious organisms are called:
a. Enrichment media
b. Differential media
c. Supportive media
d. Selective media

17. Which of the following is *not* a selective medium?
a. CNA
b. Thayer–Martin agar
c. Sheep blood agar
d. EMB

18. Which of the following is used to promote the growth of gram-negative organisms while inhibiting the growth of gram-positive organisms?
a. MacConkey agar
b. Sheep blood agar
c. Thayer–Martin agar
d. Chocolate agar

19. Which of the following is used to promote the growth of *Neisseria gonorrhoeae* and *Neisseria meningitidis?*
a. MacConkey agar
b. Sheep blood agar
c. Thayer–Martin agar
d. Phenylethyl alcohol agar

20. Use of triple-sugar iron agar or Kligler iron agar can identify all of the following characteristics of members of the Enterobacteriaceae family (common enteric intestinal pathogens) *except* which one?
a. Ability to ferment gas from sugars
b. Ability to produce hydrogen sulfide gas
c. Ability to produce ammonia
d. Ability to ferment lactose

21. Pathogenic *Shigella* spp. characteristically are:
a. Non–lactose fermenters
b. Lactose fermenters
c. Coagulase positive
d. Oxidase positive

22. MacConkey agar is quantitatively inoculated with a urine specimen and incubated appropriately. Results are 100,000 CFU/mL urine of gram-negative lactose-fermenting organisms. Which of the following would be statistically the most likely organism to cause this urinary tract infection?
a. *Escherichia coli*
b. *Proteus* spp.
c. *Staphylococcus aureus*
d. *Klebsiella* spp.

23. What color are gram-negative bacteria after the decolorizing step in the Gram stain method?
a. Purple
b. Red
c. Purple-red
d. Colorless

24. Which of the following organisms can be recognized by its spreading growth appearance on sheep blood agar?
    a. *Escherichia coli*
    b. *Proteus* spp.
    c. *Staphylococcus aureus*
    d. *Klebsiella* spp.

Urine Cultures

25. Results of a urine culture are significantly more valuable for the diagnosis of a urinary infection when in conjunction with:
    a. Red blood cells
    b. Crystals in urinary sediment
    c. Leukocytes, particularly lymphocytes
    d. Leukocytes, particularly polymorphonuclear neutrophils

Throat Cultures

26. In culturing a throat specimen for group A β-hemolytic streptococci testing, which of the following media is preferred?
    a. Sheep blood agar
    b. HE agar
    c. MacConkey agar
    d. Chocolate agar
27. What is the purpose of making cuts in the sheep blood agar when a throat culture is plated?
    a. To count the colonies growing after incubation
    b. To observe the appearance of any hemolysis present
    c. To determine whether the organism is lactose positive or negative
    d. To note the morphologic appearance of the colony growth
28. In some people, untreated pharyngitis infections with group A β-hemolytic streptococci can eventually result in:
    a. Chronic pyelonephritis
    b. Acute pyelonephritis
    c. Chronic glomerulonephritis
    d. Scarlet fever
29. In observing a sheep blood agar plate inoculated with a sputum sample showing the presence of alpha or green hemolysis after incubation, what test can be done to determine whether the organism is viridians streptococci, part of the normal respiratory flora, or *Streptococcus pneumoniae?*
    a. Bile solubility test, in which most *S. pneumoniae* colonies would be dissolved by the reagent used and inhibited by an optochin disk
    b. Bile solubility test, in which most viridians streptococci colonies would be dissolved by the reagent used and inhibited by an optochin disk
    c. Bacitracin susceptibility test, in which most *S. pneumoniae* colonies would be inhibited by the bacitracin disk
    d. Bacitracin susceptibility test, in which most viridians streptococci colonies would be inhibited by the bacitracin disk
30. In identifying the presence of most group A β-hemolytic streptococci, versus those that are non–group A, which of the following tests can be done?
    a. Bile solubility test, in which most group A β-hemolytic streptococci colonies would be inhibited by an optochin disk
    b. Bile solubility test, in which most non–group A β-hemolytic streptococci colonies would be inhibited by an optochin disk
    c. PYR test, in which most group A β-hemolytic streptococci colonies would produce a bright-red color after addition of the PYR reagent to the filter paper
    d. PYR test, in which most non–group A β-hemolytic streptococci colonies would produce a bright-red color after addition of the PYR reagent to the filter paper

Genitourinary Cultures

31. Urogenital swabs to be cultured for gonococci should be plated onto culture media:
    a. Immediately; at the bedside preferably
    b. Within 2 hours of collection
    c. Within 4 hours of collection
    d. Within 24 hours of collection
32. "Clue cells" are best seen in which of the following specimens?
    a. Wet preparation of vaginal discharge
    b. Gram stain of vaginal discharge
    c. KOH—wet preparation of vaginal discharge
    d. KOH—Gram stain of vaginal discharge
33. What are the requirements for collection of an appropriate specimen for the detection of chlamydia?
    a. Examine the collected specimen while it is still fresh, when the organisms are still motile.
    b. First use a large swab to remove any secretions present, and then use a second swab to collect the specimen.
    c. Use the cellophane tape collection procedure on the skin area around the anal opening.
    d. Culture at the bedside is preferred, using chocolate agar and sheep blood agar.
34. What are the requirements for collection of an appropriate specimen for the optimal detection of *Trichomonas vaginalis?*
    a. Examine the collected specimen while it is still fresh, when the organisms are still motile.
    b. First use a large swab to remove any secretions present, and then use a second swab to collect the specimen.
    c. Cleanse the site carefully before any collection is done.
    d. Culture at the bedside is preferred, using chocolate agar and sheep blood agar.

Enteric Disease

35. The workup for a pediatric patient with diarrhea who is otherwise healthy should include:
    a. Fungi panel by PCR
    b. Bacterial stool culture or stool bacterial PCR panel for at least *Salmonella, Shigella,* Shiga toxin, and *Campylobacter* testing
    c. Parasite panel by PCR for *Giardia lamblia, Cryptosporidium, Cyclospora cayetanensis, Dientamoeba fragilis,* and *Entamoeba*
    d. Both b and c

36. A benefit of the matrix-assisted laser desorption ionization time-of-flight mass spectrometer (MALDI-TOF) in enteric disease is:
   a. Positive pathogen identification after only 6 to 9 hours
   b. Positive pathogen identification after only 9 to 12 hours
   c. Positive pathogen identification after only 12 to 18 hours
   d. Positive pathogen identification after only 18 to 24 hours

Blood Cultures

37. Progressive syndrome, septic shock, can occur in the blood because of release of:
   a. Endotoxins
   b. Exotoxins
   c. Part of the cell wall of gram-negative bacteria
   d. Either a or c

Wound or Soft Tissue Cultures

38. Wound infections can be classified into which three major areas?
   a. Superficial, artificial, and surface wounds
   b. Superficial, subcutaneous, and deep wounds
   c. Superficial, folliculitis, and abscess
   d. Superficial, burns, and ulcer

Bacterial Disease

39. The lowest concentration of antimicrobial agent that will visibly inhibit the growth of the organism being tested is known as the:
   a. Minimum inhibitory concentration (MIC)
   b. Minimum bactericidal concentration (MBC)
   c. Agar disk diffusion test
   d. Dilution test
40. When antibiotic therapy is needed, specimens for culture and organism identification should be collected:
   a. At any time because administration of antibiotics does not affect the tests
   b. While the antibiotics are being administered
   c. Before the antibiotics have been administered
   d. After the antibiotics have been administered
41. If the antibiotic does not inhibit the growth of an organism, the organism is said to be:
   a. Susceptible
   b. Sensitive
   c. Resistant
   d. Intermediate

Quality Control in the Microbiology Laboratory

42. Every laboratory handling biological material must:
   a. Have a biological safety cabinet for handling hazardous specimens and organisms.
   b. Check the media with cultures of known stock microorganisms.
   c. Compare the staining of microorganisms with pictures in the lab manual
   d. Both a and b

Mycobacteria

43. The most sensitive staining method for acid-fast bacilli is:
   a. Ziehl–Neelsen
   b. Kinyoun
   c. Fluorochrome
   d. Gram

Tests for Fungi (Mycology)

44. Which of the following antimicrobial agents is used to inhibit nonpathogenic fungi from growing in media that have been designed to promote the growth of pathogenic fungi?
   a. Penicillin
   b. Streptomycin
   c. Chloramphenicol
   d. Cycloheximide

Tests for Parasites (Parasitology)

45. The best method for finding pinworm organisms in children is:
   a. Ova and parasite (O&P) examination
   b. Rectal swab
   c. Cellophane tape collection
   d. Blood
46. Collection of fecal samples for identification of intestinal parasites should be done:
   a. After radiologic studies using barium sulfate have been completed
   b. Before radiologic studies using barium sulfate have been done
   c. In the morning, before the patient has bathed, defecated, or urinated
   d. Before the onset of an acute phase of the intestinal disease

Tests for Viruses (Virology)

47. Viruses differ from other types of microorganisms because they:
   a. Cannot replicate outside of another living host cell.
   b. Rely on host cell machinery to reproduce the viral particles for propagation, transmission, and infection.
   c. Have anaerobic oxygen requirements
   d. Both a and b

Automation

48. Automated microbiology systems have generally been designed to replace:
   a. Manual antibiotic susceptibility procedures
   b. Manual procedures that are repetitive and that are performed daily on a large number of specimens
   c. Manual procedures that are done infrequently but are labor intensive
   d. All manual procedures done in the microbiology laboratory

Turgeon: Linné & Ringsrud's Clinical Laboratory Science, 8th Edition

STUDENT PROCEDURE WORKSHEET 15.1

Differential Staining: Gram Stain

Student Learning Outcomes

After reading Chapter 15 in *Linné & Ringsrud's Clinical Laboratory Science: Concepts, Procedures, and Clinical Applications,* 8th edition, and at the completion of the laboratory exercise and review questions, the student will be able to:

- Explain the principle of the Gram stain reaction for gram-positive and gram-negative bacteria.
- Prepare and examine a Gram-stained smear for common bacteria.
- Complete the end-of-procedure review questions with a grade of 80% or higher.

Purpose

Differentiate bacteria based on the two main chemical cellular structures (gram-positive and gram-negative) using the Gram stain technique to visualize the cellular morphology and arrangement of the organisms.

Equipment, Supplies, and Reagents

1. Microscope slide
2. Sterile loop
3. Incinerator or Bunsen burner
4. Gram stain reagents
5. Microscope slides
6. Microscope
7. Immersion oil
8. *Staphylococcus* spp. (gram-positive) overnight growth on a 5% sheep blood agar plate
9. *Escherichia coli* (gram-negative) overnight growth on a 5% sheep blood agar plate
10. Sterile water
11. 95% methanol

Instructions for the Procedure

Read the list of required equipment and supplies and the procedural steps. Follow the procedural steps in exact order.

SEQUENCE	PROCEDURAL STEP	INSTRUCTOR-OBSERVED ACCEPTABLE PERFORMANCE (CHECK IF ACCEPTABLE)
1	Label two microscope slides; one as gram positive and the other as gram negative.	
2	Place a sterile drop of water on each slide.	
3	Sterilize the inoculating loop, and then take a single colony of one organism and place it on the appropriate slide. Using the loop, spread the organism in the water until the colony is emulsified and the smear is approximately the size of a nickel. Repeat with the second organism on the appropriate slide.	
4	Allow the slides to air-dry completely; you may use heat to fix the organisms to the slide and accelerate drying; however, excessive heating can distort the cell shapes.	
5	On drying, flood the slide with 95% methanol for 60 seconds; air-dry.	
6	Flood the fixed slide with crystal-violet stain and wait 10 seconds.*	
7	Rinse with water.	
8	Flood with Gram iodine solution and wait for 10 seconds.*	
9	Rinse with water.	
10	Decolorize quickly with the alcohol-acetone solution, or with 95% alcohol if the alcohol-acetone decolorization proves to be too rapid. Continue until no more color is extracted by the solvent. This usually takes 10 to 20 seconds,* but be careful not to overdecolorize.	
11	Rinse with water.	
12	Flood with safranin for 10 seconds.*	
13	Rinse with water, air-dry, and examine using the oil-immersion lens.	

*Times may vary depending on the laboratory's procedure, either 30 or 60 seconds.

Procedural Evaluation

Student's Name ______________________ Grade ________

Instructor's Signature ______________________ Date ________

Comments:

Turgeon: Linné & Ringsrud's Clinical Laboratory Science, 8th Edition

STUDENT PROCEDURE WORKSHEET 15.1

Differential Staining: Gram Stain

Review Questions

Student's Name ______________________________ Date ________________

1. What color does a gram-positive organism stain?

2. What color does a gram-negative organism stain?

3. Gram stain results should include the gram reaction based on color, the organism's cellular shape, and any unique patterns (for example, gram-positive cocci in clusters).

   What differences can be noted between the two organisms used in this exercise?

4. List the four reagents used in the Gram stain, and state the purpose for each reagent.

5. What would happen if the alcohol reagent was left on the Gram-stained slide too long? Explain.

Turgeon: Linné & Ringsrud's Clinical Laboratory Science, 8th Edition

STUDENT PROCEDURE WORKSHEET 15.2

Quantitative Urine Streak Plate

Student Learning Outcomes

See Chapter 15 of *Linné & Ringsrud's Clinical Laboratory Science: Concepts, Procedures, and Clinical Applications*, 8th edition, for a complete discussion of this procedure.After reading Chapter 15, and at the completion of the laboratory exercise and review questions, the student will be able to:

- Select and inoculate the appropriate media for a urine specimen.
- Explain the collection of an appropriate specimen for a urine culture, quantitatively plate, and interpret the results.

Purpose

Differentiate catalase-positive micrococcal and staphyloccal species from catalase-negative streptococcal species.

Equipment, Supplies, and Reagents

1. Urine: unknown organism
2. Appropriate plates for inoculation
3. Incinerator or Bunsen burner
4. 0.001- or 0.01-mL disposable calibrated loop

Instructions for the Procedure

Read the list of required equipment and supplies and the procedural steps. Follow the procedural steps in exact order.

SEQUENCE	PROCEDURAL STEP	INSTRUCTOR-OBSERVED ACCEPTABLE PERFORMANCE (CHECK IF ACCEPTABLE)
1	Ensure that the urine specimen is well mixed.	
2	Remove the disposable calibrated inoculating loop from the package, or if using a calibrated wire loop, sterilize the loop and allow it to cool.	
3	Insert the loop into the bubble-free surface of the specimen (see Fig. 15-20).	
4	Touch the loop to the center of the sheep blood agar and spread in a line across the diameter of the plate. Without resterilizing, spread the urine by zigzagging across the inoculum. Repeat the process on a MacConkey or EMB plate (see Fig. 15-14).	
5	Incubate the culture plates at 35 °C in an inverted position, top down, for 18 to 24 hours.	
6	Interpret results.	

(Continued)

Turgeon: Linné & Ringsrud's Clinical Laboratory Science, 8th Edition

STUDENT PROCEDURE WORKSHEET 15.2

Quantitative Urine Streak Plate

Review Questions

Student's Name ______________________ Date __________

1. What specimens would be appropriate for culturing if a patient presented with frequent and painful urination?

2. What specimens would be unacceptable for culture?

3. What types of media should be used for the isolation and differentiation of the common causative agents of urinary tract infections?

4. Calculate the number of colony-forming units per milliliter from the unknown culture provided by the instructor. The CFU/mL is calculated by multiplying the number of colonies on the plate by 100 if a 0.01-mL loop was used or by 1000 for a 0.001-mL inoculating loop.

5. What is the colony count of the unknown?

6. What is the significance of the colony count?

7. What are the criteria for the workup of organisms or consideration of the organism as a contaminant in a urine specimen?

Procedural Evaluation

Student's Name ______________________ Grade__________

Instructor's Signature ______________________ Date__________

Comments:

Turgeon: Linné & Ringsrud's Clinical Laboratory Science, 8th Edition

STUDENT PROCEDURE WORKSHEET 15.3

Collecting, Processing, and Plating a Specimen for Throat Culture

Student Learning Outcomes

After reading Chapter 15 *Linné & Ringsrud's Clinical Laboratory Science: Concepts, Procedures, and Clinical Applications,* 8th edition, and at the completion of the laboratory exercise and review questions, the student will be able to:

- Properly collect a throat swab.
- Process and plate the specimen for presumptive identification of *S. pyogenes* or other throat pathogens.
- Complete the end-of-procedure review questions with a grade of 80% or higher.

Purpose

Properly collect and plate a throat culture specimen to identify the bacterial organisms associated with a sore throat, particularly either to identify or to rule out the presence of group A β-hemolytic streptococci.

Equipment, Supplies, and Reagents

1. Sterile Dacron or rayon swab with plastic shaft
2. Tongue depressor
3. 5% sheep blood agar plate
4. 0.04-unit bacitracin disk
5. Inoculating loop
6. Incinerator or Bunsen burner
7. Gloves
8. Forceps

Instructions for the Procedure

Read the list of required equipment and supplies and the procedural steps. Follow the procedural steps in exact order.

SEQUENCE	PROCEDURAL STEP	INSTRUCTOR-OBSERVED ACCEPTABLE PERFORMANCE (CHECK IF ACCEPTABLE)
1	Assemble the needed supplies so that they are easily acceptable for use; put on gloves and open the end of the sterile swab distal from the absorbent material to avoid contamination.	
2	Ask the patient to open his or her mouth.	
3	Using a sterile tongue blade to hold the tongue down and a sterile swab to collect the specimen, take the specimen directly from the back of the throat, being careful not to touch the teeth, cheeks, gums, or tongue when inserting or removing the swab (see Fig. 15-4).	
4	The tonsillar fauces and rear pharyngeal wall should be swabbed, not just gently touched, to remove organisms adhering to the membranes. White patches of exudate in the tonsillar area are especially productive for isolating the streptococcal organisms.	
5	If transporting to the laboratory, the swab containing the specimen can be placed in a special container with transport media. Commercial collection sets containing both swabs and transport media are available. Streptococci survive on dry swabs for up to 2 to 3 hours and on swabs in transport (holding) media at 4 °C for 24 to 48 hours.	
6	The specimen container must be labeled with the necessary patient identification.	
7	Using the throat swab obtained from the patient, roll the swan onto one edge of the sheep blood agar plate, being certain to transfer as much of the specimen onto the plate as possible	
8	Sterilize the inoculating loop, and use it to streak the plate out from the inoculated area. The streaking is to isolate bacterial colonies (see Fig. 15-6). Using the loop, make three or four cuts into the agar, to observe hemolysis more readily after incubation.	
9	Using a sterile forceps, place the bacitracin disk in the center of the first quadrant, area on the sheep blood plate that was streaked using the swab. Press lightly on the disk to ensure it remains adhered to the agar, but do not push the disk down into the agar.	
10	Place the sheep blood agar plate in the incubator, lid down, for 18 to 24 hours at 35 °C.	

Turgeon: Linné & Ringsrud's Clinical Laboratory Science, 8th Edition

STUDENT PROCEDURE WORKSHEET 15.3

SEQUENCE	PROCEDURAL STEP	INSTRUCTOR-OBSERVED ACCEPTABLE PERFORMANCE (CHECK IF ACCEPTABLE)
11	Following incubation examine the cultures for β-hemolytic colonies.	
12	Examine the area around the disk. If there are β-hemolytic colonies inhibited by the bacitracin disk, the organism is presumptively *S. pyogenes*.	
13	If inadequate numbers of isolated colonies are present, perform a subculture. If additional pathogens are present, do appropriate testing for identification.	

Procedural Evaluation

Student's Name ______________________________ Grade __________

Instructor's Signature ____________________________ Date ___________

Comments:

Turgeon: Linné & Ringsrud's Clinical Laboratory Science, 8th Edition

STUDENT PROCEDURE WORKSHEET 15.4

Preliminary Differentiation of *Staphylococcus* spp. from *Streptococcus* spp

Student Learning Outcomes

After reading Chapter 15 in *Linné & Ringsrud's Clinical Laboratory Science: Concepts, Procedures, and Clinical Applications,* 8th edition, and at the completion of the laboratory exercise and review questions, the student will be able to:

- Perform and interpret biochemical enzymatic tests for the preliminary differentiation of *Staphylococcus* spp. and *Streptococcus* spp.
- Interpret hemolysis on a 5% sheep blood agar plate.

Purpose

Differentiate catalase-positive micrococcal and staphyloccal species from catalase-negative streptococcal species.

Equipment, Supplies, and Reagents

1. Microscope slide
2. Sterile loop
3. Incinerator or Bunsen burner
4. 30% hydrogen peroxide (H_2O_2)
5. Microscope slides
6. Overnight pure cultures of *Staphylococcus epidermidis* and *Streptococcus pyogenes* on 5% sheep blood agar, provided by the instructor.

Instructions for the Procedure

Read the list of required equipment and supplies and the procedural steps. Follow the procedural steps in exact order.

SEQUENCE	PROCEDURAL STEP	INSTRUCTOR-OBSERVED ACCEPTABLE PERFORMANCE (CHECK IF ACCEPTABLE)
1	Examine the two pure cultures provided by the instructor. Observe colonial morphology and hemolytic patterns of the organisms on the 5% sheep blood agar plate.	
2	Label two microscope slides, one as *Staphylococcus* and the other as *Streptococcus* spp.	
3	Sterilize the inoculating loop, and then take a single colony of each organism and place on the appropriate slide.	
4	Place 1 to 2 drops of the 30% H_2O_2 on each slide.	
5	Observe the reaction for the production of oxygen from the organisms, which appears as bubbles.	

Procedural Evaluation

Student's Name ______________________________ Grade _________

Instructor's Signature ___________________________ Date ___________

Comments:

Turgeon: Linné & Ringsrud's Clinical Laboratory Science, 8th Edition

STUDENT PROCEDURE WORKSHEET 15.4

Preliminary Differentiation of *Staphylococcus* spp. from *Streptococcus* spp

Review Questions

Student's Name ______________________________ Date ________________

1. What is the principle behind the catalase test?

2. Staphylococci and streptococci are differentiated by the catalase test. What constitutes a positive and a negative test?

3. What is the mode of action of the catalase test?

4. Record your observations from this exercise in the following table:

ORGANISM	HEMOLYSIS ON BLOOD AGAR	CATALASE TEST
Staphylococcus spp.		
Streptococcus spp.		

16

Immunology and Serology

http://evolve.elsevier.com/Turgeon/clinicallab

CHAPTER CONTENTS

LEARNING OUTCOMES

Overview of Immunology and Serology
- Define the term *immunology*.

Antigens and Antibodies
- Define the terms *antigen* and *antibody*.
- Describe the general characteristics of antigens.
- Explain the general characteristics of antibodies.
- Evaluate the characteristics and clinical activities of the five classes of antibodies.
- ❖ Diagram and explain the general configuration of an immunoglobulin G (IgG) antibody molecule.
- Define the term *immune complex*.
- Compare the terms *monoclonal* and *polyclonal antibodies*.
- ❖ Describe the production of monoclonal antibodies.
- Compare the characteristics of the four phases of an immune response.

Complement
- Explain the mode of activation and consequences of complement activation.

Body Defenses Against Microbial Disease
- Define the terms, microbiota, prebiotics, probiotics, synbiotics, and pathobionts.
- Describe the first line of defense against infection.
- Name and explain the components of natural immunity.
- ❖ Contrast the functions and activities of natural immunity and *adaptive immunity*.
- ❖ Correlate the cellular and humoral components of adaptive immunity.

Hypersensitivity
- Define the term *hypersensitivity*.
- Compare the basic differences among and give examples of types I, II, III, and IV hypersensitivity reactions.
- Define the term *immune complex*.

Types of Antigens and Reactions
- Discuss various types of antigens and associated reactions.

Cells and Cellular Activities of the Immune System
- Compare the three immunologically functional groups of leukocytes.
- Describe the five steps and general activities of phagocytosis.
- Compare various types of lymphocytes, and explain the function of each type.

Immunologic Disorders
- Compare examples of primary and secondary immune deficiency disorders.

Principles of Immunologic and Serologic Methods
- Describe the characteristics of agglutination.
- Explain the mechanism of particle agglutination.
- Name and compare the principles of latex agglutination, coagglutination, liposome-mediated agglutination, direct bacterial agglutination, and hemagglutination.
- Compare the characteristics of precipitation versus flocculation.
- Explain the action and application of lysis in serologic reactions.
- Compare the features and clinical applications of immunofluorescent assays, various enzyme immunoassays, polymerase chain reaction (PCR), Western blot, and DNA chip technology.

Specimens for Serology and Immunology
- Contrast the features of the two phases of testing for antibody levels.
- Define the term *antibody titer*, explain the procedure for the serial dilution of serum, and describe the clinical application of antibody titer.

Immunologicand Serologic Testing for Bacterial and Viral Diseases
- Integrate the pathophysiology and immunologic testing in infectious mononucleosis hepatitis and acquired immunodeficiency disorder.
- Explain the rationale for and outcomes of syphilis testing.

Autoimmune Disorders
- Integrate the pathophysiology and laboratory testing for rheumatoid factor (RF) in patients with rheumatoid arthritis (RA).
- Integrate the pathophysiology and screening tests for antinuclear antibody (ANA) in systemic lupus erythematosus (SLE).
- Perform each laboratory exercise and answer related questions.

Case Studies
- ❖ Analyze the patient history, clinical signs and symptoms, and laboratory data for the stated case studies, answer the related critical thinking questions, and conclude the most likely diagnosis.

Review Questions
- Demonstrate comprehension of the chapter content by completing the end-of-chapter review questions with a grade of 80% or higher.

Note
- • indicates MLT and MLS core content.
- ❖ indicates MLT (optional) and MLS advanced content.

KEY TERMS

acquired immunity
active immunity
adaptive immunity
agglutination
allergens
allergy
anaphylactic shock
antibody
antibody titer
antigen
autoimmune disorder
cell-mediated immunity
cytolysis
first line of defense
hypersensitivity
immune complex
immune response
immunoglobulins [Ig]
immunology
immunization
lymphocytes
microbiota
monoclonal antibody (mAb)
natural immunity
pathobionts
phagocytosis
plasma cells
polyclonal antibodies
prebiotics
precipitation
probiotics
prozone
serology
synbiotics
vaccine
zone of equivalence

OVERVIEW OF IMMUNOLOGY AND SEROLOGY

Immunology is defined as the study of the molecules, cells, organs, and systems. These immunologic mechanisms are responsible for the following:

- Recognition and disposal of nonself substances
- Response and interaction of body components and related interactions
- How the immune system can be manipulated to protect against or treat diseases

Serology is a division of *immunology* that specializes in laboratory detection and measurement of a specific antibody that develops in the blood during a response to exposure to a disease-producing or other type of antigen. Blood banking techniques use serologic methods to determine blood group antigens and antibodies in the blood of a patient or blood donor (see Chapter 17).

The function of the immune system is to recognize "self" from "nonself" and to defend the body against nonself substances. Nonself materials can be as diverse as life-threatening infectious microorganisms or a lifesaving organ transplant. Desirable consequences of immunity include natural resistance to, recovery from, and acquired resistance to infectious disease. A deficiency or dysfunction of the immune system can cause many disorders, such as acquired immunodeficiency syndrome (AIDS). Undesirable consequences of immunity include allergies, rejection of transplanted organs, and development of an autoimmune disorder, a condition in which the body attacks itself as a foreign substance, as occurs in insulin-dependent (type 1) diabetes and pernicious anemia.

Many factors, including the general health and age of an individual, are important considerations in the defense against disease. The ability to respond immunologically to disease is age related. Although nonspecific and specific body defenses are present in the fetus and newborn, many defenses are incompletely developed at birth, which increases the risk of developing infectious disease. Other factors that can influence body defenses are genetic predisposition to many disorders, nutritional status, and an individual's method of coping with stress.

ANTIGENS AND ANTIBODIES

An antigen is a substance that stimulates antibody formation and has the ability to bind to an antibody. Cellular antigens of importance in immunology are major histocompatibility complex tissue antigens (or human leukocyte antigens [HLA]), autoantigens, and blood group antigens. In most cases, the normal immune system responds to foreign antigens by producing antibodies. Antibody produced in response to the foreign antigen is found in the plasma and in other body fluids and reacts with the foreign antigen in some observable way. Antibody is usually specific for the antigen against which it is formed.

The significance of antigens and antibodies is basic to the study of immunity and immunology. Various microorganisms or other antigen-bearing sources have antigenic properties and elicit an antibody response when introduced into an immunocompetent host. The antibody formed in response to a foreign antigen such as a flu vaccination can protect an individual from subsequent infections by that specific antigen.

Foreign antigenic substances are recognized by lymphocytes and plasma cells. Each specific type of antigen stimulates the production of equally specific antibodies by various body tissues. If an antibody has been formed against a foreign antigenic substance, a good way to identify the infecting organism is to identify the antibody produced in response to it. This is the basis for immunologic and serologic determinations.

Antibodies produced in response to a specific antigenic stimulus can be identified in the serum. If a known antigen is combined with a patient's serum containing antibodies against a specific antigen, a reaction will be observed. The reaction takes different forms because of variations in the technique being used and the type of antigen being assayed. If a specific antibody is not present in the patient's serum, no reaction should be observed.

Nature of Antigens

An antigen is generally described as a substance that, when injected into an animal, is recognized as foreign and, provided immunologically active cells are present, provokes an immune reaction or response. As stated previously, this immune response is the production of antibodies, substances that usually protect the body against the foreign antigen. At times, antibodies are not protective and cause allergic reactions such as hay fever or anaphylactic shock. Antigenicity is not confined exclusively to proteins. Certain nonantigenic, nonprotein substances known as *haptens* may bind themselves to protein, and the resulting hapten–protein complex is antigenic.

Antigenicity is influenced by molecular size, foreignness, shape of the molecule, and chemical composition. In addition, the antigenicity of a foreign substance is also related to the route of entry. Intravenous and intraperitoneal routes are stronger stimuli than subcutaneous and intramuscular routes.

Characteristics of Antibodies

Antibodies are proteins produced in response to foreign antigenic stimuli. Whether a cell-mediated response or an antibody response takes place depends on the way the antigen is presented to the lymphocytes; many immune reactions display both types of response.

Antibodies (immunoglobulins [Ig]) are found in the gamma globulin fraction of serum or plasma. Some antibodies occur in humans naturally as a result of exposure throughout life to bacteria and plant material through inhalation and ingestion. Antibodies can also be produced in response to natural infections, such as typhoid fever organisms, or their production can be artificially stimulated by the injection of antigens in vaccine form. Newborns do not form antibodies but may have received them passively from the mother through the placenta. Infants begin forming antibodies at about age 3 months and usually have a normal gamma globulin level by 6 months. This is important when serum from newborns is tested for antibodies, such as testing for ABO blood groups.

When antibodies result from exposure to antigenic material from another species, they are referred to as *heteroantibodies.* When antibodies result from antigenic stimulation within the same species, they are referred to as *alloantibodies* or *isoantibodies.*

Classes of Immunoglobulins (Antibodies)

Five Ig classes of antibodies with different molecular weights and biological activity occur in human blood and body fluids: IgM, IgG, IgA, IgD, and IgE (Table 16.1).

TABLE 16.1 Immunoglobulins in Serum or Plasma

Immunoglobulin Class	Molecular Weight (Daltons)	Proportion of Total Immunoglobulin
IgA	160,000–500,000	13%
IgD	180,000	1%
IgE[a]	196,000	Trace
IgG	150,000	80%
IgM	900,000	6%

[a]Associated with allergic reactions to foods, pollens, etc.

Antibody Structure

All the immunoglobulins have a similar chemical structural configuration, as shown in Fig. 16.1. The common configuration consists of a monomer composed of two identical heavy chains and two identical light chains connected by disulfide bonds or bridges in the hinge region. The chemical structure of the heavy chains is responsible for the differences in the various classes of antibodies. Light chains are of only two types, kappa (κ) and lambda (λ), and are common to all Ig classes.

Environmentally Stimulated and Immune Antibodies

Environmentally stimulated antibodies (sometimes called *natural antibodies*) appear to exist without intentional antigenic stimulus. Examples of environmentally stimulated isoantibodies in blood are the anti-A and anti-B antibodies found in the ABO blood group system (see Chapter 17). In contrast, immune antibodies are the result of stimulation by specific foreign antigens. Immune antibodies are also referred to as *unexpected antibodies* and are usually the result of specific antigenic stimulation. These antibodies can result from immunization through pregnancy, transfusion, or injection of transfused red blood cells (RBCs) bearing a foreign antigen (see Hemolytic Disease of the Fetus and Newborn, Chapter 17).

Production of Antibodies

The response to an antigenic or "foreign" substance is referred to as an *immune response.* An antibody response has the following four phases (Fig. 16.2):

1. Lag phase: no detectable antibody
2. Log phase: antibody titer increases logarithmically
3. Plateau phase: antibody titer stabilizes
4. Decline: antibody is broken down (catabolized)

Immunity is not immediate; when first infected, the person is ill or incapacitated by the disease. Antibodies require about 2 weeks to develop sufficiently, after which subsequent exposure to the antigen will elicit an effective secondary anamnestic antigen–antibody response, resulting in protective immunity.

Primary Response

When a foreign antigen is first introduced, the antibody cannot be detected immediately in the serum or plasma. It is observed about 10 to 14 days after antigenic stimulation, and the antibody titer (concentration of antibody) is greatest at about 20 days, after which it gradually decreases. This is known as the *primary response.* The subclass of antibody associated with the primary response is IgM.

Secondary Response

A second exposure to the same antigen creates a more rapid response. Detectable amounts of IgM appear first, followed by IgG antibody in the plasma or serum. A memory phenomenon elicited by the lymphocytes results in an immediate antibody response on the second exposure or subsequent exposures. This *secondary anamnestic response* also produces a higher and longer-lasting titer of IgG antibody. An anamnestic response differs from a primary antibody response in the following important aspects:

IgG
Antibody combining site
Light chain
Heavy chain
IgM

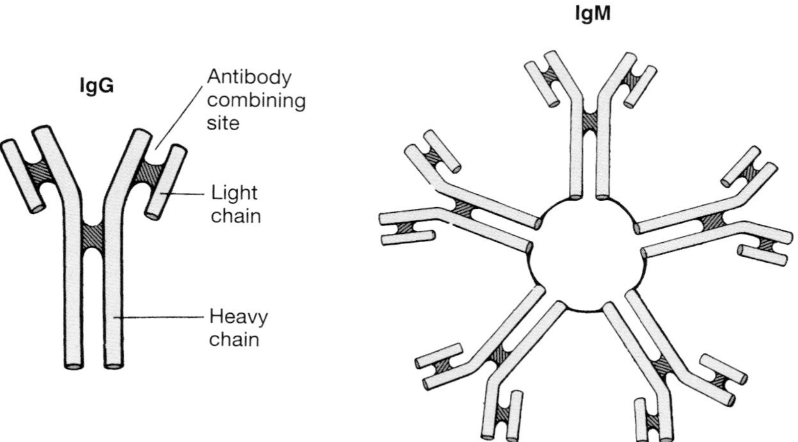

Fig. 16.1 Examples of antibody molecular structure. *Left,* Immunoglobulin G (IgG) is a simple monomer composed of two heavy chains and two light chains connected by disulfide bonds or bridges. *Right,* Immunoglobulin M (IgM) is in the form of a pentamer. Each monomer has reactive sites capable of combining with corresponding antigens.

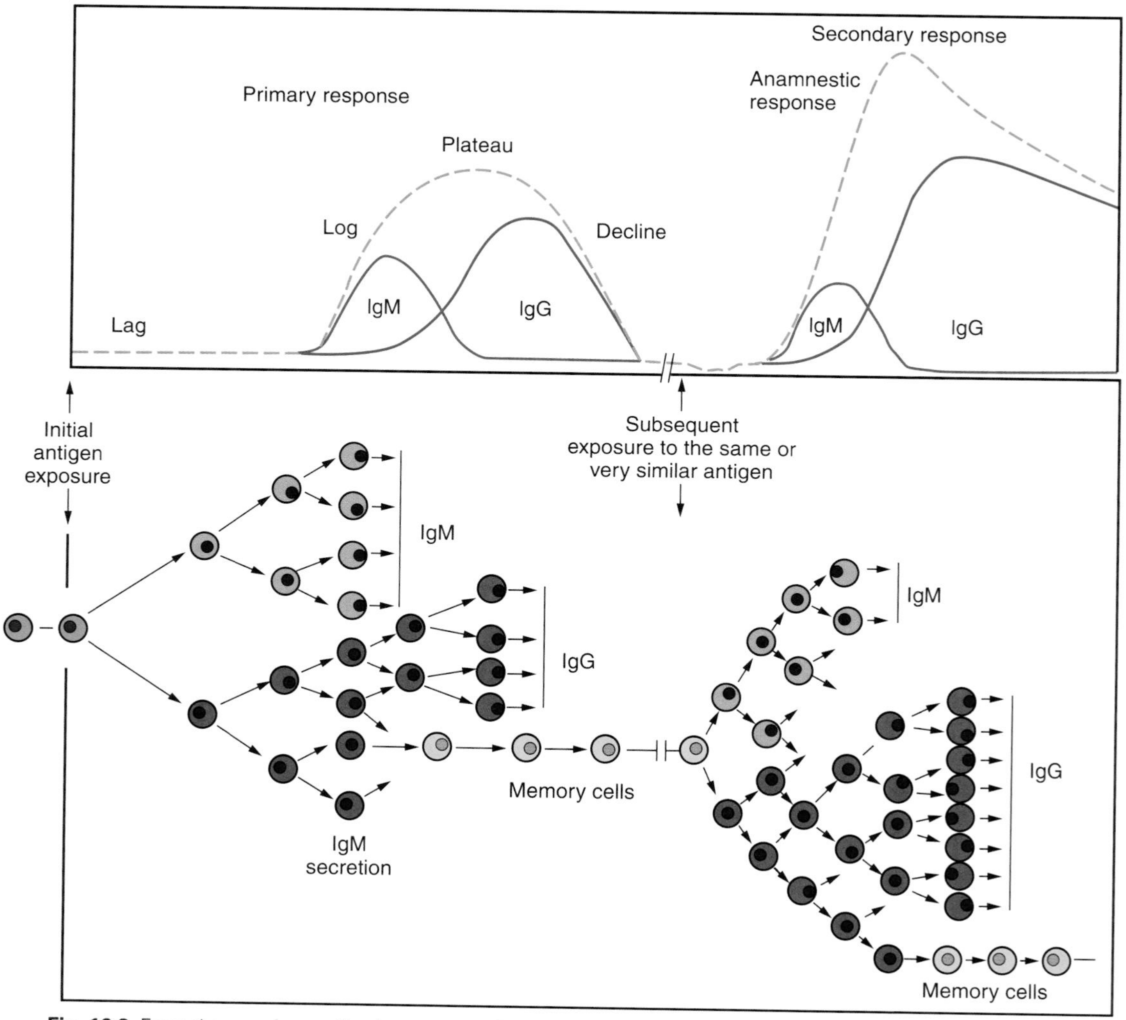

Secondary response
Anamnestic response
Primary response
Plateau
Log
Decline
IgM
IgG
Lag
IgM
IgG
Initial antigen exposure
Subsequent exposure to the same or very similar antigen
IgM
IgG
IgM
IgG
Memory cells
IgM secretion
Memory cells

Fig. 16.2 Four phases of an antibody response. Following an antigenic challenge, the antibody response in an immunocompetent person proceeds in four phases: lag, log, plateau, and decline. (Redrawn from Turgeon ML: *Fundamentals of immunohematology,* ed 2, Baltimore, 1995, Williams & Wilkins.)

- Time: a secondary response has a shorter lag phase, a longer plateau phase, and a more gradual decline in antibody titer than a primary response.
- Type of antibody: IgM-type antibodies are the principal class of antibody formed in a primary response. Although some IgM antibody is formed in a secondary response, the IgG class is the predominant type formed.
- Antibody titer: in a secondary response, antibody concentrations reach a higher titer. The plateau levels in a secondary response are typically 10-fold or more than the plateau levels in the primary response.

Immune Complexes

The noncovalent bonding of an antigen with its respective, specific antibody is called an **immune complex**. An immune complex may be small and soluble or large and precipitating, depending on the nature and proportion of antigen and antibody. Antibody can react with antigen that is fixed or localized in tissues or with antigen that is released or present in the circulation. In the circulation, an immune complex is usually removed by phagocytic cells. Under normal circumstances, this process does not lead to a pathologic consequence. In fact, it can be viewed as a major host defense against the invasion of foreign antigens. In unusual circumstances, an immune complex persists and is deposited in endothelial or vascular structures, where it causes inflammatory damage. This damage can occur in organs such as the kidneys in systemic lupus erythematosus (SLE) and other immunologic disorders.

Monoclonal and Polyclonal Antibodies

Monoclonal antibodies (mAbs) are purified antibodies cloned from a single cell. These antibodies exhibit exceptional purity and specificity; mAbs are able to recognize and bind to a specific antigen. They are secreted into the serum in large quantities when associated with a malignant proliferation of plasma cells or their precursors, as in multiple myeloma. Monoclonal antisera, produced by hybridization, are used as reagents in diagnostic testing because of their greater diagnostic precision. They are also used for cancer therapy.

Polyclonal antibodies are usually produced by immunizing animals with the antigen being studied and then isolating and purifying the antibody from the animal's serum. These antibodies are heterogeneous and lack the specificity of mAbs.

COMPLEMENT

Complement is a heat-labile series of 18 plasma proteins. Proteins of the classic activation pathway and their terminal sequence are called *components.* Normally, complement components are present in the circulation in an inactive form. When an antigen and matching antibody join one another, the classic complement activation pathway is triggered (Fig. 16.3). This cascading pathway results in the ultimate formation of the membrane attack complex, which disrupts cellular membranes.

The complement system is of importance in transfusion medicine because incompatible ABO blood transfusions can trigger complement and result in a hemolytic transfusion reaction. Complement components, such as C3 and C4, may be assayed as diagnostic testing for disorders such as SLE.

BODY DEFENSES AGAINST MICROBIAL DISEASE

Before a pathogen can invade the human body, it must overcome the general resistance provided by the body's immune system, which consists of nonspecific and specific defense mechanisms.

Microbiota

Our intestines harbor trillions of microorganisms known as **microbiota**, the human intestinal microbiome. In recent years, the enormous diversity, functional capacity , and age-associated dynamics of the human microbiome have been discovered. Various names have been given to the microbiome in human health and disease. Prebiotics are defined as nutrional substrates that promote the growth of microbes that confer health benefits in the host. Probiotics are considered to be live microbes that confer health benefits when administered in adequate amounts in the host. A combination of **prebiotics** and **probiotics** is named, **synbiotics**. In contrast, **pathobionts** are defined as typically, benigh endogenous microbies with the capacity, under altered conditions, to elicit pathogenesis.[1] Current research[1] suggests that host microbiota and the immune system interact to maintain tissue homeostasis in healthy individuals.

Microbiota regulate the following:

- Innate immune functions and homeostasis
- Adaptive immune functions in the intestines
- Systemic innate and adaptive immune functions

Disruption of the host microbiota, especially in the gut, has been shown to be associated with many autoimmune diseases

First Line of Defense

The **first line of defense** or first barrier to infection is unbroken skin and mucosal membrane surfaces (Fig. 16.4). These surfaces are extremely important because they form a physical barrier to many microorganisms. Normal biota, previously called *normal flora,* consists of bacteria that are usually found in certain parts of the body, such as the throat and intestines. These microorganisms deter penetration or facilitate elimination of foreign microorganisms from the body. Other types of first-line defenses against microbial invasion include secretions such as mucus, earwax (cerumen), lactic acid in sweat, stomach acid, saliva, and tears. The constant motion of the ciliated epithelial cells provides additional protection to the respiratory tract.

Second Line of Defense: Natural Immunity

Natural (innate or inborn) resistance is one of the two ways the body resists infection if microorganisms have penetrated the first line of defense. **Natural immunity** is characterized as a nonspecific mechanism. This second line of defense consists of particular cells (neutrophils, tissue basophils, macrophages) and soluble substances in the blood (complement, lysozyme, interferon). Neutrophils, monocytes, and macrophages can engulf invading foreign material such as bacteria. Complement proteins, soluble protein components, are the major humoral (fluid)

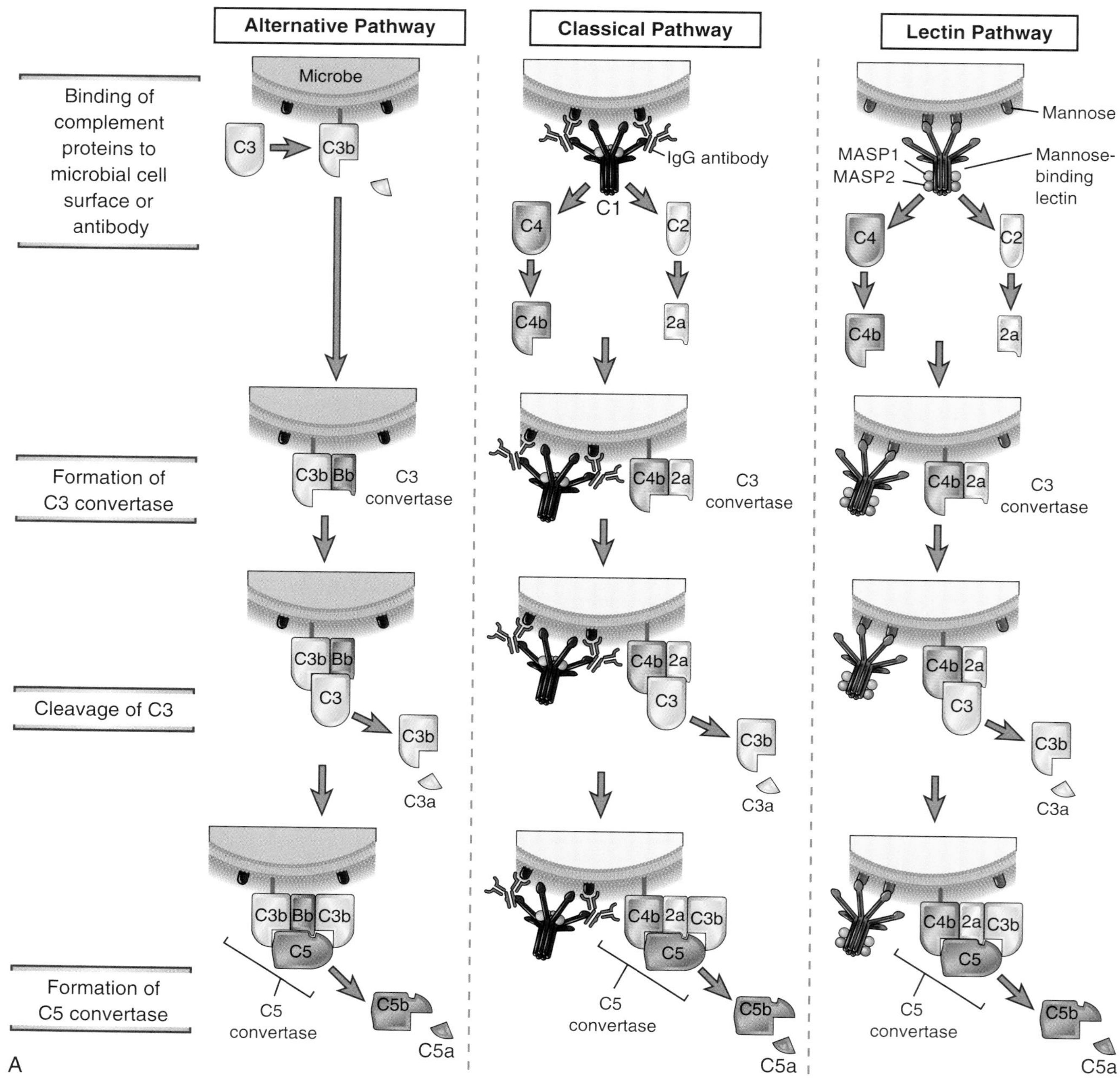

Fig. 16.3 (A) Early steps of complement activation. The steps in the activation of the alternative, classical, and lectin pathways are shown. Note that the sequence of events is similar in all three pathways, although they differ in their requirement for antibody and in the proteins used. The late steps of complement activation start after the formation of the C5 convertase and are identical in the alternative and classical pathways. Products generated in the late steps induce inflammation (C5a) and cell lysis (the membrane attack complex).

(Continued)

Protein	Serum conc. (μg/mL)	Function
C3	1000-1200	C3b binds to the surface of a microbe where it functions as an opsonin and as a component of C3 and C5 convertases. C3a stimulates inflammation.
Factor B	200	Bb is a serine protease and the active enzyme of C3 and C5 convertases.
Factor D	1-2	Plasma serine protease, which cleaves Factor B when it is bound to C3b
Properdin	25	Stabilizes the C3 convertase (C3bBb) on microbial surfaces.

B

Protein	Serum conc. (μg/mL)	Function
C1 (C1qr2s2)		Initiates the classical pathway; C1q binds to Fc portion of antibody; C1r and C1s are proteases that lead to C4 and C2 activation.
C4	300-600	C4b covalently binds to surface of microbe or cell where antibody is bound and complement is activated. C4b binds to C2 for cleavage by C1s. C4a stimulates inflammation.
C2	20	C2a is a serine protease functioning as an active enzyme of C3 and C5 convertases.
Mannose binding lectin (MBL)	0.8-1	Initiates the lectin pathway; MBL binds to terminal mannose residues of microbial carbohydrates. An MBL-associated protease activates C4 and C2, as in the classical pathway.

C

Fig. 16.3, cont'd (B) Late steps of complement activation. (C) The properties of the proteins of the late steps of complement activation are listed. Abbas AK, Lichtman AH, Pillai S: Cellular and molecular immunology ed.8, Philadelphia, 2015, Saunders.

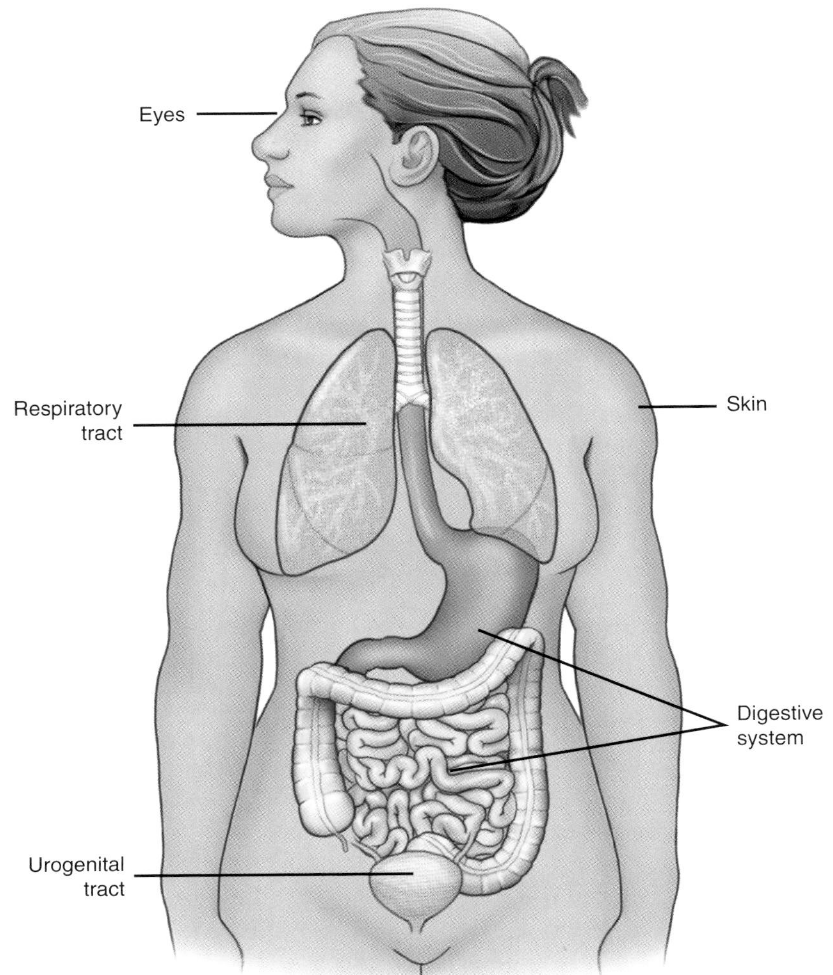

Fig. 16.4 First line of defense, nonspecific. Body fluids, specialized cells, fluids, and resident bacteria (normal biota) allow the respiratory, digestive, urogenital, integumentary, and other systems to defend the body against microbial infection. (From Turgeon ML: *Immunology and serology in laboratory medicine,* ed 5, St Louis, 2013, Mosby.)

TABLE 16.2 Acquired Immunity: Active and Passive

Type	Mode of Acquisition	Antibody Produced by Host
Active	Natural infection	Yes
	Artificial vaccination	Yes
Passive	Natural transfer in vivo or via colostrum	No
	Artificial infusion of serum or plasma	No

component of natural immunity. Lysozymes and interferon are sometimes referred to as *natural antibiotics.* Interferon is a family of proteins produced rapidly by many cells in response to viral infection; it blocks the replication of viruses in cells.

Third Line of Defense: Acquired or Adaptive Immunity

Acquired (adaptive) resistance forms a third line of defense that allows the body to recognize, remember, and respond to a specific stimulus, an antigen. The two types of acquired immunity, or adaptive immunity, are active and passive (Table 16.2). Active immunity can result from natural exposure in response to an infection or from an intentional vaccination with an antigen-bearing microorganism. Active immunity should stimulate the production of antibodies in a person with the disease.

Acquired immunity consists of cellular components (T and B lymphocytes, plasma cells) and humoral components (antibodies, cytokines) (Table 16.3). Lymphocytes selectively respond to nonself substances, or antigens such as in immunization reaction using a vaccine, which leads to immune memory and a permanently altered pattern of response or adaptation in immunocompetent individuals. The immunocompetent host is able to recognize a foreign antigen and build specific antigen-directed antibodies, retaining permanent antigenic memory.

The condition of cellular memory, acquired resistance, allows the body to respond more effectively if reinfection with the same microorganisms occurs. The actions of the adaptive response (cell-mediated immunity, humoral-mediated immunity) take place because of the interaction of antibody with complement and phagocytic cells of natural immunity and of T lymphocytes with macrophages.

Humoral-Mediated Immunity

The purpose of humoral-mediated immunity is to act as a primary defense against bacterial infection. If the reaction is natural and active, the person builds antibodies as the result of an infection with a microorganism.

The concept of vaccination, or deliberately introducing a potentially harmful microbe into a patient, promotes the building of antibodies after being vaccinated. Vaccines may be composed of living suspensions of weak or attenuated cells or viruses, killed cells or viruses, or extracted bacterial products, such as altered, formerly poisonous toxoids used to immunize against diphtheria and tetanus. Periodic booster vaccinations may be needed to expand the pool of memory cells.

If the reaction is natural and passive, a newborn receives antibodies in vivo or in colostrum produced by the mother. If the reaction is artificial and passive, a person receives antibodies by the infusion of serum or plasma made by another person.

TABLE 16.3 Acquired Immunity: Humoral and Cell Mediated

	Humoral-Mediated Immunity	Cell-Mediated Immunity
Mechanism	Antibody mediated	Cellularly mediated
Cell type	B lymphocytes	T lymphocytes
Mode of action	Antibodies in plasma soluble products	Direct cell-to-cell contact or secreted by cells

Cell-Mediated Immunity

Cell-mediated immunity is responsible for body defense (see discussion of type IV reactions in Hypersensitivity Reactions). Examples of cell-mediated immunity include the following:

- Contact sensitivity, such as poison ivy dermatitis
- Immunity to viral and fungal antigens
- Rejection of foreign tissue grafts

Under some conditions, the activities of cell-mediated immunity may not be beneficial. Immunosuppression, the suppression of the normal adaptive immune response through the use of chemotherapeutic drugs such as steroids or by other means such as radiation, may be necessary in autoimmune disorders or bone marrow transplantation.

Cell-mediated immunity is moderated by the link between T lymphocytes and phagocytic cells such as monocytes and macrophages. A T lymphocyte does not directly recognize the antigens of microorganisms. Recognition of an antigen takes place when the antigen is present on the surface of an antigen-presenting cell, such as a macrophage. Lymphocytes are immunologically active by various types of direct cell-to-cell contact and by the production of soluble factors such as cytokines.

HYPERSENSITIVITY

What Is Hypersensitivity?

Hypersensitivity can be defined as a normal but exaggerated or uncontrolled immune response to an antigen that can produce inflammation, cell destruction, or tissue injury. Immediate hypersensitivity is the basis of acute allergic reactions caused by molecules released by mast cells when an allergen interacts with membrane-bound IgE. Delayed hypersensitivity is often used synonymously with the term *cell-mediated immunity.*

The terms *immunization* and *sensitization* describe an immunologic reaction dependent on the host's response to a subsequent exposure of antigen. Small quantities of the antigen may favor sensitization. An unusual reaction, such as an allergic or hypersensitive reaction that follows a second exposure to the antigen, reveals the existence of the sensitization.

Hypersensitivity Reactions

The four types of hypersensitivity reactions are defined by the principal mechanism responsible for a specific cell or tissue injury that occurs during an immune response. Type I, II, and III reactions are antibody dependent, and type IV is cell mediated. Some overlapping occurs among the various types of hypersensitivity reactions, but there are major differences between each type.

Type I hypersensitivity reactions can range from life-threatening anaphylactic shock to milder manifestations associated with food allergies. Anaphylaxis is the clinical response to immunologic formation and fixation between a specific antigen and a tissue-fixing antibody. This reaction is usually mediated by IgE antibody. Several groups of agents cause anaphylactic reactions. The two most common agents are drugs, such as systemic penicillin, and insect stings, such as those inflicted by the common hornet, yellow hornet, and paper wasp. IgE-mediated adverse food reactions, as can occur with peanuts, can be fatal. Desensitization is a well-established technique to improve symptoms caused by specific allergens. If a patient has a history of life-threatening conditions, and if other treatment alternatives are unsatisfactory, desensitization is used to prevent anaphylaxis resulting from insect stings, such as those inflicted by yellow jackets.

Type II hypersensitivity reactions are a result of IgG or IgM binding to the surface of cells. Three different mechanisms of antibody-mediated injury exist in type II hypersensitivity, as follows:

1. Antibody-dependent, complement-mediated cytotoxic reactions are characterized by the interaction of IgG or IgM antibody to cell-bound antigen. This binding of an antigen and antibody can result in the activation of complement and destruction of the cell (cytolysis) to which the antigen is bound. Examples of antibody-dependent, complement-mediated cytotoxic reactions include immediate (acute) transfusion reactions and immune hemolytic anemias, such as hemolytic disease of the fetus and newborn.
2. Antibody-dependent, cell-mediated cytotoxicity depends on the initial binding of specific antibodies to target cell-surface antigens. Antibody binding damages solid tissues, where the antigen may be cellular or part of the extracellular matrix such as basement membrane.
3. Antireceptor antibodies disturb the normal function of receptors. Less often, antibodies may modify the function of cells by binding to receptors for hormones, such as in autoimmune thyroid disease. Hyperacute graft rejection is also an example of a type II hypersensitivity reaction.

Type III hypersensitivity reactions are caused by the deposition of immune complexes in blood vessel walls and tissues. Repeated antigen exposure leads to sensitization with the production of an insoluble antigen–antibody complex. As these complexes are deposited in tissues, the complement system is activated, macrophages and leukocytes are attracted, and immune-mediated damage occurs. Immune complexes are produced as part of the normal immune response and are usually cleared by mechanisms involving complement. The formation of immune complexes under normal conditions protects the host because these complexes facilitate the clearance of various antigens and invading microorganisms by the mononuclear phagocyte system.

Immune complexes can cause disease. SLE is an autoimmune disorder characterized by autoantibodies that form immune complexes with autoantigens, which are deposited in the renal glomeruli. As a consequence of this type III hypersensitivity reaction, inflammation of capillary vessels in the glomeruli of the kidneys develops.

Type IV hypersensitivity reactions, or cell-mediated immunity, consist of immune activities that differ from antibody-mediated immunity. Cell-mediated immunity is moderated by the link between T lymphocytes and phagocytic cells. Lymphocytes (T cells) do not recognize the antigens of microorganisms or other living cells but are immunologically active through various types of direct cell-to-cell contact and by the production of soluble factors. Cell-mediated immunologic events include the following:

- Contact sensitivity
- Delayed hypersensitivity
- Immunity to viral and fungal antigens
- Immunity to intracellular organisms
- Rejection of foreign tissue grafts
- Elimination of tumor cells bearing neoantigens

Human beings are capable of acute rejection of most transplanted foreign tissue. Acute rejection is characterized by cell mediated, possibly antibody cell-mediated cytotoxicity, rejection within 7 to 21 days as the predominant mechanism of action. The cause of rejection is development of a reaction to donor antigens from a genetically different individual of the same species, an allogeneic reaction. The major antigens to consider are A and B antigens of the ABO blood group system and the major histocompatibility complex (MHC) regions D,B,C, and A, or human leukocyte antigens (HLAs). HLA antigens are of primary importance in influencing the genetic basis of survival or rejection of transplanted organs. HLA matching is of value in organ transplantation and in the transplantation of bone marrow, peripheral blood stem cells, and umbilical cord blood cells.

No single satisfactory explanation exists for the success of tumors in escaping the immune rejection process. It is believed that early clones of neoplastic cells are eliminated by the immune response. Cells, rather than immunoglobulins, are believed to dominate tumor immunity. A tumor marker is a characteristic of a neoplastic cell that can be detected in plasma or serum. Markers may be useful in the diagnosis and selection of different treatment approaches, monitoring therapies, and determining prognosis. Tumor markers include carcinoembryonic antigen (CEA), alpha-fetoprotein, beta-human chorionic gonadotropin, neuron-specific enolase, prostatic acid phosphatase, and placental alkaline phosphatase.

Latex Sensitivity

Latex contact sensitivity in the health care setting has increased because of the increase in total exposure to latex. Latex contains low-molecular-weight soluble proteins that cause IgE-mediated allergic reactions. Once sensitized, an individual may experience allergic symptoms when exposed to any product containing latex. At-risk groups sensitized to natural rubber latex include 8% to 17% of health care workers, but less than 1% of the general US population demonstrates latex sensitivity.

Anaphylactic reactions to latex have been reported in persons who previously had experienced only irritant or allergic contact dermatitis. Direct skin contact with latex may cause a type I, or immediate-hypersensitivity, IgE-mediated reaction within 30 to 60 minutes of exposure. Certain fruits, such as bananas, chestnuts, kiwi, avocados, and tomatoes, show cross-reactivity, perhaps because of a similarity to a latex protein component. These foods have been responsible for anaphylactic reactions in latex-sensitive persons.

What Is an Allergy?

The term allergy originally meant any altered reaction to external substances. Antigens that trigger allergic reactions are called allergens. Common allergens include animal dander, pollens, foods, molds, dust, metals, drugs, and insect stings. Our basic understanding of allergies has evolved since the discovery of IgE in 1967. The most significant property of IgE antibodies is that they can be specific for hundreds of different allergens. Allergies are common and are increasing in prevalence in the United States, Western Europe, and Australia. Allergies also occur in families, although not necessarily the same allergy.

A term related to allergy, *atopy*, refers to immediate hypersensitivity mediated by IgE antibodies. The terms *allergy* and *atopy* are now often used interchangeably. Atopic allergies include hay fever, asthma, food allergies, and latex sensitivity.

TYPES OF ANTIGENS AND REACTIONS

Allergens are small-molecular-weight substances that can enter the body by being inhaled, eaten, or administered as drugs.

Hypersensitivity reactions can occur in response to different types of antigens, including environmental substances, infectious agents, food, and "self" antigens.

Environmental Substances

Environmental substances in the form of small molecules can trigger several types of hypersensitivity reactions. Dust can enter the respiratory tract, mimicking parasites, and stimulate an antibody response. An immediate hypersensitivity reaction associated with IgE, such as asthma, can result. If dust stimulates IgG antibody production, it can trigger a different type of hypersensitivity reaction, such as farmer's lung. Metals (particularly nickel) and chemicals can cause type I hypersensitivity reactions as well.

Infectious Agents

Not all infectious agents are capable of causing hypersensitivity reactions. The influenza virus can cause hypersensitivity, which results in damage to epithelial cells in the respiratory tract. Sometimes an exaggerated hypersensitivity reaction occurs, such as in the case of an influenza virus immunization.

Self-Antigens

A slight immune response to "self" antigens is normal and exists in most people. When this becomes an exaggerated response or when tolerance to other antigens breaks down, hypersensitivity reactions can occur.

Food Allergies

According to the National Institute of Allergy and Infectious Diseases (NIAID), food allergy is an important public health problem that affects adults and children and may be increasing in prevalence. The prevalence of food allergy in Europe and North America has been reported to range from 6% to 8% in children up to age 3 years. It is estimated that 5% of children younger than 5 years and 4% of teenagers and adults have food allergies.

The NIAID guidelines separate diseases defined as "food allergies" and include IgE-mediated reactions to food (food allergies), non–IgE-mediated reactions to certain foods (e.g., celiac disease), and mixed IgE and non-IgE disorders. Food allergy can cause severe allergic reactions and even death from food-induced anaphylaxis. Despite the risk, no treatment currently exists for food allergies: the disease can be managed only by allergen avoidance or treatment of symptoms. The diagnosis of food allergy may be problematic because nonallergic food reactions, such as food intolerance, are frequently confused with food allergy.

CELLS AND CELLULAR ACTIVITIES OF THE IMMUNE SYSTEM

The entire leukocyte (white blood cell [WBC]) system is designed to defend the body against disease. Each cell type has a unique function and in many cases acts in cooperation with other cell types. Leukocytes (WBCs) can be functionally divided into the general categories of (1) granulocytes, (2) monocytes and macrophages, and (3) lymphocytes–plasma cells.

Role of Granulocytes and Mononuclear Cells: Phagocytosis

The primary phagocytic cells are the granulocytic polymorphonuclear neutrophil leukocytes and cells of the mononuclear-macrophage system. Macrophages also participate in antigen presentation and induction of the immune response, as well as secretion of biologically active molecules.

The process of phagocytosis can be divided into the following steps (Fig. 16.5):

1. Chemotaxis
2. Adherence
3. Engulfment
4. Phagosome formation and fusion
5. Digestion and destruction

The physical occurrence of damage to tissues, either by trauma or microbial invasion, releases substances to initiate phagocytosis. Neutrophilic granulocytes continually circulate in the blood and can be found at the site of injury in less than 1 hour. Monocytes move more slowly; macrophages are embedded in the tissues or are wandering. Cells are guided to the site of injury by chemoattractants. Adherence brings the phagocyte in contact with the microorganism. On reaching the site of infection, phagocytes engulf the foreign matter and destroy it. Digestion is accomplished because granules of the phagocytes contain degradatory enzymes. Unfortunately, the release of digestive

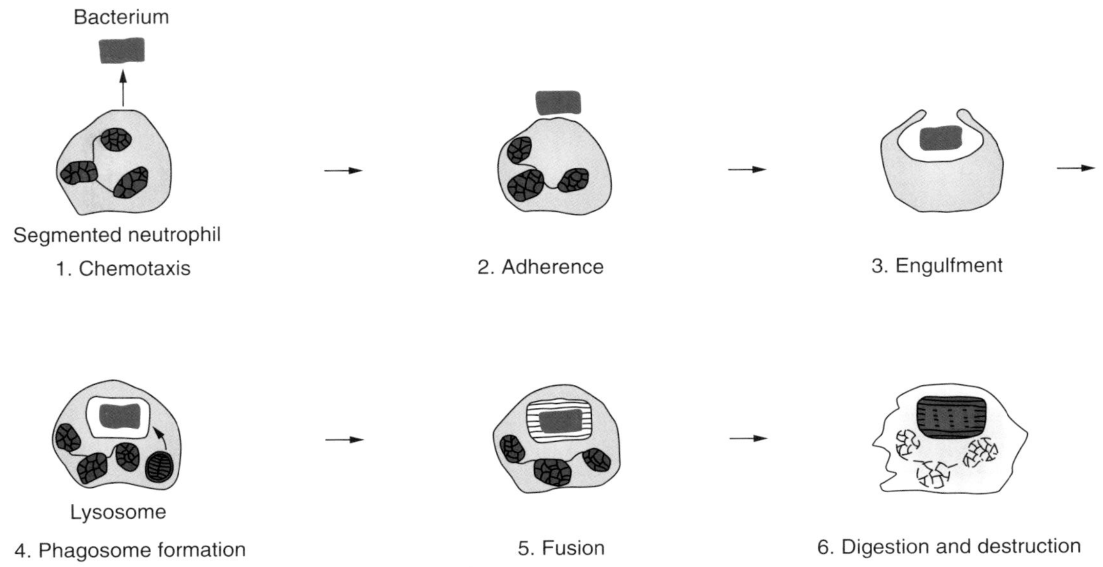

Fig. 16.5 Process of phagocytosis. (From Turgeon ML: *Clinical Hematology,* ed 5, Philadelphia, 2012, Lippincott, Williams and Wilkins.)

enzymes also kills the phagocyte in the process referred to as *cytolysis.*

If invading bacteria are not phagocytized and destroyed, they may establish themselves in secondary sites in the body, producing a secondary inflammation. If bacteria escape from secondary tissue sites, bacteremia will develop. If a patient is unresponsive to antibiotic therapy, this situation may be fatal.

Role of Lymphocytes and Plasma Cells

Lymphocytes are derived from a common stem cell in the bone marrow. T and B lymphocytes and plasma cells are the cornerstones of the immune system. Lymphocytes participate in body defenses primarily through the recognition of foreign antigen and production of antibody. About 80% of the lymphocytes circulating in the blood are T lymphocytes; about 20% of the circulating lymphocytes are B lymphocytes. Mature T lymphocytes survive for several months or years, whereas the B lymphocytes survive for only a few days. Plasma cells, not normally found in the blood, arise as the end stage of B cell differentiation into large, activated cells. The function of plasma cells is the synthesis and excretion of immunoglobulins (antibodies). Natural killer and K-type lymphocytes are a subpopulation of circulating lymphocytes.

T Lymphocytes

T cells arise in the thymus from fetal liver or bone marrow precursors that seed the thymus during embryonic development. These CD34+ progenitor cells develop in the thymic cortex. T lymphocytes function in cell-mediated immune responses such as delayed hypersensitivity, graft-versus-host reactions, and allograft rejection. They make up the majority of the lymphocytes circulating in the peripheral blood. In the periphery of the thymus, T cells further differentiate into multiple different T cell subpopulations with different functions, including cytotoxicity and the secretion of soluble factors, termed cytokines. Many different cytokines have been identified, including 25 interleukin (IL) molecules and more than 40 chemokines. Their functions include growth promotion, differentiation, chemotaxis, and cell stimulation.

B Lymphocytes

B cells are derived from hematopoietic stem cells by a complex series of differentiation events that occur in the fetal liver and, in adult life, in the bone marrow. B lymphocytes most likely mature in the bone marrow and function primarily in antibody production or the formation of immunoglobulins. B cells constitute about 10% to 30% of the blood lymphocytes. B lymphocyte differentiation is complex and ends in the generation of mature, end-stage, nonmotile cells, the plasma cells. Some activated B cells differentiate into memory B cells, long-lived cells that circulate in the blood. Memory B cells may live for years, but again, mature B cells that are not activated only live for days.

IMMUNOLOGIC DISORDERS

A breakdown in any part of the immune mechanism can lead to disease. Disorders with an immunologic origin can involve progenitor cells, phagocytosis, T cells, B cells, or complement.

Immunologic disorders can be divided into primary processes (dysfunction in the immune organ itself) and acquired, or secondary, processes (disease or therapy causing an immune defect). A third category, diseases mediated through immune mechanisms, can also be included.

Immunodeficiency disorders may be caused by defects in the quality (defects) or quantity (deficiencies) of lymphocytes and may be congenital or acquired. These conditions may be combined disorders or may involve T cells or B cells (Table 16.4).

Primary Immunodeficiency Disorders

Primary immunodeficiencies (PIDs) are rare genetic disorders of the innate and adaptive immune system. More than 120

TABLE 16.4 Disorders of T Cells and B Cells

T Cell Disorder	B Cell Disorder
Congenital	
Thymic hypoplasia (DiGeorge syndrome)	Bruton agammaglobulinemia
Acquired	
Acquired immunodeficiency syndrome	Autoimmune disorders
Hodgkin disease	Multiple myeloma
Chronic lymphocytic leukemia	
Systemic lupus erythematosus	

different gene mutations that cause impairment in the differentiation and function of immune cells have been identified, with different degrees of severity. Diseases associated with a primary defect in the immune response are the following:

- T cell disorders (40%)
- B cell disorders (50%)
- Phagocytic abnormalities (6%)
- Complement alterations (4%)

An important activity for the laboratory in this category of disorders is the measurement of IgG subclass concentrations is in the standard laboratory protocol for the investigation of a suspicious antibody deficiency. IgG is an important assay when the total IgG is with the normal age-specific reference range but the patient is symptomatic with repeated infections, particularly in pediatric patients. Measurement of IgG can support a diagnosis of specific antibody deficieny, confirm a diagnosis of common variable immunodeficiency, and facilitate risk stratification of patients with low IgA.

The most common T cell deficiency states are those associated with a concurrent B cell abnormality. Because the primary function of B cells is to produce antibody, the major clinical manifestation of a B cell deficiency is an increased susceptibility to severe bacterial infections. PID disorders are predominantly seen (75%) in children younger than 5 years.

Secondary Immunodeficiency Disorders

A secondary immunodeficiency can result from a disease process that causes a defect in normal immune function, which leads to a temporary or permanent impairment of one or multiple components of immunity in a patient. Patients with secondary immunodeficiencies, which are much more common than primary deficiencies, have an increased susceptibility to infections, as seen in the PIDs.

PRINCIPLES OF IMMUNOLOGIC AND SEROLOGIC METHODS

Principles of Agglutination

Agglutination and precipitation are the visible expression of the aggregation of antigens and antibodies through the formation of a framework in which antigen particles or molecules alternate with antibody molecules (Fig. 16.6). *Agglutination* (clumping) is the term used to describe the aggregation of particulate test antigens. *Precipitation* is the term applied to the aggregation of soluble test antigens. If a solution is allowed time

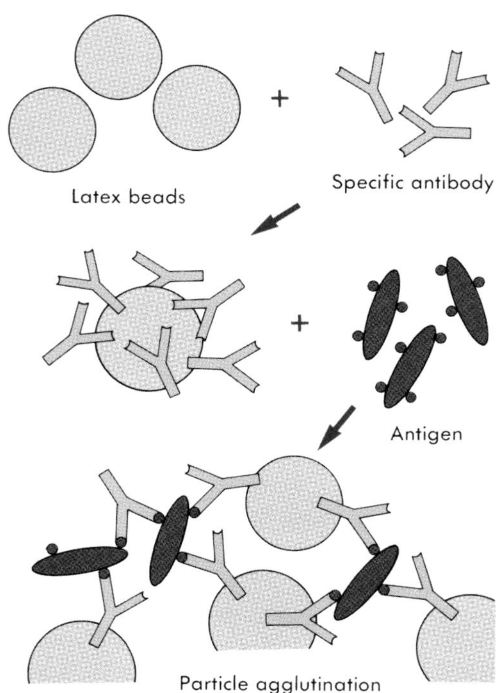

Fig. 16.6 Alignment of antibody molecules bound to the surface of a latex particle and latex agglutination reaction. (From Forbes BA, Sahm DF, Weissfeld AS: *Bailey and Scott's diagnostic microbiology,* ed 12, St Louis, 2007, Mosby.)

to settle in a test tube, precipitates (clumps) will fall to the bottom of the tube.

Agglutination occurs only if the antigen is in the form of particles such as bacteria, RBCs, latex particles (see Student Procedure Worksheet 16.1, C-Reactive Protein), WBCs, or any substance that appears cloudy when suspended in saline. Slide agglutination tests are performed less frequently than in the past and have been replaced by the immunoassay technique in most point-of-care tests.

Mechanism of Particle Agglutination

Agglutination is the clumping of particles such as erythrocytes that have antigens on their surface by antibody molecules that form bridges between the antigenic determinants. This is the endpoint for most tests involving erythrocyte antigens. Agglutination is influenced by a number of factors and is believed to occur in two stages: sensitization and lattice formation.

Sensitization

The first phase of agglutination, sensitization, represents the physical attachment of antibody molecules to antigens on the erythrocyte membrane. Physical conditions that affect the amount of antigen–antibody binding include (1) the pH, (2) temperature, (3) the length of time of incubation of the coated particles with the patient's serum (or other source of antibody), and (4) the antigen–antibody ratio.

pH (Hydrogen Ion Concentration). A pH of 7.0 is used for routine laboratory testing. It is known that some antibodies react best at a lower pH.

Temperature. The optimum temperature needed to reach equilibrium in an antibody–antigen reaction differs for different antibodies. IgM antibodies are "cold reacting," with a thermal range of 4°C to 22°C, and IgG antibodies are "warm reacting," with an optimum temperature of reaction at 37°C.

Length of Incubation. In laboratory testing, incubation times range from 15 to 60 minutes. The optimum time of incubation varies, depending on the Ig class and how tightly an antibody attaches to its specific antigen.

Lattice Formation

Lattice formation, or the establishment of cross-links between sensitized particles, such as erythrocytes, and antibodies, resulting in aggregation, is a much slower process than the sensitization phase. The formation of chemical bonds and resultant lattice formation depend on the ability of a cell with an attached antibody on its surface to come close enough to another cell to permit the antibody molecules to bridge the gap and combine with the antigen receptor site on the second cell.

Reading Agglutination Reactions

Observation of agglutination occurring in a test tube is initially made by gently shaking the test tube containing the serum and cells and viewing the lower portion, the button, with a magnifying glass as it is dispersed. Because agglutination is a reversible reaction, the test tube must be treated delicately, and hard shaking must be avoided; however, all the cells in the button must be resuspended before an accurate observation can be determined. The observer should also note whether discoloration of the fluid above the cells, the supernatant, is present. If the erythrocytes have been ruptured or hemolyzed, this observation is as important as agglutination.

The strength of agglutination, called *grading,* uses a scale of 0 or negative (no agglutination) to 4+ (all the erythrocytes are clumped) (Table 16.5 and Fig. 16.7). Pseudoagglutination, or false appearance of clumping, may rarely occur because of the presence of rouleaux formation. To disperse pseudoagglutination, a few drops of physiologic sodium chloride (saline) can be added to the reaction tube and the solution remixed and reexamined.

TABLE 16.5 Grading Agglutination Reactions

Grade	Description
Negative	No aggregates
Mixed field	Few isolated aggregates; mostly free-floating cells; supernatant appears red
Weak (+/−)	Tiny aggregates that are barely visible macroscopically; many free erythrocytes; turbid and reddish supernatant
1+	A few small aggregates just visible macroscopically; many free erythrocytes; turbid and reddish supernatant
2+	Medium-sized aggregates; some free erythrocytes; clear supernatant
3+	Several large aggregates; some free erythrocytes; clear supernatant
4+	All erythrocytes combined into one solid aggregate; clear supernatant

Microplate Agglutination Reactions

Serologic testing is now more often being performed with automated instruments as a microtechnique. Micromethods for RBC antigen and antibody testing are either hemagglutination or solid-phase adherence assays. These methods are also considered simpler to perform. Use of microplates allows for the performance of many tests on a single plate, which eliminates time-consuming steps such as labeling test tubes.

Immunofluorescent Assays

Immunofluorescent assays are popular methods for rapid antigen detection (see Chapter 6). A fluorescent substance, when absorbing light of one wavelength, emits light of another (longer) wavelength.

Fluorescent labeling is a method of demonstrating the reaction of antigens and antibodies. Fluorescent molecules are used as substitutes for radioisotope or enzyme labels. The fluorescent antibody (FA) technique consists of labeling antibody with fluorescein isothiocyanate (FITC), a fluorescent compound with an affinity for proteins, to form a conjugate. This conjugate is able to react with antibody-specific antigen. FITC emits a bright apple-green fluorescence when excited. FA techniques are extremely specific and sensitive.

Immunofluorescence can also be used to identify specific antigens on live cells in suspension (flow-cell cytometry). When a live, stained-cell suspension is put through a fluorescent active-cell sorter, which measures the fluorescent intensity of each cell, the cells are separated according to their particular fluorescent brightness. This technique permits the isolation of different cell populations with different surface antigens, such as various types of lymphocytes. Fluorescent conjugates are used in the basic methods of direct immunofluorescent assay (DFA) and indirect immunofluorescent assay (IFA).

Direct Immunofluorescent Assay

In the direct technique, a conjugated antibody is used to detect antigen–antibody reactions that can be seen with a fluorescent microscope. This technique can be applied to tissue sections or in smears for microorganisms. In DFA, the antigen-specific labeled antibody is applied to the fixed specimen, incubated, and washed. A counterstain may be applied as a last step before viewing the slide with a fluorescence microscope.

Indirect Immunofluorescent Assay

The serologic method most widely used for the detection of diverse antibodies is the IFA. The indirect method is based on the fact that antibodies (immunoglobulins) not only react with homologous antigens but also can act as antigens and react with antiimmunoglobulins.

If the specific antibody in question is present in the serum, the antibody will bind to the specific antigen. To remove any unbound antibody, the slide is washed. In the second part of this process, antihuman globulin that has been conjugated to the fluorescent dye is placed on the slide. The conjugated marker

READING AGGLUTINATION

GRADE	DESCRIPTION		APPEARANCE	
	Cells	Supernate	Macroscopic*	Microscopic†
0	No agglutinates	Dark, turbid, homogeneous	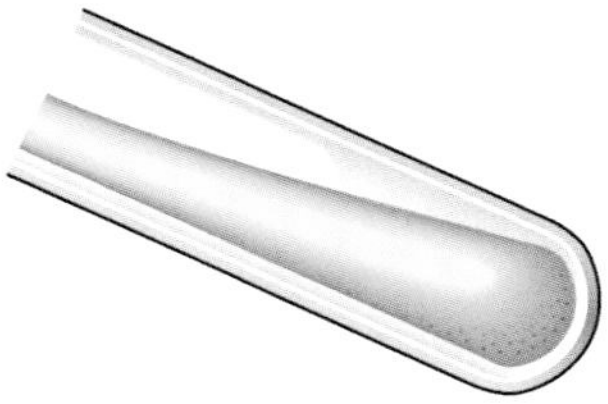	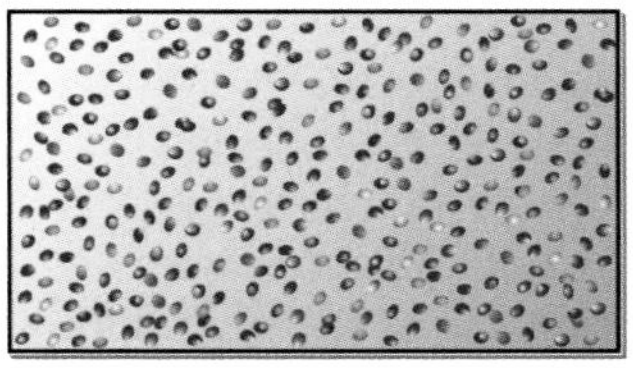
w+	Many tiny agglutinates Many free cells May not be visible without microscope	Dark, turbid	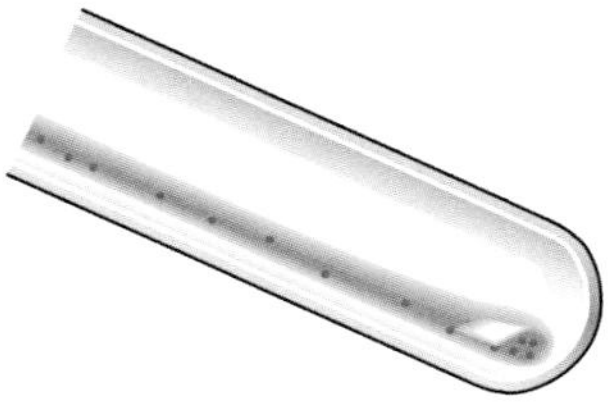	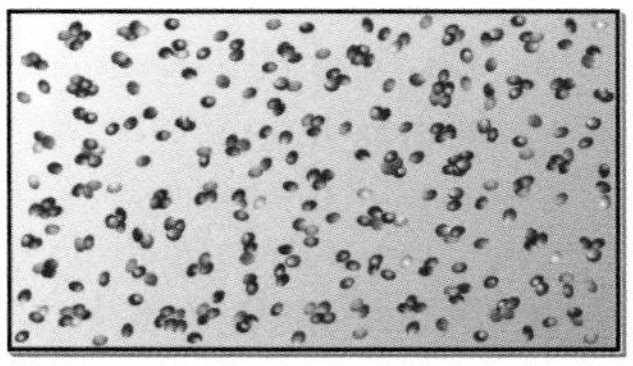
1+	Many small agglutinates Many free cells	Turbid	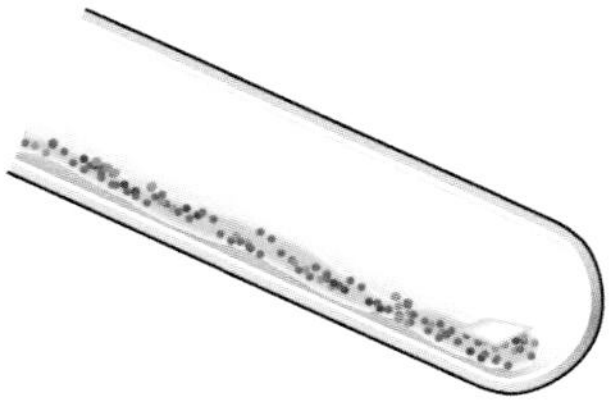	
2+	Many medium-sized agglutinates Moderate number of free cells	Clear	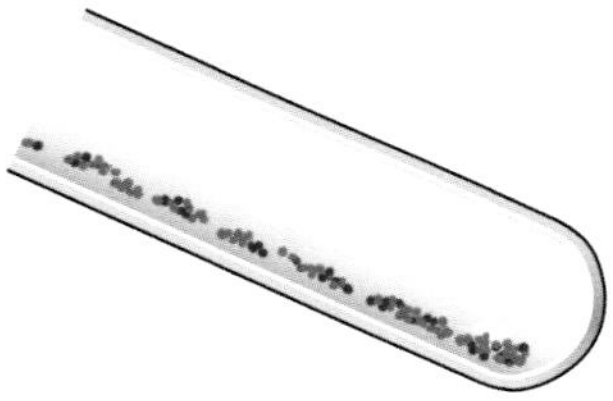	
3+	Several large agglutinates Few free cells	Clear	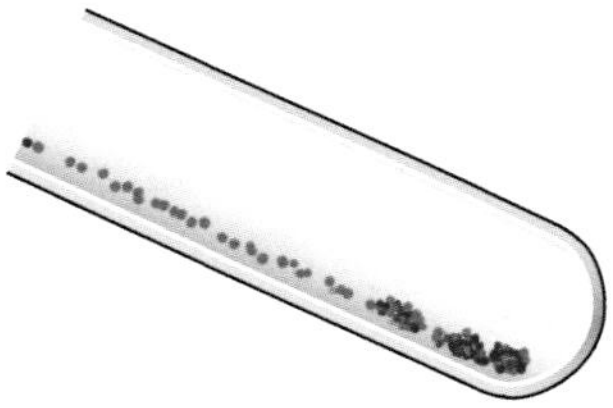	
4+	One large, solid agglutinate No free cells	Clear	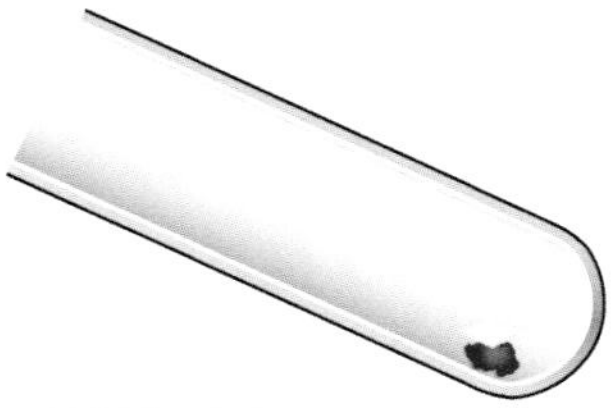	

*For any one grade, readings can be on a scale from weak + to strong + (e.g., grade 2 can be stored as 2+w, 2+, or 2+s, depending on the number and size of agglutinates).
† Microscopic readings are generally performed to differentiate pseudoagglutination (rouleaux) from true agglutination, to detect mixed-field reactions, and to confirm a negative reaction.

Fig. 16.7 Reading red blood cell agglutination reactions. (From Lehman CA: *Saunders manual of clinical laboratory science,* Philadelphia, 1998, Saunders.)

will bind to any antibody already bound to the antigen on the slide. This will serve as a marker for the antibody when the slide is viewed under a fluorescence microscope. The dye marker fluoresces apple green. If antibody is absent, the antihuman globulin dye marker will be removed during the washing procedure, and no fluorescence will be seen. As with DFA, a counterstain may be applied as a last step before viewing the slide with a fluorescence microscope. The fluorescence does not fade appreciably for a few days if the stained slides have coverslips applied with a drop of buffered glycerol and if the slides are kept refrigerated in the dark. It is best to examine the prepared slides immediately after staining.

Other Labeling Techniques

Chemiluminescence is being pursued as the technology of choice by most immunodiagnostics manufacturers. Chemiluminescence has excellent sensitivity and dynamic range. In immunoassays, chemiluminescent labels can be attached to an antigen or an antibody. Chemiluminescent labels are being used to detect proteins, viruses, oligonucleotides, and nucleic acid sequences.

Other labeling technologies include quantum dots (Q dots), squid technology, luminescent oxygen channeling immunoassay, fluorescent in situ hybridization, signal amplification techniques, and magnetic labeling technology.

Enzyme Immunoassays

Enzyme immunoassay (EIA) provides an alternative to immunofluorescent assays. Rather than tagging an antibody with a fluorochrome, EIA uses enzyme molecules that can be conjugated to specific monoclonal or polyclonal antibodies. This type of testing includes the enzyme-linked immunosorbent assay (ELISA). EIA is a popular method for waived over-the-counter testing.

The EIA method uses a nonisotopic label, which offers the advantage of safety and demonstrates specificity, sensitivity, and rapidity. Some EIA procedures provide diagnostic information and measure immune status, such as detecting either total antibody IgM or IgG. EIAs can detect extremely small quantities of antigen–antibody reactants. The conversion of a colorless substrate to a colored product allows for either visual or colorimetric detection.

Direct and Indirect Sandwich Technique

One type of EIA method involves the use of a direct or indirect sandwich technique. If the target antigen is present in a specimen, it will form a stable complex with the antibody bound to the matrix. Unbound specimen is removed by washing, and a second antibody specific for the antigen is added. In the direct method, the second antibody is conjugated to an enzyme. In the indirect method, a second nonconjugated antibody is added and washed, and a third antibody that is specific for the second antibody is added. The third antibody is conjugated to the enzyme and directed against the Fc portion of the unlabeled second antibody.

Membrane-Bound Technique

Most commercially developed EIA applications require physical separation of the specific antigens from nonspecific complexes found in clinical samples. If the antibody directed toward the agent being assayed is fixed firmly to a solid matrix, either to the inside of the wells of a microdilution tray or to the outside of a spherical plastic or metal bead or some other solid matrix, the system is called a *solid-phase immunosorbent assay (SPIA).*

A modification of SPIA uses a disposable plastic cassette consisting of the antibody-bound membrane and a small chamber to which the specimen can be added. An absorbent material is placed below the membrane to wick the liquid reactants through the membrane. This helps separate nonreacted components from the antigen–antibody complexes being studied. Flow-through EIAs are popular for influenza and group A *Streptococcus* testing because they are easy to use.

Optical Immunoassays

Optical immunoassays rely on the alteration of the thickness of inert surfaces resulting from the interaction of antigen–antibody complexes. The increased thickness causes the surface to appear a different color to the naked eye. This method of testing is used for detection of group A *Streptococcus* and influenza A.

Molecular Techniques

Beginning with polymerase chain reaction (PCR), an in vitro method to amplify low levels of specific deoxyribonucleic acid (DNA) sequences in a sample to higher quantities suitable for further analysis, molecular techniques continue to find new clinical applications. PCR analysis can lead to the detection of gene mutations that signify the early development of cancer; identification of viral DNA associated with specific cancers, such as human papillomavirus, a causative agent in cervical cancer; and detection of genetic mutations associated with a wide variety of diseases.

The *Southern blot* is used to detect DNA and ribonucleic acid (RNA), respectively. Single-base mutations that can be determined by Southern blot include sickle cell anemia and hemophilia A. The derivation of this technique from the Southern blot used for DNA detection has led to the common use of the term *Northern blot* for the detection of specific messenger RNA. The Northern blot is not routinely used in clinical molecular diagnostic techniques.

Western blot (WB) is a technique in which proteins are separated electrophoretically, transferred to membranes, and identified through the use of labeled antibodies specific for the protein of interest. WB is used to detect antibodies to specific epitopes. Specific assays using the WB technology are used to detect antibodies to human immunodeficiency virus (HIV), the causative agent of AIDS. Before an HIV result using a screening EIA is considered positive, the result should be confirmed by the use of at least one additional test. A current standard test for confirming positive HIV-1 tests uses WB technology.

Microarrays (DNA chips) are basically the product of bonding or direct synthesis of numerous specific DNA probes on a stationary, often silicon-based, support. Microarrays are miniature gene fragments attached to glass chips. These chips are used to examine the gene activity of thousands or tens of thousands of gene fragments and to identify genetic mutations using a hybridization reaction between the sequences on the microarray and a fluorescent sample. Applications of microarrays in clinical medicine include analysis of gene expression in malignancies, such as mutations in *BRCA1*, mutations of tumor-suppressor gene *p53*, genetic disease testing, and viral resistance mutation detection.

SPECIMENS FOR SEROLOGY AND IMMUNOLOGY

Immunologic testing is done in many areas of the clinical laboratory, including microbiology, chemistry, toxicology, immunology, hematology, surgical pathology, cytopathology, and immunohematology (blood banking), and a great variety of specimens are tested. With the advent of procedures devised to give rapid, accurate results, especially those based on the use of mAbs and EIA technology, many clinical constituents can be determined immunologically. Many types of body fluids can be evaluated by using immunologic technology. It is always important to determine the specimen of choice for each procedure being considered. The many commercial kits available for the various assays will state specific specimen requirements and acceptable criteria for collection.

The majority of immunology tests are done on serum. Blood is collected in a plain tube and allowed to clot completely before being centrifuged. Serum should be removed from the clot as soon as possible after processing. Lipemia, hemolysis, or any bacterial contamination can make the specimen unacceptable. Icteric or turbid serum may give valid results for some tests but may interfere with others. Blood specimens should be collected before a meal to avoid the presence of chyle, an emulsion of fat globules that often appears in serum after eating, during digestion. Contamination with alkali or acid must be avoided; these substances have a denaturing effect on serum proteins and make the specimens useless for serologic testing. Excessive heat and bacterial contamination are also avoided. Heat coagulates the proteins, and bacterial growth alters protein molecules. If the test cannot be performed immediately, the serum should be refrigerated. If the testing cannot be done within 72 hours, the serum specimen must be frozen.

For some testing, the serum complement must first be inactivated, the process that destroys complement activity. To inactivate complement, the tubes of serum are placed in a heat block at 56°C for 30 minutes. When more than 4 hours has elapsed since inactivation, a specimen can be reinactivated by heating it to 56°C for 10 minutes.

If the protein complement is not inactivated, it will promote lysis of the RBCs in some types of assays and other types of cells and can produce invalid results. Complement is also known to interfere with certain tests for syphilis and complement components. It can agglutinate latex particles and cause a false-positive reaction in certain types of latex assays.

Proper handling and storage of the specimen until testing is done are essential. Immunologic assays are also done on cerebrospinal fluid, other body fluids, and swabs of various body exudates and discharges. The established protocol for each specific assay must be followed in terms of specimen collection requirements and conditions for the assay itself.

Testing for Antibody Levels

In obtaining specimens for serologic testing, it is important to consider the phase of the disease and the condition of the patient at the time of the specimen collection. This is especially important in assays for diagnosis of infectious diseases. If serum is being tested for antibody levels for a specific infectious organism, generally the blood should be drawn during the acute phase of the illness—when the disease is first discovered or suspected—and another sample drawn during the convalescent phase, usually about 2 weeks later. Accordingly, these samples are called *acute serum* and *convalescent serum.* A difference in the amount of antibody present may be noted when the two different samples are tested concurrently. An important concept in any serologic testing is the manifestation of a rise in titer.

Antibody Titer

An antibody titer is defined as the reciprocal of the highest dilution of the patient's serum in which the antibody is still detectable. That is, the titer is read at the highest dilution of serum that gives a positive reaction with the antigen. If a serum sample has been diluted 1:64 and reacts positively with the antigen suspension used in the testing process, and the next-highest dilution of 1:128 does not give a positive reaction, the titer is read as 64. A high titer indicates that a relatively high concentration of the antibody is present in the serum. For some infections, the titer of antibody rises slowly, even months after the acute infection, as in patients with legionnaires' disease. For most pathogenic infections, an increase in the patient's titer of two doubling dilutions, or from a positive result of 1:8 to a positive result of 1:32 over several weeks, is an indication of a current infection. This is known as a "fourfold" rise in the antibody titer.

Twofold Dilutions

The standard dilution technique most frequently used in the serology laboratory is a "twofold" dilution. The basis of this type of dilution is that each tube contains half serum and half diluent, such as saline. The first tube of the twofold dilution series usually contains a specified quantity of the patient's undiluted serum. To dilute a serum specimen serially, progressive regular increments of serum are diluted (Table 16.6 and Fig. 16.8). This means each dilution is half as concentrated as the preceding one, and the total volume is the same in each tube. Serially, the second tube contains half the amount of serum and therefore half the amount of antibody; the third tube contains a quarter of the amount of antibody, the fourth tube contains an eighth, and so on. As previously noted, titers are usually reported as the reciprocal of the last dilution showing the desired reaction, such as agglutination, lysis, or a change in color.

Antigen/Antibody Ratio

The antigen/antibody ratio is the number of antibody molecules in relation to the number of antigen sites per cell. Under conditions of decreased antigen/antibody ratio, an antibody excess may exist. The outcome of excessive antibody concentration is known as the **prozone** phenomenon, which can produce a false-negative reaction (Table 16.7). This phenomenon can be overcome by serially diluting the antibody-containing serum

TABLE 16.6 Preparation of a Serial Dilution

	Tube 1	Tube 2	Tube 3	Tube 4	Tube 5	Tube 6	Tube 7	Tube 8	Tube 9	Tube 10
Saline (mL)	—	1	1	1	1	1	1	1	1	1
Serum (mL)	1	1	1 of 1:2	1 of 1:4	1 of 1:8	1 of 1:16	1 of 1:32	1 of 1:64	1 of 1:128	1:256
Final dilution	—	1:2	1:4	1:8	1:16	1:32	1:64	1:128	1:256	1:512

To prepare a twofold dilution:
1. Label tubes 1 through 10 and place in a test tube rack.
2. Add 1 mL of 0.9% saline to tubes 2 through 10.
3. Add 1 mL of patient's serum to each tube 1 and 2.
4. With the same pipette, mix the contents of tube 2 by drawing the contents up into the pipette. The process of drawing up and blowing out is considered one mixing. Repeat this process four times. Note that tube 1 contains only undiluted serum and tube 2 contains half the amount of the serum because 0.1 mL of undiluted serum was diluted with 0.1 mL saline = diluted 1:2.
5. Continue the serial diluting by transferring 1 mL of diluted serum from tube 2 to tube 3 and mixing with 1.0 mL of saline. Mix four times as described previously. Continue this dilution process until reaching tube 10. It can be extended to even higher dilutions if needed to achieve a nonreactive tube such as no agglutination or hemolysis after observing visible agglutination or hemolysis.
6. Follow-up: Specified quantities such as 0.1 mL of a specific antigen, for example, red blood cells demonstrating A antigen, would be added to each tube. The serially diluted tubes would be shaken to mix the contents, centrifuged, and finally examined for visible agglutination or hemolysis.

Note: This is a slightly different (alternate) setup of tubes with diluent than the setup in Fig. 16.8. The preparation described here has only serum in tube 1, with no diluent. The first 1:2 dilution is in tube 2.

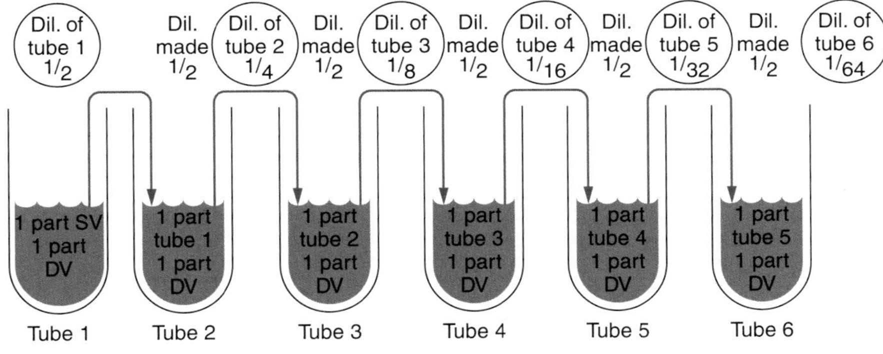

Fig. 16.8 Schematic of a twofold serial dilution. (From Turgeon ML: *Immunology and serology in laboratory medicine,* ed 5, St Louis, 2013, Mosby.)

TABLE 16.7 Prozone and Postzone Phenomenon

Zones	Prozone					Equivalence				Postzone
Serum dilution	None	1:2	1:4	1:8	1:16	1:32	1:64	1:128	1:256	1:512
Strength of agglutination	Neg	Neg	1+	2+	3+	4+	3+	2+	1+	Neg

until optimum amounts of antigen and antibody are present in the test system. The zone of equivalence is the range of dilutions where the relative concentration of antibody and antigen produce maximal binding of antigen to antibody. In the zone of equivalence, agglutination is observable. After this range of dilutions is exceeded, the postprozone range of weaker dilutions no longer exhibits visible agglutination. An excess of antigen occurs, resulting in no lattice formation in an agglutination reaction.

IMMUNOLOGIC AND SEROLOGIC TESTING FOR BACTERIAL AND VIRAL DISEASES

The advent of mAb technology has given rise to the development of many new, highly specific and sensitive immunoassays. Classic serologic testing has been an important part of some diagnostic tests in the clinical laboratory for many years. Traditional serologic tests have been done for bacterial and viral diseases or disorders.

Lyme Disease

Lyme disease (Lyme borreliosis) is caused by a spirochete bacterium, *Borrelia burgdorferi.*

Immunologic Manifestations

Cellular immune responses to *B. burgdorferi* antigens begin concurrently with early clinical illness. Mononuclear cell, antigen-specific responses develop during spirochetal dissemination,

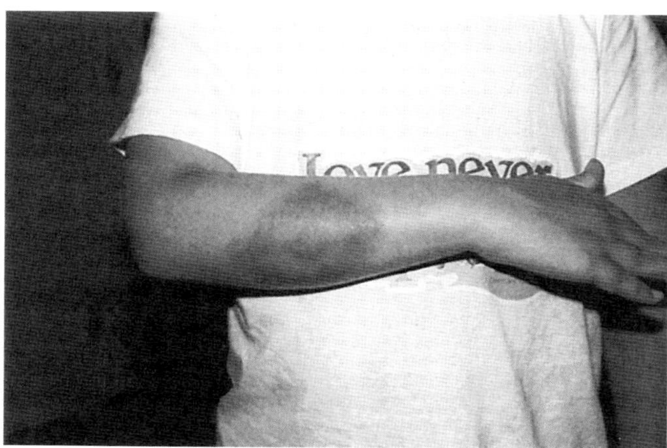

Fig. 16.9 Erythema chronicum migrans. (From Forbes BA, Sahm DF, Weissfeld AS: *Bailey and Scott's diagnostic microbiology,* ed 12, St Louis, 2007, Mosby.)

and humoral (antibody) immune responses soon follow (Fig. 16.9).

Serodiagnostic tests are insensitive during the first several weeks of infection. In the United States approximately 20% to 30% of Lyme patients have positive responses, usually of the IgM isotype, during this period, but by convalescence 2 to 4 weeks later, about 70% to 80% have seroreactivity even after antibiotic treatment. After about 1 month, most patients with an active infection have IgG antibody responses. After antibiotic treatment, antibody titers slowly fall, but IgG and even IgM responses may persist for many years after treatment. An IgM response cannot be interpreted as a manifestation of recent infection or reinfection unless the appropriate clinical characteristics are present. Antibodies formed include cryoglobulins, immune complexes, antibodies specific for *B. burgdorferi,* and anticardiolipin antibodies. Elevated titers of IgM are noted in early disease. Immunoblot analysis demonstrates that IgM antibodies form initially against the flagellar polypeptide but react later to additional cell-wall antigens. An overlapping IgG response to these antigens develops in some individuals. These antigen-specific cellular and humoral responses are not known to eradicate infection in early disease or to participate in disease pathogenesis.

Specific IgM or IgG antibodies against *B. burgdorferi* are usually not detectable in a patient's serum unless symptoms have been present for at least 2 to 4 weeks (see procedure at http://evolve.elsevier.com/Turgeon/clinicallab). In cases of Lyme arthritis, tests for serum antinuclear antibodies (ANAs) and rheumatoid factor (RF) and Venereal Disease Research Laboratories (VDRL) test results are generally negative. However, anti–*B. burgdorferi* antibodies of the IgG type should be present in the serum of patients with Lyme arthritis.

Outer surface protein A antibodies develop late in the course of human Lyme infection and then only in a subset of patients. A temporal association may exist between the onset of chronic Lyme arthritis in four patients who were HLA-DR4–positive and the development of antibodies to the outer surface protein.

Persistent organisms and spirochetal antigen deposits elicit a vigorous immune reaction, as manifested by a tissue-rich plasma-cell and lymphocytic exudate containing abundant T cells, predominantly of the helper subset, plus IgD-bearing B cells. *B. burgdorferi* antigens elicit a strong immune reaction that intensifies with chronicity of arthritis and stimulates macrophages to secrete IL-1. IL-1 is capable of stimulating synovial cells and fibroblasts to secrete collagenase and prostaglandin E2; levels of both are elevated in the synovial fluid of Lyme patients and can cause erosion of joint cartilage and bone.

Diagnostic Evaluation

In the United States the diagnosis of Lyme disease is usually based on the recognition of the characteristic clinical findings, a history of exposure in an area in which the disease is endemic, and, except in patients with erythema migrans, an antibody response to *B. burgdorferi.* In more than 50% of cases, physicians are comfortable making the diagnosis based on symptoms and patient history. Testing becomes important when the telltale bull's-eye rash or other symptoms characteristic of Lyme disease do not appear.

Antibody Detection

Assays for the detection of antibodies to *B. burgdorferi* are the most practical means for confirming infection. The Centers for Disease Control and Prevention (CDC) currently recommends a two-step process when testing blood for evidence of antibodies against the Lyme disease bacteria. Both steps can be done using the same blood sample. The first step uses EIA or rarely IFA. If the first step is negative, no further testing of the specimen is recommended. If the first step is positive or indeterminate (sometimes called *equivocal*), the second step should be performed. The second step uses an immunoblot procedure, usually a WB test. Results are considered positive only if the EIA–IFA and the immunoblot test results are both positive.

The two steps of Lyme disease testing are designed to be done together. The CDC does not recommend skipping the first test and doing only the WB test. Doing so will increase the frequency of false-positive results and may lead to misdiagnosis and improper treatment.

Enzyme-Linked Immunosorbent Assay

The ELISA is the standard test method for diagnosis of Lyme disease; it is the most widely available and frequently performed test. The sensitivities of IFA and ELISA methods are usually low during the initial 3 weeks of infection; therefore, negative results are common. The most serious disadvantages of current techniques are low sensitivity and lengthy processing time. In addition, false-positive reactions can result from cross-reactivity in tests for Lyme disease. For example, tickborne relapsing fever spirochetes, *Borrelia hermsii,* are closely related to *B. burgdorferi.* Antibodies to *B. hermsii,* an agent that coexists with the Lyme disease spirochete in portions of the western United States, strongly cross-react with *B. burgdorferi* in IFA staining and ELISA testing. Common antigens are shared among the Borrelia organisms and even with the treponemes. Serum from syphilitic patients reacts positively in assays for Lyme disease. Therefore serologic test results for antibodies to *B. burgdorferi* should be considered along with clinical data and epidemiologic information when a patient is evaluated for Lyme disease.

Western Blot Analysis

WB analysis can verify the reactivity of antibody to major surface or flagellar proteins of *B. burgdorferi.* The WB test is helpful in determining borderline negative or weakly positive results obtained from other tests, but the values are not always reliable. This procedure is more definitive in later Lyme disease, when multiple antibody bands specific for *B. burgdorferi* appear. Reported results from WB tests for Lyme disease in its late phase indicate reactive bands for IgM levels.

Polymerase Chain Reaction

The PCR assay can detect spirochetes in the synovial fluid around the joints or in other clinical samples; it looks for DNA of *B. burgdorferi.* In the past, positive PCR assay results were taken as definitive evidence that a person had an infection, but it is now known that a person can have antigens in the presence of nonviable organisms. This test amplifies small amounts of DNA that may remain, even when intact organisms are no longer present, an indication that the organism does or did exist. The PCR assay may miss the spirochete in the blood, allowing it to move into other tissues.

The PCR technique directly identifies the pathogen instead of measuring the host's immune response to it. It can detect DNA from as few as one to five organisms, even those that are nonviable. Different specific probes have been developed, and the PCR assay has been used to detect *B. burgdorferi* DNA in a variety of body fluids. The appeal of the PCR method lies in its rapid turnaround time—2 days versus 6 to 8 weeks for culture—and avoidance of the difficulties associated with culture or immunohistochemistry. It has very high specificity, but the sensitivity may be as low as 70%. The PCR test may be useful in diagnosing early Lyme disease when the patient is still seronegative.

Syphilis

Syphilis is caused by a spirochete, *Treponema pallidum.* In 1906 the first diagnostic blood procedure was developed to detect this disease. Syphilis in humans is typically transmitted by sexual contact. In male patients, the microorganism is transmitted from lesions on the penis or discharged from deeper sites with semen. Lesions in female patients are usually located in the perineal region or on the labia, vaginal wall, or cervix. In a small percentage of patients, the primary infection is extragenital, usually in or around the mouth.

Untreated syphilis is a chronic disease with subacute, symptomatic periods separated by asymptomatic intervals, during which the diagnosis can be made serologically. The progression of untreated syphilis is generally divided into three main stages from the time of contact and initial infection: primary syphilis, secondary syphilis, and late (tertiary) syphilis. A latent period may develop between the secondary and tertiary stages.

Approximately one-third of untreated individuals with primary syphilis will progress to the second stage (secondary syphilis). This usually occurs at about 2 to 8 weeks after the appearance of the original painless sore (chancre), and in some patients the chancre may still be present.

Secondary syphilis is the most contagious stage of syphilis; the bacteria have spread in the bloodstream and reached their highest numbers. The most common symptom is skin rash, but additional symptoms can be fever, malaise, loss of appetite, and swollen lymph nodes. Although it usually resolves within weeks, in some patients the second stage may last up to a year.

The serum in about a third of patients with syphilis becomes serologically reactive after 1 week and serologically demonstrable in most patients after 3 weeks. The reagin titer increases rapidly during the first 4 weeks and then remains stationary for approximately 6 months. Within 2 to 8 weeks after the appearance of the primary chancre, a patient enters the stage of secondary syphilis. Serologic tests for syphilis are positive. The late (tertiary) stage is usually seen 3 to 10 years after primary infection. In about one-fourth of untreated patients, the tertiary stage is asymptomatic and recognized only by serologic testing.

Classic serologic tests for syphilis measure the presence of two types of antibodies: treponemal and nontreponemal. Treponemal antibodies are produced against the antigens of the organisms themselves. Nontreponemal antibodies, often called *reagin antibodies,* are produced by infected patients against components of their own or other mammalian bodies. Darkfield microscopy is the test of choice for symptomatic patients with primary syphilis. The widely used nontreponemal serologic test is the rapid plasma reagin (RPR) method. The RPR procedure and the older VDRL test produce visible clumps when the particles are agglutinated by antibody. Specific treponemal serologic tests include the fluorescent treponemal antibody absorption (FTA-ABS) test and the microhemagglutination *Treponema pallidum* (MHA-TP) test. Another procedure, the *T. pallidum* immobilization test, is obsolete.

Nontreponemal Antibody Tests

Nontreponemal methods determine the presence of reagin, an antibody formed against cardiolipin. An antigen composed of cardiolipin, a lipid remnant of damaged cells; cholesterol; and lecithin is used to detect the nontreponenal reagin antibodies. Reagin antibodies are almost always produced by persons with syphilis, but they can also be produced in other infectious diseases, such as leprosy, tuberculosis, malaria, measles, chickenpox, infectious mononucleosis (IM), and hepatitis. The reagin antibodies can also be seen in noninfectious disorders such as autoimmune conditions and rheumatoid disease, as well as during pregnancy and in old age.

Rapid Plasma Reagin Card Test

The RPR test is the most widely used nontreponemal serologic procedure, although VDRL methods may be used in some clinical and reference laboratories. The RPR test is based on an agglutination or flocculation reaction in which soluble antigen particles are coalesced to form larger particles that are visible as clumps when aggregated by the antibody. This nontreponemal screening test can be confirmed by another testing method, usually the FTA-ABS or the MHA-TP test, that tests for the presence of specific treponemal antibody.

In the RPR card test, the patient's serum is mixed with an antigen suspension of a carbon-particle cardiolipin antigen on the special disposable card provided with the test kit (see procedure at http://evolve.elsevier.com/Turgeon/clinicallab). If the suspension contains reagin, the antibody-like substance present in the serum of persons with syphilis, flocculation occurs with coagglutination of the carbon particles of antigen. This flocculation appears as black clumps against the white background of the plastic-coated RPR card. This reaction is observed and graded macroscopically. A diagnosis of syphilis cannot be made solely based on a positive RPR card test, without clinical signs and symptoms or supportive history. Positive reactions are occasionally seen with other infectious conditions or inflammatory states, thus necessitating confirmation of all positive results with the qualitative RPR test. Various manufacturers produce RPR kits, and the instructions included with the kits must be followed carefully. Positive and negative control sera should be tested daily to ensure the accuracy of the test antigen reagent.

Treponemal Antibody Tests

Treponemal antibodies are produced against the antigen of the *T. pallidum* organism itself. The FTA-ABS and MHA-TP tests are used to confirm that a positive nontreponemal test result has been caused by syphilis rather than one of the other biological conditions that can also produce a positive nontreponemal test result. In the FTA-ABS test, the patient's serum is first absorbed with non–*T. pallidum* treponemal antigens to reduce any nonspecific cross-reactivity. A fluorescein-conjugated antihuman antibody reagent is then applied as a marker for specific antitreponemal antibodies in the patient's serum. The test slide is examined with a fluorescence microscope, and the intensity of fluorescence is noted.

Acquired Immunodeficiency Syndrome

HIV is the predominant virus responsible for AIDS. The replication of HIV is complicated and involves several steps (Fig. 16.10). The infectious process begins when the gp120 protein on the viral envelope binds to the protein receptor, called CD4, located on the surface of a target cell. HIV-1 has a marked preference for the CD4+ subset of T lymphocytes. In addition to T lymphocytes, macrophages, peripheral blood monocytes, and cells in the lymph nodes, skin, and other organs also express measurable amounts of the CD4 receptor and can be infected by HIV-1. About 5% of the B lymphocytes may express CD4 and may be susceptible to HIV-1 infection. Macrophages may play an important role in spreading HIV infection in the body, both to other cells and to the target organs of HIV. Monocytes/macrophages enable HIV-1 to enter the immune-protected domain of the central nervous system (CNS), including the brain and spinal cord.

The absolute number of CD4+ T lymphocytes continues to diminish as the disease progresses. When the number of cells reaches a critically low level ($<200 \times 10^9$/L), the risk of opportunistic infection increases. The progressive decline of CD4+ cells leads to a general decline in immune function and is the primary factor in determining the clinical progression of AIDS. Plasma HIV-1 RNA is a strong, CD4+ T cell–independent predictor of a rapid progression to AIDS after HIV-1 seroconversion.

Immunologic Manifestations

Cellular Abnormalities. HIV-1 has a marked subset of lymphocytes because the CD4 surface marker preference for the CD4 protein on these cells serves as a receptor site for the virus. Immunologic activation, such as participation in an immune response to HIV-1 or viruses in other cells, of CD4+ cells latently infected with HIV-1 induces the production of multiple viral particles, leading to cell death. The extensive destruction of T cells leads to the gradual depletion of the CD4+ lymphocytes. The major phenotypic cell populations affected by AIDS are CD4+ and CD8+ subsets. Both the absolute number and the percentage of CD4+ lymphocytes are important measurements. The percentage of CD4+ lymphocytes in healthy adults is between 32% and 68% of the total number of lymphocytes (CD4+, CD8+, and B lymphocytes). The CD4+ percentage is sometimes a more reliable constant measurement than the CD4+ cell count. If the CD4+ percentage remains at 21% or higher, the immune system appears to be functioning properly, regardless of the CD4+ cell count. A CD4+ percentage at or below 13% means that the immune system is challenged regardless of the CD4+ cell count. The risk of opportunistic infections becomes high, and treatment is recommended.

A diminished subpopulation of CD4+ circulating lymphocytes can also be seen in individuals with other disorders, such as cutaneous T cell lymphoma, SLE, and acute viral infection. The ratio, however, reverts to normal after recovery from a viral infection in non-AIDS patients.

Serologic Markers

Detection of Core Antigen. After initial infection, the body mounts a vigorous immune response against the viremia. The first signal of an immune response to HIV-1 infection is the appearance of acute-phase reactants, including α_1-antitrypsin and serum amyloid in plasma 3 to 5 days after transmission. Immunologic activities include the production of different types of antibodies against HIV. Some antibodies neutralize the virus, others prevent it from binding to cells, and others stimulate cytotoxic cells to attack HIV-infected cells.

The time and sequence vary for the appearance and disappearance of antibodies specific for the serologically important antigens of HIV-1 during the course of infection. A window period of seronegativity exists from the time of initial infection to 6 or 12 weeks or longer thereafter.

Antibodies to HIV-1. Antibodies to HIV-1 appear after a lag period of about 6 weeks between the time of infection and a detectable antibody response. Because of this, some virus-positive, antibody-negative individuals would be missed by initial screening assays.

In addition to a positive HIV antibody test in 85% to 90% of patients, increased antibody titers to other viruses such as cytomegalovirus (CMV), Epstein–Barr virus (EBV), hepatitis A or B, *Toxoplasma gondii* and circulating immune (antigen–antibody) complexes can be found.

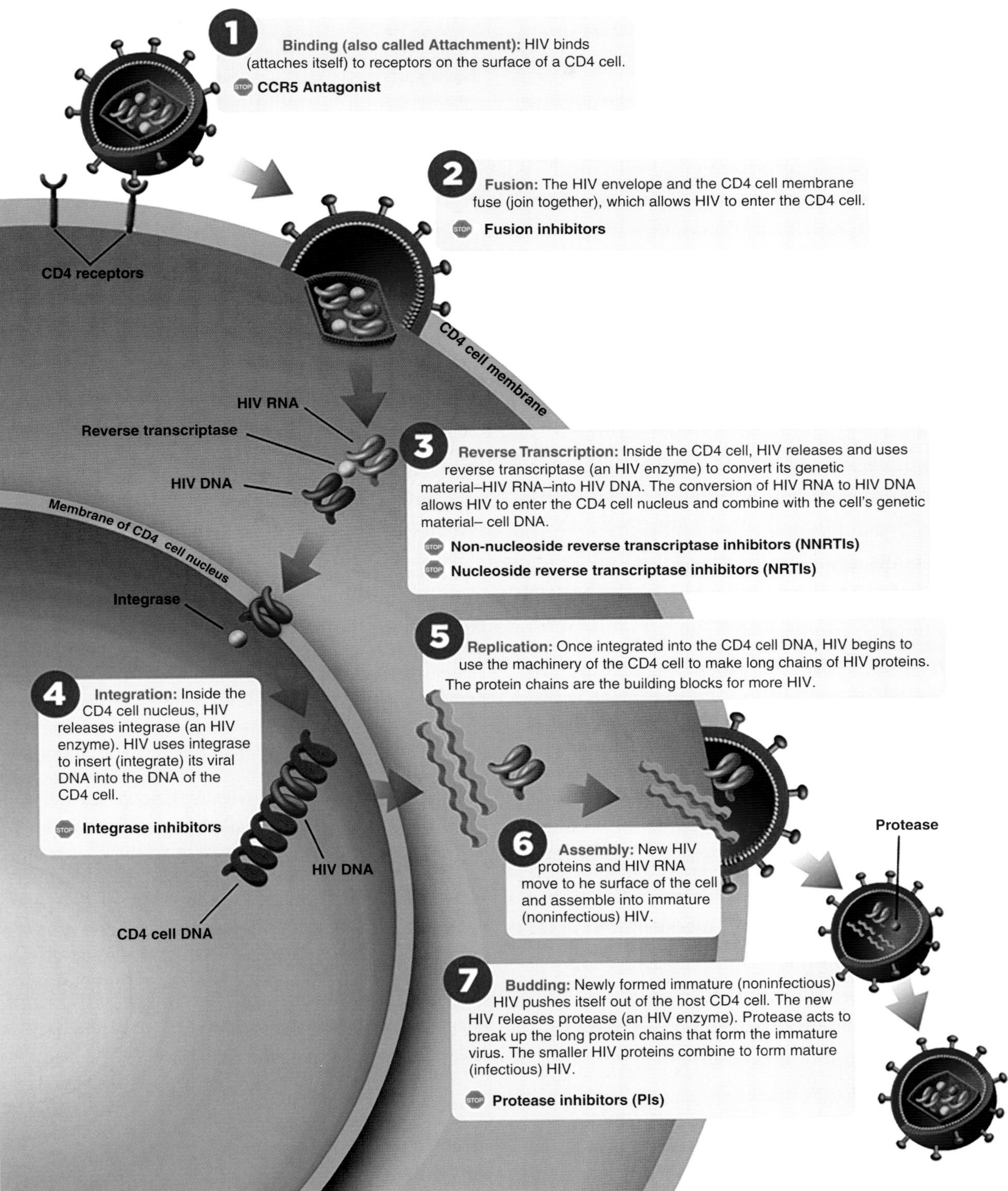

Fig. 16.10 Steps in the human immunodeficiency virus (HIV) replication cycle. (1) Fusion of the HIV cell to the host cell surface. (2) HIV ribonucleic acid (RNA), reverse transcriptase, integrase, and other viral proteins enter the host cell. (3) Viral deoxyribonucleic acid (DNA) is formed by reverse transcriptase. (4) Viral DNA is transported across the nucleus and integrates into the host DNA. (5) New viral RNA is used as genomic RNA and to make viral proteins. (6) New viral RNA and proteins move to the cell surface, and a new, immature HIV virus forms. (7) The virus matures by protease releasing individual HIV proteins. (From Turgeon ML: *Immunology and serology in laboratory medicine,* ed 5, St Louis, 2013, Mosby.)

Testing Methods

Testing assays for HIV are categorized into the following three main types:

1. Detection of HIV antibodies
2. Detection of antigens, particularly p24
3. Detection or quantification of viral nucleic acids

HIV-1 Antibodies. Detection of HIV antibodies by EIA was the first technology developed for HIV diagnosis in 1985. Diagnostic testing is classified as screening or confirmatory testing. Screening tests include traditional EIAs and newer methods. Confirmatory tests include WB, IFA, and HIV RNA detection by nucleic acid amplification testing (NAAT).

Antibodies to HIV can be detected by EIA (specificity and confirmed by immunoblot technique). Antibody testing by EIA remains the standard method for screening potential blood donors. Simultaneous testing for p24 antigenemia is considered unnecessary. Third-generation serologic assays have demonstrated that seroconversion typically occurs 3 to 12 weeks after infection, but significant delays can occur in some individuals.

Confirmatory Testing: Western Blot. Before an HIV result is considered positive, the results should be reproducible and confirmable by at least one additional test. WB analysis is currently the standard method for confirming HIV-1 seropositivity.

The WB assay is based on the recognition of the major HIV proteins (p24, gp41, gp120/160) by fractionating them according to their weight by electrophoresis and then visualizing their binding with specific antibodies over nitrocellulose sheets. A positive result is indicated by the presence of any two of these bands: p24, gp41, and gp120/160. If the test is positive for bands gp41 or p24 in conjunction with a positive EIA result, it is regarded as a confirmatory test. A negative result demonstrates the absence of bands. Indeterminate results can be found in 10% to 20% of EIA-positive tests. In general, the presence of a band at p24, p31, or p55, although still classified as indeterminate, is more indicative of true infection compared with other band patterns.

The WB appears to work best with samples that contain high levels of antibody. Antibody specificities against known viral components (generally, the core component p24 and envelope component gp41) are considered true-positive results, whereas antibodies specific against nonviral cellular contaminants are nonspecific, false-positive results.

Fourth-Generation Testing. Previously, most tests used in the diagnostic setting detected only HIV antibodies. Fourth-generation assays detect HIV-1 p24 antigen up to 20 days earlier than WB and 5 to 7 days earlier than third-generation EIAs. Levels of p24 antigen increase early after initial infection. More specific or supplemental tests for HIV-1 and HIV-2 such as NAAT, WB, or immunofluorescence must be performed to verify the presence of HIV-1 p24 antigen or antibodies to HIV-1 or HIV-2.

Fourth-generation assays allow for the differentiation between acute infection (p24 only, no HIV-1 antibody) and established infections (both p24 antigen and HIV-1 antibody). The gold standard for acute infection screening is NAAT. HIV-1 RNA can identify HIV infection as early as 5 days after exposure. In 2010 the US Food and Drug Administration (FDA) approved the first fourth-generation immunoassay that detects both antigen and antibodies to HIV (ARCHITECT HIV Ag/Ab Combo Assay, Abbott Laboratories, Abbott Park, IL). This test is a chemiluminescent microparticle immunoassay. The ARCHITECT HIV Ag/Ab Combo Assay was the first diagnostic test approved by the FDA for use in children as young as 2 years of age and pregnant women. Other fourth-generation assays such as GS HIV Combo Ag/Ab EIA (Bio-Rad Laboratories, Hercules, CA) use EIA methodology. These methods simultaneously test for HIV p24 antigen and antibodies to HIV-1 (groups M and O) and HIV-2 in human serum or plasma.

Rapid Testing for HIV. Routine HIV testing of whole blood in the emergency department has been shown to find unidentified cases. Currently, six rapid point-of-care testing (POCT) assays have FDA approval. A disadvantage of rapid tests includes lower sensitivity than third- and fourth-generation EIA assays. The sensitivity of the currently available rapid tests is similar to that of second-generation EIA assays. Currently, most protocols recommend confirming any positive rapid tests with WB or EIA. Follow-up with WB or EIA should be done 4 weeks later if confirmatory test results are negative or indeterminate.

HIV Viral Load Monitoring. Newer therapeutic agents, enabled in part by the identification of HIV-1 plasma RNA viral load as the principal marker of antiretroviral treatment (ART) effectiveness, has transformed HIV/AIDS from a previously deadly disease into a chronic condition.

Viral load monitoring is the preferred standard of care method for immunologic monitoring in developed countries compared to the use of CD4+ cell counts for monitoring clinical response to ART because it enables earlier and more accurate detection of treatment failure before immunologic decline change. In order to maintain the proper daily ART treatment of infected patients, periodic HIV viral load monitoring is essential. Monitoring is also critical for patients on pre-exposure prophylaxis. In addition, viral load monitoring is important in the prevention of disease transmission because patients with acute HIV infection, the most infectious stage of the disease with a high HIV concentration, need to be aware of their condition in order to reduce HIV transmission.

HIV-1 viral load monitoring should be conducted typically four times a year over the patient's lifetime. The results are reported as copies per mL of HIV-RNA. Viral load can be as low as 20 copies/mL or as high as 10 million copies/mL. Small increases in the number of copies can be transient or clinically significant in some patients. A result of 400 copies/mL is considered to be the threshold for likely transmission potential. The results of testing may suggest that ART treatment needs to be adjusted.

Infectious Mononucleosis

EBV, a human herpesvirus, was discovered in 1964 by Dr. M. Anthony Epstein and his colleague Yvonne Barr. It was subsequently identified as the cause of IM and several cancers, such as Burkitt lymphoma, which occurs mainly in African children, and nasopharyngeal carcinoma. EBV is widely disseminated; it is estimated that 95% of the world's population is exposed to EBV, which makes it the most ubiquitous human virus known. EBV is a DNA herpesvirus that infects B lymphocytes.

IM is usually an acute, benign, and self-limiting lymphoproliferative condition. Most individuals demonstrate antibodies to EBV without significant clinical signs or symptoms of disease. Immunocompetent persons maintain EBV as a chronic latent infection. Although this viral disorder can affect anyone, IM typically manifests in young adults.

EBV is transmitted primarily by close contact with infectious oral-pharyngeal secretions. Clinically apparent IM has an estimated frequency of 45 per 100,000 in adolescents. In immunosuppressed patients, the incidence of EBV infection ranges from 35% to 47%.

The incubation period of IM is from 10 to 50 days; once fully developed, it lasts for 1 to 4 weeks. Clinical manifestations include extreme fatigue, malaise, sore throat, fever, and cervical lymphadenopathy. Splenomegaly occurs in about 50% of patients. Jaundice is infrequent, although the most common complication is hepatitis.

Laboratory Diagnostic Evaluation

In addition to clinical signs and symptoms, laboratory testing is necessary to establish or confirm the diagnosis of IM. Hematologic studies reveal a leukocyte count ranging from 10 to 20 × 10^9/L in about two-thirds of patients; about 10% demonstrate leukopenia. A differential leukocyte count may initially disclose a neutrophilia, although mononuclear cells usually predominate as the disorder develops. Typical relative lymphocyte counts range from 60% to 90%, with 5% to 30% variant lymphocytes. These variant lymphocytes exhibit diverse morphologic features and persist for 1 to 2 months and as long as 4 to 6 months.

If the classic signs and symptoms are absent, a diagnosis of IM is more difficult to make. A definitive diagnosis can be established by serologic antibody testing. The antibodies present in IM are heterophile and EBV antibodies.

Heterophil Antibodies. In Western societies, primary exposure to EBV occurs in two waves. Approximately 50% of the population is exposed to the virus before age 5 years; a second wave of seroconversion occurs during late adolescence (age 15–24 years). Approximately 90% of adult patients demonstrate antibodies to the virus.

Within the adult population, 10% to 20% of individuals with acute IM do not produce IM heterophile antibody. The pediatric population is of particular concern because more than 50% of children younger than 4 years with IM are heterophile negative.

These antibodies represent a broad class of antibody. *Heterophil antibodies* are defined as antibodies that are stimulated by one antigen and react with an entirely unrelated surface antigen present on cells from different mammalian species. Heterophil antibodies may be present in normal individuals in low concentrations (titers), but a titer of 1:56 or greater is clinically significant in suspected cases of IM.

The IgM type of heterophil antibody usually appears during the acute phase of IM, but the antigen that stimulates its production remains unknown. IgM heterophil antibody is characterized by the following features:

1. Reacts with horse, ox, and sheep erythrocytes
2. Absorbed by beef erythrocytes
3. Not absorbed by guinea pig kidney cells
4. Does not react with EBV-specific antigens

Rapid Tests for Mononucleosis

Rapid slide tests have been developed by several manufacturers (see procedure at http://evolve.elsevier.com/Turgeon/clinicallab). Most screening tests use fine suspensions of guinea pig kidney for the rapid differential absorption.

Rapid slide tests based on the principle of agglutination of horse erythrocytes (RBCs) also are available. The use of horse RBCs appears to increase the sensitivity of the test. The Mono-Test uses stabilized horse RBCs (antigens) to demonstrate agglutination in the presence of IM heterophil antibodies through a typical antigen–antibody reaction. As a result of special processing, the horse RBCs without the need for absorption techniques will not be agglutinated by Forssman or serum sickness antibodies at the levels normally encountered in the US population.

These rapid screening tests are based on the following general principles:

1. The use of horse RBCs instead of sheep RBCs makes the test more sensitive and thus is especially valuable for low-titer serum found in the early stages of the disease.
2. The unwashed, preserved horse RBC reagent remains in a usable condition for at least 3 months and gives stronger and quicker agglutination with IM serum than horse RBCs preserved with formalin.
3. Some non-IM serum also has a high horse agglutinin titer, and therefore serologic tests cannot depend on titers alone.
4. Fine suspensions of guinea pig kidney give satisfactory instant absorption of antibodies and a clear-cut differentiation between infectious and noninfectious mononucleosis serum. Before any reagents are used for the test, the reagent test cells should be shaken well to provide a homogeneous mixture. The reagents should be used at room temperature.

For many of these rapid tests, serum, plasma, or whole blood (capillary or anticoagulated venous blood) from the patient can be used. As part of the test, it is mixed thoroughly with guinea pig kidney on one section of the slide to absorb or neutralize any Forssman antibodies present, because both IM antibodies and Forssman antibodies will agglutinate the horse RBCs in the test reagent (both are heterophil antibodies). The IM antibodies, if present, will remain reactive and will agglutinate the test horse RBCs when they are added to the absorbed serum mixture. The test reagents are available commercially as part of the specific test kit being used. Directions must always be followed carefully for each specific product. Agglutination is observed at a specific time after the final mixing, generally after 1 minute of mixing. If agglutination is observed, the test is positive. If no agglutination is observed, the test is negative. Specific instructions about the interpretation of a test are included with the product information. One commercially available test kit using this principle is MonoSlide. This product uses specially treated horse RBCs that provide color enhancement to increase the specificity, sensitivity, and readability of the test.

When serum is used for the rapid IM screening tests, the presence of hemolysis in the specimen makes it unsuitable for testing. If testing cannot be done immediately, serum or plasma may be stored at 2°C to 8°C for several days after being collected.

Most of the widely used rapid immunologic assays for IM are highly sensitive. It is still necessary, however, to use adequate and proper control programs as the only dependable method of detecting sources of technical errors. Using both a positive and negative control specimen, control sera should be tested once during each shift of use to ensure proper kit performance. When the results are not clear-cut, it is always important to repeat the test and conduct additional serologic tests if needed.

False-negative slide tests may be obtained in patients with a low heterophil titer. This can occur early, in the first 1 or 2 weeks after onset of symptoms. False-negative tests may also be seen in patients who do not mount a heterophil antibody response to the infection, especially young children. The slide test can be repeated at a later date, or an EBV titer for IgM can be performed to help establish the diagnosis for these patients.

False-positive tests for heterophil antibody have been reported in cases of CMV infections, rubella infections, leukemia, Hodgkin disease, Burkitt lymphoma, rheumatoid arthritis (RA), viral hepatitis, and multiple myeloma.

Current rapid slide tests using a variety of methods have been developed by several manufacturers. Examples of additional rapid tests for infectious mononucleosis include the following:

- The Acceava® Mono II test (Alere, Waltham, MA) is a rapid chromatographic immunoassay for the qualitative detection of infectious mononucleosis heterophil antibodies in whole blood, serum, and plasma. It is intended for use by health care professionals.
- The Acceava® Mono Cassette test (Alere) is a one-step antibody test for IgM antibodies to distinguish between active and past infections. This method uses direct solid-phase immunoassay technology to detect IM heterophile antibodies in human serum, plasma, or whole blood. It is Clinical Laboratory Improvement Amendments (CLIA) waived for whole blood specimens only; it is a CLIA moderately complex test for serum or plasma intended for use by health care professionals.
- The Clearview® MONO test (Alere) is a rapid chromatographic immunoassay used to detect infectious mononucleosis heterophile antibodies in whole blood, serum, and plasma. It is a CLIA-waived test for whole blood but nonwaived for serum or plasma and is intended for use by health care professionals.
- The QuickVue Mononucleosis Test (Quidel, San Diego, CA) uses an extract of bovine erythrocytes that gives greater sensitivity and specificity than similar extracts prepared from sheep and horse erythrocytes. It is intended for use by health care professionals.
- The MONOSPOT® Rapid latex test (Meridian BioScience, Inc., Cincinnati, OH) is used for the detection of heterophile antibodies specific to IM.
- The OSOM® Mono Test (Sekisui Diagnostics, Lexington, MA) uses color immunochromatographic dipstick technology with bovine erythrocyte extract coated on the membrane. It is CLIA waived for whole blood and CLIA moderate complexity for serum and plasma and is intended for use by health care professionals.

Epstein–Barr Virus Serology

In diagnostically inconclusive cases of IM, a more definitive assessment of immune status may be obtained through an EBV serologic panel. Candidates for EBV serology include those who do not exhibit classic symptoms of IM, who are heterophile negative, or who are immunosuppressed.

EBV-infected B lymphocytes express a variety of new antigens encoded by the virus. Infection with EBV results in corresponding antibody response to the following antigens:

- Viral capsid antigen (VCA)
- Early antigen (EA)
- Epstein–Barr nuclear antigen (EBNA)

Assays for IgM and IgG antibodies to these EBV antigens are available. EBV-specific serologic studies are beneficial in defining immune status, and their time of appearance may indicate the stage of disease (Fig. 16.11). This can provide important information for the diagnosis and management of EBV-associated disease. Patients with nasopharyngeal carcinoma have elevated titers of IgA antibodies to EBV replicative antigens, including VCA. These antibodies, which frequently precede the appearance of the tumor, serve as a prognostic indicator of remission and relapse.

Viral Capsid Antigen. VCA is produced by infected B cells and can be found in the cytoplasm. Anti-VCA IgM is usually detectable early in the course of infection but is low in concentration and disappears within 2 to 4 months. Anti-VCA IgG is usually detectable within 4 to 7 days after the onset of signs and symptoms and persists for an extended period, perhaps lifelong.

Early Antigen. EA is a complex of two components, early antigen–diffuse (EA-D), which is found in the nucleus and cytoplasm of the B cells, and early antigen–restricted (EA-R), usually found as a mass only in the cytoplasm.

Anti–EA-D of the IgG type is highly indicative of acute infection, but it is not detectable in 10% to 20% of patients with IM. EA-D disappears in about 3 months; however, a rise in titer is demonstrated during reactivation of a latent EBV infection.

Anti–EA-R IgG is not usually found in young adults during the acute phase but may be seen in the serum of very young children during the acute phase. Anti–EA-R IgG appears transiently in the later, convalescent phase. In general, anti–EA-D and anti–EA-R IgG are not consistent indicators of the disease stage.

Epstein–Barr Nuclear Antigen. EBNA is found in the nucleus of all EBV-infected cells. Although the synthesis of NA precedes EA synthesis during the infection of B cells, EBNA does not become available for antibody stimulation until after the incubation period of IM, when activated T lymphocytes destroy the EBV genome–carrying B cells. As a result, antibodies to nuclear antigen are absent or barely detectable during acute IM.

Anti-EBNA IgG does not appear until a patient has entered the convalescent period. EBNA antibodies are almost always

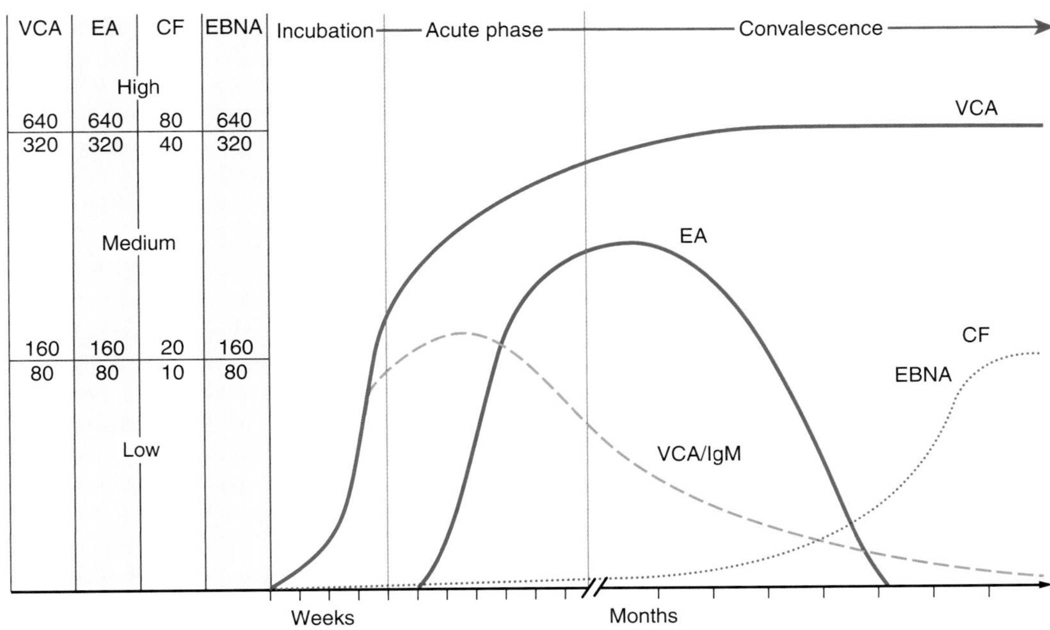

Fig. 16.11 Epstein–Barr virus (EBV) antibody response in the course of infectious mononucleosis. *CF,* Complement fixation test; *EA,* early antigen; *EBNA,* Epstein–Barr nuclear antigen; *VCA,* viral capsid antigen. (From Turgeon ML: *Immunology and serology in laboratory medicine,* ed 5, St Louis, 2013, Mosby.)

TABLE 16.8 Characteristic Antibody Formation in Infectious Mononucleosis

Parameter	VCA IgM	VCA IgG	EA-D	EA-R	EBNA IgG	Heterophile
No previous exposure	Negative	Negative	Negative	Negative	Negative	Negative
Recent (acute) infection	Positive	Positive	+/–	Negative	Negative	Positive
Past infection (convalescent period)	Negative	Positive	Negative	Negative	Positive	Negative
Reactivation of latent infection	+/–	Positive	+/–	+/–		+/–

EA-D, Early antigen–diffuse; *EA-R,* early antigen–restricted; *EBNA,* Epstein–Barr nuclear antigen; *IgG,* immunoglobulin G; *VCA,* viral capsid antigen. (From Turgeon ML: *Immunology and serology in laboratory medicine,* ed 5, St Louis, 2013, Mosby.)

present in sera containing IgG antibodies to VCA of EBV unless the patient is in the early acute phase of IM. Patients with severe immunologic defects or immunosuppressive disease may not have EBNA antibodies, even if antibodies to VCA are present.

Under normal conditions, antibody titers to EBNA gradually increase through convalescence and reach a plateau 3 to 12 months after infection. The antibody titer remains at a moderate, measurable level indefinitely because of the persistent viral carrier state established after primary EBV infection. Most healthy individuals with previous exposure to EBV have antibody titers to EBNA that range from 1:10 to 1:160. In EBV-associated malignancies, the levels of EBNA antibody are usually high in patients with nasopharyngeal carcinoma and can range from barely detectable to very high levels in patients with Burkitt lymphoma.

Test results of antibodies to EBNA should be evaluated in relation to patient symptoms, clinical history, and antibody response patterns to VCA and EA to establish a diagnosis (Tables 16.8 and 16.9). The antibody profile can be especially useful. For example, a patient with an IM-like illness caused by reactivation of a persistent EBV infection resulting from an immunosuppressive malignancy or nonmalignant disease can demonstrate high titers of IgM and IgG VCA antibodies. If the antibody to EBNA is also elevated, however, a diagnosis of primary EBV infection can be excluded.

TABLE 16.9 Characteristic Diagnostic Profile of Epstein–Barr Virus (EBV)

Stage	Description
Susceptibility	If patient is seronegative (lacks antibody to VCA)
Primary infection	Antibody (IgM) to VCA is present; EBNA is absent. High or rising titer of antibody (IgG) to VCA and no evidence of antibody to EBNA after at least 4 weeks of symptoms.
Reactivation	If antibody to EBNA and increased antibodies to EA are present, patient may be experiencing reactivation.
Past infection	Antibodies to VCA and EBNA are present.

EA, Early antigen; *EBNA,* Epstein–Barr nuclear antigen; *Ig,* immunoglobulin; VCA, viral capsid antigen.
(From Turgeon ML: *Immunology and serology in laboratory medicine,* ed 5, St Louis, 2013, Mosby.)

Hepatitis

According to the World Health Organization, almost one-third of the world's population has been infected with one of the known hepatitis viruses. In the United States acute viral hepatitis most frequently is caused by infection with hepatitis A virus, hepatitis B virus (HBV), or hepatitis C virus. These unrelated viruses are transmitted via different routes and have different epidemiologic profiles. Safe and effective vaccines have been available for hepatitis B since 1981 and for hepatitis A since 1995.

Hepatitis B is particularly important to health care professionals. HBV is the classic example of a virus acquired through blood transfusion. It serves as a model when transfusion-transmitted viral infections are considered. During the disease process, the viral DNA of HBV is actually incorporated into the host's DNA.

Hepatitis B is a complex DNA virus. Viral proteins of importance include the following:

1. The envelope protein—hepatitis B surface antigen (HBsAg)
2. A structural nucleocapsid core protein—hepatitis B core antigen
3. A soluble nucleocapsid protein—hepatitis B e antigen (HBeAg)

Hepatitis B virus does not seem capable of penetrating the skin or mucous membranes; therefore some break in these barriers is required for disease transmission. Transmission of HBV occurs by percutaneous or permucosal routes, and infective blood or body fluids can be introduced at birth, through sexual contact, or by contaminated needles. Infection can also occur in settings of continuous close personal contact.

The most frequent clinical response to HBV is an asymptomatic or subclinical infection. Diagnosis is more difficult in asymptomatic patients with negative HBV serology.

Laboratory diagnosis and monitoring of acute and chronic HBV infections involve the use of several of the following tests (Fig. 16.12):

1. HBsAg
2. HBeAg
3. Hepatitis B core antibody, total or IgM (anti-HBc)
4. Hepatitis B e antibody (anti-HBe)
5. Hepatitis B surface antibody (anti-HBs)
6. Hepatitis B viral DNA by PCR (qualitative and quantitative)

Serum testing procedures may be performed by qualitative chemiluminescent immunoassay, qualitative EIA, quantitative real-time PCR, quantitative real-time PCR–nucleic acid sequencing, or real-time PCR with reflex to genotype.

Seven drugs have been licensed in the United States for the treatment of HBV infection. Treatment for about 1 year usually results in the reduction of serum HBV DNA levels and a serum level of HBV DNA that is undetectable by PCR assay. Liver transplantation is also used for some severe cases of liver disease caused by HBV, although the new organ usually becomes infected with HBV.

AUTOIMMUNE DISORDERS

Autoimmunity represents a breakdown of the immune system's ability to discriminate between "self" and "nonself." The term

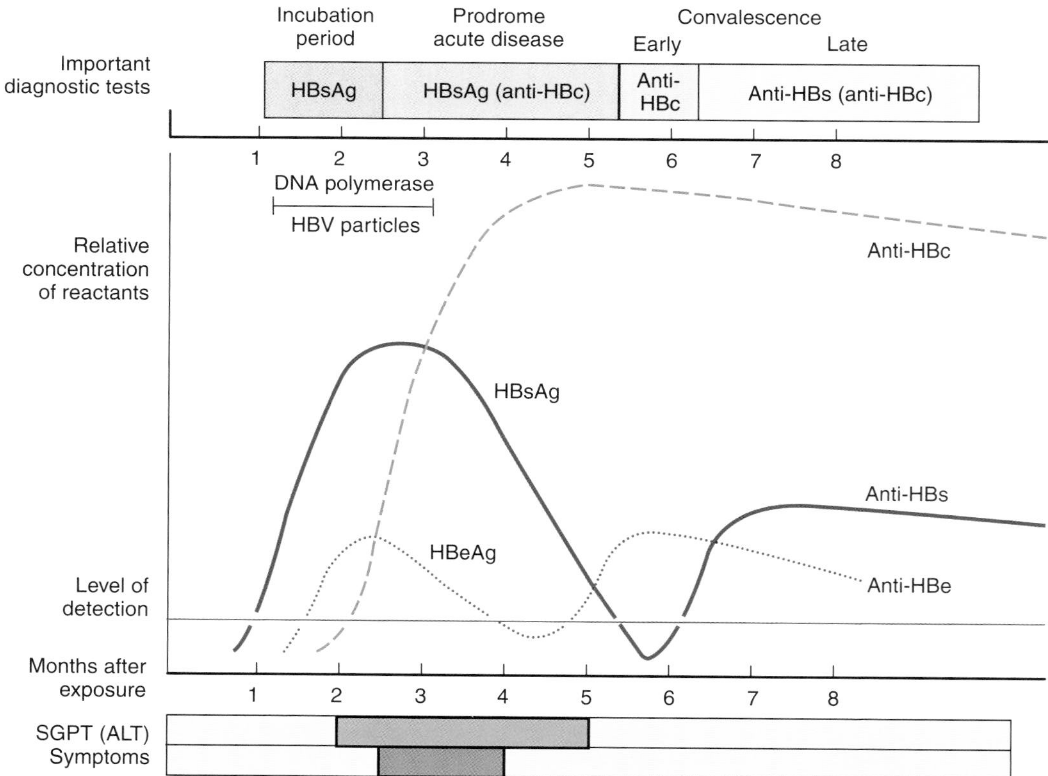

Fig. 16.12 Serologic and clinical patterns observed during acute HBV infection. (From Turgeon ML: *Immunology and serology in laboratory medicine,* ed 5, St Louis, 2013, Mosby.)

autoimmune disorder[2] refers to a varied group of chronic illnesses that involve almost every human organ system. In all these disorders, the underlying problem is similar: the body's immune system becomes misdirected, attacking the organs it was designed to protect.

Autoimmune disorder is usually prevented by the normal functioning of immunologic regulatory mechanisms. When these controls dysfunction, antibodies to "self" antigens may be produced and bind to antigens in the circulation to form circulating immune complexes or to antigens deposited in specific tissue sites.

The classification of *autoimmune disorder* is used when demonstrable immunoglobulins (autoantibodies) or cytotoxic T cells display specificity for self antigens, or autoantigens, and contribute to the pathogenesis of the disorder. The sites of organ or tissue damage depend on the location of the immune reaction.

Although a direct genetic cause has not been established in autoimmune disease,[3] there is a tendency for familial aggregates to occur. In addition, there is a tendency for more than one autoimmune disorder to occur in the same individual. Another factor related to genetic inheritance is that autoimmune disorders and autoantibodies are found more frequently in women than in men.

More than 40 autoimmune diseases occur in 5% to 10% of the general population (Box 16.1 and Fig. 16.13). The major autoimmune diseases, such as SLE, RA, diabetes type 1,[4] and multiple sclerosis, share many common features.[4] Chronic and other intermittent inflammation contribute over time to the destruction of target organs that contain inciting antigens or are the sites of immune-complex deposition. Although the adaptive immune system has long been the focus of attention, innate immune mechanisms are now viewed as central to the pathogenesis of these disorders. New genetic findings that emphasize the identification of environmental components that interact with host genetic factors are important to developing a deeper understanding of autoimmunity.

Rheumatoid Arthritis

RA is a chronic inflammatory disease primarily affecting the joints and joint tissues. Evidence indicates that immunologic factors are involved in both the articular and the extraarticular manifestations of RA. RA may represent an unusual host response to one or perhaps many etiologic agents. An infectious etiology is possible. This highly variable disease ranges from a mild illness of brief duration to a progressive, destructive polyarthritis associated with systemic vasculitis. Felty syndrome is the association of RA with splenomegaly and leukopenia. A high-titer RF assay, a positive ANA assay, and rheumatoid nodules are frequently found in patients with Felty syndrome. Patients have a propensity for bacterial infections. Juvenile rheumatoid arthritis (JRA) is a condition of chronic synovitis beginning during childhood. The etiologic hypotheses are similar to those proposed for adult RA. Subgroups of JRA include Still disease, polyarticular onset, pauciarticular onset, and RA.

Two pathogenic mechanisms have been hypothesized in RA. The extravascular immune complex hypothesis proposes an interaction of antigens and antibodies in synovial tissues and fluid. The alternate hypothesis is that RA results from cell-mediated damage because of the accumulation of lymphocytes, primarily T cells, in the rheumatoid synovium, resembling a delayed-type hypersensitivity reaction. The presence of cytokines, involved in both articular inflammation and articular destruction, supports this hypothesis.

Immunofluorescent technique reveals that the rheumatoid synovium contains large amounts of IgG and IgM, alone or together. Immunoglobulins can also be observed in synovial lining cells, blood vessels, and interstitial connective tissues. B cells make immunoglobulin in the synovium of patients with RA. As many as half the plasma cells that can be located in the synovium secrete an IgG RF that combines in the cytoplasm with similar IgG molecules (self-associating IgG). The cause of the various vascular and parenchymal lesions of RA suggests that the lesions result from injury induced by immune complexes, especially those containing antibodies to IgG.

Rheumatoid Factor

The identification of RF in the serum or synovial fluid of patients with clinical features of RA assists in confirming the diagnosis. The serum of most patients with RA has detectable soluble immune complexes. Anti–gamma globulins of the IgG and IgM classes are an integral part of these complexes. RF belongs to a larger family of antiglobulins usually defined as antibodies with specificity for antigen determinants on the Fc fragment of human or certain animal IgG. RFs have been associated with three major immunoglobulin classes: IgM, IgG, and IgA.

RF is present in many but not all persons with RA. RF can be present in other diseases such as tuberculosis, bacterial endocarditis, and hepatitis, but the highest titers are found in persons with RA. RF that appears in chronic diseases virtually disappears when the infectious process is treated with the appropriate therapy; RF that is present in RA persists indefinitely. The determination of the presence of RF is important in the prognosis and management of RA. High titers of RF indicate greater amounts of joint destruction, possibly increased systemic involvement, and generally more severe disease. RF can also be detected in synovial fluid, but its significance is little more than that of RF in serum.

The tests for RF are based on the reaction between antibodies in the patient's serum (RF) and an antigen derived from gamma globulin. Generally, all tests are designed to detect antibodies to immunoglobulins. A latex-coated suspension with albumin and chemically bonded with denatured human gamma globulin

BOX 16.1 Examples of Autoimmune Disorders

- Active chronic hepatitis
- Goodpasture syndrome
- Insulin-dependent type 1 diabetes mellitus
- Multiple sclerosis
- Pernicious anemia
- Rheumatoid arthritis
- Systemic lupus erythematosus
- Ulcerative colitis

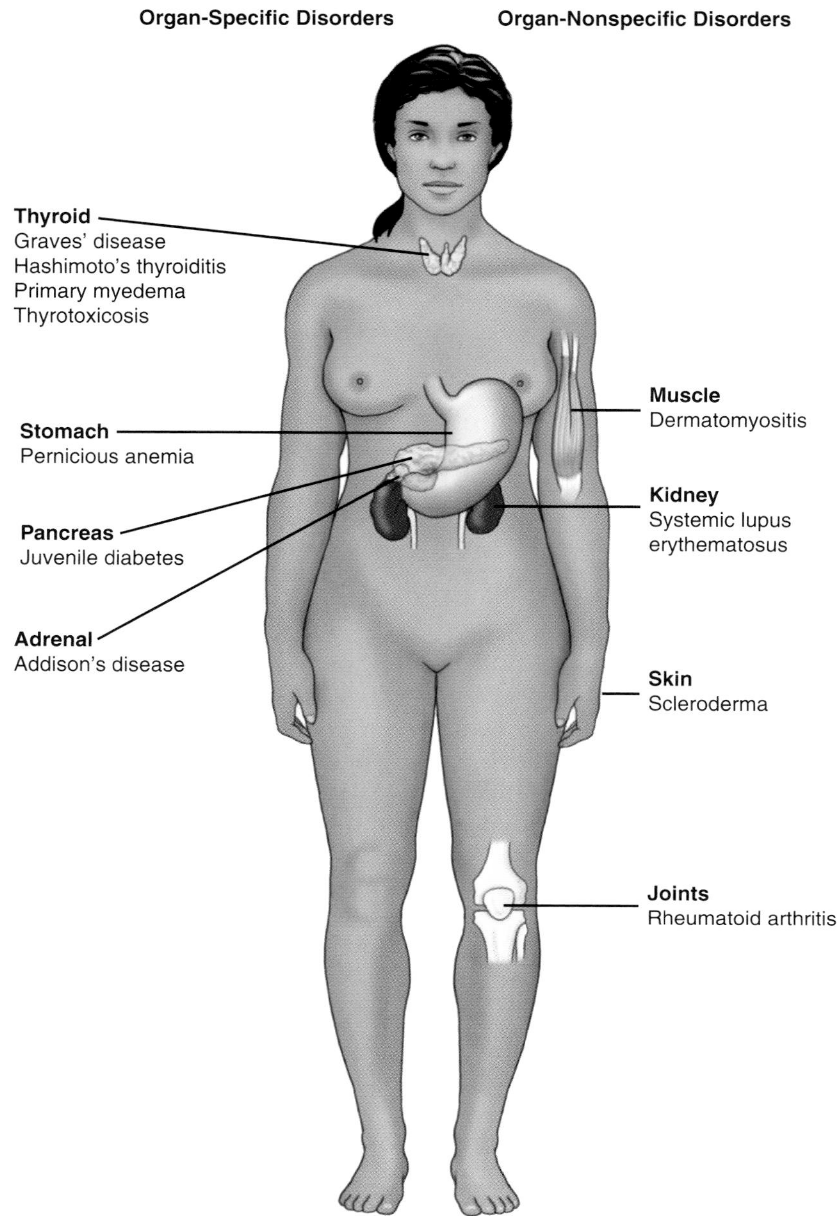

Fig. 16.13 Autoimmune disorders. (From Turgeon ML: *Immunology and serology in laboratory medicine,* ed 5, St Louis, 2013, Mosby.)

serves as the antigen in one common test for RF. If RF is present in the serum, macroscopic agglutination will be visible when the latex reagent is mixed with serum. Latex agglutination procedures have a 95% correlation with a clinical diagnosis of probable or definite RA. False-positive results may be obtained if the serum is lipemic, hemolyzed, or heavily contaminated with bacteria, or if the test result is read after the specified time (2 minutes). False-positive tests are possible with other rheumatic diseases such as SLE; in chronic infectious diseases such as hepatitis, tuberculosis, and syphilis; and in cirrhosis and sarcoidosis. Other RF tests use sensitized sheep cells in hemagglutination procedures. The latex agglutination and sheep cell agglutination tests are the most widely used routine tests for RF.

Rapid Tests for Rheumatoid Factor

Serum is usually the specimen used for the rapid latex agglutination test for RA. If the test cannot be performed immediately, the specimen should be refrigerated. If the test cannot be performed within 72 hours, the specimen should be frozen. Frozen serum should be thawed rapidly at 37°C before testing. Before the test is done, the specimen should be at room temperature. All reagents used for the rapid slide RF tests must also be at room temperature. It is always important to follow carefully all instructions provided with the testing product.

Examples of rapid rheumatoid arthritis tests are as follows:

- The Rheumatex™ RF Rapid Latex Test (Alere) detects rheumatoid factor in serum. This method uses latex particles sensitized with human gamma globulin. It is a non-CLIA-waived procedure intended for use by health care professionals.

- The Sure-Vue™ RF Rapid Latex Test (Fisher HealthCare™, Pittsburgh, PA) uses a suspension of latex particles coated with human immunoglobulin. It is a moderate complexity, non-CLIA-waived procedure intended for use by health care professionals.

Systemic Lupus Erythematosus

SLE is the classic model of autoimmune disease. The Lupus Foundation of America estimates that approximately 1.4 million Americans have a form of lupus. Lupus is most common in females during the reproductive years. No single cause has been identified for SLE, which is a disease of acute and chronic inflammation. Circulating immune complexes are the hallmark of SLE.

Demonstrable antibodies include antibodies to nuclear components; cell surface and cytoplasmic antigens of polymorphonuclear and lymphocytic leukocytes, erythrocytes, platelets, and neuronal cells; and IgG. The ANA procedure is an important screening tool for SLE. Detection of autoantibodies by immunofluorescence has become a valuable method. Immunofluorescence is extremely sensitive and may show positive results in cases where ANA procedures such as complement fixation or precipitation give negative results. At present, the immunofluorescent method is the most widely used technique for ANA screening. Serologic testing frequently reveals high levels of anti-DNA antibodies, reduced complement levels, and the presence of complement breakdown products of C3 (C3d and C3c). In addition, cryoglobulins, which represent immune complexes in some cases, are frequently present in the serum of patients with SLE. The level of cryoglobulins correlates well with the severity of SLE.

Rapid Slide Test for Antinucleoprotein

An example of a rapid slide test is the Accutex Systemic Lupus Erythematosus (SLE) Latex procedure (Thermo Scientific, Waltham, MA). It is a qualitative and semiquantitative serologic test for the detection of antinuclear antibodies in serum or plasma. This method uses a suspension of polystyrene latex particle s coated with deoxyribonucleoprotein (DNP). When the latex reagent is mixed with serum containing the ANAs, binding to the DNP-coated latex particles produces macroscopic agglutination. The procedure is positive in SLE and systemic rheumatic diseases such as RA, scleroderma, and Sjögren syndrome.

Antinuclear Antibodies

ANAs are immunoglobulins that react with the whole-cell nucleus or with nuclear components such as nuclear proteins, DNA, and histones in the tissue of the host (Fig. 16.14). ANAs are found in other diseases such as RA, are associated with the use of certain drugs, and are found in aging persons without

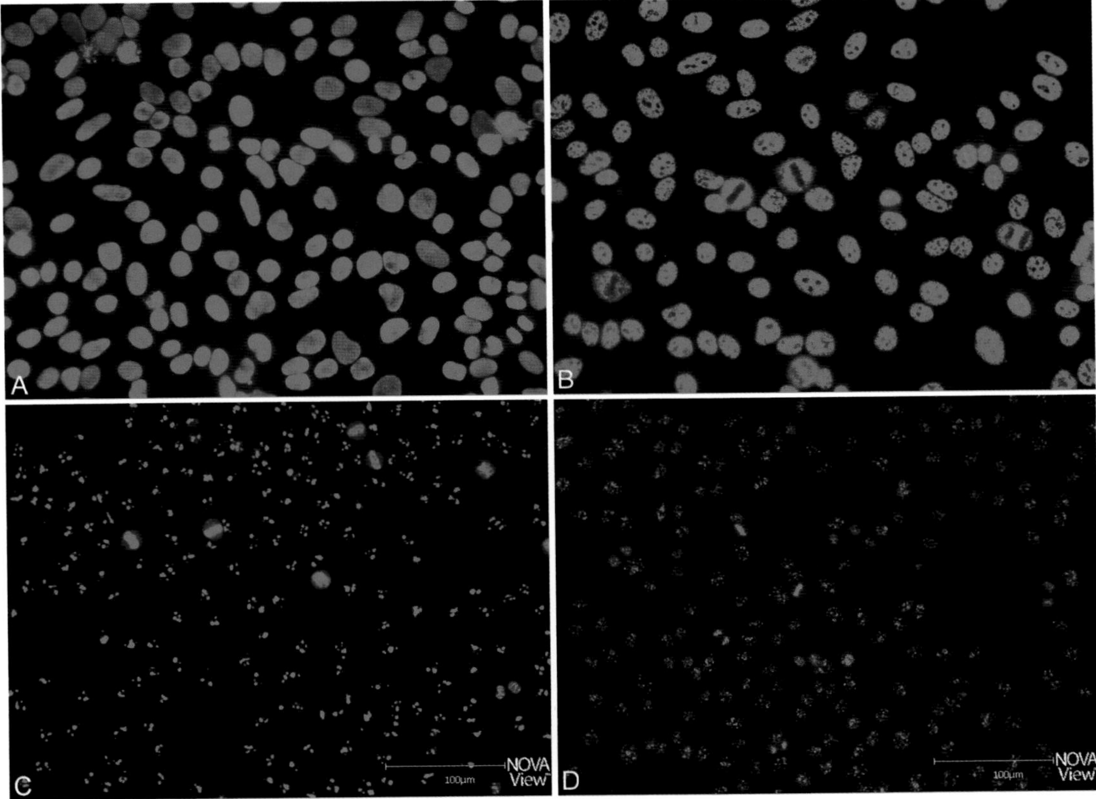

Fig. 16.14 Antinuclear antibodies (ANAs). Different patterns of nuclear fluorescent reactivity on HE_p-2 substrate demonstrate a reaction between ANAs in patient sera and the whole nucleus or nuclear components of the substrate, such as DNA, histones, or nuclear proteins. Examples of various patterns depicted in A to D. (A) ANA—homogeneous or diffused: a solid staining of the nucleus with or without apparent masking of the nucleoli. Nuclear antigens present: dsDNA, nDNA, DNP histone. Disease association: High tiers are suggestive of systemic lupus erythematosus (SLE); lower titers are suggestive of SLE or other connective tissue diseases. (B) ANA—coarse speckled. (C) ANA—nucleolar. (D) ANA—centromere. (Courtesy INOVA Diagnostics, San Diego, CA.)

disease. Thus the assays for ANAs are not specific for SLE, but ANAs are present in more than 95% of persons with SLE. Because the detection of ANAs is not diagnostic of SLE, their presence cannot confirm the disease, but their absence can be used to help rule out SLE. The significance of the presence of ANAs in a patient's serum must be considered in relation to the patient's age, gender, clinical signs and symptoms, and other laboratory findings. Fluorescent ANA techniques are often used in screening tests for SLE; many are indirect.

Indirect Immunofluorescent Tests

Indirect immunofluorescent tests for ANA are based on the use of fluorescein-conjugated antiglobulin. These methods are extremely sensitive. In one assay, the serum specimen is delivered into a well on a microscope slide that contains a mouse liver substrate. Substrates of rat or mouse liver or kidney or cell-cultured fibroblasts can also be used as the antigen and are fixed to the slides. If antibody is present in the patient's serum, the unlabeled antibody will attach to the nuclei of the cells in the substrate. After the substrate is washed in buffer, the slide is incubated with fluorescein-labeled goat antihuman immunoglobulin. If the patient antibodies have attached themselves to the nuclear antigens in the substrate, the fluorescein-tagged goat antihuman immunoglobulin will attach to these antibodies. Fluorescence will be seen microscopically using ultraviolet light. The slides should be examined as soon as possible. If immediate examination is not possible, the slides can be stored in the dark at 4°C for up to 48 hours before being read.

Several different patterns of fluorescence reactivity are seen, depending on whether the ANAs have reacted with the whole nucleus or with nuclear components, such as the nuclear proteins, DNA, or histone (a simple protein). This difference in nuclear fluorescence pattern reflects specificity for various diseases (Table 16.10). After ensuring that the results for positive and negative control specimens are giving the expected reactions, the results for the patient are reported. Results from the screening tests are reported as positive or negative. Patterns are described as being diffuse or homogeneous, peripheral, speckled, or nucleolar fluorescence.

TABLE 16.10 Antinuclear Antibody Patterns[a]

Pattern	Interpretation
Negative reaction: no green or gold fluorescence observed	Normal
Nuclear rim (peripheral)	SLE, SLE activity, and lupus nephritis
Homogeneous (diffuse)	SLE or another connective tissue disorder
Speckled	Many diseases, including SLE
Nucleolar patterns	Progressive systemic sclerosis and Sjögren syndrome

SLE, Systemic lupus erythematosus.
[a]The degree of positive fluorescence may be semiquantitated on a scale of 1+ to 4+.

Celiac Disease[5,6]

Celiac disease is a lifelong autoimmune intestinal disorder found in individuals who are genetically susceptible. There are also associated clinical disorders of an immune basis. Damage to the mucosal surface of the small intestine is caused by an immunologically toxic reaction to the ingestion of gluten and interferes with the absorption of nutrients. Celiac disease is unique in that a specific food component, gluten, has been identified as the trigger. Gluten is the common name for the offending proteins in specific cereal grains that are harmful to persons with celiac disease. These proteins are found in all forms of wheat (durum, semolina, spelt, kamut, einkorn, faro) and related grains (rye, barley, triticale) and must be eliminated from the diet.

CASE STUDIES

CASE STUDY 16.1

A 45-year-old woman comes to a clinic with complaints of morning stiffness in her ankle joints, worse on rising in the morning and improving during the day. Her discomfort is responsive to aspirin. She has also been fatigued and weak. During the last week, she has noticed that her wrist and ankle joints on both sides of her body are also painful and swollen. Blood is drawn to test for RF and antinuclear antibody. Synovial fluid is aspirated and analyzed. Results from analysis of the synovial fluid rule out crystal deposition diseases, such as gout and pseudogout, and no infectious microorganisms are seen.

Results of immunologic blood tests are as follows:

Rheumatoid factor (RF): Positive
Antinuclear antibody (ANA): Negative

Multiple Choice Questions

Answers are in Appendix A.

1. What can be the possible cause of a false-positive RF assay?
   a. Serum specimen is lipemic, hemolyzed, or heavily contaminated with bacteria.
   b. Reaction time is longer than the specified 2 minutes.
   c. The patient has systemic lupus erythematosus.
   d. All the of above are possible causes.
2. RF is *not* found in:
   a. Systemic lupus erythematosus (SLE)
   b. Bacterial endocarditis
   c. Infectious joint disease
   d. Infectious mononucleosis
3. Based on the findings, the patient is likely to have which condition?
   a. Degenerative arthritis
   b. Rheumatoid arthritis
   c. Systemic lupus erythematosus with joint involvement
   d. Joint disease from a gonococcal infection

Critical Thinking Group Discussion Questions

1. Do the patient's clinical symptoms and laboratory results support a diagnosis?
2. If so, what diagnosis would be the first choice, and why?

Note: Narrative answers published on EVOLVE instructor site.

CASE STUDY 16.2

A male college freshman is seen at the college health service complaining of general fatigue, a sore throat, and swollen lymph nodes in his neck. A throat culture is done, and blood is drawn for hematology studies and a rapid MonoSlide test. Hematology results show a normal hemoglobin value and a slight increase in the WBC count, with many large, reactive lymphocytes seen in the differential. A rapid strep test is negative, but a second swab is cultured on sheep blood and incubated, with the result to be read in 18 hours. The result of the MonoSlide test is positive.

Multiple Choice Questions

Answers are in Appendix A.

1. What result would you expect from the 18-hour incubated throat culture?
   a. Normal throat biota (flora); no β-hemolytic streptococci seen on sheep blood
   b. Only group A β-hemolytic staphylococcus seen on sheep blood
   c. Heavy growth of pathogenic *Streptococcus* on sheep blood
   d. Normal throat biota (flora) and possibly β-hemolytic streptococcus seen on sheep blood
2. What can cause agglutination of horse erythrocytes used in the rapid test?
   a. Heterophil antibodies
   b. Forssman antibodies
   c. Particles in the serum being tested
   d. All of the above
3. From these findings, what is the probable diagnosis for this patient?
   a. Systemic lupus erythematosus
   b. Infectious mononucleosis
   c. Strep throat; infection with group A β-hemolytic streptococci
   d. Parasitic infection

Critical Thinking Group Discussion Questions

1. What laboratory tests could exclude or include the possible diagnoses listed in multiple choice question 3?
2. Why did the patient have an increased WBC count with abnormal-appearing lymphocytes?

Note: Narrative answers published on EVOLVE instructor site.

REFERENCES

1. Lynch SV, Pedersen O: The human intestinal microbiome in health and disease, *N Eng J Med* 375(24):2369–2379, 2016.
2. Turgeon ML: Autoimmune disorders. In *Immunology and serology in laboratory medicine,* ed 6, St Louis, 2018, Mosby.
3. Cho JH, Gregersen PK: Genomics and the multifactorial nature of human autoimmune disease, *N Engl J Med* 365(16):1612–1623, 2011.
4. Mueller PW, et al: Type 1 diabetes autoantibodies, *Clin Lab News* 36(10):8–10, 2010.
5. Gosink J: Laboratory diagnostics for celiac disease, *MLO Med Lab Obs* 44(3):30–33, 2012.
6. Snyder MR, Murray JA: Celiac disease, *Clin Lab News* 36(9):8–10, 2010.

BIBLIOGRAPHY

Craft DW: Direct microbial antigen detection. In Mahon CR, Manuselis G, editors: *Textbook of diagnostic microbiology,* ed 2, Philadelphia, 2000, Saunders.

Donato LJ: A Game of Exclusion, Laboratory Testing for Irritable Bowel Sundrome, Cl Lab New (CLN), 43(5), 2017, 12–18.

Francois a, Milliat F, Guipand O, Benderitter M: Inflammation and Immunity in Radiation Damage to the Gut Mucosa, BioMed Research Internal, 2013, article ID 123241, 2013, https://www.hindawi.com.

Hillyard David R: The human microbiome in health and disease, http://www.arup.utah.edu. Accessed March 2017.

La Hoz RM: The Laboratory's Role in Solid Organ Transplantation, Clinical Laboratory News (CLN), 42(9), 2016, 16–22.

Lynch SV, Pedersen O: The Human Intestinal Microbiome in Health and Disease, NEJM, 375(24) pp.2369–2379, 2016.

Nakamura RM: Human autoimmune diseases: progress in clinical laboratory tests, *MLO Med Lab Obs* 32(10):32–47, 2000.

Nimmo M: Celiac disease: an update with emphasis on diagnostic considerations, *Lab Med* 36(6):2005.

Novak-Weekley S, Marlowe EM: Lab Q, No. 1611 Microbiology Am Soc of Clin Path, Clinical Laboratory, www.ascp.org. Accessed May, 2017.

Parker AR, Skold M, Ramsden DB, et. al.: The Clinical Utility of Measring IgG Subclass Investigation for Suspected Primary Antibody Deficiencies, Lab Med 48(4):314–325, 2017.

Reinhardt R: State-of-the-art allergy and autoimmune diagnostic testing, *MLO Med Lab Obs* 45(4):24–26, 2013.

Tille P: *Bailey and Scott's diagnostic microbiology,* ed 13, St Louis, 2014, Mosby.

Turgeon ML: *Fundamentals of immunohematology,* ed 2, Baltimore, 1995, Williams & Wilkins.

Turgeon ML: *Clinical hematology,* ed 6, Philadelphia, 2018, Lippincott, Williams & Wilkins.

Turgeon ML: *Immunology and serology in laboratory medicine,* ed 6, St Louis, 2018, Mosby.

Valenti WM: HIV Viral Load Monitoring, CAP TODAY, 31(2), p.2, 2017.

White A, Foley KF: Lab Q, No. 1508 Clin Chem, American Society for Clinical Pathology, Clinical Laboratory. http://www.ascp.org. Accessed May 2017.

Williamson T: Clinical utilization of anti-dsDNA and anti-chromatin assays, *Cl Lab Products* 43(4):12–14, 2013.

Wright MZ, Dearing LD: The role of HLA testing in autoimmune disease, *Adv Med Lab Prof* 13:81–84, 2001.

REVIEW QUESTIONS (ANSWERS IN APPENDIX A)

Overview of Immunology and Serology

1. Immunological mechanisms are responsible for:
   a. Recognition and disposal of nonself substances
   b. Response and interaction of body components and related interactions
   c. How the immune system can be manipulated to protect against or treat diseases
   d. All of the above

Antigens and Antibodies

2. The primary requirement for a substance to act as a foreign an antigen in a particular individual is that it must:
   a. Have a large molecular weight
   b. Be composed of protein and polysaccharide
   c. Be different from "self"
   d. Have several different combining sites
3. Which of the following immunoglobulins is found in the greatest amounts in the serum but is the smallest in size?
   a. IgA
   b. IgD
   c. IgG
   d. IgM
4. Which of the following immunoglobulins can cross the placenta and therefore provides passive immunity to the infant for the first few months of life?
   a. IgA
   b. IgD
   c. IgG
   d. IgM
5. Which of the following is an accurate statement about immunoglobulins?
   a. Produced by T lymphocytes
   b. Produced by B lymphocytes
   c. Purified (cloned) from a single ancestral cell
   d. Derived from the thymus and influenced by thymic hormones
6. Which of the following antibodies result from exposure to antigenic material from another species?
   a. Heteroantibodies
   b. Alloantibodies
   c. Isoantibodies
   d. More than one of the above
7. Which of the following substances gain antigenicity only when coupled to a large M.W. carrier molecule, e.g. protein?
   a. Agglutinins
   b. Agglutinogens
   c. Haptens
   d. Opsonins
8. In the first phase of a primary antibody response, the most notable characteristic would be:
   a. Higher titer of IgG
   b. Higher titer of IgM
   c. Long lag time
   d. Mostly IgG antibody produced

Complement

9. Complement plays an important role in immunology for all of the following reasons *except* which one?
   a. It triggers the ultimate formation of the membrane attack complex.
   b. It can result in a hemolytic transfusion reaction in an incompatible ABO transfusion.
   c. Some of the components can be assayed for diagnostic purposes.
   d. It circulates in the blood in an active form, waiting to be called into action.

Body Defenses Against Microbial Disease

10. The first line of defense in protecting the body from infection includes all of the following components *except:*
    a. Unbroken skin
    b. Normal microbiota
    c. Phagocytic leukocytes
    d. Secretions such as mucus
11. Natural immunity is characterized as being:
    a. Innate or inborn
    b. Able to recognize exogenous or endogenous agents specifically
    c. Able to eliminate exogenous or endogenous agents selectively
    d. Part of the first line of body defenses against microbial organisms
12. In acquired or adaptive immunity, one mode of acquisition of active natural immunity is:
    a. Infusion of antibody containing serum or plasma
    b. Transfer in vivo or by colostrum
    c. Vaccination
    d. A whole blood transfusion

Hypersensitivity

13. Type II hypersensitivity reactions are related to:
    a. Bee venom
    b. Antibodies (IgM, IgG)
    c. IgE antibodies
    d. Nickel allergy
14. Type III hypersensitivity reactions associated with immune complexes include:
    a. Autoimmune disorder
    b. Neoplastic disorder
    c. Infectious disease
    d. All of the above
15. A type IV hypersensitivity reaction can be caused by:
    a. Nickel
    b. Incompatible blood transfusion
    c. Bacterial contamination of water
    d. An autoimmune disorder

16. After latex exposure in a person who is allergic to latex, a reaction typically occurs within:
    a. 30 minutes
    b. 2 hours
    c. 48 hours
    d. 1 week

Types of Antigens and Reactions

17. Which agents are most commonly associated with an anaphylactic hypersensitivity reaction?
    a. A paper wasp bite
    b. A mosquito bite
    c. Goldenrod in bloom
    d. Roses

Cells and Cellular Activities of the Immune System

18. The principal type of leukocyte in the process of phagocytosis is the:
    a. Eosinophil
    b. Basophil
    c. Monocyte
    d. Neutrophil
19. A function of a subpopulation of T lymphocytes is:
    a. Primary phagocytic cells
    b. Antibody-synthesizing cells
    c. Secretion of soluble factors, cytokines
    d. Ingestion of bacteria

Immunologic Disorders

20. An acquired T lymphocyte disorder is:
    a. HIV/AIDS
    b. DiGeorge syndrome
    c. Bruton agammaglobulinemia
    d. Multiple myeloma

Principles of Immunologic and Serologic Methods

21. Which of the following is the visible result of an antigen–antibody reaction between a soluble antigen and its specific antibody?
    a. Sensitization
    b. Precipitation
    c. Agglutination
    d. Complement fixation
22. When the antigen–antibody complex occurs, agglutination takes place only if the antigen:
    a. Is in the form of particles,such as a bacterium or blood cell
    b. Is a physical attachment of antibody molecules to antigens on a surface.
    c. Both a and b
    d. Neither a nor b
23. The description of a mixed-field graded agglutination reaction is:
    a. Combination of all erythrocytes into one solid aggregate; clear supernatant
    b. Few isolated aggregates; red supernatant
    c. Medium-sized aggregates; clear supernatant
    d. Many tiny aggregates, many free cells
24. The description of a 1+ graded agglutination reaction is:
    a. Combination of all erythrocytes into one solid aggregate; clear supernatant
    b. Few isolated aggregates; red supernatant
    c. Many small aggregates, many free cells
    d. A few small aggregates; turbid and reddish supernatant
25. The description of a 2+ graded agglutination reaction is:
    a. Combination of all erythrocytes into one solid aggregate; clear supernatant
    b. Few isolated aggregates; red supernatant
    c. Medium-sized aggregates; moderate number of free cells
    d. A few small aggregates; turbid and reddish supernatant
26. The description of a 4+ graded agglutination reaction is:
    a. Combination of all erythrocytes into one solid aggregate; no free cells
    b. Few isolated aggregates; red supernatant
    c. Medium-sized aggregates; clear supernatant
    d. A few small aggregates; turbid and reddish supernatant

Specimens for Serology and Immunology

27. Factors that can denature, coagulate, or alter protein molecules include:
    a. Heat
    b. Strong acid solution
    c. Strong alkali solution
    d. All of the above
28. If testing cannot be done within ______ hours of collection, a serum specimen should be frozen at −20°C.
    a. 24
    b. 48
    c. 72
    d. 96
29. Complement can be inactivated in human serum by heating to ______°C.
    a. 25
    b. 37
    c. 45
    d. 56
30. A specimen should be reinactivated when more than how many hours have elapsed since inactivation?
    a. 1
    b. 2
    c. 4
    d. 8

Testing for Antibody Levels

31. A blood specimen collected about 2 weeks after an initial testing is what type of specimen?
    a. Acute
    b. Convalescent
    c. Reactive
    d. Delayed

Immunologic and Serologic Testing for Bacterial and Viral Disease

Lyme Disease

32 and 33. Fill in the blanks, choosing from the possible answers (a–d).
Diagnostic evaluation in Lyme disease testing screens for _______ (32) and DNA probe with patient DNA match to _______ (33) associated with the infection.
a. Antibody
b. Borrelia microorganism
c. Antigen
d. An infected tick

Syphilis

34. Which of the following is a term for nontreponemal antibodies produced by an infected patient against components of the patient's own or other mammalian cells?
a. Autoagglutinins
b. Reagin antibodies
c. Alloantibodies
d. Nonsyphilis antibodies

35. The most routinely used blood test for syphilis is:
a. VDRL
b. Darkfield microscopy
c. RPR
d. Colloidal gold

36. Which of the following is used to confirm a positive screening result when testing a patient for HIV antibody?
a. ELISA
b. Immunofluorescent assay
c. Western blot
d. Northern blot

37. The heterophil antibody produced in infectious mononucleosis is of which immunoglobulin class?
a. IgA
b. IgD
c. IgG
d. IgM

38. Which of the following is *not* a characteristic of heterophil antibodies produced in infectious mononucleosis?
a. Absorbed by guinea pig kidney cells
b. *Not* absorbed by guinea pig kidney cells
c. Absorbed by beef red cells
d. React with horse, ox, and sheep red cells

39. During the "window phase" of HBV infection, which of the following may be the only detectable marker?
a. Anti-HBc
b. Anti-HBe
c. Anti-HBs
d. HBsAg

Autoimmune Disorders

40. In certain disease states, what is the process in which antibodies are made to "self" antigens?
a. Autoimmune disease
b. Infection
c. Inflammatory response
d. Phagocytosis

41. The rheumatoid factor in rheumatoid arthritis cannot be associated with which immunoglobulin?
a. IgA
b. IgM
c. IgG
d. None of the above

42. An important screening test for systemic lupus erythematosus is for:
a. Antinuclear antibodies (ANAs)
b. C3 levels
c. C4 levels
d. Cryoglobulins

Turgeon: Linné & Ringsrud's Clinical Laboratory Science, 8th Edition

STUDENT PROCEDURE WORKSHEET 16-1

C-Reactive Protein Rapid Latex Agglutination Test

Student Learning Outcomes

See Chapter 16 of *Linné & Ringsrud's Clinical Laboratory Science: Concepts, Procedures, and Clinical Applications*, 8th edition, for a complete discussion of this procedure.After reading Chapter 16, and at the completion of the laboratory exercise and review questions, a student will be able to:

- Explain the clinical applications of the CRP assay.
- Describe specimen sources of error.
- Complete the end-of-procedure review questions with a grade of 80% or higher.

Principle

The CRP agglutination test is based on the reaction between patient serum containing CRP as the antigen and the corresponding antihuman antibody coated on the treated surface of latex particles. CRP is a direct and quantitative measure of this acute-phase reaction that reaches a peak concentration level about 48 hours after a single inflammatory stimulus) Elevations of the CRP level occur in about 70 disease states, including septicemia and meningitis in neonates, infections in immunosuppressed patients, burns complicated by infection, serious postoperative infections, myocardial infarction, malignant tumors, and rheumatic disease. Traditionally, CRP has been used clinically for monitoring these disease states. Levels of CRP parallel the course of the inflammatory response and return to lower undetectable levels as the inflammation subsides. In rheumatoid arthritis (RA), the CRP level reflects short-term and long-term disease activity. However, in some chronic inflammatory diseases, CRP is an unreliable indicator.

Specimen

No special preparation of the patient is required before specimen collection. The patient must be positively identified when the specimen is collected, and the specimen should be labeled at the bedside. Specimen labels include the patient's full name, the date, the patient's hospital identification number, and the phlebotomist's initials.

Blood should be drawn by an aseptic technique. A minimum of 2 mL of clotted blood (red-top evacuated tube) is required. The specimen should be centrifuged promptly and an aliquot of serum removed. Lipemia, hemolysis, or contamination with bacteria renders a specimen unsuitable for testing. Although icteric and turbid specimens have given valid results, fresh non–heat-inactivated serum is recommended for the test.

If the test cannot be performed immediately, the specimen should be refrigerated (2°-8 °C) for no longer than 24 hours. If additional delay occurs, the serum should be frozen at – 20 °C or below. Frozen serum should be thawed rapidly at 37 °C. Repeat freezing and thawing must be avoided. If the specimen is turbid on thawing, it should be centrifuged to clear it before use.

Preliminary Specimen Preparation

Serum must be at room temperature. Prepare a 1:5 dilution of patient serum by pipetting 0.1 mL of serum into a test tube and adding 0.4 mL of the commercially prepared glycine-saline buffer diluent. Mix the contents thoroughly.

Materials

1. Materials provided in IMMUNEX (Inverness Medical Professional Diagnostics, Princeton, NJ) kit: latex reagent, concentrated diluent 20 ×, positive control, negative control, glass slide
2. Materials required but not provided in kit: stirrers, conventional test tubes, distilled water, serologic pipettes
   NOTE: Always review the package insert for any changes in procedures. Other kit tests can be used but should be checked to align the procedural protocol of the described kit.

Reagents

1. IMMUNEX CRP Latex Reagent (latex particles sensitized with antihuman CRP [sheep]); contains buffer and preservative, sodium azide 0.1%
   Store at 2 °C to 8 °C. Do not freeze CRP latex reagent. Shake gently and thoroughly before use.
2. Concentrated diluent (glycine-saline buffer in kit); contains preservative sodium azide 2%
   Prepare a 1:20 dilution of the concentrated diluent by mixing the contents of the concentrated diluent vial with 190 mL of distilled water.
   NOTE: Store the prepared diluent at 2 °C to 8 °C. Properly stored reagent is stable until expiration date indicated on the label. Reagent that does not produce appropriate quality control results should be discarded after verification by repeat testing. Discard if contaminated (evidence of cloudiness or particulate material in solution).

Supplies and Equipment

1. Capillary pipettes
2. Applicator sticks
3. Glass slide (in kit) (Clean only with distilled water; *do not use detergent.*)
4. Stopwatch or timer
5. 12 × 75–mm test tubes
6. Serologic pipettes (1 mL graduated) and safety pipetter
7. Calibrated pipetter (optional)

Quality Control

Positive control serum (human)
Provided in kit (contains buffer, stabilizer, and preservative, sodium azide 0.1%)
Store at 2 °C to 8 °C.
NOTE: Failure to observe a positive reaction with this serum indicates deterioration of the latex reagent and/or positive control.

Negative control serum (human)
Provided in kit
Contains buffer, stabilizer, and preservative, sodium azide 0.1%
Store at 2 °C to 8 °C.
NOTE: A smooth or slightly granular reaction must be observed with the negative control. If agglutination is exhibited with this control, the test should be repeated. If repeat testing produces the same results, the reagents should be replaced.

A positive and a negative control must be tested with each unknown patient specimen.
CAUTION: Because the control sera are derived from human sources, they should be handled in the same manner as clinical serum specimens.

(Continued)

Turgeon: Linné & Ringsrud's Clinical Laboratory Science, 8th Edition

STUDENT PROCEDURE WORKSHEET 16-1

Procedure
All reagents and specimens must be at room temperature before testing.

WARNING: The latex reagent, controls, and buffer contain sodium azide as a preservative. Sodium azide may react with lead and copper plumbing to form highly explosive metal azides. On disposal, flush with a large volume of water to prevent azide buildup.

Clinical Applications
CRP is the measurement of choice in suspected inflammatory conditions. It is also a useful indicator in screening for organic diseases, both inflammatory and malignant, and in monitoring therapy or healing in patients with inflammatory conditions.

Reagent Check Test
1. Place 1 drop of the Positive Control on a section of the slide and 1 drop of the Negative Control on another section.
2. Test each control according to procedural steps below, beginning with step 4.
3. Observe results immediately at 2 minutes.
4. The Positive Control must show agglutination, whereas the Negative Control should appear uniformly turbid.

Instructions for the Procedure
Read the list of required equipment, supplies, and reagents and the procedural steps. Follow the procedural steps in exact order.

SEQUENCE	PROCEDURAL STEP	INSTRUCTOR-OBSERVED ACCEPTABLE PERFORMANCE (CHECK IF ACCEPTABLE)
1	Specimens should be tested undiluted and diluted 1:10 with the prepared diluent.	
2	Place 1 drop (~50 μL) of undiluted specimen into one of the rings on the slide and 1 drop (~50 μL) of the diluted 1:10 specimen into another ring.	
3	Place 1 drop each of Positive Control and Negative Control into two more rings on the slide.	
4	Resuspend the CRP latex reagent by gently mixing until the suspension is homogeneous. Using the dropper provided, add 1 drop of the CRP latex reagent to each serum specimen and to each control.	
5	Using separate applicator sticks, mix each specimen and each control thoroughly. The contents of the mixtures should be spread evenly over the entire area of their respective divisions on the slide.	
6	Tilt the slide back and forth, slowly and evenly, 8 to 10 times per minute, for 2 minutes. Place the slide on a flat surface and observe immediately for macroscopic agglutination using a direct light source.	

Results of Unknown Specimens

Specimen Identification ______________ Results ______________

______________ ______________

______________ ______________

______________ ______________

Instructor Initial, if acceptable ______________

(Continued)

Turgeon: Linné & Ringsrud's Clinical Laboratory Science, 8th Edition

STUDENT PROCEDURE WORKSHEET 16-1

C-Reactive Protein Rapid Latex Agglutination Test

Review Questions

Student's Name ______________________________ Date _____________

1. Name the three conditions that can be observed in a blood specimen that render it unsuitable for testing.

   a.

   b.

   c.

2. How long can a serum specimen be refrigerated?

3. Does CRP function as an antigen or an antibody in the CRP testing procedure?

4. When is the CRP assay clinically applicable?

Procedural Evaluation

Student's Name ______________________________ Grade___________

Instructor's Signature ___________________________ Date___________

Comments:

17

Immunohematology and Transfusion Medicine

http://evolve.elsevier.com/Turgeon/clinicallab

CHAPTER CONTENTS

LEARNING OUTCOMES

Overview of Blood Banking
- Define the terms *immunohematology, blood banking,* and *transfusion medicine.*

Benefits and Reasons for Transfusion
- Compare the four categories of benefits and reasons for transfusions.

Whole Blood, Blood Components, and Derivatives for Transfusion
- Correlate the various red blood cell components and derivatives used for transfusion, including packed red blood cells, plasma, and platelets, and explain the reasons for transfusion of each.

Blood Donation: Donors, Collection, Storage, and Processing
- Describe the principles of donor selection and blood processing, including assays for bloodborne infectious diseases.
- Explain proper labeling and storage of blood.

Other Types of Blood Donations
- Compare other types of blood donations.

Antigens and Antibodies in Immunohematology
- Explain the role of antigens and antibodies in immunohematology.
- Define isoantibodies and immune antibodies and their roles in transfusion medicine.
- Describe the means of detecting antigen–antibody reactions in transfusion medicine, including the role of complement.
- Discuss the preparation and requirements of antisera.
- ❖ Define *genotype* and *phenotype* as used in immunohematology.

ABO Red Blood Cell Group System
- Compare ABO red blood cell and serum typing procedures, including gel technology.
- Identify discrepancies of ABO typing results and perform tests to resolve discrepancies using appropriate methods (e.g., lectins, saline replacement, and reverse grouping with A2 and O red blood cells).
- ❖ Resolve discrepancies of ABO typing results by performing and interpreting tests using appropriate methods (e.g., lectins, saline replacement, and reverse grouping with A2 and O red blood cells).
- Explain the concept of universal donors and recipients.
- Explain Landsteiner's rule and how it applies to transfusion medicine procedures.

Rh Red Blood Cell Group System
- Differentiate what is meant by "Rh negative" and "Rh positive."
- Interpret Rh terminology and inheritance.

Other Blood Group Systems
- Name the major types of blood group systems.

Antihuman Globulin Reaction (Coombs Test)
- Discuss the principle of the direct antiglobulin test.
- ❖ Compare the principle and purposes of the direct antiglobulin test and the indirect antiglobulin test (antibody screen).

Compatibility Testing and Crossmatching
- List and explain the components of compatibility testing, including identification, ABO and Rh typing, screening for unexpected antibodies, and crossmatching.

Adverse Effects of Transfusion
- Differentiate various types of adverse effects of transfusion.

Hemolytic Disease of the Fetus and Newborn
- Integrate the pathophysiology of hemolytic disease of the fetus and newborn (HDFN) with detection and prevention.
- ❖ Calculate the number of vials of RhIg necessary for postpartum prophylaxis.

Automated Testing Technology and Systems

- Compare the applications of gel technology with solid-phase red cell adherence assays.

Case Studies

- Compare the applications of gel technology with solid-phase red cell adherence assays.
- ❖ Analyze the patient history, clinical signs and symptoms, and laboratory data for the stated case studies, answer the related critical thinking questions, and conclude the most likely diagnosis.

Review Questions

- Demonstrate comprehension of the chapter content by completing the end-of-chapter review questions with a grade of 80% or higher.

Note:

- Indicates MLT and MLS core content
- ❖ indicates MLT (optional) and MLS advanced content.

KEY TERMS

agglutination
alleles
alloantibodies
antigen
complement
genotype
hemolysis
heterozygous
homozygous
immune antibodies
isoantibodies
phenotype
Rh negative
Rh positive
universal donor
universal recipient
zeta potential

OVERVIEW OF BLOOD BANKING

The practice of transfusion medicine is regulated by several different agencies in the United States. These include the National Center for Drugs and Biologics of the US Food and Drug Administration (FDA), the Centers for Medicare and Medicaid Services, the Occupational Safety and Health Administration, and the state departments of health, which perform inspections to ensure regulatory compliance. The American Association of Blood Banks (AABB) is a professional association that provides the scientific leadership and mechanisms to deal with progress and change by providing the *AABB Technical Manual.* In addition, the AABB, the College of American Pathologists, and The Joint Commission each has written standards and conducts voluntary inspections by peers.

Therapeutic replacement of blood or its components is indicated in many cases when the potential benefit outweighs any potential harm to the patient. Potential harm includes the risk of transfusion-transmitted disease, such as viral hepatitis, human immunodeficiency virus (HIV), or acquired immunodeficiency syndrome (AIDS), which have significantly changed the practice of transfusion medicine. How blood is tested before transfusion, the way donors are selected, and the nature of the blood component or derivative used for transfusion are now vigilantly regulated for safety.

The field of immunohematology has advanced rapidly. In 1951 nine independent blood group systems were known. These historically important systems and the approximate dates of discovery are ABO (1900), MN (1927), P (1927), Rh (1939), Lutheran (1945), Kell (1946), Lewis (1946), Duffy (1950), and Kidd (1951). At present, more than 350 antigens have been identified and organized into 29 different blood group systems, more accurately referred to as *red blood cell (RBC) group systems.* The complexity of the RBC membrane and its antigenic polymorphism seems almost endless. It is expected that as the methodology for studying RBC antigen–antibody reactions improves, the boundaries of knowledge will continue to expand.

A study of the immunologic reactions of blood (RBCs) is critical when therapeutic replacement of RBCs is necessary. The many possible antigen–antibody reactions that can occur must be anticipated and tested for using the procedures available in the blood bank laboratory. Therapeutic administration of RBCs may be indicated in various clinical situations. Acute or chronic loss of blood impairs the ability of the circulatory system to deliver adequate amounts of oxygen to the body cells and critically upsets the delicate homeostatic water and acid–base balance of body fluids. RBC loss may be caused by hemorrhage, excessive destruction of RBCs, or the body's inability to replenish its own RBC supply. In specific cases, administration of blood or its components is indicated.

The procedures involved in collecting, storing, and processing blood and the distribution of RBCs and blood components are called *blood banking.* The academic knowledge and procedures involving the study of the immunologic responses to blood components are called *immunohematology.* The medical practice and techniques associated with procurement, processing, and distributing blood or blood components to patients are known as *transfusion medicine.*

Immunohematology and transfusion medicine are unlike other fields of clinical laboratory investigation. Although accuracy is critically important in the laboratory, it is absolutely essential in transfusion medicine. Even the smallest error can directly result in the death of a patient from a hemolytic transfusion reaction. As R. R. Race said, "RBC group tests are different from most other laboratory tests used in medicine in a vital way—the reported result must be correct, for the wisest physician cannot protect his patient from the consequences of a RBC grouping error."[1]

This chapter is a general introduction to the subject of blood banking and transfusion medicine.

BENEFITS AND REASONS FOR TRANSFUSION

There are many indications for the transfusion of RBCs and blood components. In general, these can be divided into the following four major categories, and the component to be transfused will depend on which category applies:

1. Transfusion may be used to restore or maintain oxygen-carrying capacity or hemoglobin. This is best done by the transfusion of RBCs with plasma-removed, packed RBCs. The most commonly used component is packed RBCs.
2. Transfusion can be used to restore or maintain blood volume. Whole-blood transfusion is now limited to situations involving massive resuscitation (trauma). This is necessary in cases of acute blood loss, as seen with massive bleeding, to prevent shock. In actively bleeding patients who have lost more than 25% to 30% of their blood volume, RBCs and a volume expander such as crystalloid (electrolyte) solutions such as 0.9% sodium chloride (isotonic saline) or thawed plasma are used. Additional needed hemoglobin can be replaced later with packed RBCs, although in most patients, about 20% of blood volume can be replaced with crystalloid solutions alone.
3. Transfusion can replace coagulation factors to maintain hemostasis. This is done with a variety of blood components, which vary with the particular situation. Components include platelet concentrates and cryoprecipitate.
4. Transfusion may be indicated to restore or maintain leukocyte functions. Although rare, this may be necessary for severely granulocytopenic patients with infections that do not respond to antibiotics.

WHOLE BLOOD, BLOOD COMPONENTS, AND DERIVATIVES FOR TRANSFUSION

Whole Blood

Whole human blood consists of the following:

- *formed elements*—RBCs, white blood cells (WBCs), and platelets—which make up about 45% of the total blood volume
- *plasma,* which makes up about 55% of the total volume

The blood volume of normal adults is approximately 5 to 6 L. In transfusion medicine, reference is often made to a "unit" of blood. For practical purposes, a unit may be considered about 450 to 500 mL of whole blood or a smaller volume of RBCs. Whole blood has been replaced with an equivalent dose of RBCs and other volume-expander solutions if needed.

A variety of preparations, including RBCs, plasma, albumin, platelet concentrates, leukocytes, and other preparations and derivatives, are harvested from a unit of whole blood (Table 17.1 and Fig. 17.1). Products prepared from whole blood by mechanical methods, especially by centrifugation, are called *components.* Products separated by more complex automated processes are called *blood derivatives* or *fractions.*

Packed Red Blood Cells

Blood component preparation begins with the separation of plasma from whole blood, leaving the RBCs. Red cells for transfusion can be prepared by sedimentation or centrifugation. The technique used must maintain the sterility of both the plasma and the RBCs. If the container is not entered when the red cells are prepared, the expiration date for the cells remains the same as for the original whole blood. If the container is entered, the RBCs are considered usable for only 24 hours. Packed RBCs are effectively used when oxygen-carrying capacity is diminished or lost, such as in treating certain anemic conditions.

Packed RBCs have essentially replaced whole blood in transfusion, except in the case of massive bleeding, when more than 25% to 30% of circulating blood volume is lost. In most cases, even in massive bleeding, RBCs together with isotonic saline or plasma substitutes are preferred.

Irradiated blood and blood components often are irradiated using cesium-137 or cobalt-60 before transfusion, to prevent the proliferation of certain types of T lymphocytes that can inhibit the immune response and cause graft-versus-host disease (GVHD). This procedure is necessary for transfusion recipients at risk for GVHD, including fetuses receiving intrauterine transfusions, select immunocompetent or immunocompromised recipients, patients undergoing hematopoietic transplantation,

TABLE 17.1 Blood Components and Derivatives

Blood Component or Derivative	Use
Packed red blood cells (RBCs)	To increase RBC mass (such as therapy for anemia); use with colloids or crystalloids in active bleeding or massive transfusion.
Leukocyte-poor red blood cells[a]	To increase RBC mass and avoid febrile and allergic reactions from leukocytes or plasma proteins; to prevent anaphylactic reactions
Deglycerolized red blood cells (frozen RBCs)	To extend storage of RBCs with rare blood types and autologous transfusion; to prevent HLA sensitization
Fresh frozen plasma	In bleeding patients with multiple coagulation defects; also for treatment of factor V or VI deficiency
Cryoprecipitate	Treatment of von Willebrand disease, factor XIII deficiency, or hypofibrinogenemia
Factor VIII concentrate	For hemophilia A (factor VIII deficiency)
Factor IX concentrate	For hereditary deficiency of factors II, VII, IX (hemophilia B), or X
Albumin/plasma protein fraction (plasma substitutes)	For volume expansion and colloidal replacement without risk of hepatitis or AIDS
Immune serum globulin	For treatment or prophylaxis of hypogammaglobulinemia; to prevent or modify hepatitis A and hepatitis C
Rh immune globulin	To prevent HDFN in Rh-negative women exposed to Rh-positive RBCs
Platelets[b]	Functional or quantitative platelet defects
Granulocytes, apheresis	Rare; for septic, severely granulocytopenic patients who do not respond to antibiotic therapy after 48 hours

[a]Irradiated.
[b]Platelet concentrates, platelet-rich plasma, or random or single donor by apheresis.
HDFN, Hemolytic disease of the fetus and newborn; *HLA,* human leukocyte antigen.

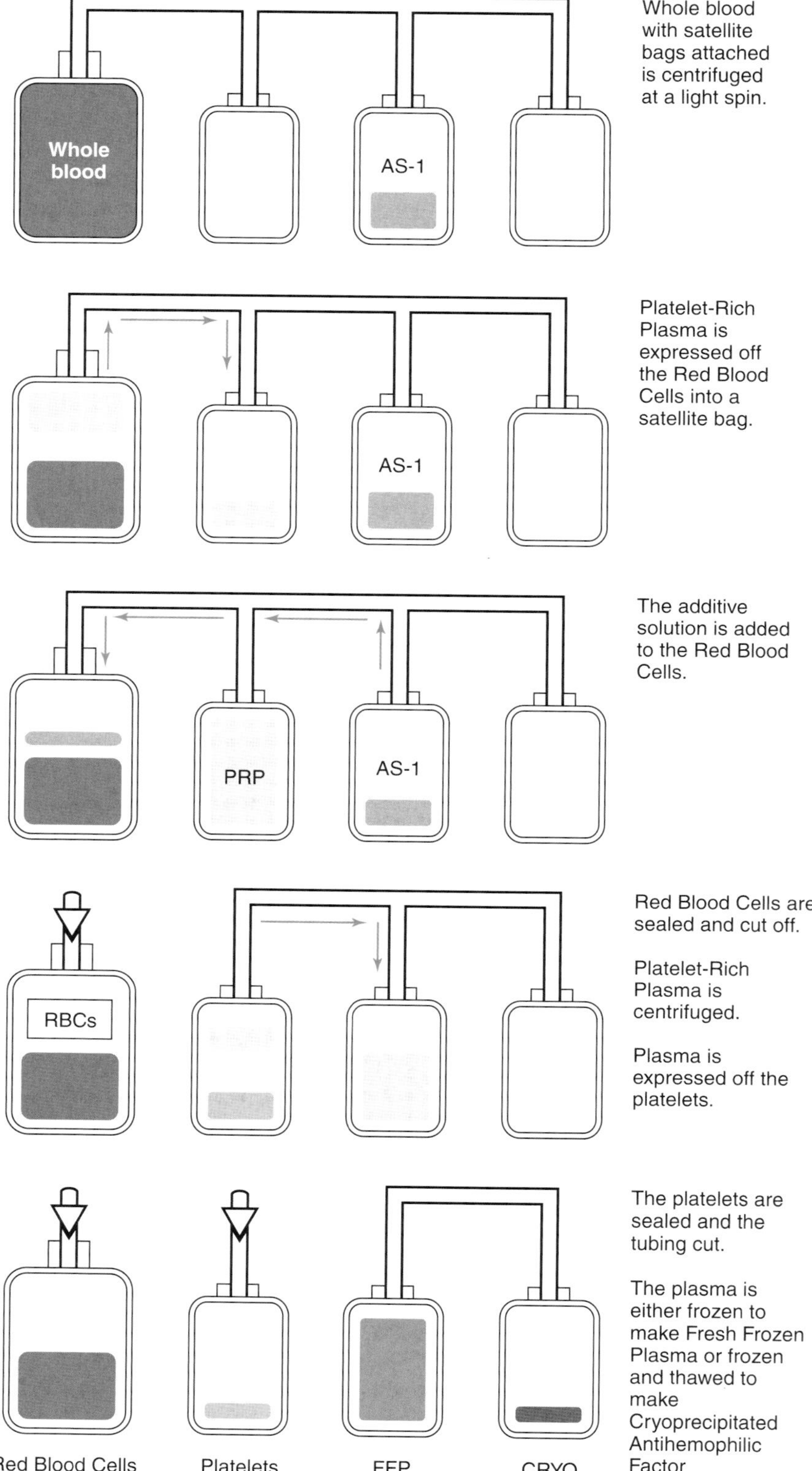

Fig. 17.1 Blood components from a unit of whole blood. Preparation of red blood cells, fresh frozen plasma, cryoprecipitate antihemophilic factor, and platelets from a whole-blood unit. *AS,* Additive solution; *CRYO,* cryoprecipitated antihemophilic factor; *FFP,* fresh frozen plasma; *PRP,* platelet-rich plasma; *RBCs,* red blood cells. (From Blaney KD, Howard PR: *Basic and applied concepts of blood banking and transfusion practices,* ed 3, St Louis, 2013, Mosby.)

individuals receiving platelets selected for human leukocyte antigen (HLA) or platelet compatibility, and individuals receiving units from blood relatives.

Plasma

When the RBCs are removed from whole blood, plasma remains. It is the liquid portion of whole blood that has been anticoagulated. Slightly more than half the volume of whole blood is plasma. Plasma should not be used to replace lost blood volume or protein because much safer products exist, including plasma substitutes such as albumin, synthetic colloids, and balanced salt solutions. These solutions have the advantage of not transmitting disease or causing allergic reactions. Plasma is appropriately used to replace coagulation factors, such as IX. Other possible plasma derivatives are serum immune globulin and Rh immune globulin (RhIg).

Fresh Frozen Plasma

When plasma is used, it is often in the form of fresh frozen plasma. Fresh frozen plasma is a good source of labile clotting factors and can be used to replace those coagulation factors. It is especially useful in treating multiple coagulation deficiencies, as seen with liver failure, disseminated intravascular coagulation (DIC), vitamin K deficiency, warfarin toxicity, or massive transfusions.

Plasma Derivatives: Factor VIII and Cryoprecipitate

Fresh frozen plasma is no longer used for the preparation of factor VIII. This blood component is now produced using monoclonal antibody technology. The use of monoclonal antibodies reduces the risk of transmission of infectious diseases, such as HIV and AIDS.

Cryoprecipitate antihemophilic factors can be extracted from frozen plasma. One unit of cryoprecipitate is 15 mL in volume and contains at least 150 mg of fibrinogen and at 80 IU of factor VIII. Von Willebrand factor is another important component of cryoprecipitate. At present, cryoprecipitate is used mainly as a replacement for fibrinogen in cases of liver failure, DIC, or massive transfusions. It can also be used when uremic patients are bleeding and when there are rare congenital deficiencies in fibrinogen.

Plasma Substitutes

Plasma substitutes include albumin and plasma protein fraction, which are prepared by the chemical fractionation of pooled plasma. These products are heat-treated to eliminate the risk of infectious diseases. They are used to treat patients who need replacement of blood volume. Alternatively, crystalloid (either saline or electrolyte) solutions are used.

Platelets

Platelets concentrates are used for patients who are bleeding as a result of low platelet counts or, occasionally, abnormally functioning platelets. Massive transfusions may also result in thrombocytopenia and require platelet concentrates. Occasionally, patients develop HLA antibodies that make transfused platelet concentrates ineffective. Crossmatched platelets are a resource for patients who are refractory to platelet transfusions. In such cases, it may be necessary to select HLA-matched donors. Platelets can be harvested by the process of plateletpheresis or from a single unit of fresh, whole blood.

Plateletpheresis

Many Red Cross Blood Centers and private donor sites use automated apheresis or plateletpheresis to collect platelets (Fig. 17.2). Plateletpheresis is a high-yield method for obtaining platelets for transfusion. Because all components, except platelets, are returned to the donor in plateletpheresis, it is possible to obtain three single donor units from one donor during a single apheresis session. Plateletpheresis allows for a yield of 200 to 500 mL of a single donor platelet unit with a minimum of 3.0×10^{11} platelets.[2]

Random-Donor Platelet Concentrates

Platelets are prepared by centrifugation and removal of plasma from a fresh unit of donor blood and subsequent separation of platelets from platelet-poor plasma. This is referred to as *random-donor platelets*. Four to six random-donor units of approximately 50 mL each are usually pooled together immediately before transfusion. Up to 8 units of individual platelets, each from a separate donor, can be pooled into a single bag for transfusion. Platelets expire 4 hours after pooling. All units are from the same ABO type. If ABO-compatible platelets are unavailable, ABO-incompatible platelets can be substituted with negligible risk. The usual adult dose is 4 to 6 units of pooled random-donor platelets.

Special Handling and Concerns

Units of platelets are stored at room temperature (20–24°C) with continuous, gentle agitation for 5 days. Bacterial contamination is a problem encountered with the platelet blood component.

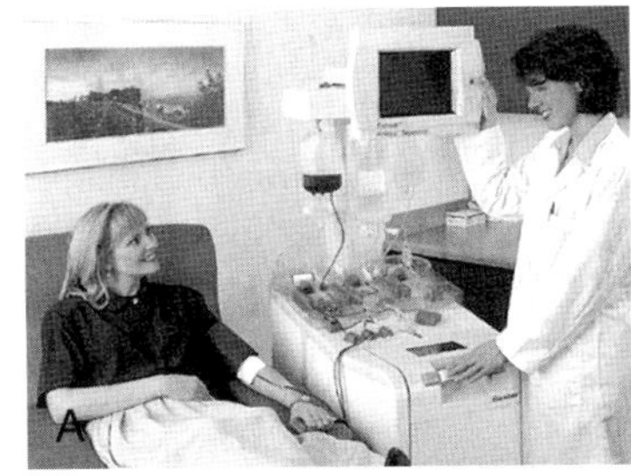

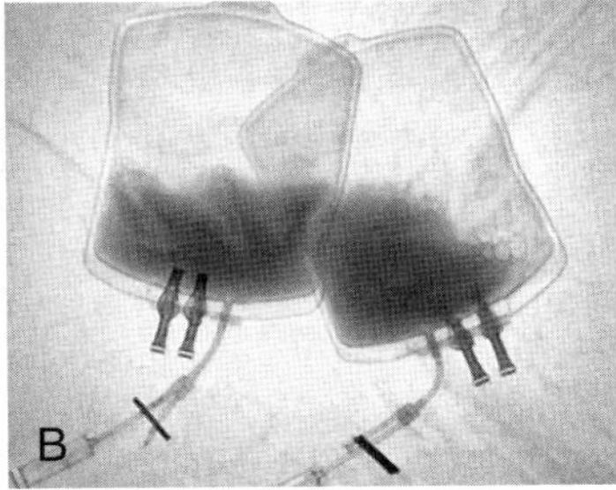

Fig. 17.2 Apheresis. (A) Instrument used for apheresis procedures. (B) Apheresis platelets. (From Blaney KD, Howard PR: *Basic and applied concepts of immunohematology*, ed 3, St. Louis, 2013, Mosby.)

BLOOD DONATION: DONORS, COLLECTION, STORAGE, AND PROCESSING

In an effort to ensure the blood supply is as safe as possible, all donors must meet specific eligibility criteria outlined by the FDA, accrediting organizations such as the AABB, and individual donation centers. To donate blood, individuals must be at least 16 years old (or the age specified by state law), healthy, and feeling well on the donation day. In addition, donors must meet weight and hemoglobin level requirements. Specific criteria exist for donors of human cells, tissue, and cellular-based and tissue-based products as well. Although the criteria are similar to those applied to blood donors, there are differences as a result of the unique patient needs for these products.

Donor Selection and Identification

The selection and proper identification of the potential blood donor are essential in ensuring that the blood collected for transfusion is safe and will be of benefit to the recipient. The most up-to-date eligibility information can be obtained by contacting the American Red Cross or visiting www.arc.com, or refer to *AABB Standards for Blood Banks and Transfusion Services* or the latest yearly edition of the Code of Federal Regulations (CFR) at 21 CFR 640.3.

The selection of the RBC donor involves a medical history and abbreviated physical examination. Two considerations must be kept in mind when selecting the donor: whether the procedure might be harmful to the donor and whether the donor's blood might be harmful to the recipient. The selection process involves a series of questions to ensure safety to both the donor and recipient.

The general guidelines to donate blood for transfusion to another person are that you must:

- Be healthy;
- Be at least 17 years old, or 16 years old if allowed by state law;
- Weigh at least 110 pounds; and
- Not have donated whole blood in the last 8 weeks (56 days) or double red cells in the last 16 weeks (112 days).

"Healthy" means that you feel well and can perform normal activities. If you have a chronic condition such as diabetes or high blood pressure, "healthy" also means that you are being treated and the condition is under control. Specific questions are asked of the donor to comply with regulations.

Other aspects of each potential donor's health history are discussed as part of the donation process before any blood is collected.

Donors also are screened for disease risk factors using a health history questionnaire (Table 17.2). Through this confidential questionnaire, donors are asked specific and direct questions regarding lifestyle, health, medical history, and travel to ensure that blood donation will not be injurious to them and that patients receive safe blood products. Table 17.3 presents examples of donor acceptability.

Each donor receives a brief examination during which temperature, pulse, blood pressure, and blood count (hemoglobin or hematocrit) are measured.

Collection of Red Blood Cells

Blood for transfusion must be collected and handled under strictly sterile conditions to prevent contamination. The collection must be aseptic, must use a sterile closed collection system, and must use a single venipuncture. If more than one venipuncture is done, a new container and donor set must be used for each skin puncture. The phlebotomist must sign or initial the donor record, whether or not a full unit is collected. The usual amount of blood drawn for 1 unit of whole blood is 450 mL. When the proper amount has been collected, extra tubes and segments must be filled with up to 30 mL of blood for the various testing procedures required before the blood can be used.

Anticoagulants and Preservatives

Infused blood, or blood that is administered by transfusion, must be anticoagulated. Blood must be collected into an FDA-approved container. The RBCs must be pyrogen-free and sterile, and they must contain anticoagulant sufficient for the amount of blood to be collected. The anticoagulant and preservative solution is generally a combination of citrate and dextrose. Citrate is used as an anticoagulant, which binds calcium, thus preventing activation of the coagulation cascade. Dextrose is used to provide an energy source for the RBCs. Inorganic phosphate buffer is added to increase adenosine triphosphate production, which increases RBC viability.

Various anticoagulant-preservative solutions in quantities of 50 to 100 mL are used to prolong the shelf life of blood cells. One solution is CPDA-1, which is FDA approved for storage of up to 35 days at 1°C to 6°C. ADSOL is another solution that extends the shelf life of stored blood to 42 days. Blood that is more than 3 weeks old is considered to be aged. Older blood may be detrimental to patients because of a deficiency in nitric oxide, a chemical messenger that relaxes blood vessels.

Once the unit has passed this date, the blood is outdated and must be removed from the blood supply.

Labeling

Conversion to the International Society of Blood Transfusion (ISBT) "128" blood labeling has begun in the United States. ISBT 128 is an international information standard for blood, tissue, and cellular therapy products.[3] In the United States, this working group is the Americas Technical Advisory Group of the International Council for Commonality in Blood Banking Automation (ICCBBA). The "United States Industry Consensus Standard for the Uniform Labeling of Blood and Blood Components Using ISBT 128" document provides specific instructions on where there is flexibility in the ISBT 128 Standard Technical Specification.

Specific information about product coding may be found in the "Product Code Structure and Labeling—Blood Components" document. Specific information about the terminology used in product coding is found in the "Standard Terminology for Blood, Cellular Therapy, and Tissue Product Descriptions" document. Version 3.0.0 of this document is considerably reorganized and expanded from Version 2.0.0. Many more examples of labels and text are included to help US users standardize labels while meeting the requirements of the FDA, the AABB,

TABLE 17.2 Abbreviated Donor History Questionnaire

	Yes	No
Date of Last Donation:		
1. Are you feeling healthy and well today?		
2. Have you read the educational materials?		
In the past 48 hours		
3. Have you taken aspirin or anything that has aspirin in it?		
In the past 6 weeks		
4. Female donors: Have you been pregnant or are you pregnant now? (Males: check "I am male.")		
In the past 8 weeks have you		
5. Donated blood, platelets, or plasma?		
6. Had any vaccinations or other shots?		
7. Had contact with someone who had a smallpox vaccination?		
In the past 16 weeks		
8. Have you donated a double unit of red cells using an apheresis machine?		
Since your last donation have you		
9. Had any new medical problems or diagnoses?		
10. Had any new medical treatments?		
11. Taken any of the medications on the Medication Deferral List?		
12. Been outside the United States or Canada?		
13. Come into contact with someone else's blood?		
14. Had an accidental needlestick?		
15. Had sexual contact with anyone who has HIV/AIDS or has had a positive test for the HIV/AIDS virus?		
16. Had sexual contact with a prostitute or anyone else who takes money or drugs or other payment for sex?		
17. Had sexual contact with anyone who has ever used needles to take drugs or steroids or anything not prescribed by their doctor?		
18. Had sexual contact with anyone who has hemophilia or has used clotting factor concentrates?		
19. Female donors: had sexual contact with a male who has ever had sexual contact with another male? (Males: check "I am male.")		
20. Had sexual contact with anyone who was born in or lived in Africa?		
21. Had sexual contact with a person who has hepatitis?		
22. Lived with a person who has hepatitis?		
23. Received money, drugs, or other payment for sex?		
24. Male donors: had sexual contact with another male, even once? (Females: check "I am female.")		
25. Had a tattoo?		
26. Had ear or body piercing?		
27. Been in juvenile detention, lockup, jail, or prison for more than 72 hours?		
28. Used needles to take drugs, steroids, or anything not prescribed by your doctor?		
29. Have any of your relatives had Creutzfeldt–Jakob disease?		

Blood and Blood Products, Product Listings and Related Information, AABB and PPTA Donor History Questionnaires, Questions about Blood https://www.fda.gov/BiologicsBloodVaccines/BloodBloodProducts/default.htm. Accessed 11.30.18.

and the ISBT 128 Standard. Documents important to ISBT 128 will be subject to a continual revision process.

At this time, both ISBT 128 and Codabar blood product–labeling formats are in use in the United States. The ABO blood group and Rh type are also shown on the label, once these tests are completed. In addition to blood group and Rh type, proper labeling of each unit of blood or blood component must include at least the following information:

- name of the product (whole blood, RBCs)
- type and amount of anticoagulant
- volume of the unit
- required storage temperature
- name address of the collecting facility, including FDA registration or license number
- expiration date
- unique donor identification number
- whether donor is a volunteer, autologous, or paid
- statements regarding recipient identification, reference to the circular of information, infectious disease risk, and prescription requirement

The pilot tubes and segments for testing must also be properly labeled. A stoppered or sealed sample of donor RBCs must be retained and properly stored by the transfusion service for at least 7 days after transfusion.

Storage of Blood

Preserved RBCs must be stored in a refrigerator with a constant temperature of 1°C to 6°C. Some type of alarm must be available that will go off whenever the temperature is not within these limits. A thermometer for recording the temperature must be

TABLE 17.3 Examples of Donor Acceptability

Condition	Comments
Acupuncture	Acceptable
Piercing (ears, body), electrolysis	Acceptable as long as the instruments used were sterile or single-use equipment
Tattoo	Wait 12 months after a tattoo if the tattoo was applied in a state that does not regulate tattoo facilities. This requirement is related to concerns about hepatitis.
Allergy	Acceptable as long as donor feels well, has no fever, and has no problems breathing through the mouth
Antibiotics	Acceptable after finishing oral antibiotics for an infection (bacterial or viral); may have taken last pill on the date of donation
	Antibiotic by injection for an infection acceptable 10 days after last injection
	Acceptable if donor is taking antibiotics to prevent an infection (such as before dental procedures or for acne)
	Some conditions that require antibiotics to prevent an infection must still be evaluated at the time of donation by the responsible medical director.
Asthma	Acceptable as long as not having difficulty breathing at the time of donation and feeling well
	Medications for asthma do not disqualify.
Birth control	Acceptable
Bleeding condition	Donors with clotting disorder from factor V who are not receiving anticoagulants are eligible to donate; all others must be evaluated by the health historian at the collection center.
Blood pressure	Acceptable as long as below 180 mm Hg systolic and below 100 mm Hg diastolic at the time of donation
	Acceptable as long as donor feels well on arrival to donate
Cancer	Depends on type of cancer and treatment history
Chronic illnesses	Acceptable as long as donor feels well
Cold, flu	Not acceptable if donor does not feel well on the day of donation
Dental procedures and oral surgery	Acceptable after dental procedures, as long as there is no infection present
	Wait until after finishing antibiotics for a dental infection.
	Wait for 3 days after having oral surgery.
Diabetes	Acceptable if well controlled on insulin or oral medications
	NOTE: Donors with diabetes who since 1980 ever used bovine (beef) insulin made from cattle from the United Kingdom are ineligible to donate. This requirement is related to concerns about bovine spongiform encephalitis.
Hormone replacement therapy (HRT)	Women receiving HRT for menopausal symptoms and prevention of osteoporosis are eligible to donate.
Immunization, vaccination	Acceptable if vaccinated for influenza, tetanus, or meningitis, provided donor is symptom-free and fever-free; includes the tetanus, diphtheria, pertussis vaccine
	Acceptable if donor received a human papillomavirus vaccine (such as Gardasil)
	Wait 4 weeks after immunizations for German measles (rubella); measles, mumps, rubella; chickenpox; and shingles.
	Wait 2 weeks after immunizations for red measles (rubeola), mumps, polio (by mouth), and yellow fever vaccine.
	Wait 21 days after immunization for hepatitis B, as long as donor is not given the immunization for exposure to hepatitis B.
	Wait 8 weeks (56 days) from the date of having a smallpox vaccination with no complications.
Malaria	Wait 3 years after completing treatment for malaria.
	Wait 12 months after returning from trip to area where malaria is found.
	Wait 3 years after living in a country or countries where malaria is found.
Pregnancy, nursing	Persons who are pregnant are not eligible to donate.
	Wait 6 weeks after giving birth.

Modified from Miller YM: *Blood eligibility guidelines, American Red Cross* (website). www.redcrossblood.org/donating-blood/eligibility-requirements/eligibility-criteria-topic#considerations_health. Accessed March 2009.

installed. Stored packed blood is inspected daily for color, turbidity, appearance of clots, and presence of hemolysis. RBC units are removed when they do not meet the appearance criteria established by the transfusion service.

Blood-Processing Tests

The FDA is responsible for ensuring the safety of the US blood supply. A blood supply with zero risk of transmitting infectious disease may not be possible, but the FDA takes several measures to protect and enhance the safety of blood products. Because of the improvements in donor-screening procedures and the use of a variety of new tests in the last few years, the blood supply is safer from infectious diseases than it has been at any other time.

The blood safety system established by the FDA depends on the following:

1. Accurate and complete educational material for donors so that they can assess their risk
2. Sensitive communication of the donor-screening questions
3. Donor understanding and honesty
4. Quality-controlled infectious marker testing procedures
5. Appropriate handling and distribution of blood and blood products for patient use

The most important consideration in ensuring that blood is free of transmissible diseases is the careful screening of a blood donor. The virtual elimination of paid blood donation in the United States has significantly decreased the risk of hepatitis. This, together with procedures to allow for self-deferral of donors who have risk factors for HIV, the causative agent of AIDS, has done much to ensure the safety of the blood supply. In addition, the following high-risk groups are usually not eligible to donate blood:

- Anyone who has ever used injection drugs not prescribed by a physician
- Men who have had sexual contact with other men since 1977
- Anyone who has ever received clotting factor concentrates such as hemophilia factor
- Anyone with a positive test for HIV or AIDS
- Men and women who have engaged in sex for money or drugs since 1977
- Anyone who has had hepatitis since his or her 11th birthday
- Anyone who has had babesiosis or Chagas disease
- Anyone who has taken etretinate (Tegison) for psoriasis
- Anyone who has risk factors for Creutzfeldt–Jakob disease (CJD) or who has a blood relative with CJD
- Anyone who has risk factors for variant CJD
- Anyone who spent 3 months or more in the United Kingdom from 1980 through 1996
- Anyone who has spent 5 years in Europe from 1980 to the present

Routine Blood Screening Tests

Transfusion-Transmitted Infection. A transfusion-transmitted infection (21 CFR 630.3[l]) means a disease or disease agent:

1. That could be fatal or life-threatening, could result in permanent impairment of a body function or permanent damage to a body structure, or could necessitate medical or surgical intervention to preclude permanent impairment of body function or permanent damage to a body structure; and
2. For which there may be a risk of transmission by blood or blood components, or by a blood derivative product manufactured from blood or blood components, because the disease or disease agent is potentially transmissible by that blood, blood component, or blood derivative product.

Blood is routinely screened for transmissible disease. The number of routine screening tests and ways of testing have increased dramatically in the past few years.

Nucleic acid amplification testing includes screening for hepatitis B, hepatitis C, HIV, and West Nile virus (WNV). In addition, donors of viable, leukocyte-rich concentrates must be tested for cytomegalovirus (CMV) with an FDA-cleared screening test for anti-CMV (total immunoglobulin [Ig]G and IgM).

Tests for Syphilis. A serologic test for syphilis continues to be required, although it has been questioned for years. It is now used as a surrogate marker for detecting donors who might be at high risk for transmitting transfusion-related disease.

Tests for Hepatitis. Transmission of hepatitis remains a risk in transfusion. From 80% to 90% of posttransfusion hepatitis is caused by the hepatitis C virus (HCV). Hepatitis B virus is responsible for about 10%, and a small percentage is caused by CMV and Epstein–Barr virus. For this reason, donated blood is screened with several tests for hepatitis virus. At present, these include a test for hepatitis B surface antigen and antibody tests for HCV and hepatitis B core antibody.

Tests for HIV/AIDS. Because of the long incubation period of HIV, donor selection methods and self-deferral of donors are essential in the screening of blood for HIV. All donated blood is tested for HIV.

Tests for Human T Cell Lymphotropic Virus. Units of blood must also be tested for human T cell lymphotropic virus types I and II antibody. A combination test is used.

West Nile Virus. Qualitative detection of WNV ribonucleic acid from volunteer blood donors is required. In addition, living organ donors and cadaveric donors must be screened.

Trypanosoma cruzi. A donor-screening test is available to detect antibodies to *Trypanosoma cruzi. T. cruzi* can be found in plasma and serum samples from infected human donors. The test is also intended for use to screen organ and tissue donors when specimens are obtained while the donor's heart is still beating.

Zika Virus

The FDA[4] has identified Zika as a transfusion-transmitted infection (TTI) under 21 CFR 630.3(l) and a relevant transfusion-transmitted infection (RTTI) under 21 CFR 630.3 (h)(2). This determination is based on the severity of the disease, risk of transfusion transmission by blood and blood components, the availability of appropriate screening measures, and significant incidence and prevalence affecting the potential donor population.

According to 21 CFR 630.3(h)(2), *relevant transfusion-transmitted infection* means a transfusion-transmitted infection not listed in 21 CFR 630.3(h)(1) when the following conditions are met: (i) Appropriate screening measures for the transfusion-transmitted infection have been developed and/or an appropriate screening test has been licensed, approved, or cleared for such use by the FDA and is available; and (ii) the disease or disease agent (a) may have significant incidence and/or prevalence to affect the potential donor population or (b) may have been released accidentally or intentionally in a manner that could place potential donors at risk of infection.

Donor-Screening Criteria

To ensure donor eligibility consistent with existing regulations, under 21 CFR 630.10(a), a blood establishment must not collect blood from a donor before determining that the donor is eligible to donate or before determining that an exception to 21 CFR 630.10 applies. Under 21 CFR 630.10(a), "to be eligible, the donor must be in good health and free from transfusion-transmitted infections as can be determined by the processes in this subchapter. A donor is not eligible if the donor is not in good health or if you identify any factor(s) that may cause the donation to adversely affect the safety, purity, or potency of the blood or blood component."

The provision of 21 CFR 630.10(e) requires blood-collection establishments to assess a donor's medical history to identify risk factors closely associated with exposure to, or clinical evidence of, an RTTI. Under 21 CFR 630.10(e)(1), "a donor is ineligible to donate when information provided by the donor or other reliable evidence indicates possible exposure to a relevant transfusion-transmitted infection if that risk of exposure is still applicable at the time of donation." Under 21 CFR 630.10(a), if a donor volunteers a recent history of Zika infection, you must not collect blood or blood components from that individual. We recommend that you defer such a donor for 120 days after a positive viral test or the resolution of symptoms, whichever timeframe is longer.

Furthermore, under 21 CFR 630.10(e)(2), a donor is ineligible to donate when donating could adversely affect the safety, purity, or potency of the blood or blood component. Under this provision, a donor must be assessed for "travel to, or residence in, an area endemic for a transfusion-transmitted infection, when such screening is necessary to assure the safety, purity, and potency of blood and blood components due to the risks presented by donor travel and the risk of transmission of that transfusion-transmitted infection by such donors" (21 CFR 630.10[e][2][iii]).

Although history of prior residence in or travel to an area with local Zika transmission or recent sexual exposure to a person who resided in or traveled to an area with local Zika transmission (with or without a diagnosis of Zika infection or suggestive symptoms) conveys increased risk of Zika, use of these risk factors to select safe donors becomes ineffective as new areas of local transmission emerge.

Laboratory Testing of Donor Blood

The FDA has concluded that it is necessary for blood establishments to implement nucleic acid testing of all donations or pathogen-reduction technology using an FDA-approved device to reduce the risk of Zika transmission by blood and blood components. The Center of Biologics Evaluation and Research at the FDA has issued alternative procedures to provide for appropriate donor testing for Zika with an investigational screening test available for use under investigational new drug applications. Alternatively, pathogen-reduction technology using an FDA-approved device as specified in the instructions for the use of the device to reduce the risk of Zika transmission may be implemented.

Federal Regulator Recommendations

1. Test all donations collected in the United States and its territories with an investigational individual donor nucleic acid test (ID-NAT) for Zika under an investigational new drug application (IND) or, when available, a licensed test; or
2. Implement pathogen-reduction technology for platelets and plasma using an FDA-approved pathogen-reduction device as specified in the instructions for the use of the device. Use of investigational pathogen reduction under an investigational device exemption (IDE) may be permitted in situations where approved technologies are unavailable. Because all donations will be tested using an investigational ID-NAT for Zika under an IND or, when available, a licensed test or pathogen-reduced using an FDA-approved pathogen-reduction device, donor educational material with respect to Zika and screening donors for Zika risk factors, such as travel history, and be discontinued.

Ebola Virus

Ebola virus (species *Zaire ebolavirus*) recommendations for assessing blood donor eligibility, donor deferral, and blood product management are directed toward an outbreak of Ebola virus disease (EVD) with widespread transmission occurring in at least one country.

Under 21 CFR 630.10(a), a donor must be in good health and free from TTIs. A donor must also have a normal temperature at the time of donation (21 CFR 630.10[f][1]). Additionally, under 21 CFR 630.10(a), a donor is not eligible if the provider identifies any factor(s) that may cause the donation to adversely affect the safety, purity, or potency of the blood or blood component. Such factors include symptoms of a recent or current illness, as well as travel to, or residence in, an area endemic for a TTI (21 CFR 630.10[e][2][i] and [iii]). Standard procedures that are already in place to assure that the donor is healthy at the time of donation serve as an effective safeguard against collecting blood or blood components from a donor who seeks to donate after the onset of clinical symptoms of EVD.

The following recommendations are intended to reduce the risks of collecting blood and blood components from potentially Ebola virus–infected persons during the asymptomatic incubation period before the onset of clinical symptoms, as well as from individuals with a history of Ebola virus infection or disease. This guidance contains a recommendation for updating donor educational materials when the Centers for Disease Control and Prevention (CDC) has classified one or more countries as having widespread transmission of Ebola virus. Recommendations should be followed for 4 weeks after the date. The CDC classifies the last affected country as a country with former widespread transmission. After this period, when there are no countries classified by the CDC as having widespread transmission of Ebola virus, it is appropriate to discontinue asking donors questions related to the risk of Ebola virus infection or disease.

Donor Educational Material and Donor History Questionnaire

In the United States it would be expected that very few individuals with a history of Ebola virus infection or disease will present as blood donors. When there are no countries classified by the CDC as having widespread transmission of Ebola virus, self-deferral of donors with a history of Ebola virus infection or disease should provide sufficient protection. Donor educational materials to instruct donors with a history of Ebola virus infection or disease to not donate blood or blood components should be regularly updated.

In the event that one or more countries are classified by the CDC as having widespread transmission of Ebola virus, the donor history questionnaire (DHQ), including full-length and abbreviated DHQs, and accompanying materials must incorporate elements to assess prospective donors for symptoms of recent or current illness with Ebola virus infection or disease and travel to, or residence in, an area endemic for Ebola virus in accordance with 21 CFR 630.10(e)(2).

The DHQ assesses donors for a history of Ebola virus infection or disease and a history of residence in or travel in the past 8 weeks to a country with widespread transmission of EVD or cases in urban areas with uncertain control measures. In addition, it assesses for a history of close contact in the past 8 weeks with a person confirmed to have Ebola virus infection or disease or a person under investigation (PUI) for Ebola virus infection or disease in whom diagnosis is pending. Close contact is defined as contact that could have resulted in direct exposure to body fluids. Individuals falling into this close-contact category include health care workers and other persons who care for, have lived with, or have otherwise been in contact with a PUI or a person confirmed to have Ebola virus infection or disease. This close-contact category includes individuals with a history of sexual contact in the past 8 weeks with a person known to have recovered from EVD before that instance of sexual contact, regardless of the time since the person's recovery.

OTHER TYPES OF BLOOD DONATIONS

Autologous Transfusions

The safest blood a recipient can receive is his or her own blood. Not only does this prevent transfusion-transmitted infectious diseases, but it also eliminates the formation of antibodies to antigens in transfused RBCs from others and the possibility of GVHD. Blood donation also stimulates erythropoiesis by repeated preoperative phlebotomy.

Patients who meet certain criteria are encouraged to donate blood for themselves before anticipated surgery if they are likely to need a transfusion. There is a significant problem with outdating of blood donated for autologous purposes because it is frequently not used. However, patients who meet donor requirements for the donation of their blood to others (an allogenic donor) can give permission for their unused units of blood to be transferred to the allogenic units of blood. Intraoperative autologous transfusion or cell-salvage techniques are alternatives to autologous donation.

Directed Transfusions

In directed transfusions, the patient directly solicits blood for transfusion from family or friends. There is no evidence that patients can select safer donors. In fact, social pressure associated with directed donations may compromise the reliability of a donor's answers to health-history questions. It is also possible that the extra paperwork and other logistics increase the probability of clerical errors.

A patient must give consent and have his or her physician submit a written request to collect blood. Directed donations are tested for transfusion-transmitted infectious diseases in the same manner as volunteer blood donations.

ANTIGENS AND ANTIBODIES IN IMMUNOHEMATOLOGY

Transfusion medicine is based on a knowledge of antigens and antibodies. An **antigen** is defined as a foreign substance or a nonself antigen. If a foreign antigen is introduced into an immunocompetent individual, an antibody can be produced.

Red Blood Cell Groups

Each species of animal, humans included, has certain antigens unique to that species and usually present on the red cell membranes of members of that species. Some blood group antigens are found not only on RBCs but also in other body fluids such as saliva and plasma.

If the RBCs are transfused into a patient who has antibodies specific to antigens on RBCs, such as cells with A antigen transfused into a patient with anti-A antibodies, the RBCs will be destroyed (hemolyzed). This cellular destruction is what is meant by an "incompatible hemolytic transfusion reaction," and it can result in the death of the recipient.

It is also known that certain antigens are more common. If RBCs containing a foreign antigen are transfused into a recipient whose red cells do not contain that antigen, the recipient can form antibodies to that specific RBC antigen. Antibodies that react with antigens from a genetically different individual of the same species are referred to as **alloantibodies**.

Antigens that exist on a person's red cells within a particular blood group system represent that person's type for that system, such as the ABO system. The number of possible types within one system varies. The more complex Rh-Hr system has more than 100 possible types. Taking all systems and type combinations into account, more than 500 billion different types of RBCs are possible.

Although no two individuals are exactly alike, except identical twins, only certain antigens are likely to create transfusion problems (incompatible adverse effects of transfusion). There is always the possibility that an unknown or untested-for antigen may create a potential problem. The antigens most likely to cause reactions are in the ABO and Rh-Hr systems and must be tested for whenever blood is administered. In certain circumstances, such as the presence of alloantibody in a patient, in specific antigens screened, or in donor RBCs, patients who receive an antigen not present on their red cells may produce an alloantibody in their plasma. These alloantibodies can react with the corresponding foreign antigen in subsequent transfusions. The presence of an alloantibody and its corresponding antigen can be demonstrated by **agglutination** in vitro or destruction of the RBC containing the foreign antigen in vivo. These two terms—*in vivo* (in the living body) and *in vitro* (in a laboratory setting)—are often used in discussing biological reactions.

Inheritance of Red Blood Cell Groups

Genes

The antigens present on an individual's RBC, WBC, and platelet membranes are inherited. Each antigen is controlled by a gene, which is the unit of inheritance. If the gene for a particular antigen is present, that antigen would be expected to be expressed.

RBC antigens and HLAs conform with Mendelian laws of inheritance and are easily identifiable. Although molecular deoxyribonucleic acid (DNA) methods are replacing antigen–antibody testing, knowledge of inheritance related to antigen inheritance is important. Genetic markers such as antigens can be used in paternity testing and exclude a man who is not the father. In direct exclusion, a child who possesses a genetic marker not possessed by either the mother or the alleged father allows for exclusion of the alleged father, as seen in this table:

	Mother	Alleged Father	Child
Phenotype	Group O	Group B	Group A
Genotype	O/O	B/B or B/O	A/O

Conclusion: The alleged father is not the father of this child.

Chromosomes

Each cell, except for mature RBCs, consists of cytoplasm and a nucleus. If the nucleus is observed under the microscope at approximately the time of cell division, several long, threadlike structures will be visible. These structures are referred to as *chromosomes*. Each species has a specific number of chromosomes, and the chromosomes occur in pairs. Humans have 46 chromosomes (23 chromosome pairs). The paired chromosomes are similar in size and shape and have their own distinct functions. A complete set of 23 chromosomes is inherited from each parent. Chromosomes occur in pairs in somatic (body) cells but not in sex cells (sperm and ovum), which contain 23 single chromosomes.

Gene Location (Linkage)

Because the gene is the unit of inheritance, it must also be located within the nucleus. Genes are exceedingly small particles that, when associated in linear form, make up the chromosome. They are too small to see under the normal brightfield microscope but together are visible as the chromosome. Genes are made up of DNA. Each trait that is inherited is controlled by the presence of a specific gene. The genes responsible for a particular trait always occur at exactly the same point or position on a particular chromosome; this position is referred to as the *locus* of the gene.

Research in the field of genetics is continually revealing new information about the location or sequence of genes on the chromosome and about diseases that are genetically inherited or environmentally induced. If genes for different inherited traits are known to be carried on the same chromosome, they are said to be *syntenic*. This term is useful in referring to genes on a single chromosome that are too far apart to display absolute linkage in inheritance. Genes that are located on the same chromosome and are normally inherited together are known as linked genes. The closer the loci of the genes, the closer is the linkage.

Alleles

Inherited traits are somewhat variable within a species. Variants of a gene for a particular trait are referred to as **alleles** for that trait. Because humans have only two genes (one pair) for any given trait, human cells will have only two alleles. However, the number of possible alleles for a trait varies. A person who has identical alleles for a trait is said to be **homozygous** for that trait. A person who has two different alleles for a trait is **heterozygous** for that trait.

Certain alleles may be stronger than or mask the presence of other alleles. In transfusion medicine, the various alleles for a particular blood group system are equally dominant, or codominant. If the gene is present (and there is a suitable testing solution available), it will be detected.

Phenotypes and Genotypes

Two other genetic terms often used in transfusion medicine are ***phenotype*** and ***genotype***. The *phenotype* is what is seen by tests made directly on the RBCs, even though other antigens may be present. The *genotype* refers to the actual total genetic makeup of an individual. It is usually impossible to determine the complete genotype in the laboratory; this usually requires additional studies, especially family studies.

Isoantibodies and Immune Antibodies

Antibody classification in immunohematology includes environmentally acquired and immune antibodies. The **isoantibodies** result from internal (such as bacterial) or external antigenic stimulus. Substances very similar to RBC group antigens A and B are so widely distributed in nature that the antibody will develop in a person if the antigen is not present. Certain bacteria and foods may have A-like or B-like antigens.

Examples of isoantibodies are the anti-A and anti-B antibodies found in the ABO blood group system. In this system, if the red cell lacks the A antigen, anti-A antibody will be found in the serum, and if the red cell lacks the B antigen, anti-B antibody will be found in the serum. Anti-A and anti-B antibodies are routinely used in testing for the ABO blood group. These antibodies are usually IgM antibodies.

In comparison, **immune antibodies** result from stimulation by specific blood group antigens. Immune antibodies are also referred to as *unexpected antibodies*. They are usually the result of specific antigenic stimulation from foreign antigens on RBCs. These antibodies are the result of immunization caused by pregnancy or prior blood transfusion. Immune antibodies are of the IgG type.

Means of Detecting Antigen–Antibody Reactions

A biological reaction that normally occurs in vivo may be demonstrated in vitro.

Antisera

To determine a person's blood type, some type of substance must be available to show what antigens are present on the red cell. The substance used for this purpose is referred to as an antiserum (plural *antisera*) or reagent. An antiserum is a prepared and highly purified solution of antibody and is named based on the antibody it contains. For example, a solution of anti-A antibodies is called *anti-A antiserum*.

Preparation of Antisera. Most of the antisera used in transfusion medicine are prepared commercially and purchased by the blood bank. In general, antiserum is prepared as follows:

1. Monoclonal antisera are produced by hybridization, a fusion of a single clone of human neoplastic antibody-producing cells with sensitized splenic lymphocytes obtained from a rodent species.
2. Animals are deliberately inoculated with antigen, and the resulting serum, which contains antibody, is purified and standardized for use as an antiserum.

Antisera Requirements. Antiserum must meet certain requirements to be acceptable for use. It must be specific for the antigen to be detected, that is, specific under the manufacturer's recommended test conditions. It must have a sufficient concentration, or titer, to detect antigen. Antiserum must have a certain avidity for, or strength of reaction with, corresponding RBC antigens. It must also be sterile, clear, provided in a good container with a dropper, and stable. Antiserum should be marked with an expiration date and must not be used after this date. In addition, it must be stored at 4°C when not in use.

Exact requirements for antisera are defined by the FDA Center for Biologics Evaluation and Research. When commercial antisera are used, the manufacturer's directions must be followed carefully and quality assurance procedures established and documented. For antisera that are produced locally and are unlicensed, there must be records of reactivity and specificity.

Reaction of Antisera with Red Cells. When antiserum is mixed with RBCs, an antigen–antibody reaction may or may not occur. If a reaction does occur, the corresponding antigen must be present on the red cell, and the result is a positive reaction. If a reaction does not occur, the antigen is absent, and the result is negative. For example, a positive reaction with anti-A antiserum demonstrates the presence of the A antigen on the red cell.

In the original definition of antibody, it was stated that antibody resulting from antigenic stimulation would react with the antigen in an observable manner. In transfusion medicine, two types of observable reactions may occur: agglutination and hemolysis.

Agglutination

Agglutination is clumping of RBCs caused by the reaction of a specific antibody and antigen on the cells. A positive antigen–antibody reaction results in an immediate combination of antibody and antigen on the red cell, followed by the visible agglutination, which takes longer to form. The IgG antibody, for example, is thought to be a somewhat Y-shaped structure with a reactive site at the end of each arm of the Y (Fig. 17.3). Each reactive site is capable of combining with corresponding antigen. Agglutination is thought to be the result of bridging of the RBCs by antibody reacting with antigen sites on adjacent RBCs. This bridging causes the RBCs to stick together. Several such bridges result in visible clumping. The degree of agglutination varies (Fig. 17.4). Very strong agglutination forms a large mass of cells that can be easily seen macroscopically. Less strong agglutination results in correspondingly smaller clumps of cells that can also be seen macroscopically, and finally in clumps of cells that can be seen only microscopically. Various strengths of agglutination can be observed.

Hemolysis

Hemolysis is the result of lysis, or destruction, of the red cell by a specific antibody. The antigen–antibody reaction causes the activation of complement, which results in the rupture of the cell membrane and the subsequent release of hemoglobin. The result is a clear, cherry-red solution, with no cloudiness because no cells are present. Hemolysis can be complete, in which no intact RBCs remain in the solution, or partial, leaving

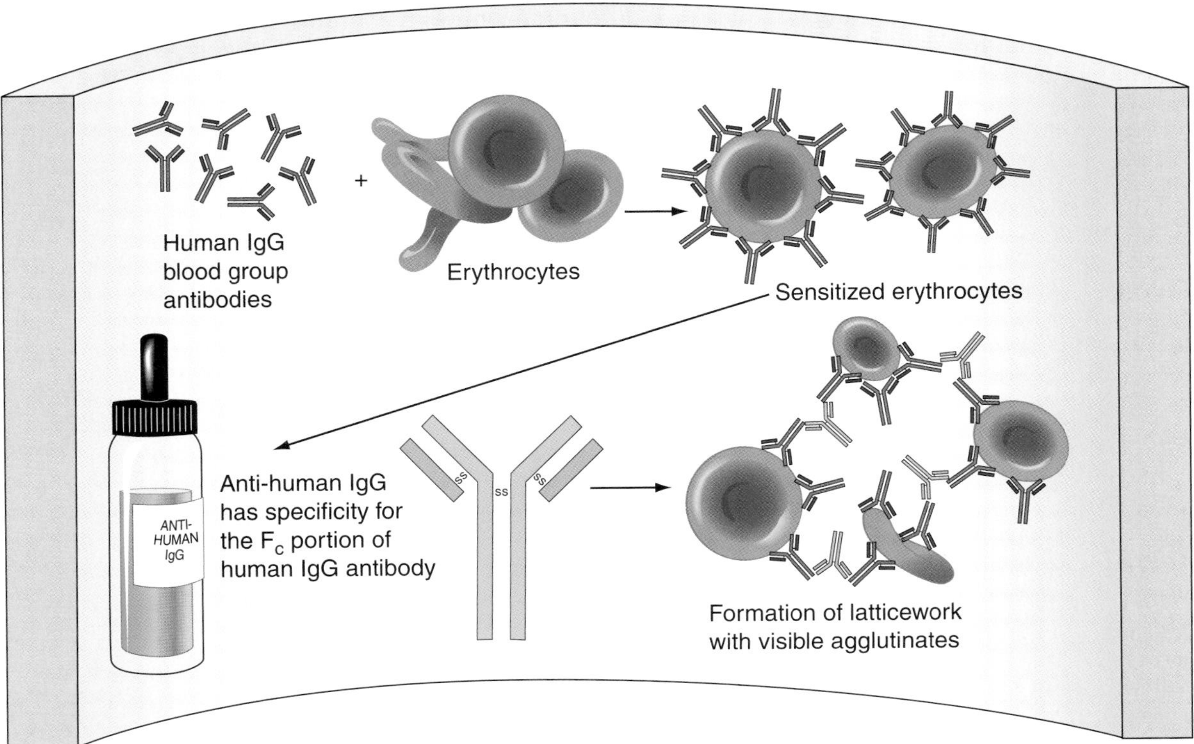

Fig. 17.3 Antihuman globulin (AHG) reaction. Antihuman globulin antibodies form a bridge between adjacent erythrocytes sensitized with human immunoglobulin (IgG) or complement components. (From Cooling L, Downs T: Immunohematology. In McPherson RA, Pincus MR, editors: *Henry's clinical diagnosis and management by laboratory methods,* ed 22, Philadelphia, 2011, Elsevier/Saunders, p. 713, Fig. 35.20.)

READING AGGLUTINATION

GRADE	DESCRIPTION		APPEARANCE	
	Cells	Supernate	Macroscopic*	Microscopic†
0	No agglutinates	Dark, turbid, homogeneous	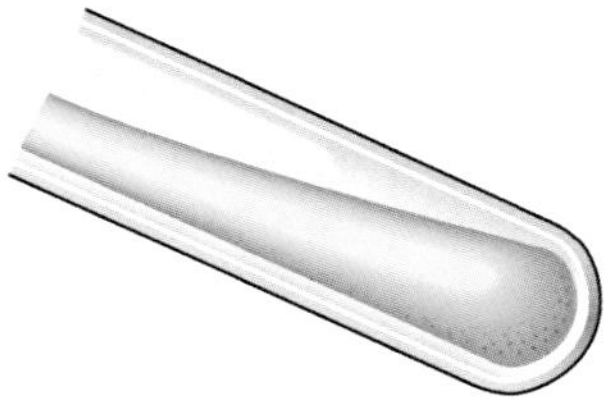	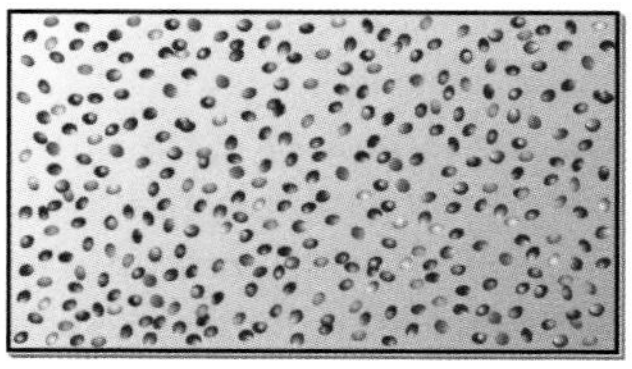
w+	Many tiny agglutinates Many free cells May not be visible without microscope	Dark, turbid	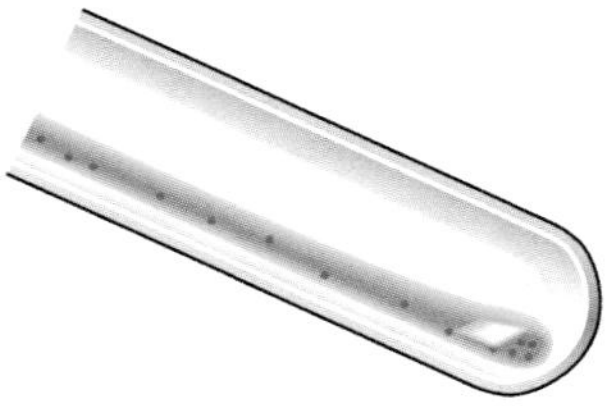	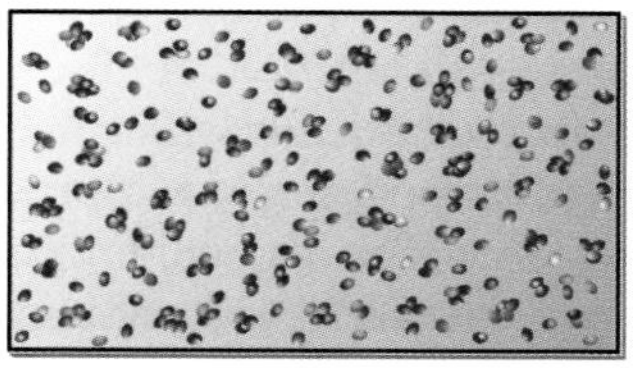
1+	Many small agglutinates Many free cells	Turbid	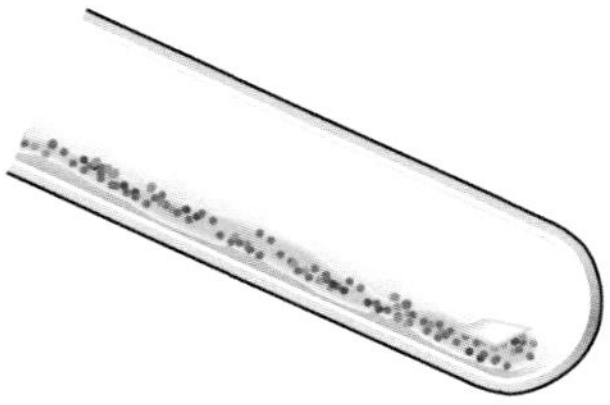	
2+	Many medium-sized agglutinates Moderate number of free cells	Clear	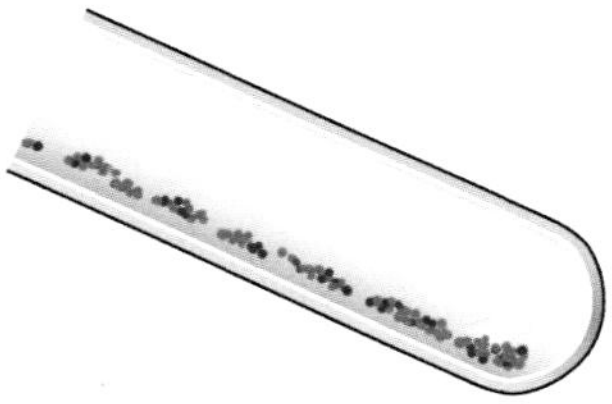	
3+	Several large agglutinates Few free cells	Clear	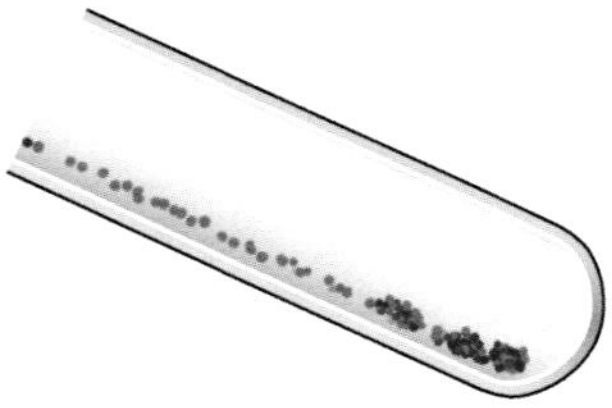	
4+	One large, solid agglutinate No free cells	Clear	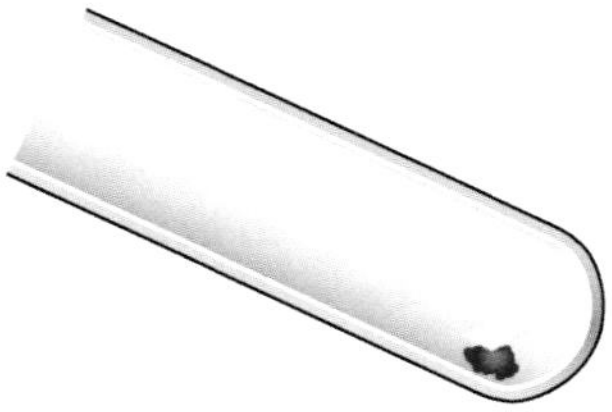	

*For any one grade, readings can be on a scale from weak+ to strong+ (e.g., grade 2 can be scored as 2+w, 2+, or 2+s, depending on the number and size of agglutinates).
†Microscopic readings are generally performed to differentiate pseudoagglutination (rouleaux) from true agglutination, to detect mixed-field reactions, and to confirm a negative reaction.

Fig. 17.4 Reading red blood cell agglutination reactions. (From Turgeon ML: *Immunology and serology in laboratory medicine,* ed 6, St Louis, 2018, Mosby.)

some RBCs intact. Partial hemolysis is particularly difficult to interpret. It is important that blood bank testing be performed on serum or plasma that is free of hemolysis and that whenever hemolysis occurs, it is interpreted as a positive reaction.

Role of Complement in Hemolysis

For hemolysis to occur, a group of protein components called *complement* must be present in the serum being tested. Complement is a complex substance with 18 plasma protein components. It is important in transfusion medicine because some antigen–antibody reactions require the presence of complement to be demonstrated in vitro. Almost all normal sera contain complement when fresh, but it is destroyed by heat. For complement to be active, serum must be either fresh or stored correctly. Complement will remain active if stored for 24 to 48 hours at 4°C or for 2 months when stored at −50°C.

If the traditional classic complement pathway is activated by an antigen–antibody reaction, complement components will react sequentially in a cascade that terminates in a membrane attack complex that punctures the cell membrane. If the cell is an RBC, hemolysis will result, with hemoglobin spilling out through the punctured membrane.

Note that it is highly questionable that any RBC antibodies will be undetectable even without active complement. That is why it is acceptable to use plasma in antibody screening, identification, and crossmatching procedures. Even without complement, it is possible to detect antibodies and incompatibility. Some antibody specificities will also bind complement, if it is present, and can cause hemolysis in vivo. These antibodies will still react at RT (ABO antibodies) or at AHG (Kidd antibodies).

Blood-Banking Techniques

The portion of blood used for testing procedures (typing and crossmatching) can be either serum (clotted) or plasma (anticoagulated). The specimen of choice for all blood bank testing has become plasma. Plasma may cause some technical problems for tube tests, such as small fibrin clots that may be present in the plasma and may be incorrectly interpreted as a positive result, but plasma is generally the sample of choice for the newer gel tests. This problem is more likely to occur in clotted specimens that are incompletely clotted or from patients on some level of anticoagulation therapy.

The detection of antigen on RBCs requires the demonstration of a positive reaction of the cells with a specific solution of antibodies (antiserum). The techniques by which RBCs and antiserum are brought together vary.

Traditionally, RBC group tests are performed in test tubes, although newer techniques, such as dextran-acrylamide gel and solid-phase technology in microplates, have become increasingly popular. When test tubes are used, they are 10 × 75 or 12 × 75 mm. Results are seen as agglutination or hemolysis, as previously described. Other methods of detecting antigen–antibody reactions include inhibition of agglutination, immunofluorescence, enzyme-linked immunosorbent assay, and solid-phase RBC adherence tests using indicator RBCs (see Chapter 16).

Many factors affect RBC agglutination, which is thought to occur in two stages: sensitization and agglutination. The first stage involves the physical attachment of antibody to RBCs and is referred to as *sensitization.* Sensitization is affected by temperature, pH, incubation time, ionic strength, and the antigen–antibody ratio. These factors are influenced by the testing medium that is employed: isotonic saline solution, low-ionic-strength saline, or albumin solution.

The second stage of agglutination involves the formation of bridges between sensitized RBCs to form the lattice that is seen as agglutination. Factors that influence this stage include the distance between the cells, the effect of enzymes, and the effect of positively charged molecules such as hexadimethrine (Polybrene).

Factors that affect the reactions used to detect an antigen–antibody reaction include the following:

- Use of adequate serum and RBCs
- Correct concentration of cell suspensions
- The testing medium
- Proper temperature and duration of incubation
- Proper use of centrifugation
- The condition and correct use of reagents
- Accurate reading and interpretation of agglutination reactions

Correct conditions are essential for reliable tests. Development of correct techniques requires thorough knowledge of these considerations as well as of the RBC groups. The technique will also depend on the brand of antiserum that is used and the manufacturer's directions.

Other Methods of Detecting Antigen–Antibody Reactions

Recent advances in technology have led to other methods besides test tube reactions to detect antigen–antibody reactions. These methods, which may be manual or automated, include gel technology, microplate testing, and solid-phase RBC adherence methods.

Gel Technology. In 1985, Yves Lapierre developed gel technology. This led to commercial development by Micro Typing Systems (Pompano Beach, FL) and FDA approval for use in 1994. Essentially, the method uses dextran acrylamide gel particles to trap agglutinated RBCs (Fig. 17.5).

Testing is performed in a prefilled card containing gel mixed with the appropriate reagent. A credit card–size gel card contains six microtubes. Each microtube contains an upper reaction chamber and a section containing predispensed gel and reagents. Individual gel cards are available for ABO and Rh typing; AHG cards are available for indirect testing, such as compatibility testing, antibody screening, and antibody identification, and direct antiglobulin testing (DAT). A foil strip on the top of the card prevents spillage or drying out of the contents.

Testing involves adding measured volumes of RBCs and plasma/serum to the reaction chamber of the microtube. Incubation allows antigen–antibody reactions to occur. Centrifugation follows to promote maximum contact between antigens and antibodies. A positive reaction demonstrates trapping of RBCs at various levels in the microtube. Larger aggregates of

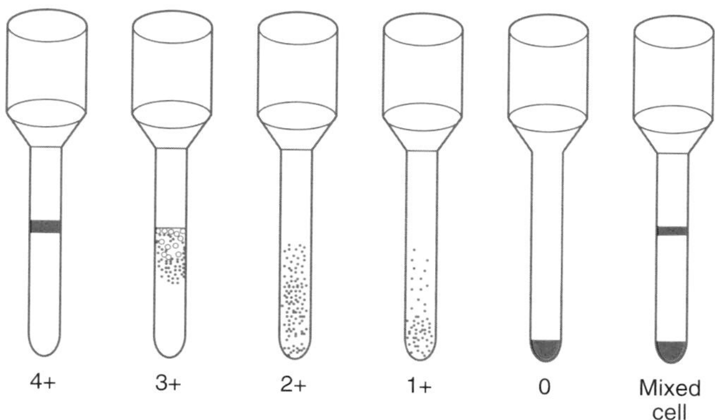

Fig. 17.5 Appearance of reaction patterns and grading for gel or column agglutination technology. (From Cooling L, Downs T: Immunohematology. In McPherson RA, Pincus MR, editors: *Henry's clinical diagnosis and management by laboratory methods*, ed 22, Philadelphia, 2011, Elsevier/Saunders, p. 719, Fig. 35.22.)

RBCs are trapped at the tip of the gel microtubes and do not travel through the gel when centrifuged. Smaller aggregates travel through the gel microtubes and may be trapped in either the top or bottom half of the tube. A negative reaction is demonstrated by the presence of a button of RBCs on the bottom of the microtube. Nonagglutinated cells travel without difficulty through the length of the tube and form a button at the tip after being centrifuges.

The ID-Micro Typing System (ID-MTS) Gel Test is suitable for a broad range of blood bank applications, including antibody screening and identification, ABO blood grouping and Rh phenotyping, compatibility testing, reverse serum grouping, and antigen typing, all using proven serologic methods. The Ortho ProVue Analyzer is a modular, microprocessor-controlled instrument designed to automate in vitro immunohematologic testing of human blood using the ID-MTS Gel Card technology.

Perceived advantages that this technology offers over tube testing are as follows:

- improved sensitivity and specificity
- no-wash antiglobulin procedure
- standardized procedures
- improved turnaround time
- enhanced regulatory compliance

Microplate Testing Methods. Automated microplate testing has been popular for routine testing in large blood donor centers. The technique can be used for RBC antigen testing and serum antibody detection. After addition of reagents, a microplate is centrifuged and resuspended to read. A positive reaction is demonstrated by a concentrated button of RBCs; a negative reaction is represented by well-dispersed RBCs throughout the well.

Solid-Phase Red Blood Cell Adherence Methods. The solid-phase RBC adherence serologic method has been available since the late 1980s. A commercially available system, Galileo, is manufactured by Immucor (Norcross, GA). Solid-phase technology is presently licensed for compatibility testing, antibody screening, and antibody identification. In this method, RBC screening cells are bound to the surface of a polystyrene microplate. When serum from a patient or donor is added, and low-ionic-strength

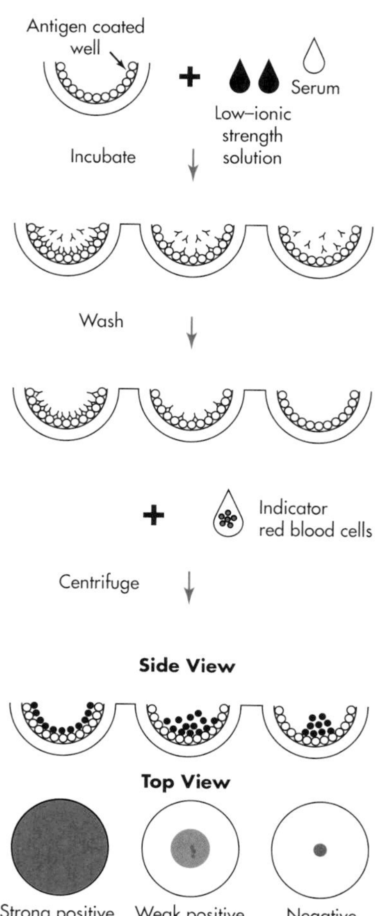

Fig. 17.6 Principles of solid-phase adherence technology with appearance of positive and negative reactions. (From Cooling L, Downs T: Immunohematology. In McPherson RA, Pincus MR, editors: *Henry's clinical diagnosis and management by laboratory methods*, ed 22, Philadelphia, 2011, Elsevier/Saunders, p. 719, Fig. 35.23.)

saline is added to the wells, the RBCs capture antibodies during the incubation phase. Subsequently, the plates are washed to remove unbound antibodies, and indicator cells are added to the wells of the microplate. The microplate is centrifuged to bring antigens and potential antibodies together (Fig. 17.6). A positive reaction is demonstrated by observing indicator RBCs being attached to the sides and bottom of the well. A negative reaction is demonstrated by the appearance of a red cell button on the bottom of the wells.

ABO RED BLOOD CELL GROUP SYSTEM

The ABO blood group system was first discovered and described in 1900 and 1901 by Karl Landsteiner, who divided RBCs into three groups: A, B, and O. In 1902 the fourth group, AB, was discovered by two of Landsteiner's pupils.

ABO Phenotypes

The ABO system consists of the groups, or phenotypes, A, B, AB, and O. These four groups may be explained by the presence or absence of two antigens on the RBC surface, the A antigen and the B antigen. If a person belongs to group A, the A antigen is present on the red cell. Group B persons have B antigen on their cells. Group AB individuals have both A and B, whereas group O people have neither A nor B.

ABO Genotypes

Genes on the chromosomes determine the antigen present on the red cell. Three allelic genes can be inherited in the ABO system: the A, B, and O genes. Because each person has two genes for any trait (one from each parent), the following combinations of alleles are possible: AA, AO, AB, BB, BO, and OO. These combinations represent the possible genotypes in the ABO system.

If the A gene is present on the chromosome, A antigen will be present on the RBCs. Presence of the B gene results in B antigen on the red cell. If both the A and B genes are present on the chromosome, A and B antigens will be expressed on the RBCs (Fig. 17.7). In addition, A substance can be demonstrated in body fluid if a person has a secretor gene, as discussed later. The presence of O gene results in neither antigen on the red cell.

In addition to the A and B genes, expression of the A and/or B antigens as A and/or B substance depends on another gene, H, at a different chromosomal location, to produce H substance, a precursor substrate for the production of the A and B antigens. Most H substance is converted to A and B antigen if the A gene and/or B gene are inherited. Group O individuals have a significant amount of H substance on their RBCs because none of the H substance is converted to A and B antigens because of the lack of A and/or B genes.

ABO Typing Procedures

When the ABO group is to be determined, both the cells and the serum should be typed as described. The antigen and antibody typing results should then be compared to be sure mistakes have not occurred and results are consistent. This is an excellent way to guard against errors in ABO grouping. ABO typing procedures are divided into front-typing and reverse-grouping procedures (Table 17.4).

Front Typing

Typing reactions that employ undetermined RBCs and known antibody or antisera are referred to as *antigen, cell, direct,* or *front-typing reactions* (Fig. 17.8; Student Procedure Worksheet 17.1).

Reverse Grouping

Testing methods that employ undetermined serum and known RBC antigens are referred to as *antibody, serum, indirect,* or *back-typing reactions* (Student Procedure Worksheet 17.2).

Red Cell Typing for Antigen

In testing RBCs for the ABO group, a suspension of RBCs in saline is prepared. This suspension is tested by mixing one portion with anti-A antiserum (anti-A antibodies), stored at 2°C to

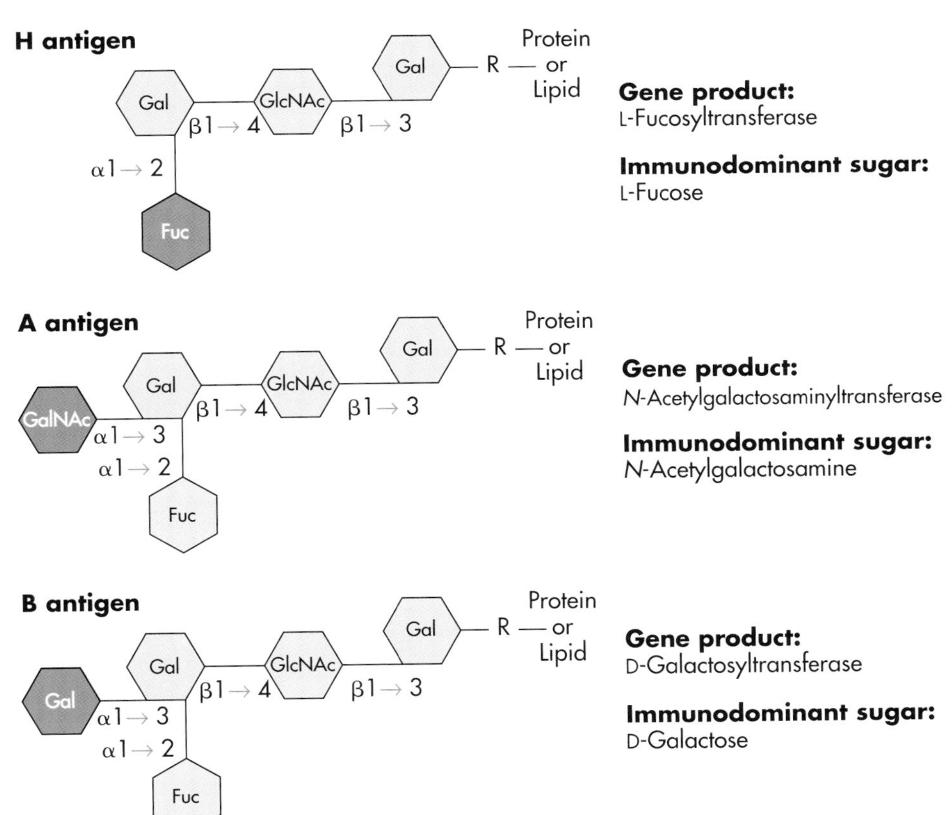

Fig. 17.7 ABH antigens. Biochemical structures of the H, A, and B antigens. *Fuc,* L-fructose; *Gal,* D-galactose; *GalNAc,* N-acetylgalactosamine; *GlcNAc,* N-acetylglucosamine. (From Blaney KD, Howard PR: *Basic and applied concepts of blood banking and transfusion practices,* ed 3, St Louis, 2013, Mosby.)

TABLE 17.4 ABO Typing Reactions

Blood Group (Phenotype)	Antigens on Red Cells	Antibody in Serum	Antigen, Front, or Direct Typing		Antibody, Back, or Indirect Typing		
			Reaction of Undetermined Cells With Anti-A Antiserum	Reaction of Undetermined Cells With Anti-B Antiserum	Reaction of Undetermined Serum With A_1 Cells	Reaction of Undetermined Serum With B Cells	Possible Genotype
A	A	Anti-B	Positive (+)	Negative (0)	Negative (0)	Positive (+)	AA, AO
B	B	Anti-A	Negative (0)	Positive (+)	Positive (+)	Negative (0)	BB, BO
AB	A and B	Neither	Positive (+)	Positive (+)	Negative (0)	Negative (0)	AB
0	Neither	Anti, A, anti-B	Negative (0)	Negative (0)	Positive (+)	Positive (+)	00

8°C. A second portion is mixed with anti-B antiserum (anti-B antibodies). The mixtures are then observed for a reaction. A positive reaction is the occurrence of agglutination or hemolysis. A negative reaction is the absence of agglutination or hemolysis. Results may be grouped as follows:

- Group A blood (RBCs): positive reaction of cells with anti-A antiserum
- Group B blood (RBCs): positive reaction of cells with anti-B antiserum
- Group O blood (RBCs): negative reaction of cells with both anti-A and anti-B antiserum
- Group AB blood (RBCs): positive reaction of cells with both anti-A and anti-B antiserum

In these typing reactions, the RBCs are merely tested for the presence or absence of A and B antigens. No direct test is made for the presence or absence of the O gene. This is phenotyping, or typing by means of tests made directly on the RBCs. Because blood is tested only for the A and B antigens, genotypes AA and AO will both type as RBC group A. Genotypes BB and BO both contain B antigen and will type as RBC group B. Genotype AB will type as group AB because both antigens are present to react with the appropriate antisera. Genotype OO will type as blood group O and will not react with either anti-A or anti-B antiserum.

Landsteiner's Rule

Corresponding antigens and antibodies cannot normally coexist in the same person's RBCs. An individual who is group A will not normally form anti-A antibodies and will not have anti-A antibodies in his or her serum. In the ABO system, unlike other blood group systems, if the A or B antigen is lacking on the red cell, the corresponding antibody will be found in the serum. These are the so-called isoantibodies. Adults lacking group A antigen will be found to have anti-A antibody in their sera. The sera of adults with RBCs lacking B antigen have anti-B antibody. This occurrence of anti-A or anti-B antibody when the corresponding antigen is lacking from the RBC is known as *Landsteiner's rule.* It exists only in the ABO system.

Serum Typing for Antibody

The presence of these environmentally stimulated anti-A and anti-B antibodies in the serum/plasma of immunocompetent individuals makes the ABO system unique among RBC groups.

The A and B antibodies are very potent, and transfusing RBCs with the antigen to a person with the antibody (ABO incompatible) would result in an immediate and severe hemolytic transfusion reaction that could result in death. It is absolutely essential that the correct ABO blood type be transfused. For these reasons, in addition to testing RBCs with known antibody, the serum is tested with known group A_1^i and group B reagent RBCs stored at 2°C to 8°C (reverse typing) to determine what antibodies are present in the serum. If there is a positive reaction with known group A_1 cells, the serum contains anti-A antibodies. If there is a positive reaction with known group B cells, the serum contains anti-B antibodies. If the serum reacts with both A_1 and B cells, both anti-A and anti-B antibodies are present. If no reaction occurs with either cell type, both antibodies are lacking. In the ABO system, the serum should contain the corresponding antibody for the A or B antigen lacking from the RBCs of the individual. [i]

The results may be grouped as follows:

- Group A blood (RBCs): positive reaction of serum with group B cells
- Group B blood (RBCs): positive reaction of serum with group A_1 cells
- Group O blood (RBCs): positive reaction of serum with both A_1 and B cells
- Group AB blood (RBCs): no reaction with either A_1 or B cells

Isoantibodies of ABO System

One cause of cell and serum discrepancies in ABO typing procedures in adults involves the expected isoantibodies. These antibodies are not manifested in newborns because infants do not normally begin to produce antibodies until they are 3 to 6 months of age. The titer (concentration) of isoantibodies normally increases gradually through adolescence and then decreases gradually. For this reason, serum grouping results may also show discrepancies in older adult patients, who may have low concentrations of antibodies.

Variation in Titer

The antibody titer varies in the population; in general, the anti-A titer is higher than the anti-B titer. In the laboratory, the anti-

[i] A_1 is a subgroup of A antigen. For this discussion, A_1 may be considered synonymous with A antigen.

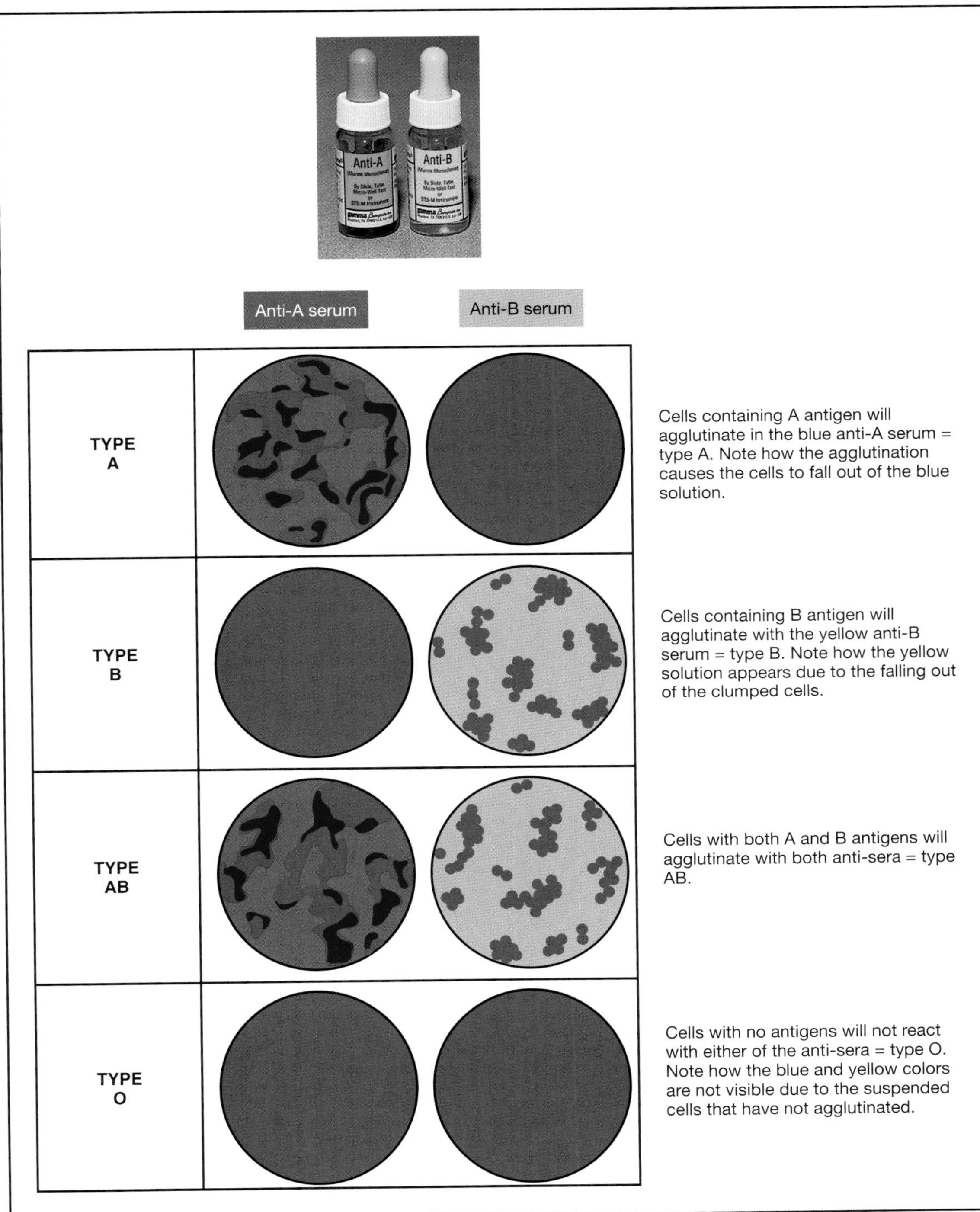

Fig. 17.8 Interpreting ABO blood typing results. **Type A:** Cells containing A antigen agglutinate with the blue anti-A serum. Agglutination causes the cells to fall out of the blue solution. **Type B:** Cells containing B antigen agglutinate with the anti-B serum. **Type AB:** Cells with both A and B antigens agglutinate with both antisera. **Type O:** Cells with no antigens do not react with either antiserum. The blue and yellow background colors of the typing sera are not visible because of the suspended cells that have not agglutinated. (From Garrels M, Oatis CS: *Laboratory testing for ambulatory settings: a guide for health care professionals,* ed 2, St Louis, 2010, Elsevier, p. 231, Procedure 6–4E.)

body titer of serum will only rarely approach the antibody titer of commercially prepared antiserum. For this reason, reactions with cell-grouping tests are generally stronger and easier to read than serum-grouping reactions.

Subgroups

The occurrence of subgroups of group A or group B antigen might also result in discrepancies between cell- and serum-grouping reactions. The classification of RBCs in the ABO system into groups A, B, AB, and O is an oversimplification. Both group A and group B may be further classified into subgroups. The most important subdivision is that of group A into A_1 and A_2. Both A_1 and A_2 cells react with anti-A antisera. However, anti-A_1 reagent can be prepared from group B human serum or with the lectin of *Dolichos biflores* seeds. Lectins are carbohydrate-binding proteins that are highly specific for sugar configurations. This anti-A_1 antibody will react with A_1 cells only. Practically, the subgroups should be kept in mind when there is difficulty in ABO grouping or compatibility testing.

H Substance

H substance is a precursor of A and B blood group antigens. The ABO system is concerned with substances A, B, and H. Genetically, the ABO system is controlled by at least three sets of genes. We have described one set—the A, A_1, B, and O gene set—which occupies a specific locus or position on corresponding chromosomes.

Another set is described as H and h, which are alleles for another locus or position. The H gene is extremely common; over 99.9% of the population inherits the H gene. Very few people carry an h allele, and the hh genotype, called Bombay or Oh, is extremely rare. It is a cause of unexpected blood-typing reactions because the cells type as group O. However, the serum of these Bombay individuals reacts strongly with group O red cells because of the presence of a potent anti-H antibody. Anti-H antisera are also prepared from the lectin of *Ulex europeaus.* Anti-H antisera will not agglutinate RBCs from Bombay individuals but will give a strong reaction with group O RBCs.

Finally, the Se and se alleles occupy a third locus. The Se and se genes regulate the presence of A, B, and H antigenic material in the body secretions. About 78% of the population has inherited the Se gene (SeSe or Sese). These persons are secretors who have H, A, or B substance produced by their secretory cells. Corresponding H, A, or B substance can be found in the saliva of these persons.

Because of the existence of subgroups, A_1 test cells must be used in ABO serum grouping. Subgrouping tests will involve the use of other reagents.

If a discrepancy is demonstrated between the results of cell and serum grouping, it must be resolved before a blood type can be determined and before type specific blood is transfused.

Immune Antibodies of ABO System

Only environmentally stimulated anti-A and anti-B antibodies have been discussed, but anti-A and anti-B antibodies may also be of the immune type. Serum may contain immune antibodies in addition to the isoantibodies. Isoantibodies are normally found in the serum of adults if the RBC lacks the corresponding antigen. These antibodies arise from the stimulation by ABH substances that are widely distributed in nature. Immune anti-A or anti-B antibodies result from specific antigenic stimulation. This stimulation may occur through incompatible transfusion, pregnancy, or injection of ABH substances or substances having ABH activity.

Physical and Chemical Properties

Immune antibodies and isoantibodies differ in physical and chemical properties and in their serologic behavior. In addition, ABO isoantibodies react best if the RBCs are suspended in saline solution. These cold antibodies react best if testing is carried out at room temperature or 4°C. Immune antibodies, warm antibodies, differ in that they react better if cells are suspended in albumin or serum and incubated at 37°C. Other differences exist in the mode of reaction in the laboratory and must be taken into account when the occurrence of an immune-type anti-A or anti-B antibody is suspected or possible—for example, in patients with HDFN who have ABO incompatibility and in screening RBCs for low titers of anti-A and anti-B.

Size and Characteristics of Antibodies

An isoantibody is a large molecule, usually IgM, with a molecular weight of about 900,000 d. The immune antibody, generally IgG, has a molecular weight of about 150,000 d. IgM antibodies are unable to cross the placental barrier, but IgG antibodies can cross the barrier. This is important in the cause of HDFN.

Universal Donors and Recipients

One concept that must be discussed in conjunction with the ABO system is that of the "universal donor" and the "universal recipient." These terms are familiar to most people, but the concept is oversimplified and used only in cases of extreme emergency.

When blood products are to be transfused, two questions must be kept in mind:

1. Does the patient's serum contain an antibody against an antigen on the transfused red cell?
2. Does the serum to be transfused contain an antibody against an antigen on the patient's red cells?

The first situation is the more serious one and must be kept in mind whenever RBCs are the transfusion product. It can result in a major reaction and in the death of the patient; the transfused RBCs will be destroyed by antibody in the patient's circulatory system, resulting in accumulation of toxic waste products and probably in severe renal failure and death.

The second situation, in which the donor serum contains antibody against the patient's RBCs, is not as serious. This situation may occur when transfusing plasma products such as fresh frozen plasma or platelet concentrates. A minor reaction might occur, depending on the amount of plasma infused and its ratio to the total blood volume of the recipient.

The terms *universal donor* and *universal recipient* pertain to the transfusion of packed RBC products in emergency situations. The universal donor is the person with group O RBCs. Group O red cells can be safely transfused into a person with any ABO blood type. This is acceptable because the donor cells do not contain the A or B antigens and will not react with the patient's A or B antibodies. The universal recipient is the patient with group AB RBCs. Their serum does not contain either anti-A or anti-B, and therefore these patients could receive RBC transfusion of any ABO blood type.

ABO type-specific RBCs should be used whenever possible. The major problem with transfusing non–type-specific RBCs is that the patient's true blood type can be obscured and can produce problems with subsequent transfusions and documentation of the patient's true blood type. Transfusion of non–type-specific RBCs includes situations in which group-specific blood is not available and RBCs must be transfused, cases where there may not be enough time to type the patient's blood and test for compatibility, and cases where the patient's RBC group cannot be accurately determined.

In patients with ABO HDFN, group O red cells are generally used. This may also be the case in unusual circumstances such as disasters or military situations in which blood cannot be typed for use before it is transfused.

Rh RED BLOOD CELL GROUP SYSTEM

Historical Background

The discovery of the Rh system was based on work by Landsteiner and Wiener in 1940 and by Levine and Stetson in 1939. A woman who delivered a stillborn fetus was studied by Levine and Stetson. The woman had never received a blood transfusion; after delivery, however, she was transfused with her husband's RBCs. Both the woman and her husband were group O. After the transfusion, the woman experienced a severe hemolytic reaction.

Similar adverse effects of transfusion had previously been known to follow the first transfusion after childbirth and did not seem to be associated with the ABO system. Levine and Stetson developed an explanation of their patient's transfusion reaction that proved to be correct. They explained the reaction by proposing that the woman's RBCs did not contain a "new" antigen. However, the child inherited this new antigen from the father, and the fetal cells containing it found their way into the mother's circulatory system. This resulted in the formation of antibody to the new antigen. When the woman was transfused with her husband's RBCs, her serum contained an antibody to the new antigen present on her husband's red cells. It was also found that the woman's serum agglutinated not only her husband's RBCs but also the red cells of 80 of 104 ABO-compatible RBCs. Levine and Stetson did not name this new antigen.

The naming of this new antigen eventually resulted from studies by Landsteiner and Wiener in 1940. They inoculated rabbits and guinea pigs with the RBCs of rhesus monkeys and found that the resulting rabbit antibody agglutinated the RBCs of rhesus monkeys and, more important, the RBCs of about 85% of samples of the white population of New York City. The 85% of the cells that were agglutinated by the antirhesus serum were called "Rh positive," and the remaining 15% not agglutinated were called "Rh negative." Later it was shown that an antibody found in the serum of certain patients who had hemolytic reactions after transfusion of ABO-compatible blood was apparently the same as the antibody in the antirhesus serum. Also, the antibody contained within the serum of the woman studied by Levine and Stetson in 1939 was similar to the antibody in the antirhesus serum.

Definition of Rh Antigens and Inheritance

Rh Antigens

The Rh blood group system is the most complex of the red cell antigen systems. More than 50 antigens are defined, and more than 150 variations of the two genes are known to control the system. However, five antigens—D, C, c, E, and e—and their corresponding antibodies are of primary importance in routine blood bank testing and transfusion medicine. Of these five, the D antigen is the most important. The presence or absence of the D antigen identifies a person's cells as being Rh positive or Rh negative.

TABLE 17.5 Comparative Nomenclature of Rh Antigens

CDe System (Fisher–Race)		Rh System (Wiener)	Numerical System (Rosenfield et al.)	
D	d	Rh_O	Hr_O	Rh1
C	c	rh′	hr′	Rh2
E	e	rh″	hr″	Rh3

Because the Rh alleles are inherited in groups of paired antigens, and each person has two chromosomes for the Rh antigens, each person has a total of five Rh antigens. This means that eight possible combinations of antigens can be carried on a particular chromosome. These possible combinations of antigens in CDE notation and the corresponding Rh notation, with their approximate frequency, are presented in Table 17.5. These frequencies are for the white population and differ for other races and ethnicities. They are included to give a general idea of the relative frequencies that might be encountered. For more definitive frequencies, consult the *AABB Technical Manual.* One of the eight possible Rh-Hr gene combinations is inherited from each parent, so the total Rh-Hr genotype for a person would be denoted as CDE/ce or CDe/cDe, and so on. In Wiener's Rh-Hr notation corresponding to the CDE system, uppercase *R* refers to the presence of D (Rh_O) antigen, and lowercase *r* refers to the absence of D. The superscript in Wiener's notation refers to the antigens C, c, E, and e.

Nomenclature

In the 1940s and 1950s, when knowledge of the new system was just forming, two different nomenclatures were developed. Each system supported the theory of inheritance put forth by the authors. Although it is now known that both early theories were incorrect, the nomenclatures have remained and are still in wide use today. The CDE system of Fisher–Race is the more preferred and is most frequently used in written text. The Rh-Hr system of Weiner easily conveys the inherited haplotype both verbally and in writing. As the complexity of the system grew and the number of antigens assigned to the system increased, a numerical system was developed by Rosenfeld in the 1960s that assigned each antigen a number based on the order in which the antigen was discovered or assigned to the system. Although not frequently used for the more common antigens, many of the high-frequency or low-frequency antigens are referred to by their numerical designation only, such as Rh23, Rh35, Rh54, and so forth (Table 17.6).

Rh System Biochemistry (Tippett)[5,6]

It is now known that there are two genes, *RHD* and *RHCE,* located closely together on chromosome 1 that encode for

TABLE 17.6 Rh Chromosomes and Approximate Frequency in the U.S. Population

		APPROXIMATE FREQUENCY IN:			
CDe Notation (Fisher–Race)	Rh-Hr NOTATION (Wiener)	White Population	Black Population	Native American Population	Asian Population
DCe	R^1	0.42	0.17	0.44	0.70
ce	r	0.37	0.26	0.11	0.03
DcE	R^2	0.14	0.11	0.34	0.21
Dce	R^o	0.04	0.44	0.02	0.03
Ce	r′	0.02	0.02	0.02	0.02
cE	r″	0.01	0.00	0.01	0.00
DCE	R^z	0.00	0.00	0.06	0.01
CE	r^y	0.00	0.00	0.00	0.00

Data from Cooling L, Downs T: Immunohematology. In McPherson R, Pincus M, editors: *Henry's clinical diagnosis by laboratory methods,* St Louis, 2011, Elsevier.

two amino acid proteins that cross through the red cell membrane multiple times (transmembrane). The *RHD* gene produces the protein on which the D antigen resides, and the *RHCE* gene produces the protein that contains the CcEe antigens in various combinations. The location of the two genes on chromosome 1 is close enough that the genes exhibit linkage, and as a result, some Rh haplotypes are more common than others. Rh-positive individuals possess at least one *RHD* gene and therefore produce the RhD protein and the D antigen on their red cells. Rh-negative individuals, on the other hand, lack the RhD protein and the D antigen. It appears that the two genes may have developed from a common ancestor gene by duplication and that many of the haplotypes seen today were produced by point mutations, recombination, and gene conversions.

A third gene, *RHAG,* located on chromosome 6, encodes for another protein, RhAG (Rh-associated glycoprotein), and is associated with the production of the Rh_{null} phenotype.

Rh-Positive and Rh-Negative Status

It is now known that the new antigen described by Levine and Stetson is the D (or Rh_O) antigen. Persons whose RBCs contain D antigen either in the homozygous or heterozygous state are now termed Rh positive; they represent approximately 85% of the population. In other words, the antibody responsible for several adverse effects of transfusion is the anti-D (anti-Rh_O) antibody. Persons whose RBCs lack the D (Rh_O) antigen are termed Rh negative; they represent about 15% of the population. The great majority of Rh-negative persons are cde/cde. The *d* notation designates the lack of D antigen in an Rh-negative person. This genotype is what is meant by a truly Rh-negative person. Other very rare genotypes that lack the D antigen must also be considered Rh negative as blood recipients.

Characteristics of Rh Antigens

C, D, E, c, and e are antigenic. This means they are capable of stimulating the production of antibodies if introduced into the body of a person whose RBCs completely lack them. The Rh antigens are permanent inherited characteristics that remain constant throughout life. However, not all the Rh antigens are equally antigenic. The D (Rh_O) antigen is the strongest and will generally result in immunization if introduced into a foreign host. For this reason, the term *Rh positive* merely refers to the presence of D antigen without respect to the other Rh antigens. The antigenic strength of D also makes it imperative that RBCs be tested for Rh type before transfusion. Rh-negative persons should not be transfused with Rh-positive (D-positive) RBCs because they are highly likely to develop anti-D antibodies. This would not be harmful at the first transfusion, but subsequent transfusions with D-positive RBCs would result in a transfusion reaction.

Although D is the most antigenic of the Rh antigens, the other antigens are also antigenic. If strength is considered in terms of antibody frequency, antic is the next most common, followed by anti-E, anti-C, and finally anti-e. Combinations of antibodies in the same RBCs are also seen.

Weak Expression of D Antigen

Not all RBCs that contain D antigen react equally well with anti-D blood grouping reagent. Some of these cells may even appear to be D negative, depending on methodology. This weak reactivity with anti-D sera is referred to as *weak D.* Weak-D red cells have the D antigen but have fewer D antigens per cell than normal Rh-positive cells.

Characteristics of Rh Antibodies

The Rh antibodies are made from the gamma globulin portion of the blood plasma and are predominantly IgG in structure. They are specific for the antigen against which they were formed. Unlike the ABO antibodies, the Rh antibodies are immune or unexpected antibodies. No environmentally stimulated antibodies occur as Rh antibodies. They result from specific antigenic stimulation, whether by transfusion, pregnancy, or injection of antigen. The typing methods in this system depend on antigen-typing or cell-typing procedures involving unknown antigen and known antiserum.

Types of Rh Typing Reagents (Antisera)

Many types of commercially available reagent antisera can be used for routine Rh testing. The reagents can be high-protein, low-protein, chemically modified, saline-reactive, monoclonal, or monoclonal blends. The most common reagents currently used are the monoclonal–polyclonal blends and monoclonal blends.

High-Protein Antisera

Commercial antisera of the high-protein variety contain IgG-type antibodies. In general, the albumin-active antisera are more avid preparations, so many of them may be used with a slide method or the rapid tube technique. In addition, the reaction takes place in less time than with saline-active antibody, and the incubation time is shortened. The high-protein reagents in rapid tube tests will generally give strong reactive results with D-positive cells at the immediate-spin, room-temperature phase. In general, most Rh antibodies are IgG in form and will not react unless the test is warmed or incubated at 37°C. High-protein reagents are labeled "for slide or rapid tube test (or modified tube test)," and it is essential to follow the manufacturer's directions.

There are several causes of false-positive results when high-protein antisera are used. A high-protein control must always be included. There may be spontaneous agglutination of IgG-coated RBCs, or factors in the patient's own serum may affect the test, which often uses unwashed RBCs suspended in the patient's own serum or plasma. Other causes of false-positive results include the following:

- Strong autoagglutinins
- Abnormal serum protein that causes rouleaux formation
- Antibodies against an additive in the reagent itself

The best control consists of an immunologically inert control reagent, generally the diluent used for manufacturing the particular antiserum. It is important to use the high-protein control provided by the same manufacturer as the maker of the antiserum.

Low-Protein Antisera

Antibody of the saline type is labeled "for saline tube tests." When this preparation is used, reactions must be carried out on saline suspensions of RBCs, and the test must be performed in a test tube. Slide tests cannot be performed.

The first Rh antibodies discovered were active in saline solution. These reagents use IgM forms of anti-D. Anti-C and anti-E antisera (in addition to anti-D) are normally available in a saline-active form. Antisera of this type will be labeled "for saline tube tests," and the tests must be performed in test tubes. Weak-D testing cannot be performed using this reagent.

Chemically Modified Antisera

These reagents use the IgG form of the antibody but are chemically modified by breaking some of the disulfide bonds at the hinge region so that the antibody molecule can stretch longer distances and cause RBC agglutination (positive reaction) in a low-protein medium. This antiserum has the advantage of a low-protein reagent with less false-positive reactions and no need for a specific Rh control reagent. In addition, these chemically modified reagents will react with the D antigen at the immediate-spin, room-temperature phase of testing and can be used for slide and tube testing.

Monoclonal Antisera

Monoclonal antisera have become the reagents of choice. They can be used in slide, tube, microplate, and automated testing methods. They have the same advantages of the chemically modified reagents, and because they are prepared from hybridoma cell cultures rather than human sources, monoclonal reagents carry no risk of disease transmission. Because of the complexity of the D antigen and the narrow specificity of the monoclonal antibodies, most commercial anti-D reagents are prepared by blending antibody from several clones.

Nature of Rh Antibody Molecule

The differences in reactivity among antibodies depend on the length of the antibody molecule. The molecules that are reactive in saline suspensions of cells are of the larger IgM type. Their length is sufficient to cause bridging of adjacent cells in suspension (agglutination). However, RBCs in suspension are known to carry an electrical charge, the zeta potential (Fig. 17.9), which causes them to repel each other. The IgM-type antibody molecules are so long that they extend beyond the range of the zeta potential and can react with antigenic sites on adjacent cells. Molecules of the smaller IgG type are so short that they do not extend beyond the zeta potential and cannot react with adjacent cells. To demonstrate the existence of IgG molecules by means of agglutination, the repulsion caused by the zeta potential must be overcome or reduced. It can be reduced by suspending the cells in a sufficiently high-protein medium (either their own serum or a commercial protein preparation, or both). Other techniques for the demonstration of IgG include high-speed centrifugation and enzyme methods.

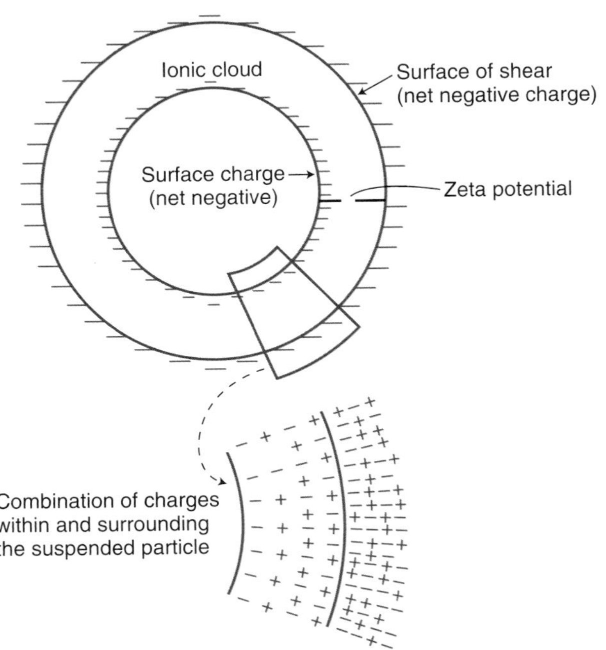

Fig. 17.9 Zeta potential. Difference in electrostatic potential between net charge at cell membrane and charge at surface of shear. (From Turgeon ML: *Immunology and serology in laboratory medicine*, ed 5, St Louis, 2013, Mosby.)

Typing Blood for Transfusion

When RBCs are to be transfused, the patient must be tested for the presence or absence of the D (Rh_O) antigen. This is because the D antigen is so antigenic that most persons who are D negative (Rh_O negative) may produce an anti-D antibody if transfused with D-positive RBCs. Individuals who are D negative (d/d) must be transfused with Rh-negative RBCs, but Rh-positive persons can be transfused with Rh-negative RBCs without adverse consequences.

Because the D (Rh_O) antigen is the most antigenic of the Rh antigens, laboratories test only for the presence or absence of this antigen and transfuse Rh-positive or Rh-negative RBCs accordingly. In most cases, this is sufficient because other Rh antibodies are comparatively rare and are tested for indirectly by compatibility testing or antibody screening techniques. RBCs that are negative at the immediate-spin phase should be further tested for the presence of weak D by means of incubation at 37°C and the antihuman globulin (AHG; Coombs) test. The use of appropriate positive and negative controls is mandatory.

By performing additional Rh tests, the complete Rh phenotype may be determined, or the most probable genotype may be determined by consulting the frequency charts available from these typing reactions. This may be useful in determining the probability of HDFN in mothers negative for an antigen that the father possesses (see later discussion). In such cases, both the mother and the father are typed, and the most probable genotypes are determined.

OTHER BLOOD GROUP SYSTEMS

Human blood groups were discovered in 1900. In addition to the antigens of the ABO and Rh systems, the ISBT has defined 30 blood group systems (Table 17.7), with numerous associated antigens in these systems (Table 17.8). Some of these antigens are common (high frequency); others are uncommon or rare (low frequency). All antigens receiving ISBT numbers must have been shown to be inherited.

ANTIHUMAN GLOBULIN REACTION

Antibodies detectable by the AHG test react with red cells, but the reaction is not observable by direct agglutination. The antibodies coat the RBCs by reacting with antigenic sites on the RBC surface, but the other arm of the antibody molecule is unable to react with antigen on an adjacent red cell to demonstrate

TABLE 17.7 Table of Blood Group Systems

No.	System Name	System Symbol	Gene Name(s)[a]	Chromosomal Location	CD Numbers
001	ABO	ABO	*ABO*	9q34.2	
002	MNS	MNS	*GYPA, GYPB, GYPE*	4q31.21	CD235
003	P	P1		22q11.2–qter	
004	Rh	RH	*RHD, RHCE*	1p36.11	CD240
005	Lutheran	LU	*LU*	19q13.32	CD239
006	Kell	KEL	*KEL*	7q34	CD238
007	Lewis	LE	*FUT3*	19p13.3	
008	Duffy	FY	*DARC*	1q23.2	CD234
009	Kidd	JK	*SLC14A1*	18q12.3	
010	Diego	DI	*SLC4A1*	17q21.31	CD233
011	Yt	YT	*ACHE*	7q22.1	
012	Xg	XG	*XG, MIC2*	Xp22.33	CD99[b]
013	Scianna	SC	*ERMAP*	1p34.2	
014	Dombrock	DO	*ART4*	12p12.3	CD297
015	Colton	CO	*AQP1*	7p14.3	
016	Landsteiner-Wiener	LW	*ICAM4*	19p13.2	CD242
017	Chido/Rodgers	CH/RG	*C4A, C4B*	6p21.3	
018	H	H	*FUT1*	19q13.33	CD173
019	Kx	XK	*XK*	Xp21.1	
020	Gerbich	GE	*GYPC*	2q14.3	CD236
021	Cromer	CROM	*CD55*	1q32.2	CD55
022	Knops	KN	*CR1*	1q32.2	CD35
023	Indian	IN	*CD44*	11p13	CD44
024	Ok	OK	*BSG*	19p13.3	CD147
025	Raph	RAPH	*CD151*	11p15.5	CD151
026	John Milton Hagen	JMH	*SEMA7A*	15q24.1	CD108
027	I	I	*GCNT2*	6p24.2	
028	Globoside	GLOB	*B3GALT3*	3q26.1	
029	Gill	GIL	*AQP3*	9p13.3	
30	Rh-associated glycoprotein	RHAG	*RHAG*	6p21-qter	CD241

[a]As recognized by the HUGO Gene Nomenclature Committee, www.genenames.org/.
[b]*MIC2* product.

TABLE 17.8 Table of Blood Group Antigens Within Systems

System	Antigen Number											
	001	002	003	004	005	006	007	008	009	010	011	012	
001	ABO	A	B	A,B	A1	—							
002	MNS	M	N	S	s	U	He	Mi^a	M^c	Vw	Mur	M^g	Vr
003	P	P1	—	—									
004	RH	D	C	E	c	e	f	Ce	C^w	C^x	V	E^w	G
005	LU	Lu^a	Lu^b	Lu3	Lu4	Lu5	Lu6	Lu7	Lu8	Lu9	—	Lu11	

From International Blood Group Reference Laboratory: *Partial listing.* http://ibgrl.blood.co.uk. Accessed August 5, 2009.

agglutination. To demonstrate the coating of RBCs by antibody, AHG reagent must be available to demonstrate that the cells have reacted with antibody, as seen previously in Fig. 17.3. These antibodies are capable of reacting in the body and, if present, may result in a severe transfusion reaction.

Developing a reagent to demonstrate the coating of antibody on RBCs is based on antibodies being some form of human globulin. The reagent need only be an antibody to human globulin. This is the basis of the antiglobulin (AHG), or Coombs, sera. The reagent is an antibody to human globulin, or AHG antibody. This antiglobulin antibody will react with any antibody coating a red cell. Because it is sufficiently long (it is actually an IgM-type antibody), it will react with antibody coating adjacent RBCs, resulting in bridging or agglutination of the RBCs. Testing with AHG is the last phase of blood compatibility testing.

Preparation and Nature of Antihuman Globulin Reagent

AHG reagent is produced commercially by the companies that produce blood group antisera. The AHG reagent may be prepared by inoculating laboratory animals (usually rabbits) with human serum or a purified globulin fraction of human serum. The laboratory animals produce an antibody to the human globulin, or AHG antibody. The animal is bled and the serum collected. This serum is purified by various techniques until it is specific for human globulin. The antihuman serum is often prepared in such a way that it reacts with both gamma globulin and complement. The antiglobulin portion of the serum is anti-IgG globulin. Some antibodies must be detected by the AHG. It has been found that some of these other antibodies use complement in their reaction or fix complement.

Monospecific and polyspecific reagents are available. Examples of monospecific reagents include anti-IgG with no anticomplement activity and anti-C3d and other complement components with no antiimmunoglobulin activity. These monospecific reagents may be produced through the injection of purified fractions of human serum into rabbits or by the production of murine (mouse) monoclonal antibodies. Monospecific antibodies may be pooled to form polyspecific reagents.

AHG reagent that contains both anti-IgG and anticomplement antibodies is called *polyspecific AHG reagent*. Currently, polyspecific AHG reagents require antibody to human IgG and the C3d component of human complement. Current polyspecific reagents are a blend of polyclonal IgG antibodies against human subclasses of IgG and monoclonal antibodies against C3b and C3d complement components.

Antihuman Globulin Test Procedures

The antiglobulin test is performed in two ways: the direct AHG and the indirect AHG methods. Neither the indirect nor the direct AHG test is specific for a particular antibody.

Direct Antihuman Globulin Test

The direct AHG test, or DAT, is performed on RBCs suspected of being coated with antibody. The DAT is used to demonstrate antibody that has coated or reacted with the RBCs in the patient's body (in vivo). RBCs coated with antibody in vivo are removed from the circulation by the mononuclear phagocytic system. The net effect is a shortened life span for the RBCs. The DAT is used to investigate adverse effects of transfusion and to diagnose autoimmune hemolytic anemia, HDFN, and drug-induced hemolytic anemia.

Indirect Antihuman Globulin Test

The indirect AHG test, or indirect antiglobulin test, is used to detect antigen–antibody reaction that occurs in the test tube (in vitro). It tests for antibodies that are freely circulating in the plasma or antisera and reacts with specific antigens on RBCs in vitro. It is used for detecting antibody in the patient/donor serum (antibody screen), identifying the presence of antibody in the patient's serum against the donor unit cells (crossmatching), and identifying antigens present on the patient's RBCs, such as weak D and Kell (phenotyping).

COMPATIBILITY TESTING AND CROSSMATCHING

Compatibility Testing: Definition and General Considerations

Whenever RBCs are to be transfused, two considerations must be kept in mind:

1. RBCs must be selected that will not be harmful to the patient or result in a transfusion reaction.
2. RBCs must be selected that will be of maximum benefit to the patient.

Whenever blood is to be transfused, it must be tested for compatibility between the donor and the recipient (patient). Compatibility testing is much more than crossmatching, which is just one part of the testing procedures. Compatibility testing involves a series of tests that must include the following:

1. Correct identification of donor and recipient
2. A review of the patient's past history and blood bank records for type and the presence of unexpected antibodies

3. ABO and Rh typing of both donor and recipient
4. Testing of serum (or plasma) of the donor and recipient for the presence of unexpected antibodies (antibody screen)
5. Identification of unexpected antibodies and management of previous antibodies identified
6. Crossmatching of the donor's RBCs with the patient's serum

In general, compatibility testing is used to help detect:

- Unexpected antibodies in the patient's serum;
- Some ABO incompatibilities; and
- Some errors in labeling, recording, or identifying patients or donors.

Unfortunately, crossmatching and compatibility testing will not prevent all transfusion problems. The most frequent causes of incompatible blood transfusions are preanalytical errors of an organizational or clerical nature. Although these errors may be detected by means of compatibility testing and the crossmatch, this is not always the case. The laboratory must always work with great care to avoid mistakes. It requires diligent effort and attention to established policies and procedures to ensure the best possible transfusion outcome for each patient.

Incompatibility in the crossmatching procedure will be discovered only if the patient's serum contains an unexpected antibody to the donor's RBCs. Compatibility testing will not prevent immunization if the patient is transfused with foreign antigen. For example, an Rh-negative person who has never been exposed to Rh-positive antigenic material will not show incompatibility if crossmatched with Rh-positive RBCs, but the person may develop an anti-D antibody. Errors of Rh typing will be detected only if the recipient's serum contains an Rh antibody.

No single crossmatching procedure or antibody screening procedure will detect all unexpected antibodies that may be present in the patient's serum. Even if the blood is found to be compatible, testing procedures will not ensure the normal survival of donor RBCs. The blood must be processed and stored correctly.

ABO and Rh Typing of Donor and Recipient

When blood is selected for transfusion, the patient and donor are tested for ABO type and the presence or absence of the D (Rh_O) antigen. The ABO group is matched and the Rh type selected with respect to the D antigen. Patients whose cells contain the D antigen are given red cells positive for the D antigen (Rh-positive RBCs), and patients who are negative for the D antigen are always given red cells negative for the D antigen (Rh-negative RBCs). The other antigens that collectively make up a person's complete blood type are not matched when RBCs are to be transfused.

Unexpected Antibody Screening and Identification

Antibody Screening

Antibodies known by various names—atypical, unexpected, or irregular antibodies—may be produced by an individual who has been exposed to foreign RBC antigens as the result of prior RBC transfusion or pregnancy. A screening procedure for such antibodies is routinely done for patients requiring transfusion, pregnant women, blood donors, and patients with a suspected transfusion reaction.

Antibody screening with known reagent RBCs allows for testing of the patient's serum in advance of the actual transfusion, allowing for selection of antigen negative donor RBCs when necessary (Figs. 17.10 and 17.11).

The group O RBCs for antibody screening are available as commercially prepared products. Each vial is from an individual donor. They are supplied in sets of two or three vials, suspended in a preservative solution, and must be stored at 2°C to 8°C when not in use. Commercial manufacturers will type for other additional antigens. To see the screening procedure, go to http://evolve.elsevier.com/Turgeon/clinicallab.

The antibody screen test is an indirect antiglobulin/Coombs test. It consists of testing two drops of patient serum and one drop from each vial of reagent RBCs. The mixture is centrifuged and observed for agglutination or hemolysis at room temperature. This is the immediate-spin, room-temperature phase, followed by the addition of an enhancement media such as low-ionic saline solution and incubation of the tubes at 37°C. After incubation, AHG antisera are added, and the tubes are centrifuged and read. Agglutination or hemolysis indicates that an antigen and its corresponding antibody are present. To screen and determine antibody identity, the antigram (a listing of the identified antigens present on the RBCs in each vial representing one donor) is consulted for the RBC antigens and the phase of reactivity (Table 17.9). Once the preliminary screening cell study has been completed and the antibody or antibodies have been preliminarily identified, a panel of RBCs (10 or more) representing multiple donors can be tested with the patient or donor's serum for antibody identification. In some cases, the patient or donor RBCs are tested to confirm the absence of the antigen on the patient's or donor's RBCs. The absence of antigen makes it feasible to build the corresponding antibody if there is a history of prior foreign RBC antigen exposure resulting from RBC transfusion or pregnancy.

Crossmatching

A well-defined compatibility testing regimen is required whenever blood is to be transfused. If compatibility testing has been performed with strict adherence to the procedures established

	Rh							MNSs				P_1	Lewis		Lutheran		Kell		Duffy		Kidd					
Cell	D	C	E	c	e	f	C^w	M	N	S	s	P_1	Le^a	Le^b	Lu^a	Lu^b	K	k	Fy^a	Fy^b	Jk^a	Jk^b				
I R1R1 (56)	+	+	0	0	+	0	0	+	+	0	+	0	+	0	0	+	+	+	+	0	+	+				
II R2R2 (89)	+	0	+	+	0	0	0	0	+	+	0	+	0	+	0	+	0	+	0	+	+	0				

Fig. 17.10 Screening cell antigram. Diagrams the antigens present on the red cells in each bottle, for the lot number indicated. *+,* Antigen present; *0,* antigen absent. (From Blaney KD, Howard PR: *Basic and applied concepts of immunohematology,* ed 3, St Louis, 2013, Mosby.)

	Result	Tentative interpretation
1.	Antibody screen	1. Alloantibody 2. IgG 3. Single specificity

Cell	IS	37° C	AHG	CC
I	0	0	0	✓
II	0	0	2+	NT

Direct antiglobulin test

Poly		IgG	C3
0	✓	NT	NT

2. Antibody screen — 1. Alloantibody 2. IgG 3. Multiple specificities

Cell	IS	37° C	AHG	CC
I	0	0	3+	NT
II	0	2+	3+	NT

Direct antiglobulin test

Poly		IgG	C3
0	✓	NT	NT

3. Antibody screen — 1. Alloantibody 2. IgM specificity 3. Single specificity showing dosage

Cell	IS	37° C	AHG	CC
I	1+	0	0	✓
II	2+	0	0	✓

Direct antiglobulin test

Poly		IgG	C3
0	✓	NT	NT

4. Antibody screen — 1. Autoantibody 2. IgM specificity 3. Cold autoantibody

Cell	IS	37° C	AHG	CC
I	1+	0	0	✓
II	1+	0	0	✓

Direct antiglobulin test

Poly	IgG		C3
2+	0	✓	1+

5. Antibody screen — 1. Autoantibody/transfusion reaction 2. IgG 3. Warm autoantibody with possible underlying alloantibodies

Cell	IS	37° C	AHG	CC
I	0	0	2+	NT
II	0	0	2+	NT

Direct antiglobulin test

Poly	IgG	C3
2+	2+	0

Fig. 17.11 Screen interpretations. Tentative interpretations that can be made after testing of the antibody screen and direct antiglobulin test. *0,* No agglutination or hemolysis; *37° C,* 37°C incubation; ✓, check cells agglutinate; *AHG,* antihuman globulin test; *C3,* anticomplement reagent; *CC,* check cells; *IS,* immediate spin; *NT,* not tested; *Poly,* polyspecific antiglobulin reagent. (From Blaney KD, Howard PR: *Basic and applied concepts of immunohematology,* ed 3, St Louis, 2013, Mosby.)

TABLE 17.9 Antibody Screening Antigram and Patient Results

Blood Group	Antigen	I R1R1	II R2R2	Patient Results
Rh	D	+	+	Neg
	C	Neg	+	Neg
	E	Neg	+	Neg
	c	+	Neg	+
	E	+	Neg	Neg
	F	Neg	Neg	Neg
	C^W	Neg	Neg	Neg
MNSs	M	+	Neg	Neg
	N	+	+	Neg
	S	Neg	+	Neg
	S	+	Neg	Neg
P_1	P_1	Neg	+	Neg
Lewis	Le^a	+	Neg	Neg
	Le^b	Neg	+	Neg
Lutheran	Lu^a	Neg	+	Neg
	Lu^b	Neg	+	Neg
Kell	K	+	Neg	Neg
	K	+	+	Neg
Duffy	Fy^a	+	Neg	Neg
	Fy^b	+	Neg	Neg
Kidd	Jk^a	+	+	Neg
	Jk^b	+	Neg	Neg

NOTE: Each vial contains the RBCs of one donor. In this example, the probable unexpected antibody is antic.
+, the antigen is present on the commercial red blood cells (RBCs); *Neg*, the antigen is absent on the commercial RBCs.

by the particular transfusion service, transfusion of RBCs can be a relatively safe procedure with tremendous benefit to the patient.

The major crossmatch involves testing the donor's RBCs with the patient's serum to detect any antibody in the patient's serum that will react with the donor's RBCs. The presence of such antibody in the patient's serum would certainly result in a major transfusion reaction because the infused donor cells would be destroyed by the patient's antibodies. Even if the patient's serum did contain an unexpected antibody, it would be detected only if the donor's cells contained the corresponding antigen. For this reason, an antibody screening is performed.

Crossmatch Procedure

The traditional crossmatch involves mixing serum and a 2% to 4% suspension of cells in saline solution in a test tube. An immediate centrifugation is performed, and the test tubes are observed for the presence of agglutination or hemolysis. At this stage, ABO incompatibility will be observable, as will incompatibility caused by antibodies of the P, MNSs, Lewis, Lutheran, or Wright systems.

If the test is negative at this point, the test tube is incubated at 37°C for a sufficient time and observed again. Saline solution–reacting antibodies of the Rh-Hr and Lewis systems will be detected, and antibodies of the P, MNSs, and Kell systems may sometimes react at this stage. If the crossmatch is still negative, it may be further tested using the AHG crossmatch.

Antihuman Globulin Crossmatch

The AHG crossmatch is an extension of the traditional crossmatch procedure. After incubation at 37°C, the cells are thoroughly washed with saline solution. The AHG serum is added and the test carried out as recommended by the manufacturer. This is an indirect test between the patient and the prospective donor. The crossmatch will detect most Rh antibodies. In addition, it may be the only means of detecting some antibodies, especially in the Duffy, Kidd, and Kell blood group systems. The AHG crossmatch is no longer necessary when the patient's serum has been previously screened for unexpected antibodies with reagent cells and has no previous history of clinically significant antibodies.

Abbreviated Crossmatch

For an abbreviated (immediate spin) crossmatch, only a crossmatch procedure designed to detect ABO incompatibility is required. This consists of testing the donor cells and patient serum (major crossmatch) at room temperature by immediate spin or by centrifugation after incubation for 5 minutes.

Other Crossmatching Techniques

Automation has assumed a significant role in blood bank testing (see Automation in Blood Banking). *Electronic crossmatching* or computer-based crossmatching refers to the issue of blood without direct serologic crossmatching (e.g., the mixing of patient plasma with donor red cells). The application of computerized crossmatching may be permissible. Computerized selection of RBCs may be used if regulatory requirements are met. In addition, patients must not have any clinically significant antibodies to qualify their blood specimen for computer-based crossmatching. Using computer-based crossmatching, the AHG phase of the crossmatch is omitted, and only a procedure to detect ABO compatibility is performed. The purpose of computer-based crossmatching is to respond faster to transfusion requests and reduce the laboratory workload.

Microplate methods for antibody detection using LIS salt solution are also used to screen large numbers of sera for unexpected antibodies. A technique that uses polyethylene glycol is also used for antibody detection and identification. This may be used as a supplement to more conventional methods when weak reactions are encountered.

ADVERSE EFFECTS OF TRANSFUSION

Although the safety of transfused blood has improved considerably over the last several decades, substantial risks associated with transfusions remain. Clinically, the result of RBC destruction is a transfusion reaction.

The signs and symptoms of a transfusion reaction vary from patient to patient. Generally, chills, high temperature, pain in the lower back, nausea, vomiting, and shock, as indicated by decreased blood pressure and rapid pulse, characterize an immediate reaction. The first effects of a transfusion reaction are rarely fatal, but the by-products of RBC destruction pose many problems, primarily severe renal involvement. A patient may eventually die of kidney failure.

TABLE 17.10 Examples of Adverse Effects of Transfusion

Type of Reaction	Examples
Immediate immune	Hemolytic, febrile, allergic, anaphylactic, and TRALI
Immediate nonimmune	Bacterial contamination, nonimmune hemolysis, circulatory overload
Delayed immune	Alloimmunization, delayed hemolytic GVHD
Delayed nonimmune	Iron overload, disease transmission

GVHD, Graft-versus-host disease; *TRALI*, transfusion-related acute lung injury.

Adverse effects of transfusion can generally be characterized as *immune* or *nonimmune* (Table 17.10). Both immunologic and nonimmunologic types can occur as immediate adverse effects of transfusion.

Immediate Immunologic Adverse Reactions

Some patients receive transfusions intended for someone else each year in the United States, and a small number of these patients die of complications.[7] Most of these errors result from clerical rather than technical errors. Radio frequency identification monitoring technology allows patients to wear wristbands that transmit their blood type by tiny radio signals. Microchips are embedded into both the wristband and the unit of blood. If sensors detect a difference between the signals coming from the wristband and from the microchip in the blood bag, a computer will flash a message. Another safety system is the bar coding of patient wristbands and blood bags (see Chapter 4).

Other immediate immunologic adverse effects of transfusion include febrile nonhemolytic reactions, usually a reaction to the donor's granulocytes. Anaphylaxis from antibody to IgA, urticaria (hives) from antibody to plasma proteins, and noncardiac pulmonary edema from antibody to leukocytes or complement activation are other immediate immunologic causes of adverse transfusion effects.

Transfusion-Related Acute Lung Injury

Transfusion-related acute lung injury (TRALI) has been identified as a life-threatening complication of transfusion, with significant morbidity and mortality. TRALI is thought to result from the interaction of donor-specific leukocyte antibodies with patient leukocytes. This transfusion-related reaction is so serious that in 2014, the AABB revised the TRALI risk reduction requirement[8] as follows:

> 5.4.1.1.1 Plasma and whole blood for allogeneic transfusion shall be from males, females who have not been pregnant, or females who have been tested since their most recent pregnancy and results interpreted as negative for HLA antibodies.

Hemolytic Transfusion Reactions

Acute Hemolytic Transfusion Reaction. Acute hemolytic transfusion reactions occur when donor RBCs are lysed intravascularly by the presence of preformed, antigen-specific antibodies in the recipient. ABO incompatibility between the donor and the recipient is the most common type of acute hemolytic reaction. Anti-Jka can also produce this type of reaction.

Under these circumstances of ABO incompatibility, if anti-A and anti-B antibodies are present in the patient, these antibodies will bind to transfused antigen bearing A- or B-incompatible donor RBCs. This specific antigen–antibody reaction activates complement and terminates in the lysis of RBCs, hemolysis. Products released from RBCs by hemolysis include interleukins 1 and 6 (IL-1, IL-6) and tumor necrosis factor. These products mediate fever, hypotension, and endothelial cell activation.[9] Symptoms occur immediately or within several hours.

Delayed Hemolytic Transfusion Reaction. The overall incidence of delayed hemolytic transfusion reactions is higher than that of immediate acute transfusion reactions. These reactions commonly reflect the reoccurrence of a non-ABO antibody that was developed previously due to exposure to a blood group antigen not possessed by the recipient as the result of pregnancy or blood transfusion. Reemergence of a hidden antibody takes, on average, 3 to 10 days. These extravascular hemolytic reactions are usually mild.

Immediate Nonimmunologic Adverse Reactions

Immediate nonimmunologic transfusion reactions include marked fever with shock from congestive heart failure caused by increased blood volume, bacterial contamination, and hemolysis of infused RBCs from the physical destruction of cells, such as from freezing or overheating or mixing of nonisotonic solutions with RBCs.

Transfusion-associated circulatory overload (TACO) has been observed as the second most common cause of transfusion-associated fatalities in the United States. Symptoms of TACO include dyspnea, tachypnea, and coughing during or within a few hours of the completion of a transfusion(s).

Septic transfusion reactions result from bacterial contamination of donor blood components. Platelets are the most frequent cause because of the need for room-temperature storage and the introduction of bacteria at the time of donation. Fever and/or chills are the most common symptoms that occur beginning during or shortly after transfusion.

Other Severe Adverse Reactions

Graft-versus-host disease (GVHD) may result from engraftment of transfused functional lymphocytes. Purpura (presence of purple patches on skin and mucous membranes) from bleeding may be caused by the development of antiplatelet antibodies. Also, the patient may be sensitized and may form antibodies to donor antigens on RBCs, WBCs, platelets, or plasma protein. Other delayed nonimmunologic adverse effects include iron overload from multiple (>100) transfusions and disease transmission as a result of transfusion as can occur with hepatitis, HIV, and protozoan infections.

HEMOLYTIC DISEASE OF THE FETUS AND NEWBORN

Pathophysiology

HDFN occurs when a baby inherits an antigen for which the mother is negative. For HDFN to occur, the fetus must be positive for an antigen and the mother must be negative for that specific antigen. HDFN most often involves antigens of the ABO or Rh blood group systems. The D antigen of the Rh system is one of the most potent antibody stimulators in a pregnant woman if the fetus is D positive (Rh positive) and the mother is D negative (Rh negative.).

This condition develops while the fetus is in the uterus (Fig. 17.12). The mechanism involves sensitization or immunization of the mother to foreign antigen present on her child's RBCs. Although the circulatory systems of a mother and her child are separate, and only small molecules such as nutrients can cross the placenta, some leaking of fetal RBCs can occur into the mother's circulatory system, most likely very late in pregnancy or at birth. If any incompatible fetal RBCs enter the mother's circulatory system, she can become sensitized to the antigen and potentially develop an antibody to the antigen on the fetal RBCs. If immunization occurs, it is permanent. The antibody formed by the mother is of the IgG type. IgG antibodies can cross the placenta into the circulatory system of the fetus, react with the corresponding antigen on the RBCs of the fetus, and result in the destruction of the fetus or newborn infant's RBCs.

Accumulation of the hemoglobin breakdown product bilirubin is not a problem for a baby before birth. However, there can be serious postpartum harm (Fig. 17.13). Bilirubin can accumulate in the lipid-rich tissue of the brain after birth and cause severe neurologic problems. Anti-D was the most common cause of HDFN before modern prophylaxis.

ABO Antigens

Most often, HDFN occurs as a result of antigens in the ABO system. In this case the mother is usually group O, and the child inherits the A or B antigen from the father. Group O individuals have a relatively high concentration of IgG anti-A and anti-B in addition to IgM anti-A and anti-B antibody. This immune IgG

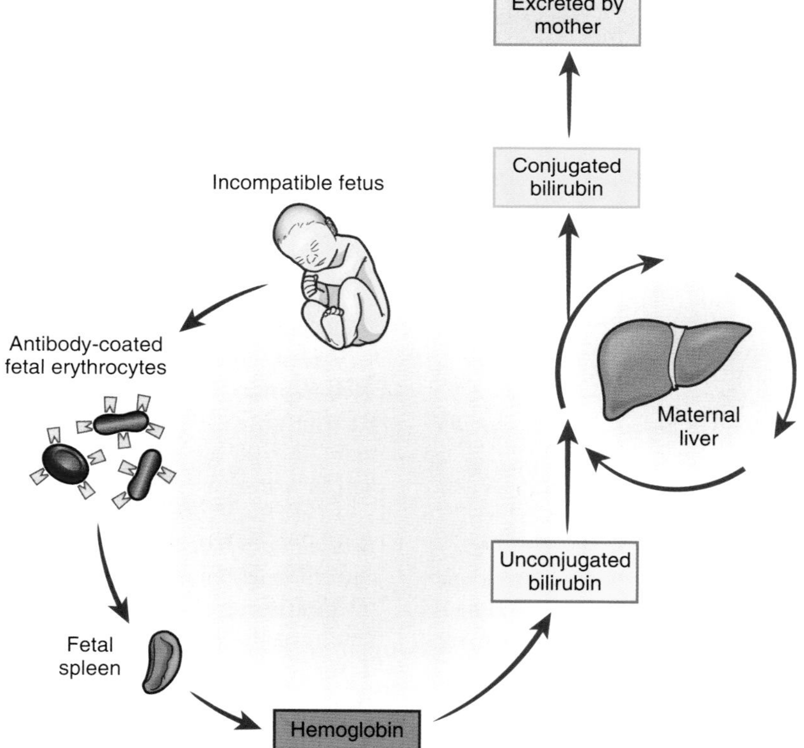

Fig. 17.12 Basic physiology of hemolytic disease of the fetus and newborn (HDFN). If Rh_O (D) antigen–bearing erythrocytes enter the maternal circulation, these erythrocytes are recognized as foreign by the Rh_O (D)–negative mother. If antigenic stimulation or an anamnestic response caused by anti-D occurs in subsequent pregnancies, high titers of anti-D are produced in the maternal circulation. These anti-D antibodies can cross the placental barrier and attach to the D-positive erythrocytes of the fetus in the current pregnancy. These antibody-coated erythrocytes have a shortened survival, and the fetus suffers from anemia. The bilirubin resulting from erythrocyte (hemoglobin) breakdown is excreted through the maternal circulation and does not injure the fetus before birth. (Redrawn from Turgeon ML: *Fundamentals of immunohematology,* ed 2, Baltimore, 1995, Williams & Wilkins.)

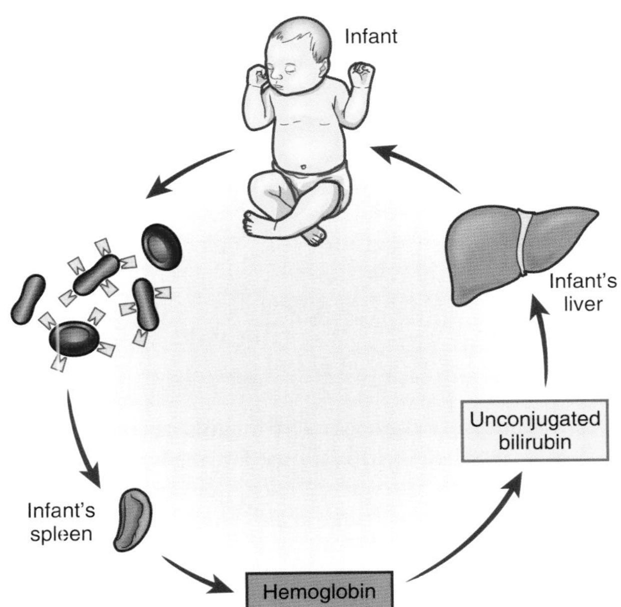

Fig. 17.13 Postpartum effects of hemolytic disease of the fetus and newborn (HDFN). After delivery, the accumulation of bilirubin can severely harm a newborn infant. The liver of the newborn does not produce the enzyme glucuronyl transferase, which is necessary for converting bilirubin to an excretable form. Consequently, bilirubin accumulates, and if not removed, it will be deposited in lipid-rich tissues such as the brain. Excessive bilirubin in the circulation also produces jaundice. (Redrawn from Turgeon ML: *Fundamentals of immunohematology*, ed 2, Baltimore, 1995, Williams & Wilkins.)

antibody can cross the placenta and react with the corresponding antigen on the RBCs of the fetus. Although ABO sensitization may occur often, hemolytic disease caused by ABO incompatibility is less severe. The child may be only mildly affected and may require minimal or no treatment.

Rh Antigens

Severe HDFN most often involves the Rh blood group system such as D antigen followed by antic and anti-Kell. In the case of Rh incompatibility, the mother is negative for D (d/d), and the father is positive for D. The child inherits this antigen from the father and is D positive (D/d). If any of the D-positive RBCs of the fetus cross into the mother's circulatory system, she may develop an immune anti-D antibody. This IgG crosses the placenta and reacts with the RBCs of the fetus.

Sensitization usually occurs only very late in pregnancy or at delivery, so the first child is rarely affected by HDFN. Subsequent pregnancies with children who are D negative theoretically are not affected by anti-D antibody in the mother's circulatory system. For this reason, determining the most probable genotype of the parents in possible cases of HDFF may be useful in predicting the chance of occurrence of the disease. For example, if the father is heterozygous for the D antigen (D/d) and the mother is D negative (d/d), the chances are that only half the children will inherit the D antigen (Fig. 17.14). On the other hand, if the father is homozygous for D (D/D), the children will inherit the D antigen, and there is a 100% chance

	D	*d*
d	*D/d*	*d/d*
d	*D/d*	*d/d*

	D	*D*
d	*D/d*	*D/d*
d	*D/d*	*D/d*

Fig. 17.14 Chance for development of hemolytic disease of the fetus and newborn (HDFN). Risk of HDFN is based on genotypes for the D antigen.

of HDFN. About 1 in 10 pregnancies involve an Rh-negative mother and an Rh-positive father.

The first child is rarely affected by HDFN. Fewer than 20% of Rh-negative women actually become immunized during pregnancy. Although a woman can have one or two children who are both Rh positive and encounter no difficulties, her immunization is permanent. Once the disease develops in one child, subsequent children positive for the antigen are likely to be affected at least as severely. If a woman has been sensitized before pregnancy as a result of transfusion of incompatible RBCs or injection of antigenic material, even the first child can be severely affected. Anti-D antibody is the most common cause of HDFN. Other antibodies causing the disease include antic, anti-K (Kell), anti-E, and even incompatibilities in the ABO system.

Routine Laboratory Prenatal and Postnatal Testing

Many laboratory tests are performed in cases of HDFN, on the parents' (primarily the mother's) RBCs before birth and on the child's RBCs after birth. The first step is to type the mother for ABO and Rh early in pregnancy. The mother's serum is usually screened by means of the indirect AHG test to see if an antibody exists. If an antibody is found, it is identified and the titer determined. This titer is rechecked throughout pregnancy as a monitor of the possible severity of the disease. An increasing titer indicates an active immune response.

After birth, several tests can be performed on the child's red cells, in addition to further tests on the maternal serum. Initially, a sample of umbilical cord RBCs is tested for ABO group and Rh type, and a direct AHG test is performed. Other laboratory tests that may be performed on the child's RBCs include hemoglobin determinations, blood smear examination and differential, reticulocyte count, and serum bilirubin determination.

The decision to perform exchange transfusion will depend on a combination of laboratory results and the clinical condition of the child. Preparation can and should be made before birth so that the exchange can be done as soon as possible if necessary.

Treatment

When HDFN does occur, it varies considerably in severity. Usually, ABO incompatibility results in a mild form of HDFN that responds to phototherapy to break down bilirubin.

In its most severe form (anti-D), the infant may be stillborn or severely affected at birth. In other cases, such as ABO incompatibility, a baby is usually mildly affected. Severely affected infants are exposed to the products of RBC destruction and develop anemia. The cell destruction results in a hemolytic anemia accompanied by abnormal levels of serum bilirubin, with the clinical appearance of jaundice. The accumulation of bilirubin can result in irreversible brain damage (kernicterus) if present in extremely elevated concentration. If the child survives and is not treated adequately, the brain damage will result in severe mental retardation.

Treatment for infants with severe HDFN includes RBC exchange transfusion. In an exchange transfusion, a significant proportion of the child's RBCs is replaced with transfused red cells. The exchange transfusion corrects the anemia and removes the abnormal levels of serum bilirubin, at least temporarily, and can prevent brain damage. The procedure may need to be repeated several times, depending on the level of bilirubin accumulation.

The type of RBCs used for transfusion depends on the antibody responsible for the disease. Use of O-negative red cells is the most common selection. The RBCs must be negative for the antigen against which the antibody has been formed. The child is given blood that is compatible with the mother. In HDFN caused by the formation of anti-D antibody in the mother's serum, the child is transfused with RBCs that are specific for the child's own ABO type but negative for the D antigen. This is because not all the child's blood is replaced at the time of exchange, and some maternal antibody is left. RBCs are given that will not react with the remaining antibody and will not harm the child. In cases of ABO incompatibility that require exchange, the mother is usually group O and the child group A or B. In such cases, the child is transfused with group O RBCs of the child's Rh type.

In cases of severe HDFN, it is sometimes necessary to attempt to treat the fetus before birth. This intrauterine transfusion may be necessary to correct severe anemia and prevent death in utero (stillbirth) when the risk of early delivery is too great. In such cases, based on maternal antibody titer, obstetric history, and ultrasound, an amniocentesis is performed. The amniotic fluid is tested for bilirubin level and fetal maturity. If the fetus is not mature enough to be delivered by cesarean birth and appears to be severely affected, an intrauterine transfusion may be indicated. In an intrauterine transfusion, packed RBCs are infused through the fetal abdominal wall into the peritoneum. Direct transfusion into the umbilical vein may also be attempted.

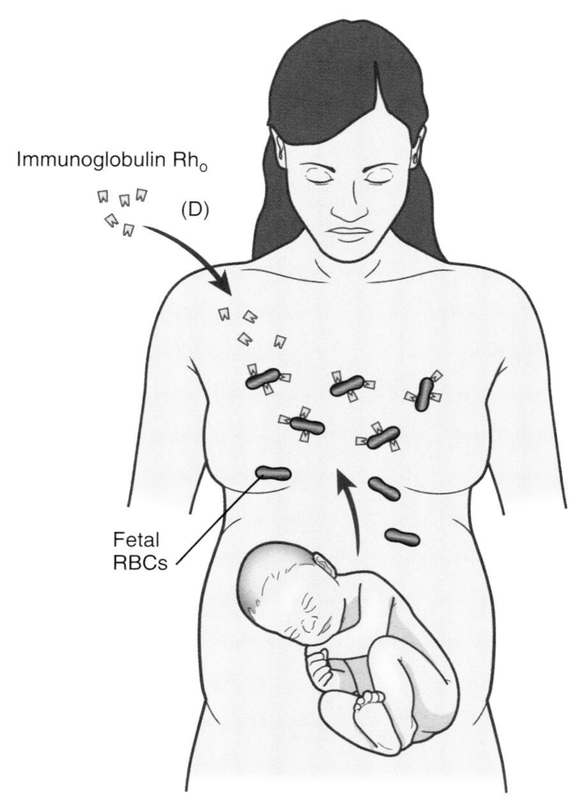

Fig. 17.15 Prevention of primary immune response to Rh_O (D)–incompatible fetus. Prevention of sensitization of a Rh_O (D)–negative mother to a Rh_O (D)–positive fetus can be accomplished by the antenatal or postnatal administration of immune globulin-D. The passively administered anti-D binds with the D antigen of the fetal erythrocytes. These cells are subsequently phagocytized and removed from the maternal circulation without foreign antigen recognition by the mother's immune system. (Redrawn from Turgeon ML: *Fundamentals of immunohematology*, ed 2, Baltimore, 1995, Williams & Wilkins.)

Prevention of Rh Immunization

In the United States antepartum RhIg is administered routinely at 28 weeks of gestation to pregnant women who have not previously formed anti-D and are carrying an RhD-positive fetus or a fetus with an undetermined RhD antigen status. If they deliver an Rh D-positive baby, they receive postpartum Rh immunoprophylaxis (Fig. 17.15). If RhIg is injected within 72 hours of delivery into an Rh-negative woman who delivered an Rh-positive baby, she should be protected against Rh problems in subsequent pregnancies.

An exception to the need for Rh immunoprophylaxis is some of the estimated 0.6% to 1.0% of white women who express a serologic weak-D phenotype. In this population of women with the weak-D phenotype, about 80% have a weak D of type 1, 2, or 3 that can be managed as if they are Rh positive. In these cases, it is recommended that Rh genotyping be performed to determine the molecular basis of serologic weak-D phenotypes to determine the need for Rh immunoprophylaxis.

Mechanism of Action

The use of RhIg is based on interference with recognition of the Rh antigen on the fetal cells by the mother's immune system. This blocking interference prevents immunization (sensitization) by the Rh-positive RBCs of the fetus. The mother is passively immunized by the administration of RhIg when recognition of foreign antigen on the maternal RBCs (sensitization) by fetal RBCs is most likely. Most exposure to fetal blood occurs at delivery.

Qualitative Screening of Fetal RBCs in Maternal Circulation

The rosette screen is a highly sensitive method to qualitatively detect 10 mL or more of fetal whole blood, or 0.2% fetal cells in the maternal circulation. It is currently the only screening test that is FDA approved for clinical use in the United States.

The rosette test is inexpensive and does not require special equipment. FDA-approved, commercially available kits include the Fetal Bleed Screening Test (ImmucorGamma, Norcross, GA) and the FetalScreen II/Fetal Maternal Screening Test (Ortho-Clinical Diagnostics, Raritan, NJ). A limitation of the rosette screening procedure is that because it relies on the presence of the D antigen to distinguish fetal from maternal cells, it cannot be used to detect FMH in D-positive mothers or in D-negative mothers carrying a D-negative fetus.

If the rosette test is negative, one vial (300 µg) of RhIg is sufficient to prevent immunization in 99% of patients. A positive rosette test, which indicates an FMH exceeding 10 mL, requires quantification of the FMH by either the Kleihauer–Betke acid-elution test or flow cytometry to determine the dose of RhIg required for prophylaxis.

Quantitative Tests for Measuring Fetal RBCs in Maternal Circulation

Fetal hemoglobin, or hemoglobin F (HbF), can be measured by various techniques; most measure the amount of HbF. The most frequently used techniques are:

- Acid-elution technique (modified Kleihauer–Betke test), and
- Flow cytometry based on antibodies against HbF.

Acid-Elution Stain (Modified Kleihauer–Betke Method). The Kleihauer–Betke acid-elution test, the most widely used confirmatory test for quantifying FMH, is based on the observation of an increased amount of HbF-bearing RBCs in a maternal blood specimen following labor and delivery. Fetal RBCs contain 20% to 25% HbF compared with the concentration of HbF in the circulating RBCs of normal adults of 0.5% to 7.0%.

The principle of the Kleihauer–Betke acid-elution test is that HbF is resistant to acid elution but adult hemoglobin is not. If a thin blood smear is exposed to an acid buffer, the adult RBC loses its hemoglobin into the buffer, leaving only the RBC stroma, but the fetal RBC is unaffected and retains its hemoglobin. The smears are examined under the microscope after staining, and the percentage of fetal cells in the maternal RBCs is used to calculate the approximate volume of fetal hemorrhage into the maternal circulation. A limitation of this procedure is a reported[10] tendency to overestimate the amount of hemorrhage.

Flow Cytometry. Although the Kleihauer–Betke test is inexpensive and requires no special equipment, it lacks standardization and precision and may not be accurate in conditions with elevated F cells. Flow cytometric analysis permits the distinction of true fetal cells, which contain HbF as the major form of hemoglobin, from maternal circulating F cells, which have lower cellular HbF content.[10]

There are two main categories of flow cytometry for the assessment of FMH depending on the target antigen of interest: HbF and RhD. FDA-approved reagents for both methods are commercially available.

Flow Cytometry Using Antifetal Hemoglobin Antibodies. Flow cytometry using monoclonal antibodies directed against HbF has some important advantages over the Kleihauer–Betke test in the quantitation of FMH. Flow cytometry can:

- Accurately distinguish adult HbF RBCs from fetal RBCs;
- Analyze more cells, which improves accuracy; and
- Produce more reproducible results.

Anti-HbF flow cytometry is a promising alternative, although its use is limited by equipment and staffing costs. Because hematology analyzers with flow-cytometry capabilities may be adapted for fetal cell detection, flow cytometry is a viable automated alternative for quantifying FMH.

Assessment Plan for Fetomaternal Hemorrhage

The concentration of postpartum prophylaxis is determined for each individual patient by a four-step procedure:

1. A rosette fetal RBC screening for fetomaternal hemorrhage
2. Quantitation of the amount fetomaternal hemorrhage by Kleihauer–Betke acid-elution assay or flow-cytometry assay
3. Estimation of the volume of fetomaternal hemorrhage (Box 17.1)
4. Calculation of the required number of vials of RhIg (Box 17.2)

BOX 17.1 Estimation of Fetomaternal Hemorrhage

Fetomaternal hemorrhage (FMH) volume (mL of whole blood) = maternal blood volume[a] × percent (%) of fetal RBCs (based on acid-elution assay).

If the results of acid-elution analysis of FMH = 1%, the volume of FMH is 50 mL.

[a]Conventionally, the maternal total blood volume is assumed to be 5000 mL. The precise maternal blood volume can be calculated based on the mother's height and weight.

From Fung MK, Grossman BJ, Hillyer C, Westhoff CM, editors: *Technical manual,* ed 18, Bethesda, MD, 2014, American Association of Blood Banks.

BOX 17.2 Calculated Required Dose of Rh Immunoglobin (RhIg)[a]

Number of vials of RhIg = volume of fetomaternal hemorrhage (FMH)/30 mL[b]

Example: If the volume of FMH is 50 mL, the required number of vials of RhIg = 1.7 + 1 = 3[c]

[a]The RhIg Dose Calculator is an online application that converts the result of an acid-elution assay or flow cytometry (% of fetal red blood cells [RBCs] among adult RBCs) to a recommended dose. The calculator assumes a maternal blood volume of 5000 mL, but the height and weight of the mother can be entered manually for increased accuracy.

[b]In this equation, 30 mL represents the volume of fetal whole blood that can be prevented from causing formation of anti-D if the mother receives a timely injection of the contents of 1 vial of RhIg (300 of µg of anti-D).

[c]Adjustments in calculating the dose of RhIg can be made as follows:

1. If the calculated number to the right of the decimal point is less than 5, round up to the next whole number. Example: If calculated dose is 1.3, round up to the next whole number. Therefore, 1.3 = 2 doses.
2. If the calculated number to the right of the decimal point is greater than or equal to 5, round up to the next whole number and add 1. Therefore, in the calculation example, 1.7 rounds up to 2, and 1 is added to the dose requirement, for a total of 3 vials.

From Fung MK, Grossman BJ, Hillyer C, Westhoff CM, editors: *Technical manual,* ed 18, Bethesda, MD, 2014, American Association of Blood Banks; Paton A: Bringing new vigor to RhIg calculations, *CAP Today* 22(1), 2008; College of American Pathologists (CAP): RhIg Dose Calculator, www.cap.org.

The amount of fetal RBCs present in the maternal circulation is important for the RhIg dosage. If the amount of Rh-positive fetal RBCs entering the mother's circulation is greater than 30 mL of whole blood, the standard dose of RhIg is not enough to prevent anti-D antibody formation. It is important to determine the presence and amount of fetomaternal hemorrhage.

Administration of Postpartum Rh Immunoprophylaxis

RhIg is injected intramuscularly within 72 hours of delivery in mothers (1) who are D negative, (2) who have no detectable anti-D antibody, and (3) whose newborns are D positive.

Antepartum treatment at 28 weeks' gestation has also been advocated by the American College of Obstetricians and Gynecologists. If done, a sample of RBCs obtained immediately before treatment should be tested for ABO group, Rh type, antibody screen, and identification of antibody, if present.

RhIg is supplied as a sterile, clear, approximately 1-mL solution to be injected intramuscularly. It is a concentrated solution (300 µg/mL) of IgG anti-D that may be derived from human plasma. It does not transmit hepatitis, HIV, or other detectable infectious diseases.

The anti-D antibody can be detected 12 to 60 hours after the administration of RhIg and is sometimes found for as long as 5 months thereafter. If it is detected 6 months after delivery, active immunization and failure of the RhIg can be assumed. Such failures are infrequent, but they can occur if RhIg is given too late or in too small a dose or if Rh immunization has already occurred during the pregnancy. Most of the D-positive fetal cells enter the maternal circulation at delivery.

AUTOMATED TESTING TECHNOLOGY AND SYSTEMS

Gel Technology

The Bio-Rad (Hercules, CA) IH-1000 system offers a gel column agglutination with an extremely broad selection of gel cards.

The test menu cards include the following:

- ABO/Rh (forward and reverse)
- Weak D/D variant
- Newborn card (anti-A, anti-B, anti-A,B)
- Phenotyping (anti-C, anti-E, anti-c, anti-e, anti-K)
- Antibody screening
- Direct AHG test (DAT)
- Crossmatching (AHG with anti-IgG or AHG with anti-IgG,-C3d)

The ORTHO VISION® Analyzer (Ortho-Clinical Diagnostics, Buckinghamshire, England) was developed to meet the unique needs of immunohematology labs through the proprietary benefits of responsive automation. The ORTHO VISION® Analyzer automates the full range of immunohematology testing, including serial dilutions for titration studies and selected cell panels, which helps to eliminate manual testing.

The menu of tests includes the following:

- ABO/Rh grouping
- ABO/Rh confirmation
- Antibody screen
- Antibody identification
- Selected cell panel
- Rh phenotype (C, c, E, e)
- Donor confirmation
- Crossmatch (AHG)
- Antigen typing
- Serial dilutions for titration studies
- Eluates
- DAT (polyspecific)
- DAT (IgG)
- Cord blood testing

The ORTHO ProVue® Analyzer is a modular, microprocessor-controlled instrument designed to automate in vitro immunohematological testing of human blood utilizing the ID-MTS™ Gel Card technology. This instrument can be used by hospital transfusion services and smaller blood banks with a small number of tests.

The test menu includes the following:

- ABO and Rh typing
- Antibody screening and identification
- Crossmatching
- Direct antiglobulin testing
- Antigen typing

Automated Solid-Phase Red Cell Adherence Assays

Automated solid-phase red cell adherence assays (SPRCAs) manufactured by Immucor have the trade names Capture-R Ready-Screen and Capture-R Ready ID. Capture-P® technology is an innovative IgG platelet antibody detection and crossmatch system. Capture-P® assays allow a laboratory to complete specialty platelet compatibility testing with the same methodology used for routine red cell antibody screening.

Instruments that support this technology include Galileo, Galileo ECHO, and NEO. Automated instruments use microplates and microwell strips to perform hemagglutination assays and SPRCAs. Hemagglutination assays are used for ABO and D antigen phenotype, antigen typing, and immediate-spin crossmatching.

The Galileo ECHO system performs ABO/Rh typing, weak-D phenotype, antibody screen and antibody identification, IgG direct antiglobulin test, and Ig crossmatch. A negative Rh test result can be reflexed to a weak-D test; a positive antibody screen can be reflexed to a panel of antigen cells for identification. Antigens are precoated on the test wells at the time of manufacture. The Echo is faster than the Galileo, so it is great for STAT orders and antibody workups, but the throughput of the Galileo is much greater than that of the Echo, so it is a workhorse for batch testing and routine work.

Echo Lumena's® broad test menu allows blood banks to automate more of their workload and provides better cost justification for an automated platform: ABO/Rh D, donor confirmation ABO retype, weak-D phenotype, antibody screen and identification, D-positive panel, D-negative panel, and IgG DAT.

NEO Iris® is Immucor's latest (sixth generation) analyzer and offers maximum productivity with the highest type and screen throughput on the market. It is ideal for large patient laboratories, clinical laboratories, and donor centers.

The test menu includes the following:

- ABO/Rh D typing, weak D
- Donor confirmation
- CMV testing
- IgG DAT
- IgG crossmatching, antigen screening
- Phenotyping of antigens Rh, Kell, Jka, Jkb, Fya, Fyb, S, s, k
- Antibody screening and identification

Antigens are precoated on the test wells at the time of manufacture.

Bio-Rad's automated systems for SPRCAs are the TANGO infinity system and TANGO optimo system. They combine Erytype S and Solidscreen II with instrumentation. The TANGO infinity system is used for routine immunohematology testing procedures, including blood grouping and antibody screening and identification for patients, donors, and cord blood specimens. The TANGO optimo system can analyze all routine testing procedures including blood grouping, antibody screening and crossmatching.

Random-access systems are used for antibody screening and identification, direct AHG, IgG crossmatch, weak D, and ABD/Kell red cell phenotyping. The technology is similar to the Immucor Capture system where the microtiter wells are designed to accommodate either antiglobulin tests or hemagglutination assays.

Erytype® S and Solidscreen® II are proprietary test systems used for blood group serology testing. Erytype® S uses microplate wells precoated with blood-grouping monoclonal antibodies. Traditional agglutination reactions result, and the agglutination patterns are captured and interpreted by the TANGO automation platforms. Assays include forward and reverse ABO group with D, ABO forward grouping, Rh typing, Rh + K phenotype, antibody screening and identification, crossmatching (anti-Ig-G), direct antihuman globulin (AHG), and weak-D testing. Solidscreen II provides a standardized method for antiglobulin testing. This method combines traditional low-ionic-strength test methods with a unique solid-phase format. The procedure uses a microwell coated with protein A, which has a high affinity for the Fc portion of antihuman globulin. The system allows for the use of the same liquid reagent red cells and low-ionic-strength solution that is used in conventional tube testing for antibody screening and identification.

CASE STUDIES

CASE STUDY 17.1

A well-hydrated male infant is 1 day old when the neonatologist observes that he is beginning to appear jaundiced. This baby is the first child of a 30-year-old computer analyst with no previous obstetric history or history of prior blood transfusion. The pregnancy had been normal.

Total bilirubin, hemoglobin/hematocrit, blood type/Rh, and direct antiglobulin tests are ordered for the baby. A cord blood sample has not been collected at delivery. Blood grouping and Rh testing and a screening test for unexpected antibodies are requested for the mother. Laboratory data are as follows:

Neonatal results

Total bilirubin: 10.8 mg/dL
Hemoglobin: 16.9 g/dL
Hematocrit: 52%
Blood group and Rh: A, Rh positive
Direct antiglobulin test: Negative

Maternal results

Blood group and Rh: O, Rh negative
Unexpected antibody screen: Negative

Treatment

The baby is immediately started on phototherapy. Subsequent total bilirubin tests are no higher than the 24-hour value and continue to decrease over the next 48 hours. At discharge, the total bilirubin is 6.9 mg/dL.

Multiple Choice Questions

Answers are in Appendix A.

1. The most probable cause of the infant's jaundice is:
   a. Prematurity
   b. Dehydration
   c. Milk allergy
   d. Blood group incompatibility between mother and baby
2. The baby's total bilirubin decreased over time because:
   a. Ultraviolet (UV) light breaks down bilirubin pigment.
   b. The baby was no longer exposed to maternal red blood cell antigens.
   c. The baby was no longer exposed to maternal antibodies.
   d. Both a and c
3. What is the most likely diagnosis?
   a. ABO incompatibility between mother and baby
   b. Rh incompatibility between mother and baby
   c. Rare blood group incompatibility between mother and baby
   d. Both a and b

Critical Thinking Group Discussion Questions

1. The mother is group O Rh negative and the baby is group A Rh positive. What are the possible consequences of the differences in blood group and Rh status?
2. Why was phototherapy selected for the baby as the treatment of choice rather than an exchange transfusion?
3. Should the mother receive prophylactic therapy, such as immune globulin D?

Note: Narrative answers published on instructor EVOLVE site.

CASE STUDY 17.2

A 17-year-old man is admitted with multiple injuries after his motorcycle crashes. The emergency department physician draws a blood sample for a STAT type and crossmatch. The motorcyclist's passenger also has blood drawn for a STAT type and screen.

An immediate-spin crossmatch is compatible between the group A patient and group A donor. The unit of blood is issued from the blood bank as an emergency release. After receiving 50 mL of the first unit of RBCs, the man develops shaking chills and becomes hypotensive with a falling blood pressure. The unit of cells is immediately discontinued, and the transfusion service is notified of the situation.

A recheck of testing is requested immediately.

Laboratory Testing

Clerical check: No evidence of clerical errors
Hemoglobinemia: Slight hemolysis observed
Direct antiglobulin test
 Patient pretransfusion: Negative
 Patient posttransfusion: Weakly positive
Recheck of blood grouping
 Patient pretransfusion: A positive
 Patient posttransfusion: O positive
 Donor: A positive
Repeat crossmatches
 Patient pretransfusion + Donor red blood cells = Compatible
 Patient posttransfusion + Donor red blood cells = Incompatible

Multiple Choice Questions

Answers are in Appendix A.

1. What is the most probable cause of the incompatible crossmatch?
   a. A mix-up in the patient specimens
   b. A mix-up in the transfused units
   c. Rh incompatibility
   d. None of the above
2. What type of transfusion reaction did the patient experience?
   a. Immediate hemolytic
   b. Delayed hemolytic
   c. Immediate nonhemolytic
   d. Delayed nonhemolytic
3. Could this type of transfusion reaction be fatal?
   a. Yes
   b. No
   c. Maybe
   d. Cannot be determined

Critical Thinking Group Discussion Questions

1. Why did this patient experience shaking chills and other adverse effects after receiving only 50 mL of red blood cells?
2. If the patient's adverse reaction to the blood transfusion had not been noted soon after the beginning of the transfusion, what physiologic changes would have occurred to the patient?

Note: Narrative answers published on instructor EVOLVE site.

REFERENCES

1. Dunsford I, Bowley CC, editors: *Techniques in blood grouping,* Edinburgh, 1955, Oliver & Boyd, preface.
2. Blaney KD, Howard PR: *Basic and applied concepts of immunohematology,* ed 3, St Louis, 2013, Mosby, p 317.
3. *International Council for Commonality in Blood Banking Automation: ISBT 128—the global information standard for medical products of human origin*, www.iccbba.org/.
4. US Department of Health and Human Services, Food and Drug Administration, Center for Biologics Evaluation and Research: *Revised recommendations for reducing the risk of Zika virus transmission by blood and blood components,* www.fda.gov/downloads/BiologicsBloodVaccines/GuidanceCompliance RegulatoryInformation/Guidances/Blood/UCM518213.pdf, accessed August 15, 2017.
5. Petrides M, et al: *Practical guide to transfusion medicine,* ed 2, Bethesda, Md, 2007, AABB Press.
6. American Association of Blood Banks (AABB): *Technical manual of the American Association of Blood Banks,* ed 16, Bethesda, MD, 2008, AABB.
7. Allen S: *System targets blood-type mix-ups*, www.boston.com. Accessed August 20, 2017.
8. American Association of Blood Banks (AABB): *Standards for blood banks and transfusion services,* ed 29, Bethesda, Md, 2014, AABB.
9. Torres R, Kenney B, Tomey CA: Diagnosis, treatment, and reporting of adverse effects of transfusion, *Lab Med* 43(5):217–230, 2012.
10. Kim YA, Mkaar RS: Detection of fetomaternal hemorrhage, *Am J Hematol* 87(4), 2012.

BIBLIOGRAPHY

Check W: Algorithm for HIV testing detects more cases, more quickly, *CAP Today* 27(12):40, 2013. 421.

Gurevitz SA: Update and utilization of component therapy in blood transfusions, *Lab Med* 42(4):235–240, 2011.

Holmberg JA: Blood group genotyping, *Adv Med Lab Prof* 25(2):26, 2013.

Howard PR: *Basic and applied concepts of blood banking and transfusion practices,* ed 4, St Louis, 2016, Elsevier/Mosby.

Immucor: Echo Compact Immunohematology automation, www.immucor.com.

McPherson RA, Pincus MR, editors: *Henry's clinical diagnosis and management by laboratory methods,* ed 22., Philadelphia, 2011, Elsevier/Saunders.

Tech guide: blood banking products, *Cl Lab Products* 43(3):18–20, 2013.

US Department of Health and Human Services: *Food and Drug Administration, Center for Biologics Evaluation and Research: Recommendations for assessment of blood donor eligibility, donor deferral and blood product management in response to Ebola virus,* www.fda.gov/BiologicsBloodVaccines/GuidanceCompliance RegulatoryInformation/Guidances/, accessed August 15, 2017.

Virk M, Sandler G: Rh immunoprophylaxis for women with a serologic weak D phenotype, *Lab Med* 46(3):190–194, 2015.

REVIEW QUESTIONS (ANSWERS IN APPENDIX A)

❖ Denotes advanced-content-level question.

Overview of Blood Banking

1. Transfusion medicine is defined as:
   - **a.** Actual genetic makeup; may not be evident by direct tests
   - **b.** RBC (blood) type, as determined by direct tests
   - **c.** The techniques and procedures involved in the study of the immunologic responses of blood (RBCs)
   - **d.** The procedures involved in collecting, storing, processing, and distributing blood and dispensing blood components to patients
2. Immunohematology is defined as:
   - **a.** Actual genetic makeup; may not be evident by direct tests
   - **b.** RBC (blood) type, as determined by direct tests
   - **c.** The techniques and procedures involved in the study of the immunologic responses of blood (RBCs)
   - **d.** Unexpected antibodies that result from specific antigenic stimulation

Benefits and Reasons for Transfusion

3. All the following are benefits of and reasons for blood transfusion *except:*
   - **a.** Restore or maintain oxygen-carrying capacity
   - **b.** Restore or maintain blood volume
   - **c.** Can replace coagulation factors to maintain hemostasis
   - **d.** Replace antibiotics in treatment of patients with granulocytic infections

Whole Blood, Blood Components, and Derivatives for Transfusion

4. Fresh frozen plasma is characterized by all of the following statements *except:*
   - **a.** A source of all coagulation factors
   - **b.** A source of heat-labile coagulation factors
   - **c.** Good for treating immune deficiencies
   - **d.** Transported with dry ice to keep frozen
5. Packed red blood cells are characterized by all of the following *except:*
   - **a.** Have the same expiration date as the original donor unit if kept sterile while being prepared
   - **b.** Good for 24 hours if the unit of blood is entered to prepare the RBCs
   - **c.** Can be used exclusively in cases of massive bleeding without any other fluids.
   - **d.** Used to restore oxygen-carrying capacity
6. Platelet concentrates are characterized by all of the following except:
   - **a.** Must be monitored for bacterial contamination
   - **b.** Are useful in cases of massive blood loss and replacement
   - **c.** Can stimulate production of HLA antibodies
   - **d.** Never need to be crossmatched

Blood Donation: Donors, Collection, Storage, and Processing

7. Which of the following tests is required in the screening of potential blood donors for transfusion-transmitted disease?
   - **a.** Hepatitis B surface antigen (HBsAg)
   - **b.** Hepatitis C antibody (HCV)
   - **c.** Hepatitis B core antibody (HBc)
   - **d.** All of the above

Other Types of Blood Donations

8. Autologous donation is characterized as:
   - **a.** Being safer than donor blood
   - **b.** Not requiring additional processing or crossmatching
   - **c.** Preventing transfusion-transmitted infectious disease from the unit of blood
   - **d.** All of the above

Antigens and Antibodies in Immunohematology

9. Genotype is the:
   - **a.** Actual genetic makeup; may not be evident by direct tests
   - **b.** RBC (blood) type, as determined by direct tests
   - **c.** Techniques and procedures involved in the study of the immunologic responses of blood (RBCs)
   - **d.** Unexpected antibodies that result from specific antigenic stimulation
10. Immune antibody is the:
    - **a.** Actual genetic makeup; may not be evident by direct tests
    - **b.** RBC (blood) type, as determined by direct tests
    - **c.** The techniques and procedures involved in the study of the immunologic responses of blood (RBCs)
    - **d.** Unexpected antibodies that result from specific antigenic stimulation
11. Phenotype is the:
    - **a.** Actual genetic makeup; may not be evident by direct tests
    - **b.** RBC (blood) type, as determined by direct testing
    - **c.** The techniques and procedures involved in the study of the immunologic responses of blood (RBCs)
    - **d.** Unexpected antibodies that result from specific antigenic stimulation

ABO Red Blood Cell Group System

12. The phenotype of genotype AO is:
    - **a.** AB
    - **b.** A
    - **c.** B
    - **d.** O
13. The phenotype of genotype BO is:
    - **a.** AB
    - **b.** A
    - **c.** B
    - **d.** O

14. The phenotype of genotype BB is:
a. AB
b. A
c. B
d. O

15. The phenotype of genotype AB is:
a. AB
b. A
c. B
d. O

Rh Red Blood Cell Group System

16. Patients are generally described as Rh positive or Rh negative based on the presence of which of the following antigens on the RBCs?
a. c
b. D
c. E
d. Kidd

Other Blood Group Systems

17. Other blood group systems include:
a. Kell
b. Duffy
c. Lewis
d. All of the above

Antihuman Globulin Reaction

18. The indirect antiglobulin test is performed:
a. On RBCs suspected of being coated with antibody
b. On serum suspected of containing antibodies
c. To determine ABO blood group antigens
d. To determine Rh blood group antigens

19. The direct antiglobulin test (DAT) is performed:
a. On RBCs suspected of being coated with antibody
b. On serum suspected of containing antibodies
c. To determine ABO blood group antigens
d. To determine Rh blood group antigens

Compatibility Testing and Crossmatching

20. When blood is to be transfused to a patient, the most important question is:
a. Does the patient's serum contain an antibody against the donor's RBCs?
b. Does the donor's serum contain an antibody against the patient's RBCs?
c. Do the patient's RBCs contain an antigen against the donor's serum?
d. Either b or c

21. If a patient is group A, what is the preferred blood group for transfusion?
a. A
b. B
c. O
d. AB

22. Crossmatching of the donor's RBCs with the patient's serum could demonstrate:
a. Major incompatibility between patient and donor
b. Minor incompatibility between patient and donor
c. Verification of correct Rh type
d. Presence of unexpected antibodies in the donor's serum

23. Testing of the patient's serum with a panel of group O cells for unexpected antibodies can demonstrate:
a. Antibodies to rare antigens in all cells of the panel
b. Rare patient antigens
c. Patient antibodies to various nonself antigens
d. Both a and c

24. Compatibility testing can help to detect:
a. Some ABO incompatibilities
b. Some errors in labeling, recording, or identification
c. Most unexpected antibodies in the patient's serum
d. All of the above

Adverse Effects of Transfusion

25. Which of the following are generally characterized as a transfusion reaction?
a. Hemolytic reactions
b. Febrile reactions
c. Allergic reactions
d. All of the above

Hemolytic Disease of the Fetus and Newborn

26. The most important reason for the decrease in the number of cases of hemolytic disease of the fetus and newborn (HDFN) is:
a. Use of the acid-elution stain
b. More correct Rh typing
c. Use of improved typing procedures
d. Use of Rh immune globulin

27. HDFN does not usually occur in the first pregnancy if the mother is D negative and the baby is D positive. Which of the following is the most likely reason for this?
a. The mother's immune system cannot build antibodies during the 9 months of her first pregnancy.
b. The baby's D antigens are poorly developed before birth.
c. The greatest exposure of the mother to the baby's RBCs with D antigens is during labor and delivery.
d. A difference in Rh status between mother and baby is not an important factor in the development of HDFN.

28. If 50 mL of fetal red blood cells are estimated to be in the maternal circulation, how many vials of RhIg will be required?
a. 1
b. 2
c. 3
d. 4

Automated Testing Technology and Systems

29. The automated blood banking testing format of the BioRad Solidscreen II test system uses:
   a. Traditional low-ionic-strength test methods and a microwell coated with protein A.
   b. Gel column technology.
   c. Microplates and microwell strips to perform hemagglutination assays.
   d. Microwell plates precoated with blood-grouping monoclonal antibodies.

Turgeon: Linné & Ringsrud's Clinical Laboratory Science, 8th Edition

STUDENT PROCEDURE WORKSHEET 17-1

ABO Blood Grouping (Forward Antigen Typing) Procedure

Student Learning Outcomes

See Chapter 17 of *Linné & Ringsrud's Clinical Laboratory Science: Concepts, Procedures, and Clinical Applications*, 8th edition, for a complete discussion of this procedure.After reading Chapter 17, and at the completion of the laboratory exercise and review questions, the student will be able to:

- Describe the forward and reverse typing for the identification of ABO blood groups.
- Complete the end-of-procedure review questions with a grade of 80% or higher.

Principle

Determination of ABO blood group status is determined by direct detection of the A and/or B blood group antigens on erythrocytes. Confirmation of ABO blood grouping can be determined by the isoantibodies synthesized in normal individuals in response to A and/or B antigenic stimulation.

Specimen

No special preparation of the patient is required before specimen collection. The patient must be positively identified when the specimen is collected, and the specimen must be labeled at the bedside. Specimen labels include the patient's full name, the date, the patient's hospital identification number, and the phlebotomist's initials. Bar coding is now a popular method of identification as well. Blood should be drawn by aseptic technique. A minimum of 2 mL of anticoagulated blood (lavender-top evacuated tube) is required. Hemolysis or contamination with bacteria renders a specimen unsuitable for testing. If the test cannot be performed immediately, the specimen should be refrigerated (2 °C–8 °C).

Equipment and Supplies

1. Centrifuge
2. Magnifier reading device
3. 10 × 75–mm test tubes
4. Normal saline (0.9% NaCl)
5. Disposable pipettes
6. Marking pen

Reagents

1. Commercial blood grouping antisera
2. Anti-A and anti-B typing sera (store at 4 °C)
3. Group A and group B reagent RBCs (store at 4 °C)
   NOTE: Reagents must be used before the expiration date published on the label.

Quality Control

Positive control: known group A reagent RBCs should demonstrate agglutination with anti-A typing serum.
Positive control: known group B reagent RBCs should demonstrate agglutination with anti-B typing serum.
Negative control: known group A reagent RBCs should not demonstrate agglutination with anti-B typing serum.
Negative control: known group B reagent RBCs should not demonstrate agglutination with anti-A typing serum.

Instructions for the Procedure

Read the list of required equipment, supplies, and reagents and the procedural steps. Follow the procedural steps in exact order.

Reporting and Interpretation of Results

Agglutination is an indication of an antigen-antibody bonding reaction.

- If anti-A yields agglutination with RBCs, the erythrocytes have the corresponding A antigen or group A.
- If anti-B yields agglutination with RBCs, the erythrocytes have the corresponding B antigen or group B.
- If anti-A yields agglutination with RBCs and anti-B yields agglutination with RBCs, the erythrocytes have both the corresponding A antigen and B antigen on the cellular membrane. This is a *group AB reaction*.
- If anti-A yields no agglutination with RBCs, the erythrocytes do not have the corresponding A antigen or group A. If anti-B yields no agglutination with RBCs, the erythrocytes do not have the corresponding B antigen or group B. This is a *group O reaction*.

AGGLUTINATION REACTIONS

ANTI-A	ANTI-B	BLOOD GROUP
Positive	Negative	A
Negative	Positive	B
Positive	Positive	AB
Negative	Negative	O

Sources of Error

Clinical Sources

Discrepancies in forward typing can result from conditions such as weak antigens, altered expression of antigens caused by disease, chimerism, or excessive blood group substances. Excess of blood group–specific substance caused by disorders such as carcinoma of stomach and pancreas that neutralize the reagent anti-A and anti-B can produces a false-negative or weak reaction in forward typing. Incorrect typing can result from additional antigens such as acquired A-like and B-like antigens or antibody-sensitized RBCs such as autoimmune disorders. If a patient has been recently transfused with non–group-specific blood, mixed-filed agglutination may be observed.

Technical Sources

- Antisera should not be cloudy, and need to be refrigerated unless being used.
- Do not rely on the color of tubes to identify reagent antisera. All tubes must be properly labeled.
- Do not perform tests at temperatures higher than room temperature.
- Observe for agglutination with a well-lit background.
- Record results immediately after observation.

Clinical Applications

Direct blood grouping is the first step in proper blood grouping. *Reverse grouping* involves using known reagent RBCs with blood serum for the detection of A or B antibodies (see Student Procedure Worksheet 17-2).

(Continued)

Turgeon: Linné & Ringsrud's Clinical Laboratory Science, 8th Edition

STUDENT PROCEDURE WORKSHEET 17-1

Limitations

Reverse cell typing using a patient's serum containing isoantibodies should be performed to verify the results.

NOTE: The Micronics ABORhCard Card is a newly FDA-approved, single-use, disposable blood typing device allows a quick determination of a person's blood type and Rh status from a fingerstick of blood. This portable credit-card-sized device eliminates the need for the instruments or other equipment, liquid typing reagents, and refrigeration traditionally used to determine a person's blood group. Additional features include long shelf life and waste containment in the card for easy disposal. The card is a qualitative in vitro agglutination test that determines both ABO blood group and Rh factor of an individual in approximately 2 minutes. The test cannot be used for blood bank processing of blood products, for determining RHD status for the purpose of administration of Rh immunoglobulin, or for blood screening before transfusion.

References

Micronics Credit-Card Size Agglutination. www.micronics.net. Retrieved July 2013.

SEQUENCE	PROCEDURAL STEP	INSTRUCTOR-OBSERVED ACCEPTABLE PERFORMANCE (CHECK IF ACCEPTABLE)
1	Check the patient's name and identification number on the blood specimen and requisition.	
2	Prepared a 2% to 5% suspension of the patient's RBCs in normal saline.	
3	Label two test tubes, one with the letter A and the other with B.	
4	To the tube labeled A, add 1 drop of anti-A antiserum.	
5	To the tube labeled B, add 1 drop of anti-B antiserum.	
6	Using a disposable pipette, add 1 drop of the cell suspension to each of the test tubes.	
7	Mix well, and centrifuge the test tubes for 15 seconds at 3400 rpm.	
8	Resuspend the cells with gentle agitation, and examine macroscopically for agglutination (see Agglutination Reactions).	

(Continued)

Turgeon: Linné & Ringsrud's Clinical Laboratory Science, 8th Edition

STUDENT PROCEDURE WORKSHEET 17-1

ABO Blood Grouping (Forward Antigen Typing) Procedure

RESULTS OF UNKNOWN SPECIMENS			
PATIENT ID	ANTI-A ANTISERA	ANTI-B ANTISERA	INTERPRETATION

Instructor Initial, if acceptable ________________

Review Questions

1. Group O blood type has ________ antigens on the red blood cell membrane.
   a. O
   b. B
   c. A
   d. No A or B

2. Describe at least three technical sources of error in direct blood grouping.

Procedural Evaluation

Student's Name ______________________________ Grade__________

Instructor's Signature __________________________ Date__________

Comments:

Turgeon: Linné & Ringsrud's Clinical Laboratory Science, 8th Edition

STUDENT PROCEDURE WORKSHEET 17-2

ABO Blood Grouping (Reverse Grouping)

Student Learning Outcomes
After reading Chapter 17 of *Linné & Ringsrud's Clinical Laboratory Science: Concepts, Procedures, and Clinical Applications,* 8th edition, and at the completion of the laboratory exercise and review questions, the student will be able to:

- Identify ABO blood groups.
- Complete the end-of-procedure review questions with a grade of 80% or higher.

Principle and Specimen
See Student Procedure Worksheet 17-1.

Equipment, Supplies, and Reagents

1. Reagent erythrocytes: A_1 and B (A_2 optional)
2. Disposable test tubes, 10×75 mm
3. Disposable pipettes, 4 -inch plastic or Pasteur
4. High-intensity lamp or optical magnifying lens
5. Centrifuge

Quality Control
Reagent erythrocytes should be tested daily with known antisera.

Sources of Error

Clinical Sources
Discrepancies in reverse blood grouping can be cause by low concentrations of isoantibodies in older adult or immunosuppressed patients. Another source of discrepancy can be seen in newborns who have not synthesized their own antibodies and may have circulating maternal antibodies.

Technical Sources

- Do not perform tests at temperatures colder or warmer than room temperature.
- Observe for agglutination with a well-lit background. Do not shake the reaction tube too hard because it will disperse agglutination.
- Record results immediately after observation.

Clinical Applications
Reverse grouping involves using known reagent RBCs with blood serum for the detection of A or B antibodies.

Reference
Turgeon ML: *Fundamentals of immunohematology,* ed 2, Baltimore, 1995, Williams & Wilkins, pp 344-346.

Instructions for the Procedure
Read the list of required equipment, supplies, and reagents and the procedural steps. Follow the procedural steps in exact order.

SEQUENCE	PROCEDURAL STEP	INSTRUCTOR-OBSERVED ACCEPTABLE PERFORMANCE (CHECK IF ACCEPTABLE)
1	Label two 10×75–mm test tubes one with the letter *A,* the other with the letter *B,* A and B. Label each with the last three digits of the laboratory number. NOTE: The letters *A* and *B* should be underlined to denote reverse grouping.	
2	To each test tube, add 2 drops of the serum or plasma to be tested, using a disposable pipette.	
3	To the tube labeled A, add 1 drop of the thoroughly mixed A_1 reagent erythrocytes.	
4	To the tube labeled B, add 1 drop of the thoroughly mixed B reagent erythrocytes.	
5	Mix well and centrifuge both test tubes for 15 seconds at 3400 rpm.	
6	Resuspend the cells by gentle agitation, and examine macroscopically for agglutination; record results.	

Turgeon: Linné & Ringsrud's Clinical Laboratory Science, 8th Edition

Results of Unknown Specimens

PATIENT ID	REAGENT CELLS A	REAGENT CELLS B	INTERPRETATION

Instructor Initial, if acceptable ___________________

Procedural Evaluation

Student's Name ___________________________________ Grade __________

Instructor's Signature ______________________________ Date ____________

Comments:

Turgeon: Linné & Ringsrud's Clinical Laboratory Science, 8th Edition

STUDENT PROCEDURE WORKSHEET 17-2

ABO Blood Grouping (Reverse Grouping)

Review Questions

1. Group O blood type has ___________ antibodies in the serum.
   a. A
   b. B
   c. Both A and B
   d. Neither A nor B
2. Describe at least three technical sources of error in reverse (antibody) testing.

A APPENDIX

Answers to Review Questions

CHAPTER 1 FUNDAMENTALS OF THE CLINICAL LABORATORY

Case Studies

Case Study 1.1

1. d

Case Study 1.2

1. c

Review Questions

1. b
2. a
3. c
4. d
5. b
6. c
7. a
8. c
9. a
10. b
11. d
12. d
13. d
14. a
15. c
16. a
17. d

Bonus Challenge Question

18. d

CHAPTER 2 SAFETY: PATIENT AND CLINICAL LABORATORY PRACTICES

Case Studies

Case Study 2.1

1. c
2. a

Review Questions

1. a
2. d
3. a
4. c
5. b
6. d
7. d
8. d
9. d
10. c
11. a
12. d
13. b
14. a
15. b
16. d
17. c
18. a
19. c
20. d
21. b
22. b
23. a
24. b
25. d
26. c
27. d
28. a
29. a

Bonus Challenge Questions

30. c
31. d
32. b
33. b
34. d

CHAPTER 3 QUALITY ASSESSMENT AND QUALITY CONTROL IN THE CLINICAL LABORATORY

Case Studies

Case Study 3.1

1. b
2. b

Review Questions

1. d
2. d
3. a
4. a

CHAPTER 3 (*CONT*)

5. d
6. b
7. c
8. b
9. b
10. b
11. a
12. b
13. a
14. c
15. a
16. a
17. b
18. d
19. b
20. d
21. b
22. a
23. d
24. b
25. d
26. b
27. a
28. d
29. a
30. b
31. a
32. c
33. b
34. b
35. a
36. c
37. a

Bonus Challenge Questions

38. b
39. c
40. a

CHAPTER 4 PHLEBOTOMY: COLLECTING AND PROCESSING PATIENT BLOOD SPECIMENS

Case Studies

Case Study 4.1

1. b
2. c

Case Study 4.2

1. a
2. b

Case Study 4.3

1. c
2. a

Review Questions

1. b
2. a
3. c
4. b
5. b
6. b
7. d
8. b
9. d
10. c
11. a
12. d
13. b
14. a
15. d
16. c
17. a
18. c
19. b
20. d
21. d
22. d
23. a
24. b
25. a
26. c
27. d
28. d

CHAPTER 5 THE MICROSCOPE

Review Questions

1. b
2. c
3. a
4. c
5. b
6. a
7. b
8. b
9. c
10. d
11. c
12. d
13. b
14. a
15. d
16. d
17. c
18. d
19. b
20. b
21. a
22. c
23. d

CHAPTER 5 (*CONT*)

24. a
25. c
26. c

CHAPTER 6 SYSTEMS OF MEASUREMENT, LABORATORY EQUIPMENT, AND REAGENTS

Review Questions

1. c
2. a
3. b
4. c
5. c
6. b
7. c
8. b
9. c
10. a
11. b
12. b
13. d
14. a
15. a
16. d
17. a
18. a

Bonus Challenge Questions

19. d
20. c
21. a
22. b

CHAPTER 7 LABORATORY MATHEMATICS AND SOLUTION PREPARATION

Review Questions

1. d
2. a
3. a
4. d
5. d
6. c
7. b
8. b
9. b
10. c
11. b
12. c
13. a
14. b
15. b
16. c
17. c
18. b
19. b
20. b
21. d
22. c
23. a
24. b
25. d
26. c
27. b
28. b
29. b

Bonus Challenge Questions

30. a
31. c
32. b
33. a

CHAPTER 8 BASIC AND CONTEMPORARY TECHNIQUES IN THE CLINICAL LABORATORY

Review Questions

1. d
2. c
3. b
4. d
5. a
6. b
7. b
8. a
9. c
10. a
11. b
12. d
13. b
14. a
15. c
16. a
17. a
18. d
19. b
20. a
21. b
22. b
23. c
24. a
25. b
26. a
27. d
28. d
29. b
30. d
31. d
32. a
33. b

CHAPTER 8 (*CONT*)

34. d
35. c
36. a
37. a
38. b
39. b
40. a
41. a
42. b
43. c
44. b
45. c
46. d
47. b
48. d
49. d
50. d
51. d
52. a
53. a

Bonus Challenge Questions

54. c
55. b
56. a

CHAPTER 9 LABORATORY TESTING: FROM POINT OF CARE TO TOTAL AUTOMATION

Case Studies

Case Study 9.1

1. c
2. a
3. b

Review Questions

1. a
2. a
3. a
4. a
5. a
6. a
7. b
8. d
9. a
10. d
11. d
12. b
13. c
14. d
15. d
16. c
17. d
18. d

Bonus Challenge Questions

19. a
20. b

CHAPTER 10 INTRODUCTION TO THE PRINCIPLES AND PRACTICE OF CLINICAL CHEMISTRY

Case Studies

Case Study 10.1

1. a
2. d

Case Study 10.2

1. b

Case Study 10.3

1. d
2. b

Case Study 10.4

1. b
2. a

Case Study 10.5

1. d
2. d

Case Study 10.6

1. c
2. c

Case Study 10.7

1. a
2. d
3. d

Review Questions

1. a
2. d
3. b
4. b
5. d
6. a
7. d
8. b
9. c
10. b
11. b
12. a
13. d
14. b
15. a
16. a

CHAPTER 10 (*CONT*)

17. b
18. c
19. d
20. d
21. d
22. d
23. d
24. a
25. a
26. d
27. b
28. a
29. d
30. c
31. d
32. a
33. a
34. c
35. c
36. d
37. a
38. a
39. d
40. a
41. c
42. c
43. c
44. b
45. a
46. c
47. b
48. a
49. c
50. b
51. a
52. a
53. d
54. d
55. b
56. c
57. a
58. d
59. a

CHAPTER 11 AN INTRODUCTION TO THE PRINCIPLES AND PRACTICE OF CLINICAL HEMATOLOGY

Case Studies

Case Study 11.1

1. a
2. a
3. a

Case Study 11.2

1. c
2. b
3. a

Case Study 11.3

1. b
2. b
3. b

Case Study 11.4

1. a
2. c
3. c

Case Study 11.5

1. b
2. c
3. c

Review Questions

1. a
2. c
3. b
4. c
5. d
6. a
7. c
8. d
9. a
10. a
11. d
12. c
13. c
14. a
15. b
16. a
17. d
18. d
19. c
20. d
21. b
22. b
23. a
24. c
25. d
26. b
27. d
28. a
29. b
30. c
31. a
32. d
33. c
34. b

CHAPTER 11 (*CONT*)

35. c
36. d
37. d
38. a
39. a
40. c
41. d
42. c
43. b
44. d
45. a
46. c
47. c
48. c
49. a
50. a
51. b
52. a
53. a
54. d
55. d
56. b
57. d
58. a
59. b
60. c

CHAPTER 12 HEMOSTASIS AND BLOOD COAGULATION

Case Studies

Case Study 12.1

1. b
2. a

Case Study 12.2

1. a
2. c

Case Study 12.3

1. a
2. d

Review Questions

1. c
2. a
3. c
4. d
5. a
6. c
7. a
8. b
9. a
10. a
11. a
12. b
13. c
14. a
15. b
16. a
17. d
18. c
19. b
20. b
21. a
22. d
23. b

CHAPTER 13 RENAL PHYSIOLOGY AND URINALYSIS

Case Studies

Case Study 13.1

1. a
2. b
3. b

Case Study 13.2

1. a
2. d
3. a

Case Study 13.3

1. d
2. b
3. c

Case Study 13.4

1. d
2. d
3. d

Case Study 13.5

1. a
2. a
3. c

Review Questions

1. d
2. b
3. d
4. a
5. c
6. d
7. b
8. a
9. c
10. a
11. c

CHAPTER 13 (*CONT*)

12. a
13. b
14. d
15. d
16. c
17. a
18. a
19. b
20. a
21. b
22. d
23. b
24. c
25. a
26. d
27. b
28. c
29. c
30. d
31. a
32. b
33. c
34. d
35. d
36. d
37. a
38. c
39. b
40. a
41. a
42. a

CHAPTER 14 EXAMINATION OF BODY FLUIDS AND MISCELLANEOUS SPECIMENS

Case Studies

Case Study 14.1

1. a
2. b
3. b

Case Study 14.2

1. a
2. c
3. b

Review Questions

1. a
2. a
3. d
4. b
5. c
6. d
7. a
8. a
9. b
10. d
11. c
12. a
13. d
14. a
15. b
16. d
17. d
18. a
19. c
20. b
21. a
22. d
23. d
24. d
25. d

CHAPTER 15 INTRODUCTION TO MEDICAL MICROBIOLOGY

Case Studies

Case Study 15.1

1. a
2. a

Case Study 15.2

1. b
2. c

Case Study 15.3

1. a
2. d

Case Study 15.4

1. b
2. c

Case Study 15.5

1. d
2. d

Case Study 15.6

1. b
2. b

Review Questions

1. a
2. a
3. c
4. a
5. c
6. c
7. c
8. c
9. d
10. c

CHAPTER 15 (*CONT*)

11. a
12. c
13. d
14. c
15. a
16. a
17. c
18. a
19. c
20. c
21. a
22. b
23. d
24. c
25. a
26. a
27. d
28. b
29. d
30. a
31. b
32. d
33. a
34. c
35. a
36. a
37. d
38. b
39. a
40. c
41. c
42. a
43. a
44. d
45. c
46. b
47. d
48. b

CHAPTER 16 IMMUNOLOGY

Case Study 16.1

1. d
2. d
3. b

Case Study 16.2

1. d
2. a
3. b

Review Questions

1. d
2. c
3. c
4. c
5. b
6. a
7. c
8. b
9. d
10. c
11. a
12. c
13. b
14. a
15. a
16. a
17. a
18. d
19. c
20. a
21. b
22. c
23. d
24. c
25. c
26. a
27. d
28. c
29. d
30. c
31. b
32. a
33. b
34. b
35. c
36. c
37. d
38. a
39. a
40. a
41. d
42. a

CHAPTER 17 IMMUNOHEMATOLOGY AND TRANSFUSION MEDICINE

Case Study 17.1

1. d
2. a
3. a

Case Study 17.2

1. a
2. a
3. a

Review Questions

1. d
2. c

CHAPTER 17 (*CONT*)

3. d
4. a
5. c
6. d
7. d
8. d
9. a
10. d
11. b
12. b
13. c
14. c
15. a
16. b
17. d
18. b
19. a
20. a
21. a
22. a
23. c
24. d
25. d
26. d
27. c
28. c
29. a

APPENDIX B

Disease/Organ Panels

http://evolve.elsevier.com/Turgeon

CHAPTER CONTENTS

AMA-DESIGNATED[1] LABORATORY TESTING PANELS

Acute Hepatitis Panel

Hepatitis A antibody, IgM (HAV Ab, IgM)
Hepatitis B surface antigen (HbsAg)
Hepatitis B core antibody, IgM (HbcAb, IgM)
Hepatitis C (HCV) antibody screen

Basic Metabolic Panel

Calcium
Carbon dioxide (CO_2)
Chloride
Creatinine
Glucose
Potassium
Sodium
Urea nitrogen (BUN)

[1]American Medical Association (AMA): AMA-recognized organ/disease panels. In *Current procedural terminology standard edition*, Chicago, 2013, AMA.

Comprehensive Metabolic Panel

Alanine aminotransferase (ALT)
Albumin
Alkaline phosphatase
Aspartate aminotransferase (AST)
Bilirubin (total)
Calcium
Carbon dioxide (CO_2)
Chloride
Creatinine
Glucose
Potassium
Sodium
Total protein
Urea nitrogen (BUN)

Electrolyte Panel

Carbon dioxide (CO_2)
Chloride
Phosphorus
Potassium

Lipid Panel

Cholesterol (total)
HDL cholesterol, direct
Non-HDL cholesterol
Triglycerides

Liver Function Panel

Alanine amino transferase (ALT)
Albumin
Alkaline phosphatase
Aspartate amino transferase (AST)
Direct bilirubin
Total bilirubin
Total protein

Obstetrics Panel

ABO/RH(D) and antibody screen
Complete blood count (CBC) with automated differential (CBCD)
Hepatitis B surface antigen (HBsAg)
Rubella IgG Ab, immune status (RUBG)
Syphilis serology (RPR)

Renal Function Panel

Albumin
Calcium
Carbon dioxide (CO_2)
Chloride
Creatinine
Glucose
Phosphorus
Potassium
Sodium
Urea nitrogen (BUN)

REPRESENTATIVE EXAMPLES OF LABORATORY TESTING RELATED TO A SPECIFIC DISORDER OR DISEASE

Anemia

Assays for B_{12} and folate
Bilirubin
Complete blood count (CBC) with red blood cell (RBC) indices
Direct antihuman globulin (AHG)
Erythrocyte sedimentation rate (ESR)
Iron studies
Reticulocyte count
Additional test options, depending on CBC, RBC indices, reticulocyte count

Arthritis

Antinuclear antibody (ANA)
C-reactive protein
Cyclic citrullinated peptide antibody
Erythrocyte sedimentation rate (ESR)
Rheumatoid factor
Uric acid

Bleeding or Coagulation Disorder

Partial thromboplastin time
Platelet count
Platelet function test
Prothrombin time
Thrombin time
Additional testing: specific blood coagulation factor deficiency

Cardiac Injury

CK-MB
Creatine kinase (CK)
Troponin-1

Collagen Disease/Systemic Lupus Erythematosus (SLE)

Antibody neutrophil cytoplasmic antibody (ANCA)
Anti-DNA
Antinuclear antibody (ANA)
C4
C-reactive protein
C3
Erythrocyte sedimentation rate (ESR)

Disseminated Intravascular Coagulation (DIC)

Complete blood count (CBC) with examination of blood film
D-dimers
Fibrinogen
Partial thromboplastin time
Platelet count
Prothrombin time
Thrombin time

Hemolysis

Bilirubin
Complete blood count (CBC)
Direct antiglobulin test
Free hemoglobin (plasma and urine)
Haptoglobin
Lactate dehydrogenase (LD)
Reticulocyte count

Hepatic Function

Alanine amino transferase (ALT)
Albumin
Alkaline phosphatase
Aspartate amino transferase (AST)
Bilirubin time (total and direct)
Gamma-glutamyl transferase (GGT)
Protein, total
Prothrombin time

Hepatitis Serology, Chronic Carrier

Hepatitis B surface Ag
Hepatitis Be Ab
Hepatitis Be Ag
Hepatitis C Ab

Human Immunodeficiency Virus

Complete blood count (CBC) with CD4 and CD8 lymphocyte subsets
HIV genotype
HIV 1 and 2 Ab (enzyme immunoassay [EIA]) with Western blot confirmation
HIV viral load

Hypertension

Basic Metabolic Panel

Renin

Thyroid Screening

Urinalysis
Urinary free cortisol
Urinary metanephrines

Iron/Hemochromatosis

Alanine amino transferase (ALT)
Ferritin
Percent (%) saturation
Serum iron
Total iron-binding capacity (TIBC)

Newborn Screening

Argininosuccinic acidemia (ASA)
Beta-ketothiolase deficiency (BIOT)
Carnitine uptake defect (CUD)
Citrullinemia (CIT)
Congenital adrenal hyperplasia (CAH)
Congenital hypothyroidism (CH)
Cystic fibrosis (CF)
Galactosemia (GALT)
Glutaric acidemia type I (GA I)
Hemoglobin sickle/beta-thalassemia (Hb S/βTh)
Hemoglobin sickle/C, disease (Hb S/C)
Homocystinuria (HCY)
Isovaleric acidemia (IVA)
Long-chain hydroxyacyl-CoA dehydrogenase deficiency (LCHAD)
Maple syrup urine disease (MSUD)
Medium-chain acyl-CoA dehydrogenase deficiency (MCAD)
Methylmalonic acidemia (Cbl A,B)
Methylmalonic acidemia (mutase deficiency) (MUT)
Multiple carboxylase deficiency (MCD)
Phenylketonuria (PKU)
Propionic acidemia (PROP)
Sickle cell anemia (Hb SS disease) (Hb SS)
3-hydroxy 3-methyl glutaric aciduria (HMG)
3-methylcrotonyl-CoA carboxylase deficiency (3MCC)
Trifunctional protein deficiency (TFP)
Tyrosinemia type I (TYR I)
Very long-chain acyl-CoA dehydrogenase deficiency (VLCAD)
Newborn testing for secondary target conditions varies by state

Pancreatic

Amylase
Calcium (total and ionized)
Glucose
Lipase
Triglycerides

Parathyroid

Albumin
Alkaline phosphatase
Calcium (total and ionized)
Creatine
Magnesium
Parathyroid (PTH) (whole molecule, amino terminal)
Phosphorus
Protein, total
Urinary calcium

Respiratory Distress

CO_2 content
O_2 saturation
$P_{A\text{-}a}O_2$
P_aCO_2
P_aO_2
pH

Thyroid Screening (Urine)

Thyroid-stimulating hormone (TSH) (third or fourth generation)
Thyroxine (free T4)

Toxicology Screening (Urine)

Amphetamines
Barbiturates
Benzodiazepines
Cocaine metabolites
Marijuana metabolites
Methadone
Methaqualone
Opiate metabolites
Phencyclidine
Propoxyphene

REFERENCES

Department of Practice Parameters: *Principles of practice parameters,* Chicago, 1995, American Medical Association, 1–18.
Glenn GC, Altschuler CH, Gambino R, et al: Practice parameter on laboratory panel testing for screening and case finding in asymptomatic adults, *Arch Pathol Lab Med* 120:929–941, 1996.

GLOSSARY

A

absolute cell count (absolute numbers): Concentration of a cell type expressed as a number per volume of whole blood, usually per liter; obtained by multiplying the relative percentage value by the total leukocyte count per liter.

absorbance: Amount of light that is absorbed or retained and therefore not able to pass through or be transmitted through a solution.

absorbance spectrophotometry: Methodology that uses Beer's law, whereby the amount of light absorbed by a solution is directly proportional to the concentration of the solution; this measurement can be made only by mathematical calculation from the transmission data obtained by use of a quantitative analytical method, such as spectrophotometry.

absorbance units: Units of measure for light that is absorbed by a colored solution.

absorbed light: Light that is not transmitted.

acceptable control range: Statistically determined range of values within which a test result must fall to be considered acceptable; it is a means of quality control or assurance.

accuracy: Correctness of a result, freedom from error, or how close the answer is to the "true" value.

accurate and precise technology (APT): "Easy" or automated quantitative tests or easy qualitative tests for which the manufacturer of the automated instrument has been granted special standing under the definitions of laboratory tests in the Clinical Laboratory Improvement Amendments of 1988 (CLIA '88).

acholic stool: Absence of bile; results in formation of colorless, chalky-appearing fecal specimens.

acid–base balance: Maintenance of a constant balance between acids and bases; maintenance of constant pH.

acid crystals: Crystals seen in urine of an acidic pH, less than pH 7.0.

acid-fast bacteria (AFB): Bacteria that retain staining dye and make the decolorization step difficult.

acid-fast stain: Used to detect organisms that are difficult to decolorize, even with acid-alcohol solutions; typical organisms are those that cause tuberculosis or leprosy.

acidophilic: "Acid-loving"; on blood films, the cell components that stain with the acidic portion of Wright or Wright–Giemsa stain, such as hemoglobin and eosinophilic granules, which stain orange to pink.

acidosis: Decrease in blood pH.

acquired immunity: Acquired (adaptive or specific) immunity is not present at birth. As a person's immune system encounters foreign substances (antigens), the components of acquired immunity recognize each antigen and begin to develop a memory for that antigen. Acquired immunity takes time to develop after initial exposure to a new antigen. Memory is formed, and subsequent responses to a previously encountered antigen are more effective.

activated partial thromboplastin time (APTT): A test sensitive to heparin; useful in detecting deficiencies in intrinsic and common pathway factors.

active immunity: A type of immunity or resistance developed by the production of antibodies in a person in response to an exposure to an antigen, a pathogen, or a vaccine.

active reabsorption: A form of reabsorption that requires the expenditure of energy. This is usually against a concentration gradient, from a region of lower to one of higher concentration.

acute glomerulonephritis (AGN): Also called *postinfectious glomerulonephritis.* A disease of the kidney glomerulus that is an immunologic sequela of a bacterial infection. Characteristics include oliguria, edema, proteinuria with red blood cell or granular casts, and hematuria.

acute interstitial nephritis (AIN): An inflammation of the interstitial tissue of the kidney that is an immunologic, adverse reaction to certain drugs, such as sulfonamide or methicillin. The condition is characterized by fever, rash, proteinuria, and the presence of eosinophils in the urine.

acute phase: Early in the course of a disease, when the disease is first suspected; blood is drawn (acute-phase serum) when little or no antibody has had time to develop and is compared with antibody level in convalescent serum.

acute-phase reactants: Group of glycoproteins associated with nonspecific inflammatory conditions.

acute pyelonephritis: An infection of the pelvis and parenchyma of the kidney; usually the result of an ascending infection from the lower urinary tract.

adaptive immunity: See *acquired immunity.*

additives, anticoagulants: Additives usually are anticoagulants that prevent coagulation of the blood specimen. Several different anticoagulants are available for different testing purposes. Some laboratory tests require the use of plasma or whole blood for the assay, and these must be anticoagulated during the collection process.

aerobes: Microbes that require oxygen for growth.

aerosols: Infectious particles that are airborne; fine mist in which particles are dispersed.

agar: A seaweed extract that is liquid when heated and solid when cooled; used as base medium for preparation of culture plates, slant tubes, and stab tubes.

agar disk diffusion tests: Tests that employ antibiotic-impregnated disks placed on an agar culture plate inoculated with the organism to be tested.

agar slant: Tubes of agar media that are solidified on a slant (the surface of the medium is on an incline); useful for particular cultures.

agglutination: Visible clumping or aggregation of red cells or any particles; used as an indication of a specific antigen–antibody reaction.

agglutinins: Antibodies that form visible clumps, or agglutinate, with their specific antigens.

agglutinogens: Antigens that form visible clumps, or agglutinate, with their specific antibodies.

aggregometer: Instrument that measures platelet aggregation in platelet dysfunction studies.

albuminemia: Decreased blood albumin.

albuminuria: Presence of albumin in the urine.

aldosterone: Hormone that controls the sodium–potassium pump, the primary mechanism for sodium reabsorption in the kidney; regulator of blood sodium and potassium levels.

algorithm: A set of steps followed to solve a problem or to reach a diagnosis by laboratory assays.

alignment: Microscope adjustment that ensures that the light path from the light source throughout the microscope and ocular is physically correct.

aliquot: One of a number of equal parts.

alkaline crystals: Crystals seen in urine of an alkaline pH; generally pH 7.0 and above.

alkalosis: Increase in blood pH.

alleles: Variants of a gene for a particular trait.

allergens: Antigens that trigger allergic reactions. Common allergens include animal dander, pollens, foods, molds, dust, metals, drugs, and insect stings.

allergy: A hypersensitivity reaction to allergens.

alloantibodies: Antibodies resulting from antigenic stimulation within the same species.

alpha hemolysis: Incomplete or partial hemolysis (appears green).

ambulatory patient: A patient not confined to bed, for example, an outpatient or clinic patient.

American Standard Code for Information Interchange (ASCII): Standardized codes allowing the keyboard of the computer to be used to enter alphanumeric as well as numerical data into the computer.

Americans with Disabilities Act (ADA): Mandates that specific plans be developed for any person with a disability employed by a clinical laboratory to ensure that the person is working in a safe atmosphere.

amniotic fluid: Watery fluid that surrounds the fetus in utero.

amorphous material: Crystalline material seen in the urine sediment as granules without shape or form.

amplicon: A section of DNA or RNA that is the source or product of natural or artificial amplification or replication.

anaerobes: Microbes that cannot grow in an atmosphere of oxygen; special steps must be taken to provide an oxygen-free atmosphere for incubation and growth of these organisms.

analog computation: Measurement derived directly from an instrument signal.

analyte: Substance being analyzed in an analytical procedure.

analytical balance: Instrument used to weigh substances to a high degree of accuracy, such as chemicals used in the preparation of standard solutions.

analytical functions: Process whereby analytical analyses are carried out; includes generating work lists, doing the analyses, entering the results, quality control measures, and results verification.

analyzer: In polarizing microscopy, a polarizing filter located above the specimen, between the objective and the eyepiece.

anaphylactic reaction: A severe hypersensitivity reaction that can result in death.

anemia: A condition in which there is a decrease in hemoglobin in the blood and therefore in the amount of oxygen reaching the tissues and organs. May be the result of a decrease in the number of erythrocytes (decreased red cell mass), decreased hemoglobin concentration, or abnormal hemoglobin.

anion gap: Concentration of unmeasured anions; calculated as the difference between measured cations and measured anions.

anisocytosis: A general term indicating increased variation in the size of red cells in the blood film.

antibiotic resistance: Exists if the growth of a microorganism is not inhibited by the presence of an antibiotic; the organism is resistant to the antibiotic.

antibiotic sensitivity or susceptibility: Ability of the antibiotic to inhibit the growth of a microorganism.

antibody: Protein substance, found in the plasma or other body fluids, that is formed as the result of antigenic stimulation and is specific for the antigen against which it is formed. In blood banking, antibodies are present in commercially prepared serum called *antiserum.*

antibody titer: Amount of antibody present or required to produce a reaction with a particular amount of another substance; concentration of antibody.

anticoagulant: Prevents coagulation of blood.

antidiuretic hormone (ADH): A hormone that regulates urine volume by increasing the amount of water reabsorbed by the kidney.

antigen: Foreign (different from "self") substance that, when introduced into the body of a person lacking the antigen, results in an immune response and formation of a corresponding antibody. In blood banking, antigens are generally but not always found on the red cell membrane.

antigen–antibody ratio: Number of antibody molecules in relation to the number of antigen sites per cell.

antihuman globulin (AHG) test (AGT) or reaction: Method of detecting the presence of all human isoantibodies by using a specially prepared antiserum to human immunoglobulin or complement. May be a direct antiglobulin test (DAT) or an indirect antiglobulin test (IAT) test. Also known as the *Coombs reaction* or *Coombs test.*

antinuclear antibodies (ANA): Circulating immunoglobulins that react with the whole nucleus or nuclear components; frequently assayed by using indirect fluorescent antibody (IFA) techniques.

antisepsis (adj., antiseptic): Antimicrobial substances are applied to living tissue or skin to reduce the possibility of infection.

antiserum: Serum containing antibodies. In blood banking, a special highly purified preparation of antibodies used as a reagent to show the presence of antigen on red blood cells.

anuria: The complete absence of urine formation.

aperture iris diaphragm: The part of the microscope located at the bottom of the Abbé condenser, under the lens but within the condenser body; controls the amount of light passing through the material under observation; can be opened or closed to adjust contrast by means of a lever.

aplastic: Condition when the bone marrow is suppressed or unable to function normally in cell production.

Apt test: Test for maternal hemoglobin ingestion in newborn infants.

arithmetic logic unit: A component of the central processing unit (CPU) of a computer.

arthrocentesis: Collection of synovial fluid from a joint by needle aspiration.

artificial neural networks (ANN): Manufactured electrical circuits that emulate the brain's thought process.

ASCII: See *American Standard Code for Information Exchange.*

ascorbic acid (vitamin C): A strong reducing substance that may interfere with several of the reagent strip tests used in urinalysis, especially tests for blood and glucose.

atherosclerosis: Condition of "hardening of the arteries" in which plaques of cholesterol, lipids, and cellular debris collect in the inner layers of the walls of large- and medium-sized arteries.

autoantibodies: Antibodies directed against self-antigens.

autoclave: Apparatus for effecting sterilization by using steam under pressure; when it is used with an automatic regulating pressure gauge, the degree of heat to which the contents are subjected is automatically regulated also.

autoimmune disorder: A condition resulting from the failure of the body's immune system to recognize self antigens.

automated cell counters: Instruments designed to repeatedly and automatically count the numbers of formed cellular elements present in a blood specimen, usually the erythrocytes, leukocytes, and platelets.

automated differential counters: Instruments designed to repeatedly and automatically determine the types and percentages of leukocytes present in a blood specimen.

automated hematocrit: The hematocrit result obtained when a multiparameter instrument is used for hematology determinations. The result is computed from the measured red cell volume.

automatic pipettes: Devices used to repeatedly and accurately measure volumes of standard solutions, reagents, specimens, or other liquid substances.

automatic pipetting devices: See *automatic pipettes.*

azotemia: Significantly increased concentrations of urea and creatinine in the blood.

B

B lymphocyte: Blood cell that matures in the bone marrow; undergoes transformation to plasma cell that produces antibodies or immunoglobulins.

bacilli: Rod-shaped bacteria.

bacteremia: Presence of bacteria in the blood; bacteria can be cultured from the blood.

bacteriology: The study of bacteria.

bacteriuria: Presence of bacteria in the urine.

balance the centrifuge: To make certain that weight is distributed evenly on opposite sides of the centrifuge to prevent breakage of contents being centrifuged.

bar-code readers: Optical reading devices that convert a series of black lines into a sequence of numbers or letters for entry into a computer; can be used to code information such as names of patients, identification numbers, and tests requested.

bar coding: A sample recognition system whereby the bar codes—a series of black lines or bars on a label, for example—can be electronically read. Bar codes contain information such as name, hospital number, date, and other patient demographic data; see *bar-code readers.*

barrier precautions: Personal protective devices such as gloves and gowns placed between blood or other body fluid specimen and the person handling it to prevent transmission of infectious agents borne by specimens. See also *personal protective equipment.*

basic first aid: Immediate care given after an injury, before treatment is started by trained medical personnel.

basophilia: An increase in the number of basophils.

basophilic: "Base-loving"; the acidic cell components, such as nuclei and cytoplasmic RNA, that stain blue-violet by methylene azure in polychrome stains.

basophilic stippling: The presence of dark blue granules evenly distributed throughout the red cell in Wright-stained blood films.

basophils: A type of leukocyte that exhibits dark blue or purple granules in the cytoplasm.

batch analyzer: Analyzer that can test a batch of samples simultaneously for one particular analyte at a time; designed to analyze a number of different analytes, but only one at a time.

batch or run: A collection of any number of specimens to be analyzed at any one time, plus control specimens, standard solutions, and so forth.

bedside testing: See *point-of-care testing (POCT).*

Beer's law, Beer–Lambert law: In a solution, color intensity at a constant depth is directly proportional to concentration.

Benedict qualitative test: A copper reduction test for reducing sugars (substances) in urine; the basis of the Clinitest Tablet Test.

beta hemolysis: Clear or complete hemolysis.

bilirubin: Vivid yellow pigment; major by-product of normal red blood cell destruction.

bilirubin glucuronide, direct bilirubin, conjugated bilirubin: Water-soluble form of bilirubin; formed by conjugation with glucuronic acid in the liver.

biochemical properties and reactions: Properties are characteristics such as molecular weight or melting point present in various types of chemicals; reactions involve the conversion of one chemical species, the reactant, to another chemical species, the product.

biohazard: A substance containing or potentially containing infectious organisms.

biohazard containers: All infectious materials are handled as potential biohazards. These special containers should be used for all blood, other body fluids and tissues, and disposable materials contaminated with them; they should be tagged "Biohazard" or bear the standard biohazard symbol.

biohazard symbol: Symbol or term denoting any infectious material or agent that presents a possible health risk.

biohazard waste: See *infectious waste.*

biometrics: The science of statistics applied to biological observations.

biosafety cabinet: Protective workplace device used to control the presence of infectious agents in the air.

birefringence: Ability of an object or crystal to rotate or polarize light.

blank solution: Solution containing all the components, including solvents and solutes, except the compound to be measured.

bleeding time (BT): No longer a frequently used procedure. The time required for cessation of bleeding after a standardized capillary puncture to a capillary bed; depends on capillary integrity, numbers of platelets, and platelet function.

blood banking: The procedures involved in collecting, storing, processing, and distributing blood.

bloodborne pathogens: Infectious agents or pathogens carried by blood and blood products.

blood spot collection: Collection of capillary blood onto a filter paper, for example, spot collections for neonatal screening programs.

blood transfusion: Technique of replacing whole blood or its components.

Board of Registry of the American Society of Clinical Pathologists (ASCP): Offers an examination and certification for medical laboratory personnel.

body cavity fluids (body fluids): Fluids normally found in small amounts in various cavities or body spaces; examples include cerebrospinal, pleural, abdominal, pericardial, peritoneal, and synovial fluid. In certain conditions, such fluid is aspirated and assayed.

body tube: The part of the microscope through which the light passes to the ocular.

brightfield illumination: An illumination system used in the common clinical microscope.

broth media: Culture media that are in a broth or liquid form in a tube.

buffer: An aqueous solution that has a highly stable pH. A buffer is highly resistant to changes in pH if an acid or basic solution is added to the solution.

buffy coat: One of the three layers of normal anticoagulated blood. A thin grayish-white layer on top of the packed red blood cells, consisting of leukocytes and platelets, which normally makes up 1% of the total blood volume.

buret: Long, cylindrical graduated tube with a stopcock delivery closing on one end, used to control the delivery of the flow of liquid from the device; used to deliver measured quantities of fluid or solutions.

C

calculi: Kidney or renal stones.

calibrated cuvettes: Tubes or cuvettes that have been optically matched so that the same solution in each will give the same reading on the photometer.

calibration: Means by which glassware or other laboratory apparatus is checked to determine the exact units it will measure or deliver by relating them to a known concentration of an analyte.

calibration mark: Mark on volumetric glassware that indicates the point from which the volume is measured.

capillary blood (peripheral blood) collection: Blood drawn from the capillary bed by means of puncturing the skin, for example, a finger or heel puncture.

capillary pipette: Small glass or plastic tube used to collect small amounts of capillary blood, usually directly from a capillary puncture.

capillary tube density gradient: Method of cell enumeration whereby cells, upon centrifugation, settle in different layers because of their different densities; they are further expanded, stained, and magnified to derive the results of the counts.

CAP quality assurance program: Provided by the College of American Pathologists (CAP) to assist a laboratory in organizing and managing its quality assurance program.

carcinogen: Substance that can cause the development of cancerous growths in living tissues.

casts: Structures that result from solidification of Tamm–Horsfall mucoprotein in the lumen of the kidney tubules; they form a mold, or cast, of the tubule and trap other material that may be present when they are formed. Several types exist. They represent a biopsy of the kidney and are clinically significant.

catabolism: The phase of metabolism in which fats are broken down for energy.

cathode ray tube (CRT), terminal, video display unit: Television-like screen device used to monitor input, output, and general status of a computer system.

cell-mediated immunity: Also called a *cell-mediated (cellular) response.* Involves actions of T lymphocytes and their subsets, together with plasma cells and macrophages.

Celsius scale: Scale used to measure temperature in the metric system; outdated term for this scale is *centigrade.*

Centers for Disease Control and Prevention (CDC): Carries out mandated public health laws and reporting requirements.

centralized laboratory: A central location in a health care facility where all laboratory testing is done.

central memory: A component of the central processing unit (CPU) of a computer; provides storage and rapid access for information (data).

central processing unit (CPU): The part of the computer that controls and performs the execution of programs or instructions.

centrifugation: Separation of a solid material from a liquid by application of increased gravitational force by rapid rotating or spinning.

cerebrospinal fluid (CSF): Extravascular fluid that surrounds the brain and spinal cord. Formed by the choroid plexus in the ventricles of the brain and found within the subarachnoid space, the central canal of the spinal cord, and the four ventricles of the brain.

cervical mucus test: See *Fern test.*

chain of custody: When results of laboratory testing are to be used in a court of law, a specific chain of documentation is required, whereby all steps of the testing are recorded, from specimen collection to the issuing of the results report.

chemical hygiene plan: Outlines the specific work practices and procedures necessary to protect workers from any health hazards associated with the use of hazardous chemicals.

chemiluminescence: an analytical method in which the emission of light (luminescence) as the result of a chemical reaction is measured.

chloride shift: When carbon dioxide leaves the plasma and chloride diffuses or shifts out of the red cells to replace it; can take place when plasma and red cells are not separated in a timely manner.

chromasia: The staining reaction of red cells in the Wright-stained blood film.

chromatography: Method of analysis in which the solutes, dissolved in a common solvent, are separated from one another by differential distribution of the solutes between two phases (a mobile phase and a stationary phase).

chromosome: Threadlike structure within the nucleus of each cell, made up of genes. Chromosomes exist in pairs in all cells except sex cells. Each species has a specific number of paired chromosomes.

chylomicrons: Small droplets of lipoproteins that give blood specimens a characteristic milky appearance when present.

CLIA '88: See *Clinical Laboratory Improvement Amendments of 1988 (CLIA '88).*

clinical assistant (CLA): A classification of laboratory personnel.

clinical immunology: Study of antigen–antibody reactions in vitro.

Clinical Laboratory Improvement Amendments of 1988 (CLIA '88): Standards set for all laboratories to ensure quality patient care; provisions include requirements for quality control and assurance, for the use of proficiency tests, and for certain levels of personnel to perform and supervise work done in the clinical laboratory.

clinical laboratory scientist (CLS): See *medical laboratory scientist (MLS).*

clinical laboratory technician (CLT): See *medical laboratory technician (MLT).*

clinical pathology: Medical discipline by which clinical laboratory science and technology are applied to the care of patients.

clinical significance: A sign or symptom that can be part of a diagnostic finding.

clone: Cell originating from a single ancestral parent cell.

clot: Formation of a fibrin network; a thrombus.

clot retraction: Clot pulls together and becomes smaller.

clue cells: Vaginal squamous epithelial cells that are covered or encrusted with *Gardnerella vaginalis.*

coagglutination: To enhance visibility of agglutination, antibodies are bound to a particle.

coagulation: Mechanism whereby after injury to a blood vessel, plasma coagulation factors, tissue factors, and calcium work together on the surface of platelets to form a fibrin clot.

coagulation cascade: Process of coagulation in which a series of biochemical reactions occurs, converting inactive substances to active forms that in turn activate other substances; carefully controlled process responding to injury while maintaining normal blood circulation.

coagulation factors: Proteins engaged in the formation of a fibrin clot from fibrinogen.

coagulation system: See *coagulation cascade.*

cocci: Bacteria that are round.

coefficient of variation (CV): Used to compare the standard deviations of two samples; in percent, the CV is equal to the standard deviation divided by the mean.

cofactors: Proteins that accelerate the reactions of the enzymes involved in the coagulation process.

College of American Pathologists (CAP): Professional organization of pathologists; one responsibility is to certify clinical laboratories.

colony-forming unit (CFU): In microbiology, colony count; in hematology, a pluripotential, undifferentiated stem cell stimulated to proliferate and differentiate into colonies of a specific cell type.

colony-forming unit, culture (CFU-C): Multipotential hematopoietic (myeloid) stem cell.

colony-forming unit, lymphoid (CFU-L): Committed lymphoid stem cell.

colony-forming unit, spleen (CFU-S): Uncommitted pluripotential stem cell; also called *colony-forming unit, lymphoid-myeloid (CFU-LM).*

colony-stimulating factor (CSF): Factor required for hematopoietic stem cells to multiply and differentiate.

colorimeter: An instrument used in chemical analyses.

colorimetry: Technique used to determine the concentration of a substance by the variation in intensity of its color.

commensal state: Situation in which parasite and host exist together with no harm coming to the host.

Commission on Office Laboratory Accreditation (COLA): Provides accreditation for physician office laboratories; has been approved by the Health Care Financing Administration.

common pathway: Final stages of the coagulation cascade, beginning with the convergence of the extrinsic and intrinsic pathways (factor X) and ending with the formation of the fibrin clot.

community-acquired infection: Infection from organisms residing or incubating in the patient before admission to a health care facility.

compatibility testing: All of the tests performed before a transfusion to ensure that the transfused blood or component will benefit and not harm the recipient. These include tests on both recipient and donor blood, including a crossmatch between patient serum and donor red blood cells.

compensated polarized light: Modification of the polarizing microscope in which a compensator (first-order red plate or filter) is inserted between the two crossed polarizing filters and positioned at 45 degrees to the crossed polarizer and analyzer to determine the type of birefringence. In the clinical laboratory, especially useful in the examination of synovial fluid.

complement: Group of serum proteins that can produce inflammatory effects and lysis of cells when activated.

complement fixation: When complement is tied up or bound (fixed) to an antigen–antibody complex, it is no longer available to be activated.

complete blood count (CBC): Hematologic tests basic to the initial evaluation and follow-up of the patient. Generally includes measurement of hemoglobin, hematocrit, red blood cell count with morphology, white blood cell count with differential, and platelet estimate; specific tests vary with the facility.

components: Portions of whole blood prepared for transfusion by physical means, especially centrifugation.

concentration of solution: The amount of solute in a given volume of solution. May be expressed in different ways, for example, moles of solute per volume of solution, with use of the liter as the reference value.

condenser: The part of the microscope that directs and focuses the beam of light from the light source onto the material under examination; positioned just under the stage and can be raised or lowered by means of an adjustment knob.

confidence limits (confidence interval): A value used to express or estimate a statistical parameter; an example is when the reference range is set using values 2 standard deviations (SDs) on either side of the mean, with 95% of the values falling above and below the mean; see also *95% confidence interval.*

conjugated bilirubin, direct bilirubin, bilirubin glucuronide: Bilirubin that has been conjugated with glucuronate in the liver; exists in plasma unbound to any protein, as contrasted to unconjugated bilirubin; is water soluble, and high blood levels are excreted in the urine.

continuous-flow analyzer: Instrument that constantly pumps reagent and sample through tubing and coil, forming a continuous stream.

continuous quality improvement (CQI): See *total quality improvement (TQI).*

control specimen: Material or solution with a known concentration of the analytes being measured; used for quality control when the test result for the control specimen must be within certain limits for the unknown values run in the same "batch" to be considered reportable.

convalescent phase: Approximately 2 weeks after the acute phase of illness, convalescent serum is tested and the antibody titer compared with that of the acute-phase serum; an important phase of serology testing is the manifestation of a rise in antibody titer during the course of a disease.

Coombs test: See *antihuman globulin test (AHG).*

cortex (kidney): Outer anatomic portion of the kidney; consists of the glomerular portions of the nephron and the proximal convoluted tubules.

coulometry: Technique in which the charge required to completely electrolyze a sample is measured.

Coulter principle: Means of counting particles and measuring their size or volume by impedance change caused by the particle in a current-conducting fluid (electrolyte); this principle is applied in many of the blood cell counters used in hematology laboratories (Coulter counter).

creatinine clearance: Estimate of the function of the glomerular filtration rate; obtained by measuring the amount of creatinine in plasma and its rate of excretion in the urine.

crenated: Appearance of red blood cells when present in a hypertonic solution, for example, in urine of a high specific gravity. The cells appear shrunken, with little spicules or projections.

critical or panic values: See *panic or critical values.*

crossmatch: A procedure used to determine the compatibility of a donor's blood with that of a recipient after the specimens have been matched for major blood type. One part of compatibility testing.

crystalluria: The presence of crystals in the urine sediment.

crystals, abnormal: Urinary crystals of metabolic or iatrogenic origin that are generally of pathologic significance and require chemical confirmation.

crystals, normal: Urinary crystals that may be found in normal urine specimens of an acid or alkaline pH; generally are not pathologic and can be reported on the basis of morphologic appearance.

culture: Growing of microorganisms or living tissue cells in special, artificial medium.
culture medium: Mixture of nutrients on which a microorganism is grown; see *culture*.
culture plate: Petri dish or plate in which the medium is placed; where a culture of an organism grows.
cuvette: Tube or receptacle used in a photometer for holding the sample to be measured.
cyanide-nitroprusside reaction: Qualitative test used to confirm the presence of cystine crystals in the urine.
cyanosis: Bluish discoloration of the skin and mucous membranes.
cylindroids: A type of hyaline cast with one end that tapers off to a tail or point.
cysts: Inactive form of a microorganism, as in parasite cyst.
cytocentrifugation: Special slow centrifugation method used to prepare permanent microscope slides of fluids such as urine or other body fluids, resulting in better morphologic preservation than by other centrifugation or preparation methods.
cytocentrifuge: Uses a slow centrifuging speed, a low inertia, which rapidly spreads monolayers of cells across a special slide; used for critical morphologic studies.
cytolysis: The rupturing of a cell.

D

data: Information or results.
database: Systematic store of information (data) that can be accessed by the operator or user of a computer system.
darkfield microscopy: A specialized type of microscopic examination.
decontamination: Process of eliminating something that has become contaminated or mixed with something that makes it impure; an example is cleaning a work surface after blood or other potentially infectious material has been spilled on it.
deionization: Process of removing ionized substances from water.
deionized water: See *deionization*.
density: Amount of matter per unit volume of a substance.
Department of Health and Human Services (HHS): Department of the US government under which the Health Care Financing Administration (HCFA) is managed. Responsible for implementation of laws and writing of regulations that provide details on how various laws are to be carried out; publishes details of proposed regulations in the *Federal Register,* an official government document.
derivatives: Blood products prepared from whole blood by more complex methods than components. Also referred to as *fractions*.
dextrose: Glucose; a simple sugar.
diabetes mellitus: Chronic metabolic syndrome of impaired carbohydrate, fat, and protein metabolism secondary to insufficiency of insulin secretion or to the inhibition of the activity of insulin; characterized by increased concentration of glucose in the blood and urine.
diabetic coma: State of unconsciousness caused by a high glucose concentration.
dialysis: The separation of fluid from molecules or cells.
diaphragm: A part of a microscope that controls the amount of light shining up into a slide.
diazo reaction: Coupling of a diazonium salt with another aromatic ring to give an azo dye.
difference check: Computer comparison of current patient result with a previous result for that same patient.
differential media: Media containing dyes, indicators, or other constituents that give colonies of particular organisms distinctive and easily recognizable characteristics.
differential stain: Stain used to differentiate specific cellular details in a microorganism; more than one stain is used to produce the end result. Gram stain is an example of a differential stain.
digital computation: Calculations that involve data available in the form of discrete units or numbers.
digital microscopy: A type of microscope that uses camera technology to capture an image without directly viewing the image through the oculars of a microscope.
dilution factor: Reciprocal of the dilution made; multiply the result by the reciprocal of the dilution to correct for the dilution used.
dilutions: Weaker solutions made from a stronger solution. The term describes the relative concentrations of the components of a mixture; the preferred method is to refer to the number of parts of the material being diluted in the total number of parts of the final product.
diopter: A metric unit of measure for the refractive power of a lens. The focus of a microscope is adjusted for the microscopist by means of the diopter adjustment in the ocular.
direct agglutination: Showing visible agglutination when the constituent (antibody) being measured is present to react with the antigen, as with antigen-coated latex particles in latex agglutination assays.
discrete sample analyzer: Instrument that compartmentalizes each sample reaction.
disinfectant: Cleaning solution that removes pathogenic organisms but not necessarily bacterial or other spores, for example, household bleach.
disinfection: A process using specialized cleansing techniques that destroys or prevents growth of organisms capable of causing an infection.
dispersion: The scattering of the values of a frequency distribution from an average.
disseminated intravascular coagulation (DIC): A dangerous situation of uncontrolled bleeding and blood clotting.
distilled water: As water is boiled, the steam is cooled, condensed, and collected as distilled water; this process removes minerals such as iron, magnesium, and calcium.
diuresis: Any increase in urine volume, even if temporary.
documentation: An important aspect of quality assurance; Clinical Laboratory Improvement Amendments of 1998 (CLIA '88) regulations mandate that any problem or situation that might affect the outcome of a test result must be recorded and reported, with follow-up monitored.
drift: Moving away from the acceptable standard deviation range.
dry-film reagent technology: Instruments or tests that use a dry-film layered device that supplies the necessary reagents for the reaction to take place when the serum sample is added to it; the specimen (serum) provides the solvent (water) necessary to rehydrate the dry reagents on the film.
duplicate determinations: Specimens are measured in duplicate to check technique used; a measure of precision or repeatability of the method.
dysmorphic: Distorted or misshapen. Red cells in the urine that are dysmorphic may indicate glomerular disease.

E

edema: The abnormal accumulation of fluid in the interstitial spaces of tissues, resulting in generalized swelling.
effusion: Abnormal accumulation of any of the extracellular fluids. Fluid escapes from the blood or lymphatic vessels into the tissues or body cavities such as serous cavities—pericardium, peritoneum, or pleura—or the joints.
Ehrlich's aldehyde reaction: Reaction of urobilinogen, porphobilinogen, and other Ehrlich-reactive compounds with *p*-dimethylaminobenzaldehyde in concentrated hydrochloric acid to form a colored aldehyde.
electrical resistance cell counter: Cell counter that uses electrical resistance. Blood cells passing through an aperture through which an electric current is being passed cause a change in the electrical resistance; this change is counted as voltage pulses.
electrolyte battery or profile: Collection of tests for common electrolytes: chloride, bicarbonate, sodium, and potassium. These four electrolytes often are measured at the same time because changes in the concentration of one almost always are accompanied by changes in one or more of the others.
electronic cell-counting device: Automatic instrument that counts cellular elements in the blood (usually erythrocytes, leukocytes, and platelets) repeatedly and accurately.
electron microscopy: A type of microscope that uses accelerated electrons as a source of illumination.
electrophoresis: Movement of charged particles in an electrical field; technique used to separate mixtures of ionic solutes by the differences in their rates of migration in an electrical field.
employee "right to know" rule: Designed to ensure that laboratory workers are fully aware of the hazardous chemicals being used in the workplace.
enrichment media: Media that permit one organism to grow rapidly while inhibiting the growth of other organisms.

enumeration of formed elements: Counting of cellular elements of the blood (usually erythrocytes, leukocytes, and platelets).

enzyme immunoassay (EIA): Uses enzymes as immunochemical labels in detection of antigen–antibody reactions.

enzyme-linked (or labeled) immunosorbent assay (ELISA): Immunoassay or test that uses an enzyme conjugated to antibodies or antigens to produce a visible end point; diagnostic test used to detect antigens or antibodies in a patient's specimen.

enzymology: The study of the various biological materials (proteins) that have catalytic activity; the study of enzymes present in the blood.

eosinopenia: A decrease in the absolute number of eosinophils below normal limits.

eosinophilia: An increase in the absolute number of eosinophils above normal limits.

eosinophils: A type of leukocyte with orange-red color granules in the cytoplasm.

epithelial cells: Cells that make up the covering of the various internal and external organs of the body, including the lining of the blood vessels.

equivalent (equiv) weight (or mass): Mass in grams that will liberate, combine with, or replace 1 g of hydrogen ion; generally is the molecular weight divided by the valence.

error analysis: The study of the kind and quantity of errors that occur in analytical examinations.

erythrocyte: Red blood cell, one of the formed elements of the peripheral blood; chief role is to transport oxygen to the tissues.

erythrocyte sedimentation rate (ESR): Rate in millimeters at which the red blood cells fall, or sediment, in a given unit of time (usually 1 hour).

ethics: The discipline dealing with good and bad or a set of moral principles.

etiologic agent: Agent causing a disease.

eukaryote: Fungi, algae, protozoa; more complex than prokaryotes; contain membrane-enclosed organelles such as mitochondria, lysosomes, and a true membrane-enclosed nucleus.

exfoliated: Sloughed off tissue or cells.

exon: Coding sequence of DNA present in mature messenger RNA; DNA initially transcribed to messenger RNA consists of coding sequences (exons) and noncoding sequences (introns).

exponents: Superscript numbers used to indicate how many times a number must be multiplied by itself.

exposures to hazardous chemicals: Occupational Safety and Health Administration (OSHA) standards seek to minimize occupational exposures of this type.

extravascular component: Tissue surrounding the blood vessels.

extravascular fluid: Body cavity fluid other than blood or urine.

extrinsic system of coagulation: Coagulation pathway that is activated by tissue thromboplastin; necessary components are factor VII and calcium.

exudate: Effusion that results from inflammatory conditions, such as infections and malignancies, that directly affect the membranes lining a cavity.

eyepiece (ocular): Microscope lens that magnifies the image formed by the objective.

F

facultative anaerobe: Organism that can grow under either aerobic or anaerobic conditions.

facultative parasite: Parasite that can exist in a free-living state, as a commensal, or as a parasite; see *commensal parasite.*

false negatives: Those subjects who have a negative test yet do have the disease.

false positives: Those subjects who have a positive test but do not have the disease.

fastidious: Said of a microorganism that is sensitive to changes; usually requires protected culture conditions.

fasting blood glucose: Blood glucose test performed on a fasting specimen; see *fasting state.*

fasting state: The patient refrains from consumption of food and liquids other than water for 8 to 12 hours. For example, blood is collected after a 12-hour fast for some tests. Additional patient restrictions are sometimes also necessary, such as no smoking or administration of certain drugs during the fasting period.

federal regulations: Standards existing to meet objectives, such as safety regulations. For the clinical laboratory, see *Clinical Laboratory Improvement Amendments of 1988 (CLIA '88).*

Fern test (cervical mucus test): Test used to determine ovulation in fertility studies and for contraception and rupture of membranes in pregnancy by observing the appearance of dried cervical mucus on a glass microscope slide.

fibrin: End product of coagulation. Forms a visible clot, a fibrin mesh, to entrap the blood cells. Is derived from fibrinogen, a plasma protein, by the action of thrombin.

fibrin clot: See *fibrin.*

fibrinogen, coagulation factor I: Plasma protein that is the substrate for thrombin action in the formation of fibrin. Manufactured by the liver; is not vitamin K–dependent; is the soluble precursor of the clot-forming protein fibrin.

fibrinolysis: Destruction of the fibrin clot by plasmin activity to keep the vascular system free from clots; under normal conditions, coagulation and fibrinolysis are kept in balance.

fibrinolytic system: Functions to keep the vascular system free of fibrin clots or deposited fibrin; see *fibrinolysis.*

fibronectin: Assists in bonding platelets to substrate; is secreted by endothelial cells.

field diaphragm: The part of the microscope through which light passes up to the condenser. Located in the light port in the base of the microscope, it controls the area of the circle of light in the field of view when the specimen and condenser have been properly focused.

first line of defense: Nonspecific immune defense in which body fluids, specialized cells, fluids, and resident bacteria (normal biota) allow the respiratory, digestive, urogenital, integumentary, and other systems to defend the body against microbial infection.

first morning urine specimen: First urine voided in the morning. It is generally the most concentrated specimen of the day because less fluid or water is excreted during the night, yet the kidney has maintained excretion of a constant concentration of solid or dissolved substances.

fistula: An abnormal connection, such as between the colon and the urinary tract.

fixed angle–head centrifuge: A centrifuge in which the cups are held in a rigid position and at a fixed angle.

flame emission photometry: Atoms of certain elements, when sprayed into a hot flame, become excited and emit energy at wavelengths characteristic for those elements (commonly lithium, sodium, and potassium). Uses a device (flame photometer) to measure the intensity of the colored flame. Solution containing metal ions is sprayed into a flame, and the intensity and color of the flame are proportional to the amount of substance present in the solution.

flame photometer: Instrument used to measure the energy emitted by certain elements when they are sprayed into a flame in the photometer; see *flame emission photometry.*

flocculation: Clumping of fine particles to form visible masses.

floppy disks or diskettes: Diskettes that can store information not needed on a hard drive.

flow cytometers: Used to identify and enumerate the blood cells in a given patient sample; see *flow cytometry.*

flow cytometry: Enumeration and differentiation of blood cells by passing them through a focused beam of a laser.

fluorescence microscopy: A microscope that uses fluorescence to generate an image.

fluorescent antibody (FA): Assay that uses antibodies labeled with fluorescein compounds, which cause microscopic fluorescence as an indication of an antigen–antibody complex being formed.

fluorescent antinuclear antibody (FANA): Screening assay for systemic lupus erythematosus (SLE); see *fluorescent antibody.*

focal length: Slightly less than the distance from an objective being examined microscopically to the center of the objective lens; practically, equal to the working distance.

Food and Drug Administration (FDA): Issues certification and licensure requirements, which are an external control for clinical laboratory standards.

Forssman antibody: A heterophil antibody.

free bilirubin, unconjugated bilirubin, indirect bilirubin: Water-insoluble form of bilirubin that is carried through the blood bound to albumin.

functionality: The range of operations that can be run on a computer system.

fungemia: Presence of fungi in the blood.

G

galactosuria: The presence of galactose in the urine.

galvanometer: Measures and records the amount of current (in the form of electrons) reaching it.

Gaussian curve or distribution: Particular symmetric statistical distribution, also known as a "normal" distribution; a statistical tool used to set reference ranges.

genitourinary tract specimens: Specimens collected from the genital or urinary tract, for example, the vaginal cervix and perineal area in women and the anterior urethra in men.

genome: The genetic material of an organism that is encoded either in DNA or, for many types of viruses, in RNA.

genotype: Actual total genetic makeup. Often impossible to determine by laboratory testing but requires additional family studies.

genus: Members of the same genus share common biological characteristics; the next larger classification after species.

germ tube: An appendage on yeast cells, the beginning of true hyphae.

gestational diabetes: Glucose intolerance that occurs during some pregnancies.

glitter cells: Large, swollen neutrophilic leukocytes that appear in hypotonic urine with a specific gravity of approximately 1.010 or less. The cells show Brownian motion of granules in the cytoplasm, giving a glittering appearance.

glomerular filtrate: Ultrafiltrate of blood formed as blood is filtered through the glomerular capillaries of the glomerulus into Bowman's capsule. First step in urine formation; basically blood plasma without protein or fat.

glomerulus: Part of the nephron; made up of a tuft of blood vessels.

gluconeogenesis: Glucose from fat and protein that is provided to the blood.

glucose oxidase: Enzyme that allows for the oxidation of glucose to gluconic acid; the basis of the reagent strip tests for glucose in the urine.

glucose tolerance test: Measures the response of the body to a challenge load of glucose; used to aid in the diagnosis of diabetes mellitus.

glucosuria, glycosuria: Abnormally high concentration of glucose in the urine.

glycated hemoglobin: Hemoglobin derivative, also known as *hemoglobin* A_{1C}; formed when glucose and hemoglobin combine; tests used to monitor long-term blood glucose concentration in the blood of diabetics to measure diabetes control.

glycogenesis: Formation of glycogen from glucose.

glycolysis: Breakdown or oxidation of glucose.

glycosuria: Presence of glucose in the urine.

grades of chemicals: Varying qualities of production criteria that are placed on the manufacture of chemicals for laboratory use, depending on the use to which the chemical is put; the grade indicates the level of quality.

graduated pipette, measuring pipette: Cylindrical tube used to deliver a measured volume of liquid between two calibration (or graduation) marks on the tube; has several graduation or calibration marks on the tube, allowing a variety of measurements with the same device.

gram-molecular weight: One gram-molecular weight equals the sum of all atomic weights in a molecule of compound, expressed in grams.

gram negative: See *Gram staining reaction.*

gram positive: See *Gram staining reaction.*

Gram-stained smear: Used routinely to determine Gram staining characteristics; see *Gram staining reaction.*

Gram staining reaction (Gram stain): With the Gram staining method, microorganisms retaining the violet (purple) color of the primary stain (crystal violet–iodine complex) are considered gram "positive"; microorganisms having the red-pink color of the counterstain (safranin) are considered gram "negative." Use of these properties serves to classify or differentiate organisms in microbiology; Gram stain is a differential stain.

granulocyte: Leukocyte that contains prominent cytoplasmic granules; neutrophils, eosinophils, and basophils.

gravimetric analysis: Analysis by measurement of mass.

Griess test: A test for nitrite that involves a diazo reaction; basis of the reagent strip tests for nitrite in the urine.

group A β-hemolytic streptococci: Microorganisms that account for most infectious "strep throat." Organisms are isolated from throat swabs by one of several methods such as culture plates and rapid slide agglutination procedures.

gum guaiac: Phenolic compound that turns blue when oxidized. Commonly used as the chromogen in tests for the detection of occult blood in feces.

H

handwashing: The most important means of interrupting the transmission of infectious pathogens.

Hansel stain: Stain containing eosin and methylene blue; used to stain for the presence of eosinophils.

hapten: Nonantigenic, nonprotein substance that binds to protein, making a hapten–protein complex that is antigenic.

haptoglobin: Protein-bound form of hemoglobin by which hemoglobin is carried through the bloodstream.

hard copy: Computer-generated data printed on paper.

hard disks or hard drive: Revolving disks in a computer with a magnetic surface that can be easily accessed; data are stored in tracks, a series of concentric circles on the disks.

hardware: Physical elements of a computer system such as the central processing unit, printer, and terminal.

Hazard Communication Standard (HCS): The Hazard Communication Standard (HCS) is now aligned with the Globally Harmonized System of Classification and Labeling of Chemicals (GHS). This update to the HCS provides a common and coherent approach to classifying chemicals and communicating hazard information on labels and safety data sheets.

hazard identification system: Provides, in words, symbols, and pictures, information on the presence of potential laboratory materials considered hazardous. Examples include materials identified as flammable, as a health risk, or as chemically reactive.

Health Care Financing Administration (HCFA): Agency of the US Department of Health and Human Services; regulates and administers funding under the Health Insurance for the Aged Act of 1965 (Medicare); regulates reimbursement for Medicare-related activities. Medicare and Medicaid amendments to the Social Security Act authorize the regulation of specific laboratory services if the government is authorized to pay for these services to the aging and needy population of the United States. HCFA coordinates its regulatory functions with the Centers for Disease Control and Prevention (CDC).

Health Level 7 (HL7) standards: Standards that define how electronic information is packaged and communicated from one party to another, sets the language, structure and data types required for seamless integration between computer systems. HL7 standards support the management, delivery, and evaluation of health services.

hemagglutination (HA): Agglutination of red cells as indicator of antibody–antigen complex formation.

hematocrit: Ratio of packed red blood cell volume to whole blood volume, expressed as a percent or ratio unit.

hematoma: Collection of blood under the skin.

hematopoiesis: Blood cell production.

hematuria: Presence of red blood cells in the urine.

heme: An iron complex containing one iron atom. The iron-containing portion of the hemoglobin molecule.

hemocytometer: Counting chamber used to perform manual cell counts.

hemoglobin: Iron-containing protein portion of the red blood cells that carries oxygen to the tissues; four globin chains, each containing a heme moiety.

hemoglobinopathies: Disorders in which the presence of structurally abnormal hemoglobins is considered to play an important role pathologically.

hemoglobinuria: The presence of free hemoglobin in the urine.

hemoglobin variants: Different structural forms of hemoglobin, which vary in the content and sequence of amino acids in the globulin chains.

hemolysis: Rupture of the red cell membrane and release of hemoglobin into the suspending medium or plasma; the plasma or serum appears reddish. In blood banking and other immunologic reactions, hemolysis is used as an indicator of an antigen–antibody reaction.

hemolysis, alpha: In microbiology, partial destruction (lysis) of red blood cells in a blood agar plate; greenish color appears around the bacterial colony producing the alpha-hemolysin.

hemolysis, beta: In microbiology, complete destruction (lysis) of red blood cells around a colony on a blood agar plate; leads to a completely clear zone surrounding the colony producing the beta-hemolysin.
hemolytic jaundice: Type of jaundice that results from increased destruction of red cells.
hemolyzed serum: Serum with lysed red blood cells in it; appears pink or red.
hemophilia: Hereditary deficiency of plasma coagulation proteins; results in varying degrees of bleeding disorders, mild to severe, depending on the specific deficiency.
hemophilia A: Classic bleeder's disease; sex-linked deficiency of the coagulant component of factor VIII (antihemophilic factor); see *hemophilia.*
hemophilia B: Christmas disease; sex-linked deficiency of factor IX; see *hemophilia.*
hemosiderin: Iron-containing granules that may occur in the urine after a hemolytic episode. Stain blue with Prussian blue stain for iron.
hemostasis/hemostatic mechanism: Cessation of blood flow from an injured blood vessel, with final intent to stop the bleeding. The state of equilibrium in which the supply is equal to the demand between all the fluid and cellular elements that make up the blood.
hemostatic plug: Result of activation of the hemostatic system; formation of platelet plug.
hepatic jaundice (hepatocellular jaundice): Jaundice that results from conditions that involve the liver cells directly and prevent normal excretion of bilirubin, including failure in conjugation and failure in transport (regurgitation).
hepatitis B virus (HBV): Virus that can be directly transmitted by the blood, causing hepatitis, an acute viral illness. Hepatitis is an inflammation of the liver that is endemic worldwide. Complete recovery is usual; some patients, however, remain carriers or can develop chronic hepatitis.
hepatitis C virus (HCV): Previously known as *non-A, non-B hepatitis virus.* Can be transmitted directly by the blood, causing acute viral hepatitis. This infection does not show the serologic markers of hepatitis A or hepatitis B.
heteroantibodies: Antibodies resulting from exposure to antigenic material from another species.
heterophil antibodies: Antibodies stimulated by one antigen that react with entirely unrelated antigens on the red cells from different mammalian species; examples are Forssman, infectious mononucleosis, and serum sickness antibodies.
heterozygous: Having different alleles for a given trait.
high-complexity tests: Clinical Laboratory Amendments of 1988 (CLIA '88) regulations define a certain group of tests in this category; they require technical personnel of the highest degree of experience and training to be responsible for the testing.
high-power objective: Usually a 40 × magnification objective, used for more detailed examination of wet preparations.
histiocyte: A cell of the reticuloendothelial system; called a *macrophage* when it has begun to phagocytose.
Hoesch test: Inverse aldehyde reaction used for the detection of porphobilinogen in the urine.
homozygous: Having identical alleles for a given trait.
horizontal-head centrifuge: A centrifuge in which cups holding tubes of material to be centrifuged occupy a vertical position when the centrifuge is at rest but assume a horizontal position when the centrifuge revolves.
hospital information system (HIS): Main hospital database; contains the base of information about the patient, established when the patient was first admitted or registered by the hospital or clinic. This database can be accessed by the laboratory information system (LIS) as necessary.
household bleach: See *disinfectant.*
human chorionic gonadotropin (hCG): Hormone produced by the placenta during pregnancy; constituent measured in most rapid pregnancy tests.
human immunodeficiency virus (HIV): Virus that can be transmitted by the blood and some body fluids; can cause HIV infection or acquired immunodeficiency syndrome (AIDS).
humoral response: Involves antibodies produced by the B lymphocytes along with complement.
hyaluronate (hyaluronic acid): High-molecular-weight mucopolysaccharide found in synovial fluid, responsible for its normal viscosity. Secreted by the synovial fluid cells that line the joint cavity.
hyperglycemia: Increase in concentration of blood glucose.
hyperkalemia: High concentration of potassium in the serum or blood.
hypernatremia: High concentration of sodium in the serum or blood.
hypersensitivity: Excessive, discomfort-producing, and sometimes fatal reactions produced by the normal immune system. Hypersensitivity reactions can be divided into four types—types I through IV—based on the mechanisms involved and time taken for the reaction to express itself.
hypertonic: Solution or diluent that is more concentrated than that inside of the red cell.
hyphae: Tubelike projections, a part of the basic structure of molds; also called *mycelia.*
hypochromia (adj., hypochromic): A condition of red blood cells with decreased hemoglobin content, which appears very pale and shows an increased area of central pallor on the peripheral blood film.
hypoglycemia: Low concentration of glucose in the blood.
hypokalemia: Low concentration of potassium in the serum or blood.
hyponatremia: Low concentration of sodium in the serum or blood.
hypotonic: Solution or diluent that is less concentrated than that inside of the red cell.
hypoxia: Lack of oxygen.

I

iatrogenic: The result of medication or treatment; inadvertently caused by the physician.
icterus: See *jaundice.*
immune antibodies: Result from stimulation by a specific foreign antigen.
immune complex: Combination of an antigen and an antibody that tends to accumulate in bodily tissue and is associated with various pathological conditions, such as glomerulonephritis and systemic lupus erythematosus (SLE).
immune response: Any reaction demonstrating a specific antibody response to antigenic stimulus.
immunization: Introducing a foreign antigen such as attenuated live polio virus into a person's immune system to protect against developing an infectious disease in the future.
immunoassays: Assays using antigen–antibody reactions to detect the presence of a specific constituent.
immunofluorescence: Technique used for rapid identification of an antigen by treating it with a known antibody tagged with a fluorescent dye and observing the resulting characteristic antigen–antibody reaction; will appear luminous in ultraviolet light projected using a fluorescent microscope.
immunoglobulins (Ig): Antibodies; proteins of the gamma globulin type; produced by B lymphocytes (plasma cells).
immunohematology: The study of antigen–antibody reactions and their effects on blood. Includes blood transfusion medicine and blood banking.
immunology: The study of the molecules, cells, organs, and systems responsible for recognition and disposal of nonself substances, response and interaction of body components and related interactions, and the way that the immune system can be manipulated to protect against or treat diseases such as in the transplantation of organs.
immunoprophylaxis: Recommended after exposure to blood that is known to contain or might contain hepatitis B antigen; immune globulin is given in a single dose as soon as possible after the exposure, within 24 hours if practical.
impaired glucose tolerance: When there is an abnormal glucose tolerance test but no measured hyperglycemia; a midway position between normal and a state of diagnosed diabetes mellitus.
incidence: The number of subjects found to have a disease within a defined period, such as within a particular year.
indirect agglutination: Assays that show agglutination when no positive constituent is present.
indwelling lines: Devices used to administer therapeutic products such as fluids, medications, and blood products to patients over long

periods. With careful training, it is also possible to collect blood samples from these lines. Also called *vascular access devices (VADs).*

infection control: Set policy or program within a health care institution to prevent exposure to biological hazards.

infection control program: Program whereby laboratory sets up specific steps to prevent contamination from biohazardous specimens in the collection steps, transportation to the laboratory, and processing and testing steps.

infectious waste: Waste that contains biohazardous specimens, such as blood and blood products, contaminated materials, or other potentially infectious products.

inflammatory reaction (inflammation): Redness, tenderness, or swelling of tissue as a response to injury or infection.

informed consent: Legal consent granted by the patient whereby he or she is made aware of, understands, and agrees to the nature of the testing or services to be done.

infusion set: Allows collection of blood from patients with small, fragile, or rolling veins.

inoculate: To place the specimen on the medium in the plate or tube.

inoculating loop or needle: Metal loop or needle attached to a long handle, used to inoculate culture media with specimens or to transfer colonies for subculture. Metal loops must be flamed between uses. Disposable varieties of these loops are available.

inoculum: What is being inoculated onto the medium—plate or tube; usually the specimen is the inoculum; in antimicrobial susceptibility tests, the isolated organism to be tested is prepared in a specific way, depending on the methodology being used.

input device: Any device allowing data or instructions to be placed into a computer system.

input devices: Allow communication between the user and the central processing unit (CPU).

in situ monitoring: Monitoring in place or on site.

insulin shock: State of unconsciousness caused by a low blood glucose concentration.

interfacing data: Communications link that allows the transfer of data between the user and the computer system or between another processor and the computer system.

interleukins (IL): Hematopoietic growth factors that contribute to the control of hematopoiesis.

internal standard: Chemical compound of known amount added to a specimen and carried through all steps of an analytical procedure to provide a basis for accurate quantitation, despite variations in the procedural steps; is similar chemically and structurally to the substance being assayed; frequently used in gas chromatography and high-pressure liquid chromatography assays.

International Bureau of Weights and Measures: Responsible for maintaining the standards on which the SI system of measurement is based; see also *International System of Units.*

International Committee on Nomenclature of Blood Clotting Factors: Establishes and maintains standardized terminology for the various coagulation factors.

international normalized ratio (INR): The prothrombin time (PT) ratio obtained if the World Health Organization (WHO) international reference standard preparation is used as the source of thromboplastin in the PT assay; compares the patient's PT to a mean, normal PT; ensures that results for PT tests done in any laboratory can be compared.

international sensitivity index (ISI): Mathematical indicator of the responsiveness of the prothrombin time (PT) testing systems to deficiencies of vitamin K coagulation factors; World Health Organization (WHO) reference standard is assigned an ISI of 1.

International System of Units: Abbreviated *SI units,* from Système International d'Unités; standard international language of measurement.

international units: An internationally accepted unit of measurement for the amount of a substance; the mass, volume, or number of cells.

interpretive report: Reporting of laboratory results in a usable format, including information about reference ranges or flagging of abnormal values, so that the physician can find the results for the requested analyses in an efficient, concise manner.

interpupillary distance: The distance between the two oculars of a binocular microscope; must be adjusted for the microscopist.

intravascular component: Platelets and coagulation proteins that circulate in the blood vessels.

intravascular devices: Devices used to obtain specimens of blood from blood vessels.

intravascular hemolysis: Hemolysis or abnormal destruction of red blood cells in the bloodstream.

intrinsic system of coagulation: Use of plasma contact factors to initiate coagulation, beginning with the activation of factor XII; all necessary factors required are contained in the circulating blood.

in vitro antigen–antibody reactions: Reactions between antigens and antibodies in a test tube or on a slide (outside the living body; *in vitro* is a Latin term meaning "in glass").

ionic concentration: In urinalysis, a measure that is related to specific gravity. The principle of the reagent strip test for specific gravity; substances must ionize to be measurable with this method.

ionized calcium: Calcium that participates in the coagulation process; necessary to activate thromboplastin and to convert prothrombin to thrombin.

ion-selective electrodes (IS): A type of electrode that converts the activity of a specific ion dissolved in a solution into an electrical potential, which can be measured by potentiometry (voltmeter or pH meter). An ISE can be used to measure ion concentrations in blood plasma or serum, water, food, and pharmaceuticals.

iris diaphragm: The part of the microscope located at the bottom of the Abbé condenser, under the lens but within the condenser body; controls the amount of light passing through the material under observation; can be opened or closed to adjust contrast by means of a lever.

ISO 15189: A standard that specifies requirements for quality and competence in medical laboratories.

isoantibodies: Antibodies resulting from antigenic stimulation within the same species.

isolated colonies: When streak plates are properly made, isolated or individual colonies may be seen in specific sections of the plate; enables pure cultures to be made.

iso-osmolar: Two solutions having the same solute concentration, such as the glomerular filtrate and plasma, are normally iso-osmolar with each other.

isotonic: Situation when the concentration of fluid or diluent outside the red cell is the same as it is inside the red cell.

J

jaundice: Accumulation of bilirubin pigment in the tissues and blood; skin and sclera of eyes become jaundiced, or yellow.

jaundiced serum: Increased concentration of bilirubin in the blood (serum) and accumulation of bilirubin pigment in the tissues; serum appears brownish yellow.

Joint Commission, The (TJC): Voluntary organization, not governmental, made up of representatives from various health care associations such as hospitals and physician and dentist offices. Mission of JCAHO is to enhance the quality of health care provided to the public, and the organization is dedicated to improving the process to carry out this mission. One important function of JCAHO is accreditation of US hospitals. Standards and guidelines are set for hospitals, and accreditation is carried out and monitored through a continual process of site visits, surveys, and reports. The organization also monitors other health care facilities, such as mental health facilities, nursing homes, home health agencies, hospices, managed care, and ambulatory care organizations.

K

kernicterus: Results when unconjugated bilirubin passes into the brain and nerve cells and is deposited in the nuclei of these cells; can result in cell damage and death.

ketoacidosis: Acidosis resulting from the presence of increased ketone bodies.

ketogenic diet: A diet containing more than 1.5 g of fat per 1 g of carbohydrate; this will result in ketone accumulation, with ketosis and ketonuria.

ketonemia: Increased concentration of ketones in the blood.

ketonuria: Increased concentration of ketones in the urine.

ketonuria: A medical condition in which abnormally high amounts of ketones and ketone bodies are excreted in the urine. This condition can be associated with out-of-control diabetes or starvation.

ketosis: Increased concentration of ketones in the blood and urine.

kilogram (kg): Standard unit for measurement of mass (and weight).

L

labile factor: Factor V; essential for prompt conversion of prothrombin to thrombin in clotting mechanism; is involved in common pathway of both intrinsic and extrinsic clotting pathways.

laboratory information system (LIS): Computer system designed for use by the clinical laboratory; includes collection of patient information, generation of test results, assembly of data output, production of ancillary reports, and storage of data.

laboratory medicine: Medical discipline by which clinical laboratory science and technology are applied to the care of patients.

laboratory procedure manual: Collection of information about the specific procedures for all analytical assays performed by the laboratory; includes information about specimen requirements and special collection or processing details, test request information, procedural information (how to perform the test, reagents used for the assay, control specimens used), calibration of instruments, quality control data, details about reference values and reporting of results, and any information about bibliographical resources.

laboratory report: Information about results of various assays performed by the laboratory; should be presented in a usable format; see *interpretive report.*

Landsteiner's rule: In the ABO blood group system, if the A or B antigen is lacking on the red cell, the corresponding antibody will be found in the serum.

larvae: Immature form, as in parasite larvae.

latex agglutination: Particles of latex are used to visualize an antigen–antibody agglutination reaction; test latex particles are coated with a specific antibody and clump together (agglutinate) when the specific antigen is present in the specimen being assayed.

latex-microparticle enzyme immunoassay (MEIA): An immunoassay technology.

lattice formation: In process of agglutination, results in the visible aggregation or clumping reaction.

LEAN: A management system that focuses on efficiency and cost savings in laboratory operations.

leukemia: Progressive malignant disease of the blood-forming organs, characterized by abnormal proliferation of leukocytes and their precursors in body tissues. Peripheral blood cells and bone marrow cells are changed quantitatively and qualitatively.

leukoblastic reaction: The presence of white blood cells forms more immature cells than bands in the peripheral blood.

leukocyte: White blood cell; one of formed elements found in peripheral blood.

leukocyte differential: Classification and recorded percentages of various types of leukocytes as seen on a stained blood film or as obtained from an electronic counting device.

leukocyte esterase: Enzyme present in the azurophilic or primary granules of the granulocytic leukocytes; presence of this enzyme in the urine indicates urinary tract infection.

leukocytosis: An increase in the white cell count above the normal upper limit.

leukoerythroblastotic reaction: The presence of younger forms of leukocytes and red cells than are normally found in peripheral blood.

leukopenia: A decrease in the white cell count below the normal lower limit.

Levey-Jennings control chart: See *quality control chart.*

light absorbed: Light that is absorbed by a colored solution; measured as absorbance units or optical density (OD).

light-emitting diode (LED): Readout device found in digital computerized equipment; a semiconductor device visualized as a glowing readout.

light transmitted: Light that passes through a colored solution; measured as percent transmittance units (%T).

linear graph paper: Graph paper with a linear scale on both axes.

linkage (linked genes): Genes for different traits located on the same chromosome, positioned so closely that they are inherited as a unit.

lipemic serum: Serum with presence of fats or lipids; appears white or milky.

lipogenesis: The creation of the biochemical class, lipids.

liter (L): Standard unit of volume.

lithiasis: Kidney stone formation.

local area network (LAN): A network of computers.

low-power objective: Usually a 10 × magnification objective; used for the initial scanning and observation in most routine microscopic work.

Lupus erythematosus (LE) factor: Present in the blood of persons with SLE; has the ability to depolymerize the nuclear chromatin of polymorphonuclear leukocytes (PMNs), making them capable of being ingested by an intact PMN (thus creating the LE cell).

lymphocytes: A type of blood cell.

lymphocytosis: An increase in the absolute number of lymphocytes above normal limits.

lysin: Antibody that causes lysis.

lysis: Hemolysis of the red cells, rupture of the red cell membrane, and release of hemoglobin; an indicator of an antigen–antibody reaction.

M

macrophage: Any phagocytic cell of the reticuloendothelial system. Thought to be derived from both monocytes and histiocytic cells.

magnification: Enlargement of an image.

malabsorption: Inadequate, incomplete, or impaired absorption from the gastrointestinal tract; may be associated with the presence of increased fat in the feces.

mass per unit mass: See *weight per unit weight.*

material safety data sheets: See *safety data sheets.*

mean (X-bar): Statistically calculated mathematical average value for a valid series of numbers, as for a series of test results, for example; the series of values is totaled and divided by the number in the series; also called the *X-bar.*

mean corpuscular hemoglobin: A calculation of the average weight of hemoglobin in the average red blood cell (RBC).

mean corpuscular hemoglobin concentration (MCHC): Calculation of the hemoglobin concentration relative to the average red blood cell (RBC).

mean corpuscular volume (MCV): A calculation to express the size of a red blood cell.

measurement of mass or weight: Gravimetric analysis; commonly, measurement of weight by using various types of balances for preparation of laboratory reagents and standard solutions.

meconium: Viscid, elastic, greenish-black material composed of amniotic fluid, biliary and intestinal secretions, and epithelial cells; passed from the intestine by newborn infants within the first 24 hours after delivery.

median: The middle value of a body of data; the point that falls halfway between the highest and lowest in position.

median cubital vein: Vein in the antecubital area, most commonly used as site for venipuncture collection of venous blood.

medical laboratory scientist (MLS): Formerly known as medical technologist (MT) or clinical laboratory scientist (CLS), usually holds a bachelor of science degree.

medical laboratory technician (MLT): Formerly clinical laboratory technician (CLT), usually holds an associate degree.

medical technologist (MT): See *clinical laboratory scientist (CLS).*

medulla (kidney): Central anatomic portion of the kidney; consists of the loop of Henle, the distal convoluted tubules, and the collecting tubules.

megakaryocytes: Also called *platelets.*

melena: Black or tarry fecal specimens; dark color is due to the presence of blood, which is changed to a black substance as it passes through the gastrointestinal tract.

meniscus: Curvature in the top surface of a liquid.

menu: Programs or functions (options) offered by a system.

meter (m): Standard unit for measurement of length or distance.

metric system: System of weights and measures based on a decimal system, or divisions and multiples of tens; based on a standard unit of length, the meter.

microalbuminuria: The presence of very small amounts of albumin in the urine.

microbiota: The microbe population living in the intestinal tract.

microorganisms: Microscopic organisms; organisms seen only with the use of a microscope; these organisms include bacteria, viruses, fungi, and protozoa.

micropipette, micropipettor: Device used to measure very precise, very small volumes; micropipettes are usually calibrated to contain a specific volume, and the entire contents is part of the measurement.

microsampling: Obtaining very small amounts of blood or other body specimens such as capillary blood or cerebrospinal fluid; usually requires micromethods for assay.

microscope objectives: The part of a microscope that holds the lens for various magnifications.

middleware: Software that connects hardware systems.

milliequivalent: Relates to the equivalent; see *milliequivalent weight.*

milliequivalent weight: The equivalent weight in milligrams equals 1 milliequivalent (mEq).

milligram-molecular weight: Molecular weight expressed in milligrams.

millimole (mmole): One milligram-molecular weight is equal to a millimole (mmole).

minimal bactericidal concentration (MBC): Minimum concentration of antimicrobial agent needed to kill an organism.

minimum inhibitory concentration (MIC): Minimum concentration of antimicrobial agent needed to prevent visually discernible growth of a bacterial or fungal suspension.

mode: The value that occurs most commonly in a mass of data.

moderate-complexity tests: Clinical Laboratory Improvement Amendments of 1988 (CLIA '88) regulations place most laboratory tests in this category. Complexity is based on the analyte tested and the method or instrumentation used to perform the test.

molality: The number of moles of solute per kilogram of solvent.

molarity: Gram-molecular mass or weight of a compound per liter of solution.

molecular diagnostics: The use of principles of basic molecular biology in the practice of laboratory medicine.

monoclonal antibody: Highly specified antibody derived entirely from a single ancestral antibody-forming parent cell. Produced by hybridization; used in diagnostic testing.

monocytes: A type of blood cell.

mononuclear phagocytic system: Formerly called the *reticuloendothelial system (RES).* A functional system of the body involved primarily in defense against infection and in disposal of the products of the breakdown of cells by phagocytosis.

multiple-reagent strips: Plastic strips that contain one or more chemically impregnated test sites on an absorbent pad. When a chemical reaction occurs, it is indicated by a color change. This is the basis for chemical screening in urinalysis, for example. Also referred to as *dipsticks.*

mycelium: See *hyphae.*

mycology: The study or science of fungi.

myeloid: Of or pertaining to the bone marrow. The granulocytic leukocytes come from the myeloid series of development and include neutrophils, eosinophils, basophils, and monocytes.

myoglobinuria: The presence of myoglobin in the urine.

N

National Bureau of Standards (NBS): Agency of the US government. Maintains and supplies standard reference materials needed for the preparation of primary standard solutions; develops reference methods and reference materials.

National Cholesterol Education Program (NCEP): Program established to set standards for the detection and classification of individuals at high risk for coronary heart disease (CHD).

National Committee for Clinical Laboratory Standards (NCCLS): Nonprofit educational organization that sets voluntary consensus standards for all areas of clinical laboratories.

natural antibodies: Exist without antigenic stimulus; examples are anti-A and anti-B in ABO groups.

natural immunity: Also called *innate immunity.* Immunity that is naturally existing. It does not require prior sensitization to an antigen.

necrosis: A condition of dead tissue.

negative birefringence: Pattern of birefringence seen when a crystal appears yellow when the long axis of the crystal is parallel to the slow wave of vibration of a full-wave compensator and blue when the long axis is perpendicular to the slow wave.

negative exponent: Indicates the number of times the reciprocal of the base is to be multiplied by itself; indicates a fraction.

negative predictive value (PV): Indicates the number of patients with a normal test result who do not have a disease compared with all patients with a normal (negative) result.

neonatal physiologic jaundice: Type of jaundice that results from an enzyme deficiency in the immature liver of the newborn.

neonatal screening programs: Approved testing laboratories test for specific diseases or pathologies in newborns; capillary blood is usually collected onto filter paper and sent to the reference laboratory for testing; see also *blood spot collections.*

nephelometry: Measurement of light that has been scattered when it strikes a particle in a liquid; the nephelometer measures the amount of light scattered.

nephron: Working unit of the kidney, where urine is formed; includes glomerulus, Bowman's capsule, proximal and distal convoluted tubules, and loop of Henle.

nephrotic syndrome: An abnormal kidney condition characterized by heavy or massive proteinuria (albuminuria), decreased blood albumin (hypoalbuminemia), and edema.

neutropenia: A reduction of the absolute neutrophil count below normal limits.

neutrophilia: An increase in the absolute number of neutrophils present in the blood above normal limits.

95% confidence interval: Numerical limits within which a sample must fall to be part of the normal distribution of values; determined statistically and is the basis for quality control "rules" for the acceptance or rejection of certain results; based on a Gaussian curve, whereby 95% of the population have observations within 2 standard deviations.

nocturia: The excretion of more than 400 mL of urine at night.

nomenclature of blood clotting factors: International Committee on Nomenclature of Blood Clotting Factors ascertains consistency in terminology used; standardizes the complex nomenclature for the various clotting factors.

nonglucose-reducing substances (NGRSs): Substances other than glucose (including several sugars) that may be present in the urine and that have the ability to reduce heavy metal from a higher to a lower oxidation state. NGRSs are not detected by the reagent strip tests specific for glucose.

normal flora (normal biota): Organisms that inhabit the human body normally and do not cause disease.

normality: Number of equivalent weights per liter of solution.

"normal" range or value: See *reference range or value.*

normochromic: Said of red cells with normal hemoglobin content.

normocytic: Refers to a normal-size cell.

nosepiece: The part of the microscope on which the objectives are mounted. Usually on a pivot to allow for a quick change of objectives.

nosocomial infection: Infection acquired in a hospital or health care facility.

numerical aperture (NA): Index or measurement of the resolving power of a microscope. Also an index of the light-gathering power of a lens that describes the amount of light entering the objective. As the numerical aperture increases, resolution decreases.

O

objective: The major part of the magnification system of the microscope. Most commonly used microscopes have three objectives: low power, high power, and oil immersion. Usually mounted in a rotating nosepiece that enables a quick change of objectives.

obligate parasite: A parasite that cannot survive without its designated host.

obstructive jaundice, posthepatic jaundice, regurgitative jaundice: Type of jaundice that results from obstruction of the common bile duct by stones, tumors, spasms, or stricture.

occult blood: Blood not observable by the naked eye; requires the use of a chemical test to be detected.

Occupational Exposure to Bloodborne Pathogens: A federal regulation of clothing and processes related to the reduction of exposure to infectious diseases.

Occupational Safety and Health Act of 1970: Created the Occupational Safety and Health Administration within the US Department of Labor to set levels of safety and health for all workers in the United States. A federal agency.

Occupational Safety and Health Administration (OSHA): See *Occupational Health and Safety Act of 1970.*

ocular (eyepiece): The part of the microscope that magnifies the image formed by the objective.

oil-immersion objective: Generally a 100× magnification lens with a relatively short working distance of 1.8 mm. Requires the addition of a special immersion oil placed between the objective and the slide or coverglass. Cannot be used with wet preparations.

oliguria: Abnormally small excretion of urine; less than 500 mL/24 hours.

opportunistic pathogen: Organism that does not usually cause disease in persons with an intact immune system but does cause disease in immunocompromised persons.

optical density (OD): Term used to express the amount of light being absorbed when being passed through a solution; see *absorbed light.*

optical methods, cell counters: Automated cell counters with focused laser beams whereby cells cause a change in the deflection of a beam of light, which is converted to measurable pulses by a photomultiplier tube.

oral glucose tolerance test (OGTT): Oral glucose is consumed and blood tested for glucose concentration; test measures the ability of a person to respond appropriately to a heavy load of glucose.

order entry: The first step in the laboratory information system is the test ordering or order entry.

organized sediment: The biological part of the urine sediment; includes cells, fat of biological origin, casts, organisms, and microorganisms.

orthostatic proteinuria: Proteinuria that is present when persons are engaged in normal activity but disappears when they lie down.

OSHA standards: See *Occupational Safety and Health Act of 1970.*

osmolality: A measurement of the concentration of all chemical substances (solutes) dissolved in the fluid part of blood (solvent).

osmolarity: Number of osmoles of solute per liter of solution.

osmosis: The passage of a solvent through a membrane from a dilute solution into a more concentrated one.

osmotic fragility: Test to determine the ability of the red blood cells to withstand hypotonic or hypoosmotic solutions. Measure of the resistance of the red cell membrane to rupture; cells with membrane defects (hereditary spherocytosis) have increased fragility.

output/output device: Any device that allows information generated by a computer system, such as results of calculations for a laboratory assay, to be used. Information output can be printed, displayed, or transferred to another processor.

ova: Eggs, as in parasite eggs.

oval fat body (OFB), renal tubular fat (RTF) body: Renal epithelial cell (and possibly macrophage) filled with fat droplets.

oxyhemoglobin: Oxygen-saturated hemoglobin.

P

packed cell volume (PCV): The hematocrit. A macroscopic measurement of the percentage volume of packed red cells.

panic or critical values: Possibly life-threatening laboratory values that must be noted and communicated to the physician as quickly as possible; automated instruments flag or highlight these results for the laboratory personnel.

parasitism: Result of parasite injuring its host by its actions.

parasitology: The study or science of parasites.

parcentric: Microscope objectives that are aligned so that a specimen centered in the field of view for one objective remains centered when the nosepiece is rotated to bring another objective into use.

parfocal: A situation when a specimen centered in the field of view for one microscope objective remains centered when the nosepiece is rotated to bring another microscope objective into use.

pathogens: Microorganisms that cause disease.

pathologist: A licensed physician with special training in clinical or anatomic pathology.

Patient Care Partnership: An understanding of the proper treatment of patients. Being considerate of this partnership constitutes good patient care. In the laboratory context, the partnership must be considered in collecting the various patient specimens needed for testing.

patient demographics: Information about the patient, such as name, gender, age, birth date, and referring or attending physician.

percent: Parts per hundred parts.

percent solution: Somewhat outdated expression of concentration based on parts per hundred parts, for example, 10% sodium chloride, which is 10 g NaCl diluted to 100 mL with deionized water; currently expressed as 10 g/dL.

percent transmittance: Amount of light that passes through a colored solution compared with the amount of light that passes through a blank solution.

percent transmittance units: Units used to measure the amount of light transmitted through a solution.

pericardial fluid: Extravascular fluid that surrounds the heart.

periodic performance review (PPR): A component of quality assurance.

peripheral blood film: Blood smear prepared on a glass microscope slide using circulating peripheral blood. Blood is usually obtained by venipuncture or finger puncture.

peritoneal fluid: Extravascular fluid that surrounds the abdominal and pelvic cavities.

peroxidase: Enzyme that catalyzes release of free oxygen from hydrogen peroxide. Peroxidase activity of the heme portion of the hemoglobin molecule is the basis of the reagent strip tests for blood.

personal protective equipment: The Occupational Safety and Health Administration (OSHA) requires facilities to provide their personnel with protective equipment, such as protective clothing, gloves, eyewear, protective shields and barriers, and respiratory devices, for their safety in the workplace.

Petri dish or plate: Shallow, flat glass or plastic plate with a loose-fitting deep cover, used to hold culture media.

pH: Unit that describes the acidity or alkalinity of a solution.

phagocytosis: A process in which a cell engulfs and disposes of foreign material.

phase contrast: Microscope illumination system that uses a special condenser with an annular diaphragm with a matched absorption ring in the corresponding objective. Used to give additional contrast in wet preparations; especially useful for counting platelets and observing urinary sediment.

phase-contrast microscopy: A type of microscope that uses a hollow cone of light instead of the solid cone of light normally used in light microscopy.

phases of testing: Three parts of laboratory testing: preanalytical (preevaluation), analytical (evaluation), and postanalytical (postevaluation).

phenotype: Observable genetic makeup that can be determined by direct testing (i.e., blood type).

phlebotomist: Person trained in drawing blood. Primarily trained to draw blood by venipuncture but also trained to perform capillary collections and to do skin punctures of various types. Drawing blood specimens from indwelling lines is an additional technique performed by a trained phlebotomist.

phlebotomy: The process of withdrawing blood from a patient.

photoelectric cell photodetector: Electronic device that measures the intensity of light being transmitted by a solution; produces electrons in proportion to the amount of light reaching it.

photometry: Technique used to determine the quantitative concentration of a substance by measuring the variation in its color intensity by use of a photometer.

physical properties: In urinalysis, color, transparency, odor, foam, and specific gravity of a urine specimen.

physician office laboratory (POL): A laboratory in a physician's office or clinic where tests are done only on the patients coming to the practice or group.

physiologic jaundice: Can result from a deficiency of an enzyme that transfers glucuronate groups onto bilirubin or from liver immaturity; can result in jaundice that occurs in some infants during the first few days of life; also called *neonatal jaundice;* see *jaundice.*

plan for evacuation: Routes for exiting the laboratory site in an emergency must be readily available to all persons working in the laboratory area.

plasma: Liquid portion of blood after it has been anticoagulated and centrifuged or otherwise allowed to settle.

plasma cell, plasmacyte: Derivative of the B lymphocyte. Large, with a round or oval eccentric nucleus. Specialized for production of antibodies; rarely is seen in the peripheral blood.

plasmin: Proteolytic enzyme that breaks down fibrin; is generated by the activation of a plasma precursor, plasminogen.

platelet adhesion, platelet adherence: Test that measures the ability of platelets to adhere to glass surfaces; essential requirement for primary hemostasis.

platelet aggregation: Massing or clumping of platelets with one another; test for platelet function.

platelet plug: Formation of an aggregate or mass of platelets that physically plug or slow down the flow of blood at the site of an injury to a blood vessel; result of activation of the hemostatic system.

platelets: Cells that facilitate blood clotting by forming a platelet plug and releasing chemicals into the coagulation cascade in the blood. Also called *thrombocytes.*

pleural fluid: Extravascular fluid that surrounds the lungs.

pluripotential stem cell (PSC): Stem cell that is uncommitted to any specific cell line; stimulation results in differentiation and maturation.

poikilocytes: Red blood cells with irregular shapes.

point-of-care testing (POCT): Tests performed at the bedside of the patient or near the site where the patient is; a decentralized form of laboratory testing—the laboratory testing comes to the patient. Capillary blood samples can be used to perform rapid testing procedures; a common test is the glucose blood test, done for management of patients with diabetes mellitus.

polarize: To bend or rotate light.

polarized light: Light that is propagated so that radiation waves occur in only one direction rather than at random.

polarizer: A filter that allows the passage of light waves in only one orientation.

polarizing microscope polarized light microscopy: Microscope illumination system that employs two crossed polarizing lenses, extinguishing the passage of light through the microscope. Used to detect objects or crystals that bend or polarize light, making them visible when viewed with crossed polarizing filters.

polychromasia: Many colors. A property of red cells that show a faint blue or blue-orange color when stained with Wright stain because of the presence of both blue RNA and red hemoglobin in young red cells.

polychromatophilia (adj., polychromatophilic): A blue color added to the normally red-staining red blood cells on a blood smear.

polyclonal antibodies: Antibodies derived from multiple ancestral clones of antibody-producing cells; characteristically produced in infectious diseases.

polydipsia: Excessive thirst.

polymerase chain reaction (PCR): A procedure to increase the number of specific DNA segments.

polyphagia: Excessive, constant hunger.

polyuria: Excessive urination.

porphobilinogen: An unstable intermediary product in the synthesis of heme; a significant increase in the urine can be seen in acute intermittent hepatic porphyria.

porphyrias: A group of inherited disorders that are characterized by an increased production of porphyrins; some forms result in the presence of porphobilinogen in the urine.

positive birefringence: Pattern of birefringence seen when a crystal appears blue when the long axis of the crystal is parallel to the slow wave of vibration of a full-wave compensator and yellow when the long axis is perpendicular to the slow wave.

positive exponent: Indicates the number of times the base is to be multiplied by itself.

positive predictive value (PV): Indicates the number of patients with an abnormal test result who have a disease compared with all patients with an abnormal result.

postanalytical function: Includes functions that occur after the analysis itself, such as generating chart reports, printing result reports as needed, archiving results, and billing.

postcoital test (PCT): Test that evaluates cervical mucus; scored on a scale of 1 to 15 by assessment of spinnbarkeit, ferning, consistency, and pH.

postexposure prophylaxis (PEP): For HIV exposure, the degree of risk for infection must be assessed and the worker followed by the health care facility's infection control department and offered postexposure prophylaxis immediately.

posthepatic jaundice: See *obstructive jaundice.*

postprandial: Directly after a meal; a postprandial blood specimen is one collected directly after a meal.

postprandial specimen, 2-hour: Blood that is drawn 2 hours after a meal.

postrenal azotemia: Azotemia resulting from obstruction whereby urea is reabsorbed into the circulation; see *azotemia.*

potentiometry: Technique in which the potential difference between two electrodes is measured under equilibrium.

pour plates: A specimen is inoculated in a liquid medium, which is then mixed and poured into a culture plate, where it solidifies.

preanalytical functions: Functions in testing protocol that occur before the actual analyses—test ordering, specimen collection, and so forth.

precipitation (precipitate): Visible result of an antigen–antibody reaction between a soluble antigen and its specific antibody.

precipitin: An antibody that reacts with a soluble antigen to form a precipitate.

precision, reproducibility: Measure of the closeness of the results obtained when analysis on the same sample is repeated; agreement between replicate measurements.

predictive value (PV): Means or ability to predict the results of an analysis of the same data by using another test instrument or measurement; contributes to the validity of a test.

prerenal azotemia: Azotemia resulting from poor perfusion of the kidneys; see *azotemia.*

prevalence: The proportion of a population that has a disease.

primary culture: The initial or first culture done with a specimen.

primary hemostasis: Involves platelets and the vascular response.

primary response: First antibody response to foreign antigen.

proenzymes: Enzyme precursors or zymogens.

proficiency testing (PT) or survey: Program under which samples are sent to a group of laboratories for analysis; results are compared with those of other laboratories participating in the program. Included as a component of quality assurance programs.

proficiency testing programs: See *proficiency testing (PT) or survey.*

program: Set of commands or steps that instruct the computer to perform a certain task.

program for infection control: See *infection control.*

prokaryote: Small bacterium containing DNA in a single, circular chromosome.

prophylaxis: To prevent exposure.

proportion: Two or more ratios having the same relative meaning but with different numbers.

proportioning: A combination of predetermined amounts of reagent and sample in an automated laboratory instrument.

protective immunity: Provided by antibodies that after formation will protect from subsequent exposure to the antigen.

protective isolation: Measures used to protect a patient from infectious agents.

protein error of pH indicators: Color change of a pH indicator caused by the presence of protein rather than hydrogen ion concentration.

protein-free filtrate: After preparation of a specimen to remove the protein, the filtrate, free from protein, remains.

proteinuria: Presence of protein, usually albumin, in the urine.

prothrombin, coagulation factor II, prethrombin: Produced by the liver; is vitamin K dependent.

prothrombin time (PT): Time it takes for the plasma to clot after an excess of thromboplastin and an optimal concentration of calcium have been added; measures functional activity of the extrinsic and common pathways of coagulation.

protoplasts: Unusually long, rod-shaped forms of bacteria with central swelling; the result of damage to the cell wall by antibiotics.

provider-performed microscopies (PPM): Specific microscopies (mostly wet mounts) usually performed by the physician or provider for his or her own patients; these tests are a special subcategory of the moderately complex Clinical Laboratory Improvement Amendments of 1988 (CLIA '88) tests.

prozone phenomenon: An excess of antibody; can result in a false-negative reaction.

pseudocasts: False casts. Structures in the urine sediment that appear similar to, and might be mistaken for, casts.

pseudohyphae: False hyphae. Elongated yeast cells that may be branched and have terminal buds and resemble the mycelia of true fungi.

Public Health Service Act: Act under which Medicare and Medicaid are licensed.

puncture-resistant sharps containers: Used for disposal of sharps such as needles, lancets, and broken glass.

pure culture: Culture in which each colony is from a single isolated originating bacterial cell.

pyuria: Presence of pus (leukocytes) in the urine; indicates a possible urinary tract infection.

Q

quality assurance (QA): Comprehensive set of policies, procedures, and practices necessary to make sure that a laboratory's results are reliable. QA includes record keeping, calibration and maintenance of equipment, quality control, proficiency testing, and training.

quality assurance indicators: Indicators that monitor the performance of a laboratory and are evaluated as part of continuous quality improvement (CQI); see *continuous quality improvement.*

quality assurance program: Plan to carry out policies and practices necessary to comply with quality assurance standards set by accreditation agencies to make certain that a laboratory's results are reliable and that these results are used in the best interest of the patient. See also *total quality improvement (TQI).*

quality control (QC): Set of laboratory procedures designed to ensure that a test method is working properly and that the results meet the diagnostic needs of the physician. QC includes testing control samples, charting the results, and analyzing them statistically.

quality control chart: Visual documentation of information derived from using control specimens; values for control specimen assays used for a particular substance are plotted on the chart on a regular basis and are statistically analyzed for trends of change.

quality control program: Plan to carry out procedures established to make certain that laboratory assay methods are working properly and that assay results meet the diagnostic needs of the physician; makes use of control specimens and standard solutions.

quality control specimen: See *control specimen.*

quantitative analysis: A very precise means of measurement of the quantity of a substance.

quantitative transfer: Process of transferring the entire amount of a weighed or measured substance from one vessel to another; usually used in the process of reagent preparation, in which the weighed substance (chemical) must be transferred in its entirety to a volumetric flask for dilution with deionized water.

quantitative urine culture methods: Traditional method of detecting urinary tract infection, in which urine is cultured on an appropriate medium and identified.

R

radio frequency identification device (RFID): An electronic form of identification.

random access analyzer: Instrument that does all the selected determinations on one sample before going on to the next sample.

random access memory (RAM): Central memory in the central processing unit (CPU) of a computer; commonly used as a means of storage of information that is frequently altered, changed, or updated.

rapid streptococcal antigen detection: Basis for rapid tests for detection of "strep throat" caused by group A β-hemolytic streptococci.

ratio: Amount of something in proportion to an amount of something else; always describes a relative amount.

reactive lymphocytes: Altered lymphocytes associated with viral infections, especially infectious mononucleosis; also referred to as *atypical* or *variant lymphocytes.*

reagent: Any substance employed to produce a chemical reaction.

reagin antibodies: Antibody-like proteins that react in some serologic tests for syphilis.

recovery solution: A measured amount of a substance being quantitated is added to a specimen; theoretically, the amount of substance added should be recovered at the end of the determination if the method is an accurate one.

red blood cell indices: In hematology, the calculated values for red cell measurements such as mean cell volume (MCV), mean cell hemoglobin (MCH), and mean cell hemoglobin concentration (MCHC).

reduced hemoglobin: A hemoglobin molecule lacking oxygen.

reducing sugars: Sugars (including glucose) that have the ability to reduce copper ions from Cu^{2+} to Cu^{+} in the presence of alkali and heat.

reference laboratory: Laboratory setting where specimens are sent that require more complex testing methodologies and for tests that are infrequently ordered.

reference range, normal range, normal values, reference values: Range of values that includes 95% of the test results for a healthy reference population; see *Gaussian curve.*

reflectance photometry or spectrophotometry: Photometric technique whereby light reflected from the surface of a colorimetric reaction is used to measure the amount of unknown colored product generated in the reaction; a beam of light is directed at a flat surface, and the amount of light reflected is measured.

refractive index: A measure of solute concentration. The ratio of the velocity of light in air to the velocity of light in solution.

refractometer: Temperature-compensated instrument used to measure refractive index.

relative centrifugal force (RCF): Expression of the number of revolutions per minute and the centrifugal force generated; method of comparing the forces generated by various centrifuges, taking into account the speed of rotation and the radius from the center of rotation.

relative numbers (cell count): The concentration of a cell type expressed as a percentage.

reliability: Ability of a laboratory assay to produce consistent results when testing is repeated successively.

renal azotemia: Azotemia resulting primarily from diminished glomerular filtration; see *azotemia.*

renal threshold: Level above which a substance cannot be reabsorbed by the renal tubules and is thus excreted into the urine.

renal tubular fat (RTF): See *oval fat bodies.*

reproducibility: See *precision, reproducibility.*

resolution: Limit of usable magnification; tells how small and how close individual objects can be and still be recognized.

reticulocyte: Young red blood cell that has just extruded its nucleus. Characterized by the presence of RNA; becomes a normal, mature red cell when all the RNA is lost; stains with a supravital stain.

rhabdomyolysis: Acute destruction of muscle fibers.

rheostat: Control used to adjust the amount of light entering a microscope.

rheumatoid factor (RF): Autoantibodies present in the serum of patients with clinical features of rheumatoid arthritis; circulating complexes of immunoglobulins, known collectively as *rheumatoid factor.*

Rh immune globulin (RhIg): Concentrated and purified form of anti-D antibody, used to immunosuppress Rh-negative women who deliver Rh-positive babies, to prevent sensitization of the mother by her child's red blood cells.

rhinitis: Inflammation of the mucous membranes of the nose, usually accompanied by swelling of the mucosa and nasal discharge.

Rh negative: Red blood cells lacking the D antigen (d/d).

Rh positive: Red blood cells containing the D antigen (D/D or D/d).

rickettsiology: The study or observation of rickettsia.

rounding off a number: To bring a digit (number) to the chosen number of significant figures.

Rous test: A wet Prussian blue stain for iron; used to confirm the presence of hemosiderin in the urine sediment.

S

safety data sheets (SDS): Formerly called *material safety data sheets (MSDS).* Information about the hazards of each chemical are provided by the supplier or manufacturer of the chemical; any hazardous chemicals used in a laboratory should be accompanied by this information.

safety manual: Current compilation of all safety practices and procedures, kept in a readily available format for use by all persons in a specific laboratory setting; anything that could pose a potential safety hazard for persons in the laboratory must be described in this manual.

safety program: Required by the Occupational Safety and Health Administration (OSHA) for every clinical laboratory.

sampling procedure: Only a very small amount of sample is usually used in laboratory measurements; sampling difficulties can lead to fluctuations and variations in results reporting; affects reliability of the procedure.

scanning electron microscope (SEM): A type of electron microscope that looks at the surface of a specimen and produces a three-dimensional image by striking the sample with a focused beam of electrons.

secondary hemostasis: Response by coagulation proteins.

secondary response: Response to second exposure to the same antigen; rapid amounts of detectable antibody in the serum or plasma.

sediment: Solid material that has settled out of suspension, for example, urinary sediment.

segmented neutrophils: A type of blood cell.

selective media: Substances present in these media selectively inhibit the growth of certain microorganisms and permit the growth of others.

semen: Sperm-containing fluid produced by fertile males.

semilogarithmic graph paper: Graph paper with a logarithmic scale on one axis and a linear scale on the other; allows the plotting of a straight line when percent transmittance readings are plotted against concentration.

sensitivity: The proportion of cases having a specific disease or condition that give a positive test result.

sensitivity to antimicrobial agents: The situation that exists when an organism's growth is inhibited in the presence of certain antibiotics (antimicrobial agents).

sensitization: Process in which an individual is made sensitive to a foreign antigen through exposure. Once sensitization has occurred, the individual responds to a repeated exposure with an accentuated immune response.

septicemia, sepsis: Bacteria in the blood or toxin produced by the bacteria is causing harm to the patient.

serial dilutions: Progressive dilutions of a substance in a series of tubes in predetermined ratios to give concentrations of a specific amount.

serologic pipette: Much like a graduated pipette but is graduated to the end of the delivery tip; allows for a faster delivery and is less precise for this reason.

serologic reaction: The observed reaction when an antigen–antibody reaction has taken place.

serology: The division of immunology specializing in detection and measurement of specific antibodies that develop in the blood (serum) during a response to exposure to a disease-producing antigen.

serotonin: Vasoconstricting substance.

serous fluids: The fluid within the closed cavities of the body, such as the pleural, pericardial, and peritoneal cavities.

serum: The fluid portion of blood that remains after coagulation. Preferable to plasma when typing or otherwise testing blood for compatibility.

serum separator collection tubes: See *serum separator gel.*

serum separator gel: Additive used to assist in obtaining serum after centrifuging a whole blood specimen. A special silicone gel layer is added to the collection tubes that moves to form a barrier between the cells and serum during centrifugation; the gel hardens to form an inert barrier, allowing easy serum separation or removal after the centrifugation process.

sharps containers: Used disposable needles and other sharp objects must be safely discarded in these containers, which are made of rigid plastic, metal, or stiff paperboard. The containers must be conveniently located, easily recognizable, and marked as a biohazard. All skin lancets, needles, scalpel blades, and bleeding-time devices must be discarded properly in a sharps container, with extreme caution.

shelf life: Expiration date of a product.

shift cells: Nucleated red cells or polychromatic macrocytes (reticulocytes) in the peripheral blood.

shift to the left: The release into the peripheral blood of immature cell forms that are normally present only in the bone marrow.

significant figures: Digits of whole numbers or in decimal form, beginning with the leftmost nonzero digit and extending to the right; numbers should contain only digits necessary for the precision of the determination or measurement; the digits of a number that are known to be reliable.

simple stain: One stain that colors everything in the cell the same color.

single dilution: When one unit of original specimen is diluted to a final volume of 2, 5, or 10, and so on; when a concentrated specimen or solution needs a single dilution, usually expressed as a ratio; examples are 1:2, 1:5, and 1:10.

Six Sigma: A management process to increase quality and efficiency and reduce costs.

skin puncture: Capillary puncture for blood microsampling, such as finger puncture or heel puncture.

slant culture, tube: The surface of the medium is inclined at an angle.

slide agglutination: Used in assay to determine antigen–antibody reaction; usually employs latex agglutination.

software: Series of instructions or commands that direct the operation of a computer system.

solute: Substance dissolved in a solution; usually the substances being measured in clinical laboratory analyses are the solutes, these being dissolved in the blood.

solvent: Substance in which a solute is dissolved; usually deionized water in laboratory reagents.

species: Basic unit of the biological world; used in nomenclature.

specific gravity: Ratio of the density of a solution to the density of an equal volume of water at a constant temperature; depends on the weight and number of particles in a solution.

specificity: The proportion of cases with absence of a specific disease or condition that gives a negative test result.

spectrophotometer: Device that quantitatively provides the relationship between the intensity of the color of an unknown solution and that of a standard solution; see *photometry.*

spectrophotometry: Quantitative measuring technique in which the color of a solution of an unknown concentration is compared with the color of a similar solution of known concentration.

spermatozoa (sperm): Mature male germ cells.

spore: An inert stage of a microorganism that the organism can revert to in a hostile environment.

spring-activated skin-puncturing device: Device used to collect capillary blood; makes a clean, rapid incision of a consistent depth.

spun microhematocrit method: Hematocrit measurement method that uses a high-speed centrifuge in a relatively short centrifugation time.

stable factor: Factor VII; presence monitored by thrombin time.

stab tube: A tube of medium that is inoculated by stabbing or passing through the medium with an inoculating needle, leaving the specimen behind in the medium.

standard calibration curve: Plotting of percent transmission or absorbance readings on graph paper for several known standard solutions of varying concentrations will enable construction of a "standard curve" for a particular assay.

standard deviation (SD): Statistical measurement of the degree of variation from the mean of a series of measurements; measure of precision or reproducibility.

Standard Precautions: Recommended safety policies used for handling all biological (patient) specimens. The potential infectivity of any patient's blood or body fluids is unknown; therefore all blood and body substances (fluids) are considered equally infectious; also called *Universal Precautions.*

standards: A uniform set of rules or regulations; see *standard solution.*

standard solution: Reference material of the substance being assayed that is of fixed and known chemical composition and can be prepared in a pure form for use in the laboratory; certified reference material that is generally accepted or officially recognized as the unique standard for the assay, regardless of the purity of the analyte content.

steatorrhea: Presence or increased quantities of fat in the feces.

stem cell: The common progenitor or uncommitted pluripotential stem cell from which all types of blood cells are derived.

stercobilin: Pigment derived from bilirubin; responsible for normal color of the feces.

stercobilinogen: Colorless degradation product of urobilinogen; is formed in the intestine and oxidized to the colored pigment stercobilin.

sterile: Free from living microorganisms.

sterilization: Killing or destroying all microorganisms.

Sternheimer–Malbin stain: A crystal violet and safranin stain commonly used in the microscopic analysis of the urine sediment.

streak plate: Culture plate prepared by inoculating so as to spread out colonies as much as possible so that single, isolated colonies may be observed after incubation.

subculture: A colony from the primary culture plate that is picked up with an inoculating loop or needle and transferred to a second medium for further culturing.
supernatant: Fluid without cellular or other types of precipitate.
supportive media: Media that contain nutrients that allow most nonfastidious organisms to grow at their normal rates.
supravital stains: A special stain used to impart color to living cells such as reticulocytes.
synovial fluid: Extravascular fluid that surrounds the joints of the body.
syringe and needle collection system: Separate syringes and needles of appropriate size and gauge are used to collect some blood specimens. Blood in the syringe is carefully added to the appropriate collection tube containing the necessary additive.

T

Tamm–Horsfall protein: Mucoprotein secreted by the renal tubular cells and not derived from the blood plasma. This protein forms the matrix of urinary casts.
taxonomy: Biological classification system of microorganisms on the basis of their natural relationships and, from this, giving them suitable names.
telescoped sediment: Urine sediment that contains all, or most, types of casts (hyaline, cellular, granular, and waxy) in one sediment.
test tube culture: Culture medium dispersed in test tubes, such as slants or liquid broth.
therapeutic drug monitoring: Testing of blood level of a drug to monitor or keep track of its medical effectiveness in treatment of a disease.
thin-layer chromatography: Method of chromatography often used to do therapeutic drug-monitoring tests; the stationary phase is a thin layer of an adsorbent coated on a glass plate or sheet of plastic; the mobile phase is a solvent or a solvent mixture.
throat swab: Sterile fibrous material (commonly Dacron or rayon) fixed to a stick; used to collect material from the back of the throat for culture or rapid-detection tests for diagnosis of "strep throat."
thrombin: Activated form of factor II that acts as a serine proteolytic enzyme to cleave fibrinogen and form fibrin; is a reagent to test platelet aggregation.
thrombin time (TT): Measurement of the time required for change of fibrinogen to fibrin.
thrombocyte, platelet: One of the formed elements in the peripheral blood; chief function is its role in coagulation of blood.
thromboplastin: Substance with ability to convert prothrombin to thrombin.
thrombosis: Formation of a thrombus or fibrin clot.
thrombus: Result of activation of the hemostatic system; formation of platelet plug.
timed urine collection: Urine collected over time, for example, 2, 12, or 24 hours. Collection commonly is preserved by refrigeration between voidings and is used when a quantitative assay is needed. It is important to adhere to specific time requirements and be certain that the collection time is noted on the container. Entire timed collection must be sent to the laboratory in the container.
titer: Concentration of a substance, such as an antibody in serum.
titration: Quantitative volumetric technique of measuring the concentration of an unknown solution by comparing it with a measured volume of a solution of known concentration.
T lymphocyte: Blood cell that is derived from the thymus; functions in cell-mediated responses; makes up the majority of the lymphocytes in the peripheral blood.
to-contain pipettes: Pipettes calibrated to contain a specific amount of liquid; to ensure that all the liquid is emptied from the pipette, it must be rinsed well with a diluting solution.
to-deliver pipettes: Pipettes calibrated to deliver a specified volume when filled properly and the liquid is allowed to drain completely into a receiving vessel.
tolerance: Form of resistance to an antimicrobial agent. In volumetric glassware, the degree of acceptable variability of volume delivery from that stated on the glassware; the tolerance increases with the capacity of the pipette.
torsion balance: Laboratory balance commonly used to weigh chemicals; is assembled as a single flexible structure by means of highly tensed torsion bands of watch-spring alloy; has no knife edges to dull or other loose parts.
total quality improvement (TQI): Internal monitoring programs to improve the quality of services performed by the clinical laboratory.
total quality management (TQM): See *total quality improvement (TQI).*
total testing process (TTP): A quality assurance method.
tourniquet: Elastic strip or cuff that can be tightened when applied around the arm, usually just above the elbow; allows the vein to become more prominent so that venipuncture can be more easily done.
toxicology: Study of the origin, nature, and effects of poison. Toxicologic analyses are used to detect the amounts of substances that could be poisonous or toxic at certain concentrations.
transfer needle: See *inoculating loop or needle.*
transfusion reaction: Any adverse effect of transfusion; generally characterized as hemolytic, febrile, allergic, or circulatory overload.
transmission-based precautions: Precautions coming from the Centers for Disease Control and Prevention (CDC) that apply to patients (1) with known specific infection or suspected to be infected with specific microorganisms spread by airborne, droplet, or contact routes or (2) during the incubation period of certain easily transmitted diseases.
transmission electron microscope (TEM): A type of microscope that illuminates the specimen with a beam of electrons produced by an electron gun; the electrons are accelerated by a high voltage potential and passed through a condenser lens system (usually two magnetic lenses). The electron microscope allows for significantly greater magnification (up to 50,000 times magnification) than the brightfield microscope.
transmitted light: Light that is not absorbed.
transudate: An effusion formed as the result of filtration through a membrane.
traumatic tap: The presence of blood in a body fluid specimen, such as cerebrospinal fluid, as a result of bleeding at the site of entry as the fluid is collected. First tube appears bloody, whereas subsequent tubes show lesser concentrations of blood.
trend: A statistical term used to indicate movement away from the mean.
triglycerides: A lipid component.
triple-beam balance, "trip" balance: Three-beamed balance. Each beam provides a different weighing scale; scales are provided with movable weights. Used commonly in preparation of laboratory reagents.
trophozoite: Motile form of a parasite.
true negatives: Those subjects who have a negative test and who do not have the disease.
true positives: Those subjects who have a positive test and who have the disease.
tuberculosis control: The Occupational Safety and Health Administration (OSHA) requires the use of special masks and respirators for persons who are exposed to patients with known or suspected pulmonary tuberculosis.
tumor-specific markers: Antigens or antibodies indicative of a disorder.
turbidimetry: Measurement of the loss in light intensity transmitted through a solution because of the light being scattered as a result of the turbidity of the solution.
type 1, or insulin-dependent, diabetes mellitus (IDDM): Insulin injection is required because insufficient amounts of insulin are secreted by the pancreas.
type 2, or non–insulin-dependent, diabetes mellitus (NIDDM): The activity of the insulin present is not sufficient; patients are usually not dependent on insulin injections.
typing: Testing of suspensions of red cells with known antibody solutions (antisera) to determine the identity of antigens, known as the *blood type.*

U

ultracentrifuge: High-speed centrifuge; generally used for research.
ultrafiltrate of plasma: Filtrate of plasma over a membrane, whereby extremely small particles such as proteins are restricted, or not filtered.
unconjugated bilirubin, indirect bilirubin, free bilirubin: Water-insoluble form of bilirubin that is formed as a breakdown product from heme by the reticuloendothelial system and carried in the bloodstream bound to albumin. Because of its insolubility, this form cannot be excreted by the kidney or found in the urine.
unexpected antibody: Antibody that results from specific antigenic stimulus. In blood banking, the result of stimulation from pregnancy, transfusion, or injection of red cells. Also referred to as an *immune antibody.*
Universal Blood and Body Substance Technique (UBBST): See *Standard Precautions.*

Universal Precautions: See *Standard Precautions.*

Unopette system: Formerly, a popular commercially available disposable self-filling pipette and diluent-reservoir system used to measure and dilute blood for testing purposes.

unorganized sediment: The chemical part of the urine sediment; includes crystals of chemicals and amorphous material.

urea nitrogen/creatinine ratio: Useful relationship in diagnosis of renal function disorders. Normal ratio for a person on a normal diet is between 12 and 20.

uremia: Abnormally high concentration of urea nitrogen in the blood.

urinalysis: The physical, chemical, and microscopic analysis of urine.

urinary system: Consists of two kidneys and two ureters plus the bladder and the urethra.

urine: Fluid composed of the waste materials of blood; formed in the kidney and excreted from the body by way of the urinary system.

urobilin: An orange-yellow pigment found in normal urine. Urobilin is an oxidation product of the colorless urobilinogen.

urobilinogen: Group of colorless chromogens that are formed in the intestine from the reduction of bilirubin by the action of bacteria present in the normal bacterial flora; normal product of bilirubin metabolism.

urochrome: A yellow pigment found in normal urine.

uroerythrin: A red pigment found in normal urine.

V

vaccination: The process of introducing a foreign antigen such as an attenuated live or killed organism into a person to stimulate immune antibodies (immunize).

vaccines: Substances such as attenuated live viruses or dead bacteria used to expose a person to an antigen possessed by the virus or bacteria to stimulate an immune process and prevent contracting a specific infectious disease.

vacuum tube and needle-collection system: Blood-collection system consisting of evacuated collection tubes with appropriate additives, double-ended needles, and needle holders; allows blood collection directly from the vein into the tube.

valence: Expression of the total combining power of an element whereby it can combine chemically with atoms of hydrogen or their equivalent.

variance (or error): Fluctuation in the measurement of a substance; factors causing variance can be limitations of the procedure itself or can be related to the sampling mechanism.

vascular: Related to blood vessels such as veins.

vascular access device (VAD): Device or indwelling line used to administer therapeutic products over a long period; see *indwelling line.*

vascular component: Activity of the blood vessels themselves.

vasoconstriction: Constriction of blood vessels; most immediate response of the body to bleeding.

venipuncture (also phlebotomy): Process of collecting blood from a vein.

venous blood: Blood collected from a vein by venipuncture.

verified: Results must be verified, or approved or reviewed, before the data are released to the patient report.

virology: The study or science of viruses.

visible spectrum: The range of light that is visible to the human eye, generally from wavelengths of 380 to 750 nm.

visual colorimetry: Determination or comparison of color intensity of a solution by use of the human eye; has all but been replaced by photoelectric colorimetry and spectrophotometry instrumentation.

voided midstream urine specimen: Noncatheterized urine specimen collected after the first few milliliters have been deposited in the urinal or toilet; the urine is free-flowing, and the midportion of the collection is saved in a specimen container.

volume per unit volume: Measured volume of a liquid added to a specific volume of another liquid (v/v); usually expressed as milliliters per milliliter (mL/mL) or milliliters per liter (mL/L).

volumetric glassware: Glassware that has been manufactured of good-quality glass and calibrated under strict conditions to hold, contain, or deliver a specific volume of liquid; examples include a volumetric pipette, a flask, and a buret.

volumetric (or transfer) pipette: Extremely accurate, single-line pipette used to measure specimens, controls, and standard solutions or anything requiring precise measurement.

von Willebrand disease (vWD): Deficiency of von Willebrand factor (vWF); prolonged bleeding time results; see *von Willebrand factor (vWF).*

von Willebrand factor (vWF): Subendothelial factor (factor VIII:vWF); acts as the glue necessary for optimal platelet–collagen binding to occur; factor is required for normal platelet adhesion to endothelium.

W

waived laboratory tests (waived testing): Clinical Laboratory Improvement Amendments of 1988 (CLIA '88) regulations specify that the Food and Drug Administration (FDA) has cleared these tests; that is, the tests are so simple that the likelihood of erroneous results is negligible, or no risk is posed to the patient if the tests are performed incorrectly.

waste disposal program: The Occupational Safety and Health Administration (OSHA) standards mandate implementation of a specific plan for disposal of medical wastes to prevent transmission of infectious agents and accidental exposure to possibly hazardous material.

Watson–Schwartz test: Test for urobilinogen and porphobilinogen, based on the Ehrlich aldehyde reaction; basis of the Multistix reagent strip test for Ehrlich-reacting substances.

wavelength of light: Linear distance traveled by one complete wave cycle of a particular beam of radiant energy.

weight (mass) per unit volume (w/v): Measured weight of a substance added to a specific volume of a diluent, usually deionized or distilled water. The usual way is as grams per liter (g/L) or milligrams per milliliter (mg/mL).

weight per unit weight (w/w): Mass per unit mass; used when the desired chemical to be weighed is a solid and is mixed with or diluted with another solid.

Western blot technology: Antigenic proteins or nucleic acids are separated by gel electrophoresis and transferred or blotted onto membrane filter paper; antiserum from the patient is allowed to react with the filter paper, and by use of labeled anti-antibody detectors, the specific antibody bound to its homologous antigen is detected.

wet-reagent chemistry: Assay using wet reagents. Traditional manual chemistry assays use wet-reagent chemistry. Compare with dry-reagent technology.

white blood cell differential: Determination of the percentage of each white blood cell type present in a peripheral blood film.

wide-area network (WAN): A network of computers.

Wintrobe hematocrit method: A macromethod for hematocrit determination; has generally been replaced by the microhematocrit or calculated hematocrit.

working distance: In microscopy, the distance from the bottom of the objective to the material being studied.

work list: Defines the workload for a laboratory for a defined period—for the day, for example.

Wright–Giemsa stain: Variation of Wright stain. See *Wright stain.*

Wright stain: A mixture of eosin and methylene blue used to observe the cellular morphology of blood cells in examination of blood films; a polychromatic Romanovsky-type stain.

X

xanthochromia: Yellowish discoloration; used to describe the supernatant spinal or other serous fluid, indicating the presence of previous hemorrhage. Strictly speaking, xanthochromia represents a yellow color; however, the term is applied to pale pink to orange or yellow in describing fluids.

xenoantibodies: Antibodies resulting from exposure to antigenic material from another species.

Z

zone of equivalence: A variable ratio of antigen and antibody that results in precipitation in which there is no unbound antibody or antigen.

zymogens: Enzyme precursors or proenzymes.

Note: Page numbers followed by *f* indicate figures, *t* indicate tables, and *b* indicate boxes.

D

F

G

H

I

J

K

L

M

N

O

P

Q

R

S